Stroke Prevention and Treatment

Second Edition

Stroke Prevention and Treatment

An Evidence-based Approach

Second Edition

Edited by

Jeffrey L. Saver
David Geffen School of Medicine, University of California

Graeme J. Hankey
Medical School, The University of Western Australia

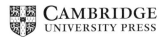
CAMBRIDGE
UNIVERSITY PRESS

CAMBRIDGE
UNIVERSITY PRESS

University Printing House, Cambridge CB2 8BS, United Kingdom

One Liberty Plaza, 20th Floor, New York, NY 10006, USA

477 Williamstown Road, Port Melbourne, VIC 3207, Australia

314–321, 3rd Floor, Plot 3, Splendor Forum, Jasola District Centre,
New Delhi – 110025, India

79 Anson Road, #06–04/06, Singapore 079906

Cambridge University Press is part of the University of Cambridge.

It furthers the University's mission by disseminating knowledge in the pursuit of
education, learning, and research at the highest international levels of excellence.

www.cambridge.org
Information on this title: www.cambridge.org/9781107113145
DOI: 10.1017/9781316286234

© Cambridge University Press 2005, 2021

First published 2005
Reprinted 2006
Second edition 2021

Printed in the United Kingdom by TJ Books Ltd, Padstow Cornwall

A catalogue record for this publication is available from the British Library.

Library of Congress Cataloging-in-Publication Data
Names: Saver, Jeffrey L., editor. | Hankey, Graeme J., editor. | Hankey, Graeme J. Stroke treatment and prevention.
Title: Stroke prevention and treatment : an evidence-based approach / edited by Jeffrey L. Saver, Graeme J. Hankey.
Other titles: Stroke treatment and prevention.
Description: Second edition. | Cambridge, United Kingdom ; New York, NY : Cambridge University Press, 2020. | Preceded by
Stroke treatment and prevention : an evidence-based approach / Graeme J. Hankey. 2005. | Includes bibliographical references and
index.
Identifiers: LCCN 2019038966 (print) | LCCN 2019038967 (ebook) | ISBN 9781107113145 (hardback) | ISBN 9781316286234
(ebook)
Subjects: MESH: Stroke – prevention & control | Stroke – therapy | Stroke Rehabilitation | Evidence-Based Medicine
Classification: LCC RC388.5 (print) | LCC RC388.5 (ebook) | NLM WL 356 |DDC 616.8/1–dc23
LC record available at https://lccn.loc.gov/2019038966
LC ebook record available at https://lccn.loc.gov/2019038967

ISBN 978-1-107-11314-5 Hardback

From Jeffrey L. Saver – I thank Don Easton, Ed Feldmann, Jose Biller, and Lou Caplan for introducing me to evidence-based stroke medicine, and my parents (Harry and Esther), wife (Kay), and son (Dash) for introducing me to the world and evidence of its wonder.

From Graeme J. Hankey – I thank Charles Warlow, Peter Sandercock and Jan van Gijn for introducing me to evidence-based stroke medicine, my parents (Jean and John) and daughters (Genevieve and Michelle), and my wife Claire for her longstanding love and support.

Contents

Part VI Stroke Rehabilitation and Recovery

Contributors

Rustam Al-Shahi Salman, MA, PhD, FRCP Edin
Centre for Clinical Brain Sciences, University of Edinburgh, Edinburgh, UK

Craig Anderson, MBBS, PhD, FRACP, FAHMS
The George Institute for Global Health, Faculty of Medicine, University of New South Wales, Sydney, Australia

Eivind Berge, MD, PhD, FESO
Department of Internal Medicine, Oslo University Hospital Oslo, and Institute of Clinical Medicine, University of Tromsø, Norway

Leo H. Bonati, MD
Department of Neurology and Stroke Center, University Hospital Basel, University of Basel, Switzerland

Marian C. Brady, BSc (Hons), PhD, FRCSLT
Nursing, Midwifery and Allied Health Professions Research Unit, Glasgow Caledonian University, Glasgow, Scotland

Sherri A. Braksick, MD
Department of Neurology, Division of Neurocritical Care, Mayo Clinic, Rochester, MN, USA

Martin M. Brown, MA, MD, FRCP
Stroke Research Centre, UCL Queen Square Institute of Neurology, University College London, London, UK

Robert D. Brown, Jr., MD, MPH
Department of Neurology, Mayo Clinic, Rochester, MN, USA

Askiel Bruno, MD, MS
Department of Neurology, Section of Vascular Neurology, Medical College of Georgia, Augusta University, Augusta, GA, USA

Salvador Cruz-Flores, MD, MPH, FAHA, FCCM, FAAN, FNCS
Department of Neurology, Paul L. Foster School of Medicine; Texas Tech University Health Sciences Center El Paso, El Paso, TX, USA

Stefan T. Engelter, MD, FESO, FEAN
Department of Neurology and Stroke Center, University Hospital Basel, Department of Clinical Research, and Neurology and Neurorehabilitation, University Department of Geriatric Medicine Felix Platter; University of Basel, Basel, Switzerland

Jonathan J. Evans, BSc (Hons), DipClinPsychol, PhD
Institute of Health & Wellbeing, University of Glasgow, Glasgow, Scotland

Larry B. Goldstein, MD, FAAN, FANA, FAHA
Department of Neurology and Kentucky Neuroscience Institute, University of Kentucky, Lexington, KY, USA

Graeme J. Hankey, MBBS, MD, FRACP, FRCP, FRCP Edin, FAHA, FESO, FWSO, FAAHMS
Professor of Neurology, Medical School, The University of Western Australia; Consultant Neurologist, Sir Charles Gairdner Hospital, Perth, Australia

James P. Klaas, MD
Department of Neurology, Mayo Clinic, Rochester, MN, USA

Gert Kwakkel, PhD, PT
Department of Rehabilitation Medicine, MOVE Research Institute Amsterdam, Amsterdam Neurosciences, Amsterdam University Medical Centre, location VUmc, The Netherlands; Rehabilitation Research Centre, Reade, The Netherlands; and Department of Physical Therapy and Human Movement Sciences, Northwestern University, Chicago, IL, USA

Peter Langhorne, PhD, FRCP
Institute of Cardiovascular and Medical Sciences, University of Glasgow, Glasgow, UK

Meng Lee, MD
Department of Neurology, Chang Gung University College of Medicine, Chang Gung Memorial Hospital, Chiayi Branch, Chiayi, Taiwan

Xinyi Leng
Department of Medicine & Therapeutics, The Chinese University of Hong Kong, Hong Kong SAR, China

Philippe A. Lyrer, MD, FESO
Department of Neurology and Stroke Center, University Hospital Basel, University of Basel, Switzerland

Jodie Marquez, BAppSc, PhD
Faculty of Health and Medicine, University of Newcastle, Callaghan, Australia

Tom Moullaali, MBBS, MRCP
Centre for Clinical Brain Sciences, University of Edinburgh, Edinburgh, UK and The George Institute for Global Health, Faculty of Medicine, University of New South Wales, Sydney, Australia

Mandy D. Müller, MD
Department of Neurology and Stroke Center, University Hospital Basel, University of Basel, Basel, Switzerland

Bruce Ovbiagele, MD
Department of Neurology, University of California, San Francisco, CA, USA

Maurizio Paciaroni, MD
Stroke Unit and Division of Cardiovascular Medicine, Santa Maria della Misericordia Hospital, University of Perugia, Perugia, Italy

Mark Parsons, BMed, PhD, FRACP
Department of Medicine and Neurology, Melbourne Brain Centre at the Royal Melbourne Hospital, Australia

Alejandro A. Rabinstein, MD
Department of Neurology, Mayo Clinic, Rochester, MN, USA

Subhashini Ramesh, MD
Department of Medicine, Section of Critical Care Medicine, Inova Fairfax Medical Campus, Inova Health System, Falls Church, VA, USA

Else Charlotte Sandset, MD, PhD, FESO
Department of Neurology, Oslo University Hospital, Oslo, Norway

Nerses Sanossian, MD
Department of Neurology, Keck School of Medicine, University of Southern California, Los Angeles, CA, USA

Jeffrey L. Saver, MD, FAHA, FAAN
Department of Neurology, David Geffen School of Medicine, University of California, Los Angeles, CA, USA

Lee H. Schwamm, MD
Department of Neurology, Massachusetts General Hospital and Harvard Medical School, Boston, MA, USA

Amytis Towfighi, MD, FAHA
Department of Neurology, Keck School of Medicine of University of Southern California, Los Angeles, CA, USA

Christopher Traenka, MD
Department of Neurology and Stroke Center, University Hospital Basel, Department of Clinical Research, and Neurology and Neurorehabilitation, University Department of Geriatric Medicine, Felix Platter, University of Basel, Basel, Switzerland

Janne M. Veerbeek, PhD, PT
Department of Rehabilitation Medicine, Amsterdam Neurosciences and Amsterdam Movement Sciences, Amsterdam, The Netherlands; Division of Vascular Neurology and Neurorehabilitation, Department of Neurology, University of Zurich and University Hospital Zurich, Zurich, Switzerland; and cereneo, center for Neurology and Rehabilitation, Vitznau, Switzerland

Joanna Wardlaw, FRCR, FRSE, FMedSci, FAHA
Centre for Clinical Brain Sciences and UK Dementia Research Institute, University of Edinburgh, Edinburgh, UK

Lawrence K.S. Wong MBBS(NSW), MHA(NSW), MD (NSW), MRCP(UK), FHKAM(Medicine), FRCP(Lond)
Department of Medicine & Therapeutics, The Chinese University of Hong Kong, Hong Kong SAR, China

Kori Sauser Zachrison, MD, MSc
Department of Emergency Medicine, Massachusetts General Hospital and Harvard Medical School Boston, MA, USA

Preface

Since the first edition of this book was published in 2005, the global burden of stroke has continued to rise. The number of new strokes each year, alive stroke survivors, disability-adjusted life-years (DALYs) lost to stroke annually, and stroke-related deaths per year have increased, despite stable or mildly declining age-adjusted stroke incidence rates and improved outcomes among individuals experiencing stroke. The increase in overall stroke numbers, despite reductions in rates, reflects global population growth, increasing life expectancy, ageing of populations in developed countries, and heightened risks of non-communicable disease in the developing world – and signals an ongoing need for this volume. The reduction in rates reflects improved prevention and treatment of stroke, which has coincided with the development, rigorous evaluation, and implementation into practice of an expanding array of effective treatments – testament to the success of the collaborative, international accumulation of evidence to support best stroke care practices collated herein.

In this second edition of *Stroke Treatment and Prevention* we aim to update stroke clinicians and practitioners with the optimal evidence for strategies and interventions to treat stroke and prevent first and recurrent stroke. Where available, randomized controlled trials (RCTs) and systematic reviews of RCTs of the interventions are described and sourced predominantly from the Cochrane Library.

We have assembled an international panel of leading experts who have kindly and generously contributed chapters in their field of expertise. We trust that you will enjoy, and be enlightened by, their appraisal of the best available evidence and their interpretation of its implications for clinical practice and future research. We are also grateful to John Wiley and Sons Limited for granting permission to reproduce the forest plot figures from the Cochrane Library.

Jeffrey L. Saver

Graeme J. Hankey

Stroke: The Size of the Problem

Graeme J. Hankey

The global and regional burden of stroke during 1990–2015 has been estimated by the Global Burden of Disease (GBD) studies of 2010, 2013, and 2015 (Krishnamurthi et al., 2013, 2015; Feigin et al., 2014, 2015; GBD 2015 Neurological Disorders Collaborator Group, 2017).

The GBD 2010 study group undertook a systematic review which identified 119 relevant studies (58 from high-income countries [HIC] and 61 from low- and middle-income countries [LMIC]) that were published between 1990 and 2010 and from which regional and country-specific estimates of the incidence, prevalence, mortality, and disability-adjusted life-years (DALYs) lost by age group (<75 years, ≥75 years, and in total) and country income level of first-ever ischaemic and haemorrhagic stroke in all 21 regions of the world for 1990, 2005, and 2010 could be calculated (Feigin et al., 2014). Pathological subtypes of stroke were confirmed by brain imaging or autopsy in at least 70% of cases.

The GBD estimates of stroke incidence in all regions were therefore obtained using a systematic approach which allows comparison across disease states. Complementary estimates of stroke incidence, based on epidemiological studies of stroke incidence using ideal methods, and also adjusted to the World Health Organization (WHO) world population figures, are provided by Thrift and Kim and colleagues (2020).

Incidence

In 2010, the age-standardized incidence rate of stroke was 258 (234–284) per 100,000 person-years (Feigin et al., 2014) (Table 1.1).

The absolute number of people who experienced a first stroke was 16.9 million in 2010; 68.6% were resident in LMIC and 62% were aged younger than 75 years (Feigin et al., 2014) (Table 1.1). In 2013, there were 10.3 million new strokes (67% ischaemic stroke [IS]) (Feigin et al., 2015).

Ischaemic Stroke

In 2010, the age-standardized incidence of IS was 176 (161–192) per 100,000 person-years (Bennett et al., 2014) (Table 1.1).

In 2010, there were approximately 11,569,000 incident IS events (63% in LMIC) (Bennett et al., 2014).

Haemorrhagic Stroke

In 2010, the overall age-standardized incidence rate of haemorrhagic stroke (HS) (intracerebral and subarachnoid haemorrhage) was 81.52 (95% confidence interval [CI]: 72.27–92.82) per 100,000 person-years globally.

In 2010, there were 5.3 million cases of HS; 80% were in LMIC (Krishnamurthi et al., 2013, 2014).

There were significant regional differences in incidence rates of HS, with the highest rates in LMIC regions such as sub-Saharan Africa and East Asia, and lowest rates in high-income North America and Western Europe.

The overall age-standardized incidence rates of HS per 100,000 person-years were 48.41 (95% CI: 45.44–52.13) in HIC and 99.43 (95% CI: 85.37–116.28) in LMIC. Hence, LMIC had a 40% higher incidence of HS than did HIC.

Trends in Stroke Incidence Rates

From 1990 to 2010, the age-standardized incidence of stroke per 100,000 person-years remained fairly stable, being 251 (95% CI: 230–273) in 1990 and 258 (95% CI: 234–284) in 2010 (Feigin et al., 2014) (Table 1.1).

However, from 1990 to 2010, the absolute number of people with a first stroke increased significantly by 68%, from 10 million to 16.9 million.

From 1990 to 2010, the age-standardized incidence of stroke per 100,000 person-years significantly decreased by 12% (95% CI: 6–17) in HIC, and increased by 12% (95% CI: –3–22) in LMIC, albeit non-significantly.

Table 1.1 Age-adjusted annual incidence and mortality rates (per 100,000 person-years), prevalence (per 100,000 people), and disability-adjusted life-years (DALYs) lost (number, and per 100,000) for all stroke, ischaemic stroke, and haemorrhagic stroke, in 1990, 2005, 2010, and 2015

All Stroke	1990		2005		2010		2015		Change from 1990–2015	
	Number of events	Rate (95% CI) per 100,000	Number of events	Rate (95% CI) per 100,000	Number of events	Rate (95% CI) per 100,000	Number of events	Rate (95% UI) per 100,000	Number of events	Rate (95% UI) per 100,000
Incidence	10,078,935	251 (230–273)	14,734,124	256 (232–284)	16,894,536	258 (234–284)	Not reported	Not reported	68%↑ (to 2010)	12% (6–17%) ↓ HIC (to 2010) 12% (−3–22%) ↑ LMIC (to 2010)
Prevalence	17,915,338	435 (389–497)	28,495,582	490 (437–558)	33,024,958	502 (451–572)	42,431,000 (42.068 m – 42.767 m)	627 (621–631)	59.2% (58–60%) ↑	9.8% (9–10%) ↓
DALYs lost	86,010,384	2063 (1950–2280)	101,951,696	1750 (1569–1831)	102,232,304	1554 (1374–1642)	118,627,000 (114.862 m – 111.627 m)	1777 (1721–1835)	21.7% (18–26%)↑	32.3% (30–34%) ↓
Deaths	4,660,449	117 (112–130)	5,684,970	99 (89–104)	5,874,182	88 (80–94)	6,326,000 (6.175 m – 6.493 m)	101 (99–104)	36.4% (32–41%) ↑	30% (28–32%) ↓

Ischaemic stroke

	Count	Rate (UI)	Count	Rate (UI)	Count	Rate (UI)	Change	Change (CI)
Incidence	7,238,758	181 (167–196)	10,097,297	175 (160–192)	11,569,538	176 (161–192)	37% ↑	13% (6–18%) ↓ HIC 6% (−7–18%) ↑ LMIC
DALYs lost	32,128,220	796 (734–906)	38,571,908	668 (617–774)	39,389,408	598 (560–692)	18% ↑	34% (16–36%) ↓ HIC 17% (−11–19%) ↓ LMIC
Mortality	2,241,077	58 (54–64)	2,701,873	47 (44–54)	2,835,419	42 (40–49)	21% ↑	37% (19–39%) ↓ HIC 14% (9–19%) ↓ LMIC

Haemorrhagic stroke

	Count	Rate (UI)	Count	Rate (UI)	Count	Rate (UI)	Change	Change (CI)
Incidence	2,840,177	69 (62–77)	4,636,828	80 (71–92)	5,324,997	82 (72–93)	47% ↑	18.5% ↑ globally 8% (1–15%) ↓ HIC 22% (5–30%) ↑ LMIC
DALYs lost	53,882,164	1267 (1068–1484)	63,379,792	1081 (935–1234)	62,842,896	956 (828–1104)	14% ↑	39% (32–44%) ↓ HIC 25% (7–38%) ↓ LMIC
Mortality	2,419,372	60 (51–70)	2,983,097	52 (45–59)	3,038,763	46 (40–53)	20% ↑	38% (32–43%) ↓ HIC 23% (−7–36%) ↓ LMIC

Source: Adapted from Krishnamurthi et al., 2013, 2014; Feigin et al., 2014; Bennett et al., 2014, and GBD 2015 Neurological Disorders Collaborator Group, 2017.
CI: confidence interval. HIC: high-income countries. LMIC: low- and middle-income countries. UI: uncertainty interval.

Ischaemic Stroke

From 1990 to 2010, the age-standardized incidence of IS per 100,000 person-years remained fairly stable, being 181 (95% CI: 167–196) in 1990 and 176 (95% CI: 161–192) in 2010

From 1990 to 2010, there was a significant increase in the absolute number of people with incident IS from 7.2 million to 11.6 million (37% increase).

Age-standardized IS incidence in HIC declined by about 13% (95% uncertainty interval [UI]: 6–18%). However, in LMIC there was a modest 6% increase in the age-standardized incidence of IS (95% UI: −7–18%).

Haemorrhagic Stroke

The age-standardized incidence of HS increased by 18.5% worldwide between 1990 and 2010, from 69 (62–77) to 82 (72–93) per 100,000 person-years.

From 1990 to 2010, there was a 47% increase worldwide in the absolute number of HS cases, from 2.8 million to 5.3 million.

In HIC, there was a reduction in incidence of HS by 8% (95% CI: 1–15%) in the past 2 decades. However, in low-income and middle-income countries there was a significant increase in the incidence of HS by 22% (95% CI: 5-30%), which is one rate that has increased over the past two decades, particularly in people younger than 75 years (19% increase in HS in past two decades, 95%CI: 5–30% increase).

Prevalence

In 2010, the prevalence of stroke survivors was 502 (451–572) per 100,000 people and the absolute number of stroke survivors was 33 million.

In 2015, the prevalence of stroke survivors was 627 (95% UI: 621–631) per 100,000 people and the absolute number of stroke survivors was 42.431 million (95% UI: 42.068–42.767 million) (GBD 2015 Neurological Disorders Collaborator Group, 2017).

Ischaemic Stroke

In 2013, in younger adults aged 20–64 years, the global prevalence of IS was 7.258 million cases (95% UI: 6.996–7.569 million) (Krishnamurthi et al., 2015).

Haemorrhagic Stroke

In 2013, in younger adults aged 20–64 years, the global prevalence of HS was 3.725 million cases (95% UI: 3.548–3.871 million) (Krishnamurthi et al., 2015).

Trends in Prevalence

From 1990 to 2010, the absolute number of stroke survivors increased significantly by 84%, from 18 million to 33 million (Feigin et al., 2014).

Between 1990 and 2015, the absolute number of stroke survivors increased globally by 59.2% (58.4–59.9%), whereas the age-standardized prevalence rate of stroke fell by 9.8% (9.4–10.3% reduction) (GBD 2015 Neurological Disorders Collaborator Group, 2017).

Ischaemic and Haemorrhagic Stroke

Between 1990 and 2013, there were significant increases in absolute numbers and prevalence rates of both HS and IS for younger adults globally (Krishnamurthi et al., 2015).

Mortality

In 2010, the age-standardized mortality rate of stroke was 88 (80–94) per 100,000 person-years, and the absolute number of stroke-related deaths was 5.9 million (Feigin et al., 2014)

In 2015, the age-standardized mortality rate of stroke was 101 (99–104) per 100,000 person-years, and the number of stroke deaths was 6.3 million (95% UI: 6.2–6.5 million) (GBD 2015 Neurological Disorders Collaborator Group, 2017).

The percentage of estimated total global mortality due to stroke in 2013 was 11.3%, which exceeds that of HIV/AIDS, tuberculosis, and malaria combined (7.2%) by more than 50% (GBD 2013 Mortality and Causes of Death Collaborators, 2015).

Ischaemic Stroke

In 2010, the age-standardized mortality rate of IS was 42 (40–49) per 100,000 person-years, and there were approximately 2.835 million deaths from IS (57% in LMIC) (Bennett et al., 2014).

Haemorrhagic Stroke

In 2010, the age-standardized mortality rate of HS was 46 (40–53) per 100,000 person-years, and there were 3.0 million deaths due to HS.

Hence, HS caused more than half (51.7%) of the 5.9 million stroke-related deaths in 2010, despite causing less than one-third of all strokes.

The largest proportion of HS deaths occurred in LMIC countries. Low- and middle-income countries had a 77% higher mortality from HS than did HIC.

The highest mortality rates in 2010 were in low-income Central Asia, Southeast Asia, and sub-Saharan Africa, whereas the lowest mortality rates were in high-income North America, Australasia, and Western Europe.

In 2013, in younger adults aged 20–64 years, the number of deaths from HS (1.047 million [95% UI: 0.945–1.184 million]) was significantly higher than the number of deaths from IS (0.436 million [95% UI: 0.354–0.504 million]) (Krishnamurthi et al., 2015).

Trends in Stroke Mortality Rates

From 1990 to 2010, mortality rates decreased significantly from 117 (112–130) to 88 (80–94) per 100,000. The fall was in both HIC (37%, 31–41) and LMIC (20%, 15–30). However, the absolute number of stroke-related deaths significantly increased by 26%, from 4.7 million to 5.9 million.

Between 1990 and 2015, the absolute number of stroke deaths increased globally by 36.4% (32.4–40.8%), whereas the age-standardized mortality rate of stroke fell by 30% (27.7–32.0% reduction) (GBD 2015 Neurological Disorders Collaborator Group, 2017).

Ischaemic Stroke

From 1990 to 2010, mortality rates due to IS decreased by one-fifth, from 58 (54–64) to 42 (40–49) per 100,000.

However, the absolute number of deaths from IS increased from 2.24 million to 2.84 million (21% increase).

Age-standardized mortality in HIC declined by about 37% (95% UI: 19–39%).

In LMIC, there were modest reductions in mortality rates.

Haemorrhagic Stroke

From 1990 to 2010, mortality rates due to HS decreased from 60 (51–70) to 46 (40–53) per 100,000.

There was a significant reduction in HS mortality by 38% (95% CI: 32–43%) in HIC and by 23% (95% CI: –3–36%) in LMIC .

However, the number of deaths globally from HS increased by 20% from 2.4 million to 3.0 million.

DALYs Lost

In 2010, the rate of DALYs lost due to stroke was 1554 (1374–1643) per 100,000, and the absolute number of DALYs lost was 102 million.

In 2015, the rate of DALYs lost due to stroke was 1777 (1721–1835) per 100,000 and the absolute number of DALYs lost was 118.627 million (114.862–122.627 million) (GBD 2015 Neurological Disorders Collaborator Group, 2017; GBD 2016 DALYs and HALE Collaborators, 2017).

Ischaemic Stroke

In 2010, there were approximately 39.4 million DALYs lost due to IS (64% in LMIC) (Bennett et al., 2014).

Haemorrhagic Stroke

In 2010, there were 62.8 million DALYs lost (86% in LMIC) due to HS.

Consequently, HS caused three-fifths (61.5%) of the 102.2 million DALYs lost due to stroke throughout the world.

Low- and middle-income countries had 65% higher DALY rates of HS than did HIC.

Trends in DALYs Lost

From 1990 to 2010, the age-standardized rate of DALYs lost per 100,000 decreased from 2063 (1950–2280) to 1554 (1374–1642), but the absolute number of DALYs lost increased by 12% from 86 million to 102 million.

Between 1990 and 2015, the age-standardized rate of DALYs lost per 100,000 decreased by 32.3% (30.0–34.4% decrease), but the absolute number of DALYs lost increased by 21.7% (17.8–25.7%) (GBD 2015 Neurological Disorders Collaborator Group, 2017).

Ischaemic Stroke

From 1990 to 2010, the age-standardized rate of DALYs lost per 100,000 decreased from 796 (734–906) to 598 (560–692), but the absolute number of DALYs lost due to IS increased by 18%, from 32 million to 39 million.

Age-standardized DALYs lost in HIC declined by about 34% (95% UI: 16–36%).

The bulk of DALYs lost were in LMIC.

Haemorrhagic Stroke

From 1990 to 2010, the age-standardized rate of DALYs lost per 100,000 decreased from 1267 (1068–1484) to 956 (828–1104). In HIC, there was a reduction in DALYs lost due to HS by 39% (95% CI: 32–44%), and in LMIC countries, there was a reduction in DALYs lost by 25% (95% CI: 7–38%).

However, from 1990 to 2010, the absolute number of DALYs lost due to HS increased by 14% from 54 million to 63 million.

Special Populations

Low- and Middle-Income Countries

In 2010, most of the burden of IS and HS was in LMIC, which accounted for

- 63% of incident IS and 80% of HS,
- 57% of deaths due to IS and 84% of deaths due to HS, and
- 64% of DALYs lost due to IS and 86% due to HS (Krishnamurthi et al., 2013).

The average age of incident and fatal IS and HS was 6 years younger in LMIC than in HIC.

The greater burden of stroke in LMIC is not simply because a larger proportion of the world's population lives in LMIC. The rates (i.e. number per 100,000 population) of stroke incidence, DALY loss, and mortality due to stroke are higher in LMIC, correlating inversely with country-level macroeconomic status indicators. Thus, not only are individuals in LMIC more likely to have strokes, but these strokes are also more likely to lead to death and disability.

The disproportionate stroke burden in LMIC is also not mediated by a greater prevalence of cardiovascular risk factors in LMIC. Cardiovascular risk is actually lower in low-income countries. However, national per capita income correlates inversely with stroke mortality and DALY loss rates independent of cardiovascular risk. It is therefore likely that suboptimal resources in LMIC to invest in stroke prevention, treatment, and rehabilitation have contributed to, and perpetuate, substantial inequities in stroke incidence and outcomes, beyond the burden of stroke risk factors.

People Younger than 75 Years of Age

In 2010, much of the burden of stroke was borne by people younger than 75 years, who accounted for

- 62.0% of new strokes,
- 69.8% of prevalent strokes,
- 45.5% of deaths from stroke, and
- 71.7% of DALYs lost because of stroke (Feigin et al., 2014) (Table 1.2).

People younger than 75 years also accounted for

- 62% of incident IS and 78% of HS, and
- 63% of DALYs lost due to IS and 83% due to HS.

Children and Young Adults

In 2010, 5.2 million (31%) strokes occurred in children (aged <20 years) and young and middle-aged adults (20–64 years).

Children from LMIC contributed almost 74,000 (89%) strokes, and young and middle-aged adults from LMIC contributed almost 4.0 million (78%) strokes.

In 2013, in younger adults aged 20 to 64 years, there were 1.483 million (95% UI: 1.340–1.659 million) stroke deaths globally (Krishnamurthi et al., 2015). The total DALYs from all strokes in those aged 20–64 years was 51.429 million (95% UI: 46.561–57.320 million) (Krishnamurthi et al., 2015).

Among younger adults, death rates for all strokes declined significantly between 1990 and 2013, in both developing countries, from 47 (95% UI: 42.6–51.7) in 1990 to 39 (95% UI: 35.0–43.8) in 2013, and in developed countries, from 33.3 (95% UI: 29.8–37.0) in 1990 to 23.5 (95% UI: 21.1–26.9) in 2013 (Krishnamurthi et al., 2015).

Summary

- In 2010, an estimated 16.9 million strokes occurred worldwide, or 1 every 2 seconds, at an incidence rate of 258 (234–284) per 100,000 persons per year. Approximately 70% of these strokes occurred in low- and middle-income countries (LMIC). The 16.9 million incident strokes were added to a pool of 33 million prevalent stroke survivors (502 [451–572) per 100,000 people). There were 5.9 million stroke-related deaths, at a rate of 88 (80–94 per 100,000 person-years), and 102 million disability-adjusted life-years (DALYs) lost due to stroke at a rate of 1554 (1374–1642) per 100,000 people.
- In 2010, stroke was the second leading cause of death and the third leading cause of DALYs worldwide.
- In 2010, most of the global burden of stroke was due to haemorrhagic stroke (HS), and most of the burden of HS was borne by LMIC. Although HS was

Table 1.2 Burden of stroke in 2010 globally, and by low and middle-income countries and people younger than 75 years. Age-adjusted annual incidence and mortality rates (per 100,000 person-years), prevalence (per 100,000 people), and disability-adjusted life-years (DALYs) lost (number, and per 100,000) for all stroke, ischaemic stroke, and haemorrhagic stroke, in 2010

All stroke	Global		Low- and middle-income countries			Age <75 years		
	Number of events	Rate (95% CI)	Number of events	%	Rate (95% CI)	Number of events	%	Rate (95% CI)
Incidence	16,894,536	258 (234–284)	11,590,294	68.6%	281 (244–322)	10,469,624	62.0%	169 (152–187)
Prevalence	33,024,958	502 (451–572)	17,238,778	52.2%	393 (330–483)	23,052,804	69.8%	367 (328–420)
DALYs lost	102,232,304	1554 (1374–1642)	79,411,312	77.7%	1821 (1589–1925)	73,293,552	71.7%	1163 (1011–1232)
Mortality	5,874,182	88 (80–94)	4,164,293	70.9%	105 (91–112)	2,668,499	45.5%	43 (38–45)
Ischaemic stroke								
Incidence	11,569,538	176 (161–192)	7,316,281	63%			67%	
DALYs lost	39,389,408	598 (560–692)	25,137,666	64%			63%	
Mortality	2,835,419	42 (40–49)	1,625,339	57%				
Haemorrhagic stroke								
Incidence	5,324,997	82 (72–93)	4,274,013	80%	99 (85–116)		78%	
DALYs lost	62,842,896	956 (828–1104)	54,273,644	86%			83%	
Mortality	3,038,763	46 (40–53)	2,538,954	84%	62 (53–72)			

Adapted from Krishnamurthi et al., 2013, 2014; Feigin et al., 2014; Bennett et al., 2014.

only half as common as ischaemic stroke (IS), constituting a third (31.5%) of the 16.9 million incident stroke events (20% in the high-income countries [HIC] and 37% in LMIC), HS caused more than half (51.7%) of the 5.9 million stroke-related deaths, and three-fifths (61.5%) of the 102.2 million DALYs lost throughout the world. The number of years of life lost were greater with HS because it affected people at a younger age (mean 65.1 years [standard deviation (SD) 0.11]) than did IS (73.1 years [0.10]) and had a higher case fatality (57% vs 25%).

- In the preceding two decades, between 1990 and 2010, the global incidence rate of stroke has remained stable but the absolute number of incident strokes has increased by 68% (from 10 million to 16.9 million); the prevalence rate has increased modestly (from 435 to 502 per 100,000), yet the absolute number of stroke survivors has nearly doubled (81% increase from 17.9 million to 33 million); the rate of DALYs lost due to stroke has decreased (from 2063 [1950–2280] to 1554 [1374–1642] per 100,000), but the absolute number of DALYs lost has increased by 12% (from 86 million to 102 million); and the age-standardized rates of stroke mortality have decreased (from 117 [112–130] to 88 [80–94] per 100,000 person-years), but the absolute number of stroke-related deaths has increased by 26% (from 4.7 million to 5.9 million).

- Over the past 2 decades (1990–2010), the worldwide burden of HS has increased in terms of absolute numbers of HS incident events. Whilst the absolute number of people with IS stroke has increased significantly by 37%, the absolute number of people with incident HS has increased by 47%.

- Although age-standardized IS mortality rates have declined over the past 2 decades, the absolute global burden of IS is increasing, with the bulk of DALYs lost occurring in LMIC. Between 1990 and 2010, there has been an increase in the number of deaths due to IS by 21% and HS by 20%, and the number of DALYs lost due to IS by 18% and HS by 14%.

- The increase in absolute numbers has arisen despite a reduction in the age-standardized incidence rates of IS by 13% and HS by 19%, a reduction in the mortality rates of IS by 37% and HS by 38%, and a reduction in DALYs lost due to IS by 34% and HS by 39%.

- The reduction in rates probably shows improved education, prevention, diagnosis, treatment, and rehabilitation of stroke. The increase in absolute numbers, despite a reduction in rates, is presumably because global population growth and increasing life expectancy have increased the denominator by a greater proportion than the increasing number of stroke events has increased the numerator.

- Most of the burden of stroke is in LMIC, which bear 63% of incident IS and 80% of IS, 57% of deaths due to IS and 84% due to HS, and 64% of DALYs lost due to IS and 86% due to HS. The average age of incident and fatal IS and HS was 6 years younger in LMIC than in HIC.

- The higher burden of stroke in LMIC is not simply because a larger proportion of the world's population lives in LMIC, as the *rates* of stroke incidence, DALY loss, and mortality due to stroke per 100,000 are higher in LMIC. It is also not mediated by a greater prevalence of cardiovascular risk factors but more so by the lower national per capita income realizing suboptimal resources to invest in stroke prevention, treatment, and rehabilitation.

- Most of the burden of IS and HS is also borne by people younger than 75 years, who bear 62% of incident IS and 78% of HS, and 63% of DALYs lost due to IS and 83% due to HS.

- Overall, despite stable age-standardized incidence rates of stroke and decreasing age-standardized mortality rates due to stroke worldwide in the past 2 decades, the global burden of stroke is great and increasing due to increases in the absolute number of (a) people who have a stroke every year, (b) stroke survivors, (c) DALYs lost due to stroke, and (d) stroke-related deaths.

References

Bennett DA, Krishnamurthi RV, Barker-Collo S, Forouzanfar MH, Naghavi M, Connor M, et al.; Global Burden of Diseases, Injuries, and Risk Factors 2010 Study Stroke Expert Group. (2014). The global burden of ischemic stroke: findings of the GBD 2010 study. *Glob Heart*, **9**, 107–12.

Feigin VL, Forouzanfar MH, Krishnamurthi R, Mensah GA, Connor M, Bennett DA, et al.; Global Burden of Diseases, Injuries, and Risk Factors Study 2010 (GBD 2010) and the GBD Stroke Experts Group. (2014). Global and regional burden of stroke during 1990–2010: findings from the Global Burden of Disease Study 2010. *Lancet*, **383**, 245–54. Erratum in *Lancet*, 2014; **383**: 218.

Feigin VL, Krishnamurthi RV, Parmar P, Norrving B, Mensah GA, Bennett DA, et al.; GBD 2013 Writing Group; GBD 2013 Stroke Panel Experts Group. (2015). Update on the global burden of ischemic and hemorrhagic stroke in 1990–2013: the GBD 2013 Study. *Neuroepidemiology*, **45**, 161–76.

GBD 2013 Mortality and Causes of Death Collaborators. (2015). Global, regional, and national age-sex specific all-cause and cause-specific mortality for 240 causes of death, 1990–2013: a systematic analysis for the Global Burden of Disease Study 2013. *Lancet*, **385**, 117–71

GBD 2015 Neurological Disorders Collaborator Group. (2017) Global, regional, and national burden of neurological disorders during 1990–2015: a systematic analysis for the Global Burden of Disease Study 2015. *Lancet Neurol*, **16**, 877–97

GBD 2016 DALYs and HALE Collaborators. (2017). Global, regional, and national disability-adjusted life-years (DALYs) for 333 diseases and injuries and healthy life expectancy (HALE) for 195 countries and territories, 1990–2016: a systematic analysis for the Global Burden of Disease Study 2016. *Lancet*, **390**, 1260–1344

GBD 2016 Disease and Injury Incidence and Prevalence Collaborators. (2017). Global, regional, and national incidence, prevalence, and years lived with disability for 328 diseases and injuries for 195 countries, 1990–2016: a systematic analysis for the Global Burden of Disease Study 2016. *Lancet*, **390**, 1211–59.

Global Stroke Statistics 2019. Kim J, Thayabaranathan T, Donnan GA, Howard G, Howard VJ, Rothwell PM, et al. Global Stroke Statistics 2019. Int J Stroke. 2020 Mar

9:1747493020909545. doi: 10.1177/1747493020909545. PMID: 32146867

Krishnamurthi RV, Feigin VL, Forouzanfar MH, Mensah GA, Connor M, Bennett DA, et al.; Global Burden of Diseases, Injuries, Risk Factors Study 2010 (GBD 2010); GBD Stroke Experts Group. (2013). Global and regional burden of first-ever ischaemic and haemorrhagic stroke during 1990–2010: findings from the Global Burden of Disease Study 2010. *Lancet Glob Health*, **1**, e259–81.

Krishnamurthi RV, Moran AE, Forouzanfar MH, Bennett DA, Mensah GA, Lawes CM, et al.; Global Burden of Diseases, Injuries, and Risk Factors 2010 Study Stroke Expert Group. (2014). The global burden of hemorrhagic stroke: a summary of findings from the GBD 2010 study. *Glob Heart*, **9**, 101–6.

Krishnamurthi RV, Moran AE, Feigin VL, Barker-Collo S, Norrving B, Mensah GA, et al.; GBD 2013 Stroke Panel Experts Group. (2015). Stroke prevalence, mortality and disability-adjusted life years in adults aged 20–64 years in 1990–2013: data from the Global Burden of Disease 2013 Study. *Neuroepidemiology*, **45**, 190–202.

Thrift AG, Thayabaranathan T, Howard G, Howard VJ, Rothwell PM, Feigin VL, et al. (2017). Global stroke statistics. *Int J Stroke*, **12**, 13–32.

Chapter 2

Understanding Evidence

Jeffrey L. Saver
Graeme J. Hankey

One of the challenges in finding effective treatments for stroke is that stroke is not a single entity. Stroke has a broad spectrum of clinical features, pathologies, aetiologies, and prognoses. Consequently, there is wide variation in the types of treatments for stroke and in the response of patients to effective treatments. This means that 'magic bullet' therapies that treat all types of stroke are likely to be limited in number and effectiveness, confined to aspects of risk factor management to prevent first or recurrent stroke, acute supportive care to prevent early complications, and rehabilitation treatments to promote neuroplasticity and stroke recovery. This diversity is analogous to that seen with infectious diseases and cancers. They also have a broad spectrum of clinical features, pathologies, causes, and outcomes. As a result, there is a range of antibiotic and antineoplastic treatments targeting different aetiologies and mechanisms of cellular injury and, even in targeted patients, their effectiveness is variable. This is because the response of patients is also determined by other genetic and acquired factors.

Given that there are likely to be different treatments for different causes and sequelae of stroke, and different responses in different patients, stroke researchers need ideally to aim to evaluate the effects of treatments for particular pathological and aetiological subtypes and sequelae of stroke, and stroke clinicians need ideally to strive to target effective treatments to appropriate patients who are likely to respond favourably.

Stroke clinicians therefore need to know which treatments for patients with particular types and sequelae of stroke are effective (or ineffective), and their respective risks and costs. Theory alone is insufficient for guiding practice; treatments should have been tested appropriately and thoroughly in clinical practice (Doust and Del Mar, 2004; Ionnadis, 2005; Djulbegovic and Guyatt, 2017). Although appropriate

evaluation usually requires enormous efforts and resources, this is several-fold less than the costs of misplaced scepticism, which leads to underuse of effective treatments, and of misplaced enthusiasm, which leads to the introduction of, and perseverance with, ineffective and dangerous treatments. Formal evaluations demonstrating the effectiveness of many therapeutic advances have led to their wide dissemination in practice, such as statins and carotid artery revascularization procedures for stroke prevention and intravenous thrombolytics and endovascular thrombectomy for acute ischaemic stroke (Sarpong and Zuvekas, 2014; Lichtman et al., 2017; Adeoye et al., 2011; George et al., 2019). Conversely, formal trials showing lack of benefit of many physiologically plausible treatments have led to reductions in use of many costly, and sometimes risky, ineffective therapies, such as extracranial–intracranial bypass surgery for atherosclerotic disease and intensive glucose control for acute ischaemic stroke (Johnston et al., 2006; Powers et al., 2011; Johnston et al., 2019). This experience confirms that it is critical to evaluate all potential therapies for stroke with formal controlled clinical trials, and to enrol eligible patients in available trials. Contrary to the commonly expressed notion that it is not ethical to enrol patients in controlled clinical trials in which they might not be allocated to a therapy in which a physician has a strong personal, but unvalidated, belief, moral imperatives support performance and offering enrolment in well-designed clinical trials as the best action that can be taken both for the individual patient being cared for and for all future patients (Ashcroft, 2000; Emanuel et al., 2000; van Gjin, 2005; Lyden et al., 2010).

Indeed, a primary reason for the wide variation in stroke management among different clinics, cities, regions, and countries, and use of ineffective and harmful treatments, is continuing uncertainty about the safety and effectiveness of many of the available

Table 2.1 Reasons for using ineffective or harmful treatments

- Lack of reliable evidence of safety and effectiveness
- Over-reliance on surrogate outcomes
- Anecdotal clinical experience
- Use of historical controls
- Unsound theoretical/physiological reasoning (e.g. enthusiasm for a particular physiological model, which is incorrect)
- Dismal natural history of the disease (poor prognosis so unwillingness not to offer some therapy)
- Patients' expectations (real or assumed)
- A desire to 'do something'
- Ritual
- No questions asked or permitted ('eminence-based' rather than 'evidence-based' medicine)

treatments due to the lack of reliable evidence of efficacy and safety (Table 2.1) (Chalmers, 2004; Doust and Del Mar, 2004; Ionnadis, 2005). Fewer than 10–25% of practice guideline recommendations in cardiovascular care are supported by high-grade randomized trial evidence (McAlister et al., 2007; Schumacher et al., 2019).

In the presence of systematic uncertainty about the relative intrinsic merits of different treatments, clinicians cannot be sure about their benefits in any particular instance – as in treating an individual patient. Therefore, it seems irrational and unethical to insist one way or another before the completion of a suitable evaluation/trial of the different treatments. Therefore, the best treatment for the patient is to participate in a relevant trial (Ashcroft, 2000; Emanuel et al., 2000; Lyden et al., 2010). Although this is experimentation, it is simply choice under uncertainty, coupled with data collection. The choice is made by random allocation, and constructive doubt is its practical counterpart, but this should not matter as there is no better mechanism for choice under uncertainty. When circumstances increase practitioner unease with random allocation, as when there is strong personal belief in a therapy even though there is community scientific equipoise or when the outcome of standard care is uniformly poor, enrolment into clinical trials can be made more appealing to clinicians and patients by use of unequal ratio randomization (e.g. 2 patients randomized to experimental therapy for every 1 to conventional care) (Broderick et al., 2013); response-adaptive randomization (dynamically changing the randomization ratio to assign more patients to more effective or safer treatment regimens based on interim data from an ongoing trial) (Hobbs et al., 2013); and

incorporation of the 'uncertainty principle' as an entry criterion. The 'uncertainty principle' approach states that a patient can be entered if, and only if, the responsible clinician is, personally, substantially uncertain which of the trial treatments would be most appropriate for that particular patient (ECST Trialists, 1998; Sackett, 2000; IST-3 Collaborative Group et al., 2012). If clinicians are inaccurate in their personal judgements of treatment benefits, trials enrolling with the 'uncertainty principle' as an added entry criterion will yield the same results as trials enrolling without this addition; however, if clinicians are accurate in their understanding of treatment benefits, enrolling under the 'uncertainty principle' will tend to bias trials toward neutral results (Vyas and Saver, 2016).

In order to assess the effects of a treatment on outcome after stroke, the treatment must be evaluated in patients, and the outcomes it yields must be compared with those in patients who have not been exposed to the treatment, but who are ideally identical in all other ways such as in prevalence and level of prognostic factors that influence outcome (i.e. a control group). A control group is needed because the outcome after stroke is neither uniformly poor nor good (i.e. it is variable), and because it is difficult to accurately predict the outcome of any individual patient (see Chapter 1).

As stroke commonly causes substantial loss of brain tissue within minutes to hours, and there are many pathogenetic pathways mediating injury in acute stroke, it is likely that individual efficacious treatments for stroke will have small to moderate benefits, rather than massively favourable effects, on patient outcome. Should a dramatically beneficial treatment exist, it could in theory exert so large a treatment effect that it could be identified reliably from observational studies of the outcome of treated patients compared with the literature or with untreated historical or concurrent controls, without the need for large randomized trials. This is because any possible modest effects of systematic or random error, either in the opposite direction to the treatment effect (i.e. reducing the true treatment effect) or in the same direction as the treatment effect (i.e. inflating the true treatment effect), are not likely to be large enough to disguise the dramatic effect of the treatment. For example, the striking effectiveness of penicillin was realized from observational studies of treated patients with hitherto uniformly fatal or disabling diseases,

Table 2.2 Common sources of error in studies of interventions for stroke

Systematic errors (biases) in the assessment of treatment effects

- Selection bias (systematic pretreatment differences in comparator groups)
- Performance bias (systematic differences in the care provided apart from the intervention being evaluated)
- Attrition bias (systematic differences in withdrawals from the treatment groups)
- Recording/detection bias (systematic differences in outcome assessment)
- Outcome reporting bias (selective reporting of some, but not other, outcomes depending on direction of the results)

Random errors in the assessment of treatment effects

- Relate to the impact of play of chance on comparisons of the outcome between those exposed and not exposed to the treatment of interest
- Are determined by the number of relevant outcome events in the study
- The potential error can be quantified by means of a confidence interval (CI) which indicates the range of effects statistically compatible with the observed results
- Can prevent real effects of treatment being detected or their size being estimated reliably

Table 2.3 Strategies to minimize systematic and random errors

Minimization of systematic error

- Proper randomization
- Analysis by allocated treatment (including all randomized patients: intention to treat)
- Outcome evaluation blind to allocated treatment
- Pre-specification of primary outcome (preventing data dredging or 'p-hacking')
- Chief emphasis on results in overall population (without undue data-dependent emphasis on particular subgroups)
- Systematic review of all relevant studies (without undue data-dependent emphasis on particular studies)

Minimization of random error

- Large numbers of participants with major outcomes (with streamlined methods to facilitate recruitment)
- Systematic search and review of all relevant studies (yielding the largest possible number of participants with major outcome events)

such as pneumococcal meningitis, who subsequently recovered dramatically after penicillin. Randomized controlled trials (RCTs) were deemed not to be required.

However, the great preponderance of (if not all) treatments for stroke are likely to have mild or moderate effects. Even relatively small benefits of a treatment for stroke are clinically worthwhile, given the frequency of morbidity and mortality and expense from the disease, particularly if the treatment is safe, inexpensive, and widely applicable (Warlow 2004; Cranston et al., 2017). In order to reliably identify such moderate, yet important, treatment effects, it is necessary to ensure that they are not underestimated or even nullified (and therefore missed) by modest systematic or random errors (false negative, or type II error) (Table 2.2) (Collins and MacMahon, 2001; Rush et al., 2018). Similarly, for treatments with no effect, it is necessary that modest systematic and random errors are minimized, and not sufficiently large to produce an erroneous conclusion that the treatment is effective (false positive, or type I error).

Strategies to Minimize Systematic and Random Errors

Reliable and accurate identification of treatment effects requires simultaneous minimization of systematic errors (bias) and random errors (Table 2.3).

Randomization is the most efficient method of minimizing systematic bias in treatment allocation; *blinded outcome evaluation* is the most efficient method of minimizing observer or recording/detection bias; *pre-specification and pre-registration* of the primary outcome and hypothesis is the most reliable method of minimizing outcome reporting bias; and registering and analysing *large numbers of participants with primary outcome events* (and therefore randomizing large numbers of patients) is the main method of minimizing random error (Collins and MacMahon, 2001; Kaplan et al., 2014; Gopal et al., 2018; Strauss et al., 2019).

Of these, random error is arguably the most important to minimize. Surprisingly large numbers of patients (often thousands or even tens of thousands) must be included in randomized trials of stroke treatments to provide really reliable estimates of effect. Trials of such size are uncommon in stroke medicine.

Different study types vary in the degree to which they restrain bias and overcome noise to provide reliable measurement of treatment effects. The best evidence about the effects of stroke treatments comes from large RCTs in which there are large numbers of

Table 2.4 Hierarchy of evidence strength supporting a therapy per evidence-based medicine

Randomized trials

1. Multiple, congruent, very large mega-trials
2. Single, very large mega-trial
3. Multiple, congruent small- to moderate-size trials
4. Multiple, mostly congruent small- to moderate-size trials
5. Single small- to moderate-size trial

Observational data

6. Large and propensity-weighted or multivariate-adjusted studies
7. Small or unadjusted studies

Physiological data

8. Studies in humans
9. Studies in other species

Authority

10. Expert opinion

outcome events, and in which outcome evaluation is undertaken by observers who are blinded to the treatment allocation. Evidence-based medicine grading classifications array granular study types in order from most to least reliable. Though the fine orderings differ modestly across different consensus groups and authors (Laika 2008; Shaneyfelt 2016), the shared overall framework is to value RCTs at the highest tier, followed by large observational studies that have made some attempts at adjusting for differences in patient groups, then physiological studies, and lastly expert opinion (Table 2.4).

Grading Systems for Recommendations in Evidence-based Guidelines

Formal grading systems have been developed to characterize the strength of evidence for diagnostic and treatment recommendations advanced in guidelines. Two systems that are commonly applied in assessing stroke prevention and treatment strategies are (1) the Grading of Recommendations Assessment, Development and Evaluation (GRADE) working group system (Table 2.5) (Guyatt et al., 2011); and (2) the American College of Cardiology/American Heart Association (American Stroke Association) (ACC/AHA) clinical practice guideline recommendation classification system (Table 2.6) (Halperin et al., 2016).

Key Elements to the Design of a Clinical Trial of a Treatment for Stroke

All clinical trials *should* be designed and reported using the CONSORT guidelines (Schulz et al., 2010). However, not all trials are reported in this way and not all journals insist on it (Blanco et al., 2018). Thus, some trials may have been carried out adequately but reported inadequately, and others may have been designed and carried out inadequately. When analysing a clinical trial, several important aspects of design, conduct, reporting, and interpretation should be considered. Several key aspects are covered in this section and, for further details of what to look for in a report of an RCT, we would recommend Lees et al. (2003), Lewis and Warlow (2004), Rothwell et al. (2005), Schulz et al. (2010), Saver (2011), Bath et al. (2012), Dahabreh et al. (2016), Hill (2018), and Higgins et al. (2018).

Hypothesis and Aim

- Are the study primary hypothesis and aim clearly stated, in a testable (falsifiable) manner? In addition, was the primary analysis to test the study hypothesis pre-specified prior to data unblinding?
- Were study secondary hypotheses and subgroup analyses clearly stated? In addition, were the analyses to test secondary hypotheses and subgroups pre-specified prior to data unblinding?

Design

- What is the study design?
- Is it a randomized trial?
- Is the method of randomization described and was it an appropriate method? (Broglio, 2018)

    Was the decision to enter each patient made irreversibly in ignorance of which trial treatment that patient would be allocated to receive? If not (e.g. if allocation was based on date of birth, date of admission, alternation [e.g. first patient receives treatment A, second receives treatment B, and alternating assignment continues thereafter]), foreknowledge of the next treatment allocation could affect the decision to enter the patient, and those allocated one treatment might then differ systematically from those allocated another.

Table 2.5 GRADE system for rating quality of evidence for evidence-based guidelines

Study design	Quality of evidence	Lower rating if ...	Higher rating if ...
Randomized trial	High	Risk of bias	Large effect
	Moderate	−1 Serious	+1 Large
		−2 Very serious	+2 Very large
Observational study	Low	Inconsistency	Dose response
	Very Low	−1 Serious	+1 Evidence of a gradient
		−2 Very serious	All plausible confounding
		Indirectness	+1 Would reduce a
		−1 Serious	demonstrated effect, or
		−2 Very serious	+1 Would suggest a
		Imprecision	spurious effect when
		−1 Serious	results show no effect
		−2 Very serious	
		Publication bias	
		−1 Serious	
		−2 Very serious	

Source: From Guyatt et al. (2011).

Table 2.6 ACC/AHA (ASA) system for rating strength of, and quality of evidence for, evidence-based guideline recommendations

Class (strength) of recommendations *Reflects the magnitude of benefit over risk*	
Class I (Strong)	Benefit>>>Risk
Class IIa (Moderate)	Benefit>>Risk
Class IIb (Weak)	Benefit>Risk
Class III: No Benefit (Moderate)	Benefit=Risk
Class III: Harm (Strong)	Risk>Benefit

Level (quality) of evidence
Reflects the certainty of the evidence supporting the recommendation

Level A
- High-quality evidence from more than 1 RCT
- Meta-analyses of high-quality RCTs
- One or more RCTs corroborated by high-quality registry studies

Level B-R (randomized)
- Moderate-quality evidence from 1 or more RCTs
- Meta-analyses of moderate-quality RCTs

Level B-NR (nonrandomized)
- Moderate-quality evidence from 1 or more well-designed, well-executed nonrandomized studies, observational studies, or registry studies
- Meta-analyses of such studies

Level C-LD (limited data)
- Randomized or nonrandomized observational or registry studies with limitations of design or execution
- Meta-analyses of such studies
- Physiological or mechanistic studies in human subjects

Level C-EO (expert opinion)
- Consensus of expert opinion based on clinical experience

Source: From Halpern et al. (2016).
RCT: randomized controlled trial.

Were adequate measures taken to conceal allocations, such as use of central internet or phone randomization assignment systems? Or were concealment methods vulnerable to potential breaching by site staff, such as use of sealed envelopes that could be held up to the light and made semi-transparent?

Patients

- Were explicit and clearly operational inclusion and exclusion criteria employed?
- Were most eligible patients enrolled? Or were many treated outside of the trial, rendering the trial population potentially not representative of the targeted patient population?

Follow-up

- Were all patients followed up prospectively at pre-specified, regular intervals?
- Was patient follow-up complete?

    If not, this can lead to attrition bias (systematic differences in withdrawals from trials), because patients who are withdrawn from, or stop participating in, a trial tend to differ from those who remain in the study (e.g. they may have a higher rate of complications or adverse effects from the disease or treatment respectively). This type of bias can be minimized by performing an 'intention-to-treat analysis' where the analysis of results at the end of the study includes every patient who was assigned to the intervention or control group, regardless of whether they received the assigned treatment or subsequently dropped out of the trial (see below).
- Was the trial stopped early? Truncated RCTs may be associated with greater effect sizes than RCTs not stopped early (Bassler et al., 2010).

Outcome measures

Is the primary measure of outcome:
- relevant to the patient (e.g. death, functional dependency, serious vascular event)?
- relevant to the intervention (i.e. potentially modifiable by the treatment, given its expected mechanism of action)?
- valid (does it actually measure what it intends to measure)?
- reliable (reproducible)?

- simple?
- communicable?

Avoid surrogate outcome measures in pivotal phase III studies:
- Surrogate outcomes may reflect only one part of the disease process and beneficial effects on them may not be associated with worthwhile improvements in survival and functional outcome. Deciding whether a treatment is safe and efficacious just on the basis of its effects on a physiological measurement, a blood test, or an imaging biomarker may be misleading.
- Basing treatment decisions on effects on surrogate outcomes may be hazardous (Fleming and Powers, 2012). Cardiac premature beats are associated with a poor prognosis and antidysrhythmic drugs can markedly reduce their frequency. However, various antidysrhythmic drugs, though they reduce the surrogate outcome (ventricular premature beats), actually increase mortality.

Outcome Evaluation

- Were the outcome events ascertained in such a way to reduce the risk of bias (i.e. blind to the assigned treatment)?

Statistical Analysis

- Is the primary analysis by intention-to-treat (i.e. is the final analysis based on the groups to which all randomized patients were originally allocated)?

    Even in a properly randomized trial, bias can be inadvertently introduced by the post-randomization exclusion of certain patients (e.g. those who are non-compliant with treatment), particularly if the outcome of those excluded from one treatment group differs from that of those excluded from another. 'On-treatment' comparisons, among only those who were compliant, are therefore potentially biased (DeMets and Cook, 2019). However, because there is always some non-compliance with allocated treatments in clinical trials, an intention-to-treat analysis tends to underestimate the effects produced by full compliance with study treatments. In order to estimate the treatment effect with full compliance, it is more appropriate to avoid using the potentially biased 'on-treatment' comparisons, and to apply the approximately level of compliance seen in the trial (e.g. 80%) to the estimate of the treatment effect provided by the intention-to-treat comparison, to yield a less-biased estimate of therapeutic effect with full compliance (e.g. a 10% absolute risk reduction with 80% compliance would suggest a 12% absolute risk reduction with 100% compliance).

- Is the point estimate for the treatment effect, and its confidence interval (CI), stated, not just p-values?

  It is important that the results are expressed to indicate the clinical magnitude of effect (treatment effect point estimate) and the uncertainty around that magnitude (CI), not just statistical significance or non-significance (p-value) (Sullivan and Feinn, 2012). Trials optimally should give a precise estimate of treatment effect and therefore have narrow CIs (e.g. absolute reduction of 25%, 95% CI: 22–28%).

- Is the result stated as an absolute effect rather than only as a relative effect?

  Large relative treatment effects can look impressive (e.g. '50% reduction'), but if event rates are low, the absolute benefit may be small (e.g. reduction from 2% to 1% of patients having an event over 10 years).

- Is the result clinically significant as well as statistically significant?

  Outcome differences that do not exceed the minimal clinically important difference (MCID), as determined by patients and clinicians, are of no important consequence. As has been said, 'A difference, to be a difference, must make a difference.'

- Do pre-specified secondary outcomes show the same general direction and degree of effect as the primary outcome?

  Consistent evidence of a treatment effect across all pre-specified endpoints that are expected to have some co-variation provides supportive evidence that the benefit or non-benefit on the primary outcome reflects a genuine biological effect and not play of chance.

- Are there safety (on-treatment) population and per-protocol population analyses, and are they appropriate?

  In addition to the primary analysis in the intention-to-treat population, it can be helpful to analyse select outcomes in predefined safety and per-protocol populations. The safety/on-treatment population will include all patients as actually treated, rather than as randomized (e.g. a patient who was randomized to treatment A but actually received treatment B will be included in the treatment A group in the intent-to-treat analysis, but in the treatment B group in the safety analysis). Analysis of the safety/on-treatment population may be of value in describing the frequency of specific adverse effects among only those who actually received the treatment. The 'per-protocol' population will include all patients in both treatment groups deemed to have been handled throughout the study in a protocol-adherent manner, including adjudicated as meeting all study entry criteria even when additional information about the patient emerges after trial enrolment and complying with the allocated treatment. Evidence that treatment benefits or harms are magnified in the per-protocol population, compared with the intention-to-treat population, provides supportive evidence that the effects are due to genuine biological activity rather than play of chance.

- Is the intervention cost-effective compared with (an)other intervention(s)?

  Given that finite societal resources are available for healthcare, it is important to quantify the relative health benefits, harms, and costs associated with alternative interventions by means of a cost-effectiveness analysis. This is an analytic approach in which the incremental financial costs and incremental changes in health outcome states of an intervention (intervention A) and at least one alternative (intervention B) are calculated. The incremental costs are the additional resources (e.g. medical care costs, costs from productivity changes) incurred from the use of intervention A over intervention B. The health outcome changes are typically the number of cases of a disease prevented or the number of quality-adjusted life-years (QALYs) gained through the use of intervention A over intervention B. The result is expressed as the difference in cost between the two interventions divided by the difference in their effect – the incremental cost effectiveness ratio (ICER) (Sanders et al., 2019). The World Health Organization has suggested that a reasonable threshold for considering an intervention cost-effective is 1–3 times the annual per capita gross domestic product (GDP) of a country per additional QALY, which for the developed nations is approximately $50,000 to $175,000 per QALY gained (WHO Commission on Macroeconomics and Health, 2001).

If there are there any subgroup analyses:

- Were they pre-specified and adjusted for multiple data looks?

    As individual patients differ from each other and treatments can have disparate effects in individuals with different clinical features, there is an understandable temptation to examine treatment effects in subgroups of interest, particularly if the overall trial is negative. However, the more subgroups that are examined the more likely that an effect will be identified due to chance (e.g. analysing 20 subgroups will lead to one being statistically significant at the $p = 0.05$ level, 1 out of 20, just due to play of chance) (Counsell et al., 1994; Munroe, 2011). Post hoc subgroup analyses cannot, therefore, be regarded as anything more than hypothesis-generating. Even pre-specified subgroup analyses, if many analytic groups were planned, must be considered hypothesis-generating unless the p-value threshold for considering a finding statistically significant has been lowered to account for the multiplicity of analyses. Any apparent treatment effect must be confirmed in a further trial in which there is an a priori hypothesis that a particular subgroup of patients will benefit while other subgroups will not.

- Are claims advanced regarding them based on evidence of differences in response between the groups?

    Individual population segments in subgroup analyses have fewer patients than in the overall trial. Consequently, analysis of an individual subgroup segment alone (e.g. only older patients) is almost always underpowered to determine the presence or absence of treatment effects, and is vulnerable to showing chance associations or non-associations. In contrast, analyses of differences across subgroup segments (e.g. older *versus* younger patients) use the full size and power of the whole sample of randomized patients. Evidence of heterogeneity of response across subgroups (e.g. an interaction between age and treatment response) provides more reliable evidence of

Table 2.7 Criteria to assess the credibility of subgroup analyses

Design

1. Is the subgroup variable a characteristic measured at baseline or after randomization?
2. Is the effect suggested by comparisons within rather than between studies?
3. Was the hypothesis specified a priori?
4. Was the direction of the subgroup effect specified a priori?
5. Was the subgroup effect one of a small number of hypothesized effects tested?

Analysis

6. Does the interaction test suggest a low likelihood that chance explains the apparent subgroup effect?
7. Is the significant subgroup effect independent?

Context

8. Is the size of the subgroup effect large?
9. Is the interaction consistent across studies?
10. Is the interaction consistent across closely related outcomes within the study?
11. Is there indirect evidence that supports the hypothesized interaction (biological rationale)?

a genuine qualitative difference in treatment effect (Table 2.7) (Sun et al., 2010; Wallach et al., 2017).

Conclusions

- Is the study conclusion supported by the trial's findings?

    Claims that a trial has shown a treatment benefit or harm should only be advanced if findings for the pre-specified primary outcome show an effect that is both statistically significant (exceeds the pre-specified p-value threshold for the trial) and clinically significant (exceeds the MCID) (Pocock and Stone, 2016b). Conversely, if a trial has not shown superiority of one treatment over another, that does not mean it has shown the two treatments are equivalent (Pocock and Stone, 2016a; Mauri and D'Agostino, 2017). Failure to demonstrate that treatment yields a large difference in outcomes does not rule out the possibility that the treatment yields a more modest, but clinically meaningful, difference in outcomes (Pocock and Stone, 2016a, 2016b). Many trials are underpowered to rule out small to moderate, but clinically meaningful, effects on outcome. Only if the trial results have demonstrated that any differences between the treatments must be less than the MCID (as is the goal of equivalence and non-inferiority trials) can a claim be advanced that there are no differences in outcome with the study intervention.

Trial Sponsorship and Competing Interests

The development of new medical interventions requires funding, and elements of a market economy are indispensable. However, capitalism should be subject to restraining forces to ensure an appropriate balance with any other endeavour in society, and especially so when individuals' lives and health are directly affected. Sponsors of trials of interventions have a right to use their knowledge regarding an intervention's effect and general principles of study design to inform trial protocols, but they also have a responsibility to study participants and future patients and prescribers of an intervention to include, in study design, conduct, analysis, and reporting, clinicians with expertise in the disease being treated and in disease-specific aspects of trial design (Donnan et al., 2003; van Gijn, 2005; Harman et al., 2015; Rasmussen et al., 2018).

Due to the potential for the best interests of patients and society to be compromised by the financial interests of the sponsors and prescribing/procedure-performing clinicians, it is essential that the highest form of honesty and integrity prevails (Shaw, 1911; Lo and Field, 2009).

To foster ethical conduct and reporting of clinical trials, several regulations and guidelines have been developed. 'Good Clinical Practice (GCP)' guidelines provide an ethical and scientific quality standard for investigators, sponsors, monitors, and institutional review boards throughout each stage of drug trials (International Council for Harmonisation, 2016). The GCP recommendations focus on diverse study aspects, including the relations between the site clinical investigator and both the patient and the sponsor, how often every value in the trial records of individual patients should be checked against source medical records, and which disciplines and stakeholders should be represented on institutional review boards/research ethics committees. In a complementary effort, the DAMOCLES consensus group has delineated the types and roles of data safety and monitoring boards tasked to perform constant oversight of the well-being and interests of trial participants during study conduct (DAMOCLES Study Group, 2005). The International Committee of Medical Journal Editors (ICMJE) have established requirements for transparent reporting of who was responsible for data storage, management, and analysis among study sponsors and academic steering committees (ICMJE, 2018). Best practices in transparent declaration and management of financial conflicts of interest among clinical investigators have been promulgated (AAMC-AAU Advisory Committee on Financial Conflicts of Interest in Human Subjects Research, 2008; Lo and Field, 2009; Stead, 2017). To prevent non-publication of unfavourable trial results (publication bias), the ICMJE, consensus groups, and governmental legislation and regulations have indicated that trials should be publicly registered before initiation, report key results in a publicly accessible manner, and work to make de-identified individual patient-level data available for external, independent analysis (Laine et al., 2007; Ali et al., 2012; Zarin et al., 2016; Taichman et al., 2018). Preliminary guidance has also been developed regarding the composition, roles, and responsibilities of academic steering committees of clinical trials (Donnan et al., 2003; van Gijn, 2005; Harman et al., 2015; Rasmussen et al., 2018).

There is evidence that research funded by pharmaceutical companies is more likely to have outcomes favouring the sponsor than research funded from other sources (Bekelman et al., 2003; Falk Delgado and Falk Delgado, 2017; Lundh et al., 2017), including for neurovascular and cardiovascular trials (Liebeskind et al., 2006; Ridker and Torres, 2006). As industry-funded trials, compared with academic sponsored trials, are on average designed with higher-quality features to reduce risk of bias (Lundh et al., 2017), the higher rate of positive findings seems likely to be due to non-reporting of nonpositive trials (publication bias), more frequent use of surrogate endpoints more likely to show treatment effect, and more favourable interpretation of study mathematical results ('spin'). Recent initiatives to mandate trial registration and reporting and to require pre-specification of primary analyses may mitigate this discrepancy, and represent appropriate regulatory supervision to ensure transparent and complete reporting of trial results regardless of sponsor type.

It is crucial that trial sponsorship and all potential competing interests are presented in any report of a study.

Limitations of RCTs

Sample Size (Random Error and Imprecise Estimates of Treatment Effects)

Although RCTs provide the least biased and hence most reliable evaluation of whether a treatment is effective and safe, they are commonly limited by sub-optimal sample size. As a result, there is potential for some random error and therefore imprecision in the estimated treatment effect.

Generalizability/External Validity

Another weakness of RCTs is limited generalizability. The results of trials conducted in a single centre, region, or country and in a single racial or ethnic group or type of patients cannot necessarily be generalized (applied) to other centres, regions, or countries and other racial or ethnic groups or types of patients. Often, patients enrolled in clinical trials are on average younger and healthier than patients encountered in clinical practice (Flather et al., 2006; Sheth et al., 2016). Even well-executed trials with sound internal validity may not necessarily inform us about the effect of a treatment among patients who were not entered into the trial (i.e. its external validity) (Rothwell, 2005; Dekkers et al., 2010).

One of the solutions to the geographical and race–ethnic limitations of RCTs conducted in individual countries is to conduct multicentre trials in multiple countries, but the disadvantages include practical difficulties, time, and cost (Senn and Lewis, 2019). Another solution, particularly if a single, large multi-national RCT is impractical, is to perform parallel trials in different regions contemporaneously, using shared methodology and data definitions to facilitate pooled analysis upon completion (Mead et al., 2015). Failing that, a further approach is to perform a systematic review and meta-analysis of independently designed and conducted trials from different localities.

Systematic Reviews and Meta-analyses of RCTs

A systematic review and meta-analysis seeks to reduce systematic error (bias) and random error by applying scientific methods to the review of all of the published and unpublished research evidence; in this case RCTs. The PRISMA statement provides consensus recommendations of best practices when reporting systematic reviews and meta-analyses (Liberati et al., 2009).

Systematic Reviews

The scientific methods or strategies of a systematic review include the following:

- Defining the *research question* to ensure the review will be relevant and reliable and guide the development of the review protocol. Most reviews define a broad question (e.g. Does thrombolysis in acute ischaemic stroke improve outcome?) which includes several pre-specified subquestions (e.g. Does thrombolysis with alteplase within 3 hours of stroke onset reduce death and dependency at 3–6 months after stroke?).
- Developing a *review protocol* based on the research question. The protocol contains specific explicit and reproducible inclusion and exclusion criteria for selecting trials for the review in order to minimize bias in trial selection. The protocol also contains explicit methods of data extraction and synthesis to minimize bias during data collection and the analysis of results.
- Undertaking a systematic and *comprehensive search* for all potentially relevant trials.
- Applying the pre-specified eligibility criteria to *select relevant trials.*
- Performing a *critical appraisal* of quality (research designs and characteristics) of the trials to ensure that most emphasis is given to the most methodologically sound trials.
- *Extracting and analysing data* using predefined, explicit methods. The statistical synthesis of analysis of the results is called a meta-analysis (see Meta-analyses section later in this chapter).
- *Interpreting* the results and drawing conclusions based on the totality of the available evidence (not a biased subset).

Therefore, a systematic review provides a method of reviewing the available evidence using explicit scientific strategies to reduce any bias (e.g. in trial selection and data extraction) in the estimate of the direction of the treatment effect from using only selected trials, and to increase the precision of the estimate of the treatment effect by examining a larger amount of data and thereby reducing random error (Higgins and Green, 2011; Murad et al., 2014; Pollock and Berge, 2018).

Sources of Bias in Systematic Reviews

There are three main sources of bias in systematic reviews: publication bias, study quality bias, and outcome recording bias.

Publication Bias

Systematic reviews aim to identify and include all trials that are relevant to the research question. However, some studies are difficult to find, and these may tend to differ from trials which are easy to find. For example, studies which have reported a 'positive' or interesting result are more likely to be published, and therefore easier to locate, than studies which have produced 'negative' (harmful or neutral) results (Liebeskind et al., 2006; Hopewell et al., 2009). The conduct of a systematic review therefore needs to engage multiple overlapping sources of study ascertainment. The search should ideally cover multiple electronic databases of published trials (e.g. Medline, Embase), mixed published and unpublished trials (e.g. the Cochrane Central Register of Controlled Trials [CENTRAL]), and trial registries (e.g. clinicaltrials.gov in the USA, the Australian New Zealand Clinical Trials Registry [ANZCTR] in Australasia, and the Chinese Clinical Trial Registry [ChiCTR] in China), as each individual database has some restrictions in scope, e.g. to a journal in certain languages. In addition, hand searching of additional sources, including additional journals, conference abstracts, theses, and unpublished trials, should be undertaken, as well as review of studies cited in initially retrieved articles (Higgins and Green, 2011; Chan, 2012; NICE, 2014).

Study Quality Bias

There is sound empirical evidence that more methodologically robust trials tend to indicate that new treatments are less effective than do less reliable trials (Savovic et al., 2018). It is therefore important that the conduct of a systematic review includes a measure of the methodological quality of the trials included, and if possible a sensitivity analysis of the results according to the methodological quality of the trials (Higgins and Green, 2011; Higgins et al., 2018).

Outcome Reporting Bias

Most clinical trials measure and analyse several outcomes. There is a tendency for some trials to publish the results of their most impressive outcomes and not to report their least impressive results. If a systematic review then combines only the published results from trial reports, there will be a bias toward overestimating the benefits of the intervention. Such outcome recording bias is minimized by (1) requiring individual trials to report results for all of their planned outcomes; (2) having all trials in a particular area agree to collect a core outcome set of shared, standardized outcomes; and (3) defining, in advance, the outcomes which are to be used in the systematic review and then collecting the relevant data consistently from each study just for those outcomes (Clarke and Williamson, 2016; Kirkham et al., 2018). Thereby, the relevant outcomes for the research question should be recorded in a similar manner among the different trials.

Meta-analyses

A *meta-analysis* is a statistical process for combining data from different trials.

Study-level and Individual Participant Data Meta-analyses

There are two broad types of meta-analysis approaches for interventional clinical trials: (1) study-level meta-analysis, and (2) individual participant-level data (IPD) meta-analysis (Jones et al., 2009). Study-level meta-analysis is the more common technique. Aggregate, summary, treatment-group level data are extracted from trial reports (e.g. the number of patients randomized to each group and the number of outcome events in each treatment group), but not individual patient-level data (e.g. which patient had or did not have an outcome event, and the particular characteristics). Study-level meta-analyses have advantages of more readily available data sources (published, and perhaps unpublished, trial-level reports), simplicity of data abstraction, and reduced analytic workload.

For individual participant data meta-analyses, data are collected on every individual participant enrolled in every trial and pooled in a unified database (Riley et al., 2010; Stewart et al., 2015). Individual participant data meta-analyses require sharing of detailed, unpublished, patient-level data from many trials, take longer to perform, and are more resource intensive. However, individual participant-level data meta-analyses can be more reliable that study-level meta-analyses, and uniquely permit analysis of detailed interactions of multiple patient baseline features and response to study treatment. In most instances (4 times out of 5), study-level and individual participant-level data meta-analyses yield similar conclusions for a primary outcome effect, but occasionally they produce different results and the individual patient data analysis will more often be correct (Tudur Smith et al., 2016).

Outcome Data Types

The type of meta-analytic statistical technique to use when analysing the data depends on the type of outcome event being evaluated. Most stroke prevention trials have recorded dichotomous outcomes (e.g. occurrence of recurrent stroke or not), and can be analysed based on how many patients had events (proportion with event) or, reflecting different durations of follow-up across and within trials, based on time to occurrence of an event (hazard ratio). Most acute stroke trials have recorded ordinal outcomes, reflecting the spectrum of disability that can result from stroke, such as the 7-level modified Rankin Scale (mRS) that assigns patients to ordered, but not equally spaced, levels of disability ranging from 0 – symptom free, through various levels of survival with disability, to 6 – dead. Ordinal scales can be analysed by dichotomizing them into binary endpoints (e.g. alive and independent [mRS 0–2] vs dependent or dead [mRS 3–6]) or by analysing shifts in the distribution of outcomes across all the scale's health states (e.g. common odds ratio) (Saver and Gornbein, 2009; Saver, 2011; Bath et al., 2012). Some trials report outcomes on continuous scales, such as walking speed or infarct volume. Continuous outcome measures can be analysed by dichotomizing them into binary endpoints (e.g. presence or absence of infarct growth) or by comparing point estimates (mean or median) and measures of dispersion (standard deviation or interquartile range) between treatment groups.

Fixed-effects and Random-effects Meta-analysis Models

If the control and treatment groups contain patients followed up in the same way for approximately the same time, the simplest study-level meta-analytic approach is to analyse dichotomous outcomes. Since each study is an independent estimate of the treatment effect with its own sampling error, one cannot just add up all the patients and all the events across the trials and use a simple mean to derive the overall estimated treatment effect. Rather, one must compute a weighted mean of the effect sizes observed in each trial, with more weight given to studies with greater precision (generally studies with larger sample sizes). There are two general approaches to assigning the weights to each study: (1) a 'fixed effect'

model and (2) a 'random effect' model (Borenstein et al., 2010; Higgins and Green, 2011). The fixed effect model assumes that there is one true effect size which is shared by all the included studies. The random effect model allows that the true effect could vary from study to study, e.g. the effect size might be a little higher if patients are older or have more severe initial deficits (Serghiou and Goodman, 2019).

When there is substantial heterogeneity in populations and modes of treatment delivery between different trials, the fixed effects model will not be fully reliable. The random effects model is more appropriate when individual trials differ considerably in study population composition or therapy approach, but it tends to overemphasize the effects of smaller trials.

Alternative Methods of Expressing Treatment Effects: RR, OR, RD, BPH, and NNT

When the outcomes are dichotomous/binary (e.g. occurrence or non-occurrence of stroke, recovery or non-recovery to functional independence), five effect measures are commonly used to express treatment effects:

- Two are measures of *relative* effect: **the risk ratio (RR)** and **the odds ratio (OR)**.
- **Three are measures of *absolute* effect: the risk difference (RD)** (also called the absolute risk reduction), the **benefit per hundred or thousand (BPH or BPT)** (also called the natural frequency), and the **number needed to treat (NNT)**. All three absolute effect measures are different ways of stating the underlying variable.

Methods of calculating these effect measures are shown in Table 2.8.

The risk ratio (or relative risk reduction) is the ratio of the rate of an event in the intervention group versus the rate of an event in the control group. The odds ratio is the ratio of the odds of an event in the intervention group versus the odds of an event in the control group. The numerical values of risk ratios and odds ratios are similar when events occur uncommonly in clinical trial treatment groups, but can differ substantially when events occur frequently (see examples in Table 2.9). Among the measures of relative treatment effect,

Table 2.8 Calculation of risk ratio (RR), odds ratio (OR), risk difference (RD), benefit per hundred (BPH), and number needed to treat (NNT) for a binary outcome from a 2 × 2 table

1. Display trial results as a 2 ×2 table:

	Individuals with unfavourable event ('Loss' = L)	Individuals without unfavourable event ('Win' = W)	Total (N)
Experimental intervention	L(E)	W(E)	N(E)
Control intervention	L(C)	W(C)	N(C)

2. From the above, calculate the following effect measures:

Effect measure	Aspect characterized	Formula
RR	= $\dfrac{\text{risk of event in experimental group}}{\text{risk of event in control group}}$	= $\dfrac{L(E)/N(E)}{L(C)/N(C)}$
OR	= $\dfrac{\text{odds of event in experimental group}}{\text{odds of event in control group}}$	= $\dfrac{L(E)/W(E)}{L(C)/W(C)}$
RD	= risk of event in experimental group – risk of event in control group	= L(E)/N(E) – L(C)/N(C)
BPT	= per hundred patients with experimental rather than control, # fewer who will have event	= RD ×100
NNT	= # patients who need to be treated with experimental rather than control prescription for 1 more patient to avoid event	= 100/RD

risk ratios are generally preferred over odds ratios when expressing relative effects observed in clinical trials, as they are easier to interpret (Sackett et al., 1996; Higgins and Green, 2011). RRs describe the multiplication of the risk that occurs with the use of the experimental intervention. Odds ratios are more challenging to interpret. ORs describe the multiplication of the odds of the outcome that occur with use of the experimental intervention (Norton et al., 2018). To understand what an odds ratio means in terms of changes in numbers of events, it is simplest to first convert it into a risk ratio, given a typical control group risk, and then interpret the risk ratio.

The risk difference is the numerical difference between the rate of an event in the intervention group versus the rate of an event in the control group. The risk difference is straightforward to interpret: it describes the actual difference in the observed rate of events between experimental and control interventions. The RD provides perspective more straightforwardly relevant to clinical decision-making than do relative measures of treatment effect (RR or OR), as it directly conveys the magnitude of benefit for an individual without

varying according to rate of events in the control group (Laupacis et al., 1988; Higgins and Green, 2011; Ranganathan et al., 2016). The benefit per hundred (BPH) and benefit per thousand (BPT) express the risk difference in an even more intuitive manner, as counts of occurrences among commonly understood base population sizes (natural frequencies) (Hoffrage et al., 2000; Saver and Lewis, 2019). For example, consider an intervention that reduces the rate of a dependent or dead outcome from acute stroke by an absolute 2% (RD = 0.02 or 2%). Then out of every 100 patients treated with the intervention rather than control, 2 fewer will have a dependent or dead outcome (BPH = 2). The number needed to treat also expresses the risk difference in a more intuitive manner. The NNT is the number of patients who need to be treated with one therapy vs another for 1 additional patient to have the desired outcome (Laupacis et al., 1988; Saver and Lewis, 2019). In the same example (RD = 0.02, or 2%), the NNT is 50, indicating that among every 50 patients treated with the intervention rather than control, 1 fewer will have dependent or dead outcome.

Table 2.9 Examples of different measures of effect in clinical trials with varying outcome rates and effect magnitudes

Example	Rates of unfavourable outcome		Risk ratio (RR)	Odds ratio (OR)	Risk difference (RD)	Benefit/harm per hundred (BPH)	Number needed to treat (NNT)
	Experimental group	Control group					
Beneficial effects							
1	0.3 (30%)	0.5 (50%)	0.6 (↓40%)	0.43 (↓57%)	0.2 (20%)	20	5
2	0.03 (3%)	0.05 (5%)	0.6 (↓40%)	0.59 (↓41%)	0.02 (2%)	2	50
Nearly neutral effects							
3	0.301 (30.1%)	0.30 (30.0%)	1.01 (↑1%)	1.01 (↑1%)	0.002 (0.2%)	0.2	500
Harmful effects							
4	0.5 (50%)	0.3 (30%)	1.67 (↑67%)	2.33 (↑133%)	−0.2 (−20%)	20	5
5	0.05 (5%)	0.03 (3%)	1.67 (↑67%)	1.70 (↑70%)	−0.02 (−2%)	2	50

Confidence Intervals to Express Precision of Treatment Effect Estimate

An effect estimate derived from a single trial or a group of trials is imperfect, as play of chance may have caused the effect to be higher or lower than the true value in the particular sample of patients in that trial or trials. The degree of imprecision can be characterized by calculating and displaying a CI. The CI indicates the degree of scatter among effect estimates around the true effect size that would be observed if many trials (or groups of trials) of the same size and combined event rates were performed. A 95% CI indicates the range of the estimates of the effect size that would be obtained 95% of the time. As the estimates of the effect size will follow a normal (bell-curve) distribution due to chance, the estimate obtained in any one trial is more likely to lie in the middle of the CI than at the extremes. Confidence intervals should always be presented along with point estimates for effect sizes, for RR, OR, RD, BPH, NNT, and other effect measures.

If the 95% CI of the effect measure does not include (i.e. does not overlap) the null effect value (e.g. 1.0 for RR and OR; 0.0 for RD, BPH, and NNT), the result is statistically significant at the $P = 0.05$ level. The larger the number of outcome events in a trial or meta-analysis, the greater the statistical power, the more precise the result, the narrower the 95% CIs, and the smaller the treatment effect can be and still reach statistical significance. This can be seen in Figure 2.1.

Presentation of Results of Systematic Reviews and Meta-analyses

The results of systematic reviews and meta-analyses are conventionally presented in the format of a graph, called a forest plot (Figure 2.1). For a designated outcome, the result of each trial is allocated a row, and the name of the study appears in the first column. The second and third columns indicate the number of patients with the outcome and the total number of patients for those randomly allocated to the experimental treatment. The fourth and fifth columns indicate the number of patients with the outcome and the total number of patients for those randomly allocated to control. The sixth column indicates the weight given to the individual trial's result in the derivation of the pooled treatment

effect estimate from all trials. The seventh column displays numerically the RR and its 95% CI calculated for each trial. The layout of the right, graphical side is described in the figure legend.

Consistency and Heterogeneity

The different trials brought together in a systematic review will generally vary somewhat in the estimates of treatment effect direction and magnitude that they provide. This heterogeneity in findings of treatment effect arises from three broad sources: clinical, methodological, and statistical (Sedgwick, 2015). Clinical heterogeneity reflects differences between studies in patient populations or in the dose, delivery method, and concomitant care that was provided. Methodological heterogeneity reflects differences between studies in design, conduct, or analysis (e.g. differences in degree of blinding, loss-to-follow-up). The presence of substantial heterogeneity across trials makes the pooled estimate of treatment effect size less reliable, and requires investigation. When heterogeneity arises from clinical factors (e.g. stronger effects in trials enrolling older compared with younger patients, or in trials in which treatment was given earlier after onset), it can provide important insight into features that determine responsiveness to the experimental intervention. However, when lack of consistency across trials does not arise from any identifiable clinical feature, and when it is associated with variations in trial quality, the pooled estimate of treatment effect is less dependable. Use of random effects rather than fixed effects meta-analysis models should be used when there is moderate or greater cross-trial heterogeneity.

As the value and reliability of systematic reviews and meta-analyses is greatest when the results of the studies include treatment effects of similar direction and magnitude, it is useful to establish objectively whether studies in the meta-analysis showed generally consistent or variable findings. A statistical test of heterogeneity is usually presented that assesses whether the differences among the studies are compatible with only arising from chance (so that the studies demonstrate homogeneity in their effect estimates), or whether the differences among the studies are large enough to be unlikely to arise from chance alone (so that the studies demonstrate heterogeneity in their effect estimates) (Higgins et al., 2003; Higgins and Green, 2011). Unless we know how consistent the results are, we cannot determine the generalizability of the results of the meta-analysis.

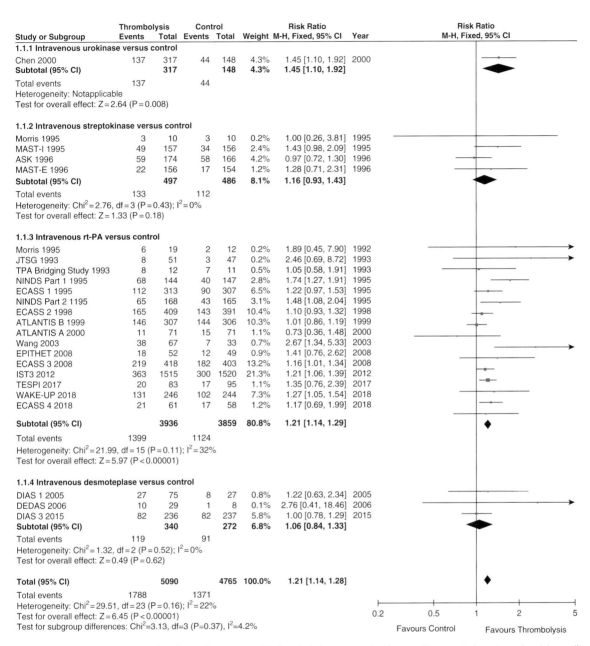

Figure 2.1 Forest plot showing the effects of *intravenous (IV) thrombolytics* compared with control in acute ischaemic stroke, trials enrolling patients with disabling deficits, only or predominantly, with treatment started within 9 h of onset, on *favourable outcome (alive and disability-free, modified Rankin Scale [mRS] 0–1) at 3–6 months*. In the left, numerical section, each individual trial has its own row, starting with trial name; Subtotal sections show numerical meta-analytic effect estimates from pooling of trials testing the same agent; and the bottom Total section shows numerical meta-analytic effect estimates from pooling of all trials. In the right, graphical section, the risk ratio (RR) for a favourable outcome in the IV lytics versus control group is plotted for each trial, including the point estimate (black square) and the 95% confidence interval (CI) (horizontal line). The size of the black squares reflects trial sample size. Black diamonds in the Subtotal sections indicate the pooled results of trials testing the same agent, centred on the RR point estimate and extending to the 95% CIs. The bottom-most black diamonds show the RR and the 95% CI of the RR from pooling of all trials. (Figure from Chapter 6.)

Two approaches to testing for heterogeneity are often performed. One is to undertake a test for heterogeneity that examines the null hypothesis that all studies are evaluating the same effect. The usual test statistic (Cochran's Q) is computed as the weighted sum of squared differences between individual study

Table 2.10 Selected sources of information about clinical trials and systematic reviews*

Cochrane Library

- Cochrane Database of Systematic Reviews (CDSR)
  - Systematic reviews/meta-analyses (more than 7900)
- Cochrane Central Register of Controlled Trials (CENTRAL)
  - Individual trials (more than 1.3 million)

Journal article databases

- Medline
  - Biomedical articles from 1950–present (more than 26 million records from more than 5600 journals) (but still does not include all trials)
- Embase
  - Biomedical articles from 1947–present (more than 32 million records from more than 8500 journals) (but still does not include all trials)
- CINAHL
  - Nursing and allied health journal articles from 1937–present (more than 6 million records from more than 5400 journals)

Clinical trial registries

- ClinicalTrials.gov
  - From 2000–present (more than 300,000 research studies)
- EU Clinical Trials Register
  - From 2004–present (more than 34,250 clinical trials)
- ISRCTN
  - From 2005–present (more than 18,000 research studies)
- Chinese Clinical Trial Registry (CHiCTR)
  - From 2005–present (more than 21,000 clinical trials)

* Values in table for numbers of records, journals, trials, and research studies reflect 2019 data.

effects and the pooled effect across studies. The power of the Q test is influenced by the number of trials in the meta-analysis, having relatively low power when the number of studies is small and sometimes too much power when the number of studies is high. In many meta-analyses, the number of studies is low, and a broader p-value threshold (e.g. $p < 0.10$ rather than $p < 0.05$) is set for considering the assessment to have indicated presence of heterogeneity.

The second approach, rather than simply testing for presence or absence of heterogeneity, quantifies the percentage of variation across studies that is due to heterogeneity rather than chance, using the I^2 statistic. The I^2 value ranges from 0% to 100%, and is not so influenced by the number of studies in the meta-analysis. A broad guide to interpreting I^2 findings is (Higgins and Green, 2011):

- 0% to 40%: might not be important
- 30% to 60%: may represent moderate heterogeneity

- 50% to 90%: may represent substantial heterogeneity
- 75% to 100%: considerable heterogeneity

Where to Find Clinical Trials and Systematic Reviews

Sources of information about clinical trials and systematic reviews are given in Table 2.10.

What If There Is No Robust Evidence from Systematic Reviews of RCTs?

For many therapeutic choices, robust evidence from RCTs to guide decision-making is not available, given that only 10–25% of practice guideline recommendations in cardiovascular care are supported by high-grade randomized trial evidence (McAlister et al., 2007; Wallis et al., 2018; Schumacher et al., 2019). Examples and recommended approaches are listed in Table 2.11.

Table 2.11 When robust evidence from RCTs for a decision regarding your patient is not available*

Reasons

- RCT(s) not feasible because the condition is so rare and the patients are so few.
- RCT(s) not undertaken due to lack of burning questions or resources.
- RCT(s) not undertaken due to lack of equipoise (and of willingness to randomize) in the clinical community.
- The intervention is new and has not had time to be evaluated.

No RCTs exist at all

- Examples
    - Different immunomodulatory regimens for cerebral angiitis (condition rare)
    - External ventricular drainage for acute hydrocephalus after subarachnoid haemorrhage (lack of equipoise)
    - Smartwatch atrial fibrillation monitoring to guide intermittent use of anticoagulants (intervention too new)
- Actions
    - Use reasoning from experience with individual patients but beware of the potential fallacies.
    - Use physiological reasoning and observations from preclinical models but beware of the potential non-applicability.
    - Plan or join (as a collaborator) an RCT, if feasible.
    - Obtain experience with any new operative/procedural intervention (e.g. run-in phase) before evaluating it in randomized comparison.

Only a single pivotal RCT exists

- Examples
    - Calcium channel blockers for vasospastic amaurosis fugax (condition uncommon, lack of resources)
    - Endovascular thrombectomy for basilar artery occlusion (lack of equipoise)
    - Low-dose (0.6 mg/kg) alteplase for acute ischaemic stroke (lack of burning question, resources)
- Actions
    - Draw upon the evidence of the single completed trial, but only partially (Could there have been a false positive or false negative result?)
        If we had relied on the results of the first trial of the NXY-059 free-radical-trapping agent for acute ischaemic stroke (Lees et al., 2006), we would have been using an agent not confirmed to be useful in a replication trial (Shuaib et al., 2007). If we had stopped testing IV alteplase for acute ischaemic stroke after the non-positive first NINDS-Study Part 1 RCT, we would not later have been able to use alteplase widely when secondary outcome beneficial signals were confirmed prospectively in the second NINDS-Study Part 2 RCT (NINDS rt-PA Stroke Study Group, 1995) and later trials (Emberson et al., 2014).
    - Plan a new RCT or join an RCT to determine the consistency of the result in another population of patients, and improve the precision of the estimate of the overall treatment effect.

Several RCTs exist, but a systematic review reveals non-significant or equivalent results

- Examples
    - Anticoagulation for cerebral venous thrombosis (Coutinho et al., 2011)
    - Statins for acute ischaemic stroke (see Chapter 12)
- Actions
    - Review the 95% CI of the overall estimate of the result and the statistical test for heterogeneity, and consider the possibility of a modest, but clinically worthwhile, treatment effect being missed (e.g. a false negative result).
    - Plan or join (as a collaborator) an RCT if a potentially important treatment effect may have been misinterpreted as a false negative result because of inadequate statistical power.
    - In the meantime, reasoning from personal experience, physiology, and preclinical studies is required, but beware of the potential fallacies of the reasoning.

RCTs exist, but certain types of patients were not included in the trials

- Examples
    - Endovascular thrombectomy for very elderly (90+ years) patients
    - Coiling (rather than clipping) for basilar artery aneurysms – these patients were not included in the International Subarachnoid Aneurysm Trial (ISAT), as these aneurysms are difficult to clip surgically and easier to coil angiographically (Molyneux et al., 2005)

Table 2.11 (cont.)

RCTs exist, but certain types of patients were not included in the trials

- Actions
  - Use reasoning from available RCT data, personal experience, and physiology when extrapolating the study findings to other patients, but beware of the potential fallacies.
  - Plan a new RCT or join an RCT to determine the consistency or heterogeneity of treatment effect in the unexplored patient population, if substantial uncertainty regarding extrapolation exists.

* Updated and modified from van Gijn (2005).

Summary

1. Almost all efficacious *stroke treatments confer moderate-to-large benefits*, but not staggeringly huge benefits. If uncertainty exists about the effect of a treatment, it is likely that the treatment effect is in fact at most moderate to large. However, moderate treatment effects can be clinically very worthwhile for the patient.

2. *To detect moderate-to-large treatment benefits, trials must avoid bias and random error.* Studies with weak designs (personal experience, observational studies with historical controls, and observational studies with concurrent, non-randomized controls) will not sufficiently control bias and random error to enable reliable discrimination of a true moderate-to-large benefit from false positives and false negatives. Randomized clinical trials are required.

3. *'Ingredients' for a good trial*

Evidence from a randomized trial is likely to be more reliable if the following exists:

- Proper randomization and concealment of allocation (i.e. clinician cannot have foreknowledge of next treatment allocation)
- Outcome evaluation blind to the allocated treatment
- Analysis by allocated treatment (including all randomized patients: intention-to-treat)
- Large numbers of major outcomes and correspondingly narrow CIs
- Conclusion based on pre-specified primary hypothesis and outcome
- Chief emphasis on findings in overall study population (without undue data-dependent emphasis on particular subgroups)

4. *Advantages of systematic reviews (over traditional unsystematic, narrative reviews)*

- Use explicit, well-developed methods to reduce bias
- Summarize large amounts of data explicitly
- Provide all available data
- Increase statistical power and precision
- Look for consistencies/inconsistencies
- Improve generalizability

5. *Cochrane Reviews*

- Generally higher quality than other systematic reviews
- Periodically updated
- Available over internet
- Abstracts available free of charge
- Full reviews available free of charge in more than 100 low- and middle-income countries and for a small fee in high-income countries

References

AAMC-AAU Advisory Committee on Financial Conflicts of Interest in Human Subjects Research. (2008). Protecting patients, preserving integrity, advancing health: accelerating the implementation of COI policies in human subjects research. www.aamc.org/download/482216/data/protectingpatients.pdf. Accessed March 2019.

Adeoye O, Hornung R, Khatri P, Kleindorfer D. (2011). Recombinant tissue-type plasminogen activator use for ischemic stroke in the United States: a doubling of treatment rates over the course of 5 years. *Stroke*, **42**, 1952–5.

Ali M, Bath P, Brady M, Davis S, Diener HC, Donnan G, et al.; VISTA Steering Committees. (2012). Development, expansion, and use of a stroke clinical trials resource for novel exploratory analyses. *Int J Stroke*, **7**, 133–8.

Ashcroft R. (2000). Giving medicine a fair trial: trials should not second guess what patients want. *BMJ*, **320**, 1686.

Bassler D, Briel M, Montori VM, Lane M, Glasziou P, Zhou Q, et al.; STOPIT-2 Study Group. (2010). Stopping randomized trials early for benefit and estimation of treatment effects: systematic review and meta-regression analysis. *JAMA*, **303**: 1180–7.

Bath PM, Lees KR, Schellinger PD, Altman H, Bland M, Hogg C, et al.; European Stroke Organisation Outcomes Working Group. (2012). Statistical analysis of the primary outcome in acute stroke trials. *Stroke*, **43**, 1171–8.

Bekelman JE, Li Y, Gross CP. (2003). Scope and impact of financial conflicts of interest in biomedical research: a systematic review. *JAMA*, **289**, 454–65.

Blanco D, Biggane AM, Cobo E; MiRoR Network. (2018). Are CONSORT checklists submitted by authors adequately reflecting what information is actually reported in published papers? *Trials*, **19**, 80. doi:10.1186/s13063-018-2475-0.

Borenstein M, Hedges LV, Higgins JP, Rothstein HR. (2010). A basic introduction to fixed-effect and random-effects models for meta-analysis. *Res Synth Methods*, **1**, 97–111.

Broderick JP, Palesch YY, Demchuk AM, Yeatts SD, Khatri P, Hill MD, et al.; Interventional Management of Stroke (IMS) III Investigators. (2013). Endovascular therapy after intravenous t-PA versus t-PA alone for stroke. *N Engl J Med*, **368**, 893–903.

Broglio K. (2018). Randomization in clinical trials: permuted blocks and stratification. *JAMA*, **319**, 2223–4.

Chalmers I. (2004). Well informed uncertainties about the effects of treatments. *BMJ*, **328**, 475–6.

Chan AW. (2012). Out of sight but not out of mind: how to search for unpublished clinical trial evidence. *BMJ*, **344**, d8013. doi:10.1136/bmj.d8013.

Clarke M, Williamson PR. (2016). Core outcome sets and systematic reviews. *Syst Rev*, **5**, 11. doi:10.1186/s13643-016-0188-6.

Collins R, MacMahon S. (2001). Reliable assessment of the effects of treatment on mortality and major morbidity I: clinical trials. *Lancet*, **357**, 373–80.

Counsell CE, Clarke MJ, Slattery J, Sandercock PA. (1994). The miracle of DICE therapy for acute stroke: fact or fictional product of subgroup analysis? *BMJ*, **309**, 1677–81.

Coutinho J, de Bruijn SF, Deveber G, Stam J. (2011). Anticoagulation for cerebral venous sinus thrombosis. *Cochrane Database Syst Rev*, 8, CD002005. doi:10.1002/14651858.CD002005.pub2.

Cranston JS, Kaplan BD, Saver JL. (2017). Minimal clinically important difference for safe and simple novel acute ischemic stroke therapies. *Stroke*, **48**, 2946–51.

Dahabreh IJ, Hayward R, Kent DM. (2016). Using group data to treat individuals: understanding heterogeneous treatment effects in the age of precision medicine and patient-centred evidence. *Int J Epidemiol*, **45**, 2184–93.

DAMOCLES Study Group, NHS Health Technology Assessment Programme. (2005). A proposed charter for clinical trial data monitoring committees: helping them to do their job well. *Lancet*, **365**, 711–22.

Dekkers OM, von Elm E, Algra A, Romijn JA, Vandenbroucke JP. (2010). How to assess the external validity of therapeutic trials: a conceptual approach. *Int J Epidemiol*, **39**, 89–94.

DeMets DL, Cook T. (2019). Challenges of non-intention-to-treat analyses. *JAMA*, **321**, 145–6.

Djulbegovic B, Guyatt GH. (2017). Progress in evidence-based medicine: a quarter century on. *Lancet* **390**, 415–23.

Donnan GA, Davis SM, Kaste M; International Trial Subcommittee of the International Stroke Liaison Committee, American Stroke Association. (2003). Stroke. Recommendations for the relationship between sponsors and investigators in the design and conduct of clinical stroke trials. *Stroke*, **34**, 1041–5.

Doust J, Del Mar C. (2004). Why do doctors use treatments that do not work? *BMJ*, **328**, 474–5.

ECST Trialists. (1998). Randomised trial of endarterectomy for recently symptomatic carotid stenosis: final results of the MRC European Carotid Surgery Trial (ECST). *Lancet*, **351**, 1379–87.

Emanuel EJ, Wendler D, Grady C. (2000). What makes clinical research ethical? *JAMA*, **283**, 2701–11.

Emberson J, Lees KR, Lyden P, Blackwell L, Albers G, Bluhmki E, et al.; Stroke Thrombolysis Trialists' Collaborative Group. (2014). Effect of treatment delay, age, and stroke severity on the effects of intravenous thrombolysis with alteplase for acute ischaemic stroke: a meta-analysis of individual patient data from randomised trials. *Lancet*, **384**, 1929–35.

Falk Delgado A, Falk Delgado A. (2017). The association of funding source on effect size in randomized controlled trials: 2013–2015 – a cross-sectional survey and meta-analysis. *Trials*, **18**, 125. doi:10.1186/s13063-017-1872-0.

Flather M, Delahunty N, Collinson J. (2006). Generalizing results of randomized trials to clinical practice: reliability and cautions. *Clin Trials*, **3**, 508–12.

Fleming TR, Powers JH. (2012). Biomarkers and surrogate endpoints in clinical trials. *Stat Med*, 31, 2973–84.

George BP, Pieters TA, Zammit CG, Kelly AG, Sheth KN, Bhalla T. (2019). Trends in interhospital transfers and mechanical thrombectomy for United States acute ischemic stroke inpatients. *J Stroke Cerebrovasc Dis*, **28**, 980–7. doi:10.1016/j.jstrokecerebrovasdis.2018.12.018. [Epub ahead of print]

Gopal AD, Wallach JD, Aminawung JA, Gonsalves G, Dal-Ré R, Miller JE, et al. (2018). Adherence to the International Committee of Medical Journal Editors' (ICMJE) prospective registration policy and implications for outcome integrity: a cross-sectional analysis of trials published in high-impact specialty society journals. *Trials*, **19**, 448. doi:10.1186/s13063-018-2825-y.

Guyatt G, Oxman AD, Akl EA, Kunz R, Vist G, Brozek J, et al. (2011). GRADE guidelines: 1. Introduction-GRADE evidence profiles and summary of findings tables. *J Clin Epidemiol*, **64**, 383–94.

Halperin JL, Levine GN, Al-Khatib SM, Birtcher KK, Bozkurt B, Brindis RG, et al. (2016). Further evolution of the ACC/AHA Clinical Practice Guideline Recommendation Classification System: a report of the American College of Cardiology/American Heart Association Task Force on Clinical Practice Guidelines. *Circulation*, **133**, 1426–8.

Harman NL, Conroy EJ, Lewis SC, Murray G, Norrie J, Sydes MR, et al. (2015). Exploring the role and function of trial steering committees: results of an expert panel meeting. *Trials*, **16**, 597. doi:10.1186/s13063-015-1125-z.

Higgins JPT, Green S, eds. (2011). *Cochrane Handbook for Systematic Reviews of Interventions Version 5.1.0* [updated March 2011]. The Cochrane Collaboration. Available from www.handbook.cochrane.org.

Higgins JPT, Savović J, Page MJ, Sterne JAC, on behalf of the ROB2 Development Group. (2018). Revised Cochrane risk-of-bias tool for randomized trials (RoB 2). www.riskofbias.info/welcome/rob-2-0-tool/current-version-of-rob-2 . Accessed March 2019.

Higgins JPT, Thompson SG, Deeks JJ, Altman DG. (2003). Measuring inconsistency in meta-analyses. *BMJ*, **327**, 557–60.

Hill MD. (2018). How to review a clinical research paper. *Stroke*, **49**, e204–e206.

Hobbs BP, Carlin BP, Sargent DJ. (2013). Adaptive adjustment of the randomization ratio using historical control data. *Clin Trials*, **10**, 430–40.

Hoffrage U, Lindsey S, Hertwig R, Gigerenzer G. (2000). Medicine: communicating statistical information. *Science*, **290**, 2261–2.

Hopewell S, Loudon K, Clarke MJ, Oxman AD, Dickersin K. (2009). Publication bias in clinical trials due to statistical significance or direction of trial results. *Cochrane Database Syst Rev*, 1, MR000006. doi:10.1002/14651858.MR000006. pub3.

International Committee of Medical Journal Editors. (2018). *Recommendations for the Conduct, Reporting, Editing, and Publication of Scholarly Work in Medical Journals.* www.icmje.org/icmje-recommendations.pdf. Accessed March 2019.

International Council for Harmonisation of Technical Requirements for Pharmaceuticals for Human Use. (2016). *Guideline for Good Clinical Practice E6 (R2).* www.ich.org/fileadmin/Public_Web_Site/ICH_Products/Guidelines/Efficacy/E6/E6_R2__Step_4_2016_1109.pdf. Accessed March 2019.

IST-3 Collaborative Group, Sandercock P, Wardlaw JM, Lindley RI, Dennis M, Cohen G, Murray G, et al. (2012). The benefits and harms of intravenous thrombolysis with recombinant tissue plasminogen activator within 6 h of acute ischaemic stroke (the third international stroke trial [IST-3]): a randomised controlled trial. *Lancet*, **379**, 2352–63.

Ioannidis JP. (2005). Why most published research findings are false. *PLoS Med*, **2**, e124.

Johnston KC, Bruno A, Paulis Q, Hall CE, Barrett KM, Barsan W, et al. (2019). Intensive versus standard treatment of hyperglycemia in acute ischemic stroke: a randomized controlled trial. *JAMA*, 322, 326–35.

Johnston SC, Rootenberg JD, Katrak S, Smith WS, Elkins JS. (2006). Effect of a US National Institutes of Health programme of clinical trials on public health and costs. *Lancet*, **367**, 1319–27.

Jones AP, Riley RD, Williamson PR, Whitehead A. (2009). Meta-analysis of individual patient data versus aggregate data from longitudinal clinical trials. *Clin Trials*, **6**, 16–27.

Kaplan RM, Chambers DA, Glasgow RE. (2014). Big data and large sample size: a cautionary note on the potential for bias. *Clin Transl Sci*, 7, 342–6.

Kirkham JJ, Altman DG, Chan AW, Gamble C, Dwan KM, Williamson PR. (2018). Outcome reporting bias in trials: a methodological approach for assessment and adjustment in systematic reviews. *BMJ*, **362**, k3802. doi:10.1136/bmj.k3802.

Laika J. (2008). Time to weed the (EBM-) pyramids?! https://laikaspoetnik.wordpress.com/2008/09/26/time-to-weed-the-ebm-pyramids/. Accessed March 2019.

Laine C, Horton R, DeAngelis CD, Drazen JM, Frizelle FA, Godlee F, et al. (2007). Clinical trial registration: looking back and moving ahead. *JAMA*, **298**, 93–4.

Laupacis A, Sackett DL, Roberts RS. (1988). An assessment of clinically useful measures of the consequences of treatment. *N Engl J Med*, **318**, 1728–33.

Lees KR, Hankey GJ, Hacke W. (2003). Design of future acute-stroke treatment trials. *Lancet Neurol*, **2**, 54–61.

Lees KR, Zivin JA, Ashwood T, Davalos A, Davis SM, Diener HC, Grotta J, Lyden P, Shuaib A, Hårdemark HG, Wasiewski WW; Stroke-Acute Ischemic NXY Treatment (SAINT I) Trial Investigators. (2006). NXY-059 for acute ischemic stroke. *N Engl J Med* **354**: 588–600.

Lewis SC, Warlow CP. (2004). How to spot bias and other potential problems in randomised controlled trials. *J Neurol Neurosurg Psychiatry*, **75**(2), 181–7.

Liberati A, Altman DG, Tetzlaff J, Mulrow C, Gøtzsche PC, Ioannidis JP, et al. (2009). The PRISMA statement for reporting systematic reviews and meta-analyses of studies that evaluate health care interventions: explanation and elaboration. *PLoS Med*, **6**, e1000100. doi:10.1371/journal.pmed.1000100.

Lichtman JH, Jones MR, Leifheit EC, Sheffet AJ, Howard G, Lal BK, et al. (2017). Carotid endarterectomy and carotid artery stenting in the US Medicare population, 1999–2014. *JAMA*, **318**, 1035–46.

Liebeskind DS, Kidwell CS, Sayre JW, Saver JL. (2006). Evidence of publication bias in reporting acute stroke clinical trials. *Neurology*, **67**, 973–9.

Lo B, Field MJ; Institute of Medicine Committee on Conflict of Interest in Medical Research, Education, and Practice. (2009). *Conflict of Interest in Medical Research, Education, and Practice.* Washington, DC: National Academies Press.

Lundh A, Lexchin J, Mintzes B, Schroll JB, Bero L5. (2017). Industry sponsorship and research outcome. *Cochrane Database Syst Rev*, **2**, MR000033. doi:10.1002/14651858.MR000033.pub3.

Lyden PD, Meyer BC, Hemmen TM, Rapp KS. (2010). An ethical hierarchy for decision making during medical emergencies. *Ann Neurol*, **67**, 434–40.

Mauri L, D'Agostino RB Sr. (201). Challenges in the design and interpretation of noninferiority trials. *N Engl J Med*, **377**, 1357–67.

McAlister FA, van Diepen S, Padwal RS, Johnson JA, Majumdar SR. (2007). How evidence-based are the recommendations in evidence-based guidelines? *PLoS Med*, **4**, e250.

Mead G, Hackett ML, Lundström E, Murray V, Hankey GJ, Dennis M. (2015). The FOCUS, AFFINITY and EFFECTS trials studying the effect(s) of fluoxetine in patients with a recent stroke: a study protocol for three multicentre randomised controlled trials. *Trials*, **16**, 369. doi:10.1186/s13063-015-0864-1.

Molyneux AJ, Kerr RS, Yu LM, Clarke M, Sneade M, Yarnold JA, et al.; International Subarachnoid Aneurysm Trial (ISAT) Collaborative Group. (2005). International subarachnoid aneurysm trial (ISAT) of neurosurgical clipping versus endovascular coiling in 2143 patients with ruptured intracranial aneurysms: a randomised comparison of effects on survival, dependency, seizures, rebleeding, subgroups, and aneurysm occlusion. *Lancet*, **366**, 809–17.

Munroe R. (2011). Significant. https://xkcd.com/882/. Accessed March 2019.

Murad MH, Montori VM, Ioannidis JP, Jaeschke R, Devereaux PJ, Prasad K, (2014). How to read a systematic review and meta-analysis and apply the results to patient care: users' guides to the medical literature. *JAMA*, **312**, 171–9.

NICE: National Institute for Health and Care Excellence. (2014). *Developing NICE guidelines: the manual.* www.nice.org.uk/media/default/about/what-we-do/our-programmes/developing-nice-guidelines-the-manual.pdf. Accessed March 2019.

NINDS (National Institute of Neurological Disorders and Stroke) rt-PA Stroke Study Group. (1995). Tissue plasminogen activator for acute ischemic stroke. *N Engl J Med*, **333**, 1581–7.

Norton EC, Dowd BE, Maciejewski ML. (2018). Odds ratios – current best practice and use. *JAMA*, **320**, 84–5.

Pocock SJ, Stone GW. (2016a). The primary outcome fails – what next? *N Engl J Med*, **375**, 861–70.

Pocock SJ, Stone GW. (2016b). The primary outcome is positive – is that good enough? *N Engl J Med*, **375**, 971–9.

Pollock A, Berge E. (2018). How to do a systematic review. *Int J Stroke*, **13**, 138–56.

Powers WJ, Clarke WR, Grubb RL Jr, Videen TO, Adams HP Jr, Derdeyn CP; COSS Investigators. (2011). Extracranial-intracranial bypass surgery for stroke prevention in hemodynamic cerebral ischemia: the Carotid Occlusion Surgery Study randomized trial. *JAMA*, **306**, 1983–92.

Ranganathan P, Pramesh CS, Aggarwal R. (2016). Common pitfalls in statistical analysis: Absolute risk reduction, relative risk reduction, and number needed to treat. *Perspect Clin Res*, **7**, 51–3.

Rasmussen K, Bero L, Redberg R, Gøtzsche PC, Lundh A. (2018). Collaboration between academics and industry in clinical trials: cross sectional study of publications and survey of lead academic authors. *BMJ*, **363**, k3654. doi:10.1136/bmj.k3654.

Ridker PM, Torres J. (2006). Reported outcomes in major cardiovascular clinical trials funded by for-profit and not-for-profit organizations: 2000–2005. *JAMA*, **295**, 2270–4.

Riley RD, Lambert PC, Abo-Zaid G. (2010). Meta-analysis of individual participant data: rationale, conduct, and reporting. *BMJ*, **340**, c221.

Rothwell PM. (2005). External validity of randomised controlled trials: 'to whom do the results of this trial apply?' *Lancet*, **365**, 82–93.

Rothwell PM, Mehta Z, Howard SC, Gutnikov SA, Warlow CP. (2005). Treating individuals 3: from subgroups to individuals: general principles and the example of carotid endarterectomy. *Lancet*, **365**, 256–65.

Rush CJ, Campbell RT, Jhund PS, Petrie MC, McMurray JJV. (2018). Association is not causation: treatment effects cannot be estimated from observational data in heart failure. *Eur Heart J*, **39**, 3417–38.

Sackett DL. (2000). Why randomized controlled trials fail but needn't. 1. Failure to gain 'coal-face' commitment and to use the uncertainty principle. *Can Med Assoc J*, **162**, 1311–14.

Sackett DL, Deeks JJ, Altman DG. (1996). Down with odds ratios! *Evid Based Med*, **1**, 164–6.

Sanders GD, Maciejewski ML, Basu A. (2019). Overview of cost-effectiveness analysis. *JAMA*, **321**, 1400–1. doi:10.1001/jama.2019.1265.

Sarpong EM, Zuvekas SH. (2014). *Changes in Statin Therapy among Adults (Age ≥ 18) by Selected Characteristics, United States, 2000–2001 to 2010–2011.* Statistical Brief #459. November. Rockville, MD: Agency for Healthcare Research and Quality. www.meps.ahrq.gov/mepsweb/data_files/publications/st459/stat459.shtml.

Saver JL. (2011). Optimal end points for acute stroke therapy trials: best ways to measure treatment effects of drugs and devices. *Stroke*, **42**, 2356–62.

Saver JL, Gornbein J. (2009). Treatment effects for which shift or binary analyses are advantageous in acute stroke trials. *Neurology*, **72**, 1310–15.

Saver JL, Lewis RJ. (2019). Number needed to treat: conveying the likelihood of a therapeutic effect. *JAMA*, **321**, 798–9. doi:10.1001/jama.2018.21971.

Savovic J, Turner RM, Mawdsley D, Jones HE, Beynon R, Higgins JPT, et al. (2018). Association between risk-of-bias assessments and results of randomized trials in Cochrane Reviews: the ROBES Meta-Epidemiologic Study. *Am J Epidemiol*, **187**, 1113–22.

Schulz KF, Altman DG, Moher D, for the CONSORT Group. (2010). CONSORT 2010 statement: updated guidelines for reporting parallel group randomised trials. *PLoS Med*, **7**, e1000251.

Schumacher RC, Nguyen OK, Desphande K, Makam AN. (2019). Evidence-based medicine and the American Thoracic Society Clinical Practice Guidelines. *JAMA Intern Med*, **179**, 584–6. doi:10.1001/jamainternmed.2018.7461. [Epub ahead of print]

Sedgwick P. (2015). Meta-analysis: what is heterogeneity? *BMJ*, **16**, h1435. doi:10.1136/bmj.h1435.

Senn SJ, Lewis RJ. (2019). Treatment effects in multicenter randomized clinical trials. *JAMA*, **321**, 1211–12. doi:10.1001/jama.2019.1480.

Serghiou S, Goodman SN. (2019). Random-effects meta-analysis: summarizing evidence with caveats. *JAMA*, **321**, 301–2.

Shaneyfelt T. (2016). Pyramids are guides not rules: the evolution of the evidence pyramid. *Evid Based Med*, **21**, 121–2.

Shaw GB. (1911). *The Doctor's Dilemma*. London: Constable and Company.

Sheth SA, Saver JL, Starkman S, Grunberg ID, Guzy J, Ali LK, et al. (2016). Enrollment bias: frequency and impact on patient selection in endovascular stroke trials. *J Neurointerv Surg*, **8**, 353–9.

Shuaib A, Lees KR, Lyden P, Grotta J, Davalos A, Davis SM, et al.; SAINT II Trial Investigators. (2007). NXY-059 for the treatment of acute ischemic stroke. *N Engl J Med*, **357**, 562–71.

Stead WW. (2017). The complex and multifaceted aspects of conflicts of interest. *JAMA*, **317**, 1765–7.

Stewart LA, Clarke M, Rovers M, Riley RD, Simmonds M, Stewart G, et al.; PRISMA-IPD Development Group. (2015). Preferred reporting items for systematic review and meta-analyses of individual participant data: the PRISMA-IPD statement. *JAMA*, **313**, 1657–65.

Straus SE, Glasziou P, Richardson WS, Haynes RB. (2019). *Evidence-Based Medicine: How to Practice and Teach EBM*, 5th ed. Edinburgh: Elsevier Limited.

Sullivan GM, Feinn R. (2012). Using effect size – or why the p value is not enough. *J Grad Med Educ*, **4**, 279–82.

Sun X, Briel M, Walter SD, Guyatt GH. (2010). Is a subgroup effect believable? Updating criteria to evaluate the credibility of subgroup analyses. *BMJ*, **340**, c117.

Taichman DB, Sahni P, Pinborg A, Peiperl L, Laine C, James A, et al. (2017). Data sharing statements for clinical trials: a requirement of the International Committee of Medical Journal Editors. *JAMA*, **317**, 2491–2.

Tudur Smith C, Marcucci M, Nolan SJ, Iorio A, Sudell M, Riley R, et al. (2016). Individual participant data meta-analyses compared with meta-analyses based on aggregate data. *Cochrane Database Syst Rev*, **9**, MR000007. doi:10.1002/14651858.MR000007.pub3 .

van Gijn J. (2005). From randomised trials to rational practice. *Cerebrovasc Dis*, **19**, 69–76.

Vyas A, Saver J. (2016). The 'uncertainty principle' as an entry criterion in stroke clinical trials: bias towards null findings. *Neurology*, **86** (16 Supplement), P2.382.

Wallach JD, Sullivan PG, Trepanowski JF, Sainani KL, Steyerberg EW, Ioannidis JP. (2017). Evaluation of evidence of statistical support and corroboration of subgroup claims in randomized clinical trials. *JAMA Intern Med*, **177**, 554–60.

Wallis CJD, Detsky AS, Fan E. (2018). Establishing the effectiveness of procedural interventions: the limited role of randomized trials. *JAMA*, **320**, 2421-2. doi:10.1001/jama.2018.16329.

Warlow C. (2004). The Willis Lecture 2003: evaluating treatments for stroke patients too slowly: time to get out of second gear. *Stroke*, **35**, 2211–19.

WHO Commission on Macroeconomics and Health & World Health Organization. (2001). *Macroeconomics and Health: Investing in Health for Economic Development.* Geneva: World Health Organization. www.who.int/iris/handle/10665/42463.

Zarin DA, Tse T, Williams RJ, Carr S. (2016). Trial reporting in ClinicalTrials.gov – the final rule. *N Engl J Med*, **375**, 1998–2004.

3

Prehospital Stroke Care and Regionalized Stroke Systems

Kori Sauser Zachrison
Lee H. Schwamm

Prehospital stroke care is the first link in the stroke chain of survival and includes symptom recognition, engagement of the Emergency Medical Services (EMS) system, timely and effective dispatcher response, and emergency medical response. Prehospital stroke screening tools are an important component in guiding the EMS response to stroke and proper triage of patients. Additionally, there is a growing body of research focused on applications for telemedicine, mobile stroke units, and diagnostic testing in the prehospital arena. Prehospital stroke care is integral to the organization of regionalized stroke systems. Implementation of stroke systems of care can lead to improved access to specialty services and improved patient health outcomes. In addition to increasing access to acute stroke care, telestroke shows great potential for integrating stroke systems of care and facilitating interactions between centres.

Prehospital Stroke Care

Achieving optimal patient health outcomes after stroke depends on effective systems of care and begins in the prehospital setting. There are many important components of prehospital stroke care, including symptom recognition, engagement of dispatch, deployment of EMS, appropriate prehospital triage, and pre-arrival notification to the receiving hospital.

Symptom Recognition

Background

Patient or bystander recognition of stroke symptoms is necessarily the first step in the stroke chain of survival (Powers et al., 2018). Once symptoms are recognized, stroke patients or bystanders must also be aware of the importance of immediately engaging the EMS system. Yet public awareness of stroke warning signs is poor (Jurkowski et al., 2010; Madsen et al., 2015); less than

60% of stroke patients use EMS (Mochari-Greenberger et al., 2015); and nearly half of calls to EMS systems for stroke events are made more than 1 hour after symptom onset (Mosley et al., 2007). For this reason, prolonged onset-to-arrival time is the greatest source of delays in care and a frequent cause of ineligibility for reperfusion therapy (Madsen et al., 2016; Matsuo, et al. 2017; Centers for Disease Control and Prevention, 2007). Improving timeliness of patient presentation depends on public awareness and symptom recognition.

Evidence

Public education programmes may be effective in improving public awareness, highlighting stroke signs and symptoms, the urgency of immediate care, and the need to call the EMS system for suspected stroke symptoms. In two studies, participants were administered structured questionnaires assessing knowledge of stroke incidence, symptoms, consequences, and behaviour in case of a stroke. The group completing the questionnaire after a widespread informational campaign demonstrated better knowledge about stroke than did the pre-initiative participants (Chiti et al., 2007; Nishikawa et al., 2016). Another study assessed the effect of a multimedia stroke education campaign and found that individuals in the intervention region demonstrated increased awareness of stroke symptoms and the importance of immediately calling 911 in case of stroke relative to individuals in a control region (Jurkowski et al. 2010). A randomized controlled trial (RCT) in Texas found that classroom instruction significantly improved middle school children's knowledge of stroke symptoms and intention to call 911 (Morgenstern et al., 2007). The FAST mnemonic (Facial droop, Arm weakness, Speech disturbance, Time to call 911) and its language-independent Stroke 112 version may also be effective (Zhao et al., 2018). A pre-post study of elementary school students found that students' knowledge of stroke symptoms substantially improved with a hip-hop curriculum incorporating the FAST components (Williams and Noble, 2008); and a FAST educational campaign directed towards adults found that nearly all participants recalled stroke warning signs at 3-month follow-up (Wall et al., 2008). Yet public education programmes must be sustained to maintain their benefit. A study using a television advertising campaign in Ontario found that public awareness of stroke warning signs increased during the period of the campaign and Emergency Department (ED) stroke presentations increased, but decreased during an advertising blackout (Hodgson et al., 2007, 2009). Public education programmes should also provide instructions to reach diverse populations. For example, the Massachusetts Department of Public Health provides stroke education written materials and videos in multiple languages including Spanish, Portuguese, and Khmer Cambodian (see Figure 3.1) (Massachusetts Health Promotions Clearinghouse, 2018). In a systematic review, among 15 studies of mass media campaigns and community initiatives aiming to reduce patient delays by promoting the signs and symptoms of a stroke, the majority showed positive intervention effects, although methodological rigour was variable (Mellon et al., 2015).

By improving public awareness and symptom recognition, such campaigns may lead to earlier ED presentation and increase the proportion of patients eligible for acute therapies. A multilevel intervention conducted in East Texas targeted public stroke identification, outcome expectations, and social norms in addition to provider norms and behaviour. In this study, rate of tissue plasminogen activator (tPA) treatment increased significantly in the intervention community and was unchanged in the comparison community (Morgenstern et al., 2002).

Comment

The available limited evidence from randomized controlled trials and prospective time series studies, and expert consensus, supports the importance of public education for stroke symptom recognition, the importance of seeking care urgently, and of engaging EMS for suspected stroke (Powers et al., 2018; Higashida et al., 2013). Such programmes should be designed to maintain efficacy and be culturally competent to reach diverse populations, especially targeting those populations at highest risk.

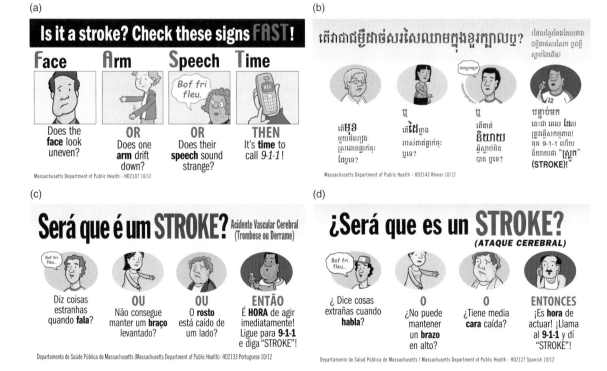

Figure 3.1 Stroke Heroes Act FAST Poster in English (a), Khmer Cambodian (b), Portuguese (c), and Spanish (d).

Figures reproduced with permission of the Massachusetts Department of Public Health.

Dispatcher Response

Background

Once stroke symptoms are recognized and patients or bystanders make the decision to call the EMS system, dispatchers must be able to recognize stroke signs and symptoms and dispatch the highest level of care available with maximal efficiency.

Evidence

The appropriate EMS response to a potential stroke call begins with dispatcher recognition. Studies of consecutive stroke dispatches found that a Medical Priority Dispatch System structured caller interview algorithm enabled dispatchers to identify stroke patients with 41–83% sensitivity (Ramanujam et al., 2008; Buck et al., 2009); and in an intervention study, the Emergency Stroke Calls: Obtaining Rapid Telephone Triage (ESCORTT) training package improved dispatcher recognition of stroke from 63% to 80–88% of cases (Watkins et al., 2014). In reviews of 911 calls and EMS run sheets of patients with calls for potential stroke, dispatchers were able to identify stroke with high reliability if the caller described facial droop, weakness/fall, or impaired communication or used the word *stroke* (Reginella et al., 2006; Richards et al., 2017). Another analysis of consecutive patients found that emergency dispatcher stroke recognition was associated with higher rates of on-scene stroke recognition and stroke scale performance by paramedics and emergency medical technicians (EMTs) (Oostema et al., 2018).

Comment

While research devoted to the role of medical dispatch is limited, available evidence and expert consensus underscore the important role that dispatchers play in the rapid recognition of potential stroke and expedient mobilization of EMS (Acker et al., 2007; Higashida et al., 2013). Suspected stroke calls should be given the highest priority dispatch and predetermined plans should guide dispatcher response with algorithms taking into account stroke severity, patient last known well time, distances to various hospitals, and capabilities of regional hospitals (Acker et al., 2007; Higashida et al., 2013; Mission: Lifeline Stroke, 2017). In order to ensure appropriate response, dispatcher guidelines should be promoted that prioritize stroke response, and call centres will require adequate funding for resources and continued training.

Emergency Medical Response

Background

The emergency medical response is a crucial component of prehospital stroke care and includes stabilization in the field, ground or air transport, and hospital pre-arrival notification. Despite significant fragmentation and regionalization in the organization of EMS systems in the USA and worldwide (Evenson et al., 2009; Higashida et al., 2013), the primary goals of emergency medical response are consistent throughout: rapid evaluation, early stabilization, and rapid transport and triage to an appropriate level facility.

Evidence

Despite the importance of timely presentation, many stroke patients still do not use EMS transportation to the hospital. In analyses of patients presenting to hospitals participating in Get with the Guidelines – Stroke, fewer than two-thirds of patients arrived by EMS (Ekundayo et al., 2013; Mochari-Greenberger et al., 2015). EMS activation was more likely among older patients, patients with Medicaid and Medicare insurance, and patients with more severe stroke; it was less likely among patients of minority race and ethnicity and those living in rural communities (Ekundayo et al., 2013; Mochari-Greenberger et al., 2015). The reasons for this observed disparity remain poorly understood.

There is a paucity of evidence to support requiring a specific level of prehospital provider response in standard ambulances for suspected stroke patients, among the options of EMTs who are basic life support (BLS) providers, paramedics who are advanced life support (ALS) providers, and, in Europe and some other regions of the world, physicians. One single-centre study of 203 patients with altered level of consciousness found no significant difference in admission rate, mortality, or disposition for patients transported by BLS versus ALS prehospital providers; however, only about 20% of the study population were stroke patients and the study did not assess other important outcomes such as time benchmarks and tPA delivery (Adams et al., 1996). In EMS systems in which BLS providers greatly outnumber ALS providers, restricting first response or transport to ALS providers would likely increase prehospital delays.

Some observational studies have considered the role for helicopter transport of patients in rural locations and in interfacility transfers. Helicopter transport has important potential to improve access to primary and comprehensive stroke centres. One study found that, in 2014, one-third of the US population did not have 60-minute drive time access to a primary stroke centre (PSC) by ground transport, but 91% of the population would have access to a PSC by air (Adeoye et al., 2014). In a large observational study of data from 32 stroke units between 2003 and 2009, patients transported by helicopter had shorter arrival times and higher thrombolysis rates when compared with patients transported by ambulance (Reiner-Deitemyer et al., 2011). Smaller studies have noted similar findings, illustrating the potential for helicopter transport to shorten transport times and extend access to thrombolytic therapy, stroke unit care, and study enrolment (Silliman et al., 2003; Hawk et al., 2016). For interhospital transfers, observational studies examining transport times and safety have found that helicopter transport was faster than ground and not associated with significant differences in complications, morbidity, or mortality (Svenson et al., 2006; Olson and Rabinstein, 2012; Hesselfeldt et al., 2014; Hutton et al., 2015). For endovascular thrombectomy, observational studies have found that helicopter transport of likely large vessel occlusion (LVO) patients directly from the field or by interfacility transfer can increase availability and timeliness of intervention to remotely located patients (Gupta et al., 2016; Regenhardt et al., 2018). Furthermore, helicopter transfer of ischaemic stroke patients for potential thrombolysis has been reported to be cost-effective ($3700 per quality-adjusted life-year [QALY]) (Silbergleit et al., 2003) and has potential to extend recruitment into acute stroke trials for patients in remote areas (Leira et al., 2006, 2009).

Several screening tools have been developed to enable accurate identification of stroke patients in the prehospital setting. The following scale and screening tools were the first to be developed and are now the most widely deployed:

- **Cincinnati Prehospital Stroke Scale (CPSS):** The CPSS is a three-item examination of facial weakness, arm strength, and speech disturbance. In a study comparing physician and paramedic scoring of 171 patients, there was high agreement for both total score (correlation: 0.89, 95% confidence interval [CI]: 0.87–0.92) as well as for each scale item (Kothari et al., 1999). Another study, examining EMS stroke recognition and accuracy, reviewed 441 EMS-transported stroke patient cases. Identification of stroke in the prehospital setting was higher among cases with CPSS documentation than in cases without (sensitivity 84.7% versus 30.9%, positive predictive value 56.2% versus 30.4%) (Oostema et al., 2015).

- **Los Angeles Prehospital Stroke Screen (LAPSS):** The LAPSS uses medical history and fingerstick glucose items to exclude acute stroke mimics (history of seizures, hypoglycaemia or hyperglycaemia, baseline ambulatory status, onset >24 hours prior), and examination for unilateral face, arm, and/or hand weakness to identify the most common types of stroke. One study retrospectively applied the LAPSS to 48 acute stroke patients and found that the LAPSS had a sensitivity of 92% (Kidwell et al., 1998). Another study assessed paramedic use of the LAPSS after a training and certification process; among 206 patients on whom the LAPSS was completed, sensitivity was 91%, specificity was 97%, positive predictive value was 86%, and negative predictive value was 98% (Kidwell et al., 2000).

Many additional stroke recognition instruments have subsequently been developed and used in the prehospital setting, generally similar in character, including the Melbourne Ambulance Stroke Screen (MASS), the Ontario Prehospital Stroke Screen (OPSS), the Medic Prehospital Assessment for Stroke Code (Med PACS), the Face Arm Speech Test (FAST), and the Recognition of Stroke in the Emergency Room (ROSIER) (Brandler et al., 2014; Rudd et al., 2016).

Systematic reviews of the performance of these stroke screens have found that most perform fairly well, with relative advantages and disadvantages to each. In one systematic review of eight studies, the LAPSS and OPSS had higher point estimates for accuracy than the CPSS (44–95%), although confidence intervals overlapped, while the MASS, Med PACS, ROSIER, and FAST had less favourable operating characteristics (Brandler et al., 2014). In another systematic analysis that included 21 studies, some not fully published, higher sensitivity point estimates were seen for the CPSS and FAST, while the LAPSS and similar instruments had higher specificity point estimates (Rudd, 2016). For the CPSS, sensitivity point estimates ranged from 44–95% and specificity from 24–79%, while for the LAPSS, sensitivity point estimates ranged from 59–91% and specificity from 48–97%.

In addition to stroke screening tools, prehospital instruments have been developed to assess stroke severity and patterns of stroke deficits in order to identify: (1) patients with LVOs among all acute cerebral ischaemia (ACI) patients (thrombectomy-capable stroke centre-appropriate patients), and (2) patients with LVO-ACI or with intracerebral haemorrhage from among all acute focal cerebrovascular disease patients (comprehensive stroke centre [CSC]–appropriate patients). The following three stroke severity scales were among the earliest developed and have undergone at least partial validation in actual prehospital settings:

- **Los Angeles Motor Scale (LAMS):** The LAMS assigns points to each of the LAPSS exam items of face, grip, and arm weakness, yielding a total score of 0–5 when there is unilateral weakness and 0–10 when there is bilateral weakness (Nazliel et al., 2008). In a field validation study, when applied by paramedics to consecutive patients enrolled at the prehospital scene in a clinical trial, a LAMS score ≥4 identified LVOs among ACI patients with 76% sensitivity and 65% specificity, and CSC-appropriate patients among all suspected focal stroke patients with 73% sensitivity and 71% specificity (Noorian et al., 2018).

- **Rapid Arterial oCclusion Evaluation (RACE) Scale:** The RACE assigns points for face, arm, and leg weakness; gaze deviation; inability to follow verbal commands; aphasia; and unawareness of limb weakness, for a total 0- to 9-point scale. In a mixed field and interfacility transfer validation study, when applied by paramedics to patients arising from these site types, a RACE score ≥5 identified LVOs among ACI patients with sensitivity of 85% and specificity of 65% (Perez de la Ossa et al., 2014).

- **Cincinnati Stroke Assessment Tool (C-STAT):** The C-STAT assigns points for arm weakness, gaze deviation, and inability to state age or month or follow verbal commands, for a total 0- to 4-point scale (Katz et al., 2015; McMullan et al., 2017). In a field validation study, when applied by prehospital personnel to a subset of transported stroke patients, a C-STAT score ≥2 identified LVOs among ACI patients with 71% sensitivity and 70% specificity, and CSC-appropriate patients among all suspected focal stroke patients with 57% sensitivity and 79% specificity (McMullan et al., 2017).

Many additional stroke severity instruments have been developed for prehospital use; they are generally similar in character to the LAMS, RACE, and C-STAT, but not yet validated in actual prehospital studies. They include the Field Assessment Stroke Triage for Emergency Destination (FAST-ED), Prehospital Acute Stroke Severity (PASS) scale, Vision-Aphasia-Neglect (VAN) scale, 3-item Stroke Scale (3i-SS), and Emergency Medical Stroke Assessment (EMSA) (Noorian et al., 2018; Gropen et al., 2018). In studies comparing simultaneous application of 5 (Zhao et al., 2017) and 7 (Noorian et al., 2018) of these scales at the same time to consecutive patients in the ED, all generally performed comparably in identifying LVO and CSC-appropriate patients.

Mobile telemedicine permitting remote stroke physicians to evaluate potential stroke patients at the scene or in standard ambulances has great potential. Studies evaluating feasibility have had mixed results; technical challenges have been frequent, but agreement on National Institutes of Health Stroke Scale (NIHSS) scores between remote and in-person examiners range from moderate to excellent (Liman et al., 2012; Van Hooff et al., 2013; Wu et al., 2014; Chapman Smith et al., 2016). A systematic review of telemedicine in prehospital care concluded that neurovascular disease was the most common focus and telemedicine improved the prehospital diagnosis of stroke (Amadi-Obi et al., 2014).

A technologically advanced approach to prehospital stroke care has been the development of mobile stroke units (MSUs), ambulances equipped with a computed tomography (CT) scanner, a CT technologist, a mobile blood laboratory, a critical care nurse, and a stroke physician either in person or via telemedicine, in addition to a paramedic or EMT (Figure 3.2). Deployment of mobile stroke units has been shown to shorten onset to thrombolysis treatment times in two cluster-controlled trials. In a single centre, 100-patient trial in Homburg, Germany, median time from dispatcher calling a stroke alarm to decision to administer intravenous thrombolysis was reduced in weeks that the MSU was active, from median 76 to 35 minutes, without differences in safety endpoints (Walter et al., 2012). In the larger Pre-Hospital Acute Neurological Treatment and Optimization of Medical care in Stroke (PHANTOM-S) trial in Berlin, comparing 3213 patients treated during MSU-active weeks and 2969

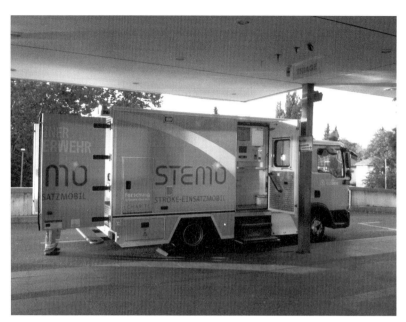

Figure 3.2 A Stroke Emergency Mobile (STEMO) unit.

Figure reproduced with permission of Heinrich Audebert, MD.

during control weeks, alarm-to-thrombolysis treatment time was reduced from 76 to 52 minutes for patients treated by a Stroke Emergency Mobile (STEMO) unit, with no increased risk for intracerebral haemorrhage (Ebinger et al., 2014). The proportion of patients receiving thrombolysis within the golden hour of 60 minutes from onset was 31% for MSU-treated patients versus 4.9% in control patients, with no difference in mortality but increased likelihood of discharge home (Ebinger et al., 2015).

All CT scanners in mobile stroke units can perform CT angiography, and some can perform perfusion CT, so that in the prehospital setting MSUs can definitively identify patients with LVOs causing ACI appropriate for direct routing to thrombectomy-capable receiving hospitals (John et al., 2016; Fassbender et al., 2017). In the PHANTOM-S trial, MSU deployment significantly shortened median alarm-to-imaging time, from 50 to 35 minutes (Ebinger et al., 2014).

An additional future potential treatment approach is paramedic delivery in standard ambulances of neuroprotective therapies that do not require brain imaging to distinguish ischaemic and haemorrhagic stroke prior to initiation. Several prehospital randomized trials have demonstrated the feasibility of prehospital start of potentially neuroprotective agents (Ankolekar et al., 2013; Hougaard et al., 2014; Saver et al., 2015). The largest was the Field Administration of Stroke Therapy-Magnesium (FAST-MAG) phase 3

trial, a multicentre, double-blind, randomized controlled study in which patients with suspected stroke in the prehospital setting were randomized to receive intravenous magnesium sulfate or placebo within 2 hours of symptom onset. Among the 1700 patients enrolled, there were no significant differences in disability at 90 days, mortality, or all serious adverse events (Saver et al. 2015). The study did, however, establish the feasibility of rapidly achieving informed consent and delivering a study agent to suspected hyperacute stroke patients in the prehospital setting, with median time from last known wellness state to start of neuroprotective agent of 45 minutes.

Arrival at the hospital by ambulance has also been associated with improved emergency treatment compared with private transport. In an analysis of 35,936 patients from Get with the Guidelines-Stroke (GWTG-S), patients arriving by ambulance were more likely to have brain imaging completed within the guideline-recommended 25-minute window (Kelly et al., 2012). This finding has been shown in other state-level analyses as well (Patel et al., 2011; Sauser et al., 2014a). In an analysis of 204,591 patients from 1563 GWTG-S hospitals, arrival by ambulance was associated with increased likelihood of tPA administration among eligible patients (odds ratio [OR] 1.47 versus non-ambulance arrival), and with increased likelihood of tPA treatment within 60 minutes (OR:

1.44) (Ekundayo et al., 2013). Arrival by ambulance has also been associated with shorter door-to-needle times for thrombolysis in Michigan's Coverdell state stroke registry data (Sauser et al., 2014b).

While ambulance arrival in itself has been associated with improved care delivery and treatment times, pre-arrival notification by prehospital providers has been shown to lead to further improvements in stroke care by enabling earlier resource mobilization. In a state-level analysis of 13,894 patients with suspected stroke, time to brain imaging and to imaging interpretation was faster in patients arriving by ambulance versus those who did not, but was fastest among those arriving by ambulance *with* hospital pre-arrival notification (Patel et al., 2011). In a single-centre review of 229 stroke patients, prehospital notification by EMS was associated with improved time to stroke team arrival and to CT scan completion and interpretation, and was associated with increased rates of intravenous thrombolysis (McKinney et al., 2013). Another single-centre review of 102 suspected stroke patients found that prehospital notification was associated with significantly shorter door-to-imaging and door-to-needle times (Bae et al., 2010). A third single-centre review of 118 acute stroke patients found improved door-to-imaging times and increased rates of thrombolysis in the patients for whom the hospital had pre-arrival notification (Abdullah et al., 2008). A review of 371,988 patients presenting to GWTG-S hospitals found that pre-arrival notification was associated with increased likelihood of tPA administration among eligible patients and shorter median door-to-imaging times, door-to-needle times for thrombolysis, and meeting national benchmarks (door-to-imaging within 25 minutes, door-to-needle within 60 minutes, onset-to-needle within 120 minutes, and tPA use within 3 hours) (Lin et al., 2012).

Comment

Prehospital care has significant downstream effects on stroke patients' care delivery and outcomes, yet many stroke patients still do not activate EMS transportation to the hospital. Stroke education campaigns need to highlight the importance of early use of EMS, especially among minorities. For patients in rural and remote settings, there is a role for helicopter transport when ground transportation would take more than 1 hour. For all potential stroke patients transported by ambulance, consistent use of a validated prehospital stroke identification tool (e.g. CPSS, LAPSS) enables early and reasonably accurate identification of patients with acute cerebrovascular disease, enabling improved hospital pre-arrival notification and timely treatment upon hospital arrival. In addition, consistent use of a validated prehospital instrument for assessing stroke severity (e.g. LAMS, C-STAT, RACE) allows reasonably accurate identification of patients with LVOs and with intracerebral haemorrhage for potential direct routing to more advanced stroke centres. Stroke severity assessments should be deployed when two-tier routing of select patients directly to thrombectomy-capable and CSCs is advantageous, and a single scale should be used consistently within regional EMS systems. More advanced diagnostics and therapeutics in the prehospital setting, including prehospital telemedicine for stroke recognition, paramedic delivery of neuroprotective therapies, and mobile stroke unit provision of CT scanning and thrombolytic therapy in the field, show substantial promise, but further research is necessary to evaluate their utility and cost-effectiveness.

Regionalized Stroke Systems
Stroke Systems of Care

Background

The American Stroke Association has highlighted the need for organized and coordinated stroke systems of care in order to promote access to evidence-based stroke care. Barriers to access are substantial, particularly in rural and neurologically underserved areas, and fragmentation in care leads to suboptimal care delivery and treatment, as well as safety concerns and inefficiencies (Schwamm et al., 2005; Acker et al., 2007). A stroke system of care is a framework that integrates regional stroke facilities, EMS, and public and governmental agencies and resources and coordinates access to the full range of stroke prevention, treatment, and rehabilitation. This may include implementation of telemedicine and aeromedical transport in order to increase access in neurologically underserved areas (Schwamm et al., 2009a).

Potential elements in a hierarchical, regional stroke system of care include hospitals of five capacity levels: non-stroke centre hospitals, Acute Stroke Ready Hospitals (ASRHs), PSCs, Thrombectomy Stroke Centres (TSCs), and CSCs (Figures 3.3 and 3.4 and Table 3.1). In the USA, ASRHs, PSCs, TSCs,

Table 3.1 Components of acute stroke ready hospitals and primary stroke centres

	ASRH	PSC	Comment
EMS training provided	+	+	≥2 h annually
ED stroke education (annual hours)	+ (4 h)	+ (8 h)	
Acute stroke team with at least 2 members	+	+	15 min response time
Stroke protocols for treatment and stabilization	+	+	Annual revisions
Laboratory testing, ECG, CXR results available within 45 min of ordering	+	+	24/7 availability
Brain imaging completed and read within 45 min of ordering	+	+	Head CT or MRI, 24/7 availability
IV tPA for eligible patients, with goal DTN ≤60 min	+	+	24/7 availability
Stroke unit, including protocols and telemetry	*	+	
Neurosurgical services available within:	3 h	2 h	Onsite or by transfer
Telestroke	Initiated within 20 min when indicated	If hub site, response within 20 min of request	
Transfer of patients if indicated	To PSC or CSC	To CSC	Within 2 hours of ED arrival

ASRH: Acute Stroke Ready Hospital. PSC: Primary Stroke Centre. EMS: Emergency Medical Services. h: hour/s. ED: Emergency Department. min: minutes. ECG: electrocardiogram. CXR: chest x-ray. tPA: tissue plasminogen activator. DTN: door-to-needle time. CSC: Comprehensive Stroke Centre.

* Only required if patients are admitted.

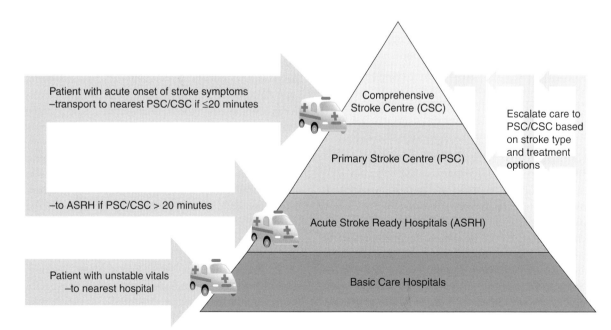

Figure 3.3 Field triage principles.

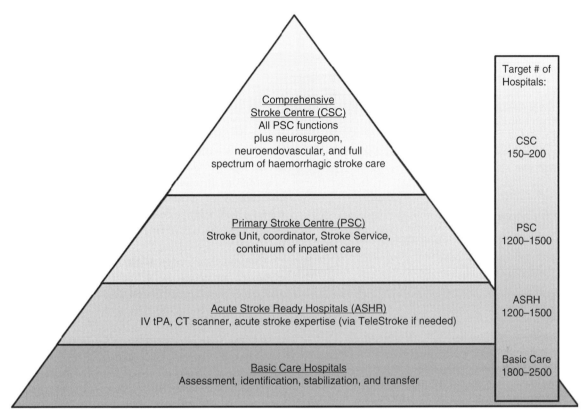

Figure 3.4 The Stroke Care Pyramid in the United States.

and CSCs are certified by the Joint Commission, by other national accrediting bodies, or by state departments of health (Powers et al., 2018).

- A non-stroke centre hospital has not made an institutional commitment to maintain a capable stroke care service 24/7/365. These hospitals should be bypassed by ambulances carrying stroke patients, and should have protocols for rapidly transferring patients who self-present with stroke or develop stroke as inpatients to facilities with stroke care capability.
- An ASRH has made an institutional commitment to provide initial emergent intravenous therapies to stroke patients and has written protocols for emergency stroke care, access to emergency brain imaging and laboratory testing at all times, the ability to administer intravenous tPA and coagulopathy reversal drugs, and written transfer agreements to efficiently send patients after initial

stabilization to more advanced stroke centres. The ASRH does not have fully organized inpatient stroke care or a stroke unit, and some resources may be via telemedicine.

- A PSC has all of the components of an ASRH; in addition, a PSC has a fully organized inpatient stroke care system or stroke unit. PSCs can provide both emergency and full inpatient care for the preponderance of stroke patients, except for those who require endovascular, neurosurgical, or neurological intensive care unit care (Higashida et al., 2013).
- A TSC has all of the components of a PSC and in addition provides around-the-clock access to endovascular mechanical thrombectomy for acute ischaemic strokes due to LVOs.
- A CSC has all of the components of a PSC and in addition has around-the-clock access to state-of-the-art care including endovascular techniques, the presence of a neurological intensive care unit,

and neurosurgical services in order to provide care for the most complex stroke patients (Higashida et al., 2013; Powers et al., 2018).

Evidence

The evidence for the hospital elements of regional stroke systems of care focuses on the distinctive advantages of PSCs and CSCs. The remaining levels are gap-fillers: ASRHs provide some of the services of PSCs in regions without a PSC, and TSCs provide some of the services of CSCs in regions without a CSC.

Primary Stroke Centres

A wide range of studies indicate that outcomes for all patients with acute ischaemic and haemorrhagic stroke are improved if care is delivered at facilities with organized inpatient stroke care. An analysis of 6223 ischaemic stroke patients in the Registry of the Canadian Stroke Network used an organized care index (OCI) to quantify the amount of hospitals' organized stroke care (namely, the presence of physical and occupational therapies, a stroke team, and a stroke unit). Patients treated at hospitals with higher OCIs had lower odds of 30-day mortality, and the number needed to treat to prevent 1 death at 30 days ranged from 4 to 9 across ischaemic stroke subtypes (Smith et al., 2010). In a German study, five network community hospitals with specialized stroke services and telemedical support from academic hospitals were matched with five community hospitals without specialized stroke care. Care delivery and outcomes of 3122 stroke patients presenting to these hospitals were studied; network hospitals were more likely to meet quality of care indicators, and patients treated in network hospitals were less likely to have poor outcomes (death, institutional care, or disability) (Audebert et al., 2006). An observational study of 30,947 ischaemic stroke patients treated at hospitals in New York State studied the relationship between admission to a stroke centre and use of thrombolytic therapy and patient mortality, finding that patients admitted to stroke centres were more frequently treated with tPA and had lower mortality (Xian, 2011). Other observational studies have also found that PSCs have a shorter time to imaging and to tPA treatment and higher tPA treatment rates (Rose et al., 2008; Sung et al., 2010).

Transitions of hospitals and regional care systems to organized inpatient care have been associated with improved patient outcomes. In the USA, a matched-hospital analysis examining 732 hospitals and 173,985 ischaemic stroke admissions found that hospital adoption of the Get with the Guidelines-Stroke hospital-based quality improvement programme was associated with reduced patient mortality and increased patient discharge to home rather than institutional care (Song et al., 2016). In London, a citywide hub-and-spoke model was implemented centred on eight hyperacute stroke units designed to treat suspected acute stroke patients during the first 72 hours of symptom duration, with faster response times and 24/7 access to specialist care. A pre–post analysis found a 12% relative reduction in deaths and a total 90-day cost savings of £5.2 million per year (Hunter et al., 2013).

Controlled clinical trials also support the benefits of organized inpatient care. A meta-analysis of 28 trials and 5855 participants found that stroke unit care reduced 1-year mortality (OR: 0.81), reduced odds of death or institutionalized care (OR: 0.78), and reduced the odds of death or dependency (OR: 0.79) (Figure 3.5) (Stroke Unit Trialists' Collaboration, 2013).

Structural aspects of stroke care (i.e. stroke centre certification) or performance recognition programmes best able to identify high-performing hospitals need consideration. In a hospital-level examination of 1356 hospitals participating in GWTG-S from 2010–2012, hospitals were classified by PSC status and by whether they had received recognition for performance with a GWTG-S achievement award. When hospitals were examined for conformity to quality of care measures for ischaemic stroke, PAA recognition was a stronger predictor of high performance than was PSC certification (Fonarow et al., 2013).

Comprehensive Stroke Centres

Care for select patients at CSCs is supported by the simple fact that many effective endovascular and neurosurgical therapies are available only at CSCs or TSCs, mandating patient access to advanced care sites. Endovascular thrombectomy for acute ischaemic stroke due to LVOs (Goyal et al., 2016), coiling or clipping of ruptured saccular aneurysms (Falk Delgado et al., 2017), minimally invasive haematoma evacuation for intracerebral haemorrhage (Tang et al., 2018), decompressive hemicraniectomy for large hemispheric infarcts (Alexander et al., 2016), and neurointensivist care of critically ill stroke patients

Review: Organised inpatient (stroke unit) care for stroke
Comparison: 1 Organised stroke unit care versus alternative service
Outcome: 3 Death or dependency by the end of scheduled follow-up

Study or subgroup	Treatment n/N	Control n/N	Peto Odds Ratio Peto, Fixed, 95% CI	Weight	Peto Odds Ratio Peto, Fixed, 95% CI
1 Stroke ward versus general medical ward					
Athens 1995	138/302	145/302		24.7 %	0.91 [0.66, 1.25]
Beijing 2004	113/195	118/197		15.6 %	0.92 [0.62, 1.38]
Dover 1984 (GMW)	54/98	50/89		7.6 %	0.96 [0.54, 1.70]
Edinburgh 1980	93/155	94/156		12.2 %	0.99 [0.63, 1.56]
Goteborg-Sahlgren 1994	108/166	54/83		8.3 %	1.00 [0.58, 1.74]
Huaihua 2004	83/324	39/73		8.3 %	0.27 [0.16, 0.47]
Joinville 2003	18/35	23/39		3.0 %	0.74 [0.30, 1.84]
Nottingham 1996 (GMW)	63/98	52/76		6.3 %	0.83 [0.44, 1.56]
Orpington 1993 (GMW)	38/53	39/48		3.0 %	0.59 [0.24, 1.48]
Orpington 1995	34/34	37/37			Not estimable
Perth 1997	10/29	15/30		2.4 %	0.54 [0.19, 1.49]
Trondheim 1991	54/110	81/110		8.6 %	0.36 [0.21, 0.61]
Subtotal (95% CI)	1599	1240		100.0 %	0.75 [0.64, 0.88]
Total events: 806 (Treatment), 747 (Control)					
Heterogeneity: Chi² = 26.73, df = 10 (P = 0.003); i² = 63%					
Test for overall effect: Z = 3.56 (P = 0.00037)					
2 Mixed rehabilitation ward versus general medical ward					
Birmingham 1972	8/29	7/23		7.4 %	0.87 [0.26, 2.89]
Helsinki 1995	47/121	65/122		41.8 %	0.56 [0.34, 0.93]
Illinois 1966	20/56	17/35		14.5 %	0.59 [0.25, 1.39]
Kuopio 1985	31/50	31/45		15.0 %	0.74 [0.32, 1.72]
New York 1962	23/42	23/40		14.1 %	0.90 [0.38, 2.13]
Newcastle 1993	26/34	28/33		7.3 %	0.59 [0.18, 1.96]
Subtotal (95% CI)	332	298		100.0 %	0.65 [0.47, 0.90]
Total events: 155 (Treatment), 171 (Control)					
Heterogeneity: Chi² = 1.26, df = 5 (P = 0.94); i² = 0.0%					
Test for overall effect: Z = 2.57 (P = 0.010)					
3 Mobile stroke team versus general medical ward					
Manchester 2003	91/157	95/151		87.1 %	0.81 [0.52, 1.28]
Montreal 1985	58/65	60/65		12.9 %	0.69 [0.21, 2.27]
Subtotal (95% CI)	222	216		100.0 %	0.80 [0.52, 1.22]
Total events: 149 (Treatment), 155 (Control)					
Heterogeneity: Chi² = 0.06, df = 1 (P = 0.81); i² = 0.0%					
Test for overall effect: Z = 1.04 (P = 0.30)					
4 Stroke ward versus mixed rehabilitation ward					
Dover 1984 (MRW)	11/18	19/28		10.3 %	0.75 [0.22, 2.56]
Nottingham 1996 (MRW)	60/78	48/63		25.4 %	1.04 [0.48, 2.27]
Orpington 1993 (MRW)	63/71	69/73		11.2 %	0.47 [0.15, 1.53]
Tampere 1993	53/98	55/113		53.2 %	1.24 [0.72, 2.13]
Subtotal (95% CI)	265	277		100.0 %	1.01 [0.68, 1.50]
Total events: 187 (Treatment), 191 (Control)					
Heterogeneity: Chi² = 2.40, df = 3 (P = 0.49); i² = 0.0%					
Test for overall effect: Z = 0.05 (P = 0.96)					
5 Stroke ward versus mobile stroke team					
Orpington 2000	61/152	73/152		100.0 %	0.73 [0.46, 1.14]
Subtotal (95% CI)	152	152		100.0 %	0.73 [0.46, 1.14]
Total events: 61 (Treatment), 73 (Control)					
Heterogeneity: not applicable					
Test for overall effect: Z = 1.38 (P = 0.17)					
6 Stroke ward versus stroke ward					
Groningen 2003	7/27	13/27		100.0 %	0.39 [0.13, 1.17]
Subtotal (95% CI)	27	27		100.0 %	0.39 [0.13, 1.17]
Total events: 7 (Treatment), 13 (Control)					
Heterogeneity: not applicable					
Test for overall effect: Z = 1.68 (P = 0.094)					
Test for subgroup differences: Chi² = 4.36, df = 5 (P=0.50), I² = 0.0%					

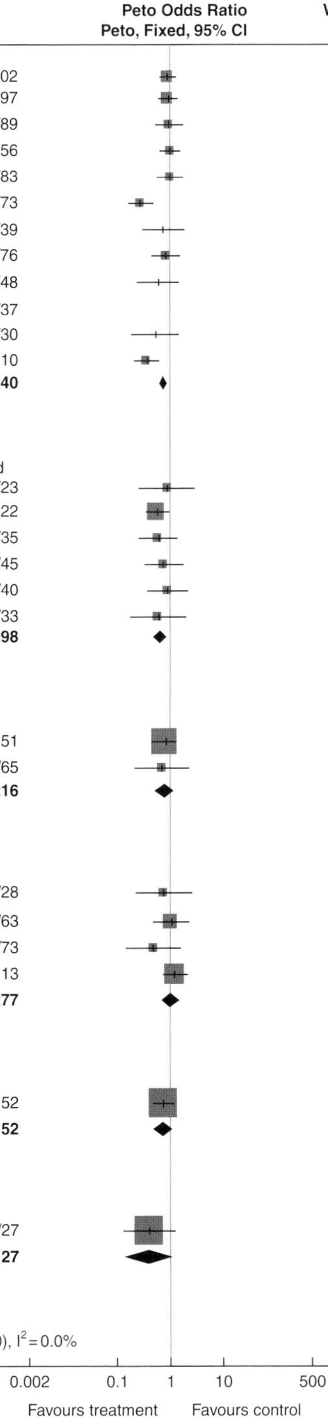

0.002   0.1   1   10   500

Favours treatment   Favours control

Figure 3.5 Organized stroke unit care versus alternative source.
Outcome: death or dependency by the end of scheduled follow-up.

Figure reproduced with permission of Cochrane Database.

(Knopf et al., 2012) are all distinctively or only available at CSCs.

In addition, multiple studies indicate that patients with complex neurovascular conditions have better outcomes when cared for at advanced care facilities with high-volume experience. For example, a relation between case volume and outcome is well-established for subarachnoid haemorrhage. In a meta-analysis of four observational studies with a total of 36,600 subarachnoid haemorrhage patients, mortality was decreased with care in high-volume hospitals: OR: 0.77, 95% CI: 0.60–0.97, $p < 0.01$ (Boogaarts et al., 2014). In an analysis of 32,336 subarachnoid haemorrhage patients in the United States Nationwide Inpatient Sample, mortality rates at hospitals with 100, 80, 60, 40, and 20 cases per year increased from 18.7% to 19.8%, 21.7%, 24.5%, and 28.4%, respectively (Pandey et al., 2015).

The relationship between high-volume centres and improved outcomes among patients with subarachnoid haemorrhage suggests that preferentially transporting certain types of suspected stroke patients to stroke centres may optimize their outcomes. An observational analysis examined 61,685 ischaemic stroke patients treated in 333 hospitals in Finland. Hospitals were classified as CSCs, PSCs, or general hospitals according to Brain Attack Coalition criteria, and patients treated at stroke centre hospitals had lower 1-year mortality and reduced institutional care compared with those treated at general hospitals, and over the 9-year follow-up median survival was increased by 1 year for patients treated in stroke centres (Meretoja et al., 2010).

Concentrating care for complex neurovascular patients at advanced stroke centres has been shown to be cost-effective from a societal perspective. One cost-utility analysis compared two scenarios for subarachnoid haemorrhage: regionalization of care in which patients at low-volume hospitals (<20 cases annually) would be transferred to hospitals with high volume (≥20 cases annually) versus a scenario in which every patient is treated at the geographically closest hospital. The study found that transferring a patient with subarachnoid haemorrhage (SAH) from a low- to high-volume hospital would gain 1.6 QALYs at a cost of $10,548/QALY (well within the generally accepted range for cost-effectiveness from the societal perspective) (Bardach et al., 2004). A similar cost-effectiveness analysis examined the role for transferring patients

with intracerebral haemorrhage from hospitals without specialized neurological intensive care units to centres with specialized units. As there are limited high-quality data on the effect of neurological intensive care units on functional outcomes, the analysis explored various favourability assumptions and found a cost of $47,000/QALY and $91,000/QALY in the favourable and moderately favourable scenarios – straddling the societal willing-to-pay threshold (Fletcher et al., 2015). Among patients with ischaemic stroke, treatment with tPA and treatment with endovascular thrombectomy have been shown to be highly cost-effective (Joo et al., 2017; Shireman et al., 2017). An analysis of endovascular thrombectomy found that catheter treatment increased QALYs by 1.74 years and decreased lifetime medical costs by $23,000 (Shireman et al., 2017). Therefore, treatment of large vessel ischaemic stroke patients at centres with higher rates of endovascular thrombectomy delivery is likely to be cost-effective.

Comment

Implementation of stroke systems of care can lead to improved access to specialty services and improved patient outcomes. By preferentially transporting all stroke patients to centres where organized inpatient care and thrombolytic therapy are more likely and more timely, and select stroke patients to centres where advanced endovascular and surgical therapies are expertly and efficiently available, regionalization of stroke care is desirable and cost-effective from both the patient and the societal perspectives. Patients should be escalated up the stroke pyramid to centres of increasing capability when needed; when appropriate, patients should also flow down the pyramid to lower-cost community centres when specialty services are no longer required. Stroke systems should also establish written protocols for interhospital patient transfers, using the trauma system as a model (Acker et al., 2007). Given the substantial international and intranational variations in rules and regulations, geography, and resources (Higashida et al., 2013; Lindsay et al., 2016), implementation of stroke systems of care will necessarily be distinct and customized for each region or locality and may encounter significant obstacles, namely substantial cost and resource constraints (Schwamm et al., 2005). While such constraints may necessitate an incremental approach to implementation of a system of care, it is important to note that such costs may be offset by the potential cost savings realized by individual hospitals and facilities (Schwamm et al., 2005). Additionally, telemedicine resources may offer a cost-effective solution for access to specialty care and keeping patients at community hospitals. Finally, PSCs, CSCs, and stroke systems of care must provide ongoing education to the public and to key personnel and continually evaluate the effectiveness of their care delivery for continuous quality improvement (Powers et al., 2018; Higashida et al., 2013).

Telemedicine

Background

Telemedicine utilizes telecommunication technologies to provide medical information and services. Telemedicine for stroke care (i.e. *telestroke*) can connect hospitals without full-time neurological or radiological services to around-the-clock acute stroke expertise. Telestroke has the potential to fill the gap that exists in many parts of the USA that otherwise lack access to acute stroke services (Schwamm et al., 2009a, 2009b; Demaerschalk et al., 2017), may allow more hospitals to become ASRHs or PSCs (Powers et al., 2018), and, in providing emergent neurological expertise, may overcome a major barrier to tPA utilization (Brown et al., 2005; Schwamm et al., 2009b; Gadhia et al., 2018). The current structure of telestroke arrangements ranges from small partnerships to large multi-hospital affiliations (hub-and-spoke model) to for-profit transactional relationships (see Figure 3.7) (Schwamm et al., 2009a).

Evidence

The utility of telestroke in the acute hospital-based evaluation of stroke patients has been demonstrated in reports from multiple countries and regions, including Ontario (Waite et al., 2006), Germany (Audebert et al., 2006), Swabia (Wiborg et al., 2003), Texas (Choi et al., 2006), Massachusetts (Schwamm et al., 2004), and rural community hospitals in Georgia (Hess et al., 2005). The most studied utilization of telestroke is with respect to thrombolysis eligibility. Telestroke has been given a Class I recommendation based on Level A evidence in support of its use for National Institutes of Health Stroke Scale (NIHSS) assessment, timely review of brain imaging, and determination of tPA eligibility (Higashida et al., 2013).

The feasibility and utility of assessing NIHSS via telestroke using high-quality, dedicated video-conferencing software has been established. Inter-rater agreement for the NIHSS between bedside examination by a stroke neurologist and remote examination through telestroke by a stroke neurologist has been found to be very high both for console telemedicine equipment, with correlation coefficients of 0.97 and 0.96 (Shafqat et al., 1999; Wang et al., 2003), and for smartphone equipment, with correlation coefficient of 0.95 and kappa of 0.98 (Demaerschalk et al., 2012; Anderson et al., 2013).

Engagement of telestroke has also been shown to increase the use of tPA in eligible patients. A review of 655 stroke patients treated at two community hospitals east of Houston found that, after implementation of a telemedicine project, the rate of tPA treatment more than quadrupled (Choi et al., 2006). Implementation of telestroke led to administration of tPA in rural or island settings where thrombolytics were not previously regularly used (Schwamm et al., 2004; Wang et al., 2004). In a controlled trial, among 234 stroke patients at four spoke sites randomly assigned to use of televideo versus telephone to determine suitability for tPA treatment, correct treatment decisions were more often made in the telemedicine group (OR: 10.9, 95% CI: 2.7–44.6) (Meyer et al., 2008).

In addition to increasing tPA utilization, telestroke may decrease treatment times for tPA administration. An analysis of 50 tPA-treated patients in the REACH telestroke network found that mean onset to treatment time was shorter than other stroke care delivery systems (127.6 minutes vs 145.9 minutes) (Switzer et al., 2009) and improved over time as the system became more efficient (Hess et al., 2005). While onset to treatment times were shorter, it is not clear whether this was also true for door-to-needle times, as this was not reported.

Telestroke is associated with similar long-term functional outcomes and mortality to traditional tPA delivery at the bedside. The STRokE DOC study found no difference in rates of intracerebral haemorrhage after tPA or in 90-day functional outcomes or mortality in telemedicine-treated patients compared with that to be expected from bedside evaluation (Meyer et al., 2008). A telestroke pilot project in Germany examined all patients receiving telemedicine-authorized thrombolysis in 12 regional centres in a telestroke network and found no significant difference in rates of symptomatic haemorrhage after thrombolysis, or in 1-week or in-hospital mortality compared with in person-authorized thrombolysis at two stroke centre hubs (Audebert et al., 2006). Long-term outcomes of 3- and 6-month mortality and functional outcomes after thrombolytic treatment were similar between patients treated at telemedicine-linked community hospitals and stroke centre hospitals (Schwab et al., 2007). In a comparison of stroke patients treated by telestroke in community hospitals and those treated at the Helsinki University Central Hospital hub, there was no significant difference in the proportion of patients with favourable outcomes (Sairanen et al., 2011).

Finally, telestroke in the acute treatment of ischaemic stroke is likely to be cost-effective. A cost-effectiveness analysis compared hub-spoke telestroke network care with treatment in remote EDs without telestroke consultation or stroke experts. The analysis found that telestroke results in a cost of $2449 per QALY over a lifetime horizon (Nelson et al., 2011).

Telemedicine also has important applications in radiological evaluation of acute stroke patients. A pilot study comparing stroke neurologists' use of telemedicine to read 72 head CT scans versus gold standard readings of hard copies found excellent reliability of stroke neurologists' reads (kappa statistic = 1.0), sensitivity of 100%, and specificity of 100% (Johnston and Worrall, 2003). A review of telestroke cases in the Partners Telestroke Network similarly found that radiology reads by telestroke were effective for identifying tPA exclusions and making decisions regarding thrombolysis administration (Schwamm et al., 2004).

In a review of 100 head CT images from patients with suspected stroke, remote image review by telestroke showed 100% agreement for images of acute ischaemic stroke, intracerebral haemorrhage, metastasis, and normal scans, but only 88% agreement (7 of 8) for cases of subarachnoid haemorrhage (Phabphal and Hirunpatch, 2008). As expected, teleradiology is subject to equipment and reader variability. In a study of 582 possible stroke patients in the Stroke Eastern Saxony Network (SOS-NET), stroke neurologists' CT reads during telemedical consultation had discrepancies from neuroradiologist reads in 43 patients (8%), 9 of which were clinically relevant (1.7%) (Puetz et al., 2013).

Studies have also indicated the feasibility of teleradiology image review via smartphones for timely and accurate interpretation of CT scans in possible cases of acute stroke. One study of 120 noncontrast head CT images and 70 CT angiography images from the Calgary Stroke Program database compared neuroradiologist reads via workstation versus smartphone and found that the sensitivity, specificity, and accuracy of detecting haemorrhage were 100% with perfect agreement (kappa = 1) (Mitchell et al., 2011). Diagnosis of acute parenchymal ischaemic change, dense vessel sign, and vessel occlusion on CT angiography were good (parenchymal ischaemic change: kappa 0.8; dense vessel sign: kappa 0.69, vessel occlusion: kappa 1.0) with no significant difference in interpretation time between devices. In another study of 74 acute ischaemic stroke patients, neuroradiologists accurately diagnosed presence or absence of LVOs on CT angiography on smartphones, with 100% agreement versus workstation diagnosis (Hidlay et al., 2018).

The use of mobile telestroke in ambulances has also been shown to be feasible. In 27 ambulance runs of standardized patients, the correlation on prehospital NIHSS scores assessed by a remote rater using tablet-based telemedicine and an in-person rater was 0.96 (Chapman Smith et al., 2016). Remote evaluation permits physicians to contribute to the assessment and routing decisions for stroke versus nonstroke and potential LVO versus non-LVO ischaemic stroke. In mobile stroke units, mobile telestroke assessment enables physicians to make decisions regarding prehospital start of intravenous thrombolysis. Among 50 consecutive mobile stroke unit patients, a remote telemedicine neurologist rendered comparable thrombolytic decisions to an in-person neurologist (Bowry et al., 2018) (see Figure 3.6).

Comment

Telestroke has important applications in the prehospital setting and acute evaluation of possible stroke patients for maximally integrating stroke systems of care. Its utility for assessing stroke severity, reviewing brain imaging, and safely increasing the use of tPA in eligible patients has been well established, and has even been shown to impact patients' long-term functional and mortality outcomes. Telestroke should be considered whenever local resources are limited and/or neurological expertise is unavailable. When telestroke is implemented, patients should be aware of indications, benefits, and risks of its applications, and regulatory oversight will be important to ensure minimum safety, efficacy, and technical standards (Schwamm et al., 2009a). Recommendations to

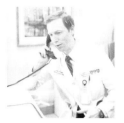
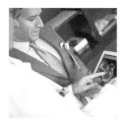
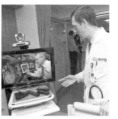
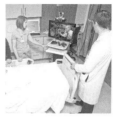

1 CONSULT REQUEST
When a patient with stroke/neurology symptoms is in need of emergent care, your team pushes the patient's imaging studies and pages the on-call TeleNeurology specialist for a consultation.

2 CASE REVIEW
The TeleNeurology specialist immediately begins the assessment of the images and returns the page by phone to review the case; the consult may transition to a videoconference call, if appropriate. Using the video connection, the specialist will review the patient's presentation with your emergency department physician and, aided by your local staff, will perform a neurological assessment and discuss the findings with you. Together you decide on the plan of care.

3 ONLINE ASSESSMENT
The TeleNeurology specialist documents the information within the TeleNeurology Web Portal. You can access the portal to retrieve your local EMR or have it sent via fax.

4 COLLABORATIVE DECISION MAKING
Upon completion of the examination, the findings will be discussed with your team. Together you decide on a plan of care.

Figure 3.6 Example of the telemedicine process.
Figure reproduced with permission of Massachusetts General Hospital TeleNeurology.

specify explicit standards for telestroke delivery have been advanced (Demaerschalk et al., 2017). Telestroke support for thrombolysis decision-making in EDs may be implemented within two different models for hospital interactions: the 'drip and ship' model, with lytics started at the telestroke hospital, followed by patient transfer to a higher level of care, and the 'drip and keep' model, in which the patient remains at the original hospital (see Figure 3.7). Future studies should also define minimum educational requirements and training necessary for telestroke utilization (Schwamm et al., 2009b).

Interactions within Systems of Care

Background

Regionalization of acute stroke care enables better coordination of regional or state health resources including EMS, stroke centres and hospitals of varying capabilities, telemedicine, and other interactions between hospitals (Higashida et al., 2013; Powers et al., 2018). Because of the substantial variation between regions in stroke population, geographical factors, and regional resources, the organization and interactions within the stroke system of care will naturally vary, and EMS plays a key role. In addition

to its roles in dissemination of public information and education, provision of professional training, and development of disaster planning, the EMS system must address issues related to communication, transportation, access to care, and patient transfer.

Evidence

There is substantial variation between hospitals in the use of tPA and endovascular therapy for stroke, and in 30-day mortality (Kleindorfer et al., 2009; Adeoye et al., 2011; Berkowitz et al., 2014; Thompson et al., 2017). A study of the 2011 US Medicare Provider and Analysis Review data set noted that 17% of all acute ischaemic stroke discharges were from hospitals that did not provide any tPA during that year and 28% were from hospitals capable of delivering both tPA and endovascular therapy (Adeoye et al., 2014). When considering geographical proximity within 60 minutes of ground transport time, the authors found that 81% of the US population had access to a hospital that had given IV tPA, 66% had access to PSCs, and 56% had access to endovascular-capable hospitals (Adeoye et al., 2014). Allowing the option of air transportation, 97% had access to hospitals that had used tPA, 91% to PSCs, and

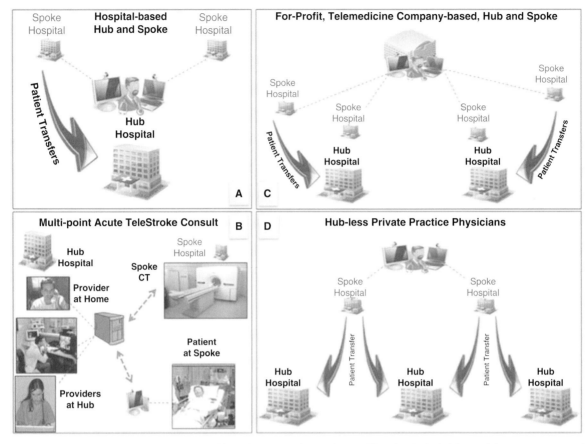

Figure 3.7 Various telestroke organizational models. A, The expert teleconsultant is affiliated with the hub hospital that receives potential postconsultation transfers; B, more detailed schematic diagram of the consult process in a model in which the teleconsultant is affiliated with the hub hospital showing the possibility of multipoint acute stroke consult; C, the teleconsultant is an employee of a for-profit telemedicine company unaffiliated with the receiving hub; D, the teleconsultant is a private practice neurologist unaffiliated with the receiving hub.

Figure reproduced with permission of Wolters Kluwer Health, Inc.

85% to endovascular capable hospitals within 60 minutes' drive time. See Figure 3.8.

Given this variation, the optimal routing for an individual stroke patient who activates the EMS system will vary based on the patient's specific condition and the particular array of available stroke centre destinations that are available nearby. Most EMS systems prefer to avoid travel times of more than 30 minutes, as lengthy transportations deprive the home catchment region of the ambulance resource for new emergencies that may arise. Within that constraint, it is desirable to transport patients to certified stroke centres over non-stroke centres, and, when equidistant, to transport patients to higher-level stroke centres over lower-level stroke centres (Higashida et al., 2013).

Since favourable outcomes for patients with acute ischaemic stroke due to LVOs are more greatly benefitted by accelerated endovascular thrombectomy than accelerated intravenous thrombolysis, real-world observations and geospatial models have indicated that it is also preferable to transport patients with likely LVO per prehospital stroke severity scales directly to more distant endovascular-capable hospitals, bypassing nearer non-endovascular stroke centres, as long as the additional distance is modest. In a multicentre registry study of 984 thrombectomy patients, patients routed directly to an endovascular-capable hospital had higher rates of functional independence at 3 months than did patients routed first to a non-endovascular hospital: 60.0% vs 52.2%, OR: 1.38 (95% CI: 1.06–1.79) (Froehler et al., 2017). In

60-minute Drive Time and Population Coverage
AHA/ASA/TJC Comprehensive and Primary Stroke Center
Certification and Acute Stroke Ready Hospital Certification

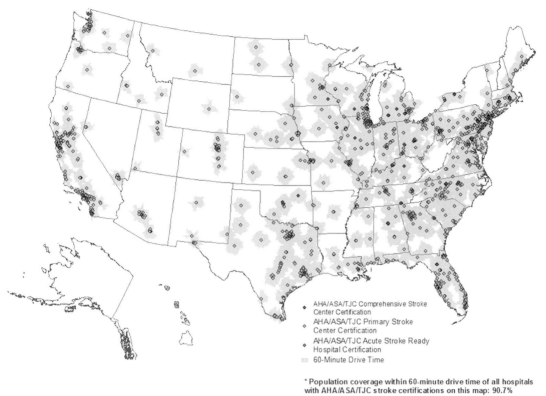

AHA/ASA/TJC Comprehensive Stroke
Center Certification
AHA/ASA/TJC Primary Stroke
Center Certification
AHA/ASA/TJC Acute Stroke Ready
Hospital Certification
60-Minute Drive Time

* Population coverage within 60-minute drive time of all hospitals
with AHA/ASA/TJC stroke certifications on this map: 90.7%

Figure 3.8 US stroke centres and population covered by 60-minute drive time.
Figure reproduced with permission of the American Heart Association.

a conditional probability model, direct routing to endovascular-capable hospitals showed better clinical outcomes with travel times up to 60 minutes longer, unless the non-endovascular hospitals had unusually fast door-to-needle and door-in–door-out performance (Holodinsky et al., 2018). Another model similarly found that best routing recommendations were sensitive to small changes in input parameters regarding processes of care at endovascular and non-endovascular centres, but that, in general, good outcomes were most often maximized with routing of patients with severe stroke directly to CSCs (Ali et al., 2018).

When patients with LVOs are brought initially to non-endovascular stroke centres, rapid identification and transfer to endovascular-capable hospitals are associated with improved outcomes. In a study of 70 patients transferred from 14 PSCs to a regional

CSC, rapid recognition of LVO and notification of the CSC for transfer was associated with a marked increase in functional independence outcome at 3 months, 50% vs 25%, $p = 0.04$ (McTaggart et al., 2017).

Comment

There is substantial variation between regions and between hospitals in the delivery of acute ischaemic stroke care, with the consequence that interactions within stroke systems of care are of great importance. The EMS system must address issues related to communication, transportation, access to care, and patient transfer. This necessitates collaboration among prehospital and hospital providers with ongoing collaborative educational activities, feedback loops, and process-improvement efforts. Transport protocols must be collaboratively developed to address routing considerations

51

for patients with suspected stroke. These must include handoff protocols for stroke patients transferred between hospitals before or after IV thrombolysis, and especially for drip-and-ship patients with tPA still infusing to ensure compliance with the post-tPA treatment protocols and accurate tPA dosing. Timely endovascular treatment for patients with LVOs ideally should not be delayed in waiting for the completion of tPA infusions. One reasonable strategy for selective routing of some prehospital stroke patients is reflected in the Mission Lifeline: Stroke consensus policy recommendation to route likely LVO patients directly to CSCs if they were no more than 15 minutes farther away (Mission: Lifeline Stroke, 2017).

Summary

In summary, prehospital stroke care and regionalization of stroke care are critical components of effective stroke systems of care. There is good observational evidence supporting the importance of symptom recognition, engagement of Emergency Medical Services, dispatcher response, and prehospital stroke screening and stroke severity tools. Research also supports the important potential of the prehospital setting for early stroke intervention and as a valuable research platform. In addition, there is a growing body of evidence for new approaches including mobile stroke units, telemedicine applications, and advanced diagnostic testing in the prehospital setting. However, more level I, randomized controlled trial evidence is needed to better understand how to achieve the best outcomes for stroke patients with maximal cost-effectiveness in the prehospital setting. Future research must also ensure that approaches lead to the best outcomes for diverse patient populations.

References

Abdullah AR, Smith EE, Biddinger PD, Kalenderian D, Schwamm LH. (2008). Advance hospital notification by EMS in acute stroke is associated with shorter door-to-computed tomography time and increased likelihood of administration of tissue-plasminogen activator. *Prehospital Emerg Care*, **12**, 426–31. doi:10.1080/10903120802290828.

Acker JE 3rd, Pancioli AM, Crocco TJ, Eckstein MK, Jauch EC, Larrabee H, et al. (2007). Implementation strategies for emergency medical services within stroke systems of care: a policy statement from the American Heart Association/American Stroke Association Expert Panel on Emergency Medical Services Systems and the Stroke Council. *Stroke*, **38**, 3097–115. doi:10.1161/STROKEAHA.107.186094.

Adams J, Aldag G, Wolford R. (1996). Does the level of prehospital care influence the outcome of patients with altered levels of consciousness? *Prehospital Disaster Med*, **11**, 101–4.

Adeoye O, Albright KC, Carr BG, Wolff C, Mullen MT, Abruzzo L, et al. (2014). Geographic access to acute stroke care in the United States. *Stroke*, **45**, 3019–24. doi:10.1161/STROKEAHA.114.006293.

Adeoye O, Hornung R, Khatri P, Kleindorfer D. (2011). Recombinant tissue-type plasminogen activator use for ischemic stroke in the United States: a doubling of treatment rates over the course of 5 years. *Stroke*, **42**,1952–5. doi:10.1161/STROKEAHA.110.612358.

Alexander P, Heels-Ansdell D, Siemieniuk R. (2016). Hemicraniectomy versus medical treatment with large MCA infarct: a review and meta-analysis. *BMJ Open*, **6**, e014390. doi:10.1136/bmjopen-2016-014390.

Ali A, Zachrison KS, Eschenfeldt PC, Schwamm LH, Hur C. (2018). Optimization of prehospital triage of patients with suspected ischemic stroke. *Stroke*, **49**, 2532–5. doi:10.1161/STROKEAHA.118.022041.

Amadi-Obi A, Gilligan P, Owens N, O'Donnell C. (2014). Telemedicine in pre-hospital care: a review of telemedicine applications in the pre-hospital environment. *Int J Emerg Med*, **7**, 29. doi:10.1186/s12245-014-0029-0.

Anderson ER, Smith B, Ido M, Frankel M. (2013). Remote assessment of stroke using the iPhone 4. *J Stroke Cerebrovasc Dis*, **22**, 340–4. doi:10.1016/j.jstrokecerebrovasdis.2011.09.013.

Ankolekar S, Fuller M, Cross I, Renton C, Cox P, Sprigg N, et al. (2013). Feasibility of an ambulance-based stroke trial, and safety of glyceryl trinitrate in ultra-acute stroke: the Rapid Intervention with Glyceryl trinitrate in Hypertensive stroke Trial (RIGHT, ISRCTN66434824). *Stroke*, **44**, 3120–8. doi:10.1161/STROKEAHA.113.001301.

Audebert HJ, Kukla C, Vatankhah B, Gotzler B, Schenkel J, Hofer S, et al. (2006). Comparison of tissue plasminogen activator administration management between telestroke network hospitals and academic stroke centers: the Telemedical Pilot Project for Integrative Stroke Care in Bavaria/Germany. *Stroke*, **37**, 1822–7. doi:10.1161/01.STR.0000226741.20629.b2.

Bae H-J, Kim D-H, Yoo N-T, et al. (2010). Prehospital notification from the emergency medical service reduces the transfer and intra-hospital processing times for acute stroke patients. *J Clin Neurol*, **6**, 138. doi:10.3988/jcn.2010.6.3.138.

Bardach NS, Olson SJ, Elkins JS, Smith WS, Lawton MT, Johnston SC, et al. (2004). Regionalization of treatment for subarachnoid hemorrhage a cost-utility analysis. *Circulation*, **109**, 2207–12. doi:10.1161/01.CIR.0000126433.12527.E6.

Berkowitz AL, Mittal MK, McLane HC, Shen GC, Muralidharan R, Lyons JL, et al. (2014). Worldwide reported use of IV tissue plasminogen activator for acute ischemic stroke. *Int J Stroke*, **9**, 349–55. doi:10.1111/ijs.12205.

Boogaarts HD, van Amerongen MJ, de Vries J, Westert GP, Veerbeek AL, Grotenhuis JA, et al. (2014). Caseload as a factor for outcome in aneurysmal subarachnoid hemorrhage: a systematic review and meta-analysis. *J Neurosurg*, **120**, 605–11. doi:10.3171/2013.9.JNS13640.

Bowry R, Parker SA, Yamal JM, Hwang H, Appana S, Rangel-Gutierrez N, et al. (2018). Time to decision and treatment with tPA (tissue-type plasminogen activator) using telemedicine versus an onboard neurologist on a mobile stroke unit. *Stroke*, **49**, 1528–30. doi:10.1161/STROKEAHA.117.020585.

Brandler ES, Sharma M, Sinert RH, Levine SR. (2014). Prehospital stroke scales in urban environments: a systematic review. *Neurology*, **82**, 2241–9. doi:10.1212/WNL.0000000000000523.

Brown DL, Barsan WG, Lisabeth LD, Gallery ME, Morgenstern LB. (2005). Survey of emergency physicians about recombinant tissue plasminogen activator for acute ischemic stroke. *Ann Emerg Med*, **46**, 56–60. doi:10.1016/j.annemergmed.2004.12.025.

Buck BH, Starkman S, Eckstein M, Kidwell CS, Haines J, Huang R, et al. (2009). Dispatcher recognition of stroke using the National Academy Medical Priority Dispatch System. *Stroke*, **40**(6), 2027–30. doi:10.1161/STROKEAHA.108.545574.

Centers for Disease Control and Prevention (CDC). (2007). Prehospital and hospital delays after stroke onset – United States, 2005–2006. *MMWR Morb Mortal Wkly Rep*, **56**, 474–8.

Chapman Smith SN, Govindarajan P, Padrick MM, Lippman JM, McMurry TL, Resler BL, et al.; as the iTREAT Investigators. (2016). A low-cost, tablet-based option for prehospital neurologic assessment: The iTREAT Study. *Neurology*, **87**(1), 19–26. doi:10.1212/WNL.0000000000002799.

Chiti, A, Fanucchi S, Sonnoli C, Barni S, Orlandi G. (2007). Stroke symptoms and the decision to call for an ambulance: turn on people's minds! *Stroke J Cereb Circ*, **38**, e58–59. doi:10.1161/STROKEAHA.107.489179.

Choi JY, Porche NA, Albright KC, Khaja AM, Ho VS, Grotta JC. (2006). Using telemedicine to facilitate thrombolytic therapy for patients with acute stroke. *Jt Comm J Qual Patient Saf*, **32**, 199–205.

Demaerschalk BM, Berg J, Chong BW, Gross H, Nystrom K, Adeoye O, et al. (2017). American Telemedicine Association: telestroke guidelines. *Telemed J E Health*, **23**, 376–89. doi:10.1089/tmj.2017.0006.

Demaerschalk BM, Vegunta S, Vargas BB, Wu Q, Channer DD, Hentz JG. (2012). Reliability of real-time video smartphone for assessing National Institutes of Health Stroke Scale scores in acute stroke patients. *Stroke J Cereb Circ*, **43**, 3271–7. doi:10.1161/STROKEAHA.112.669150.

Ebinger M, Kunz A, Wendt M, Rozanski M, Winter B, Waldschmidt C, et al. (2015). Effects of golden hour thrombolysis: a Prehospital Acute Neurological Treatment and Optimization of Medical Care in Stroke (PHANTOM-S) Substudy. *JAMA Neurol*, **72**, 25–30. doi:10.1001/jamaneurol.2014.3188.

Ebinger M, Winter B, Wendt M, Weber JE, Waldschmidt C, Rozanski M, et al. (2014). Effect of the use of ambulance-based thrombolysis on time to thrombolysis in acute ischemic stroke: a randomized clinical trial. *JAMA*, **311**, 1622–31. doi:10.1001/jama.2014.2850.

Ekundayo OJ, Saver JL, Fonarow GC, Schwamm LH, Xian Y, Zhao X, et al. (2013). Patterns of emergency medical services use and its association with timely stroke treatment: findings from Get with the Guidelines-Stroke. *Circ Cardiovasc Qual Outcomes*, **6**, 262–9. doi:10.1161/CIRCOUTCOMES.113.000089.

Evenson KR, Foraker RE, Morris DL, Rosamond WD. (2009). A comprehensive review of prehospital and in-hospital delay times in acute stroke care. *Int J Stroke*, **4**, 187–99. doi:10.1111/j.1747-4949.2009.00276.x.

Falk Delgado A, Andersson T, Falk Delgado A. (2017). Clinical outcome after surgical clipping or endovascular coiling for cerebral aneurysms: a pragmatic meta-analysis of randomized and non-randomized trials with short- and long-term follow-up. *J Neurointerv Surg*, **9**, 264–77. doi:10.1136/neurintsurg-2016-012292.

Fassbender K, Grotta JC, Walter S, Grunwald IQ, Ragoschke-Schumm A, Saver JL. (2017). Mobile stroke units for prehospital thrombolysis, triage, and beyond: benefits and challenges. *Lancet Neurol*, **16**, 227–37. doi:10.1016/S1474-4422(17)30008-X.

Fletcher JJ, Kotagal V, Mammoser A, Peterson M, Morgenstern LB, Burke JF, et al. (2015). Cost-effectiveness of transfers to centers with neurological intensive care units after intracerebral hemorrhage. *Stroke*, **46**, 58–64. doi:10.1161/STROKEAHA.114.006653.

Fonarow GC, Liang L, Smith EE, Reeves MJ, Saver JL, Xian Y, et al (2013). Comparison of performance achievement award recognition with primary stroke center certification for acute ischemic stroke care. *J Am Heart Assoc*, **2**, e000451. doi:10.1161/JAHA.113.000451.

Froehler MT, Saver JL, Zaidat OO, Jahan R, Aziz-Sultan MA, Klucznik RP, et al. (2017). Interhospital transfer before thrombectomy is associated with delayed treatment and worse outcome in the STRATIS Registry (Systematic Evaluation of Patients Treated With Neurothrombectomy Devices for Acute Ischemic Stroke). *Circulation*, **136**, 2311–21. doi:10.1161/CIRCULATIONAHA.117.028920.

Gadhia R, Schwamm LH, Viswanathan A, Whitney C, Moreno A, Zachrison KS. (2018). Evaluation of the experience of spoke hospitals in an academic telestroke network. *Telemed J E Health*, **25**. doi:10.1089/tmj.2018.0133. [Epub ahead of print]

Goyal M, Menon BK, van Zwam WH, Dippel DW, Mitchell PG, Demchuk AM, et al. (2016). Endovascular thrombectomy after large-vessel ischaemic stroke: a meta-analysis of individual patient data from five randomised trials. *Lancet*, **387**, 1723–31. doi:10.1016/S0140-6736(16)00163-X.

Gropen TI, Boehme A, Martin-Schild S, Albright K, Samai A, Pishanidar S, et al. (2018). Derivation and validation of the emergency medical stroke assessment and comparison of large vessel occlusion scales. *J Stroke Cerebrovasc Dis*, **27**, 806–15. doi:10.1016/j.jstrokecerebrovasdis.2017.10.018.

Gupta R, Manuel M, Owada K, Dhungana S, Busby L, Glenn BA, et al. (2016). Severe hemiparesis as a prehospital tool to triage stroke severity: a pilot study to assess diagnostic accuracy and treatment times. *J Neurointerv Surg*, **8**, 775–7. doi:10.1136/neurintsurg-2015-011940.

Hawk A, Marco C, Huang M2, Chow B. (2016). Helicopter scene response for stroke patients: a 5-year experience. *Air Med J*, **35**, 352–4. doi:10.1016/j.amj.2016.05.007.

Hess DC, Wang S, Hamilton W, Lee S, Pardue C, Waller JL, et al. (2005). REACH: clinical feasibility of a rural telestroke network. *Stroke*, **36**, 2018–2020. doi:10.1161/01.STR.0000177534.02969.e4

Hesselfeldt R, Gyllenborg J, Steinmetz J, Do HQ, Hejselbaek J, Rasmussen LS. (2014). Is air transport of stroke patients faster than ground transport? A prospective controlled observational study. *Emerg Med J*, **31**, 268–72. doi:10.1136/emermed-2012-202270.

Hidlay DT, McTaggart RA, Baird G, Yaghi S, Hemendinger M, Tung EL, et al. (2018). Accuracy of smartphone-based evaluation of emergent large vessel occlusion on CTA. *Clin Neurol Neurosurg*, **171**, 135–8. doi:10.1016/j.clineuro.2018.06.012.

Higashida R, Alberts MJ, Alexander DN, Crocco TJ, Demaerschalk BM, Derdeyn CP, et al. (2013). Interactions within stroke systems of care: a policy statement from the American Heart Association/American Stroke Association. *Stroke*, **44**, 2961–2984. doi:10.1161/STR.0b013e3182a6d2b2.

Hodgson C, Lindsay P, Rubini F. (2007). Can mass media influence emergency department visits for stroke? *Stroke J Cereb Circ*, **38**, 2115–22. doi:10.1161/STROKEAHA.107.484071.

Hodgson C, Lindsay P, Rubini F. (2009). Using paid mass media to teach the warning signs of stroke: the long and the short of it. *Health Promot J Aust Off J Aust Assoc Health Promot Prof*, **20**, 58–64.

Holodinsky JK, Williamson TS, Demchuk AM, Zhao H, Zhu L, Francis MJ, et al. (2018). Modeling stroke patient transport for all patients with suspected large-vessel occlusion. *JAMA Neurol*, **75**, 1477–86. doi:10.1001/jamaneurol.2018.2424.

Hougaard KD, Hjort N, Zeidler D, Sørensen L, Nørgaard A, Hansen TM, et al. (2014). Remote ischemic preconditioning as an adjunct therapy to thrombolysis in patients with acute ischemic stroke: a randomized trial. *Stroke*, **45**, 159–67. doi:10.1161/STROKEAHA.113.001346.

Hunter RM, Davie C, Rudd A, Thompson A, Walker H, Thomson N, et al. (2013). Impact on clinical and cost outcomes of a centralized approach to acute stroke care in London: a comparative effectiveness before and after model. *PloS One*, **8**, e70420. doi:10.1371/journal.pone.0070420.

Hutton CF, Fleming J, Youngquist S, Hutton KC, Heiser DM, Barton ED. (2015). Stroke and helicopter emergency medical service transports: an analysis of 25,332 patients. *Air Med J*, **34**, 348–56. doi:10.1016/j.amj.2015.06.011.

Johnston KC, Worrall BB. (2003). Teleradiology Assessment of Computerized Tomographs Online Reliability Study (TRACTORS) for acute stroke evaluation. *Telemed J E Health*, **9**, 227–233. doi:10.1089/153056203322502605.

John S, Stock S, Masaryk T, Bauer A, Cerejo R, Uchino K, et al. (2016). Performance of CT angiography on a mobile stroke treatment unit: implications for triage. *J Neuroimaging*, **26**(4), 391–4. doi:10.1111/jon.12346.

Joo H, Wang G, George MG. (2017). Age-specific cost effectiveness of using intravenous recombinant tissue plasminogen activator for treating acute ischemic stroke. *Am J Prev Med*, **53**, S205–S212. doi:10.1016/j.amepre.2017.06.004.

Jurkowski JM, Maniccia DM, Spicer DA, Dennison BA. (2010). Impact of a multimedia campaign to increase intention to call 9-1-1 for stroke symptoms, upstate New York, 2006–2007. *Prev Chronic Dis*, **7**, A35.

Katz BS, McMullan JT, Sucharew H, Adeoye O, Broderick JP. (2015). Design and validation of a prehospital scale to predict stroke severity: Cincinnati Prehospital Stroke Severity Scale. *Stroke*, **46**, 1508–12. doi:10.1161/STROKEAHA.115.008804.

Kelly AG, Hellkamp AS, Olson D, Smith EE, Schwamm LH. (2012). Predictors of rapid brain imaging in acute stroke: analysis of the Get with the Guidelines-Stroke program. *Stroke J Cereb Circ*, **43**, 1279–84. doi:10.1161/STROKEAHA.111.626374.

Kidwell CS, Saver JL, Schubert GB, Eckstein M, Starkman S. (1998). Design and retrospective analysis of the Los Angeles prehospital stroke screen (LAPSS). *Prehosp Emerg Care*, **2**, 267–73. doi:10.1080/10903129808958878.

Kidwell CS, Starkman S, Eckstein M, Weems K, Saver JL. (2000). Identifying stroke in the field. Prospective validation of the Los Angeles prehospital stroke screen (LAPSS). *Stroke J Cereb Circ*, **31**, 71–6.

Kleindorfer D, Xu Y, Moomaw CJ, Khatri P, Adeoye O, Hornung R. (2009). US geographic distribution of rt-PA utilization by hospital for acute ischemic stroke. *Stroke*, **40**, 3580–4. doi:10.1161/STROKEAHA.109.554626.

Knopf L, Staff I, Gomes J. (2012). Impact of a neurointensivist on outcomes in critically ill stroke patients. *Neurocrit Care*, **16**, 63–71. doi:10.1007/s12028-011-9620-x.

Kothari RU, Pancioli A, Liu T, Brott T, Broderick J. (1999). Cincinnati Prehospital Stroke Scale: reproducibility and validity. *Ann Emerg Med*, **33**, 373–8.

Leira EC, Ahmed A, Lamb DL, Olalde HM, Callison RC, Torner JC, et al. (2009). Extending acute trials to remote populations a pilot study during interhospital helicopter transfer. *Stroke*, **40**, 895–901. doi:10.1161/STROKEAHA.108.530204.

Leira EC, Lamb DL, Nugent AS, Azeemuddin A, Grimsman KJ, Clarke WR, et al. (2006). Feasibility of acute clinical trials during aerial interhospital transfer. *Stroke*, **37**, 2504–7. doi:10.1161/01.STR.0000239661.07675.9d.

Liman TG, Winter B, Waldschmidt C, Zerbe N, Hufnagl P, Audebert HJ. (2012). Telestroke ambulances in prehospital stroke management: concept and pilot feasibility study. *Stroke*, **43**, 2086–2090. doi:10.1161/STROKEAHA.112.657270.

Lin CB, Peterson ED, Smith EE, Saver JL, Liang L, Xian Y, et al. (2012). Emergency medical service hospital prenotification is associated with improved evaluation and treatment of acute ischemic stroke. *Circ Cardiovasc Qual Outcomes*, **5**, 514–22. doi:10.1161/CIRCOUTCOMES.112.965210.

Lindsay MP, Norrving B, Furie KL, Donnan G, Langhorne P, Davis S, on behalf of the World Stroke Organization Global Stroke Quality and Guidelines Advisory Committee. (2016). Global stroke guidelines and action plan: a road map for quality stroke care. www.world-stroke.org/images/GSGAAP/Global_Stroke_Guidelines_and_Action_Plan_All_in_one.pdf. Accessed December 2018.

Madsen TE, Baird KA, Silver B, Gjelsvik A. (2015). Analysis of gender differences in knowledge of stroke warning signs. *J Stroke Cerebrovasc Dis*, **24**(7), 1540–7. doi:10.1016/j.jstrokecerebrovasdis.2015.03.017.

Madsen TE, Sucharew H, Katz B, Alwell KA, Moomaw CJ, Kissela BM, et al. (2016). Gender and time to arrival among ischemic stroke patients in the Greater Cincinnati/Northern Kentucky Stroke Study. *J Stroke Cerebrovasc Dis*, **25**(3), 504–10. doi:10.1016/j.jstrokecerebrovasdis.2015.10.026.

Massachusetts Health Promotions Clearinghouse. (2018). https://massclearinghouse.ehs.state.ma.us/mm5/merchant.mvc?Session_ID=77925787535d2a643e9b77bc3fe1539d&Screen=SRCH. Accessed December 2018.

Matsuo R, Yamaguchi Y, Matsushita T, Hata J, Kiyuna F, Fukuda K, et al.; Fukuoka Stroke Registry Investigators.

(2017). Association between onset-to-door time and clinical outcomes after ischemic stroke. *Stroke*, **48**, 3049–56. doi:10.1161/STROKEAHA.117.018132.

McKinney JS, Mylavarapu K, Lane J, Roberts V, Ohman-Strickland P, Merlin MA. (2013). Hospital prenotification of stroke patients by emergency medical services improves stroke time targets. J *Stroke Cerebrovasc Dis*, **22**, 113–18. doi:10.1016/j.jstrokecerebrovasdis.2011.06.018.

McMullan JT, Katz B, Broderick J, Schmit P, Sucharew H, Adeoye O. (2017). prospective prehospital evaluation of the Cincinnati Stroke Triage Assessment Tool. *Prehosp Emerg Care*, **21**, 481–8. doi:10.1080/10903127.2016.1274349.

McTaggart RA. Yagh S, Cutting SM, Hemendinger M, Baird GL, Haas RA, et al. (2017). Association of a primary stroke center protocol for suspected stroke by large-vessel occlusion with efficiency of care and patient outcomes. *JAMA Neurol*, **74**, 793–800. doi:10.1001/jamaneurol.2017.0477.

Mellon L, Doyle F, Rohde D, Williams D, Hickey A. (2015). Stroke warning campaigns: delivering better patient outcomes? A systematic review. *Patient Relat Outcome Meas*, **6**, 61–73. doi:10.2147/PROM.S54087.

Meretoja A, Roine RO, Kaste M, Linna M, Roine S, Juntunen M, et al. (2010). Effectiveness of primary and comprehensive stroke centers PERFECT stroke: a nationwide observational study from Finland. *Stroke*, **41**, 1102–1107. doi:10.1161/STROKEAHA.109.577718.

Meyer BC, Raman R, Hemmen T, Obler R, Zivin JA, Rao R, et al. (2008). Efficacy of site-independent telemedicine in the STRokE DOC trial: a randomised, blinded, prospective study. *Lancet Neurol*, **7**, 787–95. doi:10.1016/S1474-4422(08)70171-6.

Mission: Lifeline Stroke. (2017). Severity-based stroke triage algorithm for EMS. www.heart.org/idc/groups/ahaecc-public/@wcm/@gwtg/documents/downloadable/ucm_498615.pdf. Accessed December 2018.

Mitchell JR, Sharma P, Modi J, Simpson M, Thomas M, Hill MD, et al. (2011). A smartphone client-server teleradiology system for primary diagnosis of acute stroke. *J Med Internet Res*, **13**, e31. doi:10.2196/jmir.1732.

Mochari-Greenberger H, Xian Y, Hellkamp AS, Schulte PJ, Bhatt DL, Fonarow GC, et al. (2015). Racial/ethnic and sex differences in emergency medical services transport among hospitalized US stroke patients: analysis of the National Get with the Guidelines-Stroke registry. *J Am Heart Assoc*, **4**, e002099. doi:10.1161/JAHA.115.002099.

Morgenstern LB, Gonzales NR, Maddox KE, Brown DL, Karim AP, Espinosa N, et al. (2007). A randomized, controlled trial to teach middle school children to recognize stroke and call 911: the kids identifying and defeating stroke project. *Stroke J Cereb Circ*, **38**, 2972–8. doi:10.1161/STROKEAHA.107.490078.

Morgenstern LB, Staub L, Chan W, Wein TH, Bartholomew LK, King M, et al. (2002). Improving delivery of acute stroke therapy: the TLL Temple Foundation Stroke Project. *Stroke J Cereb Circ*, **33**, 160–6.

Mosley I, Nicol M, Donnan G, Dewey H. (2007). Stroke symptoms and the decision to call for an ambulance. *Stroke*, **38**, 361–366. doi:10.1161/01.STR.0000254528.17405.cc.

Nazliel B, Starkman S, Liebeskind DS, Ovbiagele B, Kim D, Sanossian N, et al. (2008). A brief prehospital stroke severity scale identifies ischemic stroke patients harboring persisting large arterial occlusions. *Stroke*, **39**, 2264–7. doi:10.1161/STROKEAHA.107.508127.

Nelson RE, Saltzman GM, Skalabrin EJ, Demaerschalk BM, Majersik JJ. (2011). The cost-effectiveness of telestroke in the treatment of acute ischemic stroke. *Neurology*, **77**, 1590–8. doi:10.1212/WNL.0b013e318234332d.

Nishikawa T, Okamura T, Nakayama H, Miyamatsu N, Morimoto A, Toyoda K, et al. (2016). Effects of a public education campaign on the association between knowledge of early stroke symptoms and intention to call an ambulance at stroke onset: the Acquisition of Stroke Knowledge (ASK) Study. *J Epidemiol*, **26**(3), 115–22. doi:10.2188/jea.JE20150040.

Noorian AR, Sanossian N, Shkirkova K, Liebeskind DS, Eckstein M, Stratton SJ, et al.; FAST-MAG Trial Investigators and Coordinators. (2018). Los Angeles Motor Scale to Identify Large Vessel Occlusion: prehospital validation and comparison with other screens. *Stroke*, **49**, 565–72. doi:10.1161/STROKEAHA.117.019228.

Olson MD, Rabinstein AA. (2012). Does helicopter emergency medical service transfer offer benefit to patients with stroke? *Stroke*, **43**, 878–80. doi:10.1161/STROKEAHA.111.640987.

Oostema JA, Chassee T, Reeves M. (2018). Emergency dispatcher stroke recognition: associations with downstream care. *Prehosp Emerg Care*, **22**, 466–471. doi:10.1080/10903127.2017.1405131.

Oostema JA, Konen J, Chassee T, Nasiri M, Reeves MJ. (2015). Clinical predictors of accurate prehospital stroke recognition. *Stroke*, **46**, 1513–17. doi:10.1161/STROKEAHA.115.008650.

Pandey AS, Gemmete JJ, Wilson TJ, Chaudhary N, Thompson BG, Morgenstern LB, et al. (2015). High subarachnoid hemorrhage patient volume associated with lower mortality and better outcomes. *Neurosurgery*, **77**, 462–70; doi:10.1227/NEU.0000000000000850.

Patel MD, Rose KM, O'Brien EC, Rosamond WD. (2011). Prehospital notification by emergency medical services reduces delays in stroke evaluation: findings from the North Carolina Stroke Care Collaborative. *Stroke*, **42**, 2263–8. doi:10.1161/STROKEAHA.110.605857.

Perez de la Ossa N, Carrera D, Gorchs M, Querol M, Millan M, Gomis M, et al. (2014). Design and validation of a prehospital stroke scale to predict large arterial occlusion: the Rapid Arterial Occlusion Evaluation Scale. *Stroke*, **45**, 87–91. doi:10.1161/STROKEAHA.113.003071.

Phabphal K, Hirunpatch S. (2008). The effectiveness of low-cost teleconsultation for emergency head computer tomography in patients with suspected stroke. *J Telemed Telecare*, **14**, 439–42. doi:10.1258/jtt.2008.080603.

Powers WJ, Rabinstein AA, Ackerson T, Adeoye OM, Bambakidis NC, Becker K, et al.; American Heart Association Stroke Council. (2018). 2018 Guidelines for the early management of patients with acute ischemic stroke: a guideline for healthcare professionals from the American Heart Association/American Stroke Association. *Stroke*, **49**, e46–e110.

Puetz V, Bodechtel U, Gerber JC, Dzialowski I, Kunz A, Wolz M, et al. (2013). Reliability of brain CT evaluation by stroke neurologists in telemedicine. *Neurology*, **80**, 332–8. doi:10.1212/WNL.0b013e31827f07d0.

Ramanujam P, Guluma KZ, Castillo EM, Chacon M, Jensen MB, Patel E, et al. (2008). Accuracy of stroke recognition by emergency medical dispatchers and paramedics – San Diego experience. *Prehosp Emerg Care*, **12**, 307–13. doi:10.1080/10903120802099526.

Regenhardt RW, Mecca AP, Flavin SA, Boulouis G, Lauer A, Zachrison KS, et al. (2018). Delays in the air or ground transfer of patients for endovascular thrombectomy. *Stroke*, **49**, 1419–25. doi:10.1161/STROKEAHA.118.020618.

Reginella R, Crocco T, Tadros A, Shackleford A, Davis SM. (2006). Predictors of stroke during 9-1-1 calls: opportunities for improving EMS response. *Prehosp Emerg Care*, **10**, 369–73.

Reiner-Deitemyer V, Teuschl Y, Matz K, Reiter M, Eckhardt R, Seyfang L, et al. (2011). Helicopter transport of stroke patients and its influence on thrombolysis rates: data from the Austrian Stroke Unit Registry. *Stroke*, **42**, 1295–1300. doi:10.1161/STROKEAHA.110.604710.

Richards CT, Wang B, Markul E, Albarran F, Rottman D, Aggarwal NT, et al. (2017). Identifying key words in 9-1-1 calls for stroke: a mixed methods approach. *Prehosp Emerg Care*, **21**, 761–766. doi:10.1080/10903127.2017.1332124.

Rose KM, Rosamond WD, Huston SL, Murphy CV, Tegeler CH. (2008). Predictors of time from hospital arrival to initial brain-imaging among suspected stroke patients: the North Carolina Collaborative Stroke Registry. *Stroke*, **39**, 3262–7. doi:10.1161/STROKEAHA.108.524686.

Rudd M, Buck D, Ford GA, Price CI. (2016). A systematic review of stroke recognition instruments in hospital and prehospital settings. *Emerg Med J*, **33**, 818–822. doi:10.1136/emermed-2015-205197.

Sairanen T, Soinila S, Nikkanen M, et al. (2011). Two years of Finnish Telestroke Thrombolysis at spokes equal to that at the hub. *Neurology*, **76**, 1145–52. doi:10.1212/WNL.0b013e318212a8d4.

Sauser K, Burke JF, Levine DA, Scott PA, Meurer WJ. (2014a). Time to brain imaging in acute stroke is improving:

secondary analysis of the INSTINCT trial. *Stroke J Cereb Circ*, **45**, 287–9. doi:10.1161/STROKEAHA .113.003678

Sauser K, Levine DA, Nickles AV, Reeves MJ. (2014b). Hospital variation in thrombolysis times among patients with acute ischemic stroke: the contributions of door-to-imaging time and imaging-to-needle time. *JAMA Neurol*, **71**, 1155. doi:10.1001/jamaneurol.2014.1528.

Saver JL, Starkman S, Eckstein M, Stratton SJ, Pratt FD, Hamilton S, et al. (2015). Prehospital use of magnesium sulfate as neuroprotection in acute stroke. *N Engl J Med*, **372**, 528–536. doi:10.1056/NEJMoa1408827.

Schwab S, Vatankhah B, Kukla C, Hauchwitz M, Bogdahn U, Furst A, et al. (2007). Long-term outcome after thrombolysis in telemedical stroke care. *Neurology*, **69**, 898–903. doi:10.1212/01.wnl.0000269671.08423.14.

Schwamm LH, Audebert HJ, Amarenco P, Chumbler NR, Frankel MR, George MG, et al. (2009a). Recommendations for the implementation of telemedicine within stroke systems of care: a policy statement from the American Heart Association. *Stroke*, **40**, 2635–60. doi:10.1161/STROKEAHA .109.192361.

Schwamm LH, Holloway RG, Amarenco P, Audebert HJ, Bakas T, Chumbler NR, et al. (2009b). A review of the evidence for the use of telemedicine within stroke systems of care: a scientific statement from the American Heart Association/American Stroke Association. *Stroke*, **40**, 2616–34. doi:10.1161/STROKEAHA.109.192360.

Schwamm LH, Pancioli A, Acker JE 3rd, Goldstein LB, Zorowitz RD, Shephard TJ, et al. (2005). Recommendations for the establishment of stroke systems of care recommendations from the American Stroke Association's Task Force on the Development of Stroke Systems. *Stroke*, **36**, 690–703. doi:10.1161/01.STR.0000158165.42884.4F.

Schwamm LH, Rosenthal ES, Hirshberg A, Schaefer PW, Little EA, Dvedar JC, et al. (2004). Virtual TeleStroke support for the emergency department evaluation of acute stroke. *Acad Emerg Med*, **11**, 1193–1197. doi:10.1197/j. aem.2004.08.014.

Shafqat S, Kvedar JC, Guanci MM, Chang Y, Schwamm LH. (1999). Role for telemedicine in acute stroke feasibility and reliability of remote administration of the NIH Stroke Scale. *Stroke*, **30**, 2141–5. doi:10.1161/01.STR.30.10.2141.

Shireman TI, Wang K, Saver JL, Goyal M, Bonafe A, Diener HC, et al. (2017). Cost-effectiveness of solitaire stent retriever thrombectomy for acute ischemic stroke: results from the SWIFT-PRIME Trial (Solitaire With the Intention for Thrombectomy as Primary Endovascular Treatment for Acute Ischemic Stroke). *Stroke*, **48**, 379–87. doi:10.1161/ STROKEAHA.116.014735.

Silbergleit R, Scott PA, Lowell MJ, Silbergleit R. (2003). Cost-effectiveness of helicopter transport of stroke patients for thrombolysis. *Acad Emerg Med Off J Soc Acad Emerg Med*, **10**, 966–72.

Silliman SL, Quinn B, Huggett V, Merino JG. (2003). Use of a field-to-stroke center helicopter transport program to extend thrombolytic therapy to rural residents. *Stroke J Cereb Circ*, **34**, 729–33. doi:10.1161/01.STR.0000056529 .29515.B2.

Smith EE, Hassan KA, Fang J, Selchen D, Kapral MK, Saposnik G, et al. (2010). Do all ischemic stroke subtypes benefit from organized inpatient stroke care? *Neurology*, **75**, 456–62. doi:10.1212/WNL.0b013e3181ebdd8d.

Song S, Fonarow GC, Olson DM, Liang L, Schulte PG, Hernandez AF, et al. (2016). Association of Get with the Guidelines-Stroke Program participation and clinical outcomes for Medicare beneficiaries with ischemic stroke. *Stroke*, **47**, 1294–302. doi:10.1161/STROKEAHA.115.011874.

Stroke Unit Trialists' Collaboration. (2013). Organised inpatient (stroke unit) care for stroke. *Cochrane Database Syst Rev*, 9. CD000197. doi:10.1002/14651858.CD000197.pub3.

Sung S-F, Ong C-T, Wu C-S, Hsu YC, Su YH. (2010). Increased use of thrombolytic therapy and shortening of in-hospital delays following acute ischemic stroke: experience on the establishment of a primary stroke center at a community hospital. *Acta Neurol Taiwanica*, **19**, 246–52.

Svenson JE, O'Connor JE, Lindsay MB. (2006). Is air transport faster? A comparison of air versus ground transport times for interfacility transfers in a regional referral system. *Air Med J*, **25**, 170–2. doi:10.1016/j. amj.2006.04.003.

Switzer JA, Hall C, Gross H, Waller J, Nichols FT, Wang S, et al. (2009). A web-based telestroke system facilitates rapid treatment of acute ischemic stroke patients in rural emergency departments. *J Emerg Med*, **36**, 12–18. doi:10.1016/j.jemermed.2007.06.041.

Tang Y, Yin F, Fu D, Gao X, LV Z, LI X, et al. (2018). Efficacy and safety of minimal invasive surgery treatment in hypertensive intracerebral hemorrhage: a systematic review and meta-analysis. *BMC Neurol*, **18**, 136. doi:10.1186/ s12883-018-1138-9.

Thompson MP, Zhao X, Bekelis K, Gottlieb DJ, Fonarow GC, Schulte PJ, et al. (2017). Regional variation in 30-day ischemic stroke outcomes for Medicare beneficiaries treated in Get With the Guidelines-Stroke Hospitals. *Circ Cardiovasc Qual Outcomes*, **10**. pii: e003604. doi:10.1161/ CIRCOUTCOMES.117.003604.

Van Hooff R-J, Cambron M, Van Dyck R, De Smedt A, Moens M, Espinoza AV, et al. (2013). Prehospital unassisted assessment of stroke severity using telemedicine: a feasibility study. *Stroke*, **44**, 2907–9. doi:10.1161/STROKEAHA .113.002079.

Waite K, Silver F, Jaigobin C, Black S, Lee L, Murray B, et al. (2006). Telestroke: a multi-site, emergency-based telemedicine service in Ontario. *J Telemed Telecare*, **12**, 141–5.

Wall HK, Beagan BM, O'Neill HJ, Foell KM, Boddie-Willis CL. (2008).Addressing stroke signs and symptoms through public education: the Stroke Heroes Act FAST Campaign. *Prev Chronic Dis*, **5**, A49.

Walter S, Kostopoulos P, Haass A, Keller I, Lesmeister M, Schlechtriemen T, et al. (2012). Diagnosis and treatment of patients with stroke in a mobile stroke unit versus in hospital: a randomised controlled trial. *Lancet Neurol*, **11**, 397–404. doi:10.1016/S1474-4422(12)70057-1.

Wang S, Gross H, Lee SB, Pardue C, Waller J, Nichols FT 3rd, et al. (2004). Remote evaluation of acute ischemic stroke in rural community hospitals in Georgia. *Stroke*, **35**, 1763–8. doi:10.1161/01.STR.0000131858.63829.6e.

Wang S, Lee SB, Pardue C, Ramsingh D, Waller J, Gross H, et al. (2003). Remote evaluation of acute ischemic stroke: reliability of National Institutes of Health Stroke Scale via telestroke. *Stroke J Cereb Circ*, **34**, e188–91. doi:10.1161/01.STR.0000091847.82140.9D.

Watkins CL, Jones SP, Leathley MJ, et al. Emergency Stroke Calls: Obtaining Rapid Telephone Triage (ESCORTT) – a programme of research to facilitate recognition of stroke by emergency medical dispatchers. Southampton (UK): NIHR Journals Library; February 2014.

Wiborg A, Widder B; Group for the TS. (2003). Teleneurology to improve stroke care in rural areas: the Telemedicine in Stroke in Swabia (TESS) Project. *Stroke*, **34**, 2951–6. doi:10.1161/01.STR.0000099125.30731.97.

Williams O, Noble JM. (2008). 'Hip-Hop' stroke: a stroke educational program for elementary school children living in a high-risk community. *Stroke*, **39**, 2809–16. doi:10.1161/STROKEAHA.107.513143.

Wu T-C, Nguyen C, Ankrom C, Yang J, Persse D, Vahidy F, et al. (2014). Prehospital utility of rapid stroke evaluation using in-ambulance telemedicine: a pilot feasibility study. *Stroke*, **45**, 2342–7. doi:10.1161/STROKEAHA.114.005193.

Xian Y. (2011). Association between stroke center hospitalization for acute ischemic stroke and mortality. *JAMA*, **305**, 373. doi:10.1001/jama.2011.22.

Zhao H, Coote S, Pesavento L, Churilov L, Dewey HM, Davis SM, Campbell BC. (2017). Large vessel occlusion scales increase delivery to endovascular centers without excessive harm from misclassifications. *Stroke*, **48**, 568–73. doi:10.1161/STROKEAHA.116.016056.

Zhao J, Eckenhoff MF, Sun WZ, Liu R. (2018). Stroke 112: a universal stroke awareness program to reduce language and response barriers. *Stroke*, **49**, 1766–9. doi:10.1161/STROKEAHA.118.021729.

Organized Stroke Care

Peter Langhorne

The principles of management of patients with a suspected acute stroke are to:

- make an accurate diagnosis of stroke, its pathological type (i.e. infarct or haemorrhage), and aetiological subtype (cause of the infarct or haemorrhage);
- accurately assess the patient's limitations in terms of impairments, activities, and participation and compare these with previous limitations;
- estimate the prognosis for survival, recurrent vascular events, and recovery of impairments, activities, and participation;
- provide access to acute interventions to improve recovery if eligible;
- discuss the prognosis with the patient and family (if possible), and set shared, common short- and long-term goals;
- consider which services are required to meet the shared common goals and how to access and deliver them;
- optimize survival free of limitations by immediate brain reperfusion strategies in appropriate patients with ischaemic stroke, optimize physiological homoeostasis, anticipate and prevent complications of stroke, prevent recurrence of stroke and other major vascular events, begin rehabilitation immediately, and continue longer-term rehabilitation and support.

The management of stroke patients (and their carers and families) requires an integrated, comprehensive, and coordinated stroke service which meets the needs (and wishes) of patients and carers in an effective, efficient, and equitable manner.

The major components of an organized stroke service are as follows:

1. *A fast-track outpatient service*: To provide rapid assessment, diagnosis, and secondary prevention measures for patients with suspected transient ischaemic attack (TIA) and non-disabling stroke.

2. *Hyperacute reperfusion*: To provide rapid thrombolysis and/or mechanical thrombectomy for eligible patients with acute ischaemic stroke.

3. *A comprehensive stroke unit service*: To provide rapid assessment, diagnosis and intervention by a specialist multidisciplinary team.

4. *Early supported discharge (ESD) service*: To facilitate earlier discharge from hospital with enhanced support and rehabilitation input in the home setting.

5. *Longer-term support and rehabilitation*: To review continued progress, and new and ongoing needs, and maintain rehabilitation and support (Langhorne et al., 2011).

Management of Stroke Patients at Home (vs in Hospital)

Evidence

In a generic review of hospital at home services, two randomized controlled trials compared the effect of routine processes of caring for stroke patients (often involving admission to hospital) with the effect of caring for stroke patients by means of a multidisciplinary domiciliary team aiming to provide care in the home (Shepperd et al., 2008). The trials used a range of services to serve as their control (or comparison) group, but always involving care in a general medical ward (GMW), sometimes with support of a mobile stroke team in the hospital. Overall, there was no significant difference in the proportion of patients who had died by 6 months after stroke onset among the home-based care group compared with the conventional hospital-based care group (Figure 4.1) (Shepperd et al., 2008). A similar analysis of the outcomes of death or requiring institutional care at 6 months after stroke also shows no statistically significant difference (odds ratio [OR]: 0.58, 95% confidence interval [CI]: 0.21–1.58).

Table 4.1 The type of stroke patients who should be managed in hospital

- Patients who may benefit from organized care by a multidisciplinary team in a stroke unit (most stroke patients)
- Patients who may benefit from appropriate and effective acute medical and surgical therapies such as aspirin (ischaemic stroke), intravenous (IV) thrombolysis, clot retrieval, craniectomy (cf. cerebellar infarction and oedema; malignant middle cerebral artery syndrome)
- Patients who are at risk of life-threatening, preventable, or treatable complications such as airway obstruction and respiratory failure; swallowing problems causing aspiration, dehydration, and malnutrition; epileptic seizures; venous thromboembolism; and infections

Table 4.2 The type of stroke patients who might be managed at home

- Patients who are not disabled, or do not have significant new disability and are well cared for (e.g. in a nursing home)
- Patients who can be diagnosed accurately (including stroke pathology, aetiology, and prognosis) as an outpatient
- Patients who can be cared for at home, including appropriate secondary stroke prevention and, where appropriate, domiciliary rehabilitation

Review: Hospital at home admission avoidance
Comparison: 1 Admission avoidance hospital at home versus inpatient care
Outcome: 19 Mortality at 6 months using published data

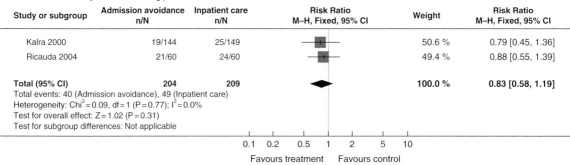

Study or subgroup	Admission avoidance n/N	Inpatient care n/N	Risk Ratio M–H, Fixed, 95% CI	Weight	Risk Ratio M–H, Fixed, 95% CI
Kalra 2000	19/144	25/149		50.6 %	0.79 [0.45, 1.36]
Ricauda 2004	21/60	24/60		49.4 %	0.88 [0.55, 1.39]
Total (95% CI)	**204**	**209**		**100.0 %**	**0.83 [0.58, 1.19]**

Total events: 40 (Admission avoidance), 49 (Inpatient care)
Heterogeneity: Chi^2 = 0.09, df = 1 (P = 0.77); I^2 = 0.0%
Test for overall effect: Z = 1.02 (P = 0.31)
Test for subgroup differences: Not applicable

0.1   0.2   0.5   1   2   5   10
Favours treatment   Favours control

Figure 4.1 Forest plot showing the proportional effects (OR and its 95% CI) of home-based stroke services compared with conventional hospital-based stroke services on a general medical ward on death at 6 months for each individual trial (each single line), and as a pooled summary estimate of the results of all trials at the bottom (black diamond).

Reproduced from Shepperd et al. (2008) with permission from the authors and John Wiley & Sons Limited. Copyright Cochrane Library, reproduced with permission.

These trials had practical problems. First, the comparator, care in a GMW, is no longer considered to be optimal stroke care. Second, in the larger trial (Kalra et al., 2000), a large proportion of patients allocated at random to care at home had eventually to be admitted to the stroke unit. Understandably, there was a trend for greater resource consumption among those randomized to home-based care.

Comment

Interpretation of the Evidence

The debate about hospital vs home care for acute stroke patients was previously relevant in the UK. The above data provide no evidence to support a radical change in policy from hospital- to home-based acute stroke care.

Admission to a properly run stroke unit is now seen as optimal care.

Implications for Practice

All stroke patients should have immediate and equitable access to appropriate assessment and management, and most should be admitted to hospital.

The type of patients who should probably be managed in hospital are listed in Table 4.1 and those who can possibly be managed at home listed in Table 4.2.

Implications for Research

The debate about hospital vs home care has largely been superseded by the compelling evidence for organized care in a stroke unit in optimizing survival and functional outcome after stroke (see below). However,

Table 4.3 The three main models of organized stroke care that have been tested in trials

- Care in a *geographically dedicated stroke ward (stroke unit)* by a multidisciplinary team. Within the geographically dedicated stroke ward, there are three models:

    (i) Acute stroke unit: provides stroke unit care in the first few hours/days after stroke. Patients are admitted directly to the unit for acute assessment, investigation, and intervention. In some countries, this model is now called a Hyperacute Stroke Unit (HASU).
    (ii) Rehabilitation stroke unit: admits patients 1–2 weeks after stroke onset and continues rehabilitation for several weeks to months as required.
    (iii) Comprehensive stroke unit: combines both acute care and rehabilitation.

- Care in several wards by a *mobile stroke team*.
- Care in a *mixed assessment/rehabilitation unit*: a generic unit which specializes in the management of disabled patients, irrespective of the cause.

there is increasing evidence that home rehabilitation does have an important role in post-acute care, and in facilitating accelerated discharge from hospital to home (Langhorne et al., 2017) (see below).

Hospital-based Care

Terminology

The term *stroke unit* encompasses the provision and coordination of multidisciplinary stroke care in a geographically defined area, such as a stroke ward (Langhorne and Dennis, 1998). The core disciplines involved are usually medical, nursing, speech and swallowing therapy/pathology, physiotherapy, occupational therapy, social work, and dietetics. Information regarding patient assessment, goals, interventions, progress, and discharge planning are coordinated by regular (at least weekly) multidisciplinary meetings.

Types of Organized (Stroke Unit) Care

The three main models of organized stroke care are listed in Table 4.3.

Evidence

Death

A systematic review of 28 randomized controlled trials (RCTs) involving 5855 patients in 12 countries included 23 trials (4591 patients) that compared organized inpatient care (stroke unit care) with care in

a general ward, usually a GMW. Organized care was associated with a statistically significant reduction in the odds of death recorded at final follow-up (median 1 year) by about 19% (OR: 0.81, 95% CI: 0.769–0.94; $P = 0.005$) from 23% (488/2090) to 18% (458/2501) (Figure 4.2) (Stroke Unit Trialists' Collaboration, 2013). This is an adjusted absolute risk reduction of 3% (1–6%), indicating that for every 100 patients assigned to organized (stroke unit) care, there were 3 fewer deaths at final follow-up compared with care in a GMW.

Death or Institutionalization

Random allocation to organized (stroke unit) care was associated with a statistically significant reduction in the odds of the combined outcome of death or institutionalization at final follow-up by about 22% (OR: 0.78, 95% CI: 0.68–0.89; $P = 0.0003$) from 40% (766/1894) to 35% (718/2046) (Figure 4.3), indicating that for every 100 patients assigned to organized care in a stroke unit, there were 5 fewer patients who died or were institutionalized at final follow-up compared with care in a GMW (Stroke Unit Trialists' Collaboration, 2013).

Death or Dependency

Random allocation to organized care in a stroke unit was associated with a statistically significant reduction in the odds of the combined outcome of death or dependency by 21% (OR: 0.79, 95% CI: 0.68–0.90; $P = 0.0007$), from 62% (1034/1681) to 56% (1027/1829), indicating that for every 100 patients assigned to organized care in a stroke unit, there were 6 fewer patients who died or were dependent at final follow-up compared with care in a GMW (Figure 4.4) (Stroke Unit Trialists' Collaboration, 2013).

Absolute Effects of Organized Care on Death, Institutional Care, and Dependency

Estimates across all the trials suggest that overall, for every 100 stroke patients randomly allocated organized (stroke unit) care, three additional patients survived, two avoided long-term care in an institution, and an additional six returned home, of whom one was physically or cognitively dependent and five were independent (Stroke Unit Trialists' Collaboration, 2013). However, there could be a wide range of results, as the 95% CI of these estimates and the absolute outcome rates varied considerably (Stroke Unit Trialists' Collaboration, 2013).

Review: Organised inpatient (stroke unit) care for stroke
Comparison: 2 Organised stroke unit care versus general medical wards
Outcome: 1 Death by the end of scheduled follow-up

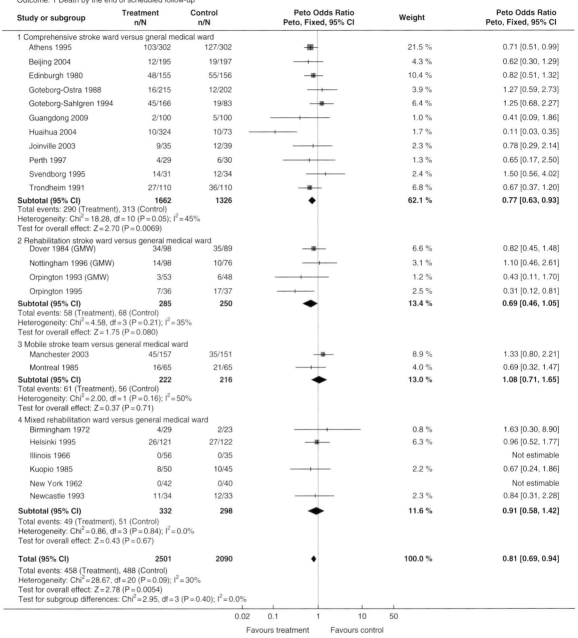

Figure 4.2 Forest plot showing the proportional effects of organized inpatient care (stroke unit care) with care in a general ward on *death* at the end of the scheduled follow-up period among individual trials (each line) and pooled (summary at the bottom). The OR for death in the organized stroke unit care group compared with that in the alternative services group is plotted for each trial (black square), along with its 95% CI (horizontal line). Meta-analysis of the pooled results of all trials is represented by a black diamond showing the OR and the 95% CI of the OR.

Reproduced from the Stroke Unit Trialists' Collaboration (2013), with permission from the authors and John Wiley & Sons Limited. Copyright Cochrane Library, reproduced with permission.

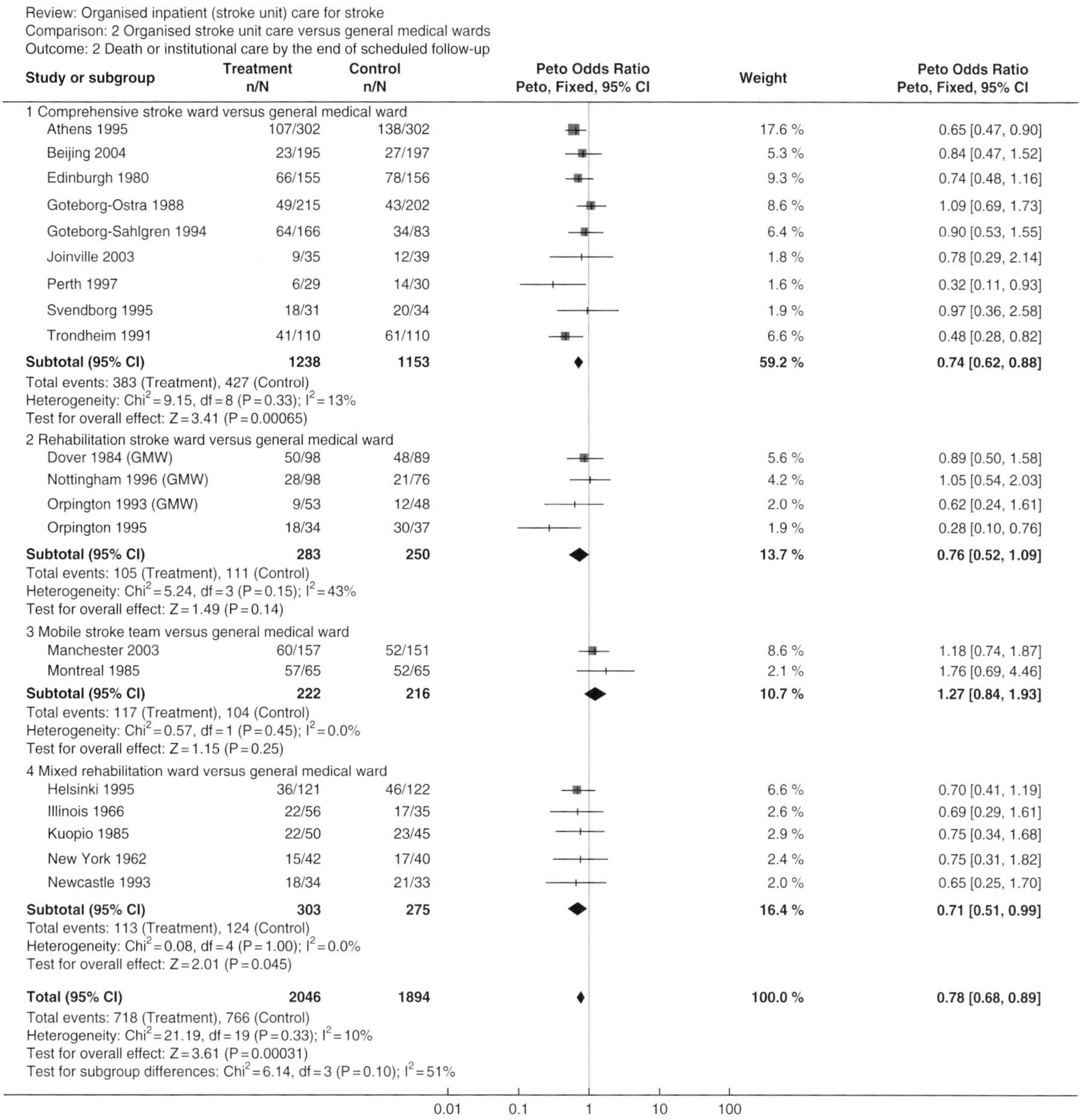

Review: Organised inpatient (stroke unit) care for stroke
Comparison: 2 Organised stroke unit care versus general medical wards
Outcome: 2 Death or institutional care by the end of scheduled follow-up

Study or subgroup	Treatment n/N	Control n/N	Peto Odds Ratio Peto, Fixed, 95% CI	Weight	Peto Odds Ratio Peto, Fixed, 95% CI
1 Comprehensive stroke ward versus general medical ward					
Athens 1995	107/302	138/302		17.6 %	0.65 [0.47, 0.90]
Beijing 2004	23/195	27/197		5.3 %	0.84 [0.47, 1.52]
Edinburgh 1980	66/155	78/156		9.3 %	0.74 [0.48, 1.16]
Goteborg-Ostra 1988	49/215	43/202		8.6 %	1.09 [0.69, 1.73]
Goteborg-Sahlgren 1994	64/166	34/83		6.4 %	0.90 [0.53, 1.55]
Joinville 2003	9/35	12/39		1.8 %	0.78 [0.29, 2.14]
Perth 1997	6/29	14/30		1.6 %	0.32 [0.11, 0.93]
Svendborg 1995	18/31	20/34		1.9 %	0.97 [0.36, 2.58]
Trondheim 1991	41/110	61/110		6.6 %	0.48 [0.28, 0.82]
Subtotal (95% CI)	**1238**	**1153**		**59.2 %**	**0.74 [0.62, 0.88]**
Total events: 383 (Treatment), 427 (Control)					
Heterogeneity: Chi² = 9.15, df = 8 (P = 0.33); I² = 13%					
Test for overall effect: Z = 3.41 (P = 0.00065)					
2 Rehabilitation stroke ward versus general medical ward					
Dover 1984 (GMW)	50/98	48/89		5.6 %	0.89 [0.50, 1.58]
Nottingham 1996 (GMW)	28/98	21/76		4.2 %	1.05 [0.54, 2.03]
Orpington 1993 (GMW)	9/53	12/48		2.0 %	0.62 [0.24, 1.61]
Orpington 1995	18/34	30/37		1.9 %	0.28 [0.10, 0.76]
Subtotal (95% CI)	**283**	**250**		**13.7 %**	**0.76 [0.52, 1.09]**
Total events: 105 (Treatment), 111 (Control)					
Heterogeneity: Chi² = 5.24, df = 3 (P = 0.15); I² = 43%					
Test for overall effect: Z = 1.49 (P = 0.14)					
3 Mobile stroke team versus general medical ward					
Manchester 2003	60/157	52/151		8.6 %	1.18 [0.74, 1.87]
Montreal 1985	57/65	52/65		2.1 %	1.76 [0.69, 4.46]
Subtotal (95% CI)	**222**	**216**		**10.7 %**	**1.27 [0.84, 1.93]**
Total events: 117 (Treatment), 104 (Control)					
Heterogeneity: Chi² = 0.57, df = 1 (P = 0.45); I² = 0.0%					
Test for overall effect: Z = 1.15 (P = 0.25)					
4 Mixed rehabilitation ward versus general medical ward					
Helsinki 1995	36/121	46/122		6.6 %	0.70 [0.41, 1.19]
Illinois 1966	22/56	17/35		2.6 %	0.69 [0.29, 1.61]
Kuopio 1985	22/50	23/45		2.9 %	0.75 [0.34, 1.68]
New York 1962	15/42	17/40		2.4 %	0.75 [0.31, 1.82]
Newcastle 1993	18/34	21/33		2.0 %	0.65 [0.25, 1.70]
Subtotal (95% CI)	**303**	**275**		**16.4 %**	**0.71 [0.51, 0.99]**
Total events: 113 (Treatment), 124 (Control)					
Heterogeneity: Chi² = 0.08, df = 4 (P = 1.00); I² = 0.0%					
Test for overall effect: Z = 2.01 (P = 0.045)					
Total (95% CI)	**2046**	**1894**		**100.0 %**	**0.78 [0.68, 0.89]**
Total events: 718 (Treatment), 766 (Control)					
Heterogeneity: Chi² = 21.19, df = 19 (P = 0.33); I² = 10%					
Test for overall effect: Z = 3.61 (P = 0.00031)					
Test for subgroup differences: Chi² = 6.14, df = 3 (P = 0.10); I² = 51%					

0.01 0.1 1 10 100

Figure 4.3 Forest plot showing the proportional effects of organized stroke unit care compared with alternative services on *death or institutionalization* at the end of the scheduled follow-up period among individual trials (each line) and pooled (summary at the bottom). Reproduced from the Stroke Unit Trialists' Collaboration (2013), with permission from the authors and John Wiley & Sons Limited. Copyright Cochrane

Length of Stay

Length of stay data were available for 18 individual trials which compared organized inpatient (stroke unit) care with an alternative service. Mean (or median) length of stay ranged from 11 to 162 days in the stroke unit groups and from 12 to 129 days in controls. The calculation of a summary result for length of stay was subject to major methodological limitations; length of stay was calculated in different ways (e.g. acute hospital stay, total stay in hospital or institution), two trials recorded median rather than mean length of stay, and in two trials the standard deviation had to be inferred from the *P*-value or from the results of similar trials. Overall, using a random effects

Review: Organised inpatient (stroke unit) care for stroke
Comparison: 2 Organised stroke unit care versus general medical wards
Outcome: 3 Death or dependency by the end of scheduled follow-up

Study or subgroup	Treatment n/N	Control n/N	Peto Odds Ratio Peto, Fixed, 95% CI	Weight	Peto Odds Ratio Peto, Fixed, 95% CI
1 Comprehensive stroke ward versus general medical ward					
Athens 1995	138/302	145/302		19.1 %	0.91 [0.66, 1.25]
Beijing 2004	113/195	118/197		12.0 %	0.92 [0.62, 1.38]
Edinburgh 1980	93/155	94/156		9.5 %	0.99 [0.63, 1.56]
Goteborg-Sahlgren 1994	108/166	54/83		6.4 %	1.00 [0.58, 1.74]
Joinville 2003	18/35	23/39		2.3 %	0.74 [0.30, 1.84]
Perth 1997	10/29	15/30		1.9 %	0.54 [0.19, 1.49]
Trondheim 1991	54/110	81/110		6.6 %	0.36 [0.21, 0.61]
Subtotal (95% CI)	**992**	**917**		**57.8 %**	**0.82 [0.68, 0.98]**
Total events: 534 (Treatment), 530 (Control)					
Heterogeneity: Chi² = 11.69, df = 6 (P = 0.07); I² = 49%					
Test for overall effect: Z = 2.13 (P = 0.033)					
2 Rehabilitation stroke ward versus general medical ward					
Dover 1984 (GMW)	54/98	50/89		5.9 %	0.96 [0.54, 1.70]
Nottingham 1996 (GMW)	63/98	52/76		4.9 %	0.83 [0.44, 1.56]
Orpington 1993 (GMW)	38/53	39/48		2.3 %	0.59 [0.24, 1.48]
Orpington 1995	34/34	37/37			Not estimable
Subtotal (95% CI)	**283**	**250**		**13.1 %**	**0.83 [0.57, 1.23]**
Total events: 189 (Treatment), 178 (Control)					
Heterogeneity: Chi² = 0.76, df = 2 (P = 0.69); I² = 0.0%					
Test for overall effect: Z = 0.92 (P = 0.36)					
3 Mobile stroke team versus general medical ward					
Manchester 2003	91/157	95/151		9.4 %	0.81 [0.52, 1.28]
Montreal 1985	58/65	60/65		1.4 %	0.69 [0.21, 2.27]
Subtotal (95% CI)	**222**	**216**		**10.7 %**	**0.80 [0.52, 1.22]**
Total events: 149 (Treatment), 155 (Control)					
Heterogeneity: Chi² = 0.06, df = 1 (P = 0.81); I² = 0.0%					
Test for overall effect: Z = 1.04 (P = 0.30)					
4 Mixed rehabilitation ward versus general medical ward					
Birmingham 1972	8/29	7/23		1.4 %	0.87 [0.26, 2.89]
Helsinki 1995	47/121	65/122		7.7 %	0.56 [0.34, 0.93]
Illinois 1966	20/56	17/35		2.7 %	0.59 [0.25, 1.39]
Kuopio 1985	31/50	31/45		2.7 %	0.74 [0.32, 1.72]
New York 1962	23/42	23/40		2.6 %	0.90 [0.38, 2.13]
Newcastle 1993	26/34	28/33		1.3 %	0.59 [0.18, 1.96]
Subtotal (95% CI)	**332**	**298**		**18.4 %**	**0.65 [0.47, 0.90]**
Total events: 155 (Treatment), 171 (Control)					
Heterogeneity: Chi² = 1.26, df = 5 (P = 0.94); I² = 0.0%					
Test for overall effect: Z = 2.57 (P = 0.010)					
Total (95% CI)	**1829**	**1681**		**100.0 %**	**0.79 [0.68, 0.90]**
Total events: 1027 (Treatment), 1034 (Control)					
Heterogeneity: Chi² = 15.31, df = 17 (P = 0.57); I² = 0.0%					
Test for overall effect: Z = 3.40 (P = 0.00067)					
Test for subgroup differences: Chi² = 1.55, df = 3 (P = 0.67); I² = 0.0%					

0.02   0.1   1   10   50
Favours treatment   Favours control

Figure 4.4 Forest plot showing the proportional effects of organized stroke unit care compared with alternative services on *death or dependency* at the end of the scheduled follow-up period among individual trials (each line) and pooled (summary at the bottom).

Reproduced from the Stroke Unit Trialists' Collaboration (2013), with permission from the authors and John Wiley & Sons Limited. Copyright Cochrane Library, reproduced with permission.

model, there was no significant reduction in the length of stay in the stroke unit group (standardized mean difference: –0.15, 95% CI: –0.32–0.02; *P* = 0.09) (Figure 4.5) (Stroke Unit Trialists' Collaboration, 2013). The summary estimates were complicated by considerable heterogeneity, which limits the extent to which more general conclusions can be drawn.

Longer-term Outcomes after Stroke

Three trials (1139 patients) carried out supplementary studies extending patient follow-up. At 5-year follow-up, care in a stroke unit was associated with a 26% reduction in odds of death (OR: 0.74, 95% CI: 0.59–0.94; *P* = 0.01), and non-significant reductions in death or institutional care (OR: 0.59, 95% CI:

Review: Organised inpatient (stroke unit) care for stroke
Comparison: 2 Organised stroke unit care versus general medical wards
Outcome: 4 Length of stay (days) in a hospital or institution

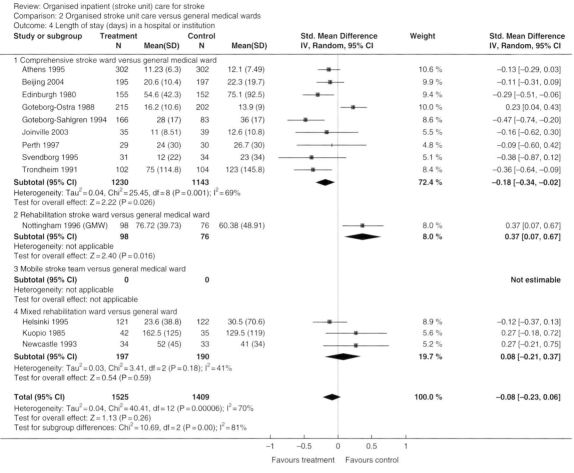

Figure 4.5 Forest plot showing the effects of organized stroke unit care compared with alternative services on *length of hospital stay (days, mean)* at the end of the scheduled follow-up period among individual trials (each line) and pooled (summary at the bottom).

Reproduced from the Stroke Unit Trialists' Collaboration (2013), with permission from the authors and John Wiley & Sons Limited. Copyright Cochrane Library, reproduced with permission.

0.33–1.05; $P = 0.07$) and death or dependency (OR: 0.54, 95% CI: 0.22–1.34; $P = 0.18$). The pattern of results was similar at 10-year follow-up, but results were no longer statistically significant (Stroke Unit Trialists' Collaboration, 2013) (Figure 4.6).

Patient Satisfaction and Quality of Life

Only two trials recorded outcome measures related to patient quality of life (Nottingham Health Profile). In both cases, there was significantly improved quality of life among survivors of care in a stroke unit. There was no systematically gathered information on patient preferences (Stroke Unit Trialists' Collaboration, 2013).

Subgroup Analyses by Trial Characteristics

In view of the variety of trial methodologies, a sensitivity analysis was undertaken based only on those trials with the lowest risk of bias that employed (a) secure randomization procedures, (b) unequivocally blinded outcome assessment, and (c) a fixed 1-year period of follow-up. Among the seven trials that met all of these criteria, stroke unit care was associated with a statistically non-significant reduction in the odds of death (OR: 0.82, 95% CI: 0.64–1.05; $P = 0.12$) and statistically significant reductions in the odds of death or institutional care (OR: 0.77, 95% CI: 0.63–0.96; $P = 0.02$) and death or dependency (OR: 0.76, 95% CI: 0.62–0.93; $P = 0.009$) (Stroke Unit Trialists' Collaboration, 2013).

Subgroup Analyses by Patient Characteristics

Predefined subgroup analyses including data from at least nine trials were carried out based on the patients' age, sex, and initial stroke severity and stroke type. The results are summarized in Table 4.4.

These subgroup analyses should be interpreted with caution, however, as they are based on a smaller number of outcome events and are, therefore, imprecise and not statistically robust. Also, the results may vary according to the outcome measure chosen. For example, patients with stroke of mild severity did not

appear to benefit from stroke unit care in terms of a reduced risk of death but did have a reduced risk of death or institutional care, and death or dependency (Stroke Unit Trialists' Collaboration, 2013).

Organized (Stroke Unit) Care vs General Medical Wards

Three different models of organized stroke unit care (comprehensive stroke ward, rehabilitation stroke ward, and mixed assessment/rehabilitation ward) tended to be more effective than GMW care. There were insufficient data to draw conclusions on the comparison of mobile team care (peripatetic service) vs GMWs. The apparent benefits of stroke unit care were seen in units with both an acute admission policy and a delayed admission policy. We could not identify any randomized trials of hyperacute stroke units (HASUs).

Different Types of Organized Stroke Unit Care: Direct Comparisons

An important question for service planning is whether the benefits of stroke unit care depend upon the establishment of a ward dedicated only to stroke care (stroke ward) or could be achieved in other ways. Three different types of organized (stroke unit) care could be compared, all of which met the basic descriptive criteria of stroke unit care (multidisciplinary staffing coordinated through regular team meetings), that is care:

1. in a ward dedicated only to stroke care (dedicated stroke ward),
2. by a mobile stroke team, or

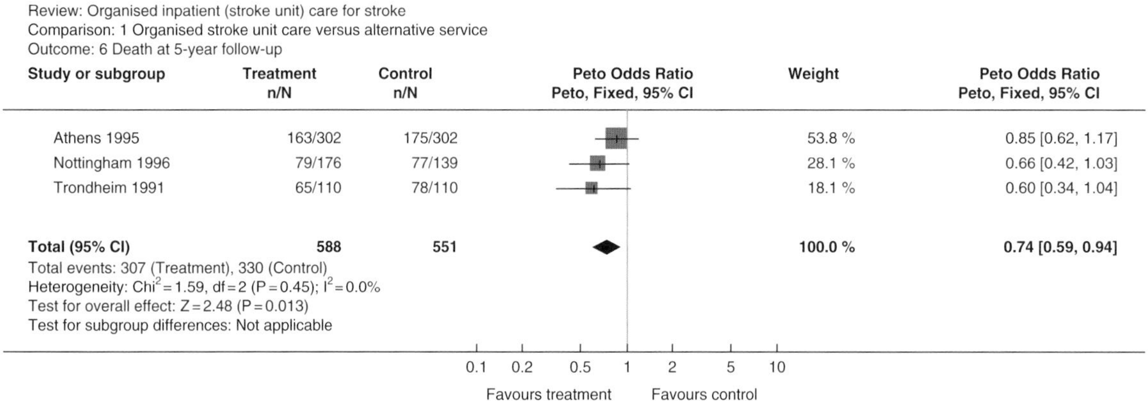

Table 4.4 OR (95% CI) for death or institutional care among patients randomly assigned to care in a stroke unit, compared with a general ward, according to the patients' age, sex, stroke severity at the time of randomization and stroke type

Patient characteristics		OR (95% CI)
Age	Age up to 75 years	0.71 (0.43–1.16)
	Age more than 75 years	0.71 (0.51–0.99)
Sex	Male	0.75 (0.54–1.04)
	Female	0.57 (0.41–0.79)
Stroke severity	Mild stroke	0.76 (0.52–1.11)
	Moderate stroke	0.81 (0.66–0.99)
	Severe stroke	0.48 (0.33–0.70)
Stroke type	Ischaemic stroke	0.63 (0.49–0.81)
	Haemorrhagic stroke	0.71 (0.27–1.87)

OR: odds ratio. CI: confidence interval.

Review: Organised inpatient (stroke unit) care for stroke
Comparison: 1 Organised stroke unit care versus alternative service
Outcome: 6 Death at 5-year follow-up

Study or subgroup	Treatment n/N	Control n/N	Peto Odds Ratio Peto, Fixed, 95% CI	Weight	Peto Odds Ratio Peto, Fixed, 95% CI
Athens 1995	163/302	175/302		53.8 %	0.85 [0.62, 1.17]
Nottingham 1996	79/176	77/139		28.1 %	0.66 [0.42, 1.03]
Trondheim 1991	65/110	78/110		18.1 %	0.60 [0.34, 1.04]
Total (95% CI)	**588**	**551**		100.0 %	0.74 [0.59, 0.94]

Total events: 307 (Treatment), 330 (Control)
Heterogeneity: Chi^2 = 1.59, df = 2 (P = 0.45); I^2 = 0.0%
Test for overall effect: Z = 2.48 (P = 0.013)
Test for subgroup differences: Not applicable

0.1 0.2 0.5 1 2 5 10
Favours treatment   Favours control

Figure 4.6 Forest plot showing the proportional effects of organized stroke unit care compared with alternative services on *death at 5-year follow-up* among individual trials (each line) and pooled (summary at the bottom).

Reproduced from the Stroke Unit Trialists' Collaboration (2013), with permission from the authors and John Wiley & Sons Limited. Copyright Cochrane Library, reproduced with permission.

3. by a generic disability service (mixed rehabilitation unit) which specializes in the management of disabling illness including stroke.

Acute Stroke Ward vs Alternative Service

In two trials, patients admitted to acute units did not have statistically significant different odds of death, death or requiring institutional care, or death or dependency when compared with a comprehensive or mixed rehabilitation ward. There was no evidence of a systematic change in length of stay.

Rehabilitation Stroke Ward vs Alternative Service

There was a pattern of improved outcomes in patients admitted to a stroke rehabilitation ward compared with either a GMW or mixed rehabilitation ward with statistically significantly fewer deaths ($P = 0.02$) and a statistically non-significant trend for fewer participants with the composite endpoints of death or requiring institutional care and death or dependency. However, the numbers were small and interpretation of length of stay data was complicated by substantial heterogeneity. There was no evidence of a systematic increase in length of stay.

Comprehensive Stroke Unit vs Alternative Service

One trial compared a comprehensive stroke ward (providing acute care and rehabilitation) with admission to GMWs where care was provided by a mobile stroke team (Kalra et al., 2000). They found statistically significant ($P < 0.001$) reductions in death and the combined outcome of death or institutional care among the comprehensive stroke ward group. There was no significant difference in length of stay.

Different Processes of Care: Indirect Comparisons

The improved functional outcome at the time of discharge of patients cared for in a stroke ward compared with a GMW or a mobile stroke team was associated with fewer systemic complications, which may be attributable to different processes of care (Evans et al., 2001; Govan et al., 2007). Patients in stroke wards were monitored more frequently and more patients received oxygen, antipyretics, measures to reduce aspiration, and early nutrition than those in general wards (Evans et al., 2001; Govan et al., 2007).

The characteristic processes of care in a stroke unit are listed in Table 4.5 (Indredavik et al., 1999; Langhorne and Pollock, 2002; Langhorne and Dennis, 2004; Langhorne et al., 2012).

Three small clinical trials have tested the conventional stroke unit (featuring systemic early assessment of problems, provision of intravenous [IV] fluids, team rehabilitation, and weekly multidisciplinary team meetings) with a more intensive programme of monitoring physiological variables (same model of care but also providing continuous monitoring of oxygen saturation, electrocardiogram, temperature, blood pressure, and glucose level with intervention for abnormalities) (Ciccone et al., 2013). There was a suggestion that continuous monitoring of physiological variables for the first two to three days may help improve outcomes and prevent complications, but the results were not conclusive.

Care Pathways

A care pathway (or clinical pathway, or critical pathway, or integrated care pathway) can be defined as a plan of care that is developed and used by a multidisciplinary team, and is applicable to more than one aspect of care (Kwan and Sandercock, 2004; Allen et al., 2009). Care pathways are intended to assist healthcare professionals in clinical decision-making (Allen et al., 2009). Despite their popularity, the evidence to support their use is weak. In trials across a range of conditions, integrated care pathways were found to be most effective in contexts where the patient's progress was predictable, where deficiencies in services were identified, and where professional working was not well established (Allen et al., 2009).

Evidence

A systematic review identified three RCTs (total of 340 patients) and 12 non-randomized studies (total of 4081 patients) which compared the effects of care pathways with standard medical care among patients admitted to hospital with acute stroke (Kwan and Sandercock, 2004). There was no significant difference between care pathway and control groups in terms of death or discharge destination. However, patients managed with a care pathway were more dependent at discharge ($P = 0.04$). More reliable data, from RCTs, are required.

Implications for Clinical Practice

There is currently insufficient evidence to justify routine implementation of care pathways for acute stroke management or stroke rehabilitation in hospital.

Implications for Research

Further research by means of well-conducted randomized and non-randomized studies and qualitative research are needed, particularly addressing the effects of care pathways on processes of care, implementation of evidence-based practice, functional outcomes, quality of life, patient and carer satisfaction, and hospital cost.

Comment

Interpretation of the Evidence

These data indicate that patients who receive organized inpatient (stroke unit) care are more likely to survive, regain independence, and return home than those receiving a less organized service. The benefit for stroke unit patients appears to be sustained for several years.

The apparent benefits were consistent among men and women; those aged above and below 75 years; those with mild, moderate, and severe strokes; and those with ischaemic or haemorrhagic stroke. Patients with more severe stroke symptoms are at greater risk of death or requiring institutional care and, hence, for these outcomes stand to gain more from treatment.

The benefits were observed in all types of stroke units which were able to provide a period of care lasting several weeks if necessary (i.e. comprehensive stroke units and rehabilitation stroke units), and were most apparent in units based in a dedicated ward (rather than a mobile stroke team). Effective units were operational in a variety of departments including neurology, geriatric medicine, general/internal medicine, and rehabilitation medicine. What they had in common was similar processes of care (Table 4.5). The more recent introduction of hyperacute stroke units (with immediate admission and discharge within 1–3 days) is not based on evidence from RCTs. In principle, they would be expected to improve care if they facilitate improved processes of care (Ramsay et al., 2015) and provide a seamless entrance to more prolonged stroke unit rehabilitation where this is required.

The *specific* processes of care which produce the benefits in saving lives (which develops mainly in the first 4 weeks after stroke) and reducing dependency after stroke are not clear (Langhorne and Pollock, 2002; Langhorne et al., 2012). The stroke units included in the systematic review did not regularly use thrombolytic agents or other acute specific treatments, and they did not provide intensive (automated) monitoring of physiological variables. Other features of care must be important in reducing the risks of complications and in identifying and treating complications early. The number of potential post-stroke physiological abnormalities, neurological and general complications that need to be expected, prevented, detected, and effectively treated to optimize the outcome for the patient is likely to be very extensive, but much of the benefit may be attributable to:

1. coordinated care by a multidisciplinary team;
2. awareness, anticipation, and prevention of complications of stroke in high-risk individuals (e.g. aspiration pneumonia, pulmonary embolism, pressure sores);
3. maintenance of physiological homoeostasis (Evans et al., 2001; Langhorne and Pollock, 2002; Govan et al., 2007; Ciccone et al., 2013).

There is also evidence that some of the beneficial effect of care in a stroke unit may be attributable to patients in a stroke ward receiving greater amounts of therapy (Kalra et al., 2000). Augmented exercise therapy may have a small but favourable effect on activities of daily living (ADL) (Veerbeek et al., 2014), but would not be expected to influence survival.

The crucial ingredients, therefore, appear to be coordinated multidisciplinary assessment, intervention, and optimization of physiological homoeostasis; measures to risk stratify, record, and prevent complications; active rehabilitation; education and training in stroke care; and specialization of all staff in the team. It is uncertain whether more intensive medical monitoring is beneficial.

As the major direct healthcare costs of acute stroke management are from nursing care and hospital overheads, length of hospital stay is an important determinant of initial costs. In the longer term, direct costs are more determined by residual disability and the care of dependent individuals in hospitals and nursing homes. Economic analyses suggest that stroke unit care is likely to be associated with a modest increase in cost, but it improves outcomes and saves resources (Major and Walker, 1998; Saka et al., 2009).

Implications for Practice

Generalizability

Evidence from large prospective observational studies of stroke patient cohorts admitted to hospitals

Table 4.5 Features of stroke units studied in randomized trials

Assessment and monitoring

Medical	Systematic clinical history and examination
	Routine investigations
	Computed tomography (CT) brain scan
	Blood tests: haematology and serum biochemistry
	Electrocardiogram
	Investigations in selected patients
	Carotid ultrasound
	Echocardiogram
	Magnetic resonance imaging (MRI) or CT angiogram
Nursing	General care needs
	Vital signs
	Swallow assessment
	Fluid balance
	Neurological monitoring
Therapy	Assessment of impairments and function

Early management

Physiological management	Careful management of food and fluids (often IV saline over the first 12–24 h)
	Monitoring and treatment of infection, pyrexia, hypoxia, and hyperglycaemia
Early mobilization	Early measures to get patient sitting up, standing, and walking
Nursing care	Careful positioning and handling, and pressure-area care
	Management of swallowing problems
	Avoidance of urinary catheters if possible

Multidisciplinary team rehabilitation

Rehabilitation process	Formal multidisciplinary meetings once a week (plus informal meetings)
	Early rehabilitation, goal setting, and involvement of carers
	Close linking of nursing with other multidisciplinary care
	Provision of information on stroke, recovery, and services
Discharge planning	Early assessment of discharge needs
	Discharge plan involving patient and carers

Source: Langhorne and Pollock (2002), Langhorne and Dennis (2004), Langhorne et al. (2012).

indicates that the results of the systematic review of RCTs are reproducible in routine clinical settings (Seenan et al., 2007; Ingeman et al., 2008; Saposnik et al., 2008; Terent et al., 2009; Turner et al., 2015). In particular, a recent study (Langhorne, O'Donnell et al., 2018) found that evidence-based treatments, diagnostics, and stroke units were less commonly available or used in low- and middle-income countries. However, access to stroke units and appropriate use of antiplatelet treatment were associated with improved recovery. Although biases are inherent in such observational data, patients admitted to a stroke unit had increased chances of survival, discharge home, and independence after stroke. The absolute benefits of organized inpatient (stroke unit) care appear to be similar to those in the RCTs.

Structure of the Stroke Unit

Stroke ward or mobile team? Acute stroke patients should be offered organized inpatient (stroke unit) care that is typically provided by a coordinated multidisciplinary team operating within a discrete stroke ward, which can offer a substantial period of rehabilitation if required (Kalra et al., 2000; Langhorne et al., 2005).

However, if a geographically dedicated stroke unit is not feasible, it is important to establish a multidisciplinary stroke team that meets regularly and follows the principles of regular patient assessment, goal setting, intervention, re-assessment, and re-intervention. Telemedicine also has the potential to facilitate organized stroke care in rural and remote areas through links with more specialized urban units.

Acute stroke ward or rehabilitation ward? The benefit of admitting all patients immediately to an acute stroke unit is that it facilitates the early implementation of a uniform and standardized approach to assessment, goal setting, intervention (including rehabilitation), discharge planning, and research. Transfer to a rehabilitation stroke ward (which ideally is linked with the acute stroke ward) is then seamless, continuous, and consistent.

Stroke unit size The size of the stroke unit will vary according to the incidence of stroke in the catchment population of the service and the activity of the hospital. A stroke unit should generally be large enough so that it is flexible in being able to accommodate fluctuating demands; the number, gender ratio, severity, and length of stay of patients will not be constant throughout the year.

Stroke Unit Staffing

Stroke units require a multidisciplinary team, which is made up of one or more doctors (e.g. stroke consultant, registrar, and resident), nurses (including specialist stroke liaison nurse), physiotherapists, occupational therapists, a speech and language therapist, and social worker as a basic minimum. A number of other health professionals also have an important role in the management of some stroke patients, such as a dietician, pharmacist, clinical neuropsychologist, specialist in orthotics/prosthetics, neuroradiologist, neurosurgeon, and vascular surgeon.

The core features of these staff are that they are interested in stroke and have been trained in stroke management. Therefore, they have the necessary knowledge and enthusiasm.

The stream of basic training of doctors (i.e. neurology, geriatric, general medical) is not as important as the interest of the doctors and the comprehensiveness of their subsequent training in stroke medicine. Consequently, stroke units are managed effectively by neurologists, geriatricians, general physicians, and rehabilitation specialists around the world, all of whom have been well trained in stroke medicine (Donnan and Davis, 2003).

Patient Selection Criteria

There are no firm grounds for restricting access according to a patient's age, sex, stroke type, or stroke severity. Local conditions often dictate whether a geriatric service is a better option for the very elderly, particularly those with pre-existent handicaps and important comorbidities.

However, when demand for beds exceeds supply, there are two options. The ideal is to reconfigure the beds and training staff to allow care of all stroke patients in a stroke unit. This requires flexibility, which may not be practical or possible. The other alternative is to prioritize patients according to different needs and services. In this case, it is important to establish local agreement about appropriate triage.

Duration of Stay

A defined maximum length of stay should not be needed if the unit:

- is of sufficient size for the population needs,
- works flexibly,
- is efficient in discharging patients when ongoing stroke unit care is no longer needed.

Ideally, an appropriately sized stroke unit should be allowed flexibility with its operating procedures and have the facility to provide care until discharge from hospital to home, to an ongoing rehabilitation facility, or to placement in appropriate alternative care. Wherever the patient is discharged or transferred, it is important to ensure a seamless/continuous transition of care.

General Processes of Care in the Stroke Unit (Care Pathways)

Stroke units should aim to replicate those core service characteristics identified in the randomized trials (Table 4.5).

Assessment Patients are assessed as soon as possible by all core and relevant members of the stroke unit.

The medical assessment comprises a relevant and targeted clinical history and examination, documenting the nature of the symptoms and physical impairments, the timing of the onset, any precipitating factors, and the subsequent course. In addition, relevant aetiological (e.g. vascular risk factors), social, vocational, and emotional factors are recorded. Initial assessments and investigations are directed to answering the following questions:

1. **Is it a stroke?** (*clinical diagnosis*)
2. **Where is the lesion?** (*anatomical diagnosis*: which part of the brain is affected and what vascular territory?)
3. **What is the cause of the stroke?** (*ischaemic or haemorrhagic*, and causes of the ischaemia or haemorrhage)
4. **What is the impact on the patient?** (impairments, activities, participation)
5. **What are the patient's prognosis and goals?**
6. **How should the patient be treated?** (to minimize brain damage, prevent recurrent stroke and complications, optimize physiological homeostasis, and rehabilitate)

The nursing assessment includes the patient's neurological status, impairments, activities, and function; swallowing function; bladder and bowel function; skin status; psychosocial status; and risk of complications (e.g. aspiration pneumonia, venous thromboembolism, urinary tract infection, and skin pressure sores), followed by a plan of general care needs of the patient.

The speech and swallowing therapist (speech pathologist) assesses communication, receptive and expressive language skills, articulation, swallowing function, and risk of aspiration by means of clinical skills, sometimes supplemented by videofluoroscopy.

The physiotherapist assesses the patient's respiratory function, muscle tone, movement, and mobility. This includes an assessment of the recovery level of the arm(s), trunk, and leg(s) and the assistance required with bed mobility and to sit up from a lying position. Sitting balance is evaluated with the patient sitting on the edge of the bed. If the patient is medically stable and not drowsy, then standing balance, ability to transfer (e.g. to commode and chair), and ambulation are evaluated if appropriate.

The occupational therapist assesses the patient's functional impairments, activities, and participation, and the abilities to perform ADL, work, and leisure activities.

The social worker assesses the patient's social situation, support from family and friends, accommodation and financial status, occupational status and goals, and access to community resources (e.g. home help, Meals on Wheels).

The dietician assesses the dietary habits and nutritional needs of the patient and, together with the swallowing therapist, recommends an appropriate diet.

Goal setting (including discharge planning) In every stroke patient, intermediate and long-term goals should be agreed on and described so that progress towards them can be measured. Moreover, everyone will feel a sense of achievement when the goals are met.

Where a patient is failing to achieve his or her goals (or milestones) then it is crucial to identify the cause and, if possible, do something about it. The reasons for failure to achieve goals are many. They may be medical (e.g. a recurrent stroke, pneumonia, or depression and loss of interest and motivation) or may reflect an inaccuracy in the team's understanding of the patient's pathology and likely clinical course (e.g. being over-optimistic about progress).

Goal setting may sometimes involve just an individual professional, but more often it needs to involve the rest of the team, the patient, and sometimes the patient's family.

It is important to know the home and social circumstances of a stroke patient for early decision-making (such as the desirability of emergency operation) and for later rehabilitation and discharge from hospital.

Goals should be meaningful and challenging, but achievable.

Communication A distinctive finding of the systematic review by the Stroke Unit Trialists' Collaboration is that stroke units are uniformly characterized by a multidisciplinary team which is coordinated/chaired by a leader (usually the senior doctor or other senior member of staff), and meets at least once a week to discuss all of the patients. Although the team is multidisciplinary, the interaction is interdisciplinary. The meeting is structured so that a doctor summarizes the key features of the patient (age, date of stroke, clinical syndrome, pathology, aetiology, key treatments, major problems, and goals), and then a brief (1–2 min) report on the progress of each patient in the preceding few days or week is given by the nurse, speech and swallowing therapist, physiotherapist, occupational therapist, and social worker. If relevant, the dietician and pharmacist also report.

The patient's progress is matched with the original short- and long-term goals. If progress is not as good as expected, reasons are sought for failure to achieve goals, such as recurrent stroke, intercurrent medical problems, depression, incorrect original diagnosis, inaccurate team assessment, and so on. Goals are reset and a future management plan detailed.

Besides a formal weekly meeting, which normally lasts about 60–90 minutes encompassing 15 patients, team members communicate directly on the ward (or through the written medical record) with each other during the week about the patient. Many units also hold informal meetings on other occasions to ensure effective multidisciplinary operation and involvement of family and carers. Key decisions are not made without widespread team consultation and approval.

Another key feature of stroke unit care is the early involvement of carers in the assessment and rehabilitation process, including the provision of appropriate information regarding the nature and cause of the stroke, and its management.

Intervention Despite some recent concerns about very early, active mobilization (AVERT Trial Collaboration Group, 2015; Langhorne, Collier et al., 2018), most believe that gentle rehabilitation should begin on day 1, following initial assessments. It is essential that rehabilitation techniques being taught in the therapy areas are carried over into everyday practice on the ward (and at home) by the nurses and carers. Carers are therefore encouraged to attend therapy sessions, and nurses are encouraged to reinforce these behaviours in the everyday handling of the patient.

Discharge planning and post-discharge support After a short period in hospital, during which the patient's status and progress have been documented, it is possible to re-assess goals, re-assess future management, and plan for ESD home (Langhorne et al., 2017), to another stroke rehabilitation facility, or to longer-term care.

Implications for Research

Future trials should focus on direct comparisons of different models of organized stroke unit care, examining the potentially important components of stroke unit care, such as intensive monitoring of physiological abnormalities, early mobilization, novel strategies to detect and prevent complications, acute supportive therapies, and systems of rehabilitation (Langhorne and Dennis, 2004).

Early Supported Discharge

Evidence

There have been 17 RCTs randomizing stroke for a total of 2422 patients in hospital to either conventional care or any ESD service intervention providing rehabilitation and support in a community setting with an aim of reducing the duration of hospital care (Langhorne et al., 2017). Overall, the ORs (95% CI) were 1.04 (0.77–1.40) for death, 0.75 (0.59–0.96) for death or institutionalization, and 0.80 (0.67–0.95) for death or dependency (Figure 4.7). Apparent benefits were more evident in the trials evaluating a coordinated multidisciplinary ESD team and in stroke patients with mild-to-moderate disability (Table 4.6). The ESD group showed significant reductions ($P < 0.001$) in the length of hospital stay, equivalent to approximately 6 days.

Comment

These data suggest that appropriately resourced ESD services provided for a selected group of stroke patients can reduce the length of hospital stay and improve functional outcomes in the longer term with lower rates of dependency and admission to institutional care (Langhorne et al., 2017). A recent large trial of a low resource intervention focusing on family training in India (ATTEND Collaborative Group 2017) could not replicate the benefits of multidisciplinary ESD services.

Therapy-based Rehabilitation for Stroke Patients Living at Home

Evidence

A systematic review of 14 RCTs of therapy-based rehabilitation services (defined as input from physiotherapy, occupational therapy, or a multidisciplinary team) targeted to a total of 1617 stroke patients living at home revealed that patients allocated therapy-based rehabilitation services were less likely to deteriorate in ability to perform ADL (OR: 0.72, 95% CI: 0.57–0.92; $P = 0.009$; absolute risk reduction: 7%) and more likely to be able to perform personal ADL (Legg and Langhorne, 2004). However, this review is now rather out of date and a more recent analysis of therapy-based rehabilitation

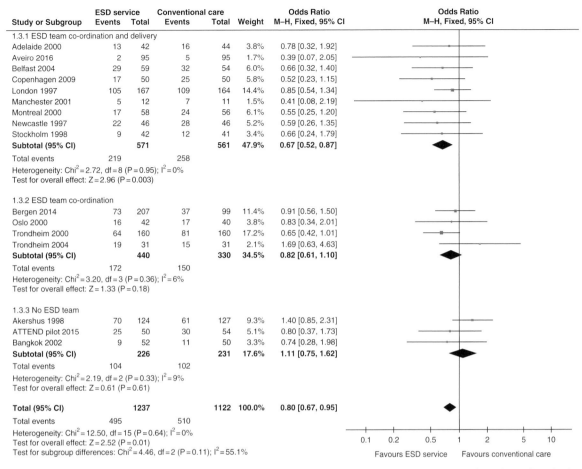

Study or Subgroup	ESD service Events	Total	Conventional care Events	Total	Weight	Odds Ratio M–H, Fixed, 95% CI
1.3.1 ESD team co-ordination and delivery						
Adelaide 2000	13	42	16	44	3.8%	0.78 [0.32, 1.92]
Aveiro 2016	2	95	5	95	1.7%	0.39 [0.07, 2.05]
Belfast 2004	29	59	32	54	6.0%	0.66 [0.32, 1.40]
Copenhagen 2009	17	50	25	50	5.8%	0.52 [0.23, 1.15]
London 1997	105	167	109	164	14.4%	0.85 [0.54, 1.34]
Manchester 2001	5	12	7	11	1.5%	0.41 [0.08, 2.19]
Montreal 2000	17	58	24	56	6.1%	0.55 [0.25, 1.20]
Newcastle 1997	22	46	28	46	5.2%	0.59 [0.26, 1.35]
Stockholm 1998	9	42	12	41	3.4%	0.66 [0.24, 1.79]
Subtotal (95% CI)		571		561	47.9%	**0.67 [0.52, 0.87]**
Total events	219		258			

Heterogeneity: Chi² = 2.72, df = 8 (P = 0.95); I² = 0%
Test for overall effect: Z = 2.96 (P = 0.003)

Study or Subgroup	ESD service Events	Total	Conventional care Events	Total	Weight	Odds Ratio M–H, Fixed, 95% CI
1.3.2 ESD team co-ordination						
Bergen 2014	73	207	37	99	11.4%	0.91 [0.56, 1.50]
Oslo 2000	16	42	17	40	3.8%	0.83 [0.34, 2.01]
Trondheim 2000	64	160	81	160	17.2%	0.65 [0.42, 1.01]
Trondheim 2004	19	31	15	31	2.1%	1.69 [0.63, 4.63]
Subtotal (95% CI)		440		330	34.5%	**0.82 [0.61, 1.10]**
Total events	172		150			

Heterogeneity: Chi² = 3.20, df = 3 (P = 0.36); I² = 6%
Test for overall effect: Z = 1.33 (P = 0.18)

Study or Subgroup	ESD service Events	Total	Conventional care Events	Total	Weight	Odds Ratio M–H, Fixed, 95% CI
1.3.3 No ESD team						
Akershus 1998	70	124	61	127	9.3%	1.40 [0.85, 2.31]
ATTEND pilot 2015	25	50	30	54	5.1%	0.80 [0.37, 1.73]
Bangkok 2002	9	52	11	50	3.3%	0.74 [0.28, 1.98]
Subtotal (95% CI)		226		231	17.6%	**1.11 [0.75, 1.62]**
Total events	104		102			

Heterogeneity: Chi² = 2.19, df = 2 (P = 0.33); I² = 9%
Test for overall effect: Z = 0.61 (P = 0.61)

Study or Subgroup	ESD service Events	Total	Conventional care Events	Total	Weight	Odds Ratio M–H, Fixed, 95% CI
Total (95% CI)		1237		1122	100.0%	**0.80 [0.67, 0.95]**
Total events	495		510			

Heterogeneity: Chi² = 12.50, df = 15 (P = 0.64); I² = 0%
Test for overall effect: Z = 2.52 (P = 0.01)
Test for subgroup differences: Chi² = 4.46, df = 2 (P = 0.11); I² = 55.1%

Favours ESD service   Favours conventional care

Figure 4.7 Forest plot showing a comparison of the effects of an early supported discharge service vs conventional care (control) on *death* or *dependency* in activities of daily living (ADL) at the end of scheduled follow-up.

Reproduced from Langhorne et al. (2017), with permission from John Wiley & Sons Limited. Copyright Cochrane Library, reproduced with permission.

services provided more than one year after stroke (Aziz et al., 2008) did not identify significant benefits.

Comment

Further research is needed to define the most effective interventions, their functional and economic benefit, and the most appropriate level and means of service delivery.

Summary

Most patients with suspected stroke should not be managed at home, but should be transported without delay to a hospital which has access to the required diagnostic tests and appropriate hyperacute treatments 24 hours/day and 7 days/week.

Once admitted, patients should be managed in a stroke unit rather than a general medical ward.

Geographically defined stroke units, dedicated to organized stroke care, appear to be more effective than stroke care on general wards with input from a mobile stroke team. There appears to be no systematic increase in length of hospital stay associated with organized (stroke unit) care. The recent development of hyperacute stroke units is not based on evaluation within randomized controlled trials (RCTs) but appears to improve processes of care in the acute phase.

In order to meet the needs of the local stroke population (which are likely to increase), and the anticipated increasing role of acute diagnostic techniques and interventions, it is crucial that future

Table 4.6 Subgroup analysis of various patient and service characteristics. Analyses show a comparison of the effects of early supported discharge vs conventional care on *death or dependency* at the end of the scheduled follow-up period

Subgroups		OR (95% CI)
Patient characteristics		
Age	Age up to 75 years	0.82 (0.60–1.12)
	Age more than 75 years	0.90 (0.61–1.31)
Sex	Male	0.73 (0.54–1.01)
	Female	0.98 (0.68–1.40)
Stroke severity	Mild/moderate stroke	0.77 (0.61–0.98)
	Severe stroke	1.40 (0.83–2.36) *
Carer status	Carer present	0.85 (0.65–1.11)
	No carer	0.90 (0.61–1.32)
Service characteristics		
ESD design	Community inreach	0.72 (0.53–0.96)
	Hospital outreach	0.71 (0.53–0.94)
MDT coordination	MDT present	0.73 (0.60–0.89)
	No MDT	1.11 (0.75–1.62)
Hospital service	Stroke unit	0.83 (0.68–1.02)
	Other ward	0.72 (0.52–0.95)

Source: From Langhorne et al. (2017).

* Denotes a significant difference between subgroups

plans anticipate the requirements for trained staff and adequate numbers of stroke unit beds for acute stroke.

Processes of care on a stroke unit should mirror those found to be effective in RCTs. Stroke care should be specialized, organized, and multidisciplinary (i.e. provided by medical, nursing, physiotherapy, occupational therapy, speech therapy, and social work staff who are interested and trained in stroke care). The multidisciplinary stroke team should meet at least once weekly to discuss patient assessments, goals, progress and management, and discharge plans.

The other beneficial components of organized stroke care are likely to be many, but it remains uncertain which are the most effective. Future research should be directed at identifying the crucial ingredients in this 'black box', so that they can be the focus of future care and optimize judicious use of resources.

Early discharge from the stroke unit with support from a domiciliary rehabilitation team (coordinated by the stroke unit) promises to reduce hospital length of stay (and thus increase turnover in the stroke unit) and improve rehabilitation in the home and patient outcome.

References

Allen D, Gillen E, Rixson L. (2009). The effectiveness of integrated care pathways for adults and children in health care settings: a systematic review. *JBI Reports*, 7(3), 80–129.

ATTEND Collaborative Group. Family-led rehabilitation after stroke in India (ATTEND): a randomised controlled trial. Lancet. 2017; 390: 588–599.

AVERT Trial Collaboration Group. (2015). Efficacy and safety of very early mobilisation within 24 h of stroke onset (AVERT): a randomised controlled trial. *Lancet*, **386**, 46–55. pii: S0140-6736(15)60690-0.

Aziz NA, Leonardi-Bee J, Phillips MF, Gladman J, Legg LA, Walker M. (2008). Therapy-based rehabilitation services for patients living at home more than one year after stroke. *Cochrane Database Syst Rev*, 2, CD005952. doi:10.1002/14651858.CD005952.pub2.

Ciccone A, Celani MG, Chiaramonte R, Rossi C, Righetti E. (2013). Continuous versus intermittent physiological monitoring for acute stroke. *Cochrane Database Syst Rev*, 5, CD008444. doi:10.1002/14651858.CD008444.pub2.

Donnan GA, Davis SM. (2003). Neurologist, internist, or strokologist? *Stroke*, 34(11), 2765.

Evans A, Perez I, Harraf F, Melbourn A, Steadman J, Donaldson N, et al. (2001). Can differences in management processes explain different outcomes between stroke unit and stroke-team care? *Lancet*, **358**(9293), 1586–92.

Govan L, Langhorne P, Weir C, for the Stroke Unit Trialists' Collaboration. (2007). Does the prevention of complications explain the survival benefit of organised inpatient (stroke unit) care? Further analysis of a systematic review. *Stroke*, **38**, 2536–40.

Indredavik B, Bakke F, Slordahl SA, Rokseth R, Haaheim L. (1999). Treatment in a combined acute and rehabilitation stroke unit. *Stroke*, **30**, 917–23.

Ingeman A, Pedersen L, Hundborg HH, Petersen P, Zielke S, Mainz J, et al. (2008).Quality of care and mortality among patients with stroke: a nationwide follow-up study. *Med Care*, **46**(1), 63–9.

Kalra L, Evans E, Perez I, Knapp M, Donaldson N, Swift C. (2000). Alternative strategies for stroke care: a prospective randomised controlled trial. *Lancet*, 356, 894–9.

Kwan J, Sandercock P. (2004). In-hospital care pathways for stroke. *Cochrane Database Syst Rev*, 4, CD002924.

Langhorne P, Baylan S; Early Supported Discharge Trialists. (2017). Services for reducing duration of hospital care for acute stroke patients. *Cochrane Database Syst Rev*, 7, CD000443. doi:10.1002/14651858. CD000443.pub4.

Langhorne P, Bernhardt J, Kwakkel G. (2011). Stroke rehabilitation. *Lancet*, **377**, 1693–702.

Langhorne P, Collier JM, Bate PJ, Thuy MNT, Bernhardt J. (2018). Very early versus delayed mobilisation after stroke. *Cochrane Database Syst Rev*, 10, CD006187.

Langhorne P, Dennis MS. (1998). *Stroke Units: An Evidence-Based Approach*. London: BMJ Publishing.

Langhorne P, Dennis MS. (2004). Stroke units: the next 10 years. *Lancet*, **363**, 834–5.

Langhorne P, de Villiers L, Pandian JD. (2012). Applicability of stroke-unit care to low-income and middle-income countries. *Lancet Neurol*, **11**, 341–8.

Langhorne P, Dey P, Woodman M, Kalra L, Wood-Dauphinee S, Patel N, et al. (2005). Is stroke unit care portable? A systematic review of the clinical trials. *Age Ageing*, **34**, 324–30.

Langhorne P, O'Donnell MJ, Chin SL, Zhang H, Xavier D, Avezum A, et al.; INTERSTROKE Collaborators. (2018).Practice patterns and outcomes after stroke across countries at different economic levels (INTERSTROKE): an international observational study. *Lancet*, **391**(10134), 2019–27.

Langhorne P, Pollock A, in conjunction with the Stroke Unit Trialists' Collaboration. (2002). What are the components of effective stroke unit care? *Age Ageing*, **31**(5), 365–71.

Legg L, Langhorne P; Outpatient Service Trialists. (2004). Rehabilitation therapy services for stroke patients living at home: systematic review of randomised trials. *Lancet*, **363** (9406), 352–6.

Major K, Walker A. (1998). Economics of stroke unit care. In P Langhorne, M Dennis, eds., *Stroke Units: An Evidence Based Approach*. London: BMJ Books, pp. 56–65.

Ramsay AI, Morris S, Hoffman A, Hunter RM, Boaden R, McKevitt C, et al. (2015). Effects of centralizing acute stroke services on stroke care provision in two large metropolitan areas in England. *Stroke*, **46**(8), 2244–51. doi:10.1161/STROKEAHA.115.009723.

Saka O, McGuire A, Wolfe C. (2009). Cost of stroke in the United Kingdom. *Age Ageing*, **38**(1), 27–32. doi:10.1093/ageing/afn281.

Saposnik G, Hill MD, O'Donnell M, Fang J, Hachinski V, Kapral MK. (2008). Variables associated with 7-day, 30-day, and 1-year fatality after ischemic stroke. *Stroke*, **39**, 2318–24.

Seenan P, Long M, Langhorne P. (2007). Stroke units in their natural habitat. *Stroke*, **38**, 1886–92.

Shepperd S, Doll H, Angus RM, Clarke MJ, Iliffe S, Kalra L, et al. (2008). Hospital at home admission avoidance. *Cochrane Database Syst Rev*, 4, CD007491. doi:10.1002/14651858.CD007491.

Stroke Unit Trialists' Collaboration. (2013). Organised inpatient (stroke unit) care for stroke. *Cochrane Database Syst Rev*, 9, CD000197. doi:10.1002/14651858.CD000197.pub3.

Terent A, Asplund K, Farahmand B, Henriksson KM, Norrving B, Stegmayr B, et al. (2009). Stroke unit care revisited: who benefits the most? A cohort study of 105 043 patients in Riks-Stroke, the Swedish Stroke Register. *J Neurol Neurosurg Psychiatry*, **80**, 881–7.

Turner M, Barber M, Dodds H, Dennis M, Langhorne P, Macleod MJ; on behalf of the Scottish Stroke Care Audit. (2015). The impact of stroke unit care on outcome in a Scottish stroke population, taking into account case mix and selection bias. *J Neurol Neurosurg Psychiatry*, **86**, 314–8. doi:10.1136/jnnp-2013-307478.

Veerbeek JM, van Wegen E, van Peppen R, van der Wees PJ, Hendriks E, Rietberg M, et al. (2014).What is the evidence for physical therapy poststroke? A systematic review and meta-analysis. *PLoS One*, **9**(2), e87987. doi:10.1371/journal.pone.0087987. eCollection 2014.

Supportive Care during Acute Cerebral Ischaemia

Askiel Bruno

Subhashini Ramesh

Jeffrey L. Saver

Introduction

Whereas nearly 10% of all acute ischaemic stroke patients presenting to Emergency Departments are eligible to receive specialized thrombolytic and thrombectomy treatments, all acute stroke patients can benefit from optimized supportive care. After a specialized brain reperfusion therapy for qualified patients, and after admission to a stroke unit, optimal management of multiple supportive care issues can enhance the functional outcome. In this chapter we discuss the management of commonly encountered supportive care issues. The ultimate goal in the management of these issues is to minimize acute stroke complications and enhance stroke recovery.

Respiration and Oxygenation

Background

Patients with acute stroke often have breathing disturbances leading to hypoxaemia (Sulter et al., 2000; Roffe et al., 2003). Severe hypoxaemia can result in cerebral hypoxia, which can exacerbate the ischaemic brain injury and cause new brain injury. Therefore, it is important to monitor breathing and oxygenation and prevent or correct hypoxaemia promptly.

Common causes of hypoxaemia during acute stroke include partial airway obstruction, hypoventilation, aspiration, atelectasis, and pneumonia. Patients with decreased consciousness or brainstem dysfunction are at increased risk of airway compromise because of impaired oropharyngeal mobility and loss of protective reflexes. In addition to airway obstruction, some acute stroke patients develop irregular breathing patterns, such as Cheyne–Stokes respirations, that further compromise blood oxygenation. Some acute stroke patients have dysphagia, placing them at risk for aspiration and further hypoxaemia. Hypoxaemia is also common during

seizures, which can be a complication of acute stroke. Also, head of bed (HOB) position has been suggested to affect oxygenation in acute stroke patients.

Evidence

A total of at least 11 randomized trials have studied normobaric oxygen supplementation to non-hypoxaemic acute stroke patients, without strong evidence of beneficial effects (Ding et al., 2018). The largest randomized trial of prophylactic low-dose oxygen supplementation randomized 8003 acute stroke patients to one of three groups: control, nocturnal oxygen only, or continuous oxygen (Roffe et al., 2017). Nasal oxygen was administered within 24 hours of hospital admission at 2 L/min when the oxygen saturation was above 93% and at 3 L/min when it was at or below 93%. Protocol treatment continued for 72 hours. The primary functional clinical outcome, ordinal modified Rankin Scale (mRS) of global disability at 3 months, was similar in the three treatment groups, with odds ratio (OR) for better outcome of 0.97 (95% CI: 0.89–1.05; $p = 0.47$) for any oxygen versus control, and OR of 1.03 (95% CI: 0.93–1.13; $p = 0.61$) for continuous vs nocturnal oxygen. A meta-analysis adding to this trial the 4 additional small trials with mRS distribution data also showed no beneficial effect of continuous oxygen supplementation, with a mean difference in mRS scores of 0.00 (95% CI: –0.15–0.14; $p = 0.97$).

Similarly, trials have not demonstrated a benefit of hyperbaric oxygen therapy in acute ischaemic stroke, although studies have been small in size. Among 11 randomized trials enrolling a total of 705 patients, mortality at 6 months did not differ with hyperbaric oxygen therapy, with risk ratio (RR) of 0.97 (95% CI: 0.34–2.75; $p = 0.96$) (Bennett et al., 2014). Functional outcome scales varied widely across trials, precluding pooled analysis, but the available data, though not excluding a therapeutic effect, were not strongly suggestive.

One early systematic review of HOB positioning in early stroke patients included 4 studies enrolling 183 patients. Different endpoints prevented formal meta-analysis, but individual study results indicated that head position does not affect blood oxygenation in stroke patients without respiratory disorders, while in patients with respiratory disorders HOB elevation is likely to improve oxygenation (Tyson et al., 2004). A large, international, cluster-randomized crossover trial of HOB position with 11,093 acute stroke (85% ischaemic) patients tested horizontal (supine) versus a 30° reclining position maintained for 24 hours (Anderson et al., 2017) (also see section on HOB position in this chapter). This study found no difference in oxygenation status or the primary functional outcome between the two treatment groups.

Comment

While management of non-hypoxaemic acute stroke patients may consist of only monitoring, hypoxaemia should be corrected promptly. Continuous pulse oximetry is a standard, simple, and reliable method to monitor blood oxygenation (Sulter et al., 2000; Kim et al., 2017). In addition to oximetry, periodic assessment of breathing pattern, breathing rate, and breath sounds can detect impending respiratory insufficiency. Blood gas analysis and end tidal CO_2 monitoring help to confirm and define respiratory insufficiency and to guide further treatment. Any effect of HOB position on oxygenation should be noted and used to optimize oxygenation.

Blood oxygen saturation should be maintained above 94%. Noninvasive measures should be considered first, such as nasal cannula, Venturi mask, non-rebreather mask, bilevel positive airway pressure, and continuous positive airway pressure.

Endotracheal intubation with mechanical ventilation should be reserved for patients who do not respond sufficiently to the noninvasive measures or are in need of airway protection from aspiration. Mechanical ventilation can also be useful in the management of stroke patients with malignant cerebral oedema (see Chapter 11). In addition to supplemental oxygen and ventilation assistance, the causes of hypoxaemia should be investigated and treated urgently. The timing of initiation of mechanical ventilation is important. Once a clear indication for mechanical ventilation is identified, urgent endotracheal intubation should be done in order to enhance oxygenation and minimize complications (Steiner et al., 1997).

Head of Bed Positioning

Background

Head positioning can potentially modify acute ischaemic stroke outcome through multiple mechanisms. During acute ischaemic stroke, cerebral autoregulation is impaired in the vicinity of the ischaemic zone, and changes in blood pressure (see blood pressure section in this chapter) as well as HOB position may affect cerebral perfusion and the ultimate fate of the brain region at risk (cerebral penumbra). Also, in patients with large strokes and significant brain oedema, the effect of intracranial pressure on cerebral perfusion needs to be considered when altering HOB position. In addition, head position may affect saliva pooling and aspiration risk. In many clinical situations, the risks and benefits of HOB recommendations need to be balanced with limited data.

Evidence

Multiple small studies of head positioning in acute stroke found a decrease in middle cerebral artery blood flow velocity with HOB elevation from 0° to 30° or 0° to 45° (Schwarz et al., 2002; Wojner-Alexandrov et al., 2005; Aries et al., 2013). In one study, these changes were similar between the stroke and the unaffected hemisphere, and between stroke patients and healthy controls (Aries et al., 2013). One small study measured cerebral perfusion pressure (CPP) in acute stroke patients and found a decrease with head position elevation and associated falls in mean arterial pressure and intracranial pressure (Schwarz et al., 2002).

Multiple studies measured frontal lobe blood flow in acute stroke patients with a transcranial optical spectroscopy method (Durduran et al., 2009; Aries et al., 2013; Favilla et al., 2014) and found a decrease with HOB elevation. However, a considerable heterogeneity in response was noted (Aries et al., 2013).

In a large, international, cluster-randomized crossover trial of head positioning, 11,093 acute stroke (85% ischaemic) patients were allocated to either lying flat or sitting up with at least 30° elevation soon after hospital admission and maintained for 24 hours (Anderson et al., 2017). Patients in this study had relatively mild strokes with median baseline National Institutes of Health Stroke Scale (NIHSS) score of 4. The median time from stroke onset to initiation of head positioning was 14 hours. There was no significant difference in the primary functional outcome of shift of disability level on the modified

Rankin Scale at 90 days, lying flat versus sitting-up: OR 1.01 (95% CI: 0.92–1.10; $p = 0.84$). Similarly, no differences were seen in the rate of functional independence (mRS: 0–2) at 90 days, lying flat versus sitting-up: 38.9% versus 39.7%, OR 0.94 (95% CI: 0.85–1.02; $p = 0.25$).

Comment

The numerous small studies of cerebral haemodynamics in acute stroke suggest potentially important effects of head positioning on regional cerebral blood flow (CBF) in some patients, and they also indicate considerable variability in responses to head position. These findings, together with the neutral result from the large randomized trial (Anderson et al., 2017) and the heterogeneous nature of ischaemic stroke, suggest that HOB position does not have a major effect upon most patients. The possibility remains that in a small subset of exquisitely collateral-dependent hyperacute stroke patients, head positioning importantly alters course, but this requires rigorous studies to confirm or discount.

Blood Pressure

Background

Normally, CBF is maintained relatively constant during arterial blood pressure fluctuations by a physiological system termed *cerebral autoregulation*. Cerebral autoregulation occurs as the cerebral blood vessels dilate (creating decreased resistance to blood flow) in response to falls in pressure and constrict (creating increased resistance to blood flow) in response to increases in pressure. However, cerebral autoregulation has upper and lower blood pressure limits. Below certain blood pressures the cerebral autoregulation is exceeded and CBF falls, with possible brain ischaemia. Also, above certain blood pressures the cerebral autoregulation is exceeded and the CBF rises, with possible brain oedema. The limits of cerebral autoregulation are related to baseline blood pressures (Strandgaard et al., 1973; Schmidt et al., 1990; Donnelly et al., 2016). The lower limits of cerebral autoregulation are approximately 60–85 mm Hg mean pressure in normotensive individuals and approximately 110–120 mm Hg mean pressure in uncontrolled hypertensive individuals.

In the vulnerable region of an acute ischaemic stroke, the cerebral penumbra, cerebral autoregulation is impaired and the CBF is directly related to changes in blood pressure (Dirnagl and Pulsinelli, 1990; Donnelly et al., 2016). Therefore, blood pressure reductions during acute ischaemic stroke may decrease the CBF and extend the ischaemic injury in the cerebral penumbra. During acute ischaemic stroke, the blood pressure is naturally elevated to various degrees above usual. Observational acute ischaemic stroke studies have found a U-shaped relation between the acute blood pressure and clinical outcomes (Castillo et al., 2004; Ahmed et al., 2009). Clinical outcomes were worse at the extremes of blood pressures than at the in-between ranges. In one large study, a systolic blood pressure range of 141–150 mm Hg was associated with best functional outcome (Ahmed et al., 2009). Blood pressure management during the acute period of ischaemic stroke has been the focus of multiple clinical trials.

Evidence

Blood Pressure Lowering

A Cochrane systematic review identified 10 randomized trials of blood pressure lowering in acute ischaemic stroke, enrolling 11,238 patients (Bath and Krishnan, 2014). Tested agents included angiotensin-converting enzyme (ACE) inhibitors, angiotensin receptor antagonists, beta-blockers, nitric oxide donors, and other agents used at physician discretion. No net effect on death by end of trial follow-up was noted, 6.0% versus 6.3%, OR 0.95 (95% CI: 0.78–1.16). In addition, in the 8 randomized trials reporting death or dependency at end of trial, no effect was observed between blood pressure lowering versus control, 41.1% versus 41.0%, OR 1.00 (95% CI: 0.92–1.08) (Figure 5.1). A subsequent systematic review identifying additional studies, with 13 trials enrolling 12,703 patients, similarly showed no effect of early blood pressure lowering upon death or dependency at 3 months, RR of 1.04 (95% CI: 0.96–1.13) (Lee et al., 2015).

In most of the blood pressure lowering trials, treatment started in the late acute period, a median of 11 to 58 hours after stroke onset. The effects of blood pressure lowering in the early acute period, the first 0–12 hours after stroke onset, have not been as well studied in randomized trials and may differ from later timepoints, since substantial ischaemic tissue at risk (penumbra) is often still present and could be jeopardized by collateral blood flow reduction with blood pressure lowering. In the RIGHT-2 trial of a mixed blood pressure lowering and neuroprotective

Review: Interventions for deliberately altering blood pressure in acute stroke
Comparison: 1 Blood pressure lowering therapy in acute stroke
Outcome: 2 Death or dependency, end of trial by stroke type

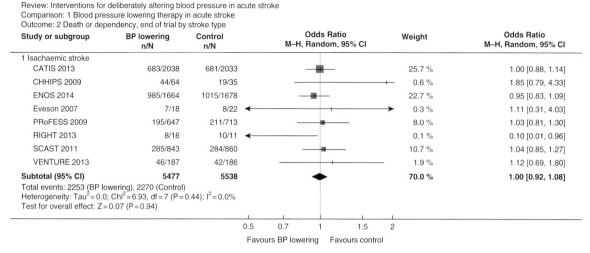

Study or subgroup	BP lowering n/N	Control n/N	Odds Ratio M–H, Random, 95% CI	Weight	Odds Ratio M–H, Random, 95% CI
1 Isachaemic stroke					
CATIS 2013	683/2038	681/2033		25.7 %	1.00 [0.88, 1.14]
CHHIPS 2009	44/64	19/35		0.6 %	1.85 [0.79, 4.33]
ENOS 2014	985/1664	1015/1678		22.7 %	0.95 [0.83, 1.09]
Eveson 2007	7/18	8/22		0.3 %	1.11 [0.31, 4.03]
PRoFESS 2009	195/647	211/713		8.0 %	1.03 [0.81, 1.30]
RIGHT 2013	8/16	10/11		0.1 %	0.10 [0.01, 0.96]
SCAST 2011	285/843	284/860		10.7 %	1.04 [0.85, 1.27]
VENTURE 2013	46/187	42/186		1.9 %	1.12 [0.69, 1.80]
Subtotal (95% CI)	**5477**	**5538**		**70.0 %**	**1.00 [0.92, 1.08]**

Total events: 2253 (BP lowering), 2270 (Control)
Heterogeneity: Tau^2=0.0; Chi^2=6.93, df=7 (P=0.44); I^2=0.0%
Test for overall effect: Z=0.07 (P=0.94)

0.5   0.7   1   1.5   2
Favours BP lowering   Favours control

Figure 5.1 Forest plot showing the effects of *more intensive blood pressure lowering therapy* in acute ischaemic stroke patients on *death or dependency*. Reproduced from Bath et al. (2014), with permission from John Wiley & Sons Limited.
Copyright Cochrane Library.

agent (glyceryl trinitrate) begun hyperacutely in the prehospital setting (median 70 min after onset), the common odds ratio point estimates for shift in 3-month disability outcome were non-significantly unfavourable for both ischaemic stroke (580 patients, common odds ratio [cOR]: 1.15, 95% CI: 0.85–1.54) and transient ischaemic attack (105 patients, cOR: 1.57, 95% CI: 0.74–3.35) (RIGHT-2 Investigators, 2019).

Gentle blood pressure lowering to systolic blood pressure (SBP) less than 185 and diastolic blood pressure (DBP) less than 110 in acute ischaemic stroke patients eligible for intravenous (IV) tissue plasminogen activator (tPA) therapy was required in the IV tPA treatment trials, and is currently recommended as a concomitant therapy in lytic-treated patients in national guidelines. However, the optimal blood pressure target for acute ischaemic stroke patients treated with IV tPA has not been conclusively defined by controlled clinical trials.

Blood Pressure Elevation

Two randomized trials have tested induced hypertension as a therapeutic intervention to augment collateral blood flow in acute ischaemic stroke patients with evidence of collateral dependency. In a small trial, 16 patients with substantial diffusion–perfusion mismatch persisting 5 hours to 4 days after stroke onset

were randomized to standard care or treatment with phenylephrine until neurological improvement occurred or mean arterial pressure reached 130–140 (Hillis et al., 2003). Patients undergoing blood pressure augmentation had reduced neurological deficits 6–8 weeks after stroke (mean NIHSS score 2.8 vs 9.7, p < 0.04). In a multicentre trial in Korea, 153 patients with non-cardioembolic stroke ineligible for recanalization therapy were randomized to conventional care or treatment with phenylephrine until the NIHSS score improved or the SBP reached 200 mm Hg (Chung et al., 2018). Induced hypertension patients showed improvement in NIHSS score by 2 or more points more often, 57.9% versus 31.2%, OR 3.04 (95% CI: 1.56–5.89; p = 0.001) and a trend towards improved functional independence (mRS 0–2) at 3 months, 75.0% versus 63.2%, OR 1.75 (95% CI: 0.-87–3.52; p = 0.12).

Comment

Avoiding extremes of blood pressure, including frank hypotension (SBP < 90 mm Hg) and hypertension sufficient to induce hypertensive encephalopathy (SBP > 220 mm Hg), seems prudent in acute ischaemic stroke patients to avoid deleterious effects on the brain and other organs. So far, there is no convincing evidence that blood pressure adjustments within this broad range during acute ischaemic stroke are beneficial.

A reasonable general strategy for patients with persisting vessel occlusions is to avoid lowering the blood pressure during the first 24 hours after stroke onset, unless a strong indication is present. During the first few hours after stroke onset, collateral blood flow to penumbral brain regions is most critical, and randomized trials have not specifically tested therapies in the hyperacute period. Thereafter, gradual blood pressure lowering may be safely started, and long-term, secondary prevention blood pressure targets eventually attained. There is little evidence to recommend a specific blood pressure lowering drug class during acute stroke. However, drugs that can control the blood pressure with minimal fluctuations may be preferred.

In patients in whom IV thrombolysis is initiated, stricter control of blood pressure during the first 24 hours is recommended to reduce risk of haemorrhagic transformation in accord with regimens used in lytic trials. In patients in whom partial reperfusion has been achieved with IV thrombolysis or endovascular thrombectomy, an individual judgement needs to be made about the best blood pressure target that balances the countervailing physiological goals of lowering blood pressure to reduce risk of reperfusion haemorrhage versus maintaining an elevated blood pressure to support residual hypoperfused fields.

Induced hypertension to enhance collateral flow in select patients with persisting vessel occlusions is a strategy that has shown promise in small trials, but has not been confirmed in definitive larger studies. Blood pressure augmentation might be used cautiously when there is evidence of persisting penumbral tissue in jeopardy of infarction or fluctuating stroke deficits in patients without congestive heart failure or coronary artery disease.

Liquids and Electrolytes

Dehydration

Both dehydration and overhydration can have detrimental effects during acute ischaemic stroke. Dehydration can lead to hypotension and subsequent hypoperfusion of vulnerable ischaemic brain regions, thus worsening a stroke. Overhydration can lead to congestive heart failure, especially in the elderly and those with renal or cardiac insufficiencies. In addition, volume overload may exacerbate ischaemic brain oedema.

Hydration status can be assessed by monitoring the mucous membranes, skin turgor, blood haematocrit, blood urea nitrogen/creatinine ratio, serum sodium, urine osmolarity, and body weight. For some critically ill stroke patients, more definitive measurements, such as central venous pressure or pulmonary capillary wedge pressure, are needed.

Evidence

Dehydration is common in acute ischaemic stroke patients. In a study of 2158 consecutive acute ischaemic stroke patients, 61% were dehydrated on presentation or at some point during their hospital course, as assessed by a blood urea nitrogen/creatinine ratio greater than 80 (Rowat et al., 2012). Patients with dehydration substantially more often died in hospital or were discharged to institutional care.

Two randomized trials have evaluated liquid support regimens in acute ischaemic stroke. In one trial, a broad population of 120 acute ischaemic stroke patients presenting within 72 hours of acute ischaemic stroke onset were randomized to a 0.9% NaCl solution at 100 mL/h for 3 days or to no IV liquids (Suwanela et al., 2017). There was no difference in the rates of freedom from disability (mRS 0–1) at 3 months with IV liquids versus control (83.3% vs 80.0%, $p = 0.64$). However, early neurological deterioration (NIHSS worsening by 3 or more points during the first 3 days), not of metabolic or haemorrhagic origin, occurred less often in the patients receiving IV liquids (3% vs 15%, $p = 0.02$).

In another trial, 212 diabetic patients presenting with acute ischaemic stroke and chronic hyperglycaemia (HBA1c $\geq$ 7.0) were randomized to moderate versus minimal IV hydration with normal saline (Lin et al., 2018). The moderate hydration group received 300–500 mL bolus followed by 40–80 mL/h for 72 hours, while the minimal hydration group received 40–60 mL/h for the first 24 hours and 0–60 mL/h during 25 to 72 hours. Long-term outcomes were not assessed. However, early neurological deterioration (total NIHSS worsening by $\geq$2 points, consciousness or motor score worsening by $\geq$1 point, or any new neurological deficit) was less frequent with moderate than minimal hydration, 10.5% versus 33.6%, OR 0.21 (95% CI: 0.10–0.44, $p < 0.05$).

Comment

Liquids

Hydration management in acute ischaemic stroke should generally aim for normovolaemia. Many acute stroke patients cannot eat or drink initially and require enteral or IV hydration. The usual daily liquid volume requirement for maintenance of normovolaemia is 25–30 mL/kg. Isotonic IV solutions, such as 0.9% NaCl or other solutions containing plasma electrolytes, are preferred over hypotonic solutions, such as 0.45% NaCl or 5% dextrose, to limit brain oedema. Hypertonic IV solutions may occasionally be useful to treat advanced ischaemic cerebral oedema, but substantial brain oedema generally does not develop until 2 to 5 days after stroke onset, so hypertonic solutions are not the initial support liquids of choice. With careful attention to intake and output of liquids, insensible losses, and diuretics, significant fluctuations in intravascular volume can be avoided, although the maintenance of euvolaemia can be challenging, especially in patients with severe renal or cardiac insufficiency.

Electrolytes

Serious electrolyte abnormalities are uncommon at presentation in patients with ischaemic stroke, unless they were pre-existing (e.g. hypokalaemia due to diuretics). Serum electrolytes should be assessed at baseline, and subsequently if the patient deteriorates or has prolonged hospital course. Causes of electrolyte disturbances should be treated, and the electrolytes replaced. Hyponatraemia is a relatively common complication during the initial hospitalization for ischaemic stroke. In one series of 47 ischaemic stroke patients with hyponatraemic or eunatraemic course, hyponatraemia developed in 34%, usually due to cerebral salt wasting (CSW) and rarely due to the syndrome of inappropriate secretion of antidiuretic hormone (SIADH) (Kalita et al., 2017). Treatment with hypertonic liquids, such as 3% NaCl, is generally indicated for hyponatraemia, as it will be effective for both CSW and SIADH (Manzanares et al., 2015).

Blood Glucose

Background

Blood glucose can fluctuate extensively during acute stroke, especially in patients with diabetes mellitus.

Both extreme hypoglycaemia and hyperglycaemia can cause neurological dysfunction and seizures. Hyperglycaemia is considerably more common and persistent than hypoglycaemia during acute stroke. Approximately 40% of acute ischaemic stroke patients have hyperglycaemia above 130 mg/dL on admission (Williams et al., 2002). There is considerable evidence linking hyperglycaemia during acute stroke with worse functional outcomes (Capes et al., 2001; McCormick et al., 2008). However, hyperglycaemia during acute ischaemic stroke may be only a marker of more severe illness and underlying insulin resistance. Clinical trials to improve functional outcomes by reducing hyperglycaemia during acute ischaemic stroke have not demonstrated efficacy.

Evidence

A systematic review identified 11 randomized controlled trials enrolling 1583 patients to greater versus lesser control of hyperglycaemia during acute ischaemic stroke using different glucose-monitoring frequencies and insulin regimens (Bellolio et al., 2014). There was no difference between the intervention and control groups in the death or dependency outcome, OR 0.99 (95% CI: 0.79 to 1.23) (Figure 5.2). The rate of symptomatic hypoglycaemia was higher in the intervention group, OR 14.6 (95% CI: 6.6–32.2). Similar findings were observed in patient subgroups with and without diabetes mellitus.

More than half of the patients in the meta-analysis were enrolled in the Glucose Insulin Stroke Trial – United Kingdom (GIST-UK), in which 933 acute ischaemic stroke patients with mild-to-moderate hyperglycaemia were randomly assigned to treatment with IV insulin or saline (control) (Gray et al., 2007). There was no evidence of efficacy from the IV insulin treatment. However, the mean blood glucose was only 10 mg/dL lower in the intervention group than in the control group, and 84% of the subjects did not have diabetes mellitus, suggesting that undertreatment and enrolment of patients with stress hyperglycaemia rather than underlying diabetes mellitus or prediabetes may have masked a potential treatment benefit.

The Stroke Hyperglycemia Insulin Network Effort (SHINE) trial (Bruno et al., 2014), enrolled 1151 hyperglycaemic acute stroke patients, randomized to standard subcutaneous insulin (target blood glucose <80–179 mg/dL) or intensive IV insulin (target blood glucose 80–130 mg/dL) therapy for the initial

Review: Insulin for glycaemic control in acute ischaemic stroke
Comparison: 1 Dependency or death
Outcome: 1 Dependency or death at the end of the follow-up

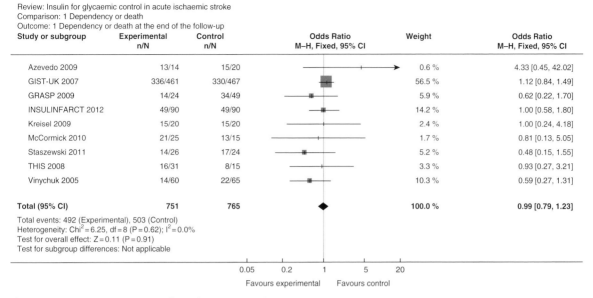

Figure 5.2 Forest plot showing the effects of *insulin therapy for glycaemic control* compared with control treatment in acute ischaemic stroke patients on *death or dependency*. Reproduced from Bellolio et al. (2014), with permission from the authors and John Wiley & Sons Limited. Copyright Cochrane Library.

72 hours after stroke onset. Eighty percent of patients had a history of diabetes mellitus type 2. The mean blood glucose level in the standard treatment group was 179 mg/dL and in the intensive group it was 118 mg/dL during the treatment period. The rates of favourable functional outcome at 3 months were similar in the two treatment groups, 21.6% in standard and 20.5% in intensive, RR 0.97 (95% CI: 0.87–1.08) (Johnston et al., 2019). Occasional severe hypoglycaemia (<40 mg/dL) occurred only in the intensive group, in 2.6% of patients.

Comment

Extremely low and high blood glucose deviations should be avoided in patients with acute ischaemic stroke. Peripheral nervous manifestations of hypoglycaemia (tremulousness, palpitation, diaphoresis, paraesthesia) usually begin to appear when the blood glucose drops below 70 mg/dL (Cryer et al., 2003). Central nervous manifestations of hypoglycaemia (generalized weakness, fatigue, confusion, and eventually seizures) usually begin to appear when the blood glucose drops below 55 mg/dL (Cryer et al., 2003). The blood glucose threshold for developing manifestations of hypoglycaemia varies between patients, and those with diabetes tend to develop manifestations at higher glucose levels than those

without diabetes. Treatment of mild-to-moderate hypoglycaemia could consist of juice consumption if not contraindicated by dysphagia. Otherwise, and to treat severe hypoglycaemia, IV 50% dextrose should be administered urgently to prevent seizures or hypoglycaemic neurological injury.

There is no agreed-on definition of hyperglycaemia during acute illness. Patients with type 2 diabetes mellitus rarely develop diabetic ketoacidosis. However, blood glucose levels above 260 mg/dL have been reported to cause focal neurological deficits resembling stroke, some with non-convulsive focal seizures. Non-convulsive hyperglycaemic hemianopia (Stayman et al., 2013; Strowd et al., 2014), aphasia (Huang et al., 2014), and mild hemiparesis (Hansford et al., 2013) have been reported.

Tight control of hyperglycaemia with IV insulin to a blood glucose range of 80–110 mg/dL is challenging and carries a significant risk of dangerous hypoglycaemia. A less-stringent control of hyperglycaemia is more feasible and less risky.

Based upon current clinical data, initial treatment of hyperglycaemia during acute ischaemic stroke using a subcutaneous regular insulin sliding scale of moderate intensity is appropriate. With current knowledge, a target blood glucose of less than 200 mg/dL during acute ischaemic stroke seems reasonable. If subcutaneous insulin treatment is insufficient to control an individual patient's hyperglycaemia, IV insulin may be used, accompanied by more intensive blood glucose and patient monitoring. As the daily insulin requirement becomes more consistent, long-acting (basal) insulin doses may be introduced to minimize blood glucose fluctuations. After establishing regular oral or tube feeding diets, oral hypoglycaemic agents may be used more safely. Monitoring the blood glucose 4 times daily should be sufficient for most acute stroke patients with diabetes.

Dysphagia and Nutrition

Dysphagia

Background

Using video fluoroscopic examination, dysphagia has been identified in 64% of acute stroke patients (Mann et al., 1999). Dysphagia in acute stroke patients results from weakness and incoordination of the oral, pharyngeal, and laryngeal muscles involved in swallowing. Presence, severity, and duration of dysphagia depend on location of the brain injury and level of consciousness. Clinical factors associated with dysphagia include decreased gag reflex, impaired voluntary cough, dysphonia, incomplete oral-labial closure, stroke severity (high NIHSS score), and lower cranial nerve palsies (Daniels et al., 2000). A relatively simple bedside water swallow test is quite sensitive in identifying dysphagia (Edmiaston et al., 2014; Chen et al., 2016). Initial swallowing function can be screened by various healthcare providers without specialized training, but an appropriate specialist can more accurately characterize impairments.

Dysphagia increases the risk of chest infections and death and limits oral nutrition (Mann et al., 1999; Joundi, et al., 2017). In particular, delayed or absent swallowing reflex increased the risk of chest infections over the subsequent 6 months nearly 12-fold. In a magnetic resonance imaging (MRI) analysis of patients with acute supratentorial stroke, acute aspiration was associated with involvement of the internal capsule or the insular cortex (Galovic et al., 2013). In the same study, extended risk of aspiration (≥ 7 days) was associated with stroke involving both the insular cortex and the frontal operculum.

Evidence

Randomized trials of dysphagia screening prior to start of oral feeding in acute ischaemic stroke patients have not been conducted, but multiple observational studies are supportive. In an analysis of 15 hospitals with 2532 acute ischaemic stroke patients, the 6 hospitals that routinely used a formal dysphagia screen before oral feeding had significantly lower rates of in-hospital pneumonia (2.4% vs 4%, $p = 0.002$) (Hinchey et al., 2005).

In a before–after study of 384 acute stroke patients, introduction of a formal 24/7 dysphagia screening by bedside nurses compared with prior weekday-only screening by speech and language pathologists was associated with earlier determination of swallowing safety (median 7 vs 20 hours) and significantly lower pneumonia rates (3.8% vs 11.6%, $p = 0.004$) (Palli et al., 2017).

A cluster-randomized trial of a nursing quality improvement intervention targeting fever, glucose management, and dysphagia screening reduced death and dependency, but without reducing the pneumonia rate (Middleton et al., 2011).

Another small cluster-controlled trial evaluated 162 acute stroke patients cared for on 2 wards, one implementing a formal swallow screen protocol and the other continuing with physician clinical assessment of swallowing (Rai et al., 2016). Stroke patients who received the formal swallow evaluations tended to have less aspiration pneumonia than the conventional care patients (6.5% vs 15.3%, $p = 0.06$).

Behavioural therapies to treat dysphagia, including swallowing exercises, oral stimulation, and oral care led by speech and language pathologists or nurses, have been tested in several randomized trials, generally comparing more intensive to less intensive therapies or standard care (Bath et al., 2018). Patients predominantly had ischaemic stroke, but some had haemorrhagic strokes. Across 6 randomized trials enrolling 511 patients, more active behavioural therapies were associated with less persistent dysphagia, 34.5% versus 53.5%, OR 0.45 (95% CI: 0.28–0.74); and across 6 randomized trials enrolling 473 patients, more active behavioural therapies were associated with reduced pneumonia, 20.3% versus 34.2%, OR 0.56 (95% CI: 0.31–1.00) (Figure 5.3).

Acupuncture to treat dysphagia after stroke has been evaluated in numerous small randomized trials. A systematic review identified 59 randomized trials enrolling 4809 patients, most ischaemic but some

Review: Swallowing therapy for dysphagia in acute and subacute stroke
Comparison: 1 Swallowing therapy
Outcome: 7 Chest infection or pneumonia

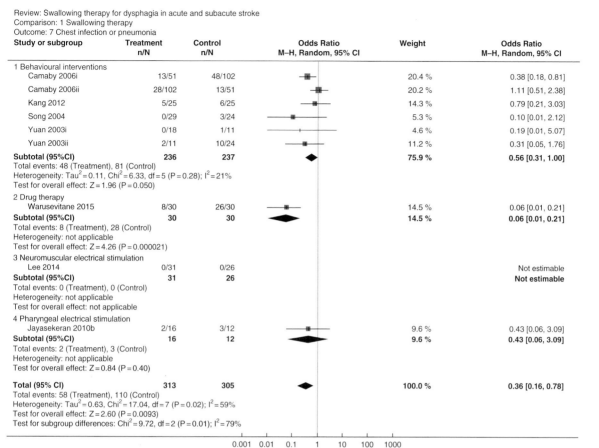

Study or subgroup	Treatment n/N	Control n/N	Odds Ratio M–H, Random, 95% CI	Weight	Odds Ratio M–H, Random, 95% CI
1 Behavioural interventions					
Camaby 2006i	13/51	48/102		20.4 %	0.38 [0.18, 0.81]
Camaby 2006ii	28/102	13/51		20.2 %	1.11 [0.51, 2.38]
Kang 2012	5/25	6/25		14.3 %	0.79 [0.21, 3.03]
Song 2004	0/29	3/24		5.3 %	0.10 [0.01, 2.12]
Yuan 2003i	0/18	1/11		4.6 %	0.19 [0.01, 5.07]
Yuan 2003ii	2/11	10/24		11.2 %	0.31 [0.05, 1.76]
Subtotal (95%CI)	**236**	**237**		**75.9 %**	**0.56 [0.31, 1.00]**

Total events: 48 (Treatment), 81 (Control)
Heterogeneity: Tau^2 = 0.11, Chi^2 = 6.33, df = 5 (P = 0.28); I^2 = 21%
Test for overall effect: Z = 1.96 (P = 0.050)

2 Drug therapy					
Warusevitane 2015	8/30	26/30		14.5 %	0.06 [0.01, 0.21]
Subtotal (95%CI)	**30**	**30**		**14.5 %**	**0.06 [0.01, 0.21]**

Total events: 8 (Treatment), 28 (Control)
Heterogeneity: not applicable
Test for overall effect: Z = 4.26 (P = 0.000021)

3 Neuromuscular electrical stimulation					
Lee 2014	0/31	0/26			Not estimable
Subtotal (95%CI)	**31**	**26**			**Not estimable**

Total events: 0 (Treatment), 0 (Control)
Heterogeneity: not applicable
Test for overall effect: not applicable

4 Pharyngeal electrical stimulation					
Jayasekeran 2010b	2/16	3/12		9.6 %	0.43 [0.06, 3.09]
Subtotal (95%CI)	**16**	**12**		**9.6 %**	**0.43 [0.06, 3.09]**

Total events: 2 (Treatment), 3 (Control)
Heterogeneity: not applicable
Test for overall effect: Z = 0.84 (P = 0.40)

Total (95% CI)	**313**	**305**		**100.0 %**	**0.36 [0.16, 0.78]**

Total events: 58 (Treatment), 110 (Control)
Heterogeneity: Tau^2 = 0.63, Chi^2 = 17.04, df = 7 (P = 0.02); I^2 = 59%
Test for overall effect: Z = 2.60 (P = 0.0093)
Test for subgroup differences: Chi^2 = 9.72, df = 2 (P = 0.01); I^2 = 79%

```
        0.001  0.01   0.1    1    10   100  1000
              Therapy better    Therapy worse
```

Figure 5.3 Forest plot showing the effects of *various swallowing therapies* in acute and subacute stroke patients on *pneumonia rates*. Reproduced from Bath et al. (2018), with permission from the authors and John Wiley & Sons Limited.

Copyright Cochrane Library.

haemorrhagic (Ye et al., 2017). Acupuncture was associated with more frequent improvement in swallowing function compared with standard therapies, 92% versus 77%, RR 1.17 (95% CI: 1.1–1.21). However, many studies had risk of bias due to incomplete blinding of patients and evaluators.

Pharyngeal electrical stimulation therapy to treat dysphagia, including electrical stimulation applied via electrodes implanted in a nasogastric tube, has been evaluated in at least 6 randomized trials (Suntrup et al., 2015; Bath et al., 2018; Dziewas et al., 2018). In 4 trials enrolling 177 patients, pharyngeal electrical stimulation was associated with non-significantly improved scores on the penetration-aspiration scale (Bath et al., 2018). A more recent multicentre trial, enrolling 69 severely dysphagic patients with

tracheostomy, was stopped early for efficacy when readiness for decannulation (removal of tracheostomy) 24–72 hours after treatment occurred more frequently in the pharyngeal stimulation group, 49% versus 9%, OR 7.00 (95% CI: 2.41–19.88; p = 0.0008) (Dziewas et al., 2018).

Transcranial direct current and magnetic stimulation therapies added to standard therapies have been evaluated as dysphagia treatments in several trials. In a study-level meta-analysis of 8 randomized trials of transcranial magnetic stimulation, enrolling 141 patients, stimulation improved scores on swallowing scales (Bath et al., 2018). Analysis of 2 randomized trials of transcranial direct current stimulation, enrolling 34 patients, showed a lesser, non-significant, but directionally favourable effect (Bath et al., 2018).

Nutrition

Under-nutrition is present in 8–25% of acute stroke patients during the first week and is associated with worse functional outcomes and higher mortality (FOOD Trial Collaboration, 2003; Yoo et al., 2008).

The largest clinical study evaluating nutritional support strategies in acute stroke patients was the Feed Or Ordinary Diet (FOOD) study, which comprised a family of 3 multicentre randomized trials. One trial included acute stroke patients without dysphagia (FOOD Trial Collaboration, 2005a), and two included patients with dysphagia (FOOD Trial Collaboration, 2005b).

In the nutrition trial in individuals without dysphagia, 4023 acute stroke patients were randomized to eat either a regular hospital diet or a hospital diet supplemented with protein (FOOD Trial Collaboration, 2005a). At 6 months, there was no significant difference in the rates of dependency or death (mRS scores 3–6) between the two treatment groups (58% vs 59%).

One trial in patients with dysphagia compared early (≤7 days from hospital admission) versus late (>7 days from hospital admission) start of enteral tube feeding. Among 859 randomized patients, earlier feeding was associated with a trend toward reduced mortality at 6 months (42% vs 48%, $p = 0.09$), but with no increase in the rate of being capable of bodily self-care (mRS scores 0–3) (21% vs 20%, $p = 0.7$) (FOOD Trial Collaboration, 2005b). The rate of gastrointestinal bleeding was higher in the early feeding group (5.1% vs 2.6%, $p = 0.04$).

The second trial in dysphagia patients compared initial nasogastric (NG) versus initial percutaneous endoscopic gastrostomy (PEG) tube feeding. Among 321 randomized patients, allocation to NG versus PEG tube feeding was associated with higher rates of being alive and capable of bodily self-care at 6 months (mRS scores 0–3) (89% vs 81%, $p = 0.05$). Also, gastrointestinal bleeding was less frequent in the NG tube group (3.1% vs 11.3%, $p = 0.005$).

Comment

Observational and limited controlled trial data support performing simple, formal swallow screening early in all ischaemic stroke patients, with initiation of oral intake in patients with retained swallowing ability, and referral to speech therapists for more detailed assessment of patients with evidence of potential dysphagia. Beginning oral feeding only in patients cleared by a careful swallowing assessment will minimize aspiration complications. Based on the findings by a specialist in swallow evaluation, some acute stroke patients with mildly impaired swallow may be cleared initially to eat only mechanically modified foods, such as puréed foods, before advancing to regular food.

When swallowing is impaired so that adequate oral feeding is unsafe, initiating feeding via NG tube is reasonable within the first 2 or 3 days after stroke onset. If swallowing function has not improved sufficiently for adequate oral intake after 1 or 2 weeks, converting to PEG tube feeding is reasonable, as NG tube irritation of nasal mucosa becomes more likely. Tube feeding during acute stroke can be continuous or by periodic bolus, depending partly on patient tolerance. If swallowing improves during stroke rehabilitation, removal of the PEG tube should be considered. Behavioural swallowing rehabilitation therapies likely hasten resolution of dysphagia. Electrical pharyngeal stimulation may be of benefit for patients with prolonged dysphagia and tracheotomy.

Fever

Background

Fever is commonly defined as core body temperature at or above 37.5°C (99.5°F) and is relatively common during acute stroke (Grau et al., 1999; Middleton et al., 2011). Fever may be a sign of infection, evidence of other medical complications, or due to the stroke itself by a variety of mechanisms. Large areas of tissue necrosis can elevate body temperature (Reith et al., 1996). Extensive preclinical data indicate that fever enhances ischaemic brain injury, in part by accelerating the biochemical reactions mediating molecular cellular damage. Accordingly, lowering the body temperature to normal might slow deleterious biochemical reactions during acute ischaemic stroke and improve outcome. Furthermore, induced hypothermia is a potential neuroprotective intervention in acute ischaemic stroke (see Chapter 12).

Evidence

Patients with fever during acute stroke have worse outcomes than do patients without fever (Reith et al., 1996; Castillo et al., 1998; Prasad and Krishnan, 2010). The relationships between fever and stroke outcome or fever and infarct volume are strongest within the initial 6- to 24-hour period (Castillo et al., 1998), while in the first 3 hours after stroke onset, lower body temperatures are actually associated with worse outcome, likely from sympathetic hyperactivity initially lowering the hypothalamic thermoregulatory setpoint (Kim and Saver, 2015). Fever may be a marker of stroke severity or a contributor to brain injury, or both.

A systematic review identified 7 randomized trials testing prophylactic versus reactive administration of pharmacological agents that reduce fever and maintain normothermia in acute stroke patients, predominantly patients with ischaemic stroke (den Hertog et al., 2009). Among 280 randomized patients, 61% were enrolled in 5 trials testing acetaminophen (paracetamol), 24% in 1 trial testing metamizol, and 16% in 1 trial testing ibuprofen. Overall, no differences were observed in the rate of dependency or death (mRS 3–6) between prophylactic and reactive pharmacotherapy, 50% versus 51%, OR 0.89 (95% CI: 0.54–1.48). In a larger, more recent trial, among 256 acute stroke patients randomized to high-dose paracetamol (6 g/day) or placebo for 3 days, body temperature from baseline to 24 hours in the control group increased by 0.18°C and in the intervention group decreased by 0.09°C (de Ridder et al., 2017). However, no benefit in global disability across mRS levels at 3 months was observed, with a common odds ratio of 1.02 (95% CI: 0.66–1.58).

While prophylactic antipyretic therapy has not been supported, a cluster-randomized trial provided support for close monitoring for fever development and aggressive reactive therapy for temperature elevation. In a cluster-controlled trial of a combined nursing quality improvement intervention targeting fever, glucose management, and dysphagia screening, the temperature intervention consisted of monitoring body temperature every 4 hours for the first 72 hours after admission and starting paracetamol if temperature was above 37.5°C (Middleton et al., 2011). A total of 19 acute stroke units were randomized, and 1696 patients enrolled. Patients in the intervention units were less likely to be dead or disabled (mRS scores 2–6) at 90 days (42% vs 58%, $p = 0.002$).

Comment

It is essential to monitor patients with acute ischaemic stroke for fever development. In patients developing hyperthermia, antipyretic therapy should be started immediately, whatever the cause. In addition, the underlying cause of the temperature elevation should be urgently investigated and directly treated. Usual treatments of fever include antipyretic medications

and surface cooling devices (cooling blankets and pads). In addition, endovascular cooling devices are available. Further studies are needed to determine or clarify the degree to which fever is a contributor to poor outcomes versus a marker of more severe illness and to define optimal temperature targets.

Antibiotics

Background

Urinary tract and chest infections are the most common infections during acute stroke (Aslanyan et al., 2004; Indredavik et al., 2008; Vermeij et al., 2009). Urinary tract infections (UTIs) occur in approximately 15–20% of patients. Risk of UTI during acute stroke is higher in women than in men and increases with age and with stroke severity (Aslanyan et al., 2004). Risk of UTI is also related to bladder dysfunction that sometimes occurs after stroke and to the use of indwelling urinary catheters (Poisson et al., 2010). Although indwelling bladder catheters can decrease nursing effort, they are not always necessary to treat bladder dysfunction in acute stroke. Thus, many hospital-acquired UTIs are likely preventable.

Chest infections occur in approximately 10–15% of acute stroke patients. Risk of pneumonia during acute stroke is higher in men than in women, in patients with diabetes, and in those with large hemispheric strokes, and the risk increases with age and with stroke severity (Aslanyan et al., 2004). In addition, risk of aspiration pneumonia is increased in acute stroke patients with dysphagia (Galovic et al., 2013) or with decreased consciousness, as their natural airway protection mechanisms are impaired (see section on dysphagia in this chapter).

Immune system suppression has been identified in acute stroke patients, and this may predispose patients to infections (Famakin, 2014). Both UTIs and chest infections increase the risk of poor functional outcomes (Aslanyan et al., 2004; Vermeij et al., 2009).

Evidence

A systematic review identified 8 randomized trials of preventive antibiotic therapy in acute stroke, enrolling 4488 patients (Vermeij et al., 2018). Preventive antibiotic regimens reduced the frequency of all-cause infections in stroke patients, 19% versus 26%, RR 0.71 (95% CI: 0.58–0.88). However, there was no beneficial effect on death or dependency, 53% versus

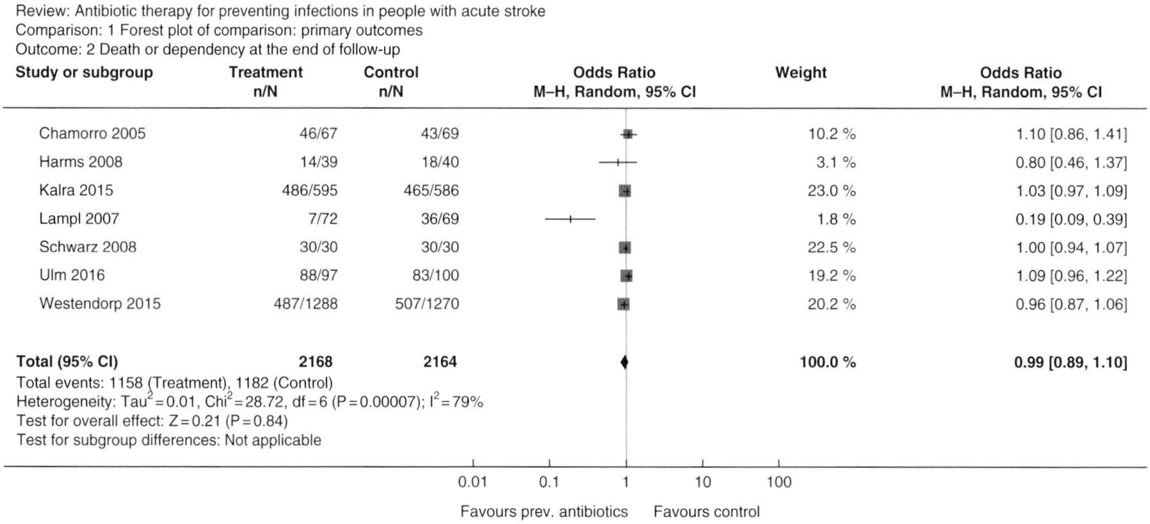

Review: Antibiotic therapy for preventing infections in people with acute stroke
Comparison: 1 Forest plot of comparison: primary outcomes
Outcome: 2 Death or dependency at the end of follow-up

Study or subgroup	Treatment n/N	Control n/N	Odds Ratio M–H, Random, 95% CI	Weight	Odds Ratio M–H, Random, 95% CI
Chamorro 2005	46/67	43/69		10.2 %	1.10 [0.86, 1.41]
Harms 2008	14/39	18/40		3.1 %	0.80 [0.46, 1.37]
Kalra 2015	486/595	465/586		23.0 %	1.03 [0.97, 1.09]
Lampl 2007	7/72	36/69		1.8 %	0.19 [0.09, 0.39]
Schwarz 2008	30/30	30/30		22.5 %	1.00 [0.94, 1.07]
Ulm 2016	88/97	83/100		19.2 %	1.09 [0.96, 1.22]
Westendorp 2015	487/1288	507/1270		20.2 %	0.96 [0.87, 1.06]
Total (95% CI)	**2168**	**2164**		**100.0 %**	**0.99 [0.89, 1.10]**

Total events: 1158 (Treatment), 1182 (Control)
Heterogeneity: Tau^2=0.01, Chi^2=28.72, df=6 (P=0.00007); I^2=79%
Test for overall effect: Z=0.21 (P=0.84)
Test for subgroup differences: Not applicable

0.01   0.1   1   10   100
Favours prev. antibiotics   Favours control

Figure 5.4 Forest plot showing the effects of *preventive antibiotics* in acute and subacute stroke patients on *death or dependency*. Reproduced from Verrmeij et al. (2018), with permission from the authors and John Wiley & Sons Limited.
Copyright Cochrane Library.

55%, RR 0.99 (95% CI: 0.89–1.10) (Figure 5.4) or upon mortality, 17% versus 16%, RR 1.03 (95% CI: 0.87–1.21).

Comment

Although prophylactic antibiotics reduce the overall infection rate, they do not improve patient functional outcome and they may contribute to the development of more virulent nosocomial infections. Accordingly, antibiotic therapy is best employed in response to specific signs of infection. Fevers, leucocytosis, and local organ signs should be aggressively evaluated for potential infections. Identified infections should be treated urgently with antimicrobial agents that are optimized to the source of the infection and the local bacterial sensitivities.

Bladder Function

Bladder Function

The most common cause of bladder dysfunction after stroke is detrusor hyper-reflexia as a direct result of the stroke, which may be compounded by immobility (e.g. unable to sit or stand), UTI, and pre-stroke bladder outflow obstruction (e.g. prostate enlargement). Detrusor hyper-reflexia tends to cause urge incontinence and frequency of micturition.

Incontinence

Incontinence of urine is common in the first few days after stroke and provokes considerable distress among patients and their carers. It is usually due to a combination of factors, such as detrusor hyper-reflexia, impaired sphincter control, pre-existing bladder outflow obstruction (e.g. prostate enlargement, gynaecological problems), constipation, immobility, inability to communicate, delayed care provider responses, confusion, impaired consciousness, and UTI (Panfili et al., 2017).

Management of incontinence aims to identify and rectify the underlying cause (e.g. infection, outflow obstruction) and exacerbating factors (excessive liquids, uncontrolled hyperglycaemia, diuretics), and commence bladder 'retraining' wherein patients are prompted to void regularly. A bedside ultrasound scan can identify a postmicturition residual volume of 100 mL or more. If present, an anticholinergic drug (e.g. oxybutynin) may help (if there are no contraindications, such as closed angle glaucoma), coupled with regular bladder emptying by intermittent catheterization.

Indwelling catheters should be restricted to patients in whom the above measures are impractical, such as those who are difficult to transfer or in whom pressure areas are a concern. Indwelling catheters can produce urinary tract trauma and infection. In one small randomized trial, external (condom) catheters reduced the occurrence of urinary infections when compared with indwelling bladder catheters (Saint et al., 2006). Also, as the duration of bladder catheterization increased, the risk of UTI increased (Saint et al., 2006; Al-Hazmi, 2015). Because incontinence of urine frequently resolves spontaneously during the first or second week after stroke, it is important to remove indwelling catheters for a 'trial of voiding' and re-assessment of bladder function as soon as the patient's condition begins to improve.

For patients with persisting incontinence, cystoscopy and urodynamic investigations may be indicated to assess bladder contractility and outflow.

Retention

Urinary retention is common, especially in men with pre-existing bladder outflow obstruction, and must be anticipated and excluded in patients with dribbling incontinence, agitation, impaired consciousness, or communication difficulties, particularly if they have been exposed to precipitants, such as drugs (e.g. tricyclic antidepressants which have antimuscarinic effects), immobility, and constipation.

A urethral catheter provides prompt relief, and in men with benign prostatic hypertrophy, alpha-blocking agents (e.g. prazosin), or finasteride (which inhibits the metabolism of testosterone to dihydrotestosterone in the prostate) may enable catheter removal without recurrent retention.

Comment

Bladder function should be assessed soon after stroke onset. The patient's abdomen should be palpated for a distended bladder. After attempted voiding, a bladder ultrasound can assess the residual bladder urine volume. If the residual volume is more than 100 mL, the bladder should be emptied regularly by attempted voiding followed by an 'in and out' urinary catheter, and the process repeated every 6–8 hours until the residual urine volume is less than 100 mL.

An indwelling catheter should be avoided if possible because it makes resolution of urinary incontinence impossible to detect and may lead to infections. If required at first, indwelling bladder catheters should be discontinued as soon as possible.

Venous Thromboembolism

Background

Largely due to impaired mobility, acute stroke patients are at risk for deep vein thrombosis (DVT). DVT can lead to pulmonary embolism (PE), which can be fatal. Development of a DVT after acute stroke can be as early as the second day, peaking between days 2 and 7 (Khan et al., 2017). Leading risk factors for DVT include impaired mobility, increasing age, and greater stroke severity. DVT above the knee (proximal) is considerably more likely to result in PE than DVT below the knee (distal). The majority of DVTs in acute stroke patients are asymptomatic (subclinical). However, both subclinical and clinical DVTs can lead to PE.

The clinical diagnosis of symptomatic DVT is often difficult due to the nonspecific nature of the symptoms and signs. The symptoms and signs of extremity DVT include local pain and tenderness, swelling, warmth, superficial venous distention, and low-grade fever. Clinical monitoring for the symptoms, high index of suspicion, and judicious use of confirmatory diagnostic tests will likely result in the highest diagnostic yield.

An accurate estimate of the prevalence of DVT in acute stroke is elusive because the reported studies include a heterogeneous group of stroke patients, diagnostic tests with diverse sensitivities and specificities, and varied prophylactic treatments. In stroke patients with immobility, reported asymptomatic DVT rates range from 10–70%, and clinically evident DVT from 2–10%. In two large British DVT prophylaxis trials where acute ischaemic stroke patients were treated primarily with stockings and aspirin, the clinical DVT rate (distal or proximal) was approximately 5% and the PE rate was approximately 1.3% (CLOTS Trials Collaboration, 2009, 2013). However, in the Get with the Guidelines-Stroke registry where 95% of acute ischaemic stroke patients received either intermittent leg compression devices or some form of prophylactic anticoagulation, the combined clinical DVT (distal or proximal) and PE rate was only 3% (Douds et al., 2014).

Evidence

Strategies to prevent DVT in acute stroke include early mobilization (including regular passive and active joint movements), hydration, compression stockings, intermittent leg compression devices, and antithrombotic drug therapy (anticoagulants and antiplatelet agents).

Compression Stockings

Two randomized trials enrolling 2615 acute stroke patients evaluated graduated thigh length compression stockings to avert DVT, with 96% of the data contributed by the large CLOTS 1 trial (CLOTS Trials Collaboration, 2009; Naccarato et al., 2010). The compression stockings did not show a statistically significant reduction in DVT compared with controls not using stockings, 15.7% versus 18.2%, OR 0.88 (95% CI: 0.72–1.08).

Intermittent Pneumatic Compression

Intermittent pneumatic compression (IPC) has been tested in 3 trials (1 large, 2 small), enrolling a total of 3053 patients (Dennis et al., 2016). IPC reduced the rate of any (asymptomatic and symptomatic) DVT, OR 0.73 (95% CI: 0.61–0.88), and tended to reduce the rate of symptomatic DVT, OR 0.73 (95% CI: 0.53–1.01). Moreover, IPC was associated with reduced mortality through 6 months, hazard ratio 0.86 (95% CI: 0.74–0.99). However, skin breaks on the legs were increased with IPC, OR 2.15 (95% CI: 1.31–3.53).

Antiplatelet Therapy

While evaluating antiplatelet therapy to prevent early progression and recurrence of acute ischaemic stroke, randomized trials have also assessed the effect of antiplatelet therapy on DVT and PE rates (Sandercock et al., 2014). DVT was assessed in 2 small trials enrolling a total of 133 patients, one assessing aspirin with dipyridamole and the other ticlopidine versus control. Early antiplatelet therapy did not statistically alter DVT rates, 24% versus 29%, OR 0.78 (95% CI: 0.36–1.67). PE was assessed in 7 trials enrolling 41,042 patients, with aspirin being the tested agent in more than 99%. PE frequency was reduced slightly with early antiplatelet therapy, 0.35% versus 0.49%, OR 0.71 (95% CI: 0.53–0.96).

Anticoagulant Therapy

Low-dose prophylactic anticoagulation versus no anticoagulation in acute ischaemic stroke patients to avert DVT or PE has been studied in 14 randomized trials, including 5 trials of unfractionated heparin (UFH), 8 trials of low-molecular-weight heparin (LMWH), and 1 trial of a heparinoid (Dennis et al., 2016). About 90% of the data are from one large trial

of UFH in which patients were enrolled regardless of mobility status. Studies did not report symptomatic DVT rates in a standardized manner. Rates of any DVT, predominantly asymptomatic, were reported in 9 small trials enrolling 785 patients, and were reduced with prophylactic anticoagulation from 50% to 17%, OR 0.21 (0.15–0.29). Rates of PE showed heterogeneity of effect by anticoagulation agent, with a smaller effect in the trial testing UFH regardless of patient mobility. In 7 trials of prophylactic dose LMWH enrolling 1090 patients, PE was reduced, 1.3% versus 3.9%, OR 0.34 (95% CI: 0.16–0.71).

Rates of symptomatic intracranial haemorrhage and extracranial bleeding were increased with anticoagulation, but nominally less so with LMWH. In 7 trials of LMWH enrolling 970 patients, increases in symptomatic intracranial haemorrhage did not reach statistical significance, 2.7% versus 1.9%, OR 1.36 (95% CI: 0.58–3.18); and in 5 LMWH trials enrolling 429 patients, no difference in extracranial bleeding was observed, 0.5% versus 0.5%, OR 1.04 (95% CI: 0.06–16.75). Although death was not altered across all trials, in 6 LMWH trials enrolling 479 patients, mortality was non-significantly increased, 11.2% versus 6.5%, OR 1.72 (95% CI: 0.92–3.37) (Dennis et al., 2016).

Newer LMWH or heparinoid agents' prophylactic doses have been compared with prophylactic UFH in 7 randomized trials in acute stroke patients. Studies did not report symptomatic DVT rates in a standardized manner. Rates of any DVT, predominantly asymptomatic, were reported in 7 trials enrolling 2585 patients, and were reduced with the newer agents compared with UFH, OR 0.55 (95% CI: 0.44–0.70). Rates of PE were evaluated in 6 trials enrolling 1250 patients and were not significantly different between LMWH and UFH, 1.2% versus 2.1%, OR 0.57 (95% CI: 0.23–1.41). Rates of symptomatic intracranial haemorrhage did not differ, but major extracranial haemorrhage was somewhat more frequent with the newer agents than UFH, 0.76% versus 0.14%, OR 3.79 (95% CI: 1.30–11.06).

In the course of evaluating high- and medium-dose anticoagulation therapy as a treatment to prevent early progression and recurrence of acute ischaemic stroke, randomized trials have also assessed the effect of these higher-dose anticoagulant regimens on venous thromboembolism outcomes (Sandercock et al., 2015). By far the largest trial was the International

Stroke Trial 1 (IST 1) (International Stroke Trial Collaborative Group, 1997). Among 14,574 randomized acute ischaemic stroke patients, 4856 were allocated to 25,000 units of UFH given subcutaneously as a fixed daily dose, and 9717 allocated to avoid heparin. DVTs were not assessed, but this medium dose UFH group had fewer PEs: 0.4% versus 0.8%, OR 0.49 (95% CI: 0.30–0.80; $p = 0.005$).

Combined use of IPC and anticoagulation for DVT prophylaxis has been shown superior to either treatment alone in high-risk general medical and surgical populations (Kakkos et al., 2016), but has not been studied in acute ischaemic stroke patients with randomized trials.

Comment

Early rehydration and passive and active movement of paretic extremities are important steps in preventing venous thromboembolism in all acute stroke patients. In patients with reduced mobility, IPC devices are beneficial in averting combined asymptomatic and symptomatic DVT and should generally be employed, though with strict surveillance of lower extremity skin integrity. IPCs are a useful component of initial therapy in both haemorrhagic and ischaemic stroke. Graduated compression stockings should be avoided, as they do not clearly confer protection against DVT and often cause patient discomfort.

Use of prophylactic, low-dose anticoagulants to avert venous thromboembolism is not recommended broadly for acute ischaemic stroke patients in current guidelines (Dennis et al., 2016; Powers et al., 2018). Beneficial effects in reducing DVT and PE are offset by increasing intracranial and extracranial haemorrhages. It is reasonable to use pharmacological thromboprophylaxis in patients who are at high risk of DVT (e.g. immobile, history of prior venous thromboembolism) and low risk of intracranial haemorrhage (e.g. small infarct less than 3 cm in diameter, no microhaemorrhages on susceptibility-weighted MRI of the brain). Subcutaneous LMWHs appear to be somewhat more effective than UFH in this setting, and may be added to hydration, passive and active limb movement, IPCs, and antiplatelet therapy.

When DVT or PE occurs, standard treatment includes full-dose anticoagulation to minimize the risk of clot propagation and embolization. However, anticoagulation therapy may be too risky for some acute stroke patients, and a risk versus benefit assessment should be carefully considered. When full-dose anticoagulation is needed but is not advisable, inferior vena cava filters can be inserted to block clots in the lower extremities from reaching the lungs. Also, pulmonary emboli can sometimes be treated with endovascular approaches, and local endovascular management may be safer than systemic anticoagulation in acute stroke.

Worsening Neurological Deficits

Worsening of neurological deficits after admission for acute ischaemic stroke occurs in approximately 10–43% of patients (Sumer et al., 2003; Weimar et al., 2005; Karepov et al., 2006; Ali and Saver, 2007). Both the multiple reasons for such worsening and the evidence supporting the different causes of worsening are shown in Table 5.1. It is useful to classify the reasons for neurological worsening as either cerebral or systemic. The cerebral causes include expanding or recurrent ischaemic stroke, malignant brain oedema, haemorrhagic conversion of an infarct, and seizure.

Expansion of brain ischaemia reflects collateral failure, clot propagation, or embolism from the initial thrombosis site, while recurrent infarction in a new territory usually reflects recurrent thromboembolism. Expansion or recurrence of brain ischaemia can be suspected by worsening of previous neurological deficits or by new neurological deficits, accompanied by evidence of new ischaemic injury within the initial vascular territory or a new vascular territory on reimaging. Malignant ischaemic brain oedema causing worsening is seen with large infarcts and is discussed in Chapter 11.

Cerebral haemorrhage after an initial infarct is confirmed by reimaging, and a useful anatomical classification includes 8 subtypes falling within 3 categories (von Kummer et al., 2015). Category 1 comprises haemorrhagic transformation within the infarcted brain tissue with no or only mild mass effect, and includes 3 subtypes: haemorrhagic infarction type 1 (HI1) – small scattered petechiae; haemorrhagic infarction type 2 (HI2) – confluent petechiae without mass effect; and parenchymal haematoma type 1 (PH1) – dense ball of blood confined to less than 30% of infarcted tissue, with no more than mild mass effect.

Category 2 comprises haemorrhagic transformation within the infarcted brain tissue, but with significant mass effects beyond the infarcted tissue. Category 2 has no subtypes: parenchymal haematoma type 2

Table 5.1 Considerations for worsening of the initial neurological deficits in acute ischaemic stroke, sometimes including a decreased level of consciousness

Causes	Examples of supportive evidence
Cerebral	
Enlarged region of brain ischaemia	New neurological deficits, increased diffusion restriction on MRI reimaging.
Brain oedema compressing nearby brain/herniation	Mass effect on brain reimaging.
Haemorrhagic transformation if infarct with mass effect	Brain haemorrhage and mass effect on reimaging.
Seizures	Rhythmic twitching or unusual behaviour, biting, incontinence, EEG showing seizure or interictal discharges; MRI may show diffusion restriction mimicking ischaemia, but the distribution is not in a defined vascular territory.
Systemic	
Infections	Fever, leucocytosis, chest or bladder symptoms, lung infiltrate on x-ray, urinalysis with high white blood cell count.
Sedating medications	Benzodiazepines, opioids.
Metabolic derangements	Hypoxaemia, hypoglycaemia, severe hyperglycaemia, severe azotaemia, hyponatraemia, hypercalcaemia.

MRI: magnetic resonance imaging. EEG: electroencephalogram.

(PH2) – dense ball of blood occupying 30% or more of the cerebral infarct, with significant mass effect.

Category 3 comprises intracranial haemorrhage outside the infarcted brain tissue and has 4 subtypes: remote intracerebral haemorrhage (RIH), intraventricular haemorrhage, subarachnoid haemorrhage, and subdural haemorrhage.

Seizures, especially new onset seizures, occur in 3–10% of patients with acute ischaemic stroke. Many seizures are manifested by obvious convulsions or rhythmic twitching movements. However, if the motor seizure activity is not witnessed and the patient is found in an impaired postictal state, the correct diagnosis can be challenging. Sometimes in a postictal state there is subtle twitching of the fingers, the face, or the eyes. Also, some seizures are non-convulsive and manifest with intermittent alterations of consciousness and unusual behaviours. Electroencephalographic monitoring in patients with unexplained confusion or stupor and suspected seizures is useful.

Many systemic or metabolic derangements, depending partly on their severity, can result in the worsening of neurological deficits (see Table 5.1). Since they often produce additional physiological stress for neuronal systems that are mediating initial reorganization and recovery, often there is worsening of the pre-existing deficits along with some decrease in level of consciousness. However, new focal neurological deficits generally do not occur.

The occurrence of neurological worsening should prompt a detailed diagnostic evaluation to determine the cause or causes, generally with immediate reimaging of brain and cerebral blood vessels as a key component. Therapy is tailored to the specific aetiologies revealed by the evaluation.

Sedation and Delirium

Background

Sedating medications should be avoided during acute stroke, as they interfere with monitoring of neurological deficits and potentially with the biology of neural reorganization. However, sedation is sometimes needed to calm patients who are on respirators, to limit motion during neuroimaging, and to manage delirium. When sedation is necessary, medication doses should be limited, and drugs with short duration of action or those that can be reversed are preferred.

Delirium, or acute confusional state, is an inability to maintain a coherent stream of thought and action. The hallmark of delirium is poor attention, and it may occur in the setting of either behavioural hyperactivity (excited delirium) or hypoactivity (quiet delirium). Agitated, hyperactive delirium represents only 25% of cases, and carries a greater risk of patient injury (Marcantonio, 2017). Delirium is distressing not only to patients but also to family and care providers and can lead to other medical complications. In a systematic review of 10 studies assessing 2004 acute stroke patients, delirium rates in individual studies ranged from 10–48%, and it was associated with a 4.7-fold increased mortality, 3.4-fold increase in discharge to long-term care institutions, and an additional 9 days added to the hospital stay (Shi et al., 2012).

Many mechanisms can contribute to delirium, including focal brain lesions disrupting alertness and attention networks, a variety of metabolic and toxic derangements, altered circadian rhythm, and pre-stroke cognitive impairment.

Evidence

There are no randomized controlled trials on the prevention and treatment of delirium specifically in acute stroke patients. However, in a broader population of hospitalized medical and surgical patients, 39 randomized trials enrolling 16,082 patients have analysed 22 interventions for delirium prevention (Siddiqi et al., 2016). Multicomponent behavioural interventions were effective in preventing delirium in hospitalized patients, while there was no clear evidence that cholinesterase inhibitors, antipsychotic medications, or melatonin reduced the occurrence of delirium.

Comment

Monitoring for the development of delirium and prompt intervention are crucial in minimizing delirium and its potential complications. Brief, validated delirium assessment measures, such as the Confusion Assessment Method (CAM), may be helpful in the intensive care unit setting. The initial management of delirium should include non-pharmacological behavioural measures, including periodic verbal reassurances and reorientation, providing rooms with windows and clocks, facilitating sensory input by using eyeglasses and hearing aids, and promoting the maintenance of a usual sleep–wake cycle to the greatest extent possible. Also, all potential reversible medical causes of delirium should be identified and corrected as soon as possible.

If behavioural management of delirium is insufficient to ensure patient protection, more intensive measures are indicated. Physical restraints, though often intended to reduce the risk of patient self-harm, are actually associated with increased injury and should be minimized. In the intensive care unit, restraints may be required to prevent the removal of endotracheal tubes and other tubes and catheters. If restraints are applied, they should be carefully monitored to reduce the risk of patient injury and discontinued as soon as the delirium has sufficiently improved.

Pharmacological therapy also may be helpful for delirium with agitation or distressing perceptual disturbances or delusional thoughts. High-potency antipsychotic agents are most commonly employed. Haloperidol is the least sedating, but confers greater risk of extrapyramidal symptoms, while olanzapine and quetiapine are more sedating, but have fewer extrapyramidal effects. Benzodiazepines, such as lorazepam, are sometimes used alone or in combination with antipsychotics. Pharmacological treatment of delirium should be initiated on an as needed basis with minimal effective drug doses. It is important to promptly discontinue the pharmacological treatments for delirium once the causes have been corrected and the delirium has resolved.

Summary

The array of supportive care therapies for stroke, delivered in an organized, systematic manner, can substantially improve outcome.

Blood oxygenation should be monitored continuously with pulse oximetry and maintained at 95% or above, using supplemental oxygen delivered noninvasively or, if needed, via mechanical ventilation. Causes of hypoxaemia should be investigated and corrected.

In the preponderance of acute stroke patients, management with head position at 30° or greater versus lying flat does not influence outcome.

In acute ischaemic stroke patients, during the first 24 hours after onset, avoiding blood pressure (BP) extremes (systolic BP [SBP] <90 mm Hg or >220 mm Hg) is prudent. More aggressive BP control (SBP ≤180 mm Hg) is appropriate for patients treated with intravenous thrombolysis. After 24 hours, gradual BP lowering towards normal range may be pursued.

Liquid management should target maintaining normovolaemia, generally with isotonic intravenous infusions initially. Hypertonic intravenous solutions may be useful in large infarcts if substantial brain oedema has developed 2–5 days post-onset, and for hyponatraemia due to cerebral salt wasting.

Moderate-intensity regulation of serum glucose levels is helpful to avert hyperglycaemic exacerbation of ischaemic injury, targeting 80–200 mg/dL. If subcutaneous insulin provides insufficient control, intravenous insulin may be used.

Bedside screening for dysphagia by nurses or physicians is recommended for all stroke patients, with initiation of oral intake in patients with retained swallowing ability, and referral to speech therapists for more detailed assessment of patients with evidence of potential dysphagia. When swallowing impairments are present, starting feeding via nasogastric tube within the first 2–3 days post-onset is reasonable. If swallowing function does not improve by 1–2 weeks, converting to percutaneous endoscopic gastrostomy (PEG) tube feeding is reasonable.

Patient temperature should be regularly monitored, and antipyretic therapy started immediately if fever is detected, with antipyretic medications and, if necessary, surface or endovascular cooling devices. Causes of fever should be investigated and redressed. Prophylactic antibiotics are not recommended, but prompt antibiotic treatment should be applied in response to specific signs of infection.

Bladder function should be monitored and, if post-void residual volume is more than 100 mL, 'in and out' urinary catheter every 6–8 hours employed. An indwelling catheter should be avoided if possible, and used for the shortest possible time if needed, to reduce infection risk.

In patients with reduced mobility, to avert deep vein thrombosis (DVT), intermittent pneumatic compression devices should generally be employed. Graduated compression stockings should be avoided. Pharmacological thromboprophylaxis is best reserved for patients with both particularly high risk of DVT (e.g. immobile, history of DVT) and low risk of intracerebral haemorrhage (e.g. small infarct, no MRI microhaemorrhages). Subcutaneous low-molecular-weight heparins (LMWHs) appear somewhat more effective than unfractionated heparin.

Should delirium, a common acute complication, develop, patients should be treated first with non-pharmacological behavioural measures. For delirium with agitation, distressing perceptual disturbances, or delusional thoughts, pharmacotherapy with high-potency antipsychotic agents, such as olanzapine or quetiapine, may be necessary, but employed for the briefest period possible.

References

Ahmed N, Wahlgren N, Brainin M, Castillo J, Ford GA, Kaste M, et al., for the SITS Investigators. (2009). Relationship of blood pressure, antihypertensive therapy, and outcome in ischaemic stroke treated with intravenous thrombolysis: retrospective analysis from Safe Implementation of Thrombolysis in Stroke-International Stroke Thrombolysis Register (SITS-ISTR). *Stroke*, **40**, 2442–9.

Al-Hazmi H. (2015). Role of duration of catheterization and length of hospital stay on the rate of catheter-related hospital-acquired urinary tract infections. *Res Rep Urol*, **7**, 41–7

Ali L, Saver JL. (2007). The ischemic stroke patient who worsens: new assessment and management approaches. *Rev Neurol Dis*, **4**, 85–91.

Anderson CS, Arima H, Lavados P, Billot L, Hackett ML, Olavarria VV, et al. (2017). Cluster-randomized, crossover trial of head positioning in acute stroke. *New Engl J Med*, **376**, 2437–47.

Aries MJ, Elting JW, Stewart R, De Keyser J, Kremer B, Vroomen P. (2013). Cerebral blood flow velocity changes during upright positioning in bed after acute stroke: an observational study. *BMJ Open*, **3**:e002960. doi:10.1136/bmjopen-2013-002960.

Aslanyan S, Weir CJ, Diener HC, Kaste M, Lees KR; GAIN International Steering Committee and Investigators. (2004). Pneumonia and urinary tract infection after acute ischemic stroke: a tertiary analysis of the GAIN International trial. *Eur J Neurol*, **11**, 49–53.

Bath PMW, Krishnan K. (2014). Interventions for deliberately altering blood pressure in acute stroke (Review). *Cochrane Database Syst Rev*, 10, CD000039. doi:10.1002/14651858.CD000039.pub3.

Bath PM, Lee HS, Everton LF. (2018). Swallowing therapy for dysphagia in acute and subacute stroke. *Cochrane Database Syst Rev*, 10. CD000323. doi:10.1002/14651858.CD000323.pub3.

Bellolio MF, Gilmore RM, Ganti L. (2014). Insulin for glycaemic control in acute ischaemic stroke. *Cochrane Database Syst Rev*, 1, CD005346. doi:10.1002/14651858.CD005346.pub4.

Bennett MH, Weibel S, Wasiak J, Schnabel A, French C, Kranke P. (2014). Hyperbaric oxygen therapy for acute ischaemic stroke. *Cochrane Database Syst Rev*, 11, CD004954. doi:10.1002/14651858.CD004954.pub3.

Bruno A, Durkalski VL, Hall CE, Juneja R, Barsan WG, Janis S, et al., on behalf of the SHINE Investigators. (2014). The Stroke Hyperglycemia Insulin Network Effort (SHINE) Trial protocol; a randomized, blinded, efficacy trial of standard versus intensive hyperglycemia management in acute stroke. *Int J Stroke*, **9**, 246–51.

Capes SE, Hunt D, Malmberg K, Pathak P, Gerstein HC. (2001). Stress hyperglycemia and prognosis of stroke in nondiabetic and diabetic patients: a systematic overview. *Stroke*, **32**, 2426–32.

Castillo J, Davalos A, Marrugat J, Noya M. (1998). Timing for fever-related brain damage in acute ischemic stroke. *Stroke*, **29**, 2455–60.

Castillo J, Leira R, García MM, Serena J, Blanco M, Dávalos A. (2004). Blood pressure decrease during the acute phase of ischemic stroke is associated with brain injury and poor stroke outcome. *Stroke*, **35**, 520–6.

Chen PC, Chuang CH, Leong CP, Guo SE, Hsin YJ. (2016). Systematic review and meta-analysis of the diagnostic accuracy of the water swallow test for screening aspiration in stroke patients. *J Adv Nurs*, **72**, 2575–86.

Chung HW, Kim SK, Kim SJ, Lee MJ, Hwang J, Seo WK, et al. (2018). Therapeutic induced hypertension in acute stroke patients with non-cardioembolic stroke: a multicenter, randomized controlled trial. *Eur Stroke J*, **3**, 7.

CLOTS Trials Collaboration. (2009). Effectiveness of thigh-length graduated compression stockings to reduce the risk of deep vein thrombosis after stroke (CLOTS trial 1): a multicenter, randomized controlled trial. *Lancet*, **373**, 1958–65.

CLOTS Trials Collaboration. (2013). Effectiveness of intermittent pneumatic compression in reduction of risk of deep vein thrombosis in patients who have had a stroke (CLOTS 3): a multicenter randomized controlled trial. *Lancet*, **382**, 516–24.

Cryer PE, Davis SN, Shamoon H. (2003). Hypoglycemia in diabetes. *Diabetes Care*, **26**, 1902–12.

Daniels SK, Ballo LA, Mahoney M-C, Foundas AL. (2000). Clinical predictors of dysphagia and aspiration risk: outcome measures in acute stroke patients. *Arch Phys Med Rehabil*, **81**, 1030–3.

den Hertog HM, van der Worp HB, Tseng MC, Dippel DWJ. (2009). Cooling therapy for acute stroke. *Cochrane Database Syst Rev*, 1, CD001247. doi:10.1002/14651858.CD001247.pub2.

Dennis M, Caso V, Kappelle LJ, Pavlovic A, Sandercock P, for the European Stroke Organisation. (2016). European Stroke Organisation (ESO) guidelines for prophylaxis for venous thromboembolism in immobile patients with acute ischaemic stroke. *Eur Stroke J*, **1**, 6–19.

de Ridder IR, den Hertog HM, van Gemert HM, Schreuder AH, Ruitenberg A, Maasland EL, et al; Trial Organization. (2017). PAIS 2 (Paracetamol [Acetaminophen] in Stroke 2): results of a randomized, double-blind placebo-controlled clinical trial. *Stroke*, 48, 977–82.

Ding J, Zhou D, Sui M, Meng R, Chandra A, Han J, et al. (2018). The effect of normobaric oxygen in patients with acute stroke: a systematic review and meta-analysis. *Neurol Res*, **40**, 433–44. doi:10.1080/01616412.2018.1454091.

Dirnagl U, Pulsinelli W. (1990). Autoregulation of cerebral blood flow in experimental focal brain ischemia. *J Cereb Blood Flow Metab*, **10**, 327–36.

Donnelly J, Budohoski KP, Smielewski P, Czosnyka M. (2016). Regulation of the cerebral circulation: bedside assessment and clinical implications. *Crit Care*, **20**, 129.

Douds GL, Hellkamp AS, DaiWai M, Olson DM, Fonarow GC, Smith EE, et al. (2014). Venous thromboembolism in the Get with the Guidelines-Stroke

acute ischemic stroke population: incidence and patterns of prophylaxis. *J Stroke Cerebrovasc*, **23**, 123–9.

Durduran T, Zhou C, Edlow BL, Yu G, Choe R, Kim MN, et al. (2009). Transcranial optical monitoring of cerebrovascular hemodynamics in acute stroke patients. *Opt Express*, **17**, 3884–902.

Dziewas R, Stellato R, van der Tweel I, Walther E, Werner CJ, Braun T, et al. (2018). Pharyngeal electrical stimulation for early decannulation in tracheotomised patients with neurogenic dysphagia after stroke (PHAST-TRAC): a prospective, single-blinded, randomised trial. *Lancet Neurol*, **17**, 849–59.

Edmiaston J, Connor LT, Steger-May K, Ford AL. (2014). A simple bedside dysphagia screen, validated against videofluoroscopy, detects dysphagia and aspiration with high sensitivity. *J Stroke Cerobrovasc Dis*, **23**, 712–16.

Famakin BM. (2014). The immune response to acute focal cerebral ischemia and associated post-stroke immunodepression: a focused review. *Aging Dis*, **5**, 307–26.

Favilla CG, Mesquita RC, Mullen M, Durduran T, Lu X, Kim MN, et al. (2014). Optical bedside monitoring of cerebral blood flow in acute ischemic stroke patients during head-of-bed manipulation. *Stroke*, **45**, 1269–74.

FOOD Trial Collaboration. (2003). Poor nutritional status on admission predicts poor outcomes after stroke: observational data from the FOOD trial. *Stroke*, **34**, 1450–6.

FOOD Trial Collaboration. (2005a). Routine oral nutritional supplementation for stroke patients in hospital (FOOD): a multi centre randomized controlled trial. *Lancet*, **365**, 755–63.

FOOD Trial Collaboration. (2005b). Effect of timing and method of enteral tube feeding for dysphagic stroke patients (FOOD): a multicentre randomized controlled trial. *Lancet*, **365**, 764–72.

Galovic M, Leisi N, Müller M. (2013). Lesion location predicts transient and extended risk of aspiration after supratentorial ischemic stroke. *Stroke*, **44**, 2760–7.

Grau AJ, Buggle F, Schnitzler P, Spiel M, Lichy C, Hacke W. (1999). Fever and infection early after ischemic stroke. *J Neurol Sci*, **171**, 115–20.

Gray CS, Hildreth AJ, Sandercock PA, O'Connell JE, Johnston DE, Cartlidge NE, et al.; GIST Trialists Collaboration. (2007). Glucose-potassium-insulin infusions in the management of post-stroke hyperglycaemia: the UK Glucose Insulin in Stroke Trial (GIST-UK). *Lancet Neurol*, **6**, 397–406.

Hansford BG, Albert D, Yang E. (2013). Classic neuroimaging findings of nonketotic hyperglycemia on computed tomography and magnetic resonance imaging with absence of typical movement disorder symptoms (hemichorea-hemiballism). *Radiology Case*, 7, 1–9.

Hillis AE, Ulatowski JA, Barker PB, Torbey M, Ziai W, Beauchamp NJ, et al. (2003). A pilot randomized trial of induced blood pressure elevation: effects on function and focal perfusion in acute and subacute stroke. *Cerebrovasc Dis*, **16**, 236–46.

Hinchey JA, Shephard T, Furie K, Smith D, Wang D, Tonn S, for the Stroke Practice Improvement Network Investigators. (2005). Formal dysphagia screening protocols prevent pneumonia. *Stroke*, 36, 1972–6.

Huang L-C, Ruge D, Tsai C-L, Wu MN, Hsu CY, Lai CL, et al. (2014). Isolated aphasic status epilepticus as initial presentation of nonketotic hyperglycemia. *Clin EEG Neurosci*, **45**, 126–8.

Indredavik B, Rohweder G, Naalsund E, Lydersen S. (2008). Medical complications in a comprehensive stroke unit and an Early Supported Discharge Service. *Stroke*, **39**, 414–20.

International Stroke Trial Collaborative Group. (1997). The International Stroke Trial (IST): a randomised trial of aspirin, subcutaneous heparin, both, or neither among 19435 patients with acute ischaemic stroke. *Lancet*, **349**, 1569–81.

Johnston KC, Bruno A, Paulis Q, Hall CE, Barrett KM, Barsan W, et al. (2019). Intensive versus standard treatment of hyperglycemia and functional outcomes in patients with acute ischemic stroke: the SHINE randomized clinical trial. *JAMA*, **322**, 326–35.

Joundi RA, Martino R, Saposnik G, Giannakeas V, Fang J, Kapral MK. (2017). Predictors of outcomes of dysphagia screening after acute ischemic stroke. *Stroke*, **48**:900–6.

Kakkos SK, Caprini JA, Geroulakos G, Nicolaides AN, Stansby G, Reddy DJ, et al. (2016). Combined intermittent pneumatic leg compression and pharmacological prophylaxis for prevention of venous thromboembolism. *Cochrane Database Syst Rev*, 9. CD005258.DOI:10.1002/14651858.CD005258.pub3.

Kalita J, Singh RK, Misra UK. (2017). Cerebral salt wasting is the most common cause of hyponatremia in stroke. *J Stroke Cerebrovasc Dis*, **26**, 1026–32.

Karepov VG, Gur AY, Bova I, Aronovich BD, Bornstein NM. (2006). Stroke-in-evolution: infarct-inherent mechanisms versus systemic causes. *Cerebrovasc Dis*, **21**, 42–6.

Khan MT, Ikram A, Saeed O, Afridi T, Sila CA, Smith MS, et al. (2017). Deep vein thrombosis in acute stroke – a systemic review of the literature. *Cureus*, **9**, e1982. doi:10.7759/cureus.1982.

Kim SH, Saver JL. (2015). Initial body temperature in ischemic stroke: nonpotentiation of tissue-type plasminogen activator benefit and inverse association with severity. *Stroke*, **46**, 132–6.

Kim TJ, Ko SB, Jeong HG, Kim CK, Kim Y, Nam K, et al. (2017). Nocturnal desaturation is associated with neurological deterioration following ischemic stroke: a retrospective observational study. *J Clin Sleep Med*, **13**, 1273–9.

Lee M, Ovbiagele B, Hong KS, Wu YL, Lee JE, Rao NM, et al. (2015). Effect of blood pressure lowering in early ischemic stroke: meta-analysis. *Stroke*, **46**, 1883–9.

Lin J, Weng Y, Li M, Mo Y, Zhao J. (2018). Hydration prevents chronic hyperglycaemic patients from neurological deterioration post-ischaemic stroke. *Acta Neurol Scand*, **137**, 557–65

Mann G, Hankey GJ, Cameron D. (1999). Swallowing function after stroke: prognosis and prognostic factors at 6 months. *Stroke*, **30**, 744–8.

Manzanares W, Aramendi I, Langlois PL, Biestro A. (2015). Hyponatremia in the neurocritical care patient: an approach based on current evidence. *Med Intensiva*, **39**, 234–43.

Marcantonio ER. (2017). Delirium in hospitalized older adults. *N Engl J Med*, **377**, 1456–66.

McCormick MT, Muir KW, Gray CS, Walters MR. (2008). Management of hyperglycemia in acute stroke: how, when, and for whom? *Stroke*, 39, 2177–85.

Middleton S, McElduff P, Ward J, Grimshaw JM, Dale S, D'Este C, et al., on behalf of the QASC Trialists Group. (2011). Implementation of evidence-based treatment protocols to manage fever, hyperglycemia, and swallowing dysfunction in acute stroke (QASC): a cluster randomized controlled trial. *Lancet*, **378**, 1699–706.

Naccarato M1, Chiodo Grandi F, Dennis M, Sandercock PA. (2010). Physical methods for preventing deep vein thrombosis in stroke. *Cochrane Database Syst Rev*, 8, CD001922. doi:10.1002/14651858.CD001922.pub3.

Palli C, Fandler S, Doppelhofer K, Niederkorn K, Enzinger C, Vetta C, et al. (2017). Early dysphagia screening by trained nurses reduces pneumonia rate in stroke patients: a clinical intervention study. *Stroke*, **48**, 2583–5.

Panfili Z, Metcalf M, Griebling TL. (2017). Contemporary evaluation and treatment of poststroke lower urinary tract dysfunction. *Urol Clin North Am*, **44**, 403–14.

Poisson SN, Johnston SC, Josephson SA. (2010). Urinary tract infections complicating stroke: Mechanisms, consequences, and possible solutions. *Stroke*, **41**, e180–4.

Powers WJ, Rabinstein AA, Ackerson T, Adeoye OM, Bambakidis NC, Becker K, et al.; American Heart Association Stroke Council. (2018). 2018 Guidelines for the early management of patients with acute ischemic stroke: a guideline for healthcare professionals from the American Heart Association/American Stroke Association. *Stroke*, **49**, e46–e110.

Prasad K, Krishnan PR. (2010). Fever is associated with doubling of odds of short-term mortality in ischemic stroke: an updated meta-analysis. *Acta Neurol Scand*, **122**, 404–8.

Rai N, Prasad K, Bhatia R, Vibha D, Singh MB, Rai VK, Kumar A. (2016). Development and implementation of acute stroke care pathway in a tertiary care hospital in India: a cluster-randomized study. *Neurol India*, **64**(suppl), S39–S45.

Reith J, Jorgensen HS, Pedersen PM, Nakayama H, Raaschou HO, Jeppesen LL, et al. (1996). Body temperature in acute stroke: relation to stroke severity, infarct size, mortality, and outcome. *Lancet*, **347**, 422–5.

RIGHT-2 Investigators. (2019). Prehospital transdermal glyceryl trinitrate in patients with ultra-acute presumed stroke (RIGHT-2): an ambulance-based, randomised, sham-controlled, blinded, phase 3 trial. *Lancet*, **393**, 1009–20.

Roffe C, Sills S, Halim H, Wilde K, Allen MB, Jones PW, et al. (2003). Unexpected nocturnal hypoxia in patients with acute stroke. Stroke, **34**, 2641–5.

Roffe C, Nevatte T, Sim J, Bishop J, Ives N, Ferdinand P, et al. (2017). Effect of routine low-dose oxygen supplementation on death and disability in adults with acute stroke: The Stroke Oxygen Study randomized clinical trial. *JAMA*, **318**, 1125–35.

Rowat A, Graham C, Dennis M. (2012). Dehydration in hospital-admitted stroke patents: Detection, frequency, and association. *Stroke*, **43**, 857–9.

Saint S, Kaufman SR, Rogers MAM, Baker PD, Ossenkop K, Lipsky BA. (2006). Condom versus indwelling urinary catheters: a randomized trial. *J Am Geriatr Soc*, **54**, 1055–61.

Sandercock PAG, Counsell C, Kane EJ. (2015). Anticoagulants for acute ischaemic stroke. *Cochrane Database Syst Rev*, 3, CD000024. doi:10.1002/14651858.CD000024.pub4.

Sandercock PAG, Counsell C, Tseng MC, Cecconi E. (2014). Oral antiplatelet therapy for acute ischaemic stroke. *Cochrane Database Syst Rev*, 3, CD000029. doi:10.1002/14651858.CD000029.pub3.

Schmidt JF, Waldemar G, Vorstrup S, Andersen AR, Gjerris F, Paulson OB. (1990). Computerised analysis of cerebral blood flow autoregulation in humans: validation of a method for pharmacologic studies. *J Cerebrovasc Pharmacol*, **15**, 983–8.

Schwarz S, Georgiadis D, Aschoff A, Schwab S. (2002). Effects of body position on intracranial pressure and cerebral perfusion in patients with large hemispheric stroke. *Stroke*, 33, 497–501.

Shi Q, Presutti R, Selchen D, Saposnik G. (2012). Delirium in acute stroke: a systematic review and meta-analysis. *Stroke*, **43**, 645–9.

Siddiqi N, Harrison JK, Clegg A, Teale EA, Young J, Taylor J, et al. (2016). Interventions for preventing delirium in hospitalised non-ICU patients. *Cochrane Database Syst Rev*, 3, CD005563. doi:10.1002/14651858.CD005563.pub3.

Stayman A, Abou-Khalil BW, Lavin P, Azar NJ. (2013). Homonymous hemianopia in nonketotic hyperglycemia is an ictal phenomenon. *Neurol Clin Pract*, **3**, 392–7.

Steiner T, Mendoza G, De Georgia M, Schellinger P, Holle R, Hacke R. (1997). Prognosis of stroke patients requiring mechanical ventilation in a neurological critical care unit. *Stroke*, 28, 711–15.

Strandgaard S, Olesen J, Skinhøj E, Lassen NA. (1973). Autoregulation of brain circulation in severe arterial hypertension. *Br Med J*, **1**, 507–10.

Strowd RE, Wabnitz A, Balakrishnan N, Craig J, Tegeler CH. (2014). Clinical reasoning: acute-onset homonymous hemianopia with hyperglycemia. *Neurology*, **82**, e129–33.

Sulter G, Elting JW, Stewart R, den Arend A, De Keyser J. (2000). Continuous pulse oximetry in acute hemiparetic stroke. *J Neurol Sci*, **179**, 65–9.

Sumer M, Ozdemir I, Erturk O. (2003). Progression in acute ischemic stroke: frequency, risk factors and prognosis. *J Clin Neurosci*, **10**, 177–80.

Suntrup S, Marian T, Schroder JB, Suttrup I, Muhle P, Oelenberg S, et al. (2015). Electrical pharyngeal stimulation for dysphagia treatment in tracheotomized stroke patients: a randomized controlled trial. *Intensive Care Med*, **41**, 1629–37.

Suwanwela NC, Chutinet A, Mayotarn S, Thanapiyachaikul R, Chaisinanunkul N, Asawavichienjinda T, et al. (2017). A randomized controlled study of intravenous fluid in acute ischemic stroke. *Clin Neurol Neurosurg*, **161**, 98–103.

Tyson SF, Nightingale P. (2004). The effects of position on oxygen saturation in acute stroke: a systematic review. *Clin Rehabil*, **18**, 863–71.

Vermeij FH, Scholte op Reimer WJM, de Man P, van Oostenbrugge RJ, Franke CL, de Jong G, et al., and the Netherlands Stroke Survey Investigators. (2009). Stroke-associated infection is an independent risk factor for poor outcome after acute ischemic stroke: data from the Netherlands Stroke Survey. *Cerebrovasc Dis*, **27**, 465–71.

Vermeij JD, Westendorp WF, Dippel DW, van de Beek D, Nederkoorn PJ. (2018). Antibiotic therapy for preventing infections in people with acute stroke. *Cochrane Database Syst Rev*, 1, CD008530. doi:10.1002/14651858.CD008530.pub3.

von Kummer R, Broderick JP, Campbell BC, Demchuk A, Goyal M, Hill MD, et al. (2015). The Heidelberg Bleeding Classification: classification of bleeding events after ischemic stroke and reperfusion therapy. *Stroke*, **46**, 2981–6.

Weimar C, Mieck T, Buchthal J, Ehrenfeld CE, Schmid E, Diener H-C, MD, for the German Stroke Study Collaboration. (2005). Neurologic worsening during the acute phase of ischemic stroke. *Arch Neurol*, **62**, 393–7.

Williams LS, Rotich J, Qi R, Fineberg A, Espay A, Bruno SE, et al. (2002). Effects of admission hyperglycemia on mortality and costs in acute ischemic stroke. *Neurology*, **59**, 67–71.

Wojner-Alexandrov AW, Garami Z, Chernyshev OY, Alexandrov AV. (2005). Heads down: flat positioning improves blood flow velocity in acute ischemic stroke. *Neurology*, **64**, 1354–7.

Ye Q, Xie Y, Shi J, Xu Z, Ou A, Xu N. (2017). Systematic review on acupuncture for treatment of dysphagia after stroke. *Evid Based Complement Alternat Med*, 6421852. doi:10.1155/2017/6421852.

Yoo SH, Kim JS, Kwon SU, Yun SC, Koh JY, Kang DW. (2008). Undernutrition as a predictor of poor clinical outcomes in acute ischemic stroke patients. *Arch Neurol*, **65**, 39–43.

Chapter 6

Reperfusion of Ischaemic Brain by Intravenous Thrombolysis

Jeffrey L. Saver

Joanna Wardlaw

Rationale

About 70% of all strokes worldwide are caused by occlusion of a cerebral artery, resulting in focal brain infarction (ischaemic stroke) (Feigin et al., 2017). The obstruction is usually a thrombus that has formed *in situ* on an atherosclerotic plaque or a thrombus that has embolized from a proximal source such as the extracranial neck vessels, the aortic arch, the heart, and the leg and pelvic veins.

When a thrombus forms or lodges in an artery, plasminogen, a precursor of plasmin, binds to the fibrin strands encasing the platelets and red blood cells in the clot. Endogenous tissue plasminogen activator (tPA), which is naturally made by endothelial cells, cleaves local plasminogen, thereby releasing active plasmin. The plasmin, in turn, breaks down cross-linked fibrin into soluble fibrin degradation products, lysing the clot. Frequently, however, such spontaneous lysis of the thrombus and recanalization of the artery do not occur until after the ischaemic brain has become fully infarcted.

Exogenous thrombolysis (or, more correctly, fibrinolysis) aims to rapidly restore blood flow by lysing fresh thrombi (*in situ* or embolic) which underpin many, but not all, ischaemic strokes, before all the ischaemic brain in the territory supplied by the artery has become infarcted. However, although some emboli consist of fresh thrombus, which is highly lysable by fibrinolysis, others are older, organized thrombi, which are less responsive, and others are non-lysable substances such as calcium, bacteria, tumour, and prosthetic material. Hence, not all ischaemic stroke is likely to respond to reperfusion by thrombolysis.

Evidence

Study Designs and Patients

A total of 29 randomized controlled trials (RCTs) comparing intravenous (IV) fibrinolytic treatment with non-fibrinolytic management within the first hours after onset of ischaemic stroke, in 10,903 patients, were reported between 1995 and 2019 (Wardlaw et al., 2014; von Kummer et al., 2016; Lorenzano and Toni, 2017; Khatri et al., 2018; Ma et al., 2019). All patients underwent computed tomography (CT) or magnetic resonance imaging (MRI) brain scan before randomization to exclude non-stroke disorders and haemorrhagic stroke, including 2994 patients (15 trials) treated identifiably within 3 hours and 6221 patients (10 trials) treated identifiably between 3 and 6 hours of stroke onset.

The RCT data with supportive care control arms were acquired over a broad, 25-year period, during which supportive medical management was evolving, including increasing delivery of supportive medical care on dedicated stroke units. More than one-quarter of the patients, and the preponderance of patients over 80 years of age, come from the later Third International Stroke Trial (IST-3). While several trials were fully double-blind, others used open label treatment with outcome assessment by blinded observers. The great preponderance of studies (28 trials, 10,589 patients) enrolled only or predominantly patients with disabling deficits at presentation; a single trial (313 patients) evaluated only patients with non-disabling deficits at presentation.

In addition to trials with non-lysis control arms, 20 RCTs, enrolling 6873 patients, have compared different IV fibrinolytic agents or doses against one another (Pancioli et al., 2008, 2013; Wardlaw et al., 2013; Saqqur et al., 2014; Mori et al., 2015, Anderson et al., 2016; Huang et al., 2016; Logallo et al., 2017; Campbell and E-IT Investigators, 2018), and 9 trials, enrolling 2269 patients, have compared therapies to enhance thrombolysis, including adding antithrombotics or ultrasound to IV fibrinolytics versus IV fibrinolytics alone (Pancioli et al., 2008, 2013; Saqqur et al., 2014; Wardlaw et al., 2014; Alexandrov et al., 2016; Anderson et al., 2016; Huang et al., 2016; Nacu et al., 2017).

Complementing broad study-level meta-analyses, an individual patient-level data systematic analysis, permitting more detailed adjustment for prognostic variables, has analysed 9 trials of IV tPA versus non-lytic controls, enrolling 6756 patients (Emberson et al., 2014; Lees et al., 2016).

Interventions

In trials with non-lysis control arms, the thrombolytic agents tested were urokinase (UK), streptokinase (SK), recombinant tissue plasminogen activator (rt-PA), and desmoteplase. About three-quarters of the patients come from the 18 RCTs testing IV rt-PA.

In trials comparing different doses, IV rt-PA was the most studied agent, investigated in 6 trials. Agents tested in trials comparing one fibrinolyic agent against another included UK, tissue-cultured UK, rt-PA, and tenecteplase. Agents tested in RCTs evaluating fibrinolytic-enhancing concomitant therapies included aspirin, the glycoprotein IIb/IIIa agent eptifibatide, the direct thrombin inhibitor argotroban, and external ultrasound with or without ultrasound-responsive lipid microspheres.

Results for Patients with Disabling Deficits, Only or Predominantly: All Thrombolytic Agents against Non-lysis Controls

Alive and Disability-free at (or near) 3–6 Months

Overall, among patients with only or predominantly disabling deficits treated up to 9 hours after ischaemic stroke, random allocation to thrombolytic therapy was associated with an increase in alive and disability-free outcome (modified Rankin Scale [mRS] 0–1) at (or near) 3–6 months after randomization (35.1% thrombolysis, 28.8% control; risk ratio [RR] 1.21, 95% confidence interval [CI]: 1.14–1.28; $P < 0.00001$. This represents 63 more disability-free patients per 1000 treated with thrombolysis compared with control (Figure 6.1). There was low heterogeneity of treatment effect across the 4 different agents ($I^2 = 4.2\%$, $P = 0.37$), indicating that the favourable treatment effect was qualitatively similar in all 4 agent

subgroups. There was mild heterogeneity of treatment effect among the individual trials ($I^2 = 19\%$, $P = 0.20$) that visual inspection suggested was driven by larger treatment effects in trials with earlier start of thrombolytic therapy.

Alive and Functionally Independent at (or near) 3–6 Months

Thrombolysis within 9 hours after ischaemic stroke was also associated with an increase in alive and functional independent outcome (mRS 0–2) at (or near) 3–6 months after randomization (47.5% thrombolysis, 43.0% control; RR 1.09, 95% CI: 1.04–1.13; $P < 0.0001$). This represents 45 more functionally independent patients per 1000 treated with thrombolysis compared with control (Figure 6.2). There was no significant heterogeneity of the treatment effect, either across the 4 different agents ($I^2 = 0\%$, $P = 0.67$) or across individual trials ($I^2 = 2\%$, $P = 0.44$).

Death by 3–6 Months

By (or near) 3–6 months, patients allocated thrombolytic therapy had an increased frequency of death (18.3% thrombolysis, 17.3% control; RR 1.13, 95% CI: 1.02–1.25; $P = 0.02$), representing an extra 10 deaths per 1000 patients treated with thrombolysis compared with control (Figure 6.3). There was moderate heterogeneity across the 4 agent groups ($I^2 = 36.0\%$, $P = 0.20$) and among individual trials ($I^2 = 35\%$, $P = 0.04$) (see agent comparison section below for more details). Across all 17 trials using IV rt-PA, no excess of mortality was noted (RR 1.07, 95% CI: 0.95–1.20). In the trials using SK, there was an excess of deaths (RR 1.43, 95% CI: 1.10–1.88) (further discussed in the section on different agents below).

Early Symptomatic Intracranial Haemorrhage

Thrombolytic therapy was associated with an increase in early symptomatic intracranial haemorrhage, within 7–10 days of treatment (7.2% thrombolysis, 1.9% control; RR 3.79, 95% CI: 3.06–4.70; $P < 0.00001$), equivalent to an excess of 53 symptomatic intracranial haemorrhages per 1000 patients treated (Figure 6.4). There was moderate heterogeneity between thrombolytic agent classes ($I^2 = 57.2\%$, $P = 0.07$) and individual trials ($I^2 = 40\%$, $P = 0.02$) (further discussed in the section on different agents below).

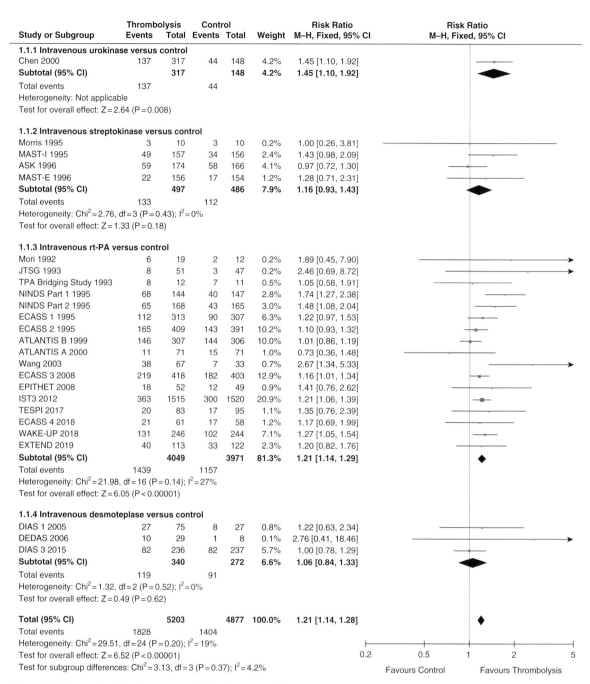

Figure 6.1 *Alive and disability-free outcome (mRS 0–1) at 3–6 months, IV Lytics vs Controls,* all trials enrolling patients with disabling deficits, only or predominantly, and treatment start within 9 hours (h) of onset.

Degree of Disability at (or near) 3–6 Months

Analyses of dichotomized outcomes consider only a single health state transition that treatment may affect. For example, the outcome of being alive and disability-free *counts* only transitions across the border between mRS level 2 and mRS level 1, while the outcome of being alive and independent counts only transitions between mRS level 3 and

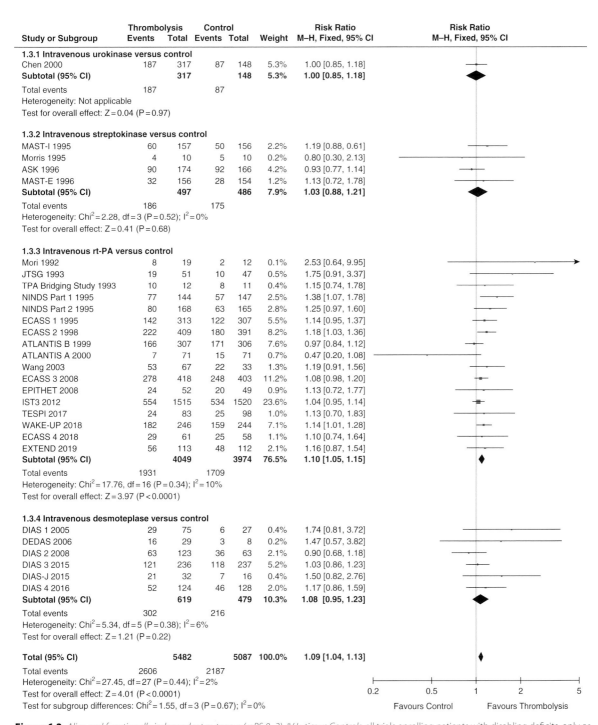

Study or Subgroup	Thrombolysis Events	Total	Control Events	Total	Weight	Risk Ratio M–H, Fixed, 95% CI
1.3.1 Intravenous urokinase versus control						
Chen 2000	187	317	87	148	5.3%	1.00 [0.85, 1.18]
Subtotal (95% CI)		317		148	5.3%	1.00 [0.85, 1.18]
Total events	187		87			
Heterogeneity: Not applicable						
Test for overall effect: Z = 0.04 (P = 0.97)						
1.3.2 Intravenous streptokinase versus control						
MAST-I 1995	60	157	50	156	2.2%	1.19 [0.88, 0.61]
Morris 1995	4	10	5	10	0.2%	0.80 [0.30, 2.13]
ASK 1996	90	174	92	166	4.2%	0.93 [0.77, 1.14]
MAST-E 1996	32	156	28	154	1.2%	1.13 [0.72, 1.78]
Subtotal (95% CI)		497		486	7.9%	1.03 [0.88, 1.21]
Total events	186		175			
Heterogeneity: Chi² = 2.28, df = 3 (P = 0.52); I² = 0%						
Test for overall effect: Z = 0.41 (P = 0.68)						
1.3.3 Intravenous rt-PA versus control						
Mori 1992	8	19	2	12	0.1%	2.53 [0.64, 9.95]
JTSG 1993	19	51	10	47	0.5%	1.75 [0.91, 3.37]
TPA Bridging Study 1993	10	12	8	11	0.4%	1.15 [0.74, 1.78]
NINDS Part 1 1995	77	144	57	147	2.5%	1.38 [1.07, 1.78]
NINDS Part 2 1995	80	168	63	165	2.8%	1.25 [0.97, 1.60]
ECASS 1 1995	142	313	122	307	5.5%	1.14 [0.95, 1.37]
ECASS 2 1998	222	409	180	391	8.2%	1.18 [1.03, 1.36]
ATLANTIS B 1999	166	307	171	306	7.6%	0.97 [0.84, 1.12]
ATLANTIS A 2000	7	71	15	71	0.7%	0.47 [0.20, 1.08]
Wang 2003	53	67	22	33	1.3%	1.19 [0.91, 1.56]
ECASS 3 2008	278	418	248	403	11.2%	1.08 [0.98, 1.20]
EPITHET 2008	24	52	20	49	0.9%	1.13 [0.72, 1.77]
IST3 2012	554	1515	534	1520	23.6%	1.04 [0.95, 1.14]
TESPI 2017	24	83	25	98	1.0%	1.13 [0.70, 1.83]
WAKE-UP 2018	182	246	159	244	7.1%	1.14 [1.01, 1.28]
ECASS 4 2018	29	61	25	58	1.1%	1.10 [0.74, 1.64]
EXTEND 2019	56	113	48	112	2.1%	1.16 [0.87, 1.54]
Subtotal (95% CI)		4049		3974	76.5%	1.10 [1.05, 1.15]
Total events	1931		1709			
Heterogeneity: Chi² = 17.76, df = 16 (P = 0.34); I² = 10%						
Test for overall effect: Z = 3.97 (P < 0.0001)						
1.3.4 Intravenous desmoteplase versus control						
DIAS 1 2005	29	75	6	27	0.4%	1.74 [0.81, 3.72]
DEDAS 2006	16	29	3	8	0.2%	1.47 [0.57, 3.82]
DIAS 2 2008	63	123	36	63	2.1%	0.90 [0.68, 1.18]
DIAS 3 2015	121	236	118	237	5.2%	1.03 [0.86, 1.23]
DIAS-J 2015	21	32	7	16	0.4%	1.50 [0.82, 2.76]
DIAS 4 2016	52	124	46	128	2.0%	1.17 [0.86, 1.59]
Subtotal (95% CI)		619		479	10.3%	1.08 [0.95, 1.23]
Total events	302		216			
Heterogeneity: Chi² = 5.34, df = 5 (P = 0.38); I² = 6%						
Test for overall effect: Z = 1.21 (P = 0.22)						
Total (95% CI)		5482		5087	100.0%	1.09 [1.04, 1.13]
Total events	2606		2187			
Heterogeneity: Chi² = 27.45, df = 27 (P = 0.44); I² = 2%						
Test for overall effect: Z = 4.01 (P < 0.0001)						
Test for subgroup differences: Chi² = 1.55, df = 3 (P = 0.67); I² = 0%						

Favours Control   Favours Thrombolysis

Figure 6.2 *Alive and functionally independent outcome (mRS 0–2), IV Lytics vs Controls,* all trials enrolling patients with disabling deficits, only or predominantly, and treatment start within 9 h of onset.

mRS level 2. In contrast, analyses of ordinal outcomes consider simultaneously multiple valuable health state transitions that treatment may affect (Saver, 2011; Bath et al., 2012). For example, analyses of the distribution of outcomes over the entire mRS count all transitions across all 7 degrees of

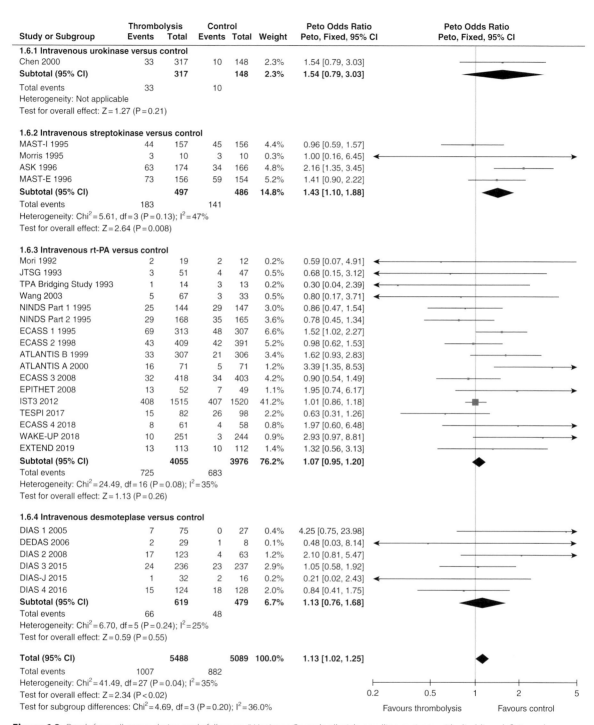

Figure 6.3 *Death from all causes during study follow-up, IV Lytics vs Controls,* all trials enrolling patients with disabling deficits, only or predominantly, and treatment start within 9 h of onset.

post-stroke disability that the scale assesses, from asymptomatic, through varying degrees of impairment, to death. While systematic analyses of the distribution of disability outcomes have not been performed for all lytic agents, an analysis is available for IV rt-PA (discussed below).

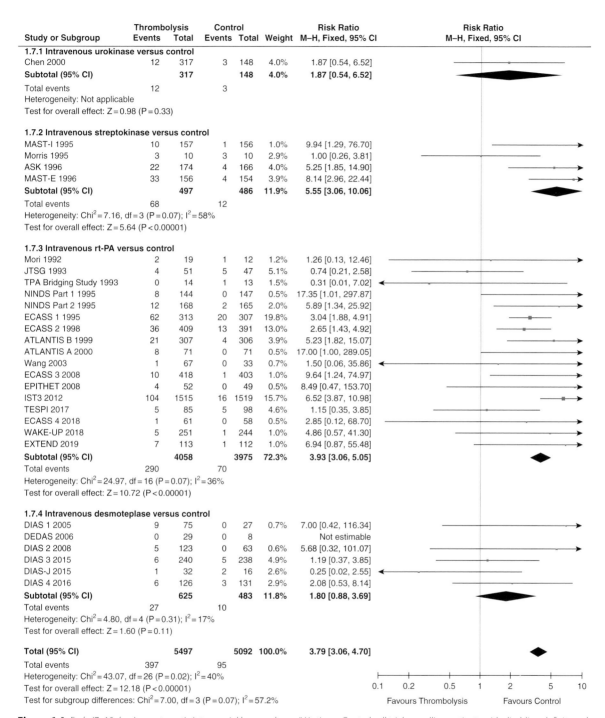

Figure 6.4 *Early (7–10 days) symptomatic intracranial haemorrhage, IV Lytics vs Controls,* all trials enrolling patients with disabling deficits, only or predominantly, and treatment start within 9 h of onset.

Results for Patients with Non-disabling Deficits: All Thrombolytic Agents against Non-lysis Controls

The single RCT enrolling only patients with non-disabling deficits at presentation (PRISMS) tested IV rt-PA versus control in 313 patients who started treatment within 3 hours (Khatri et al., 2018). The control patients had generally very good outcomes at 3 months, limiting the opportunity for lytic intervention to improve outcome. No differences were noted with IV rt-PA for freedom from disability (mRS 0–1) at 90 days, 78.2% versus 81.5%, RR 0.98 (95% CI: 0.81–1.18, $P = 0.81$); mortality, 0.6% versus 0.0% ($P = 0.50$); or symptomatic intracerebral haemorrhage, 1.3% versus 0.0% ($P = 0.30$).

Results for Patients Treated with Different Thrombolytic Drugs, Doses, or Concomitant Therapies

Results for Patients Treated with Different Thrombolytic Drugs

Different IV thrombolytic agents have been compared against control and against one another. Direct, head-to-head comparisons of agents (rt-PA vs UK; tissue-cultured UK vs conventional UK; tenecteplase vs rt-PA) were undertaken in 8 trials, enrolling 2281 patients (Wardlaw et al., 2013; Huang et al., 2016; Logallo et al., 2017; Campbell and E-IT Investigators, 2018). Overall, no statistically significant difference was shown between different thrombolytic drugs tested. However, among patients with CT- or MR-confirmed large or medium artery target occlusions, tenecteplase, compared with rt-PA, was associated with higher rates of reperfusion and reduced death or disabled outcomes (as detailed below).

Indirect comparisons of outcomes in 11 RCTs of different thrombolytic agents (urokinase, SK, rt-PA, and desmoteplase) versus control also found no significant between-agent difference in the effect of the thrombolytic drugs on death or disability (mRS 2–6) or death or dependence (mRS 3–6) (Wardlaw et al., 2014). In indirect comparisons, for death by 3–6 months there was moderate heterogeneity across the 4 agent groups ($I^2 = 37.5\%$, $P = 0.19$) and among individual trials ($I^2 = 37\%$, $P = 0.03$) (see Figure 6.3).

Visual inspection suggested the heterogeneity arose from an increased mortality rate with active treatment in SK trials. The other 3 agents had formally neutral effect on mortality, while in the trials using SK there was an excess of deaths (RR 1.43, 95% CI: 1.10–1.88). Similarly, SK produced the greatest increase in symptomatic intracerebral haemorrhage (see Figure 6.4). Although potentially related to intrinsic properties of SK, these disparate safety effects may well instead be related to the higher relative dosages employed and the more frequent use of concomitant antiplatelet and anticoagulant therapy in the SK trials.

Recombinant Tissue Plasminogen Activator

Recombinant tissue plasminogen activator is a recombinant protein corresponding to a natural plasminogen activator found on human endothelial cells. It has high fibrin specificity, and free rt-PA in the serum has a short, 4-minute half-life, though bound rt-PA is active substantially longer.

Intravenous rt-PA has been compared with non-lytic controls in 18 trials (n = 8347 patients) enrolling acute ischaemic stroke patients treated up to 9 hours, including 17 trials (8034 patients) enrolling only or predominantly patients with disabling deficits at presentation, and a single trial (313 patients) enrolling only patients with non-disabling deficits at presentation. Among patients presenting only or predominantly with disabling deficits, treatment with IV rt-PA was associated with increased alive and disability-free (mRS 0–1) outcome, RR 1.21 (95% CI: 1.14–1.29, $P < 0.00001$), increased alive and independent (mRS 0–2) outcome, RR 1.10 (95% CI: 1.05–1.15, $P < 0.0001$), no alteration in deaths, RR 1.07 (95% CI: 0.95–1.20), and an increase in symptomatic intracerebral haemorrhages, RR 3.93 (95% CI: 3.06–5.05, $P < 0.00001$). This represents, per 1000 patients treated with rt-PA compared with control, 64 more patients alive and disability-free at long-term follow-up, 45 more patients alive and independent at long-term follow-up, no significant change in death, and 54 more patients with early symptomatic haemorrhage. There was mild heterogeneity across individual trials for alive and disability-free ($I^2 = 27\%$, $P = 0.14$), death ($I^2 = 35\%$, $P = 0.08$), and symptomatic haemorrhage ($I^2 = 36\%$, $P = 0.07$), which visual inspection suggested was driven by larger benefits and fewer harms in trials with earlier start of thrombolytic therapy.

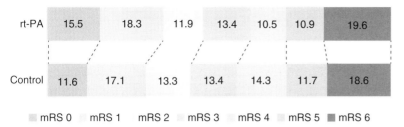

| rt-PA | 15.5 | 18.3 | 11.9 | 13.4 | 10.5 | 10.9 | 19.6 |
| Control | 11.6 | 17.1 | 13.3 | 13.4 | 14.3 | 11.7 | 18.6 |

■ mRS 0　　■ mRS 1　　■ mRS 2　　■ mRS 3　　■ mRS 4　　■ mRS 5　　■ mRS 6

Figure 6.5 *Level of disability at 3–6 months, IV rt-PA versus Control,* pooled trial analysis.
Outcome distribution is based on a pooled analysis of 6756 patients (3391 rt-PA, 3365 control), adjusted for age, presenting deficit severity, and onset to treatment time.

An analysis has been conducted of the effect of rt-PA on the distribution of patient outcomes across all 7 levels of disability assessed by the mRS, incorporating individual participant-level data on 6756 patients from 9 randomized trials (Lees et al., 2016) (Figure 6.5). In these trials, allocation to IV tPA resulted in increased nominal proportions of patients at long-term follow-up who were asymptomatic (mRS 0), alive and disability-free (mRS 0–1), alive and independent (mRS 0–2), and alive and ambulatory (mRS 0–3), with no change in the proportions of patients who were alive and not requiring continuous care (mRS 0–4) or alive (mRS 0–5) (Figure 6.5). Overall, treatment with IV rt-PA yielded a lower final degree of disability compared with control (Mann–Whitney test, $P < 0.004$). Using the automated algorithmic min–max joint outcome table method (Saver et al., 2009), the treatment group outcomes indicate that, for every 1000 patients treated with IV tPA, a net of 121 patients will have a lower level of long-term disability as a result.

Desmoteplase

Recombinant desmodus salivary plasminogen activator a-1 (desmoteplase) is a recombinant protein corresponding to a natural plasminogen activator from the vampire bat (*Desmodus rotundus*). It is theoretically attractive because of its high fibrin specificity, nonactivation by 13-amyloid, long terminal half-life, and absence of neurotoxicity compared with rt-PA (Liberatore et al., 2003; Reddrop et al., 2005). Desmoteplase has been evaluated compared with non-fibrinolytic controls in 6 trials enrolling 1108 patients, predominantly later than 3 hours after onset, with imaging findings suggesting still-salvageable tissue based on relatively small infarct cores accompanied by larger regions of hypoperfusion or evidence of large or medium artery occlusion. Over the full 7-level mRS, a non-significant favourable trend was noted toward reduced level of disability with desmoteplase therapy (3 trials, common odds ratio [cOR] 1.19, 95% CI: 0.92–1.53; $P = 0.18$). Dichotomous endpoints did not show major differences for outcomes of alive and disability-free (mRS 0–1), RR 1.06 (95% CI: 0.84–1.33), alive and independent (mRS 0–2), RR 1.07 (95% CI: 0.93–1.23), or mortality, RR 1.13 (95% CI: 0.76–1.68) (see Figures 6.1, 6.2, 6.3). A non-significant trend towards increased symptomatic intracranial haemorrhage was present, RR 3.76 (95% CI: 3.03–4.66; $P = 0.11$) (see Figure 6.4).

Tenecteplase

Tenecteplase is a genetically engineered variant of the rt-PA molecule, with three mutations introduced to yield increased plasma half-life, resistance to plasminogen-activator inhibitor 1, and fibrinolytic potency against platelet-rich thrombi. Compared with rt-PA, tenecteplase has greater fibrin specificity and can be delivered as a single bolus IV injection, rather than continuous infusion. Five randomized trials, enrolling a total of 1593 acute ischaemic stroke patients, have compared tenecteplase at varying doses with rt-PA. The largest trial, NOR-TEST, compared tenecteplase at a dose of 0.4 mg/kg to rt-PA in 1107 acute ischaemic stroke patients within 4.5 hours of symptom onset (Hughes, 2017). No difference was noted in outcomes of alive and disability-free (mRS 0–1) at 3 months (tenecteplase 64.5%, alteplase 62.6%, OR 1.08, 95% CI: 0.84–1.38) or in symptomatic intracerebral haemorrhage (2.7% vs 2.4%, OR 1.16, 95% CI: 0.51–2.68). However, enrolled patients had quite mild deficits at entry (median National Institutes of Health Stroke Scale [NIHSS] score 4.0), placing a ceiling on attainable improvements and also indicating that many patients likely had small vessel occlusions with minimal target clot volumes, likely to respond well to any lytic agent. Patients in whom CT or MR angiography confirms the presence of a large or medium vessel occlusion (LVO or MVO) prior to therapy start may be more likely to exhibit differential responses to different lytic agents. Three trials have enrolled 271 such patients, allocated to a lower tenecteplase dose of 0.25 mg/kg (138 patients) compared with standard-dose rt-PA (133 patients) (Bivard et al., 2017; Campbell and E-IT Investigators, 2018). In fixed effects combined analysis, tenecteplase was associated with increased revascularization, (34.8% vs 17.3%, OR 2.55, 95% CI: 1.44–4.51); reduced death and disability (51.6% vs 63.2%, OR 0.62, 95% CI: 0.38–1.00); reduced death and dependency (38.5% vs 54.7%, OR 0.51, 95% CI 0.32–0.83); reduced mortality (11.0% vs 17.4%, OR 0.58, 95% CI: 0.29–1.17); and unchanged low symptomatic haemorrhage rate (0.7% vs 1.5%, OR 0.48, 95% CI: 0.04–5.34).

Results for Patients Treated with Different Thrombolytic Doses

Different doses (of rt-PA, UK, desmoteplase, or tenecteplase) were compared in 15 trials (n = 4775 patients), including one large trial enrolling 3310 patients that compared a standard 0.9 mg/kg dose of rt-PA with a lower 0.6 mg/kg dose (Wardlaw et al., 2013; Anderson et al., 2016). Since all trials testing SK used the same dose, it was not possible to compare doses for SK. A higher dose of thrombolytic therapy, compared with a lower dose of the same agent, was associated with higher rates of symptomatic intracerebral haemorrhage (2.9% vs 1.6%, OR 1.78, 95% CI: 1.19–2.66; $P = 0.006$) and death by end of follow-up (10.0% vs 8.2%, OR 1.25, 95% CI: 1.02–1.53; $P = 0.03$), but no difference in rates of combined death or dependency (mRS 3–6) (58.6% vs 58.6%, OR 1.00, 95% CI: 0.88–1.14; $P = 1.00$). These analyses confirm that higher doses of thrombolytic agents lead to higher rates of bleeding and increased fatal outcome.

The ENCHANTED trial, comparing standard-dose (0.9 mg/kg) to low-dose (0.6 mg/kg) rt-PA, suggests that, within the range of effective doses, higher doses may have a bidirectional effect, increasing good outcomes (presumably by increasing reperfusion rates) but also increasing poor outcomes (through increased major intracerebral haemorrhage). With standard dose compared with low dose, rates of alive and disability-free outcome at 3 months were non-significantly increased, 48.9% versus 46.8% (OR 1.09, 95% CI: 0.95–1.25), but rates of death were also non-significantly increased, 10.3% versus 8.5% (OR 1.25, 95% CI: 0.99–1.58).

Results for Patients Treated with Different Concomitant Therapies

Antithrombotic Therapy Started at Same Time as Thrombolysis

Concomitant antithrombotic drugs given at the same time, or soon after, IVT potentially can improve recanalization and deter re-occlusion, but also can increase bleeding complications. Randomized trials have evaluated antiplatelet (aspirin, eptifibatide) and anticoagulant (argatroban) agents as concomitant therapies with fibrinolysis.

Aspirin added to IVT has been evaluated in two randomized trials. In the MAST-I trial, under a 2×2 factorial design, patients were randomized within 6 hours of onset to SK plus aspirin, SK alone, aspirin alone, or neither. Among 156 SK plus aspirin patients versus 157 SK alone patients, no benefit was noted in functional independence (mRS 0–2) at 6 months (37% vs 38%). Conversely, harm was observed in death by 6 months (44% vs 28%, RR 1.56, 95% CI: 1.14–2.12; $P = 0.005$), likely related to an increase in haemorrhagic transformation (not able to be fully assessed due to patient deaths before re-imaging) (Ciccone et al., 2000). In the ARTIS trial, 640 patients were randomized to added IV aspirin 300 mg within 90 minutes of start of standard-dose rt-PA or rt-PA alone. Aspirin did not change the frequency of alive and independent outcome (54.0% with ASA+IV rt-PA vs 57.2% with IV tPA alone, OR 0.91, 95% CI: 0.66–1.26; $P = 0.58$) or death (11.2% vs 9.7%, OR 1.17, 95% CI: 0.71–1.95; $P = 0.54$), but did increase the frequency of symptomatic intracranial haemorrhage (4.3% vs 1.6%, OR 2.86, 95% CI: 1.02–8.05; $P = 0.04$) (Zinkstok et al., 2012). These findings support the avoidance of routine aspirin therapy for the first 24 hours after fibrinolytic treatment.

Eptifibatide, a platelet glycoprotein 2b/3a inhibitor antiplatelet agent, was studied as a concomitant therapy to IV rt-PA in 3 trials, 2 randomized and 1 with historic controls, assigning 197 patients to combined therapy and 50 to IV rt-PA alone (Pancioli et al., 2008, 2013; Adeoye et al., 2015). The studies compared escalating doses of eptifibatide (75 μg/kg bolus or 135 μg/kg bolus, followed by 0.75 μg/kg infusion for 2 h) combined with escalating doses of IV rt-PA (0.3, 0.45, 0.6, and 0.9 mg/kg) versus standard-dose IV rt-PA (0.9 mg/kg). The regimen judged most promising to proceed to future larger trials was eptifibatide at the higher bolus dose added to standard-dose IV rt-PA (at a median 37 min after start of IV rt-PA), which had an acceptable symptomatic intracerebral haemorrhage (SICH) rate compared with historic IV rt-PA only controls (3.7% vs 10.0%, OR 0.35, 95% CI: 0.38–3.13).

Argatroban, a direct thrombin inhibitor anticoagulant, was studied in a pilot, dose-escalation randomized trial comparing low- and high-dose argatroban added to standard-dose IV rt-PA to IV rt-PA alone (Barreto et al., 2012). Argatroban was given as a 100 μg/kg bolus (median 60 min after IV rt-PA), followed by a 48-hour infusion adjusted to achieve a partial thromboplastin time of 1.75 × baseline in the low-dose group and 2.25 × baseline in the high-dose group. Among the 61 patients in the two argatroban plus rt-PA arms, compared with the 29 patients in the rt-PA alone arm, argatroban added to rt-PA was associated with non-significantly higher rates of alive and disability-free (mRS 0–1) outcome (31% vs 21%, R 1.57, 95% CI: 0.7–3.3; $P = 0.24$) but also higher SICH (4.9% vs 0%, $P = 0.55$).

Previous Antithrombotic Therapy at Time of Start of Thrombolysis

Different manners of reporting preclude formal meta-analysis of patients taking antiplatelet therapy at baseline prior to onset of ischaemic stroke and enrolment in a randomized trial of IV fibrinolysis (Wardlaw et al., 2014). However, salient information is available from individual trials. In the two NINDS-tPA Study trials, the ECASS 3 trial and the IST-3 trial, a total of 2037 of 4466 (56.6%) enrolled patients were taking antiplatelet therapy prior to stroke onset, predominantly aspirin. In each trial, pretreatment antiplatelet therapy did not modify the effect of alteplase upon rates of alive and independent outcome (NINDS t-PA Stroke Trial Study Group, 1997; Bluhmki et al., 2009; Lindley et al., 2015). While pretreatment antiplatelet therapy did not increase the risk of ICH in the 3 early window trials, NINDS-tPA Part 1, NINDS-tPA Part 2, and ECASS 3, it was associated with increased SICH in the 6-hour window IST-3 trial (interaction P-value = 0.02). In IST-3, among patients without pretreatment antiplatelet therapy, SICH occurred in 4.6% treated with rt-PA versus 1.4% of patients treated without IV rt-PA (OR 3.46, 95% CI: 1.35–8.86). Among patients with pretreatment antiplatelet therapy, SICH occurred in 9.0% treated with rt-PA versus 0.8% of patients treated without IV rt-PA (OR 13.26, 95% CI: 4.38–40.14). In the ECASS 3 trial, pretreatment antiplatelet therapy did not modify the risk of death at end of follow-up.

These findings from individual trials are supported by a meta-analysis of 7 confounder-adjusted observational studies, analysing 58,059 patients treated with IV rt-PA, among whom 47.6% had prior antiplatelet therapy. Prior antiplatelet therapy was associated with increased SICH (OR 1.21, 95% CI: 1.02–1.44), but no change in favourable functional outcome (OR 1.09, 95% CI: 0.96–1.24) or death at end of follow-up (OR 1.02, 95% CI: 0.98–1.07) (Luo et al., 2016). Accordingly, both trial and observational data indicate that, although patients with prior antiplatelet therapy have a potentiated risk of SICH associated with IV rt-PA within 4.5 hours of onset, they nonetheless experience the same long-term benefit upon favourable functional outcomes and the same neutral effect upon death at the end of follow-up from fibrinolysis as do antiplatelet-naïve patients.

Patients with prior anticoagulant therapy in therapeutic range at time of stroke onset were generally excluded from clinical trials testing IV thrombolysis (IVT), due to concern regarding elevated bleeding risk. Observational series have compared IVT among patients not taking warfarin and patients taking warfarin but with subtherapeutically achieved anticoagulation, generally international normalized ratio below 1.7. In unadjusted analysis of 11 studies analysing 79,357 patients, patients receiving prior subtherapeutic warfarin therapy (present in 5%), compared with no prior warfarin therapy, had increased frequency of SICH (5.7% vs 4.3%, OR 1.33, 95% CI: 1.16–1.53; $P < 0.0001$) (Diener et al., 2013; Seiffge et al., 2015; Xian et al., 2017a). But patients taking oral anticoagulants differ in several other features from non-anticoagulated patients. In each of the three largest studies, collectively enrolling 74,769 IV fibrinolysis patients, the increased risk of SICH among patients with subtherapeutic anticoagulation disappeared when adjustment was made for other prognostic features (Xian et al., 2012; Seiffge et al., 2015; Xian et al., 2017a).

No trials have addressed risk of IV rt-PA among patients who were taking non-vitamin-K oral anticoagulants (NOACs) prior to stroke onset. In two observational series, 666 of 50,083 IV fibrinolysis patients were on unreversed NOACs prior to therapy, and NOACs were associated with increased SICH in unadjusted analysis (5.9% vs 4.1%, OR 1.47, 95% CI:

1.06–2.04; $P = 0.02$) (Seiffge et al., 2015; Xian et al., 2017a). However, in each study, the increased risk of SICH among patients with NOACs disappeared when adjustment was made for other prognostic features. For the direct thrombin inhibitor NOAC, dabigatran, several small series and case reports have described reversing anticoagulant effect with the humanized monoclonal antibody idarucizumab, followed by administration of IV rt-PA. Among 40 patients treated with rt-PA following idarucizumab, symptomatic haemorrhagic transformation occurred in 1 (2.5%) and the great preponderance of patients had a favourable clinical course (Kermer et al., 2017; Pikija et al., 2017).

Concomitant Transcranial Doppler Ultrasound

In model systems, ultrasound has direct mechanical thrombolytic capacity at low frequencies (8–10 kilohertz [kHz]), enhances enzymatic fibrinolysis at high frequencies (including the 2-megahertz [MHz] frequency of diagnostic transcranial Doppler ultrasound), and may further augment pharmacological fibrinolysis when co-administered with ultrasound contrast gaseous microspheres, which oscillate and burst under the ultrasound beam (Saqqur et al., 2014). Low-frequency ultrasound added to IV rt-PA has been tested in only one small trial (26 patients); after it found high rates of haemorrhagic transformation, further development was not pursued (Daffertshofer et al., 2005). In contrast, high-frequency ultrasound, with or without microspheres, added to IV rt-PA has been compared with IV rt-PA alone in 5 randomized trials enrolling 1046 patients (Saqqur et al., 2014; Alexandrov et al., 2016; Nacu et al., 2017). In 3 proof of target activity trials, enrolling a total of 197 patients with confirmed target large vessel occlusions, sonothrombolysis was associated with increased early complete recanalization (42.9% vs 18.5%, OR 3.31, 95% CI: 1.72–6.36) and reduced death or disability (50.0% vs 75.8%, OR 0.38, 95% CI: 0.20–0.70). However, in 2 pivotal, pragmatic trials, enrolling ischaemic stroke patients and stroke mimics without a confirmed target vessel occlusion, benefit was not seen. Combining all 5 trials, among 1046 patients, sonothrombolysis, compared with IV tPA alone, was associated with no alteration in death or disability (61.9% vs 65.9%, OR 0.88, 95% CI: 0.67–1.14), death or dependency (47.7% vs 52.0%, OR 0.86, 95% CI: 0.67–1.10), mortality (15.8% vs 15.1%, OR 1.05, 95% CI: 0.75–1.49), or symptomatic haemorrhage (3.4% vs 2.5%, OR 1.37, 95% CI: 0.66–2.83).

In contrast to these studies of high-frequency ultrasound combined with IV rt-PA, one small trial (26 patients) evaluated low-frequency ultrasound added to IV rt-PA and found high rates of haemorrhagic transformation, and has not undergone further development (Daffertshofer et al., 2005).

Concomitant Neuroprotection

Neuroprotective (NP) agents block the molecular elaboration of injury in hypoxic environments, enabling brain tissue to tolerate ischaemia for longer periods. As NP drugs are often safe in haemorrhagic as well as ischaemic stroke, they could be given early after onset to stabilize threatened tissues, allowing more salvageable brain to be present at the time of later reperfusion by IVT (Fisher and Saver, 2015). Initial trials testing NP agents added to IVT began the NP agents in hospital, but only after thrombolysis had been started. For example, in two early randomized trials of NP agents added to IV fibrinolysis, the NP drugs (lubeluzole and clomethiazole) were started only well after the start of IV rt-PA, 45 minutes later in one trial and more than 140 minutes later in the other (Grotta, 2001; Lyden et al., 2001). However, more recent trials have tested NP agent start by paramedics in the field, before hospital arrival and fibrinolysis initiation. In 3 trials of different prehospital NP agents (remote ischaemic preconditioning, glyceryl trinitrate, and magnesium), 43% (188/433), 24% (10/41), and 27% (452/1700) of enrolled patients subsequently received IV rt-PA after hospital arrival (Ankolekar et al., 2013; Hougaard et al., 2014; Sanossian, 2017). In the FAST-MAG trial testing magnesium sulfate, prehospital study drug start preceded IV rt-PA start by a median of 95 minutes (Sanossian, 2017). These studies demonstrate that delivery of bridging neuroprotection in the ambulance prior to reperfusion therapy is a feasible strategy.

Concomitant Mechanical Clot Disruption

As IV delivery yields relatively modest fibrinolytic drug concentration arriving at target thrombi, it is more effective at digesting the smaller clots that obstruct small- and medium-size vessels, and less effective for LVOs with sizeable clot burdens (Legrand et al., 2013). In contrast, mechanical thrombectomy devices are highly efficient at recanalizing large proximal occlusions that have been unresponsive to IV fibrinolysis, and less effective for small distal occlusions in vessels too small for easy device access. In a pooled meta-analysis of individual patient-level data from the first 5 trials of modern endovascular reperfusion (ERT) devices, ERT added to IV rt-PA compared with IV rt-PA alone increased alive and independent (mRS 0–2) outcome at 3 months (46.4% vs 27.0%, RR 1.67, 95% CI: 1.37–2.05; $P < 0.00001$) and improved disability levels over the entire mRS (common OR 2.45, 95% CI: 1.68–3.57), and was associated with a non-significant reduction in death by 3 months (13.7% vs 18.4%, RR 0.75, 95% CI: 0.50–1.12) (Goyal et al., 2016).

In these completed randomized trials, all IVT-eligible patients were treated with IVT, and, among IVT-eligible patients, ERT plus IVT was found superior to IVT alone. However, an important additional consideration is whether, among IVT-eligible patients, ERT alone is better or worse than IVT plus ERT. IVT before ERT might improve outcomes, compared with ERT alone, by producing reperfusion before ERT, pre-conditioning clots to yield better recanalization with ERT, and providing lysis of distal thrombi after ERT. But IVT before ERT may also worsen outcomes by slowing start of ERT and promoting intracranial haemorrhage (Fischer et al., 2017). Randomized trials have not yet compared ERT alone versus IVT plus ERT. Conversely, one pilot trial compared different agents for IVT, tenecteplase versus standard rt-PA, as bridging therapy to ERT, and found that tenecteplase yielded higher rates of early reperfusion

with IVT alone, making ERT unnecessary (22% vs 10%, adjusted OR 2.6, 95% CI: 1.1–5.9) (Campbell et al., 2018).

Results for Different Treatment Times, Treatment Settings, and Types of Patients

A meta-analysis of pooled individual patient-level data was undertaken to explore for heterogeneity of treatment effect according to time from onset to treatment start, age, and presenting deficit severity (Emberson et al., 2014; Lees et al., 2016; Whiteley et al., 2016). The analysis included 6756 patients from 9 randomized trials of IV rt-PA, among whom 1549 (23%) were treated within 3 hours of onset, 2768 (41%) between 3 and 4.5 hours, 2196 (33%) between 4.5 and 6 hours, and 198 (3%) beyond 6 hours.

Effect of Onset to Treatment Time

Alive and Disability-free at the End of Patient Follow-up

Earlier treatment with rt-PA was associated with greater benefit of therapy in increasing the proportion of patients alive and disability-free (mRS 0–1) at the end of follow-up ($I^2 = 75\%$, $P_{interaction} = 0.02$) (Figure 6.6) (Emberson et al., 2014). Among patients treated within 3 hours of onset, allocation to rt-PA was associated with more frequent alive and non-disabled outcome (32.9% thrombolysis, 23.1% control; RR 1.42, 95% CI: 1.21–1.68; $P = 0.00002$) (Figure 6.6). This represents 98 more alive and non-disabled patients per 1000 treated

Study or Subgroup	rt-PA Events	Total	Control Events	Total	Risk Ratio M-H, Fixed, 95% CI
Treatment time					
1-3.0 h	259	787	176	762	1.42 [1.21, 1.68]
3.01 - 4.5 h	485	1375	432	1437	1.17 [1.05, 1.31]
More than 4.5 h	401	1229	357	1166	1.07 [0.95, 1.20]
Heterogeneity: Chi² = 7.98, df = 2 (P = 0.02); I² = 75%					
Age					
18-80	990	2512	853	2515	1.16 [1.08, 1.25]
81 and over	155	879	112	850	1.34 [1.07, 1.67]
Heterogeneity: Chi² = 1.39, df = 1 (P = 0.24); I² = 28%					
0-4	237	345	189	321	1.17 [1.04, 1.31]
5-10	611	1281	538	1252	1.11 [1.02, 1.21]
11-15	198	794	175	808	1.15 [0.96, 1.38]
16-21	77	662	55	671	1.42 [1.02, 1.97]
Heterogeneity: Chi² = 7.15, df = 4 (P = 0.13); I² = 44%					

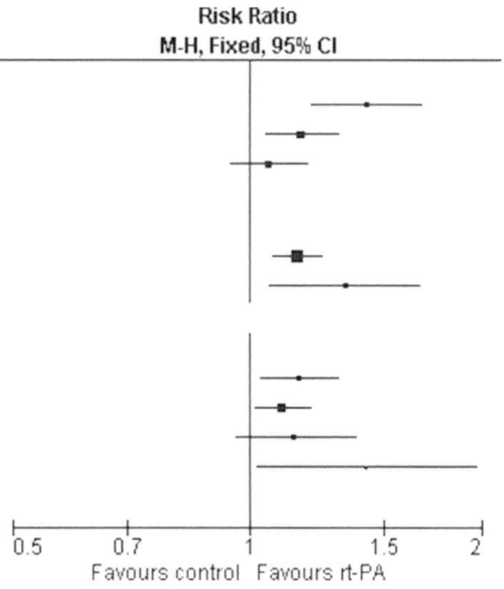

Figure 6.6 Effect of treatment time, age, and baseline NIHSS score on *alive and disability-free (mRS 0–1) outcome at 3–6 months with IV rt-PA vs Control.* Forest plot shows findings of individual patient, pooled data analysis, with findings for each subgroup adjusted for the other two. Data abstracted from Emberson et al. (2014).

with thrombolysis compared with control. Among patients treated beyond 3 but within 4.5 hours of onset, rt-PA therapy increased alive and disability-free outcome to a lesser degree (35.3% thrombolysis, 30.1% control; RR 1.17, 95% CI: 1.05–1.31; $P = 0.003$). This represents 52 more alive and non-disabled patients per 1000 treated with thrombolysis compared with control. Among patients treated beyond 4.5 hours of onset, rt-PA was not associated with a statistically significant increase in the proportion of patients alive and disability-free (32.6% thrombolysis, 30.6% control; RR 1.07, 95% CI: 0.95–1.20; $P = 0.29$).

Considering time as a continuous variable, the benefit of treatment declined with later onset to treatment time. The increased odds of an alive and non-disabled outcome with rt-PA therapy declined from about 1.86 with treatment at 1 hour to about 1.52 at 3 hours and about 1.28 at 4.5 hours. The point estimate for time at which treatment benefit entirely disappeared was 6.3 hours, and the time at which the lower 95% CI for treatment benefit first crossed neutral was at 5.1 hours (Figure 6.7A). Among 1000 patients, every 15-minute delay in rt-PA start meant approximately 7 fewer patients would achieve an alive and disability-free outcome.

Degree of Disability at the End of Patient Follow-up

In ordinal analysis, earlier treatment was associated with greater improved outcomes across all 7 disability

levels of the mRS (Figure 6.7B) (Lees et al., 2016). Using the automated algorithmic min–max joint outcome table derivation techniques (Saver et al., 2009), among patients treated within 3 hours of onset, allocation to rt-PA was associated with reduced disability levels in approximately 178 of every 1000 patients treated. Among patients treated beyond 3 but within 4.5 hours of onset, rt-PA therapy reduced disability in 66 of every 1000 patients treated.

Considering time as a continuous variable, the benefit of treatment in reducing degree of disability declined with later onset to treatment time ($P = 0.04$) (Figure 6.7B) (Lees et al., 2016). The increased odds of a less-disabled late outcome with rt-PA therapy declined from about 1.45 with treatment at 1 hour to about 1.28 at 3 hours and about 1.18 at 4.5 hours. The point estimate for time at which treatment benefit entirely disappeared was 6.1 hours and the time at which the lower 95% CI for treatment benefit first crossed neutral was at 4.6 hours. Among 1000 patients in whom treating physicians were confident of benefit, with every 15-minute delay in rt-PA start, approximately 13 patients had a more disabled outcome (Lansberg et al., 2009).

Death at the End of Patient Follow-up, and Early Major Haemorrhage

Treatment delay was associated with a non-significant increase in the nominal hazard of death by the end of

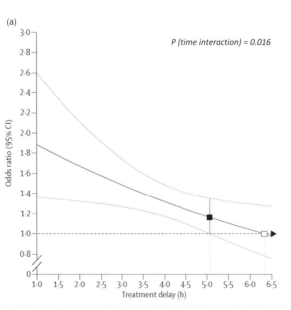

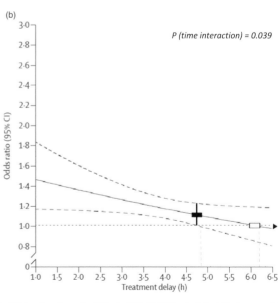

Figure 6.7 Modification of IV rt-PA benefit by onset to treatment time, for (A) *freedom from disability (mRS 0–1)*; (B) *level of disability (across all 7 ranks of the mRS)*.

follow-up (P = 0.22) (Emberson et al., 2014). For different time windows, with treatment with rt-PA rather than control, hazard ratios for death were the following: under 3 hours: hazard ratio (HR) 1.00 (95% CI: 0.81–1.24); 3–4.5 hours: HR 1.14 (0.95–1.36); and more than 4.5 hours: 1.22 (0.99–1.50). The excess of SICH was similar in all onset-to-treatment time windows (Wardlaw et al., 2014; Whiteley et al., 2016).

Effect of Age

Randomized trials have shown that older patients compared with younger patients have worse functional outcomes from acute ischaemic stroke regardless of treatment with or without IVT, but benefit to the same relative degree from thrombolytic treatment (Grotta, 2001; Wardlaw et al., 2014). Among 6756 patients enrolled in 9 pooled IV rt-PA trials, 74% were up to age 80 and 26% over age 80 (Emberson et al., 2014). Thrombolytic therapy up to 6 hours after onset increased the rate of alive and disability-free outcome (mRS 0–1) to a similar relative degree in both age groups, though with worse overall outcomes in older patients (up to age 80: 39.4% vs 33.9%, RR 1.16, 95% CI: 1.08–1.25; over age 80: 17.6% vs 13.2%, RR 1.34, 95% CI: 1.07–1.67) (see Figure 6.6). However, the similar relative benefit translates into a higher absolute benefit for older patients, since their absolute risk is higher to start with. Older patients had similar rates of SICH to younger patients regardless of treatment with or without IVT, and experienced the same relative degree of increased SICH from thrombolytic treatment: (up to age 80: 3.5% vs 0.6%, RR 6.29, 95% CI: 3.59–11.03; over age 80: 4.1% vs 0.6%, RR 7.95, 95% CI: 2.79–22.60; subgroup difference P = 0.83) (Whiteley et al., 2016).

Effect of Presenting Deficit Severity

Randomized trials have shown that patients presenting with more severe, compared with less severe, deficits have worse functional outcomes from acute ischaemic stroke regardless of treatment with or without IVT, but generally benefit to the same relative degree from thrombolytic treatment (Pancioli et al., 2008). Thrombolytic therapy up to 6 hours after onset increased the rate of alive and disability-free outcome (mRS 0–1) to a similar relative degree across 5 levels of presenting deficit severity (NIHSS ranges of 0–4, 5–10, 11–15, 16–21, and ≥22), though with worse overall outcomes in patients with worse initial severity

(see Figure 6.6). For example, rates of alive and non-disabled outcome among mild deficit patients (NIHSS score 0–4) were 68.7% versus 58.9% (RR 1.17, 95% CI: 1.04–1.31) and among severe deficit patients (NIHSS score 16–21) rates were 11.6% versus 8.2% (RR 1.42, 95% CI: 1.02–1.97). A non-significant trend towards a greater relative degree of increased SICH from thrombolytic treatment in patients with greater presenting deficits was noted (subgroup difference P = 0.27) (Whiteley et al., 2016). For example, rates of SICH among mild deficit patients (NIHSS score 0–4) were 1.7% versus 0.3%, and among severe deficit patients (NIHSS score 16–21) were 3.9% versus 0.1%.

Among patients with low initial deficit severity scores, it is important to distinguish those patients in whom the deficits, though delimited, are causing a potentially disabling functional loss (e.g. severe pure motor hemiparesis) and those patients in whom the deficits are non-disabling (e.g. pure hemisensory loss). Patients with non-disabling deficits, as assessed by treating physicians, were generally not enrolled in early trials of IV fibrinolysis. However, observational series noted that some patients in whom thrombolysis was withheld because their deficits were so mild subsequently had stroke progression in the next hours and days, with poor final outcome. Accordingly, a randomized trial, PRISMS, was undertaken, enrolling only patients ineligible for standard therapy, as their deficits were non-disabling, evaluating whether up-front IV rt-PA would avert subsequent stroke progression and improve final outcome. PRISMS enrolled 313 patients and found no improvement in disability-free (mRS 0–1) outcome at 3 months (78.2% vs 81.5.5%, RR 0.98, 95% CI: 0.81–1.18), with a low rate of stringently defined symptomatic haemorrhage (1.3% vs 0.0%) (Khatri et al., 2018). Accordingly, current data suggest that, among patients with low NIHSS deficits, only the subset in whom the deficits are disabling benefit from IV rt-PA therapy.

Imaging Findings on Noncontrast CT

The extent of likely irreversible infarct injury on initial noncontrast CT, evident as loss of grey–white matter distinction or presence of definite hypodensity (hypoattenuation), has been evaluated for potential influence upon response to fibrinolytic therapy. Among patients with no, small, and moderate early infarct signs on CT, randomized trials have shown that participants with more, compared with less, extensive early infarct changes have worse functional outcomes from acute ischaemic stroke regardless of treatment with or without IVT, but generally benefit to the same relative degree from thrombolytic treatment (Emberson et al., 2014), similar to the effect seen for stroke severity. The extent of early ischaemic injury changes on initial noncontrast brain CT scans has been most often quantified using the Alberta Stroke Program Early CT Score (ASPECTS). Among 4 trials enrolling 4413 patients testing IV rt-PA, 74% had mild early infarct changes (ASPECTS 8–10) and 26% had moderate early infarct changes (ASPECTS 0–7, but predominantly 5–7) (Wardlaw et al., 2014). Thrombolytic therapy increased alive and disability-free (mRS 0–1) outcome to a similar relative degree in both small and moderate infarct change patients (subgroup difference I^2 = 0%, P = 0.62), though patients with less-extensive infarcts had better outcomes in both treatment groups: no or small infarct signs, mRS 0–1: 43.6% versus 39.3%, RR 1.11, 95% CI: 1.02–1.20; moderate infarct signs, 22.7% versus 19.1%, RR 1.18, 95% CI: 0.94–1.48 (Figure 6.8).

While patients with no, mild, and moderate infarct signs have been well-studied, patients were generally not enrolled in initial RCTs if they had very large, evident infarcts on initial CT, such as occupying more than one-third of the territory of the middle cerebral artery, exceeding 100 mL in volume, or having

an ASPECTS score of 0–4. In the early trials, these patients were presumed to have limited potential to benefit from reperfusion, given their large, apparently established, infarct, and to be at elevated risk of haemorrhagic transformation. Patients with extensive early infarct signs are very uncommon within the first 3 hours of stroke onset, but proportionally increase as time from onset increases thereafter. The later IST-3 trial, undertaken to map more fully the range of therapy benefit, did include patients with very large infarcts. However, the sample size of this subgroup did not afford sufficient power to reliably determine whether very large baseline infarct size modified the effects of IV rt-PA on efficacy and safety outcomes. Among 250 patients with very large infarcts, allocation to IV rt-PA versus control yielded rates of functional independence (Oxford Handicap Scale 0–2) at 6 months of 9.4% versus 8.0% (adjusted OR 1.41, 95% CI: 0.36–5.54), and of symptomatic intracranial haemorrhage of 10.9% versus 3.6% (adjusted OR 3.24, 95% CI: 0.72–14.60) (IST-3 Collaborative Group, 2015). Accordingly, more randomized data in patients with very large infarct are needed before definitive recommendations can be given.

Additional findings evident on baseline noncontrast CT affect patient prognosis but not degree of benefit from fibrinolysis. Among the 3017 patients in the IST-3 trial, poorer functional outcome was

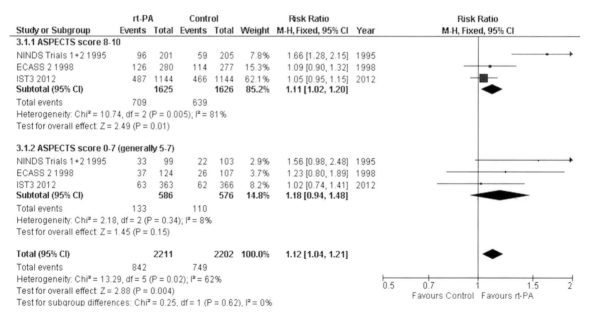

Figure 6.8 Effect of extent of established infarct extent (based on ASPECTS score) on *alive and disability-free outcome (mRS 0–1) at 3–6 months with IV rt-PA vs Control*.

associated not only with early ischaemic changes, but also with presence of a hyperattenuated artery sign (a marker of LVO) and the degree of pre-stroke leukoaraiosis and brain atrophy (markers of lower resilience); and SICH was associated not only with extent of early ischaemic changes but also with presence of old infarct and of a hyperattenuated artery sign. But none of these imaging findings, individually or in combination, modified the relative effect of rt-PA on functional independence or SICH (IST-3 Collaborative Group, 2015).

Late-presenting Patients with Imaging Evidence of Salvageable Tissue on MRI or CT

In acute cerebral ischaemia, when an artery is abruptly occluded, collateral vessels provide compensating blood flow to the supplied region. The robustness of the collateral supply varies widely from individual to individual, depending on variations in circle of Willis anatomy, stenoses and occlusions in the alternative channels themselves, the site of the new occlusion, and systemic blood pressure. Shortly after the inciting vascular occlusion, a small brain region within the supplied field may experience complete loss of blood flow, causing cellular death within 1 to a few minutes. But a much larger, surrounding zone will experience moderate reductions in blood flow that the brain cells can tolerate for tens of minutes to several hours. As time from onset lengthens, the zone of the completed, irreversible infarction – the core – expands and the rim of threatened but still salvageable tissue – penumbra – shrinks.

CT and MRI techniques indexing core and penumbra volume permit identification of the two subsets of patients in later post–last known well time windows who still harbour rescuable tissue (Wheeler et al., 2015): 'actual recent onsetters' and 'slow progressors'. Actual recent onsetters are patients in whom the stroke really began more recently than the determinable last known well time, but the exact time of onset cannot be determined by history, either because it occurred while the patient was asleep or occurred while the patient was awake but alone and neurological deficits impaired the patient's own ability to perceive or report the onset time. Slow progressors are patients in whom the pace of infarct growth is less rapid than average due to good collateral flow and/or greater parenchymal tolerance of ischaemia. With CT, perfusion CT imaging identifies as core regions with extreme reduction in blood flow or blood volume, and as penumbra regions with moderate blood flow reduction (perfusion–core mismatch). With MRI, diffusion MR sequences identify as core regions with substantial diffusion abnormality, indicating advanced bioenergetic compromise, and perfusion MRI sequences identify as penumbra regions with moderate-to-severe blood flow reduction not yet showing diffusion abnormality (perfusion–diffusion mismatch). Alternative, though less precise but more readily obtained, CT and MR approaches to identifying patients with penumbra estimate the volume of perfusion reduction using the presence of LVO (vessel–core mismatch), the extent of collateral vessels (collateral–core mismatch), or the severity of neurological deficits (clinical–core mismatch). An additional MR imaging selection approach is to estimate the physiological time since onset by comparing tissue volumes indicating bioenergetics compromise (any diffusion abnormality) and final infarct signature (FLAIR hyperintensity) – diffusion–FLAIR mismatch.

Using advanced imaging evidence of persisting salvageable tissue to select a subset of late-presenting patients has been tested in 7 randomized trials comparing IVT to non-thrombolytic therapy (including 4 rt-PA trials and 3 desmoteplase trials), and 1 pilot randomized trial comparing one thrombolytic agent against another.

The 4 IV rt-PA trials included 3 trials using a penumbral imaging selection strategy, including two using penumbral MR imaging (EPITHET among patients 3–9 h from stroke, ECASS 4 among patients 4.5–9 h from stroke) and one using penumbral MR or penumbral CT imaging (EXTEND among patients 4.5–9 h from stroke). The remaining trial (WAKE-UP) used an MR diffusion–FLAIR mismatch imaging selection strategy among patients 4.5 hours or longer after stroke (Davis et al., 2008; Picanco et al., 2014; Bendszus et al., 2018; Thomalla et al., 2018; Ma et al., 2019). Considering only imaging-selected patients enrolled 4.5 hours or longer after onset across all 4 trials (n = 897), allocation to IV rt-PA was associated with increased alive and disability-free outcome (mRS 0–1), thrombolysis 48.8%, control 39.6%, RR 1.23, 95% CI: 1.06–1.43, $P = 0.005$ (Figure 6.9).

In the 3 trials evaluating demoteplase versus placebo among perfusion–core mismatch-selected patients in the 3- to 9-hour post-onset window, 216 patients were enrolled with MR penumbral imaging and 64 with early-generation CT penumbral imaging (Warach et al., 2012). None of the trials was individually positive. However, among the MR-imaged

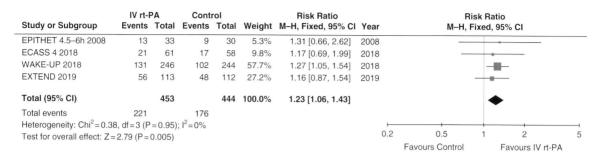

Figure 6.9 *Alive and disability-free outcome (mRS 0–1) at 3–6 months, IV rt-PA vs Controls,* in patients enrolled late, 4.5–9 h, after last known well with imaging evidence of persisting salvageable tissue.

patients, the presence of substantial penumbral volume (>60 mL), rather than modest penumbral volume (≤60 mL), was associated with a beneficial increase with desmoteplase therapy in the proportion of patients achieving good clinical outcome (concurrent success on 3 outcome scales, including functional independence [mRS 0–2]). Good outcome rates were the following: substantial penumbral volume: 43% versus 21% (OR 2.83, 95% CI: 1.16–6.94); modest penumbral volume: 57% vs 61% (OR 0.87, 95% CI: 0.34–2.27).

In the pilot trial comparing different lytic agents, tenecteplase and rt-PA were compared in 75 patients in the 3- to 6-hour window who had CT penumbral imaging evidence of persisting salvageable tissue. Tenecteplase was associated with a non-significant increase in alive and disability-free (mRS 0–1) outcome (54% vs 40%, OR 1.76, 95% CI: 0.66–4.67; P = 0.25) and an increase in alive and independent (mRS 0–2) outcome, 72% versus 44% (OR 2.97, 95% CI: 1.10–8.03; P = 0.03) (Parsons et al., 2012).

Collectively, these trials indicate that, among later-presenting patients, CT and MR penumbral and other imaging techniques can identify a subset still harbouring substantial salvageable tissue who can benefit from IV thrombolytic therapy. For IV rt-PA, while chronological time from last known well remains a simple and speedy means of patient selection up to 4.5 hours, there is now substantial evidence that treatment is also beneficial for the subset of 4.5- to 9-hour patients with CT/MR evidence of rescuable tissue.

Thrombolysis in Clinical Practice

Efficacy and Safety in Routine Practice

Multinational and national registries have prospectively evaluated whether efficacy and safety outcomes with IV thrombolytic therapy in routine practice are similar to the outcomes in the pivotal randomized trials. Considering the largest registries, a substantial worldwide experience has been catalogued with administration of IV rt-PA in the 0- to 4.5-hour window, in over 225,000 patients at over 3800 hospitals in 77 countries on 6 continents (Table 6.1). Compared with the 2162 patients allocated to IV rt-PA in the 0- to 4.5-hour window in the pooled RCTs, patients treated in regular practice were similar in character, with average age 71, NIHSS score of 11, and onset to treatment time 2 hours 25 minutes. The dose of IV rt-PA employed was 0.9 mg/kg to a maximum of 90 mg in 96% of patients and a lower dose, generally 0.6 mg/kg, in 4%, reflecting practice patterns in Asian countries. Outcomes in routine practice have been comparable or better in routine practice compared with randomized trials, including alive and non-disabled outcome at 3 months (40.1% in practice vs 31.0% in trials), SITS-MOST defined SICH (1.8% vs 1.8%), NINDS-defined SICH (5.5% vs 6.1%), and death by 3 months (16.3% vs 18.4%).

Uncommon Adverse Events: Angioedema and Systemic Haemorrhage

Large registries enable more precise characterization of the frequency, spectrum, and outcomes of adverse medication effects that occur too infrequently to be well delineated by randomized trials. Angioedema after IV rt-PA was reported in 15/1135 (1.3%) of patients in a Canadian multicentre study (Hill and Buchan, 2005). Among 41 cases collated from multiple case series, mean age was 69, 63% were female, onset began 47±32 minutes after rt-PA start, and 59% of patients were taking an angiotensin-converting enzyme inhibitor prior to lytic therapy (Yayan, 2013). The typical presentation was mild bilateral or

Table 6.1 National and multinational registries of intravenous rt-PA therapy up to 4.5 hours after onset, including pooled registry comparison with pooled trials

Feature	Registries of regular practice							Combined registries	Combined trials (STTC)*
Data source	SITS (Wahlgren and Ahmed, 2016)	RCSN (Saposnik et al., 2013; Shobha et al., 2013)	J-MARS (Nakagawara et al., 2010)	TIMS-China (Tong et al., 2016)	TTT-AIS II (Chao et al., 2014)	KNR (Kim et al., 2015)**	GWTG-Stroke		
Countries	Multinational (74)	Canada	Japan	China	Taiwan	Korea	United States	Multinational (77)	Multinational (>23)
Continents	6	1	1	1	1	1	1	6	3
Years	2002–2016	2003–2008	2005–2007	2007–2012	2004–2011	2009–2013	2009–2015	2002–2016	1991–2011
Performance sites	1216	12	942	67	23	15	1545	3820	>171
Patients	128,516	1689	7492	953	1004	1122	85,072	225,848	2162 (active arms)
Age (median, or mean)	71	72	72	63	67	69	70.2	71	71*
NIHSS (median, or mean)	11	--	15	12	15	9	10	11	12*
rt-PA Dose, mg/kg	0.9	0.9	0.6	0.9 in 69%; <0.9 in 31%	0.9 in 42%; <0.9 in 58%	0.9 in 82%; 0.6 in 18%	0.9	0.9 in 96%; 0.6 in 4%	0.9 in 86%; 1.1 in 14%
Onset to Treatment (min) (median, or mean)	150	--	133	170	141	122	138	145	≤180 min, 36%; 181–270 min, 64%
SICH SITS-MOST Defn	1.7%	--	3.5%	--	2.2%	--	--	1.8%	1.8%
NINDS Defn	6.3%	6.9%	--	7.1%	6.8%	--	4.3%	5.5%	6.1%
Other Defn	--	--	--	--	--	6.1%	6.1%	6.1%	--
Death – Early	--	16.5%	--	--	--	--	7.3%	7.5%	--
Death – by 3 min	16.6%	--	13.1%	10.8%	9.1%	13.7%	--	16.3%	18.4%
Alive and Disability-Free (mRS 0–1) – Early	--	17.7%	--	--	--	--	26.1%	25.9%	--
Alive and Disability-Free (mRS 0–1) – 3 min	40.6%	--	33%	43.4%	30.6%	38.3%	--	40.1%	31.0%

STTC: Stroke Thrombolytic Trialists Collaboration. SITS: Safe Implementation of Treatments in Stroke. RCSN: Registry of the Canadian Stroke Network. TIMS: Thrombosis Implementation and Monitor of Acute Ischemic Stroke. KNR: Korea National Registry. J-MARS: Japan Post-Marketing Alteplase Registration Study. GWTG-Stroke: Get with the Guidelines-Stroke.

* STTC publications provide some data separately for patients treated 0–4.5 h and other data only for patients treated 0–6 h. Values in this column are for only 0–4.5 h patients when available. Values with asterisks are for all patients (64% of patients were treated 0–4.5 h, 25% 4.5–6 h, and 1% with exact time missing)

SICH: SITS-MOST defn: Parenchymal haematoma type 2 and NIHSS worsening ≥ 4; NINDS defn: Any intracerebral haemorrhage and any worsening; Other defn: Korea National Registry definition of SICH was any intracerebral haemorrhage associated with NIHSS worsening ≥ 4.

** KNR data shown are only for the patients treated with IV alteplase alone (n = 1122), and not patients treated with combined IV alteplase and endovascular reperfusion (n = 404).

unilateral swelling of the lips and tongue, with the orolingual oedema persisting for 29 hours post-onset, but one case was associated with fatal ventricular tachycardia.

Serious systemic, extracranial haemorrhage occurred in 0.9% of 85,072 IV rt-PA patients in the US Get with the Guidelines-Stroke registry, and was more common among patients taking antiplatelet therapy prior to stroke onset (1.2% vs 0.7%, adjusted OR 1.45 (1.23–1.72) (Xian et al., 2017a).

Importance of Time to Treatment on Outcome

Registry studies have demonstrated that, in regular practice, time from onset to treatment is an important determinant of outcome from IV thrombolytic therapy. In studies of 58,353 and 65,384 patients treated with IV rt-PA in the Get with the Guidelines (GWTG) – Stroke registry, every 15-minute reduction in onset to treatment time was associated with increased independent ambulation at discharge (OR 1.04, 95% CI: 1.03–1.05; $P < 0.001$), increased discharge to home (OR 1.03, 95% CI: 1.02–1.04; $P < 0.001$), reduced in-hospital mortality (OR 0.96, 95% CI: 0.95–0.98; $P < 0.001$), and reduced symptomatic intracranial haemorrhage (OR 0.96, 95% CI: 0.95–0.98; $P < 0.001$) (Figure 6.10) (Saver et al., 2013; Kim et al., 2017).

Faster in-hospital processes of care are associated with improved outcomes from IV thrombolytic therapy. Among 25,504 IV rt-PA patients in the GWTG-Stroke registry treated between 2003 and 2009, the median 'door-to-needle' (DTN) time (time from hospital arrival to start of IV fibrinolytic infusion) was 78 minutes (IQR 60–98), and 26.6% of patients were treated within the national DTN target of 60 minutes. DTN times within 60 minutes were associated with a reduction in in-hospital mortality (adjusted OR 0.78, 95% CI: 0.69 to 0.90; $P < 0.0003$) and a non-significant reduction in SICH (4.7% vs 5.6%, OR 0.88, 95% CI: 0.75–1.02; $P = 0.09$) (Fonarow et al., 2011b).

Methods to Accelerate Treatment Speed

National and local quality improvement programmes can accelerate DTN times and improve patient outcomes. In the US, the national Target: Stroke initiatives disseminated 16 best practice strategies, clinical decision support tools, a comprehensive implementation manual, education, sharing of best practices, performance feedback, and new hospital recognition goals to more than 1397 hospitals. The best practice strategies were selected based on an analysis of 31 candidates, identifying 14 that independently contributed to shortened DTN times (Table 6.2). In multivariate analysis, strategies with the greatest impact for every 20% increase in adoption were the following: (1) initiating rt-PA while patient still in brain-imaging suite (DTN reduction 3.5 min, 95% CI: 2.8–4.2); (2) pre-mixing rt-PA before final treatment decision

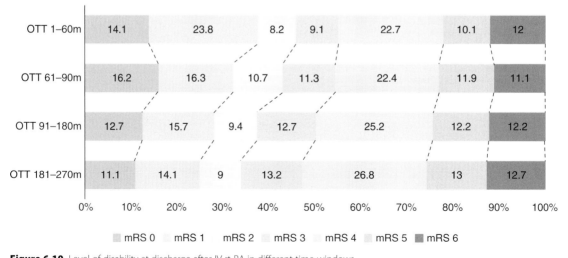

Figure 6.10 Level of disability at discharge after IV rt-PA in different time windows.

OTT indicates onset to treatment; m indicates minutes; mRS indicates modified Rankin Scale.
Data from 65,384 IV rt-PA patients in the GWTG-Stroke registry.

Table 6.2 Strategies that independently contributed to faster door-to-needle rt-PA times

Strategy		Reduction in DTN times per 20% increase in strategy use minutes (95% CI)	P-value
1	Start of IV rt-PA bolus while patient still in brain-imaging suite	3.4 (2.7–4.1)	<0.001
2	Rapid triage protocol and stroke team notification	2.5 (1.2–3.9)	<0.001
3	Prompt patient-specific data feedback to ED staff + stroke team	1.6 (1.0–2.3)	<0.001
4	Brain imaging read immediately by stroke team members	1.6 (1.1–2.0)	<0.001
5	INR and platelet count not required before rt-PA start	1.2 (0.7–1.6)	<0.001
6	Treatment decision by neurologist attending / trainee after in-person evaluation	1.2 (0.7–1.7)	<0.001
7	Trainees (residents and fellows) involved in stroke team and perform initial assessment	1.1 (0.6–1.5)	<0.001
8	Premix of rt-PA ahead of time	1.1 (0.7–1.6)	<0.001
9	Single-call activation system	1.1 (0.3–1.9)	0.006
10	Prompt patient-specific data feedback to EMS providers	1.0 (0.5–1.5)	<0.001
11	EMS uses prehospital stroke-screening tool	0.9 (0.2–1.5)	0.008
12	Written informed consent not required (only verbal) before rt-PA start	0.8 (0.3–1.3)	0.001
13	Transport of patients by Emergency Medical Services directly to CT/MRI scanner	0.7 (0.2–1.1)	0.005
14	Timer/clock attached to a chart/patient's bed to track time	0.6 (0.0–1.2)	0.04

(DTN reduction 2.6 min, 95% CI: 0.6–4.7), and (3) formal protocol for stroke patient triage and stroke team notification (DTN reduction 2.5 min, 95% CI: 1.2–3.9) (Xian et al., 2017b). From programme launch in 2010 through 2015, among 99,176 IV rt-PA treated patients, the proportion treated within time targets increased, including for DTN times 60 minutes or less (from 27% to 61%, $P < 0.0001$), DTN 45 minutes or less (from 10% to 33%, $P < 0.0001$), and DTN 30 minutes or less (from 3% to 10%, $P < 0.0001$) (Figure 6.11) (Fonarow et al., 2017).

Comment

Interpretation of the Data

These data indicate that IV thrombolytic therapy for acute ischaemic stroke is of substantial net benefit when used early after onset. The magnitude of the improvements in functional outcome conveyed by thrombolytic treatment decline sharply as time from onset increases, while the harm, chiefly SICH, persists at a low, steady level regardless of time since onset. As a result, IV thrombolytic therapy confers substantial net benefit when delivered within the first 3 hours of onset, and modest net benefit between 3 and 4.5 hours after onset. Beyond 4.5 hours, the benefits do not clearly outweigh the harm, except in patients selected for persisting salvageable tissue on imaging.

The pattern of adverse outcomes in the controlled trials provides important pathophysiological insights. With agent start within the first 3 hours of onset, early symptomatic haemorrhagic transformation occurs more often among patients treated with thrombolytics than controls, but death at the end of follow-up is not different. Patient deaths from herniation and medical complications of large bland infarcts occur more often in the control group, offsetting patient deaths from herniation and medical complications of haemorrhagic infarcts in the thrombolytic group.

The greatest amount of data is available for IV rt-PA (0.9 mg/kg over 1 h). Among patients treated with IV rt-PA under 3 hours, 178 out of 1000 will have a less disabled outcome, including 98 more being alive and free of disability, with no change in the mortality rate.

However, uncertainties remain regarding:

- whether clinical and imaging criteria can identify additional subsets of patients more than 4.5 hours

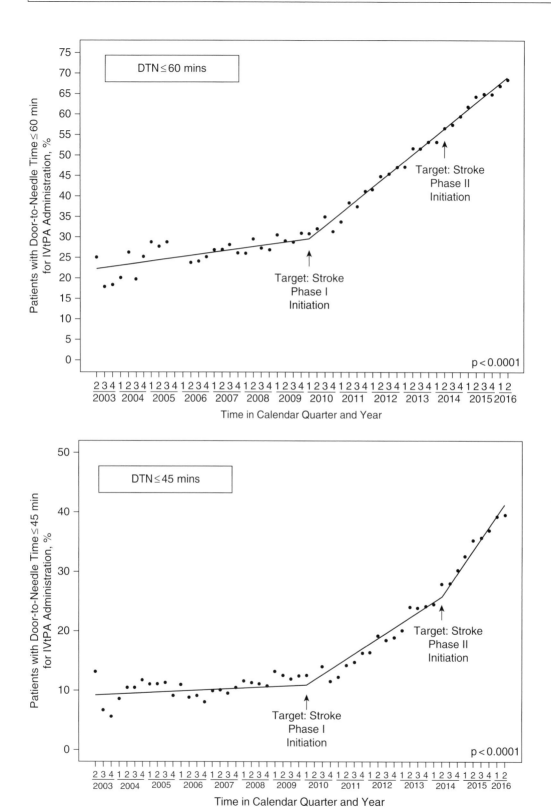

Figure 6.11 Door-to-needle times within 60 and 45 min: before, after Phase I, and after Phase II of US national Target: Stroke thrombolysis care quality improvement programme.

after onset who may benefit substantially from therapy despite late presentation;

- the optimal thrombolytic agent and dose;
- the role (if any) and timing of concomitant antithrombotic pharmacological therapy;
- whether IV thrombolytic therapy improves, worsens, or does not alter outcomes from endovascular thrombectomy in patients with large vessel occlusions.

Implications for Clinical Practice

Based on the considerable trial evidence, practice guidelines worldwide, including North America, South America, Europe, Asia, and Africa, recommend the use of IV alteplase up to 4.5 hours after stroke onset in patients meeting treatment eligibility criteria (Sharma et al., 2005; National Institute for Health and Clinical Excellence (NICE) – National Health Services, 2007; European Stroke Organization Executive Committee and the ESO Writing Committee, 2008; Lindsay et al., 2008; Bryer et al., 2010; Atallah, 2012; Cho et al., 2012; DeMers et al. 2012; Wright et al., 2012; American College of Emergency Physicians et al., 2013; Jauch et al., 2013). In some jurisdictions, the patients appropriate for alteplase delineated in the therapeutic licence approved by regulatory authorities differ in modest ways from national clinical guidelines in the same countries. For example, in the US, the national guidelines recommend alteplase up to 4.5 after onset, while the licence indicates up to 3 hours after onset; in Europe, guidelines recommend alteplase in patients both over and under 80 years old, while the licence is restricted to patients under 80 years old. The evidence from the randomized trials does support following the guidelines in these instances, providing evidence of benefit through 4.5 hours and in patients over age 80 (Hacke et al., 2018).

As thrombolytic therapy has risks as well as benefits, it is a treatment that requires continuous quality monitoring in routine practice. It should be administered only to patients without contraindications, and in organized and experienced stroke care centres with staff and facilities for rapid and accurate assessment, monitoring, and management of any complications in accordance with current guidelines (Alberts et al., 2011; Jauch et al., 2013). Active stroke centres should participate in prospective, systematic, and rigorous audit as part of a national or international registry, such as GWTG-Stroke or SITS-ISTR. This will ensure that stroke patients have access to this effective, but not risk-free, treatment; that stroke physicians, nurses, and hospital teams deepen experience and expertise in its use; and that quality control and patient selection continue to be optimized by contrasting baseline demographic, clinical, imaging, and treatment data, and early and long-term patient outcome, with contemporaneous care at comparator facilities.

The efficient and equitable delivery of thrombolysis also must overcome several prehospital and in-hospital barriers, including education of the public to recognize symptoms of stroke and to seek urgent help by calling the ambulance first rather than the family doctor (Higashida et al., 2013; Jauch et al., 2013); ambulance dispatcher and paramedic training in stroke recognition and routing (Acker et al., 2007; Higashida et al., 2013); geographically optimized regional stroke care systems that deliver patients with suspected acute stroke to stroke-capable hospitals quickly (Higashida et al., 2013); optimal communication along the whole stroke chain of care; efficient, well-trained 'Code Stroke' teams to manage patients immediately upon arrival; use of telemedicine and teleradiology to provide immediate neurological and imaging expertise to patients in remote community hospitals (Audebert et al., 2006; Wechsler et al., 2017); decision aids to enable patients and families to rapidly understand the benefits and risks of therapy (Figure 6.12) (Gadhia et al., 2010; Flynn et al., 2015; Whiteley et al., 2016; Montero et al., 2017); and optimized protocols and processes of care to enable patient assessment, imaging interpretation, and start of infusion no more than 60 minutes, and optimally within 30 minutes, of patient arrival in the Emergency Department (Fonarow et al., 2011a; Meretoja et al., 2012).

Regional and hospital-level systems that are most effective in rapid, appropriate delivery of rt-PA may vary by the country's general healthcare system. Knowledge of what works in other countries and healthcare models provides highly valuable information for development and improvement of local best practices. However, two points are probably useful everywhere. First, regular review of actual times to different stages within the stroke chain of care can be highly instructive about where delays are occurring and focus teams' efforts on problem solving to improve each step to accelerate care. Second, communication among the multidisciplinary team, from the

tPA for Cerebral Ischaemia within 3h of Onset
Changes in Outcome Due to Treatment

tPA for Cerebral Ischaemia between 3 and 4.5h after Onset
Changes in Outcome Due to Treatment

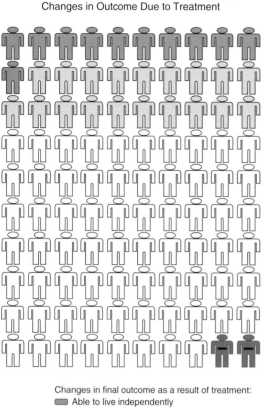

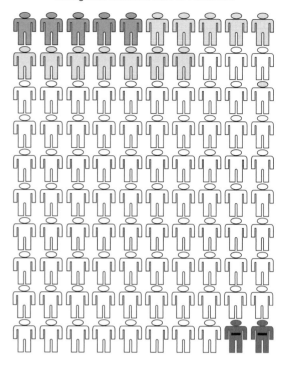

Changes in final outcome as a result of treatment:
■ Able to live independently
▢ Other improvement
▢ No major changes
■ Other worsening
■ Severely disabled or dead
Early course:
— Early worsening with brain bleeding (SICH)

Changes in final outcome as a result of treatment:
■ Able to live independently
▢ Other improvement
▢ No major changes
■ Other worsening
■ Severely disabled or dead
Early course:
— Early worsening with brain bleeding (SICH)

Figure 6.12 Visual decision aids for IV rt-PA in acute ischaemic stroke.

patient's initial contact with the ambulance through to hospital arrival, imaging, and stroke unit, is absolutely essential, may involve tens of providers from diverse disciplines, and has to run like clockwork every time to avoid delays. Advance notice from the ambulance staff that they are bringing a probable stroke patient to the hospital enables pre-arrival alerting of all multidisciplinary stroke team members, fostering rapid emergency department medical assessment, imaging suite availability, drug preparation, and inpatient care unit readiness.

Implications for Researchers

The burning question is no longer whether IVT is effective, but how to make it *more* effective. Six broad avenues of further advancement may be envisioned

and are being explored in current trials: faster treatment, more reperfusion, more salvageable brain, less bleeding, more patients, and improved systems of care.

(a) Faster treatment: As the benefit of thrombolysis is so strongly time-dependent, innovative delivery methods that enable faster start of therapy will substantially improve patient outcomes. Mobile stroke units, ambulances equipped with CT scanners, permit imaging and thrombolytic treatment to start in the prehospital setting and have been shown to accelerate infusion start in controlled trials. Much larger trials are needed to determine whether this delivery strategy is cost-effective.

(b) More reperfusion: It is critical to improve the frequency of reperfusion achieved by IV fibrinolysis. Current regimens open only 40–50% of target occlusions, sharply limiting the scope of therapeutic benefit. Further trials of newer fibrinolytic agents, and of varying combinations of reduced or full-dose fibrinolytic drugs co-administered with traditional and emerging classes of antiplatelets and anticoagulants, ultrasound, or other agents, are needed to identify regimens that can substantially enhance reperfusion efficacy without increasing haemorrhage.

(c) More salvageable brain: Reperfusion is likely to be of benefit only to still-salvageable tissues, not brain parenchyma that has already progressed to irreversible infarction by the time of lytic therapy start. Neuroprotective and collateral enhancement therapies, started prehospital in standard paramedic ambulances or upon Emergency Department arrival in advance of brain imaging, could stabilize ischaemic tissues, so that a greater proportion of the tissue at risk is still rescuable at the time that lytic therapy is started in hospital.

(d) Less bleeding: Reducing the frequency of symptomatic haemorrhagic transformation would increase the benefit–risk ratio of lytic therapy by mitigating the most common cause of harm. Agents that stabilize the blood–brain barrier and provide endothelial protection, such as matrix metalloproteinase inhibitors, are desirable concomitant treatments for thrombolytic therapy. In addition, agents that deter reperfusion injury may both reduce haemorrhagic transformation and increase brain tissue salvage.

(e) More patients: The chronological time since last known well is only a crude index of how much salvageable tissue a patient may be harbouring. The 1 in 5 ischaemic stroke patients whose deficits are first observed on awakening often actually have had ischaemia for only a short period just before waking, rather than throughout the entire time since they were last known well at sleep onset. Among patients with witnessed onset time, some are 'slow progressors', in whom the pace of infarct growth is protracted due to substantial collateral flow or parenchymal tolerance of hypoxia, so that they may also still have predominantly salvageable tissue and minimal core infarct 4.5–24 hours after symptom onset. More imaging selection studies are needed, in the wake of the WAKE-UP trial, to determine the optimal imaging algorithms for identifying patients who will benefit from therapy in the 4.5- to 9-hour window and to investigate if imaging selection can further extend the time window by identifying patients in the 9- to 24-hour window who will benefit.

(f) Improved systems of care: There are many options for arranging for delivery of thrombolytic therapy in a distributed stroke care network within a geographical region, including telemedicine support for treatment start at small frontline hospitals, one-tiered ambulance routing of patients to centres capable of providing IVT, two-tiered ambulance routing, with select patients potentially harbouring large vessel occlusions being diverted directly to endovascular-capable hospitals ('drip and ship' vs 'mothership'), and use of mobile stroke units (mobile CT ambulances) capable of delivering thrombolytic therapy in the field (Fassbender et al., 2017). The optimal organization and calibration of regional stroke systems of care, to ensure efficient thrombolytic therapy start and optimal outcomes at the population level, requires refinement in pragmatic controlled, service delivery trials.

Summary

Thrombolysis with intravenous (IV) recombinant tissue-plasminogen activator (alteplase; 0.9 mg/kg over 1 h) is beneficial for acute ischaemic stroke patients with potentially disabling neurological deficits, and without contraindications, when started within 4.5 hours of onset of symptoms. The degree of benefit is time dependent. Among 1000 patients, within 3 hours lessens long-term disability in 178 patients, while treatment between 3 and 4.5 hours lessens long-term disability in 66 patients. Though thrombolytic therapy under 4.5 hours is associated with an increased rate of symptomatic haemorrhage, treatment is not associated with an increase in death or severe disability at end of trial follow-up.

Based on the trial evidence, intravenous thrombolytic therapy within 3 hours of onset is strongly endorsed, and between 3 and 4.5 hours of onset moderately endorsed, by guidelines on 5 continents. Benefit is evident in patients under and over age 80, and in patients with up to moderate, but not extensive (more than 100 mL), early ischaemic changes on initial computed tomography (CT) or magnetic resonance imaging (MRI).

Intravenous thrombolytic therapy is also beneficial for patients 4.5 or more hours after onset found to have substantial salvageable tissue on penumbral CT and MR imaging. Systems of care should be optimized to start thrombolytic therapy no more than 60 minutes, and optimally under 30 minutes, after Emergency Department arrival.

Large-scale trials are needed, and under way, seeking to enhance intravenous thrombolytic therapy, including by testing: faster treatment start in mobile stroke units (mobile CT ambulances); the best fibrinolytic agent and concomitant lytic-enhancing combinations; bridging neuroprotection and collateral enhancement to preserve more brain tissue for lytic salvage; and the optimal way to combine intravenous thrombolytic therapy and endovascular mechanical thrombectomy in patients with large vessel occlusions.

References

Acker JE III, Pancioli AM, Crocco T J, Eckstein MK, Jauch EC, Larrabee H, et al. (2007). Implementation strategies for emergency medical services within stroke systems of care: a policy statement from the American Heart Association/ American Stroke Association Expert Panel on Emergency Medical Services Systems and the Stroke Council. *Stroke*, **38**(11), 3097–115.

Adeoye O, Sucharew H, Khoury J, Vagal A, Schmit PA, Ewing I, et al. (2015). Combined approach to lysis utilizing eptifibatide and recombinant tissue-type plasminogen activator in acute ischemic stroke-full dose regimen stroke trial. *Stroke*, **46**(9), 2529–33.

Alberts,MJ, Latchaw RE, Jagoda A, Wechsler LR, Crocco T, George MG, et al. (2011). Revised and updated recommendations for the establishment of primary stroke centers: a summary statement from the brain attack coalition. *Stroke*, **42**(9), 2651–65.

Alexandrov AV, Kohrmann M, Soinne L, Mandava P, Barreto AD, Demchuk AM, et al. (2016). Ultrasound enhanced thrombolysis for ischemic stroke: results of a multi-national phase iii trial – CLOTBUSTER. Paper presented at the European Stroke Organization Conference, Barcelona, Spain.

American College of Emergency Physicians; American Academy of Neurology (2013). Clinical policy: use of intravenous tPA for the management of acute ischemic stroke in the emergency department. *Ann Emerg Med*, **61**, 225–43.

Anderson CS, Robinson T, Lindley RI, Arima H, Lavados PM, Lee TH, et al.; Investigators and Coordinators. (2016). Low-dose versus standard-dose intravenous alteplase in acute ischemic stroke. *N Engl J Med*, **374**(24), 2313–23.

Ankolekar S, Fuller M, Cross I, Renton C, Cox P, Sprigg N, et al. (2013). Feasibility of an ambulance-based stroke trial, and safety of glyceryl trinitrate in ultra-acute stroke: the Rapid Intervention with Glyceryl Trinitrate in Hypertensive Stroke Trial (RIGHT, ISRCTN66434824). *Stroke*, **44**(11), 3120–8.

Atallah AM. (2012). Consensus on Diagnosis and Treatment of Acute Ischemic Stroke Council – Argentine Society of Cardiology. *Argentine J Cardiol*, **80**, 389–404.

Audebert HJ, Schenkel J, Heuschmann PU, Bogdahn U, Haberl RL. (2006). Effects of the implementation of a telemedical stroke network: the Telemedic Pilot Project for Integrative Stroke Care (TEMPiS) in Bavaria, Germany. *Lancet Neurol*, **5**(9), 742–8.

Barreto AD, Alexandrov AV, Lyden P, Lee J, Martin-Schild S, Shen L, et al. (2012). The argatroban and tissue-type plasminogen activator stroke study: final results of a pilot safety study. *Stroke*, **43**(3), 770–5.

Bath PM, Lees KR, Schellinger PD, Altman H, Bland M, Hogg C, et al. (2012). Statistical analysis of the primary outcome in acute stroke trials. *Stroke*, **43**(4), 1171–8.

Bendszus M, Donnan G, Hacke W, Molina C, Leys D, Ringleb P, et al.; ECASS-4 Collaborators. (2018). ECASS-4: EXTEND: Extending the Time for Thrombolysis in Emergency Neurological Deficits. *Eur Stroke J*, **3**(Suppl 1), 4 (abstract).

Bivard A, Huang X, Levi CR, Spratt N, Campbell BCV, Cheripelli BK, et al. (2017). Tenecteplase in ischemic stroke offers improved recanalization: analysis of 2 trials. *Neurology*, **89**(1), 62–7.

Bluhmki E, Chamorro A, Davalos A, Machnig T, Sauce C, Wahlgren N, et al. (2009). Stroke treatment with alteplase given 3.0–4.5 h after onset of acute ischaemic stroke (ECASS III): additional outcomes and subgroup analysis of a randomised controlled trial. *Lancet Neurol*, **8**(12), 1095–1102.

Bryer A, Connor M, Haug P, Cheyip B, Staub H, Tipping B, et al. (2010). South African guideline for management of ischaemic stroke and transient ischaemic attack 2010: a guideline from the South African Stroke Society (SASS) and the SASS Writing Committee. *S Afr Med J*, **100**(11 Pt 2), 747–78.

Campbell BC; E-IT Investigators. (2018). Tenecteplase versus alteplase before endovascular thrombectomy (EXTEND-IA TNK): a multicenter, randomized, controlled trial. Paper presented at the International Stroke Conference, Los Angeles, CA.

Chao AC, Liu CK, Chen CH, Lin HJ, Liu CH, Jeng JS, et al. (2014). Different doses of recombinant tissue-type plasminogen activator for acute stroke in Chinese patients. *Stroke*, **45**(8), 2359–65.

Cho KH, Ko SB, Kim SH, Park HK, Cho AH, Hong KS, et al. (2012). Focused update of Korean Clinical Practice

Guidelines for the Thrombolysis in Acute Stroke Management. *Korean J Stroke*, **14**, 95–105.

Ciccone A, Motto C, Aritzu E, Piana A, Candelise L. (2000). Negative interaction of aspirin and streptokinase in acute ischemic stroke: further analysis of the Multicenter Acute Stroke Trial – Italy. *Cerebrovasc Dis*, **10**(1), 61–4.

Daffertshofer M, Gass A, Ringleb P, Sitzer M, Sliwka U, Els T, et al. (2005). Transcranial low-frequency ultrasound-mediated thrombolysis in brain ischemia: increased risk of hemorrhage with combined ultrasound and tissue plasminogen activator: results of a phase II clinical trial. *Stroke*, **36**(7), 1441–6.

Davis SM, Donnan GA, Parsons MW, Levi C, Butcher KS, Peeters A, et al. (2008). Effects of alteplase beyond 3 h after stroke in the Echoplanar Imaging Thrombolytic Evaluation Trial (EPITHET): a placebo-controlled randomised trial. *Lancet Neurol*, **7**(4), 299–309.

DeMers G, Meurer WJ, Shih R, Rosenbaum S, Vilke GM. (2012). Tissue plasminogen activator and stroke: review of the literature for the clinician. *J Emerg Med* **43**(6): 1149–1154.

Diener HC, Foerch C, Riess H, Rother J, Schroth G, Weber R. (2013). Treatment of acute ischaemic stroke with thrombolysis or thrombectomy in patients receiving anti-thrombotic treatment. *Lancet Neurol*, **12**(7), 677–88.

Emberson J, Lees KR, Lyden P, Blackwell L, Albers G, Bluhmki E, et al. (2014). Effect of treatment delay, age, and stroke severity on the effects of intravenous thrombolysis with alteplase for acute ischaemic stroke: a meta-analysis of individual patient data from randomised trials. *Lancet*, **384**, 1929–35.

European Stroke Organization Executive Committee and the ESO Writing Committee. (2008). Guidelines for the Management of Ischaemic Stroke and Transient Ischemic Attack 2008. www.eso-stroke.org/pdf/ESO08_Guidelines_Original_english.pdf. Accessed July 2013.

Fassbender K, Grotta JC, Walter S, Grunwald IQ, Ragoschke-Schumm A, Saver J. (2017). Mobile stroke units for prehospital thrombolysis, triage, and beyond: benefits and challenges. *Lancet Neurol*, **16**(3), 227–37.

Feigin VL, Norrving B, Mensah GA. (2017). Global burden of stroke. *Circ Res*, **120**(3), 439–48.

Fischer U, Kaesmacher J, Mendes Pereira V, Chapot R, Siddiqui AH, Froehler MT, et al. (2017). Direct mechanical thrombectomy versus combined intravenous and mechanical thrombectomy in large-artery anterior circulation stroke: a topical review. *Stroke*, **48**(10), 2912–18.

Fisher M, Saver JL. (2015). Future directions of acute ischaemic stroke therapy. *Lancet Neurol*, **14**(7), 758–67.

Flynn D, Nesbitt DJ, Ford GA, McMeekin P, Rodgers H, Price C, et al. (2015). Development of a computerised decision aid for thrombolysis in acute stroke care. *BMC Med Inform Decis Mak*, **15**(1), 6.

Fonarow GC, Cox M, Smith E, Saver J, Reeves M, Bhatt D, et al. (2017). Abstract 86: progress in achieving more rapid door-to-needle times in acute ischemic stroke: interim findings from target: stroke phase II. *Stroke*, **48**(Suppl 1), A86.

Fonarow GC, Smith EE, Saver JL, Reeves MJ, Bhatt DL, Grau-Sepulveda MV, et al. (2011a). Timeliness of tissue-type plasminogen activator therapy in acute ischemic stroke: patient characteristics, hospital factors, and outcomes associated with door-to-needle times within 60 minutes. *Circulation*, **123**(7), 750–8.

Fonarow GC, Smith EE, Saver JL, Reeves MJ, Hernandez AF, Peterson ED, et al. (2011b). Improving door-to-needle times in acute ischemic stroke: the design and rationale for the American Heart Association/American Stroke Association's Target: Stroke initiative. *Stroke*, **42**(10), 2983–9.

Gadhia J, Starkman S, Ovbiagele B, Ali L, Liebeskind D, Saver JL. (2010). Assessment and improvement of figures to visually convey benefit and risk of stroke thrombolysis. *Stroke*, **41**(2), 300–6.

Goyal M., Menon BK, van Zwam WH, Dippel DW, Mitchell PJ, Demchuk AM, et al. (2016). Endovascular thrombectomy after large-vessel ischaemic stroke: a meta-analysis of individual patient data from five randomised trials. *Lancet*, **387**(10029), 1723–31.

Grotta J. (2001). Combination therapy stroke trial: recombinant tissue-type plasminogen activator with/without lubeluzole. *Cerebrovasc Dis*, **12**(3), 258–63.

Hacke W, Lyden P, Emberson J, Baigent C, Blackwell L, Albers G, et al; Stroke Thrombolysis Trialists' Collaborators. (2018). Effects of alteplase for acute stroke according to criteria defining the European Union and United States marketing authorizations: Individual-patient-data meta-analysis of randomized trials. *Int J Stroke*, **13**(2), 175–89.

Higashida R, Alberts MJ, Alexander DN, Crocco TJ, Demaerschalk BM, Derdeyn CP, et al. (2013). Interactions within stroke systems of care: a policy statement from the American Heart Association/American Stroke Association. *Stroke*, **44**(10), 2961–84.

Hill MD, Buchan AM. (2005). Thrombolysis for acute ischemic stroke: results of the Canadian Alteplase for Stroke Effectiveness Study. *CMAJ*, **172**(10), 1307–12.

Hougaard KD, Hjort N, Zeidler D, Sorensen L, Norgaard A, Hansen TM, et al. (2014). Remote ischemic perconditioning as an adjunct therapy to thrombolysis in patients with acute ischemic stroke: a randomized trial. *Stroke*, **45**(1), 159–67.

Huang X, MacIsaac R, Thompson JL, Levin B, Buchsbaum R, Haley EC Jr., Levi C, et al. (2016). Tenecteplase versus alteplase in stroke thrombolysis: an individual patient data meta-analysis of randomized controlled trials. *Int J Stroke*, **11**(5), 534–43.

Hughes, S. (2017). *NOR-TEST: tenecteplase similar to alteplase in stroke*. Medscape.

IST-3 Collaborative Group. (2015). Association between brain imaging signs, early and late outcomes, and response to intravenous alteplase after acute ischaemic stroke in the third International Stroke Trial (IST-3): secondary analysis of a randomised controlled trial. *Lancet Neurol*, **14**(5), 485–96.

Jauch EC, Saver JL, Adams HP Jr., Bruno A, Connors JJ, Demaerschalk BM, et al. (2013). Guidelines for the early management of patients with acute ischemic stroke: a guideline for healthcare professionals from the American Heart Association/American Stroke Association. *Stroke*, **44**(3), 870–947.

Kermer P, Eschenfelder CC, Diener HC, Grond M, Abdalla Y, Althaus K, et al. (2017). Antagonizing dabigatran by idarucizumab in cases of ischemic stroke or intracranial hemorrhage in Germany – a national case collection. *Int J Stroke*, **12**(4), 383–91.

Khatri P, Kleindorfer DO, Devlin T, Sawyer RN Jr, Starr M, Mejilla J, et al.; P. Investigators. (2018). Effect of alteplase vs aspirin on functional outcome for patients with acute ischemic stroke and minor nondisabling neurologic deficits: the PRISMS randomized clinical trial. *JAMA*, **320**(2), 156–66.

Kim BJ, Han MK, Park TH, Park SS, Lee KB, Lee BC, et al. (2015). Low-versus standard-dose alteplase for ischemic strokes within 4.5 hours: a comparative effectiveness and safety study. *Stroke*, **46**(9), 2541–8.

Kim JT, Fonarow GC, Smith EE, Reeves MJ, Navalkele DD, Grotta JC, et al. (2017). treatment with tissue plasminogen activator in the golden hour and the shape of the 4.5-hour time-benefit curve in the national United States Get with the Guidelines-Stroke population. *Circulation*, **135**(2), 128–39.

Lansberg MG, Schrooten M, Bluhmki E, Thijs VN, J. L. Saver JL. (2009). Treatment time-specific number needed to treat estimates for tissue plasminogen activator therapy in acute stroke based on shifts over the entire range of the modified Rankin Scale. *Stroke*, **40**(6), 2079–84.

Lees KR, Emberson J, Blackwell L, Bluhmki E, Davis SM, Donnan GA, et al.; Stroke Thrombolysis Trialists' Collaborators. (2016). Effects of alteplase for acute stroke on the distribution of functional outcomes: a pooled analysis of 9 trials. *Stroke*, **47**(9), 2373–9.

Legrand L, Naggara O, Turc G, Mellerio C, Roca P, Calvet D, et al. (2013). Clot burden score on admission T2*-MRI predicts recanalization in acute stroke. *Stroke*, **44**(7), 1878–84.

Liberatore GT,. Samson A, Bladin C, Schleuning WD, Medcalf RL. (2003). Vampire bat salivary plasminogen activator (desmoteplase): a unique fibrinolytic enzyme that does not promote neurodegeneration. *Stroke*, **34**(2), 537–43.

Lindley RI, Wardlaw JM, Whiteley WN, Cohen G, Blackwell L, Murray GD, et al.; ISTC Group (2015). Alteplase for acute ischemic stroke: outcomes by clinically important subgroups in the Third International Stroke Trial. *Stroke*, **46**(3), 746–56.

Lindsay P, Bayley M, McDonald A, Graham ID, Warner G, Phillips S. (2008). Toward a more effective approach to stroke: Canadian Best Practice Recommendations for Stroke Care. *CMAJ*, **178**(11), 1418–25.

Logallo N, Novotny V, Assmus J, Kvistad CE, Alteheld L, Ronning OM, et al. (2017). Tenecteplase versus alteplase for management of acute ischaemic stroke (NOR-TEST): a phase 3, randomised, open-label, blinded endpoint trial. *Lancet Neurol*, **16**(10), 781–8.

Lorenzano S, Toni D, (2017). TESPI (Thrombolysis in elderly stroke patients in Italy). Paper presented at the European Stroke Organization Conference, Prague, Czech Republic.

Luo S, Zhuang M, Zeng W, Tao J. (2016). Intravenous thrombolysis for acute ischemic stroke in patients receiving antiplatelet therapy: a systematic review and meta-analysis of 19 studies. *J Am Heart Assoc*, **5**(5), e003242.

Lyden P, Jacoby M, Schim J, Albers G, Mazzeo P, Ashwood T, et al. (2001). The Clomethiazole Acute Stroke Study in tissue-type plasminogen activator-treated stroke (CLASS-T): final results. *Neurology*, **57**, 1199–1205.

Ma H, Campbell BCV, Parsons MW, Churilov L, Levi CR, Hsu C, et al.; EXTEND Investigators. (2019). Thrombolysis guided by perfusion imaging up to 9 hours after onset of stroke. *N Engl J Med*, **380**(19), 1795–1803.

Meretoja A, Strbian D, Mustanoja S, Tatlisumak T, Lindsberg PJ, Kaste M. (2012). Reducing in-hospital delay to 20 minutes in stroke thrombolysis. *Neurology*, **79**(4), 306–13.

Montero M, Tokunboh I, Sharma L, Szeder SV, AM LD, Lansberg M, et al. (2017). Harmonized visual decision aids to expedite physician, patient, and family decision-making regarding intravenous tPA for acute ischemic stroke in different time windows. *Eur Stroke J*, **2**(IS), 155.

Mori E, Minematsu K, Nakagawara J, Hasegawa Y, Nagahiro S, Okada Y, Truelsen T, et al.; D.-J. Investigators (2015). Safety and tolerability of desmoteplase within 3 to 9 hours after symptoms onset in Japanese patients with ischemic stroke. *Stroke*, **46**(9), 2549–54.

Nacu A, Kvistad CE, Naess H, Oygarden H, Logallo N, J. Assmus J, et al. (2017). NOR-SASS (Norwegian Sonothrombolysis in Acute Stroke Study): randomized controlled contrast-enhanced sonothrombolysis in an unselected acute ischemic stroke population. *Stroke*, **48**(2), 335–41.

Nakagawara J, Minematsu K, Okada Y, Tanahashi N, Nagahiro S, Mori E, et al. (2010). Thrombolysis with 0.6 mg/kg intravenous alteplase for acute ischemic stroke in routine clinical practice: the Japan post-Marketing Alteplase Registration Study (J-MARS). *Stroke*, **41**(9), 1984–9.

National Institute for Health and Clinical Excellence (NICE) – National Health Services. (2007). Final appraisal determination: alteplase for the treatment of acute ischaemic stroke. www.nice.org.uk/nicemedia/pdf/StokeAt eplFAD.pdf. Accessed October 2009.

NINDS t-PA Stroke Trial Study Group. (1997). Generalized efficacy of t-PA for acute stroke. Subgroup analysis of the NINDS t-PA Stroke Trial. *Stroke*, **28**(11), 2119–25.

Pancioli AM, Adeoye, O, Schmit PA, Khoury J, Levine SR, Tomsick TA, et al.; and C.-E. Investigators. (2013). Combined approach to lysis utilizing eptifibatide and recombinant tissue plasminogen activator in acute ischemic stroke – enhanced regimen stroke trial. *Stroke*, **44**(9): 2381–7.

Pancioli AM, Broderick J, Brott T, Tomsick T, Khoury J, Bean J, et al. (2008). The combined approach to lysis utilizing eptifibatide and rt-PA in acute ischemic stroke: the CLEAR stroke trial. *Stroke*, **39**(12), 3268–76.

Parsons M, Spratt N, Bivard A, Campbell B, Chung K, Miteff F, et al. (2012). A randomized trial of tenecteplase versus alteplase for acute ischemic stroke. *N Engl J Med*, **366** (12), 1099–1107.

Picanco MR, Christensen S, Campbell BC, Churilov L, Parsons MW, Desmond PM, et al. (2014). Reperfusion after 4.5 hours reduces infarct growth and improves clinical outcomes. *Int J Stroke*, **9**(3), 266–9.

Pikija S, Sztriha LK, Sebastian Mutzenbach J, Golaszewski SM, Sellner J. (2017). Idarucizumab in dabigatran-treated patients with acute ischemic stroke receiving alteplase: a systematic review of the available evidence. *CNS Drugs*, **31**(9), 747–57.

Reddrop C, Moldrich RX, Beart PM, Farso M, Liberatore GT, Howells DW, et al. (2005). Vampire bat salivary plasminogen activator (desmoteplase) inhibits tissue-type plasminogen activator-induced potentiation of excitotoxic injury. *Stroke*, **36**(6), 1241–6.

Sanossian N. (2017). Before the angiography suite: prehospital stroke identification, routing, and treatment. *Endovascular Today*, **16,** 45–52.

Saposnik G, Gladstone D, Raptis R, Zhou L, Hart RG; Investigators of the Registry of the Canadian Stroke Network and the Stroke Outcomes Research Canada Working Group. (2013). Atrial fibrillation in ischemic stroke: predicting response to thrombolysis and clinical outcomes. *Stroke*, **44**(1), 99–104.

Saqqur M, Tsivgoulis G, Nicoli F, Skoloudik D, Sharma VK, Larrue V, et al. (2014). The role of sonolysis and sonothrombolysis in acute ischemic stroke: a systematic review and meta-analysis of randomized controlled trials and case-control studies. *J Neuroimaging*, **24**(3), 209–20.

Saver JL. (2011). Optimal end points for acute stroke therapy trials: best ways to measure treatment effects of drugs and devices. *Stroke*, **42**(8), 2356–62.

Saver JL, Fonarow GC, Smith EE, Reeves MJ, Grau-Sepulveda MV, Pan W, et al. (2013). Time to treatment with

intravenous tissue plasminogen activator and outcome from acute ischemic stroke. *JAMA*, **309**(23), 2480–8.

Saver JL, Gornbein J, Grotta J, Liebeskind D, Lutsep H, Schwamm L, et al. (2009). Number needed to treat to benefit and to harm for intravenous tissue plasminogen activator therapy in the 3- to 4.5-hour window: joint outcome table analysis of the ECASS 3 trial. *Stroke*, **40**(7), 2433–7.

Seiffge DJ, Hooff RJ, Nolte CH, Bejot Y, Turc G, Ikenberg B, et al. (2015). Recanalization therapies in acute ischemic stroke patients: impact of prior treatment with novel oral anticoagulants on bleeding complications and outcome. *Circulation*, **132**(13), 1261–9.

Sharma M, Clark H, Armour T, Stotts G, Coté R, Hill MD, et al. (2005). Acute stroke: evaluation and treatment. *Evid Rep Technol Assess (Summ)*, **127**, 1–7.

Shobha N., Fang J, Hill MD. (2013). Do lacunar strokes benefit from thrombolysis? Evidence from the Registry of the Canadian Stroke Network. *Int J Stroke*, **8**(Suppl A100), 45–49.

Thomalla G, Simonsen CZ, Boutitie F, Andersen G, Berthezene Y, Cheng B, et al.; W.-U. Investigators. (2018). MRI-guided thrombolysis for stroke with unknown time of onset. *N Engl J Med*, **379**(7), 611–22.

Tong X, Liao X, Pan Y, Cao Y, Wang C, Liu C, et al. (2016). Intravenous thrombolysis is more safe and effective for posterior circulation stroke: Data from the Thrombolysis Implementation and Monitor of Acute Ischemic Stroke in China (TIMS-China). *Medicine (Baltimore)*, **95**(24), e3848.

von Kummer R, Mori E, Truelsen T, Jensen JS, Gronning BA, Fiebach JB, et al. (2016). Desmoteplase 3 to 9 hours after major artery occlusion stroke: the DIAS-4 Trial (efficacy and safety study of desmoteplase to treat acute ischemic stroke). *Stroke*, **47**(12), 2880–87.

Wahlgren N, Ahmed N. (2016). *SITS Report 2016*. Stockholm: SITS International Coordination Team.

Warach S, Al-Rawi Y, Furlan AJ, Fiebach JB, Wintermark M, Lindsten A, et al. (2012). Refinement of the magnetic resonance diffusion-perfusion mismatch concept for thrombolytic patient selection: insights from the desmoteplase in acute stroke trials. *Stroke*, **43**(9), 2313–18.

Wardlaw JM, Koumellis P, Liu M. (2013). Thrombolysis (different doses, routes of administration and agents) for acute ischaemic stroke. *Cochrane Database Syst Rev*, 5, CD000514.

Wardlaw JM, Murray V, Berge E, del Zoppo GJ. (2014). Thrombolysis for acute ischaemic stroke. *Cochrane Database Syst Rev*, 7, CD000213.

Wechsler LR, Demaerschalk BM, Schwamm LH, Adeoye OM, Audebert HJ, Fanale CV, et al. (2017). Telemedicine quality and outcomes in stroke: a scientific statement for healthcare professionals from the American Heart Association/American Stroke Association. *Stroke*, **48** (1), e3–e25.

Wheeler HM, Mlynash M, Inoue M, Tipirnini A, Liggins J, Bammer R, et al. (2015). The growth rate of early DWI lesions is highly variable and associated with penumbral salvage and clinical outcomes following endovascular reperfusion. *Int J Stroke*, **10**(5), 723–9.

Whiteley WN, Emberson J, Lees KR, Blackwell L, Albers G, Bluhmki E, et al; Stroke Thrombolysis Trialists. (2016). Risk of intracerebral haemorrhage with alteplase after acute ischaemic stroke: a secondary analysis of an individual patient data meta-analysis. *Lancet Neurol*, **15**(9), 925–33.

Wright L, Hill KM, Bernhardt J, Lindley R, Ada L, Bajorek BV, et al. (2012). Stroke management: updated recommendations for treatment along the care continuum. *Intern Med J*, **42**(5), 562–9.

Xian Y, Federspiel JJ, Hernandez AF, Laskowitz DT, Schwamm LH, Bhatt DL, et al. (2017a). Use of intravenous recombinant tissue plasminogen activator in patients with acute ischemic stroke who take non-vitamin K antagonist oral anticoagulants before stroke. *Circulation*, **135**(11), 1024–35.

Xian Y, Liang L, Smith EE, Schwamm LH, Reeves MJ, Olson DM, et al. (2012). Risks of intracranial hemorrhage among patients with acute ischemic stroke receiving warfarin and treated with intravenous tissue plasminogen activator. *JAMA*, **307**(24), 2600–8.

Xian Y, Xu H, Lytle B, Blevins J, Peterson ED, Hernandez AF, et al. (2017b). Use of strategies to improve door-to-needle times with tissue-type plasminogen activator in acute ischemic stroke in clinical practice: findings from Target: Stroke. *Circ Cardiovasc Qual Outcomes*, **10**(1).

Yayan J. (2013). Onset of orolingual angioedema after treatment of acute brain ischemia with alteplase depends on the site of brain ischemia: a meta-analysis. *N Am J Med Sci*, **5**(10), 589–93.

Zinkstok SM, Roos YB; ARTIS Investigators. (2012). Early administration of aspirin in patients treated with alteplase for acute ischaemic stroke: a randomised controlled trial. *Lancet*, **380**(9843), 731–7.

Reperfusion of the Ischaemic Brain by Endovascular Thrombectomy and Thrombolysis

Meng Lee

Jeffrey L. Saver

Rationale

About 70% of all strokes worldwide are caused by occlusion of a cerebral artery, resulting in focal brain infarction (ischaemic stroke) (Feigin et al., 2017). The obstruction is usually a thrombus that has formed *in situ* on an atherosclerotic plaque or a thrombus that has embolized from a proximal source such as the extracranial neck vessels, the aortic arch, the heart, or the leg and pelvic veins.

Endovascular treatments aim to rapidly restore blood flow, before all the ischaemic brain in the territory supplied by the artery has become infarcted, by using catheter-delivered strategies to remove or disrupt fresh thrombi or other occlusive material. Endovascular therapies encompass mechanical and pharmacological approaches. Endovascular mechanical thrombectomy uses catheter-delivered devices, including retrievers and aspirators, to capture and extract the target thrombus. Endovascular mechanical angioplasty uses expandable balloons and implanted stents to restore the arterial lumen by pushing thrombus and atherosclerotic plaque against the arterial wall. Endovascular pharmacological thrombolysis (or, more correctly, fibrinolysis) lyses fresh thrombi by using intra-arterial infusions to deliver thrombolytic drugs at high concentration directly to, and within, the target clot.

Endovascular reperfusion is a complementary strategy to intravenous (IV) thrombolysis. As IV delivery yields relatively modest fibrinolytic drug concentration arriving at target thrombi, IV thrombolysis is more effective at digesting the smaller clots that obstruct small- and medium-size vessels, and less effective for large vessel occlusions (LVOs) with sizeable clot burdens (Legrand et al., 2013). In contrast, mechanical thrombectomy devices are highly efficient at recanalizing large proximal occlusions and less effective for small distal occlusions in vessels too small for easy device access.

Evidence

Study Designs and Patients

A total of 17 randomized controlled trials (RCTs) have compared endovascular recanalization therapy added to non-endovascular therapy (supportive care or intravenous fibrinolysis [IVT]) with non-endovascular therapy alone in 3361 highly selected patients (O'Rourke et al., 2010; Wardlaw et al., 2014; Badhiwala, et al., 2015; Bendszus et al., 2016; Rodrigues et al., 2016; Muir et al., 2017). The great preponderance of patients underwent vessel imaging to confirm presence of a target LVO prior to enrolment, including 2355 patients (12 trials) qualifying by computed tomography or magnetic resonance angiography (CTA or MRA, 12 trials) and 350 patients (4 trials) qualifying by catheter angiography. Another 656 patients (1 trial) were enrolled based on having substantial deficits likely to reflect LVO presence. Patients almost entirely had proximal intracranial occlusions in the anterior circulation, generally in the intracranial internal carotid artery or the M1 segment of the middle cerebral artery (MCA), and less often in the M2 MCA. Posterior circulation and more distal anterior circulation occlusions were rarely enrolled.

The endovascular therapies tested in these trials evolved over time, from moderately effective reperfusion techniques, including intra-arterial fibrinolysis, and coil retriever and combined aspiration–maceration devices (1994–2012: 7 trials, 1486 patients) to highly effective reperfusion techniques, including stent retriever and large-bore aspiration devices (2010 forward: 10 trials, 1875 patients) (Saver, 2013).

Standard care therapy, administered to participants in both endovascular and non-endovascular study arms, included IVF for all enrolled patients in 6 trials (1480 patients); IVF for all IVF-eligible and supportive care for IVF ineligible patients in 6 trials (1527 patients); supportive care with enrolment of only internationally IVF-ineligible patients in 4 trials (240 patients); and supportive care with enrolment of only nation-specific IVF-ineligible patients in 1 trial (114 patients).

In addition to trials with non-endovascular control arms, 5 randomized controlled trials, enrolling 1140 patients, have compared different endovascular mechanical thrombectomy devices against one another (Nogueira et al., 2012; Saver et al., 2012; Lapergue et al., 2017; Mocco et al., 2018; Nogueira et al., 2018); and 3 trials, enrolling 443 patients, have compared endovascular reperfusion therapies alone against IV reperfusion strategies alone (Ducrocq et al., 2005; Ciccone et al., 2010, 2013).

Complementing broad study-level meta-analyses, an individual patient-level data systematic analysis, permitting more detailed adjustment for prognostic variables, has analysed the first 5 trials of highly effective mechanical reperfusion devices versus non-endovascular controls, enrolling 1287 patients (Goyal et al., 2016; Saver et al., 2016).

Interventions

In randomized trials of intra-arterial administration of fibrinolytics, agents tested were urokinase, pro-urokinase, recombinant tissue plasminogen activator (rt-PA), and rt-PA with enhancement by ultrasound emitted from the catheter tip. In randomized trials of early generation mechanical thrombectomy, devices tested coil retrievers to physically enclose and remove the entire target thrombus and combined aspiration–maceration devices to break up and aspirate the thrombus without capturing it whole. In randomized trials of later generation mechanical thrombectomy, devices tested were (1) stent retrievers to physically enclose, trap, and retrieve the entire target thrombus; (2) large-bore aspiration catheters to physically suction the entire target thrombus; (3) large-bore aspiration catheters to engage the proximal clot by suction and then retrieve the entire the target thrombus; and (4) simultaneous, combined endovascular mechanical thrombectomy with both retriever and aspiration for clot extraction (EMBRACE technique). The later generation devices, alone and combined, were superior to lytic and early

generation mechanical techniques, as confirmed in head-to-head randomized trials (Nogueira et al., 2012; Saver et al., 2012). Accordingly, later generation, highly effective recanalization devices are the mainstay of current clinical practice, and the evidence from trials testing these devices is a special focus of this chapter.

Results for All Endovascular Interventions against Non-Endovascular Controls

Overall, across all trials and all forms of endovascular intervention, random allocation to endovascular reperfusion therapy was associated with increased freedom from disability (modified Rankin score [mRS] 0–1 at 3–6 months, 29.1% vs 17.3%; relative risk [RR] 1.72, 95% confidence interval [CI]: 1.44–2.06; $p < 0.00001$) and increased functional independence (mRS 0–2 at 3–6 months, 44.8% vs 29.3%; RR 1.58, 95% CI: 1.34–1.86; $p < 0.00001$) (Figures 7.1 and 7.2). In addition, patients allocated to endovascular therapy had reduced mortality (16.8% vs 19.3%; RR 0.84, 95% CI: 0.73–0.98; $p = 0.02$), and a non-significantly higher symptomatic haemorrhage rate (5.6% vs 4.1%; RR 1.24, 95% CI: 0.90–1.7; $p = 0.19$) (Figures 7.3 and 7.4).

Results for Patients Treated with Different Endovascular Recanalization Therapies

In the trials of endovascular recanalization therapy against non-endovascular controls, there was evidence that different endovascular treatment approaches differed in their effect upon freedom from disability (mRS 0–1) (heterogeneity $p = 0.005$), functional independence (mRS 0–2) (heterogeneity $p = 0.0001$), and mortality (heterogeneity $p = 0.02$), though not symptomatic haemorrhage. For both functional outcomes and for all-cause mortality, the highly effective mechanical thrombectomy reperfusion interventions had the greatest benefit, with lesser benefits with intra-arterial fibrinolysis, and no benefit with moderately effective mechanical thrombectomy reperfusion techniques.

These findings were confirmed in two randomized trials that directly compared stent retrievers, a highly effective endovascular mechanical thrombectomy technique, against coil retrievers, an earlier, moderately effective recanalization technique. Study-level meta-analysis of these two trials indicates that highly effective reperfusion therapies, compared with moderately effective therapies, are

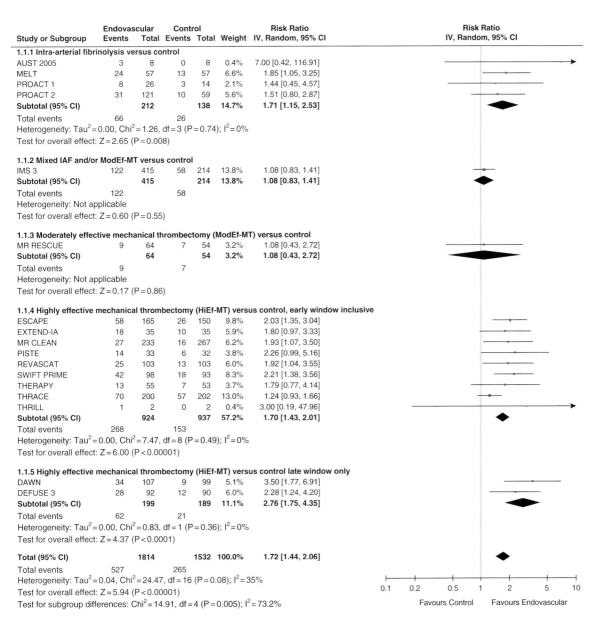

Figure 7.1 *Disability-free outcome (mRS 0–1) at 3 months – endovascular reperfusion therapy vs controls.*

associated with increased achievement of substantial reperfusion (original thrombolysis in cerebral infarction [oTICI] scale 2b or 3 – Hi-Eff devices 68.3%, Mod-Eff devices 39.2%; RR 1.70, 95% CI: 1.35–2.15; $p < 0.0001$). This improved reperfusion was associated with more disability-free outcomes at 3 months (Hi-Eff devices 26.4%, Mod-Eff devices 16.3%; RR 1.61, 95% CI: 1.01–2.58), more functional independence at 3 months (Hi-Eff devices 38.6%, Mod-Eff devices 23.9%; RR 1.56, 95% CI: 1.09–2.24),

without alterations in death or symptomatic intracranial haemorrhage.

Three randomized trials have compared different highly effective devices against one another, including stent retrievers versus aspiration devices (Lapergue et al., 2017; Mocco et al., 2018), and combined stent retrievers and aspiration devices versus aspiration devices alone (Nogueira et al., 2018). The different techniques performed roughly comparably in achieving substantial reperfusion and disability-free and

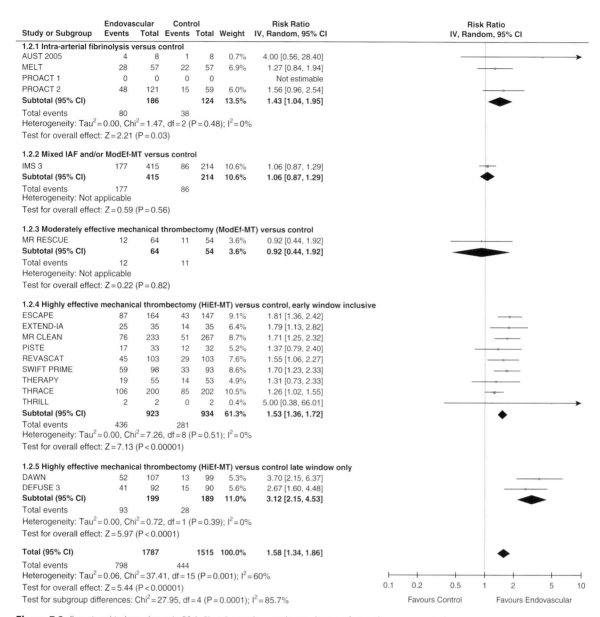

Figure 7.2 *Functional independence (mRS 0–2) at 3 months – endovascular reperfusion therapy vs controls.*

independent functional outcomes, with low mortality and symptomatic haemorrhage rates.

Results for Highly Effective Endovascular Interventions against Non-Endovascular Controls, among Broadly Selected Patients Early after Onset

A total of 9 trials enrolling 1849 patients tested highly effective endovascular interventions against non-

endovascular controls among relatively broadly selected patients presenting early after stroke onset. Permitted time windows, target occlusion locations, and degree of early ischaemic changes on presenting imaging varied across the trials, but the great preponderance of enrolled patients were within 6 hours of last known well, had intracranial internal carotid artery (ICA) or M1 segment MCA occlusions, and modest ischaemic changes on brain imaging (Alberta Stroke Program Early CT Score [ASPECTS] scale 7–10).

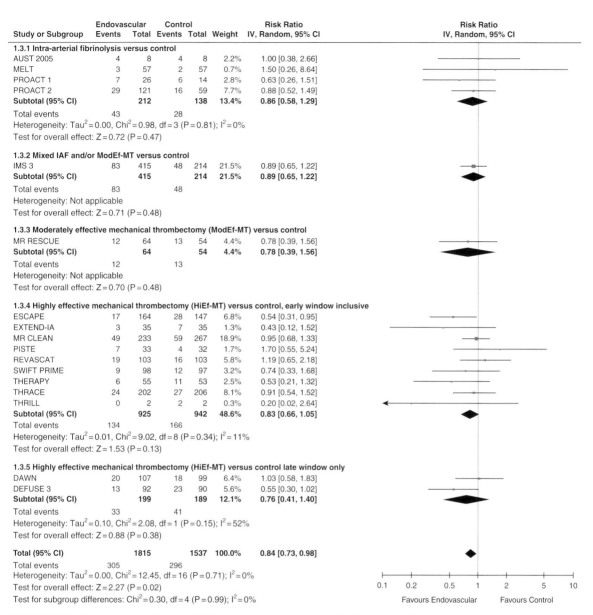

Study or Subgroup	Endovascular Events	Total	Control Events	Total	Weight	Risk Ratio IV, Random, 95% CI
1.3.1 Intra-arterial fibrinolysis versus control						
AUST 2005	4	8	4	8	2.2%	1.00 [0.38, 2.66]
MELT	3	57	2	57	0.7%	1.50 [0.26, 8.64]
PROACT 1	7	26	6	14	2.8%	0.63 [0.26, 1.51]
PROACT 2	29	121	16	59	7.7%	0.88 [0.52, 1.49]
Subtotal (95% CI)		**212**		**138**	**13.4%**	**0.86 [0.58, 1.29]**
Total events	43		28			

Heterogeneity: Tau^2=0.00, Chi^2=0.98, df=3 (P=0.81); I^2=0%
Test for overall effect: Z=0.72 (P=0.47)

1.3.2 Mixed IAF and/or ModEf-MT versus control						
IMS 3	83	415	48	214	21.5%	0.89 [0.65, 1.22]
Subtotal (95% CI)		**415**		**214**	**21.5%**	**0.89 [0.65, 1.22]**
Total events	83		48			

Heterogeneity: Not applicable
Test for overall effect: Z=0.71 (P=0.48)

1.3.3 Moderately effective mechanical thrombectomy (ModEf-MT) versus control						
MR RESCUE	12	64	13	54	4.4%	0.78 [0.39, 1.56]
Subtotal (95% CI)		**64**		**54**	**4.4%**	**0.78 [0.39, 1.56]**
Total events	12		13			

Heterogeneity: Not applicable
Test for overall effect: Z=0.70 (P=0.48)

1.3.4 Highly effective mechanical thrombectomy (HiEf-MT) versus control, early window inclusive						
ESCAPE	17	164	28	147	6.8%	0.54 [0.31, 0.95]
EXTEND-IA	3	35	7	35	1.3%	0.43 [0.12, 1.52]
MR CLEAN	49	233	59	267	18.9%	0.95 [0.68, 1.33]
PISTE	7	33	4	32	1.7%	1.70 [0.55, 5.24]
REVASCAT	19	103	16	103	5.8%	1.19 [0.65, 2.18]
SWIFT PRIME	9	98	12	97	3.2%	0.74 [0.33, 1.68]
THERAPY	6	55	11	53	2.5%	0.53 [0.21, 1.32]
THRACE	24	202	27	206	8.1%	0.91 [0.54, 1.52]
THRILL	0	2	2	2	0.3%	0.20 [0.02, 2.64]
Subtotal (95% CI)		**925**		**942**	**48.6%**	**0.83 [0.66, 1.05]**
Total events	134		166			

Heterogeneity: Tau^2=0.01, Chi^2=9.02, df=8 (P=0.34); I^2=11%
Test for overall effect: Z=1.53 (P=0.13)

1.3.5 Highly effective mechanical thrombectomy (HiEf-MT) versus control late window only						
DAWN	20	107	18	99	6.4%	1.03 [0.58, 1.83]
DEFUSE 3	13	92	23	90	5.6%	0.55 [0.30, 1.02]
Subtotal (95% CI)		**199**		**189**	**12.1%**	**0.76 [0.41, 1.40]**
Total events	33		41			

Heterogeneity: Tau^2=0.10, Chi^2=2.08, df=1 (P=0.15); I^2=52%
Test for overall effect: Z=0.88 (P=0.38)

Total (95% CI)		**1815**		**1537**	**100.0%**	**0.84 [0.73, 0.98]**
Total events	305		296			

Heterogeneity: Tau^2=0.00, Chi^2=12.45, df=16 (P=0.71); I^2=0%
Test for overall effect: Z=2.27 (P=0.02)
Test for subgroup differences: Chi^2=0.30, df=4 (P=0.99); I^2=0%

Favours Endovascular   Favours Control

Figure 7.3 *Death from all causes during study follow-up – endovascular reperfusion therapy vs controls.*

Freedom from Disability at 3 Months

Among these generally early-presenting acute ischaemic stroke (AIS) – LVO patients participating in trials predominantly testing highly effective reperfusion devices, random allocation to endovascular intervention was associated with an increase in disability-free outcome (mRS, 0–1) at 3 months after randomization (29.0% thrombolysis, 16.3% control; RR 1.72, 95% CI: 1.44–2.06; $p < 0.00001$). This represents 127 more disability-free patients per 1000 treated with endovascular reperfusion compared with control (see Figure 7.1). There was no heterogeneity across individual trials (heterogeneity $p = 0.49$), indicating consistency in evidence of treatment benefit.

Functional Independence at 3 Months

Endovascular therapy predominantly with highly effective mechanical devices was also associated with an increase in functional independence (mRS 0–2) at 3 months after randomization (47.2%

131

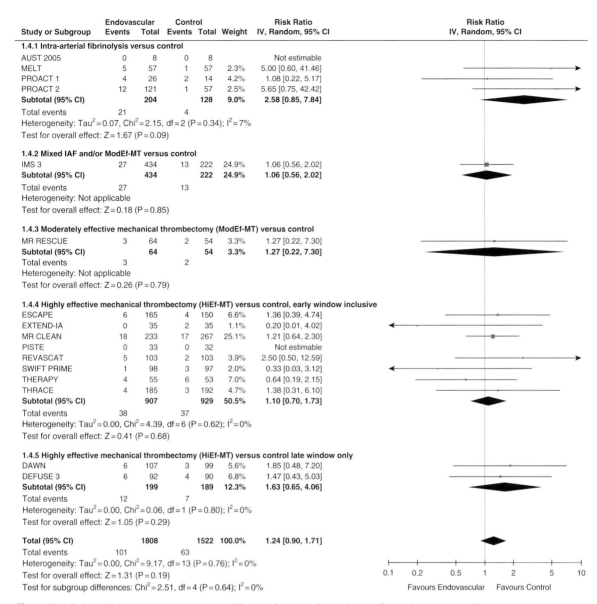

Figure 7.4 *Early (7–10 days) symptomatic intracranial haemorrhage – endovascular reperfusion therapy vs controls.*

endovascular therapy, 30.1% control; RR 1.58, 95% CI: 1.34–1.86; $p < 0.00001$). This represents 171 more functionally independent patients per 1000 treated with endovascular reperfusion compared with control (see Figure 7.2). Indications of benefit were consistent across studies, without evidence of variability (heterogeneity $p = 0.51$).

Death by 3 Months

By 3 months, patients allocated to endovascular therapy predominantly with highly effective devices had a non-significant trend toward lower mortality (14.5% endovascular therapy, 17.6% control; RR 0.83, 95% CI: 0.66–1.05; $p = 0.13$), representing a potential 31 fewer deaths per 1000 patients treated with endovascular therapy compared with control (see Figure 7.3). Signals of benefit were consistent across studies (heterogeneity $p = 0.34$).

Early Symptomatic Intracranial Haemorrhage

Endovascular therapy predominantly with highly effective devices was not associated with alteration in rates of early symptomatic intracranial haemorrhage within 7–10 days of treatment (4.2% endovascular therapy,

4.0% control; RR 1.10, 95% CI: 0.70–1.73; $p < 0.68$) (see Figure 7.4). Effect findings were consistent across trials (heterogeneity $p = 0.68$).

Other Complications

Endovascular therapy with highly effective thrombectomy devices is associated with additional, less-common complications, including, most notably, infarcts in new territories and femoral artery access site haematoma or pseudoaneurysm. These were not uniformly recorded in all the major randomized trials, but information on their frequency is available from subsets of the trials. An infarct in a new territory most commonly arises when control is lost over a thrombus or a fragment of a thrombus being retrieved from the cerebral circulation, and the released thrombus embolizes to a new territory. For example, a clot grasped and withdrawn from the M1 MCA may escape device control during passage through the ICA siphon and embolize to the anterior cerebral artery, causing ischaemia and infarction in the previously uninvolved anterior cerebral artery. Across 2 of the trials, infarcts in a new territory occurred in 5.4% (18/336) of endovascular versus 0.3% (1/370) of medical patients, RR 19.8, 95% CI: 2.7–147.7; $p = 0.004$ (Berkhemer et al., 2015; Jovin et al., 2015). A haematoma or pseudoaneurysm at the femoral arterial access site is a potential complication of all endovascular procedures. With endovascular thrombectomy, across 2 of the trials, femoral artery haematoma or pseudoaneurysm occurred in 5.6% (15/268) of endovascular versus 0% (0/253) of medical patients, RR 29.3, 95% CI: 1.8–486.7; $p = 0.02$ (Goyal et al., 2015; Jovin et al., 2015).

Degree of Disability at 3 Months

Analyses of dichotomized outcomes consider only a single health state transition that treatment may affect. For example, the outcome of being alive and disability-free counts only transitions across the border between mRS level 2 and mRS level 1, while the outcome of being alive and independent counts only transitions between mRS level 3 and mRS level 2. In contrast, analyses of ordinal outcomes consider simultaneously multiple valuable health state transitions that treatment may affect (Saver, 2011; Bath et al., 2012). For example, analysis of the distribution of outcomes over the entire mRS counts all transitions across all seven degrees of post-stroke disability the scale assesses, from asymptomatic, through varying degrees of impairment, to death.

An analysis has been conducted of the effect of highly effective reperfusion devices on the distribution of patient outcomes across all 7 levels of disability assessed by the mRS using participant-level data from the first 5 completed trials, enrolling 1287 patients (Goyal et al., 2016) (Figure 7.5). In these trials, allocation to endovascular thrombectomy resulted in increased proportions of patients at all disability ranks, including more patients who are asymptomatic (mRS 0), disability-free (mRS 0–1), functionally independent (mRS 0–2), ambulatory (mRS 0–3), not needing continuous care (mRS 0–4), and alive (mRS 0–5). Overall, treatment with highly effective endovascular thrombectomy versus control increased the odds of a better (less disabled) outcome state, adjusted common odds ratio (cOR) 2.49 (95% CI: 1.76–3.53). Using the automated algorithmic min–max joint outcome table method, for every 1000 patients treated with endovascular thrombectomy, a net of 423 patients will have a lower level of disability as a result of treatment (Tokunboh et al., 2018).

Results for Highly Effective Endovascular Interventions against Non-Endovascular Controls, among Imaging-Selected Patients Late after Onset

In acute cerebral ischaemia, when an artery is abruptly occluded, collateral vessels provide compensating blood flow to the supplied region. The robustness of

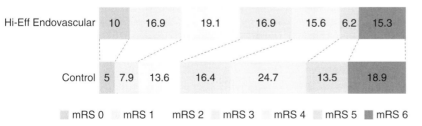

Figure 7.5 *Level of disability at 3–6 months, endovascular thrombectomy with highly effective devices versus control*, pooled trial analysis, based on data in Goyal et al. (2016).

the collateral supply varies widely from individual to individual, depending on variations in circle of Willis anatomy, stenoses and occlusions in the alternative channels themselves, the site of the new occlusion, and systemic blood pressure. Shortly after the inciting vascular occlusion, a small brain region within the supplied field may experience complete loss of blood flow, causing cellular death within 1 to a few minutes. But a much larger, surrounding zone will experience moderate reductions in blood flow that the brain cells can tolerate for tens of minutes to several hours. As time from onset lengthens, the zone of the completed, irreversible infarction – the core – expands and the rim of threatened but still salvageable tissue – the penumbra – shrinks.

CT and MRI techniques indexing core and penumbra volume permit identification of the subset of patients with well-defined onset times who are 'slow progressors' and still harbour rescuable tissue in later time windows (Wheeler et al., 2015). They also enable assessment of tissue status in patients with uncertain onset times, due to stroke onset some time during sleep or awake onset in an unaccompanied patient, with aphasia or confusion precluding patient report or observation of onset time. With CT, perfusion CT imaging identifies as core regions with extreme reduction in blood flow or blood volume, and as penumbra regions with moderate blood flow reduction (perfusion–core mismatch). With MRI, diffusion MR sequences identify as core regions with substantial diffusion abnormality, indicating advanced bioenergetic compromise, and perfusion MRI sequences identify as penumbra regions with moderate-to-severe blood flow reduction not yet showing diffusion abnormality (perfusion–diffusion mismatch). Alternative, less precise but more readily obtained, approaches to identifying patients with penumbra estimate the volume of perfusion reduction using the presence of LVO (vessel–core mismatch), the extent of collateral vessels (collateral–core mismatch), or the severity of neurological deficits (clinical–core mismatch).

Using imaging evidence of persisting salvageable tissue to select a subset of late-presenting patients has been tested in 2 trials comparing highly effective endovascular reperfusion devices with non-endovascular treatment. Across both trials, random allocation to endovascular reperfusion therapy was associated with increased freedom from disability (mRS 0–1 at 3–6 months, 31.2% vs 11.1%; RR 2.76, 95% CI: 1.75–4.35; $p < 0.0001$) and increased functional independence (mRS 0–2 at 3–6 months, 46.7% vs 14.8%; RR 3.12,

95% CI: 2.15–4.53: $p < 0.00001$) (see Figures 7.1 and 7.2). In addition, patients allocated to endovascular therapy had no alteration in mortality (16.6% vs 21.7%; RR 0.76, 95% CI: 0.41–1.40; $p = 0.38$), or symptomatic haemorrhage rate (6.3% vs 3.7%; RR 1.63, 95% CI: 0.65–4.06; $p = 0.29$) (see Figures 7.3 and 7.4).

Results for Different Treatment Times, Treatment Settings, and Types of Patients, among Broadly Selected Patients Early after Onset

A pooled, individual-level patient data meta-analysis was undertaken to explore for heterogeneity of treatment effect according to time from onset to treatment start, age, and presenting deficit severity (Goyal et al., 2016). The analysis included 1287 patients from 5 randomized trials of highly effective endovascular reperfusion devices. Among the 634 patients allocated to the endovascular arm, 558 (88.0%) actually underwent endovascular intervention; the most common reasons for not pursuing intervention were clinical improvement, clot resolution, and inability to access the target vessel. Among patients undergoing an endovascular intervention, a stent retriever device was employed in 532 (95.3%).

Effect of Onset to Treatment Time and Door-to-Treatment Time

Among the 1287 patients, 194 (15.1%) were treated within between 0.5 and 2 hours of onset, 657 (51.0%) between 2 and 4 hours, 352 (27.4%) between 4 and 6 hours, and 79 (6.1%) between 6 and 12 hours.

Alive and Functionally Independent at the End of Patient Follow-up

Earlier treatment was associated with greater benefit in increasing functional independence (mRS 0–2) at 3 months. With time from onset (last known well) to arterial puncture of 2 hours, allocation to endovascular reperfusion therapy was associated with more frequent alive and independent outcome (52.0% endovascular therapy, 27.0%, control; RR 1.93, intercept of full population ordinal model) (Figure 7.6). This represents 250 more alive and functionally independent patients per 1000 treated with endovascular reperfusion compared with control. In contrast, with time from onset (last known well) to arterial puncture of 5 hours, allocation to endovascular reperfusion therapy increased alive and independent outcome to a lesser degree (43.8% endovascular therapy, 27.0% control; RR 1.62). This represents 168 more alive and non-disabled patients per 1000 treated with endovascular therapy compared with control.

Functionally independent outcome declined more steeply with each delay during the interval from Emergency Department (ED) arrival to puncture (door to puncture) than from last known well to puncture (onset to puncture). Each 60-minute delay in onset to puncture was associated with a reduction in likelihood of functionally independent (mRS 0–2) outcome of OR 0.87 (0.78–0.96), while each 60-minute delay in door to puncture was associated with a reduction of OR 0.55 (0.43–0.71). Likely the faster decline in independent outcome with longer door to puncture than onset to puncture intervals was related to (1) a more accurately identifiable start time for the interval (ED arrival vs last known well), and (2) the screening out from some trials of patients with very rapid progression during the onset to door interval, due to entry criteria in requiring absence of substantial infarct extent upon arrival.

Degree of Disability at the End of Patient Follow-up

Considering time as a continuous variable, the benefit of treatment in reducing degree of disability tended to decline with later onset to treatment time ($p = 0.07$) (see Figure 7.6). The increased odds of a less disabled late outcome with endovascular recanalization therapy nominally declined from about 3.1 with arterial puncture at 2 hours to about 2.3 at 5 hours and about 1.8 at 8 hours. The point estimate for time at which treatment benefit for functional independence entirely disappeared was 12.2 hours, and the time at which the lower 95% CI for treatment benefit first crossed neutral was at 7.3 hours.

Time delay was associated with a steeper decline in odds of reduced final disability level across all 7 mRS ranks during the door to puncture than onset to puncture interval. Each 60-minute delay in onset to puncture was associated with a reduction in likelihood of functionally independent (mRS 0–2) outcome of OR 0.88 (0.81–0.96), while each 60-minute delay in door to puncture was associated with a reduction of OR 0.56 (0.47–0.67).

In the subset of 390 endovascular arm patients in whom substantial perfusion was achieved, there was a steep decline in final level of disability over 6 mRS ranks with longer door to reperfusion time. Among 100 treated patients, with every 15-minute decrease

in ED door-to-reperfusion time, an estimated 39 more patients have a less disabled mRS outcome at 3 months (including 25 more achieving functional independence [mRS 0–2]). For every 4-minute acceleration in ED door-to-reperfusion time, 1 of every 100 treated patients has a less disabled outcome.

Death at the End of Patient Follow-up, and Early Major Haemorrhage

Earlier treatment was associated with greater benefit in reducing mortality at 3 months ($p < 0.02$). With onset to puncture of 2 hours, allocation to endovascular reperfusion therapy was associated with reduced mortality (6.2% endovascular therapy, 17.9% control; RR 0.35, intercept of full population ordinal model) (see Figure 7.6). This represents 117 more alive and functionally independent patients per 1000 treated with endovascular reperfusion compared with control. In contrast, with onset to puncture of 5 hours, allocation to endovascular reperfusion therapy was associated with a mortality reduction of a lesser degree (9.9% endovascular therapy, 17.9% control; RR 0.55). This represents 80 more alive and non-disabled patients per 1000 treated with endovascular therapy compared with control. In contrast, earlier onset to puncture was not associated with differences in symptomatic haemorrhage rate between thrombectomy and control patients ($p = 0.40$).

Effect of Age

Randomized trials have shown that older patients compared with younger patients have worse functional outcomes from acute ischaemic stroke but benefit to the same relative degree from endovascular therapy over a wide range of ages, from 50 to over 80 years old. A tendency to a lesser degree of benefit was noted, however, for young adults aged 18 to 49, among whom control group patients have good outcomes related to greater capacity for neural repair and recovery. Among 5 pooled trials of highly effective reperfusion devices, enrolling 1287 patients, 12% were aged 18 to 49, 72% were aged 50 to 79, and 15% were 80 years and older.

Endovascular thrombectomy among broadly selected patients early after onset tended to reduce final level of disability (over 6 levels of the mRS) to a lesser degree among patients aged 18 to 49 (common odds ratio 1.36) than among patients aged 50 to 80 and above (cORs ranging from 2.41–3.68, heterogeneity $p = 0.07$). Over the broad range from age 50 to 80 and

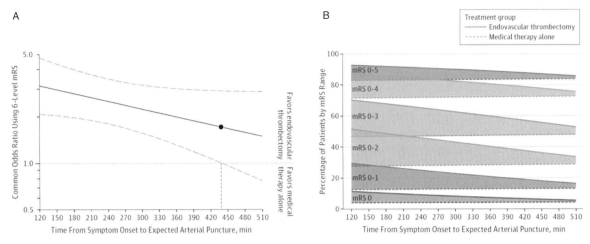

A

Common Odds Ratio Using 6-Level mRS

Favors endovascular thrombectomy   Favors medical therapy alone

Time From Symptom Onset to Expected Arterial Puncture, min

B

Percentage of Patients by mRS Range

Treatment group
—— Endovascular thrombectomy
----- Medical therapy alone

mRS 0–5
mRS 0–4
mRS 0–3
mRS 0–2
mRS 0–1
mRS 0

Time From Symptom Onset to Expected Arterial Puncture, min

Figure 7.6 Modification of endovascular thrombectomy benefit by onset to expected arterial puncture. (A) Common odds ratio for *reduced level of disability at 3 months*; (B) *3-month outcome rates for each of the 7 levels of the mRS*. Reproduced from Saver et al. (2016), with permission from the American Medical Association.

above, the relative benefit was similar in degree in different age groups but with worse overall outcomes in older patients. For example, for ages 60 to 69, functional independence (mRS 0–2) was 51.9% with endovascular therapy, 27.9% with control, OR 1.78 (95% CI: 1.25–2.55); while for age 80 and above, functional independence was 29.8% with endovascular therapy, 13.9% with control (OR 2.09, 95% CI: 1.03–4.25). Considering mortality, endovascular thrombectomy was associated with reduced death among the oldest old (aged ≥80: OR 0.60, 95% CI: 0.36–0.99) but not younger individuals (aged 18–79: OR 0.95, 95% CI: 0.69–1.37).

Effect of Presenting Deficit Severity

Randomized trials have shown that severe, compared with moderate, presenting neurological deficits are a prognostic, but not a treatment benefit-modifying, patient feature. Across a broad range of presenting deficit severity, patients with more severe deficits benefit to the same relative degree from highly effective endovascular thrombectomy, without evidence of heterogeneity (heterogeneity $p = 0.45$), but absolute rates of good outcome are lower when initial deficits are greater. The odds of a better level of disability across the entire mRS were improved by endovascular thrombectomy to a similar relative degree across 4 levels of presenting deficit severity (National Institutes of Health Stroke Scale [NIHSS] ranges of ≤10, 11–15, 16–20, and ≥21) (heterogeneity $p = 0.45$) (Figure 7.7). For example, rates of functional independence among moderate deficit patients (NIHSS 11–15) were 58.1% versus 27.1% (OR

1.70, 95% CI: 1.19–2.43), and among severe deficit patients (NIHSS ≥21) were 23.0% versus 13.8% (OR 1.80, 95% CI: 1.09–2.96).

Patients with mild initial presenting deficits have not been enrolled in substantial numbers in trials of highly effective endovascular thrombectomy. Among the first five trials, three formally excluded patients with NIHSS scores of less than 6 or less than 8, and the remainder enrolled very few patients in this range. However, observational series have noted that patients with initially mild deficits associated with LVOs have a substantial rate of subsequent stroke progression and poor outcome (Rajajee et al., 2006). Randomized trials in these patients are needed.

Effect of Imaging Findings on Noncontrast CT

Randomized trials have suggested that endovascular thrombectomy benefits both patients with mild and patients with moderate early infarct changes on initial brain imaging to the same relative degree, but may benefit patients with extensive early infarct changes less or not at all. The extent of early ischaemic injury changes on initial brain CT and MRI scans has been most often quantified using the Alberta Stroke Program Early CT Score (ASPECTS). Among 5 trials enrolling 1278 patients testing highly effective mechanical thrombectomy, 53% had mild early infarct changes (ASPECTS 9–10), 37% moderate (ASPECTS 6–8), and 9% severe early infarct changes (ASPECTS 0–5, but predominantly 4–5). The odds of a better level of disability across the entire mRS were improved by

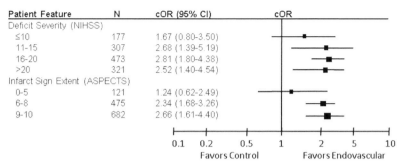

Figure 7.7 *Common odds ratio for more favourable 3-month disability level* in patient subgroups of differing presenting deficit severity and differing extent of infarct signs on first imaging. Figure based on data from Goyal et al. (2016).

endovascular thrombectomy to a similar relative degree at each of these 3 levels of presenting deficit severity (heterogeneity $p = 0.49$) (see Figure 7.7), though patients with less extensive infarcts had better outcomes in both treatment arms: no or small infarct signs (ASPECTS 9–10), 49.7% versus 30.2%, OR 0.84, 95% CI: 0.73–0.96; moderate infarct signs (ASPECTS 6–8), 44.4% vs 23.3%, OR 0.81 (0.61–1.08); extensive infarct signs (ASPECTS 0–5), 23.3% versus 13.3% (see Figure 7.7).

Late-presenting Patients with Substantial Penumbra on CT or MR Multimodal Imaging

In acute ischaemic stroke patients, time since last known well is a readily available but highly imprecise indicator of the degree to which threatened tissues are still salvageable or already irreversibly infarcted. Among patients presenting late after last known well time, there are two broad subgroups of patients who may still benefit from reperfusion therapy because they actually harbour substantial volumes of salvage brain tissue:

1. **Slow progressors**: Slow progressors are patients whose actual time of stroke onset was well defined by the clinical history, but was followed by a slower pace of infarct growth because of robust collateral flow or greater parenchymal tolerance of ischaemia.
2. **Actual recent starters**: In certain patients, the clinical history is unable to pinpoint the actual stroke onset time. In some, stroke onset occurred at some time during sleep, with symptoms first noted on awakening. In these individuals, the stroke may actually have started soon after going to sleep, in the middle of the sleep period, or just before waking up. But neither time last known well nor time symptoms first discovered coincides with time of actual stroke onset. In other patients, the stroke onset occurred while the patient was

awake, but rendered the patient unable to report what time that was, because of aphasia, confusion, anosognosia, or other deficits. In these patients, neither time last known well nor time symptoms were first discovered by other witnesses coincides with time of actual stroke onset. Among patients in whom the clinical history is insufficient to define the moment of stroke onset, 'actual recent starters' are patients in whom stroke onset was actually soon before symptoms were first discovered, on awakening or by other observers.

Both of these subgroups of late-presenting patients can be identified by multimodal CT and MRI imaging techniques that assess (1) the size of the ischaemic core – tissues that have already progressed to irreversible infarction – and (2) the size of the ischaemic penumbra – tissues that are threatened, but still salvageable. In acute cerebral ischaemia, when an artery is abruptly occluded, collateral vessels provide compensating blood flow to the supplied region. The robustness of the collateral supply varies widely from individual to individual, depending on variations in circle of Willis anatomy, stenoses and occlusions in the alternative channels themselves, the site of the new occlusion, and systemic blood pressure. Shortly after the inciting vascular occlusion, a small brain region within the supplied field may experience complete loss of blood flow, causing cellular death within 1 to a few minutes. But a much larger surrounding zone will experience moderate reductions in blood flow that the brain cells can tolerate for tens of minutes to several hours. As time from onset lengthens, the zone of the completed, irreversible infarction – the core – expands and the rim of threatened but still salvageable tissue – the penumbra – shrinks.

With CT, perfusion CT imaging identifies as core regions with extreme reduction in blood flow or blood volume, and as penumbra regions with moderate blood flow reduction (perfusion–core mismatch). With MRI, diffusion MR sequences identify as core regions with substantial diffusion abnormality, indicating advanced bioenergetic compromise, and perfusion MRI sequences identify as penumbra regions with moderate-to-severe blood flow reduction not yet showing diffusion abnormality (perfusion–diffusion mismatch). Alternative, less precise but more readily obtained, CT and MR approaches to identifying patients with persisting penumbral tissue estimate the volume of perfusion reduction using the presence of LVO (vessel–core mismatch); the extent of collateral vessels (collateral–core mismatch); or the severity of neurological deficits (clinical–core mismatch).

Two randomized trials have assessed endovascular mechanical thrombectomy with highly effective thrombectomy devices among late-presenting patients with imaging evidence of persisting salvageable tissue. One trial enrolled 189 patients with clinical–core mismatch on CT or MR 6–24 hours after last known well time, and the other trial enrolled 199 patients with perfusion–core mismatch on CT or MR 6–16 hours after last known well time. Among these imaging-selected patients, in crude combined analysis, endovascular thrombectomy compared with non-endovascular medical care increased 3-month disability-free (mRS 0–1) outcome (29.4% vs 10.6%, RR 2.75, 95% CI: 1.73–4.40; $p = 0.000007$) and increased 3-month alive and independent (mRS 0–2) outcome (46.9% vs 14.7%, RR 3.15, 95% CI: 2.17–4.58; $p < 0.000007$), without altering 3-month mortality (16.7% vs 21.7%, RR 0.76, 95% CI: 0.51–1.16; $p = 0.24$) or symptomatic intracranial haemorrhage (6.0% vs 3.7%, RR 1.63, 95% CI: 0.65–4.05; $p = 0.35$).

Endovascular Thrombectomy in Clinical Practice

Efficacy and Safety in Routine Practice

Multicentre and national registries have prospectively evaluated whether efficacy and safety outcomes with highly effective endovascular thrombectomy devices in routine practice are similar to the outcomes in the pivotal randomized trials. Considering the largest registries, a substantial worldwide experience has been catalogued, encompassing treatment with highly

effective thrombectomy in 2217 patients at over 75 hospitals in two countries on two continents (Table 7.1). Compared with the 634 patients allocated to endovascular thrombectomy in the pooled RCTs, patients treated in regular practice were similar in character, with average age 68, NIHSS score of 16, and onset to treatment time 4 hours 11 minutes. The great preponderance of devices employed were stent retrievers. Outcomes have generally been comparable or better in routine practice compared with randomized trials, including alive and disability-free outcome (37.5% vs 26.9%), alive and independent outcome at 3 months (50.8% in practice vs 46.0% in trials), symptomatic intracerebral haemorrhage (4.2% vs 4.4%), and death by 3 months (17.2% vs 15.3%).

Comment

Interpretation of the Data

These data indicate that endovascular treatment with highly effective thrombectomy devices is of substantial net benefit in acute ischaemic stroke. It is beneficial among a broad range of patients with anterior circulation LVOs in the first 6 hours after onset, both when used in tandem with IVF among lytic-eligible patients and when used as standalone therapy among lytic-ineligible patients. The magnitude of the improvements in functional outcome conveyed by endovascular thrombectomy treatment in broadly selected patients declines sharply as time from onset increases, while the harm, chiefly symptomatic intracerebral haemorrhage, persists at a low, steady level regardless of time since onset. In addition, between 6 and 24 hours after last known well time, advanced CT or MR imaging can identify a subset of patients who still harbour substantial salvageable tissues and will benefit from mechanical thrombectomy.

Among highly effective device classes, the greatest amount of randomized trial evidence is for stent retrievers, but accumulating data suggest that aspiration devices are improving and reaching or nearly reaching the same performance level, and that combined use of stent retrievers and aspiration sometimes is advantageous. The magnitude of benefit conferred is substantial: among generally broadly selected patients predominantly treated within 6 hours of last known well, 423 out of 1000 will have a less disabled outcome, including 171 more being alive and functionally independent, with no increase in the mortality rate.

Table 7.1 Multicentre and national registries of endovascular thrombectomy, including pooled registry comparison with pooled trials

Feature	Registries of regular practice			Combined registries	Combined trials
Data source	STRATIS	SITS-TBY CR	TRACK		HERMES
Countries	US	Czech Republic	US	Multinational (2)	Multinational (15)
Continents	1	1	1	2	4
Years	2014–2016	2016	2013–2915	2013–2016	2010–2014
Performance sites	55	14	23	~75	~85
Patients	984	604	629	2217	634 (570)*
Age (median, or mean)	68	71	66	68	68
NIHSS (median, or mean)	17	15	17	16	17
Devices	Stent retriever 1st	"2nd generation devices"	Stent retriever 1st		Stent retriever in 93.6%
Onset to puncture, months (m) (median, or mean)	226	175	363	251	238
Substantial reperfusion (mTICI 2b-3)	87.9% (724/824)	74.1% (433/584)	80.3% (505/629)	81.5% (1662/2037)	71% (390/549)
SICH SWIFT PRIME Defn	1.4% (12/841)				
SITS-MOST PH2 Defn		5.7% (26/460)			
Mixed Defns			7.1% (44/629)	4.2% (82/1930)	4.4% (28/634)
Death – by 3 m	14.4% (142/984)	24.9% (95/382)	19.8% (106/629)	17.2% (343/1995)	15.3% (97/634)
Alive and Disability-Free (mRS 0-1) – 3 m	43.2% (391/906)	35.9% (137/382)	30.3% (191/629)	37.5% (719/1917)	26.9% (170/633)
Alive and Independent (mRS 0-2) – 3 m	56.5% (512/906)	48.2% (184/382)	47.9% (277/629)	50.8% (973/1917)	46.0% (291/633)

HERMES: Highly Effective Reperfusion evaluated in Multiple Endovascular Stroke. STRATIS: Systematic Evaluation of Patients Treated with Neurothrombectomy Devices for Acute Ischemic Stroke. SITS-TBY CR: Safe Implementation of Treatments in Stroke – Thrombectomy, Czech Republic. TRACK: Trevo Stent-Retriever Acute Stroke Registry.

SICH: SWIFT PRIME defn: any parenchymal haematoma type 1 or 2, remote intraparenchymal haematoma, subarachnoid haemorrhage, or intraventricular haemorrhage associated with a four-point or more worsening on the NIHSS within 24 h; SITS-MOST defn: Parenchymal haematoma type 2 and NIHSS worsening ≥ 4.

* In the trials pooled in HERMES, 634 patients were randomized to the pursue-thrombectomy group, among whom 570 had persistent and accessible occlusions at the catheterization and actually underwent thrombectomy.

However, uncertainties and need for further therapeutic advance remain regarding:

- whether additional populations would benefit from endovascular thrombectomy, including patients with:

  - posterior circulation occlusions – vertebral, basilar, and posterior cerebral arteries
  - more distal anterior circulation occlusions – M2–M4 middle cerebral and anterior cerebral arteries) occlusions
  - large ischaemic cores of irreversible infarction on initial imaging
  - last known well time over 24 hours but favourable penumbral imaging profile
  - mild presenting neurological deficits

- the optimal concomitant IVF agent in lytic-eligible patients, as well as whether select populations can be identified whose outcomes are better if concomitant IV fibrinolysis is avoided
- the best intra-procedural sedation strategy, among general anaesthesia, procedural sedation, and no sedation
- the best post-procedure blood pressure management strategies, when complete, partial, and no reperfusion has been achieved
- device designs that enable achievement of complete or near complete reperfusion in 100%, rather than 70–90%, of patients.

Implications for Clinical Practice

Based on the considerable trial evidence, practice guidelines worldwide recommend the use of endovascular thrombectomy in carefully selected acute ischaemic stroke patients meeting treatment eligibility criteria (Casaubon et al., 2015; Hong et al., 2016; Wahlgren et al., 2016; Pontes-Neto et al., 2017; Powers et al., 2018). In many jurisdictions, the therapeutic licences issued by regulatory authorities include separate broad clearance of devices as general tools to clear thrombus from the neurovasculature, as well as more focused approval as treatments to improve outcome of more narrowly delineated patients; the tool clearance enables clinicians to flexibly use the device in broader populations, in accord with national guidelines and best clinical judgement.

As endovascular thrombectomy has risks as well as benefits, it is a treatment that requires continuous quality monitoring in routine practice. It should be administered only to selected patients, and in organized and experienced stroke care centres with staff and facilities for rapid and accurate assessment, monitoring, and management of any complications in accordance with current guidelines (Casaubon et al., 2015; Hong et al., 2016; Wahlgren et al., 2016; Pontes-Neto et al., 2017; Powers et al., 2018). Active stroke centres should participate in prospective, systematic, and rigorous audit as part of a national or international registry, such as GWTG-Stroke or SITS-TBY. This will ensure that stroke patients have access to this effective, but not risk-free, treatment, that stroke physicians, nurses, and hospital teams deepen experience and expertise in its use, and that quality control and patient selection continue to be optimized by contrasting baseline demographic, clinical, imaging, and treatment data, and early and long-term patient outcome, with contemporaneous care at comparator facilities.

The efficient and equitable delivery of thrombolysis also must overcome several prehospital and in-hospital barriers, including education of the public to recognize symptoms of stroke and seek urgent help by calling the ambulance first rather than the family doctor (Higashida et al., 2013; Jauch et al., 2013); ambulance dispatcher and paramedic training in stroke recognition and routing (Acker et al., 2007; Higashida et al., 2013); paramedic training in use of validated tools that further identify patients likely to have strokes due to LVO who may benefit from direct routing to a thrombectomy-capable centre (Noorian et al., 2018; Smith et al., 2018); geographically optimized regional stroke care systems that quickly deliver patients with suspected acute stroke to the appropriate tier receiving facility among general stroke-capable and advanced thrombectomy-capable hospitals (American Heart/Stroke Association Mission Lifeline Stroke Committee, 2017; Milne et al., 2017); efficient, well-trained, expanded 'Code Stroke' teams, that include neuro-interventional physicians and neuro-catheterization suite personnel, to manage patients immediately upon arrival (Kim et al., 2018); decision aids to enable patients and families to rapidly understand the benefits and risks of therapy (Figures 7.8A and 7.8B) (Tokunboh et al., 2018); and optimized protocols and processes of care to enable patient assessment, imaging interpretation, arterial puncture, and first device placement within 90 minutes of arrival for direct-arriving patients and within 60 minutes for transfer patients (Goyal et al., 2014; Wang et al., 2017; Kim et al., 2018).

Implications for Researchers

With endovascular thrombectomy now well established as an effective therapy, the next generation of research studies would best be focused upon how to make it *more* effective. Six broad avenues of further advance may be envisioned, and are being explored in current trials: faster treatment, more reperfusion, more salvageable brain, more patients, best concomitant therapy, and improved systems of care.

a. Faster treatment: As the benefit of endovascular thrombectomy is so strongly time dependent, innovative delivery methods that enable faster start of therapy will substantially improve patient outcomes. In the prehospital setting, studies to optimize identification and routing of patients likely to be harbouring LVOs for direct transfer to a thrombectomy-capable stroke centre are desirable. Cluster control trials, comparing outcomes during weeks using one identification and/or routing strategy versus outcomes during weeks using another strategy, are under way (Ribo and RACECAT Trialists, 2017). Within thrombectomy hospitals, the strategy of bringing patients directly to the catheterization suite for parenchymal imaging (CT imaging by rotational angiography systems) and immediate endovascular intervention, rather than first to a separate neuroimaging suite, merits further study (Jadhav et al., 2017).

b. More reperfusion: It is critical to improve further the frequency of reperfusion achieved by endovascular thrombectomy. While current devices achieve substantial reperfusion, thrombosis in cerebral infarction (TICI) scale grades 2b–3, in 70–90% of cases, that means that 10–30% of patients are not at all adequately reperfused. Further, complete or near complete reperfusion, TICI 2c–3, is currently achieved by procedure end in only 40–76% of patients, and achieved immediately on first pass in only 25–40%. Further innovations in thrombectomy device design are being evaluated to identify even more effective options. In addition, thrombus imaging to identify target clot features indicating

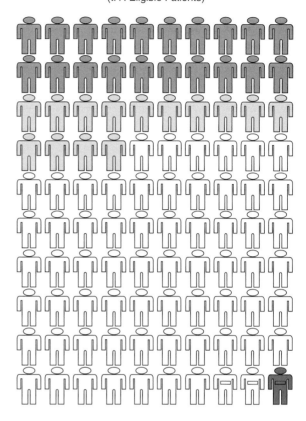

Thrombectomy Plus tPA vs tPA Alone
(tPA-Eligible Patients)

Changes in final outcome as a result of treatment:
- Able to live independently
- Other improvement
- No major changes
- Other worsening
- Severely disabled or dead

Early course:
- New territory infarct
- Early worsening with brain bleeding (SICH)*

(*No differences observed in the rate of SICH due to thrombectomy)

Figure 7.8A Visual decision aid to help patients, families, and providers rapidly understand benefits and risks of endovascular reperfusion intervention among patients who have already been treated with IV tPA. (Figure freely available, from Tokunboh et al., 2018, under a Creative Commons 3.0 Use Freely with Attribution license.)

better response to one device type than another merits further study (Zaidat et al., 2018a, 2018b).

c. More salvageable brain: Reperfusion is only of benefit to still-salvageable tissues, not brain parenchyma that has already progressed to irreversible infarction by the time of endovascular thrombectomy start. Prehospital, or ED arrival, start of neuroprotective and collateral

141

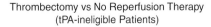

Thrombectomy vs No Reperfusion Therapy
(tPA-ineligible Patients)

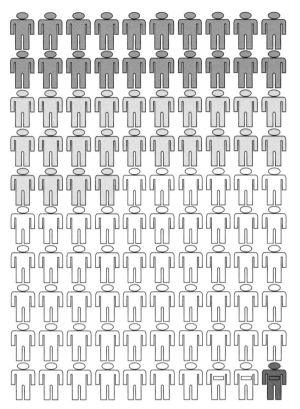

Changes in final outcome as a result of treatment:
▬ Able to live independently
▬ Other improvement
▢ No major changes
▬ Other worsening
▬ Severely disabled or dead

Early course:
▭ New territory infarct
— Early worsening with brain bleeding (SICH)*

(*No differences observed in the rate of SICH due to thrombectomy)

Figure 7.8B Visual decision aid to help patients, families, and providers rapidly understand benefits and risks of endovascular reperfusion intervention among patients who are ineligible for IV tPA. (Figure freely available, from Tokunboh et al., 2018, under a Creative Commons 3.0 Use Freely with Attribution license.)

enhancement therapies could stabilize ischaemic tissues so that a greater proportion of the tissue at risk is still rescuable at the time that the thrombectomy device is actually deployed in the target occlusion.

d. More patients: 'Minesweeper'-type basket trials are needed to efficiently determine which additional groups of patients will and will not benefit from

endovascular thrombectomy, including evaluating patients with posterior circulation occlusions (vertebral, basilar, and posterior cerebral arteries); more distal anterior circulation occlusions (M2–M4 middle cerebral and anterior cerebral arteries); larger ischaemic cores of irreversible infarction on initial imaging; last known well time of more than 24 hours but favourable penumbral imaging profile; and mild presenting neurological deficits (Ventz et al., 2017).

e. Concomitant therapies: Larger, multicentre trials are desirable, and under way, to evaluate the best form of intra-procedure sedation during endovascular thrombectomy (among general anaesthesia, procedural sedation, and no sedation). Trials are also needed to identify the best blood pressure management strategy after completion of endovascular thrombectomy, and to evaluate the potential benefit of treatments that target the molecular elaboration of post-reperfusion injury, now that reperfusion is often being achieved (Nour et al., 2013; Goyal et al., 2017; Al-Mufti et al., 2018).

f. Systems of care: There are many options for organizing routing policies for patient transport to thrombectomy-capable centres in regional stroke systems of care, including one-tiered ambulance routing of patients to centres capable of providing IV thrombolysis, and two-tiered ambulance routing, with select patients potentially harbouring LVOs being diverted directly to endovascular-capable hospitals ('drip and ship' vs 'mothership'). The best way to identify likely LVO in the field requires study, comparing different paramedic stroke severity scales, physician virtual presence by mobile telemedicine; ultrasound, electroencephalogram (EEG), microwave and other 'stroke helmets', and ambulances equipped with CT scanners (mobile stroke units) (Herzberg et al., 2014; Persson et al., 2014; Chapman Smith et al., 2016; Fassbender et al., 2017). In addition, the optimal calibration of when to bring patients to nearer PSCs or divert past them to further endovascular-capable stroke centres, to yield best outcomes at the population level, requires refinement in pragmatic controlled, service delivery trials.

Summary

Endovascular thrombectomy with highly effective reperfusion devices is beneficial for (1) relatively broadly selected acute ischaemic stroke patients with anterior circulation large vessel occlusions, who have failed or are ineligible for intravenous fibrinolysis, up to 7 hours after last known well time; and (2) imaging-selected patients found to have a favourable penumbral profile (small core and substantial still salvageable tissue) between 6 and 24 hours after last known well time. Among the broadly selected patients presenting within 6–8 hours, the benefit is strongly time dependent; for every 4-minute delay in emergency department door-to-reperfusion time, 1 of every 100 treated patients has a worse disability outcome.

Based on the trial evidence, endovascular thrombectomy with highly effective reperfusion devices in patients with large vessel anterior circulation occlusions is strongly endorsed by guidelines worldwide. Within the first 7 hours after last known well, benefit is evident in patients under and over age 80, and in patients with up to moderate early ischaemic changes on initial computed tomography or magnetic resonance imaging, with more study needed of patients with extensive early ischaemic change (ASPECTS 0–5). Systems of care should be optimized to deliver patients likely harbouring large vessel occlusions to endovascular-capable stroke centres, first device placement to occur within 90 minutes of arrival for direct-arriving patients and within 60 minutes for transfer patients.

Large-scale trials are needed, and under way, seeking to enhance endovascular thrombectomy, including by testing: alternative processes for prehospital recognition and routing of large vessel occlusion patients; novel device designs potentially more effective in achieving reperfusion in large and also medium vessel occlusions; bridging neuroprotection and collateral enhancement to preserve more brain tissue for endovascular reperfusion salvage; potential benefit in patients with larger cores and modest volumes of still salvageable tissue; and best concomitant therapies, including mode of sedation and post-procedural blood pressure management.

References

Acker JE III, Pancioli AM, Crocco TJ, Eckstein MK, Jauch EC, Larrabee H, et al. (2007). Implementation strategies for emergency medical services within stroke systems of care: a policy statement from the American Heart Association/American Stroke Association Expert Panel on Emergency Medical Services Systems and the Stroke Council. *Stroke*, **38**(11), 3097–115.

Al-Mufti F, Amuluru K, Roth W, Nuoman R, El-Ghanem M, Meyers PM. (2018). Cerebral ischemic reperfusion injury following recanalization of large vessel occlusions. *Neurosurgery*, **82**(6), 781–9.

American Heart/Stroke Association Mission Lifeline Stroke Committee. (2017). Severity-based stroke triage algorithm for EMS. www.heart.org/idc/groups/ahaecc-public/@wcm/@gwtg/documents/downloadable/ucm_492025.pdf. Accessed March 2017.

Badhiwala JH, Nassiri F, Alhazzani W, Selim MH, Farrokhyar F, Spears J, et al. (2015). Endovascular thrombectomy for acute ischemic stroke: a meta-analysis. *JAMA*, **314**(17), 1832–43.

Bath PM, Lees KR, Schellinger PD, Altman H, Bland M, Hogg C, et al. (2012). Statistical analysis of the primary outcome in acute stroke trials. *Stroke*, **43**(4), 1171–8.

Bendszus M, Thomalla G, Hacke W, Knauth M, Gerloff C, Bonekamp S, et al.; THRILL Investigators. (2016). Early termination of THRILL, a prospective study of mechanical thrombectomy in patients with acute ischemic stroke ineligible for i.v. thrombolysis. *Clin Neuroradiol*, **26**(4), 499–500.

Berkhemer OA, Fransen PSS, Beumer D, van den Berg LA, Lingsma HF, Yoo AJ, et al. (2015). A randomized trial of intraarterial treatment for acute ischemic stroke. *N Engl J Med*, **372**(1): 11–20.

Casaubon L, Boulanger J, Blacquiere D, Bucher S, Brown K, Goddard T, et al.; Heart and Stroke Foundation of Canada Canadian Stroke Best Practices Advisory Committee. (2015). Canadian Stroke Best Practice Recommendations: Hyperacute Stroke Care Guidelines, update 2015. *Int J Stroke*, **10**(6), 924–40.

Chapman Smith SN, Govindarajan P, Padrick MM, Lippman JM, McMurry TL, Resler BL, et al. (2016). A low-cost, tablet-based option for prehospital neurologic assessment: The iTREAT Study. *Neurology*, **87**(1), 19–26.

Ciccone A, Valvassori L, Nichelatti M, Sgoifo A, Ponzio M, Sterzi R, et al. (2013). Endovascular treatment for acute ischemic stroke. *N Engl J Med*, **368**(10), 904–13.

Ciccone A, Valvassori L, Ponzio M, Ballabio E, Gasparotti R, Sessa M, et al. (2010). Intra-arterial or intravenous thrombolysis for acute ischemic stroke? The SYNTHESIS pilot trial. *J Neurointerv Surg*, **2**(1), 74–9.

Ducrocq X, Bracard S, Taillandier L, Anxionnat R, Lacour JC, Guillemin F, et al. (2005). Comparison of intravenous and intra-arterial urokinase thrombolysis for acute ischaemic stroke. *J Neuroradiol*, **32**(1), 26–32.

Fassbender K, J. C. Grotta JC, S. Walter S, Grunwald IQ, Ragoschke-Schumm A, Saver JL. (2017). Mobile stroke units for prehospital thrombolysis, triage, and beyond: benefits and challenges. *Lancet Neurol*, **16**(3), 227–37.

Feigin VL, Norrving B, Mensah GA. (2017). Global burden of stroke. *Circ Res*, **120**(3), 439–48.

Goyal M, Demchuk AM, Menon BK, Eesa M, Rempel JL, Thornton J, et al.; ESCAPE Trial Investigators. (2015). Randomized assessment of rapid endovascular treatment of ischemic stroke. *N Engl J Med*, **372**(11), 1019–30.

Goyal M, Menon BK, Hill MD, Demchuk A. (2014). Consistently achieving computed tomography to endovascular recanalization <90 minutes: solutions and innovations. *Stroke*, **45**(12), e252–6.

Goyal M, Menon BK, van Zwam WH, Dippel DW, Mitchell PJ, Demchuk AM, et al.; HERMES Collaborators. (2016). Endovascular thrombectomy after large-vessel ischaemic stroke: a meta-analysis of individual patient data from five randomised trials. *Lancet*, **387**(10029), 1723–31.

Goyal N, Tsivgoulis G, Pandhi A, Chang JJ, K. Dillard K, Ishfaq MF, et al. (2017). Blood pressure levels post mechanical thrombectomy and outcomes in large vessel occlusion strokes. *Neurology*, **89**(6), 540–7.

Herzberg M, Boy S, Holscher T, Ertl M, Zimmermann M, Ittner KP, et al. (2014). Prehospital stroke diagnostics based on neurological examination and transcranial ultrasound. *Crit Ultrasound J*, **6**(1), 3.

Higashida R, Alberts MJ, Alexander DN, Crocco TJ, Demaerschalk BM, Derdeyn CP, et al. (2013). Interactions within stroke systems of care: a policy statement from the American Heart Association/American Stroke Association. *Stroke*, **44**(10), 2961–84.

Hong KS, Ko SB, Yu KH, Jung C, Park SQ, Kim BM, et al. (2016). Update of the Korean Clinical Practice Guidelines for Endovascular Recanalization Therapy in Patients with Acute Ischemic Stroke. *J Stroke*, **18**(1), 102–13.

Jadhav AP, Kenmuir CL, Aghaebrahim A, Limaye K, Wechsler LR, Hammer MD, et al. (2017). Interfacility transfer directly to the neuroangiography suite in acute ischemic stroke patients undergoing thrombectomy. *Stroke*, **48**(7), 1884–9.

Jauch EC, Saver JL, Adams HP Jr., Bruno A, Connors JJ, Demaerschalk BM, et al. (2013). Guidelines for the early management of patients with acute ischemic stroke: a guideline for healthcare professionals from the American Heart Association/American Stroke Association. *Stroke*, **44**(3), 870–947.

Jovin TG, Chamorro A, Cobo E, de Miquel MA, Molina CA, Rovira A, et al.; REVASCAT Trial Investigators. (2015). Thrombectomy within 8 hours after symptom onset in ischemic stroke. *N Engl J Med*, **372**(24), 2296–306.

Kim DH, Kim B, Jung C, Nam HS, Lee JS, Kim JW, et al.; Korean Society of Interventional Neuroradiology and Korean Stroke Society Joint Task Force Team. (2018). Consensus statements by Korean Society of Interventional

Neuroradiology and Korean Stroke Society: hyperacute endovascular treatment workflow to reduce door-to-reperfusion time. *J Korean Med Sci*, **33**(19), e143.

Lapergue B, Blanc R, Gory B, Labreuche J, Duhamel A, Marnat G, et al.; ASTER Trial Investigators. (2017). Effect of endovascular contact aspiration vs stent retriever on revascularization in patients with acute ischemic stroke and large vessel occlusion: the ASTER randomized clinical trial. *JAMA*, **318**(5), 443–52.

Legrand L, Naggara O, G. Turc G, Mellerio C, Roca P, Calvet D, et al. (2013). Clot burden score on admission T2*-MRI predicts recanalization in acute stroke. *Stroke*, **44**(7), 1878–84.

Milne MS, Holodinsky JK, Hill MD, Nygren A, Qiu C, Goyal M, et al. (2017). Drip 'n' ship versus mothership for endovascular treatment: modeling the best transportation options for optimal outcomes. *Stroke*, **48**(3), 791–4.

Mocco J, Siddiqui A, Turk A. (2018). A comparison of direct aspiration vs. stent retriever as a first approach (COMPASS): a randomized trial. Paper presented at the International Stroke Conference, Los Angeles, CA. https://professional.heart.org/idc/groups/ahamah-public/@wcm/@sop/@scon/documents/downloadable/ucm_498785.pdf. Accessed June 2018.

Muir KW, Ford GA, Messow CM, Ford I, Murray A, Clifton A, et al.; PISTE Investigators. (2017). Endovascular therapy for acute ischaemic stroke: the Pragmatic Ischaemic Stroke Thrombectomy Evaluation (PISTE) randomised, controlled trial. *J Neurol Neurosurg Psychiatry*, **88**(1), 38–44.

Nogueira RG, Frei D, Kirmani JF, Zaidat O, Lopes D, Turk AS 3rd, et al.; Penumbra Separator 3D Investigators. (2018). Safety and efficacy of a 3-dimensional stent retriever with aspiration-based thrombectomy vs aspiration-based thrombectomy alone in acute ischemic stroke intervention: a randomized clinical trial. *JAMA Neurol*, **75**(3), 304–11.

Nogueira RG, Lutsep HL, Gupta R, Jovin TG, Albers GW, Walker GA, et al. (2012). Trevo versus Merci retrievers for thrombectomy revascularisation of large vessel occlusions in acute ischaemic stroke (TREVO 2): a randomised trial. *Lancet*, **380**(9849), 1231–40.

Noorian AR, Sanossian N, Shkirkova K, Liebeskind DS, Eckstein M, Stratton SJ, et al.; FAST-MAG Trial Investigators and Coordinators. (2018). Los Angeles Motor Scale to identify large vessel occlusion: prehospital validation and comparison with other screens. *Stroke*, **49**(3), 565–72.

Nour M, Scalzo F, Liebeskind DS. (2013). Ischemia-reperfusion injury in stroke. *Interv Neurol*, **1**(3–4), 185–99.

O'Rourke K, Berge E, Walsh CD, Kelly PJ. (2010). Percutaneous vascular interventions for acute ischaemic stroke. *Cochrane Database Syst Rev*, 10, CD007574.

Persson M, Fhager A, Trefna HD, Yu Y, McKelvey T, Pegenius G, et al. (2014). Microwave-based stroke diagnosis making global prehospital thrombolytic treatment possible. *IEEE Trans Biomed Eng*, **61**(11), 2806–17.

Pontes-Neto OM, Cougo P, Martins SC, Abud DG, Nogueira RG, Miranda M, et al. (2017). Brazilian guidelines for endovascular treatment of patients with acute ischemic stroke. *Arq Neuropsiquiatr*, **75**(1), 50–6.

Powers WJ, Rabinstein AA, Ackerson T, Adeoye OM, Bambakidis NC, Becker K, et al.; American Heart Association Stroke Council. (2018). 2018 Guidelines for the early management of patients with acute ischemic stroke: a guideline for healthcare professionals from the American Heart Association/American Stroke Association. *Stroke*, **49** (3), e46–110.

Rajajee V, Kidwell C, Starkman S, Ovbiagele B, Alger JR, Villablanca P, et al. (2006). Early MRI and outcomes of untreated patients with mild or improving ischemic stroke. *Neurology*, **67**(6), 980–4.

Ribo M.; RACECAT Trialists. (2017). Direct transfer to an endovascular center compared to transfer to the closest stroke center in acute stroke patients with suspected large vessel occlusion (RACECAT). NCT02795962. https://clinicaltrials.gov/ct2/show/NCT02795962. Accessed June 2018.

Rodrigues FB, Neves JB, Caldeira D, Ferro JM, Ferreira JJ, Costa J. (2016). Endovascular treatment versus medical care alone for ischaemic stroke: systematic review and meta-analysis. *BMJ*, **353**, i1754.

Saver JL. (2011). Optimal end points for acute stroke therapy trials: best ways to measure treatment effects of drugs and devices. *Stroke*, **42**(8), 2356–62.

Saver JL. (2013). The 2012 Feinberg lecture: treatment swift and treatment sure. *Stroke*, **44**(1), 270–7.

Saver JL, Goyal M, van der Lugt A, Menon BK, Majoie CB, Dippel DW, et al.; HERMES Collaborators. (2016). Time to treatment with endovascular thrombectomy and outcomes from ischemic stroke: a meta-analysis. *JAMA*, **316**(12), 1279–88.

Saver JL, Jahan R, Levy EI, Jovin TG, Baxter B, Nogueira RG, et al. (2012). Solitaire flow restoration device versus the Merci Retriever in patients with acute ischaemic stroke (SWIFT): a randomised, parallel-group, non-inferiority trial. *Lancet*, **380**(9849), 1241–9.

Smith EE, Kent DM, Bulsara KR, Leung LY, Lichtman JH, Reeves MJ, et al.; American Heart Association Stroke Council. (2018). Accuracy of prediction instruments for diagnosing large vessel occlusion in individuals with suspected stroke: a systematic review for the 2018 Guidelines for the Early Management of Patients with Acute Ischemic Stroke. *Stroke*, **49**(3), e111–22.

Tokunboh I, Vales Montero M, Zopelaro Almeida MF, Sharma L, Starkman S, Szeder V, et al. (2018). Visual aids for patient, family, and physician decision making about endovascular thrombectomy for acute ischemic stroke. *Stroke*, **49**(1), 90–7.

Ventz S, Barry WT, Parmigiani G, Trippa L. (2017). Bayesian response-adaptive designs for basket trials. *Biometrics*, **73**(3), 905–15.

Wahlgren N, Moreira T, Michel P, Steiner T, Jansen O, Cognard C, et al. (2016). Mechanical thrombectomy in acute ischemic stroke: consensus statement by ESO-Karolinska Stroke Update 2014/2015, supported by ESO, ESMINT, ESNR and EAN. *Int J Stroke*, **11**(1), 134–47.

Wang H, Thevathasan A, Dowling R, Bush S, Mitchell P, Yan B. (2017). Streamlining workflow for endovascular mechanical thrombectomy: lessons learned from a comprehensive stroke center. *J Stroke Cerebrovasc Dis*, **26** (8), 1655–62.

Wardlaw JM, Murray V, Berge E, del Zoppo GJ. (2014). Thrombolysis for acute ischaemic stroke. *Cochrane Database Syst Rev*, 7, CD000213.

Wheeler HM, Mlynash M, Inoue M, Tipimini A, Liggins J, Bammer R, et al.; DEFUSE 2 Investigators. (2015). The growth rate of early DWI lesions is highly variable and associated with penumbral salvage and clinical outcomes following endovascular reperfusion. *Int J Stroke*, **10**(5), 723–9.

Zaidat OO, Bozorgchami H, Ribo M, Saver JL, Mattle HP, Chapot R, et al. (2018a). Primary results of the multicenter ARISE II study (Analysis of Revascularization in Ischemic Stroke with EmboTrap). *Stroke*, **49**(5), 1107–15.

Zaidat OO, Castonguay AC, Linfante I, Gupta R, Martin CO, Holloway WE, et al. (2018b). First pass effect: a new measure for stroke thrombectomy devices. *Stroke*, **49** (3): 660–6.

Collateral Flow Enhancement: Blood Pressure Lowering and Alteration of Blood Viscosity

Else Charlotte Sandset

Eivind Berge

Professor Eivind Berge passed away before the publication of this book. His contributions to stroke science through large clinical trials, major international collaboration and broad experience with systematic reviews have improved the treatment and prognosis of stroke patients. In addition, his unique combination of wisdom, kindness, and determination made him a wonderful colleague and mentor.

Blood Pressure Management

Background

Cerebral autoregulation ensures near constant brain perfusion, despite large variations in systemic blood pressure. In acute ischaemic stroke, the autoregulatory mechanisms may be disrupted in the affected hemisphere and, in certain situations, also in the opposite hemisphere, so that the cerebral perfusion becomes reliant on the systemic blood pressure (Strandgaard and Paulson, 1984; Immink et al., 2005). Blood pressure that is too low may lead to progression of the infarction and blood pressure that is too high may cause cerebral oedema or haemorrhagic transformation of the infarct.

Up to 75% of acute ischaemic stroke patients have blood pressure over 140 mm Hg within the first 24 hours of symptoms, and a spontaneous decline usually occurs within 7–10 days (Wallace and Levy, 1981; Qureshi et al., 2007). There are many contributing factors to high blood pressure in the acute phase, such as pre-existing, underdiagnosed, or undertreated hypertension; stress; urinary retention; and activation of sympathetic, adrenocorticotropic hormone (ACTH)–cortisol and renin–angiotensin systems (Qureshi, 2008). In patients with high intracranial pressure secondary to cerebral oedema, the Cushing reflex may also be a factor.

Low-to-normal blood pressure is uncommon in acute stroke. It is most commonly caused by hypovolaemia due to dehydration, or by coexisting disease, for example acute myocardial infarction, arrhythmias, heart failure, or sepsis (Vemmos et al., 2004).

Blood Pressure and Outcome

High blood pressure in the acute phase is associated with higher risks of early death and stroke recurrence, and worse functional outcome (Willmot et al., 2006). A U-shaped relationship between blood pressure in the acute phase and long-term outcome has been identified in several populations, with poorer outcomes in patients with the highest and lowest blood pressures in the acute phase (Leonardi-Bee et al., 2002; Vemmos et al., 2004). In the International Stroke Trial, systolic blood pressure in the range of 140 to 179 mm Hg was associated with the best outcome (Leonardi-Bee, 2002).

Effects of Blood Pressure Lowering Treatment

A systematic review of 16 trials involving 15,489 patients with either ischaemic, haemorrhagic, or mixed stroke found no beneficial effect of blood pressure lowering in the acute phase on death or dependency at the end of follow-up (odds ratio [OR] 0.98, 95% confidence interval [CI]: 0.92–1.05). Blood pressure lowering treatment was given within 7 days of symptom onset, and at the end of trial treatment the overall achieved systolic blood pressure reduction was 6.7 mm Hg (95% CI: 4.1–9.4 mm Hg reduction) (Bath and Krishnan, 2014).

Stroke Subtype and Location

In the same review, a subgroup analysis of 11,015 ischaemic stroke patients from 8 trials found no effect of blood pressure lowering treatment on the risk of death or dependency (OR 1.00, 95% CI: 0.92–1.08) (Bath and Krishnan, 2014) (Figure 8.1).

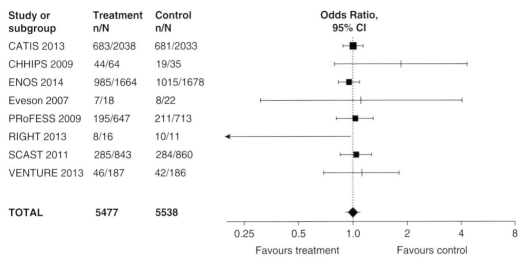

Study or subgroup	Treatment n/N	Control n/N	Odds Ratio, 95% CI
CATIS 2013	683/2038	681/2033	
CHHIPS 2009	44/64	19/35	
ENOS 2014	985/1664	1015/1678	
Eveson 2007	7/18	8/22	
PRoFESS 2009	195/647	211/713	
RIGHT 2013	8/16	10/11	
SCAST 2011	285/843	284/860	
VENTURE 2013	46/187	42/186	
TOTAL	5477	5538	

Figure 8.1 Forest plot showing the effects of any blood pressure lowering treatment pre-stroke antihypertensives on the risk of death or dependency in patients with acute ischaemic stroke. Modified from Bath and Krishnan (2014).

Similar results were found in a subgroup analysis of patients with different stroke locations, from 4 trials. Among 6180 patients with cortical stroke, the OR was 0.94 (95% CI: 0.81–1.09), and the OR was 0.98 among 2383 patients with subcortical stroke (95% CI: 0.76–1.27) (Bath and Krishnan, 2014).

Blood pressure lowering treatment in patients with intracerebral haemorrhage is discussed in Chapter 13.

Time to Treatment

Data from 16 trials involving 15,489 patients with ischaemic, haemorrhagic, or mixed stroke found a significant reduction in death or dependency if treatment was administered within 6 hours of symptom onset (OR 0.87, 95% CI: 0.76–0.99). No beneficial effects of blood pressure lowering treatment with glyceryl trinitrate were seen in the prehospital Rapid Intervention with Glyceryl Trinitrate in Hypertensive Stroke Trial-2, where patients were randomized a median 71 minutes after symptom onset (RIGHT-2 Investigators, 2019). Treatment administered later than 6 hours showed no effect on death or dependency (Bath and Krishnan, 2014).

Agent

Data from 16 trials involving 15,489 patients with ischaemic, haemorrhagic, or mixed stroke found no significant differences in the risk of death or dependency when comparing drug classes or blood pressure lowering strategies (Bath and Krishnan, 2014).

Continuing versus Stopping Pre-stroke Antihypertensives

Data from two trials involving 2860 patients with ischaemic, haemorrhagic, or mixed stroke found that continuing pre-stroke antihypertensives in the acute phase had no effect on death or dependency. Instead, there was an increased risk of disability (measured by the Barthel Index) and of poor quality of life (measured by EuroQoL) (Bath and Krishnan, 2014; Woodhouse et al., 2017; Anderson et al., 2019) (Figure 8.2).

Patients Receiving Thrombolytic Treatment

In the setting of reperfusion therapy for acute ischaemic stroke, high blood pressure is associated with an increased risk of intracerebral haemorrhage. Similar findings have been found with spikes in blood pressure during or following the administration of thrombolytic drugs.

There are limited data on the effect of blood pressure lowering in the setting of thrombolytic treatment. In a secondary analysis of observational data from the third International Stroke Trial (IST-3) of intravenous recombinant tissue plasminogen activator (rt-PA) vs control, active blood pressure lowering within the first 24 hours was associated with a significantly reduced risk of poor functional outcome at 6 months, both in the rt-PA and control groups (Berge et al., 2015). The randomized controlled Enhanced Control of Hypertension and Thrombolysis Stroke Study (ENCHANTED) assessed whether intensive

147

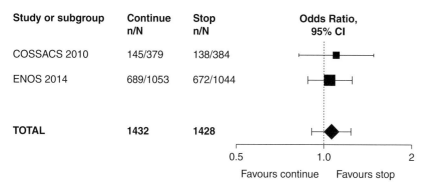

Study or subgroup	Continue n/N	Stop n/N	Odds Ratio, 95% CI
COSSACS 2010	145/379	138/384	
ENOS 2014	689/1053	672/1044	
TOTAL	1432	1428	

0.5   1.0   2

Favours continue   Favours stop

Figure 8.2 Forest plot showing the effects of continuing versus stopping pre-stroke antihypertensives on the risk of death or dependency. Modified from Bath and Krishnan (2014).

Copyright Cochrane Database of Systematic Reviews, reproduced with permission.

blood pressure lowering (systolic target 130–140 mm Hg) is beneficial in patients eligible for thrombolysis, compared with guideline treatment (target < 180 mm Hg), and the overall results were neutral, but there was less intracranial haemorrhage in the intensive group (Anderson et al., 2019).

Recommendations

Despite large-scale, acute phase trials of blood pressure lowering, definitive results are lacking. Strong recommendations can therefore not be made (Bath et al., 2018; Sandset et al., 2018).

- In patients with blood pressure at or above 220/ 120 mm Hg who do not receive intravenous thrombolysis, the benefit of initiating or reinitiating treatment of hypertension within the first 48–72 hours is uncertain. It might be reasonable to lower blood pressure by 15% during the first 24 hours after stroke onset (American Heart Association [AHA]/American Stroke Association [ASA] guidelines 2018: Class II; Level of Evidence B) (Powers et al., 2018).
- Patients who have elevated blood pressure and are otherwise eligible for treatment with intravenous rt-PA should have their blood pressure lowered so that systolic blood pressure is below 185 mm Hg and their diastolic blood pressure is below 110 mm Hg before thrombolytic treatment is administered (AHA/ASA guidelines 2018 Class I; Level of Evidence B) (Powers et al., 2018).
- No recommendations can be made regarding drug classes; however, intravenous calcium channel antagonists can cause abrupt and large reductions in blood pressure and should only be used

cautiously. Intravenous labetalol or urapidil is commonly used. Sodium nitroprusside can be recommended in cases of resistant hypertension. There is no evidence to support continuation of prestroke antihypertensive drugs. Treatment may be restarted once the patient is medically and neurologically stable and once safe feeding and enteral access is available.

- Acute stroke patients should be assessed for dehydration, and a fluid balance chart should be kept. Underlying causes of hypotension should be treated rapidly.

Alteration of Blood Viscosity Haemodilution

Therapeutic haemodilution reduces blood cell volume and viscosity, and may thereby increase blood flow to hypoperfused brain tissue.

Evidence

A systematic review identified 21 randomized controlled trials of haemodilution for acute ischaemic stroke. Twelve trials used plasma volume expanders alone (hypervolaemic haemodilution), in 8 trials the use of plasma volume expanders was combined with venesection (isovolaemic haemodilution), and in 1 trial venesection was only performed if there were signs of volume overload. The plasma volume expander was plasma alone in 1 trial, dextran in 12 trials, hydroxyethyl starch (HES) in 5 trials and albumin in 3 trials. Two trials tested haemodilution in combination with another therapy (Chang and Jensen, 2014).

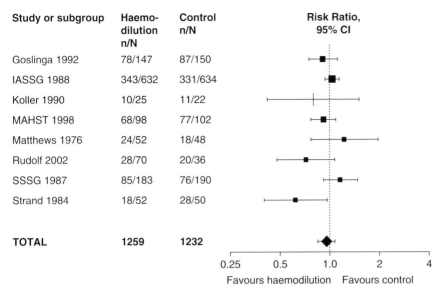

Study or subgroup	Haemo-dilution n/N	Control n/N	Risk Ratio, 95% CI
Goslinga 1992	78/147	87/150	
IASSG 1988	343/632	331/634	
Koller 1990	10/25	11/22	
MAHST 1998	68/98	77/102	
Matthews 1976	24/52	18/48	
Rudolf 2002	28/70	20/36	
SSSG 1987	85/183	76/190	
Strand 1984	18/52	28/50	
TOTAL	**1259**	**1232**	

0.25 0.5 1.0 2 4
Favours haemodilution   Favours control

Figure 8.3 Forest plot showing the effects of haemodilution on the risk of death or dependency in patients with acute ischaemic stroke. Modified from Chang and Jensen (2014).

Copyright Cochrane Database of Systematic Reviews, reproduced with permission.

There was no effect of haemodilution on death within 4 weeks or within 3–6 months, or on death or dependency or institutionalization at the end of follow-up (risk ratio [RR] 0.96, 95% CI: 0.85–1.07). The results were similar in trials of isovolaemic and hypervolaemic haemodilution. In subgroup analysis of different haemodilution strategies on functional outcome, trials of hydroxyethyl starch, including 306 patients, showed non-significantly better outcomes in patients treated with hydroxyethyl starch (RR 0.87, 95% CI: 0.71–1.07). No effects were seen for the other haemodilution strategies (Chang and Jensen, 2014) (Figure 8.3).

Six trials reported venous thromboembolic events at late follow-up. There was no beneficial effect of haemodilution (RR 0.68, 95% CI: 0.37–1.24) and no effect on the risk of serious cardiac events (RR 1.15, 95% CI: 0.66–2.05) (Chang and Jensen, 2014).

Eight trials reported anaphylactic/anaphylactoid reactions. Anaphylactic reactions occurred in 0.6% of patients treated with dextran, which was non-significantly higher than in non-treated patients (RR 3.89; 95% CI: 0.83–18.3). None of the events was fatal (Chang and Jensen, 2014).

Effect of Time to Treatment

Four trials recruited patients within 6 hours of symptom onset and 5 trials recruited patients within 6 hours or 12 hours. There was a small difference in 2 trials favouring early treatment; however, this was not seen in the other trials (Asplund, 1991; Chang and Jensen, 2014).

Recommendations

There is no beneficial effect of haemodilution treatment for acute ischaemic stroke on survival or functional outcome, and haemodilution cannot be recommended as part of routine acute management of ischaemic stroke.

Fibrinogen-depleting Agents

Fibrinogen-depleting agents are purified extracts from pit viper venom. They cleave circulating fibrinogen, leading to reduced plasma viscosity and thereby an increase in blood flow. Potential additional beneficial effects include prevention of clot extension and an indirect thrombolytic effect by promoting release of endogenous tissue plasminogen activator from the endothelium.

Evidence

A systematic review identified 8 randomized controlled trials of fibrinogen depleting agents involving 5701 patients. Six trials used ancrod and 2 trials used defibrase (Hao et al., 2012).

There was a small beneficial effect of treatment with fibrinogen-depleting agents on death or dependency at the end of follow-up (RR 0.95; 95% CI: 0.90–0.99). No differences were seen with specific

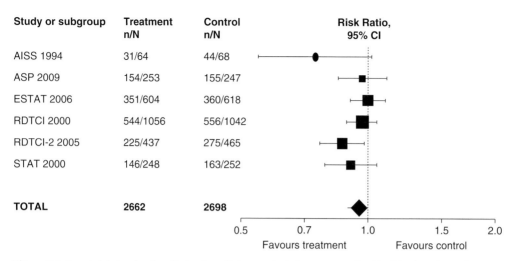

Figure 8.4 Forest plot showing the effects of any fibrinogen-depleting agent on the risk of death or dependency in patients with acute ischaemic stroke. Modified from Hao et al. (2012).

Copyright Cochrane Database of Systematic Reviews, reproduced with permission.

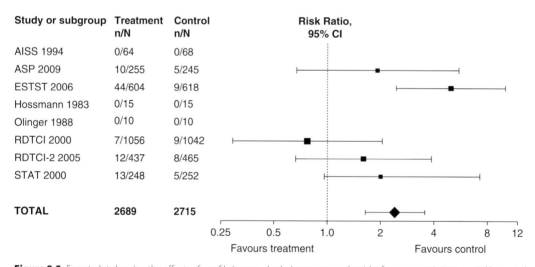

Figure 8.5 Forest plot showing the effects of any fibrinogen-depleting agent on the risk of symptomatic intracranial haemorrhage in patients with acute ischaemic stroke. Modified from Hao et al. (2012).

Cochrane Database of Systematic Reviews, reproduced with permission.

types of fibrinogen-depleting agents (Hao et al., 2012) (Figure 8.4).

Fibrinogen-depleting agents had no effect on death from all causes during the scheduled treatment period (RR 1.00, 95% CI: 0.70–1.43) or at the end of follow-up (RR 1.07, 95% CI: 0.94–1.22). The results were similar regardless of the type of fibrinogen-depleting agent used (Hao et al., 2012).

Eight trials involving 5404 patients reported symptomatic intracranial haemorrhage during the

treatment period. Fibrinogen-depleting agents were associated with a significantly increased risk of symptomatic haemorrhage (RR 2.42, 95% CI: 1.65–3.56), with an absolute difference of 2% between treatment and control. The risk appeared to be higher in ancrod-treated patients (RR 3.56, 95% CI: 2.15–5.87) than in defibrase-treated patients (RR 1.15, 95% CI: 0.60–2.20) (Hao et al., 2012) (Figure 8.5).

Four trials involving 2674 patients reported recurrent stroke (of ischaemic or unknown type) at the end

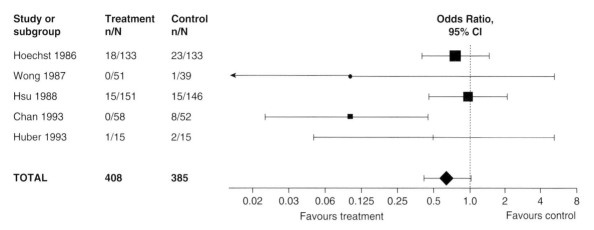

Study or subgroup	Treatment n/N	Control n/N	Odds Ratio, 95% CI
Hoechst 1986	18/133	23/133	
Wong 1987	0/51	1/39	
Hsu 1988	15/151	15/146	
Chan 1993	0/58	8/52	
Huber 1993	1/15	2/15	
TOTAL	408	385	

Figure 8.6 Forest plot showing the effects of methylxanthine derivatives on the risk of early death. Modified from Bath and Bath-Hextall (2004).

of follow-up. Treatment with fibrinogen-depleting agents was associated with fewer recurrent strokes (RR 0.67, 95% CI: 0.49–0.92). The results were similar regardless of the type of fibrinogen-depleting agent used (Hao et al., 2012).

Effect of Time to Treatment

There was no difference in treatment effects on death or dependency, death from all causes, or symptomatic intracranial haemorrhage between trials recruiting within 3 hours and trials recruiting within 6 hours. The results must be interpreted with caution, as separate trials contributed to the different time windows (Hao et al., 2012).

Recommendation

Treatment with fibrinogen-depleting agents in acute ischaemic stroke may have a marginally beneficial effect on the risk of death or dependency and on the risk of recurrent stroke. This effect is, however, outweighed by a significant increased risk of symptomatic intracranial haemorrhage. Therefore, there is no place for routine use of fibrinogen-depleting agents in the acute phase of ischaemic stroke.

Methylxanthine Derivatives

Methylxanthine derivatives such as pentoxifylline, pentifylline, and propentofylline have several potential beneficial actions in acute stroke. They increase blood flow by promoting vasodilation and inhibiting platelet aggregation, and may also decrease the release of free oxygen radicals.

Evidence

A systematic review identified 5 randomized controlled trials of methylxanthine derivatives involving 793 patients. Four trials used pentoxifylline and 1 trial used propentofylline (Bath and Bath-Hextall, 2004).

Two trials including 200 patients reported death or disability. There was no beneficial effect of treatment with methylxanthine derivatives (OR 0.49, 95% CI: 0.20–1.20) (Bath and Bath-Hextall, 2004).

Five trials including 793 patients reported early death (within 4 weeks). There was a non-significant difference in favour of treatment with methylxanthine derivatives on death (OR 0.64, 95% CI: 0.41–1.02). The results were driven by one trial of pentoxifylline including only 110 patients, which reported a significant reduction of the risk of early death. Only one trial involving 30 patients reported death beyond 4 weeks, and found no significant difference in late deaths (OR 0.70, 95% CI: 0.13–3.68) (Bath and Bath-Hextall, 2004) (Figure 8.6).

Recommendation

There is insufficient evidence to make recommendations regarding treatment with methylxanthine derivatives in acute ischaemic stroke.

Summary

In acute ischaemic stroke, cerebral blood flow autoregulatory mechanisms may be disrupted so that cerebral perfusion becomes reliant on systemic blood pressure. Too low blood pressure may lead to progression of the infarction and too high blood pressure may cause cerebral oedema or haemorrhagic transformation of the infarct. In patients with blood pressure at or above 220/ 120 mm Hg who do not receive intravenous thrombolysis, it is reasonable to lower blood pressure by 15% during the first 24 hours after stroke onset. Patients who have elevated blood pressure and are otherwise eligible for treatment with intravenous recombinant tissue plasminogen activator (rt-PA) should have their blood pressure lowered so that systolic blood pressure is lower than 185 mm Hg and their diastolic blood pressure is lower than 110 mm Hg before thrombolytic treatment is administered. Acute stroke patients should be assessed for dehydration and a fluid balance chart should be kept. Underlying causes of hypotension should be treated rapidly. There is no beneficial effect of haemodilution treatment for acute ischaemic stroke. Fibrinogen-depleting agents that reduce viscosity may marginally reduce risk of recurrent ischaemic stroke, but more greatly increase symptomatic intracranial haemorrhage. Methylxanthine derivatives such as pentoxifylline and propentofylline that reduce viscosity and produce vasodilation have insufficient evidence to support their use.

References

Anderson CS, Huang Y, Lindley RI, Chen X, Arima H, Chen G, et al.; ENCHANTED Investigators and Coordinators. (2019). Intensive blood pressure reduction with intravenous thrombolysis therapy for acute ischaemic stroke (ENCHANTED): an international, randomised, open-label, blinded-endpoint, phase 3 trial. *Lancet*, **393**(10174), 877–88.

Asplund, K. (1991). Hemodilution in acute stroke. *Cerebrovasc Dis*, **1**(Suppl. 1), 129–38.

Bath PM, Appleton JP, Krishnan K, Sprigg N. (2018). Blood pressure in acute stroke: to treat or not to treat: that is still the question. *Stroke*, **49**(7), 1784–90.

Bath PM, Bath-Hextall FJ. (2004). Pentoxifylline, propentofylline and pentifylline for acute ischaemic stroke. *Cochrane Database Syst Rev*, 3. CD000162.

Bath PM, Krishnan K. (2014). Interventions for deliberately altering blood pressure in acute stroke. *Cochrane Database Syst Rev*, 10. CD000039.

Berge E, Cohen G, Lindley RI, Sandercock P, Wardlaw JM, Sandset EC, et al. (2015). Effects of blood pressure and blood pressure-lowering treatment during the first 24 hours among patients in the third International Stroke Trial of thrombolytic treatment for acute ischemic stroke. *Stroke*, **46**(12), 3362–9.

Chang TS, Jensen MB. (2014). Haemodilution for acute ischaemic stroke. *Cochrane Database Syst Rev*, 8. CD000103.

Hao Z, Liu M, Counsell C, Wardlaw JM, Lin S, Zhao X. (2012). Fibrinogen depleting agents for acute ischaemic stroke. *Cochrane Database Syst Rev*, 3. CD000091.

Immink RV, van Montfrans GA, Stam J, Karemaker JM, Diamant M, van Lieshout JJ. (2005). Dynamic cerebral autoregulation in acute lacunar and middle cerebral artery territory ischemic stroke. *Stroke*, **36**(12), 2595–2600.

Leonardi-Bee J, Bath PM, Phillips SJ,. Sandercock PA. (2002). Blood pressure and clinical outcomes in the International Stroke Trial. *Stroke*, **33**(5), 1315–20.

Powers, WJ, Rabinstein AA, Ackerson T, Adeoye OM, Bambakidis NC, Becker K, et al.; American Heart Association Stroke Council. (2018). 2018 Guidelines for the early management of patients with acute ischemic stroke: a guideline for healthcare professionals from the American Heart Association/American Stroke Association. *Stroke*, **49**(3), e46–e110.

Qureshi AI. (2008). Acute hypertensive response in patients with stroke: pathophysiology and management. *Circulation*, **118**(2), 176–87.

Qureshi AI, Ezzeddine MA, Nasar A, Suri MF, Kirmani JF, Hussein HM, et al. (2007). Prevalence of elevated blood pressure in 563,704 adult patients with stroke presenting to the ED in the United States. *Am J Emerg Med*, **25**(1), 32–8.

RIGHT-2 Investigators. (2019). Prehospital transdermal glyceryl trinitrate in patients with ultra-acute presumed stroke (RIGHT-2): an ambulance-based, randomised, sham-controlled, blinded, phase 3 trial. *Lancet*, **393**(10175), 1009–20.

Sandset EC, Sanossian N, Woodhouse LJ, Anderson C, Berge E, Lees KR, et al.; Blood Pressure in Acute Stroke Collaboration Investigators. (2018). Protocol for a prospective collaborative systematic review and meta-analysis of individual patient data from randomized controlled trials of vasoactive drugs in acute stroke: the Blood Pressure in Acute Stroke Collaboration, stage-3. *Int J Stroke*, **13**(7), 759–65.

Strandgaard S, Paulson OB. (1984). Cerebral autoregulation. *Stroke*, **15**(3), 413–16.

Vemmos KN, Tsivgoulis G, Spengos K, Zakopoulos N, Synetos A, Manios E, et al. (2004). U-shaped relationship between mortality and admission blood pressure in patients with acute stroke. *J Intern Med*, **255**(2), 257–65.

Wallace JD, Levy LL. (1981). Blood pressure after stroke. *JAMA*, **246**(19), 2177–80.

Willmot M, Ghadami A, Whysall B, Clarke W, Wardlaw J, Bath PM. (2006). Transdermal glyceryl trinitrate lowers blood pressure and maintains cerebral blood flow in recent stroke. *Hypertension*, **47**(6), 1209–15.

Woodhouse LJ, Manning L, Potter JF, Berge E, Sprigg N, Wardlaw J, et al; Blood Pressure in Acute Stroke Council. (2017). Continuing or temporarily stopping prestroke antihypertensive medication in acute stroke: an individual patient data meta-analysis. *Hypertension*, **69**(5), 933–41.

Acute Antiplatelet Therapy for the Treatment of Ischaemic Stroke and Transient Ischaemic Attack

Jeffrey L. Saver

Rationale

The purpose of antiplatelet therapy, like that of anticoagulation (Chapter 10), in patients with acute ischaemic stroke or transient ischaemic attack (TIA) is to prevent ischaemic stroke progression, recurrent ischaemic stroke, and other serious vascular events.

Antiplatelet and anticoagulant agents target two complementary segments of the haemostatic system. Platelet adhesion and aggregation particularly tends to occur when blood passes rapidly over irregular surfaces, causing high-speed, dyslaminar flow – the resulting 'white thrombi' are platelet-rich. In contrast, coagulation proteins particularly tend to precipitate when blood flow slows or stops altogether, in low-perfusion pressure settings – the resulting 'red thrombi' are rich in interlinked fibrin and trapped erythrocytes. Consequently, antiplatelet agents are often more effective for thrombi arising from arteriopathies like atherosclerosis, while anticoagulants are often more effective for thrombi arising from venous disease and the cardiac atria.

Antiplatelet agents may be broadly defined as agents whose principal effects are to inhibit platelet adhesion and aggregation. Classes of antiplatelet agents include:

- Cyclo-oxygenase inhibitors (e.g. acetylsalicylic acid [ASA], triflusal)
- Thienopyridine derivatives (e.g. clopidogrel, prasugrel)
- Phosphodiesterase inhibitors (e.g. dipyridamole, cilostazol)
- Glycoprotein (GP) IIb/IIIa receptor inhibitors (e.g. abciximab, eptifibatide)
- P2Y12 inhibitors (e.g. ticagrelor)
- Thromboxane inhibitors

Antiplatelet Therapy vs Control

Evidence

In patients with definite or presumed acute cerebral ischaemia, early antiplatelet therapy (started within 72 hours [h] of onset) has been compared with no antithrombotic therapy in 11 randomized trials enrolling 42,852 patients (Abciximab in Ischemic Stroke Investigators, 2000; Siebler et al., 2011; Ciccone et al., 2014; Sandercock et al., 2014).

Antiplatelet Regimens Tested

Antiplatelet agents tested included aspirin, ticlopidine, and two glycoprotein IIb/IIIa receptor inhibitors, abciximab, and tirofiban. However, two aspirin megatrials, testing aspirin 160–300 mg daily started within 48 hours of onset, contributed 95% of the data (CAST [Chinese Acute Stroke Trial] Collaborative Group, 1997; International Stroke Trial Collaborative group [IST], 1997).

Time from Onset to Inclusion or Treatment

Permitted time windows for trial enrolment included patients randomized within 6 hours (MAST-I, 1995; AbESTT, 2005), 12 hours (Ciufetti et al., 1990), 24 hours (Abciximab in Ischemic Stroke [AIST] Investigators, 2000), 48 hours (CAST, 1997; IST, 1997), and 72 hours (Roden-Jullig et al., 2003), between 3 and 22 hours (SaTIS – Siebler et al., 2011), and, in one study, 3 separate populations within 5 hours, between 5 and 6 hours, and greater than 6 hours but within 3 hours of awakening (AbESTT-II – Adams et al., 2008). Actual median or mean onset to enrolment or treatment times ranged from 3.7 hours (AbESTT II/Primary) and between 3 and 6 hours (MAST-I), through 5.1 hours (AbESTT II/Companion), 9.8 hours (AbESTT II/Wake-up), 12 hours (AIST), 13 hours (SaTIS), 19 hours (IST), and 25 hours (CAST).

Brain Imaging of Qualifying Event

Nine of the eleven trials performed computed tomography (CT) scans in all patients prior to entry to exclude individuals with intracranial haemorrhage (ICH) from entry into the trial. Two trials (CAST, 1997; IST, 1997) performed a CT scan in almost all patients; in these trials, clinicians had to have a low threshold of suspicion of ICH prior to randomization. In the Chinese Acute Stroke Trial (CAST), 87% had a CT scan prior to randomization; by discharge, this number had risen to 94%. In the International Stroke Trial (IST), 67% were scanned before randomization and 29% after randomization, so that, overall, 96% of patients were scanned.

Stroke Severity at Entry

The two large aspirin trials, CAST and IST, enrolled patients without requiring a minimum initial neurological deficit to be present. Several of the other trials did require a minimal degree of deficits, including at least 1 point on the Scandinavian Stroke Scale (Roden-Jullig et al., 2003) or at least 4 points on the National Institutes of Health Stroke Scale (NIHSS) (AIST 2000; AbESTT 2005; AbESTT-II 2008; SaTIS 2011).

Scheduled Duration of Trial Treatment

The scheduled duration of treatment varied from one-time bolus (lower-dose tiers of AIST 2000), to be continued until 12 hours (higher-dose tiers of AIST 2000; AbESTT 2005; AbESTT-II 2008), 48 hours (SaTIS 2011), 5 days (Roden-Jullig et al., 2003), 10 days (MAST-I 1995), up to 2 weeks or discharge if earlier (IST 1997), 3 weeks (Ciufetti et al., 1990), and up to 4 weeks or discharge if earlier (CAST 1997).

Death or Dependency

Data regarding death or dependency at final follow-up were available from 9 trials, including 4 trials of aspirin enrolling 41,291 patients and 5 trials of abciximab enrolling 1275 patients (Figure 9.1). Overall, random allocation to antiplatelet therapy was associated with a decrease in death or dependency at the end of follow-up, relative risk (RR) 0.98, 95% confidence interval (CI): 0.96–0.99; $p = 0.01$.

Although formal testing did not show heterogeneity among agents, assessment power was limited by the large discrepancy in sample sizes between the aspirin and the abciximab groups, suggesting that consideration of each agent class separately is warranted. For aspirin, random allocation to active treatment was associated with a decrease in death or dependency at the end of follow-up, 45.0% versus 46.2% (RR 0.97, 95% CI: 0.96–0.99; $p = 0.01$). In absolute terms, 12 more patients were functionally independent at the end of follow-up for every 1000 patients treated with aspirin. For abciximab, random

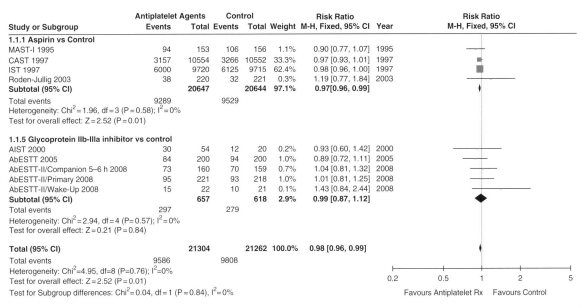

Figure 9.1 *Dependency or death (modified Rankin Scale [mRS] 3–6 or nearest equivalent) at 1–6 months, early antiplatelet agents vs avoid early antiplatelet agents.*

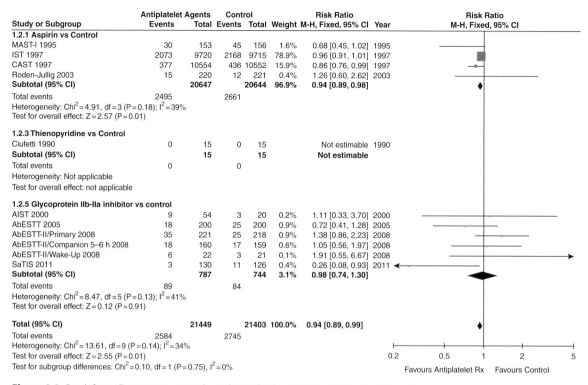

Figure 9.2 *Death from all causes at 1–6 months, early antiplatelet agents vs avoid early antiplatelet agents.*

allocation to active treatment was not associated with an alteration in death or dependency outcomes (RR 0.99, 95% CI: 0.87–1.12; *p* = 0.84).

Death

Data regarding death at final follow-up (or end of treatment if later data not available) were available from 11 trials, including 4 trials of aspirin enrolling 41,291 patients, 1 trial of a thienopyridine (ticlopidine) enrolling 30 patients, and 6 trials of glycoprotein IIb/IIIa receptor inhibitors (abciximab and tirofibran) enrolling 1531 patients (Figure 9.2). By the end of follow-up (or end of treatment period if later data not available), antiplatelet therapy was associated with a decrease in mortality (RR 0.94, 95% CI: 0.89–0.99; *p* = 0.01).

The preponderance of patients in the aspirin group limited the power of tests for heterogeneity, supporting consideration of each agent class separately. For aspirin, random allocation to active treatment was associated with a decrease in death, 12.1% versus 12.9% (RR 0.94, 95% CI: 0.89–0.98; *p* = 0.01). In absolute terms, there were 8 more patients alive at the end of follow-up for every 1000 patients treated with

aspirin. For abciximab, random allocation to active treatment was not associated with an effect on mortality (RR 0.98, 95% CI: 0.74–1.30; *p* = 0.91).

Progressive/Recurrent Ischaemic Stroke

The composite of progressive and recurrent ischaemic stroke usefully captures post-onset events that antithrombotics may in part beneficially avert. Early non-haemorrhagic progression of neurological deficits may be due to several mechanisms. Two are potentially modifiable by antithrombotic treatment – further propagation of the initial thrombus or a new cerebral thromboembolic event causing recurrent ischaemic stroke. Several other mechanisms are not modifiable by antithrombotic treatment, including haemodynamic-collateral failure, oedema, seizure, and infection. Recognition of recurrent ischaemic stroke is more straightforward, between 5 days to 6 months after onset of an initial cerebral ischaemic event.

Antiplatelet therapy was associated with a reduction in progressive or recurrent ischaemic stroke (RR 0.80, 95% CI: 0.72–0.89; *p* < 0.0001) (Figure 9.3). There was evidence of benefit both for aspirin and for glycoprotein IIb/IIIa receptor inhibitors. For aspirin,

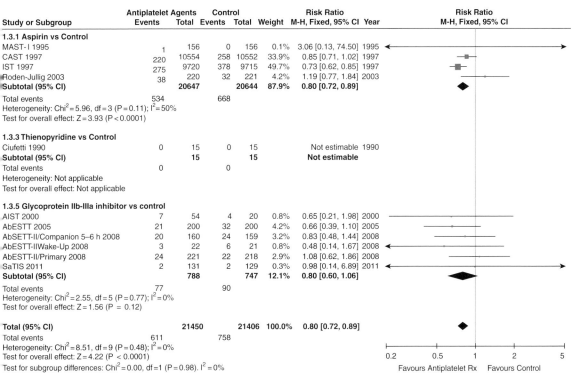

Study or Subgroup	Antiplatelet Agents Events	Total	Control Events	Total	Weight	Risk Ratio M-H, Fixed, 95% CI	Year	Risk Ratio M-H, Fixed, 95% CI
1.3.1 Aspirin vs Control								
MAST-I 1995	1	156	0	156	0.1%	3.06 [0.13, 74.50]	1995	
CAST 1997	220	10554	258	10552	33.9%	0.85 [0.71, 1.02]	1997	
IST 1997	275	9720	378	9715	49.7%	0.73 [0.62, 0.85]	1997	
Roden-Jullig 2003	38	220	32	221	4.2%	1.19 [0.77, 1.84]	2003	
Subtotal (95% CI)		**20647**		**20644**	**87.9%**	**0.80 [0.72, 0.89]**		
Total events	534		668					
Heterogeneity: Chi² = 5.96, df = 3 (P = 0.11); I² = 50%								
Test for overall effect: Z = 3.93 (P < 0.0001)								
1.3.3 Thienopyridine vs Control								
Ciufetti 1990	0	15	0	15		Not estimable	1990	
Subtotal (95% CI)		**15**		**15**		**Not estimable**		
Total events	0		0					
Heterogeneity: Not applicable								
Test for overall effect: Not applicable								
1.3.5 Glycoprotein IIb-IIIa inhibitor vs control								
AIST 2000	7	54	4	20	0.8%	0.65 [0.21, 1.98]	2000	
AbESTT 2005	21	200	32	200	4.2%	0.66 [0.39, 1.10]	2005	
AbESTT-II/Companion 5–6 h 2008	20	160	24	159	3.2%	0.83 [0.48, 1.44]	2008	
AbESTT-IIWake-Up 2008	3	22	6	21	0.8%	0.48 [0.14, 1.67]	2008	
AbESTT-II/Primary 2008	24	221	22	218	2.9%	1.08 [0.62, 1.86]	2008	
SaTIS 2011	2	131	2	129	0.3%	0.98 [0.14, 6.89]	2011	
Subtotal (95% CI)		**788**		**747**	**12.1%**	**0.80 [0.60, 1.06]**		
Total events	77		90					
Heterogeneity: Chi² = 2.55, df = 5 (P = 0.77); I² = 0%								
Test for overall effect: Z = 1.56 (P = 0.12)								
Total (95% CI)		**21450**		**21406**	**100.0%**	**0.80 [0.72, 0.89]**		
Total events	611		758					
Heterogeneity: Chi² = 8.51, df = 9 (P = 0.48); I² = 0%								
Test for overall effect: Z = 4.22 (P < 0.0001)								
Test for subgroup differences: Chi² = 0.00, df = 1 (P = 0.98). I² = 0%								

0.2 0.5 1 2 5
Favours Antiplatelet Rx Favours Control

Figure 9.3 *Death from all causes at 1–6 months: early antiplatelet agents vs avoid early antiplatelet agents.*

random allocation to active treatment was associated with a decrease in progressive/recurrent ischaemic stroke, 2.6% versus 3.2% (RR, 0.80, 95% CI: 0.72–0.89; $p < 0.0001$). In absolute terms, 6 progressive/recurrent ischaemic strokes were avoided for every 1000 patients treated. For abciximab, random allocation to active treatment was also associated with progressive/recurrent ischaemic stroke rates of 9.8% versus 12.0% (RR 0.80, 95% CI: 0.60–1.06; $p = 0.12$).

Symptomatic Intracranial Haemorrhage

Antiplatelet therapy was associated with an increase in symptomatic intracranial haemorrhage (SICH) (RR 1.33, 95% CI: 1.09–1.61; $p = 0.005$) (Figure 9.4). There was evidence of heterogeneity by agent class, with more magnified increase in SICH with glycoprotein IIb/IIIa receptor inhibitors than with aspirin, $p_{(heterogeneity)} = 0.006$, $I^2 = 86.6\%$. For aspirin, random allocation to active treatment was associated with an increase in SICH, 1.0% versus 0.8% (RR 1.22, 95% CI: 1.00–1.49; $p = 0.05$). In absolute terms, 2 additional symptomatic intracranial haemorrhages occurred for every 1000 patients treated. For glycoprotein IIb/IIIa receptor inhibitors, random allocation to active

treatment was associated with an increase in SICH, 3.4% versus 0.8% (RR 4.30, 95% CI: 1.78–10.35; $p = 0.001$).

Major Extracranial Haemorrhage

Antiplatelet therapy was associated with an increase in major extracranial haemorrhage (RR 1.72, 95% CI: 1.39–2.13; $p < 0.0001$) (Figure 9.5). There was evidence of heightened extracranial haemorrhage rates for both aspirin and for glycoprotein IIb/IIIa receptor inhibitors. For aspirin, random allocation to active treatment was associated with an increase in major extracranial haemorrhage, 1.0% versus 0.6% (RR 1.70, 95% CI: 1.36–2.1; $p < 0.00001$). In absolute terms, 4 more major extracranial haemorrhages occurred for every 1000 patients treated. For abciximab, random allocation to active treatment was also associated with major extracranial haemorrhage, RR 1.84, 95% CI: 1.02–3.32; $p = 0.04$.

Symptomatic Pulmonary Embolism

For symptomatic pulmonary embolism, events occurred infrequently, so that among agent classes, only aspirin, investigated in large mega-trials, had sample sizes

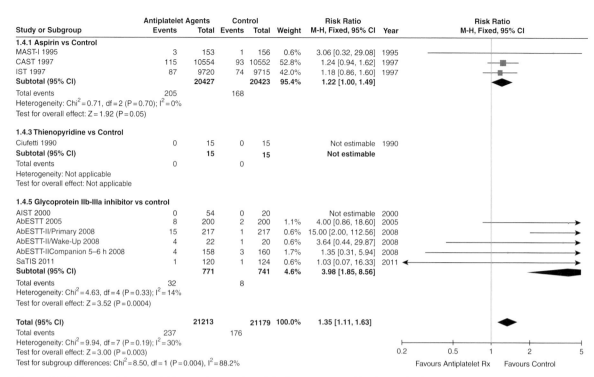

Figure 9.4 *Symptomatic intracranial haemorrhage, early antiplatelet agents vs avoid early antiplatelet agents.*

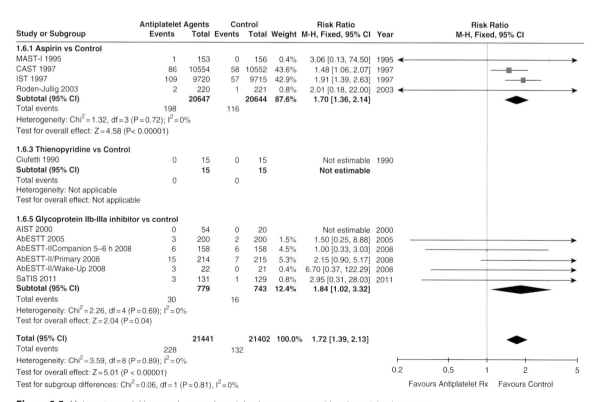

Figure 9.5 *Major extracranial haemorrhage, early antiplatelet agents vs avoid early antiplatelet agents.*

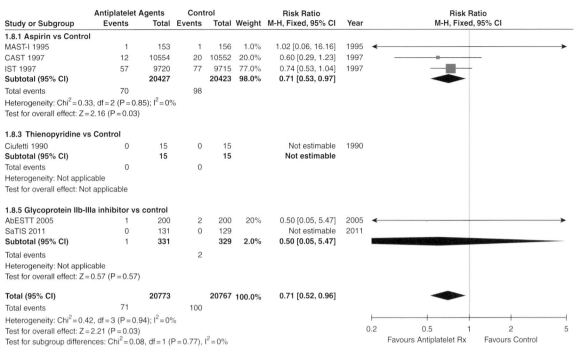

Study or Subgroup	Antiplatelet Agents		Control			Risk Ratio		Risk Ratio
	Events	Total	Events	Total	Weight	M-H, Fixed, 95% CI	Year	M-H, Fixed, 95% CI
1.8.1 Aspirin vs Control								
MAST-I 1995	1	153	1	156	1.0%	1.02 [0.06, 16.16]	1995	
CAST 1997	12	10554	20	10552	20.0%	0.60 [0.29, 1.23]	1997	
IST 1997	57	9720	77	9715	77.0%	0.74 [0.53, 1.04]	1997	
Subtotal (95% CI)		**20427**		**20423**	**98.0%**	**0.71 [0.53, 0.97]**		
Total events	70		98					
Heterogeneity: Chi² = 0.33, df = 2 (P = 0.85); I² = 0%								
Test for overall effect: Z = 2.16 (P = 0.03)								
1.8.3 Thienopyridine vs Control								
Ciufetti 1990	0	15	0	15		Not estimable	1990	
Subtotal (95% CI)		**15**		**15**		**Not estimable**		
Total events	0		0					
Heterogeneity: Not applicable								
Test for overall effect: Not applicable								
1.8.5 Glycoprotein IIb-IIIa inhibitor vs control								
AbESTT 2005	1	200	2	200	20%	0.50 [0.05, 5.47]	2005	
SaTIS 2011	0	131	0	129		Not estimable	2011	
Subtotal (95% CI)		**331**		**329**	**2.0%**	**0.50 [0.05, 5.47]**		
Total events	1		2					
Heterogeneity: Not applicable								
Test for overall effect: Z = 0.57 (P = 0.57)								
Total (95% CI)		**20773**		**20767**	**100.0%**	**0.71 [0.52, 0.96]**		
Total events	71		100					
Heterogeneity: Chi² = 0.42, df = 3 (P = 0.94); I² = 0%								
Test for overall effect: Z = 2.21 (P = 0.03)								
Test for subgroup differences: Chi² = 0.08, df = 1 (P = 0.77), I² = 0%								

0.2   0.5   1   2   5
Favours Antiplatelet Rx   Favours Control

Figure 9.6 *Pulmonary embolism, early antiplatelet agents vs avoid early antiplatelet agents.*

sufficient to be informative (Figure 9.6). Aspirin therapy was associated with a reduction in pulmonary embolism, 0.34% versus 0.48% (RR 0.71, 95% CI: 0.53–0.97; $p = 0.03$). In absolute terms, 1.5 pulmonary emboli were avoided for every 1000 patients treated with antiplatelet agents. Few trials reported results for deep vein thrombosis or for asymptomatic pulmonary embolism, so the profile of antiplatelet agent effect on venous thrombosis complications after acute cerebral ischaemia is incomplete.

Full Recovery and Shift in Levels of Disability

Two large trials examined the effect of early aspirin versus control on shift in functional outcomes across 4 levels of disability – fully recovered, independent but not fully recovered, dependent, and dead – at 1 month (CAST, 1997) or 6 months (IST, 1997) in a total of 39,866 randomized patients. Combining the trial data without adjustment, aspirin was associated with a favourable shift to less disabled outcomes across the 4 disability-level states, Mann–Whitney $p = 0.02$ (Figure 9.7). Using algorithmic joint outcome table analysis, aspirin yielded a lower disability level for a net 22 of every 1000 patients treated. For the best

outcome, aspirin versus no aspirin was associated with increased attainment of full recovery, 27.8% versus 26.7% (RR 1.04, 95% CI: 1.01–1.07; $p = 0.01$).

Patient Subgroups

Analyses for differential treatment response have been conducted among nearly 40,000 patients enrolled in 3 trials of aspirin versus no aspirin, evaluating 28 patient subgroups defined by single baseline characteristics (Chen et al., 2000), and 3 patient subgroups defined by models predicting risk of thrombotic, haemorrhagic, and poor final functional outcomes (Thompson et al., 2015). No patient profile was identified that predicted a heightened or reduced benefit of aspirin therapy.

Comment

Antiplatelet therapy with aspirin 160–300 mg daily, given orally (or per nasogastric tube or rectum in patients unable to swallow), and started within 48 hours of onset of acute cerebral ischaemia is associated with a modest reduction in recurrent ischaemic stroke and pulmonary embolism, and this benefit is partially offset by a small risk of bleeding. Overall, among every 1000 patients treated, 6 fewer will have

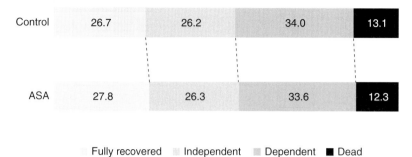

Control	26.7	26.2	34.0	13.1
ASA	27.8	26.3	33.6	12.3

Fully recovered   Independent   Dependent   ■ Dead

Figure 9.7 *Level of disability at 1–6 months, early antiplatelet agents vs avoid early antiplatelet agents,* pooled data from IST (1997), CAST (1997).

progressive/recurrent ischaemic stroke and 1.5 fewer will have pulmonary embolism, 2 more will have SICH, and 4 more will have major extracranial haemorrhage.

Through these contrasting, overtly recognizable effects, and others, aspirin confers an overall net benefit, modest in degree, upon final outcome. For every 1000 patients treated early with aspirin, compared with no aspirin, 22 have reduced disability, including 11 more who are fully recovered and 8 more alive. For reduced disability, the number needed to treat for 1 patient to benefit is 47.

The only other antiplatelet agent class with any substantial data against control in the early setting is the glycoprotein IIb/IIIa receptor inhibitors, with most of the data arising from abciximab trials. Reflecting trial design (earlier start of therapy, greater deficit severity) and more powerful pharmacological effects, both beneficial ischaemic event reductions and adverse bleeding events were more pronounced with glycoprotein IIb/IIIa receptor inhibitors. Among every 1000 patients treated, 23 fewer had progressive/recurrent ischaemic stroke but 26 more had symptomatic ICH and 17 more had major extracranial haemorrhage, with overall no net positive or negative effect on final functional independence or survival.

Implications for Practice

In acute cerebral ischaemia patients not being treated with intravenous thrombolytics, aspirin 160–300 mg is a beneficial regimen when started within the first 48 hours of onset and continued as a daily dose.

In patients who are unable to swallow safely, aspirin may be given via a nasogastric tube, per rectum as a suppository, or, in countries where available, intravenously (as 100 mg of the lysine salt of ASA).

In patients with aspirin allergy, an alternative antiplatelet agent from a class that has comparable potency and effects to aspirin should be considered. Glycoprotein IIb/IIIa receptor inhibitors are not good alternative choices based on completed studies. Randomized trials of other agents given acutely are lacking, but thienopyridines (e.g. clopidogrel) and phosphodiesterase inhibitors (e.g. dipyridamole) are potential options.

In patients who are being treated with intravenous fibrinolytic therapy, aspirin should be avoided for the first 24 hours after lytic start, given its known potentiation of bleeding risk (see Chapter 6).

The long-term antithrombotic regimen eventually finalized for a patient will depend upon findings from the diagnostic workup regarding ischaemic stroke mechanism (large artery atherosclerotic [LAA], cardioembolic, small vessel disease, etc), indications or contraindications arising in other vascular beds, and patient passage through the initial several days poststroke, when risk of haemorrhagic conversion is highest. Initial daily aspirin is a net beneficial regimen that can be deployed during the first hours and days after onset, while information is being gathered to guide the eventual selection of the final long-term regimen.

Implications for Research

The overall magnitude of clinical benefit of antiplatelet therapies alone in acute ischaemic stroke is modest (Cranston et al., 2017). Reperfusion therapies have far greater benefits for the patients eligible for them, with intravenous tissue plasminogen activator (tPA) improving the outcomes of 10-fold more patients, and endovascular mechanical thrombectomy 20-fold more cerebral ischaemia patients. This limited impact reflects the fact that the preponderance of brain injury and functional disability in acute cerebral ischaemia arises from the initial occlusion and the initially threatened brain parenchyma, which are addressed directly with reperfusion interventions. Delayed clot propagation causing stroke progression and new thromboembolism causing early recurrent ischaemic stroke are less frequent events that account for much less neural injury and activity impairment at the population level. As a result, stand alone antiplatelet therapy has less scope for benefit in acute cerebral ischaemia.

Using antiplatelet agents to enhance reperfusion therapies is a promising strategy meriting further investigation. If a combination of antiplatelet and fibrinolytic agents can be found that achieves more frequent and sustained recanalization than intravenous fibrinolysis alone, without increasing haemorrhagic risk, clinical benefits would be substantial. Continuous ultrasound studies in patients with acute ischaemic stroke have shown that thrombi behave dynamically after first exposure to intravenous fibrinolytics, with frequent early re-occlusion after initial recanalization, potentially avertable by concomitant antiplatelet therapy. While aspirin added to full-dose intravenous tissue plasminogen activator was not beneficial, initial small trials of various dose combinations of glycoprotein IIb/IIIa receptor inhibitors and fibrinolytics have been encouraging (Pancioli et al., 2013; Adeoye et al., 2015). In the Combined Approach to Lysis Utilizing Eptifibatide and rt-PA in Acute Ischemic Stroke-Enhanced Regimen (CLEAR-ER) trial, 101 patients treated with a combination of reduced-dose tissue plasminogen activator and eptifibatide, compared with historical controls from the NINDS rt-PA Study, had directionally favourable rates of disability-free (modified Rankin Scale [mRS] 0–1) outcome at 3 months, 49.5% versus 36.0% (odds ratio [OR] 1.74; 95% CI; 0.70–4.31; $p = 0.23$) (Pancioli et al., 2013). Bleeding rates were not increased.

With regard to preventing early recurrent ischaemic stroke, the initial large aspirin trials established aspirin as being of benefit, though modest. Accordingly, aspirin became the standard of care therapy for this target, and aspirin monotherapy, rather than no antithrombotic treatment, served as the control arm in subsequent trials of other antiplatelet agents or combinations of antiplatelet agents seeking to reduce subacute recurrent ischaemic stroke.

Comparisons of Different Antiplatelet Regimens

Evidence

In patients with acute ischaemic stroke or transient ischaemic attack early after onset (within 72 h) and of non-cardioembolic origin, different antiplatelet regimens have been compared with each other in 22 randomized trial comparisons enrolling 31,549 patients. The greatest number of studies have been on dual versus mono antiplatelet therapy regimens, evaluated in 17 trial comparisons enrolling 13,982 patients. Head-to-head comparison of one mono antiplatelet regimen versus another mono antiplatelet regimen has been studied in 3 trials enrolling 13,796 patients. In addition, 1 trial enrolling 675 patients has performed a head-to-head comparison of one dual antiplatelet regimen versus another dual antiplatelet regimen, and 1 trial enrolling 3096 patients has compared a triple antiplatelet therapy regimen versus mono and dual antiplatelet regimens.

Comparisons of Different Monotherapy Antiplatelet Regimens

Three trials have compared different monotherapy antiplatelet regimens in patients with acute non-cardioembolic ischaemic stroke or TIA early after onset (within 72 h), including two trials of the cyclopentyl-triazolo-pyrimidine ticagrelor versus aspirin, enrolling 13,349 patients, and one trial of the phosphodiesterase inhibitor agent cilostazol versus aspirin, enrolling 448 patients. The disparity in agent class sample sizes limits power to interrogate for treatment effect heterogeneity, suggesting the different regimens be evaluated separately.

For ticagrelor versus aspirin, the predominant source of data is the large SOCRATES trial, enrolling 13,199 patients (Johnston et al., 2016), with the smaller SETIS trial contributing an additional 150 patients (Torgano et al., 2010). In the large SOCRATES trial, enrolled patients had to be within 24 hours of a minor ischaemic stroke (NIHSS score of 5 or less) or high-risk TIA (ABCD2 score of 4 or higher), and 63% were enrolled between 12 and 24 hours post-onset. Patients received oral ticagrelor alone or aspirin alone for 3 months. In the smaller SETIS trial, patients were enrolled within 6 hours of a moderate-major ischaemic stroke (NIHSS score of 5–25), with mean time to enrolment of 4.4 hours, and patients received intravenous ticagrelor or aspirin for 3 days.

In combined analysis of the two trials, ticagrelor was associated with a reduction in progressive/recurrent ischaemic stroke (5.9% vs 6.7%, RR 0.88, 95% CI: 0.77–1.00; $p = 0.05$; Figure 9.8). In addition, ticagrelor did not increase SICH (0.2% vs 0.3%, RR 0.62, 95% CI: 0.31–1.24; $p = 0.18$; Figure 9.9) or major extracranial haemorrhage (0.17% vs 0.13%, RR 1.21, 95% CI: 0.54–2.58; $p = 0.69$; Figure 9.10). Mortality by 3 months did not show a treatment group difference (RR 1.15, 95% CI: 0.83–1.60; $p = 0.39$; Figure 9.11). However, in the large SOCRATES trial, for the trial's primary endpoint composite of any stroke (ischaemic or haemorrhagic), myocardial infarction, or all-cause death, directionally favourable ticagrelor effects did not reach statistical significance (6.7% vs 7.5%, hazard ratio [HR] 0.89, 95% CI: 0.78–1.01; $p = 0.07$). The SETIS trial did not report data for this composite endpoint. Also, in SOCRATES, ticagrelor versus aspirin was associated with more combined major or minor bleeding events (1.1% vs 0.7%, $p = 0.005$) and more dyspnoea events (1.4% vs 0.3%, $p = 0.0001$).

For cilostazol, the single CAIST trial enrolled 458 patients with mild-to-moderate, but not severe, ischaemic stroke (NIHSS score up to 15) within 48

Study or Subgroup	Novel Antiplatelet Events	Novel Antiplatelet Total	Aspirin Events	Aspirin Total	Weight	Risk Ratio M-H, Fixed, 95% CI	Year
1.3.1 Cilostazol vs Aspirin							
CAIST 2011	45	228	40	219	8.4%	1.08 [0.74, 1.59]	2011
Subtotal (95% CI)		**228**		**219**	**8.4%**	**1.08 [0.74, 1.59]**	
Total events	45		40				
Heterogeneity: Not applicable							
Test for overall effect: Z = 0.40 (P = 0.69)							
1.3.2 Ticagrelor vs Aspirin							
SETIS 2010	5	75	6	75	1.2%	0.83 [0.27, 2.61]	2010
SOCRATES 2016	385	6589	441	6610	90.4%	0.88 [0.77, 1.00]	2016
Subtotal (95% CI)		**6664**		**6685**	**91.6%**	**0.88 [0.77, 1.00]**	
Total events	390		447				
Heterogeneity: $Chi^2 = 0.01$, df = 1 (P = 0.93); $I^2 = 0\%$							
Test for overall effect: Z = 1.99 (P = 0.05)							
Total (95% CI)		**6892**		**6904**	**100.0%**	**0.89 [0.79, 1.01]**	
Total events	435		487				
Heterogeneity: $Chi^2 = 1.05$, df = 2 (P = 0.59); $I^2 = 0\%$							
Test for overall effect: Z = 1.79 (P = 0.07)							
Test for subgroup differences: $Chi^2 = 1.04$, df = 1 (P = 0.31), $I^2 = 3.7\%$							

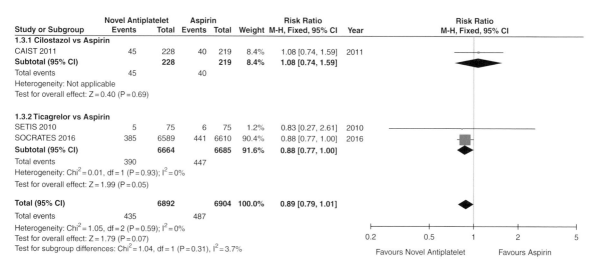

Figure 9.8 *Progressive/recurrent ischaemic stroke, head-to-head comparisons of early single antiplatelet agents.*

Study or Subgroup	Novel Antiplatelet Events	Novel Antiplatelet Total	Aspirin Events	Aspirin Total	Weight	Risk Ratio M-H, Fixed, 95% CI	Year
1.4.1 Cilostazol vs Aspirin							
CAIST 2011	0	225	2	224	10.7%	0.20 [0.01, 4.12]	2011
Subtotal (95% CI)		**225**		**224**	**10.7%**	**0.20 [0.01, 4.12]**	
Total events	0		2				
Heterogeneity: Not applicable							
Test for overall effect: Z = 1.04 (P = 0.30)							
1.4.2 Ticagrelor vs Aspirin							
SETIS 2010	1	75	3	75	12.8%	0.33 [0.04, 3.13]	2010
SOCRATES 2016	12	6589	18	6610	76.5%	0.67 [0.32, 1.39]	2016
Subtotal (95% CI)		**6664**		**6685**	**89.3%**	**0.62 [0.31, 1.24]**	
Total events	13		21				
Heterogeneity: $Chi^2 = 0.34$, df = 1 (P = 0.56); $I^2 = 0\%$							
Test for overall effect: Z = 1.35 (P = 0.18)							
Total (95% CI)		**6889**		**6909**	**100.0%**	**0.58 [0.30, 1.12]**	
Total events	13		23				
Heterogeneity: $Chi^2 = 0.86$, df = 2 (P = 0.65); $I^2 = 0\%$							
Test for overall effect: Z = 1.62 (P = 0.11)							
Test for subgroup differences: $Chi^2 = 0.51$, df = 1 (P = 0.47), $I^2 = 0\%$							

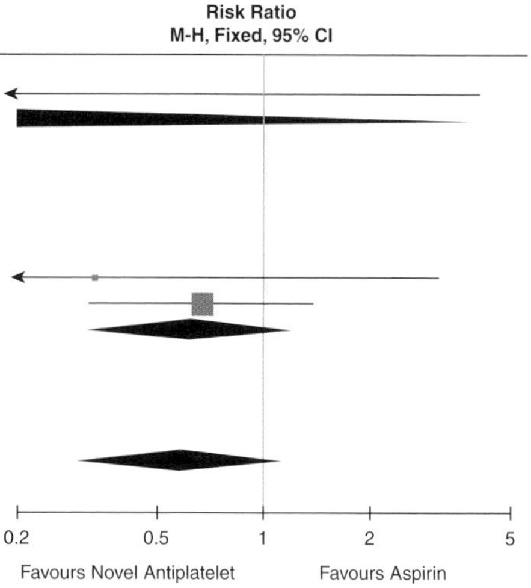

Figure 9.9 *Symptomatic intracranial haemorrhage, head-to-head comparisons of early single antiplatelet agents.*

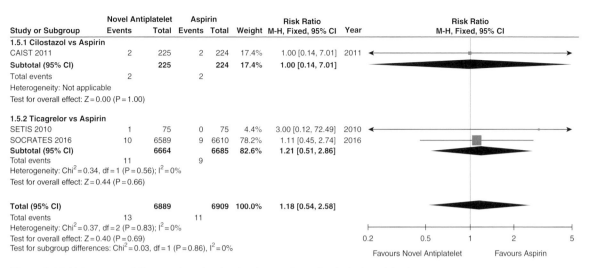

Figure 9.10 *Major extracranial haemorrhage, head-to-head comparisons of early single antiplatelet agents.*

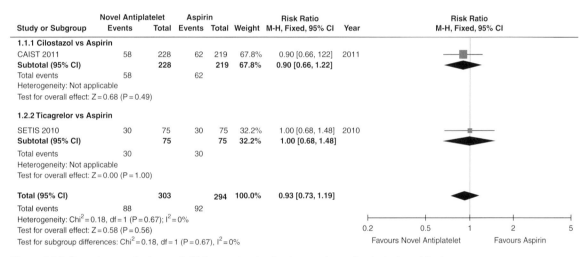

Figure 9.11 *Dependency or death at end of follow-up, head-to-head comparisons of early single antiplatelet agents.*

hours of onset (mean actual time from onset 34 h), and allocated them to cilostazol or aspirin for 90 days (Lee et al., 2011). No statistically significant difference between the cilostazol and aspirin regimens was observed, including for the trial's primary endpoint of death or dependency at 3 months (RR: 0.90, 95% CI: 0.66–1.22; Figure 9.12), and for progressing/recurrent ischaemic stroke (RR: 1.08, 95% CI: 0.74–1.08; see Figure 9.8), SICH (RR: 0.20, 95% CI: 0.01–4.12; see Figure 9.9), major extracranial haemorrhage (RR: 1.00, 95% CI: 0.14–7.01; see Figure 9.10), and mortality (RR: 0.96, 95% CI: 0.14–6.73; Figure 9.12).

Comparisons of Dual vs Mono Antiplatelet Regimens

In patients with acute ischaemic stroke or TIA early after onset (within 72 h) and of non-cardioembolic origin, dual antiplatelet therapy has been compared with mono antiplatelet therapy antithrombotic therapy in 17 randomized trial comparisons enrolling 13,982 patients (Wong et al., 2013; Johnston et al., 2018; Yang et al., 2018). The comparisons include 10 from trials confined to early-presenting patients and 7 from early-presenting subgroups of trials enrolling both early- and later-presenting patients.

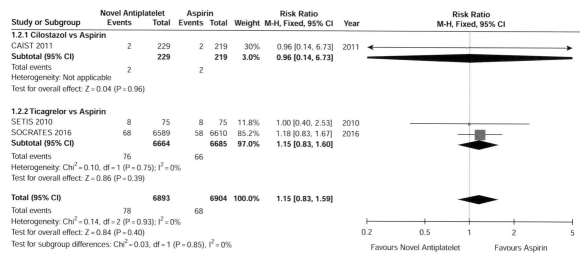

Study or Subgroup	Novel Antiplatelet Events	Total	Aspirin Events	Total	Weight	Risk Ratio M-H, Fixed, 95% CI	Year	Risk Ratio M-H, Fixed, 95% CI
1.2.1 Cilostazol vs Aspirin								
CAIST 2011	2	229	2	219	30%	0.96 [0.14, 6.73]	2011	
Subtotal (95% CI)		**229**		**219**	**3.0%**	**0.96 [0.14, 6.73]**		
Total events	2		2					
Heterogeneity: Not applicable								
Test for overall effect: Z = 0.04 (P = 0.96)								
1.2.2 Ticagrelor vs Aspirin								
SETIS 2010	8	75	8	75	11.8%	1.00 [0.40, 2.53]	2010	
SOCRATES 2016	68	6589	58	6610	85.2%	1.18 [0.83, 1.67]	2016	
Subtotal (95% CI)		**6664**		**6685**	**97.0%**	**1.15 [0.83, 1.60]**		
Total events	76		66					
Heterogeneity: Chi² = 0.10, df = 1 (P = 0.75); I² = 0%								
Test for overall effect: Z = 0.86 (P = 0.39)								
Total (95% CI)		**6893**		**6904**	**100.0%**	**1.15 [0.83, 1.59]**		
Total events	78		68					
Heterogeneity: Chi² = 0.14, df = 2 (P = 0.93); I² = 0%								
Test for overall effect: Z = 0.84 (P = 0.40)								
Test for subgroup differences: Chi² = 0.03, df = 1 (P = 0.85), I² = 0%								

0.2   0.5   1   2   5

Favours Novel Antiplatelet   Favours Aspirin

Figure 9.12 *Death at end of follow-up, head-to-head comparisons of early single antiplatelet agents.*

Antiplatelet Regimens Tested

The most common monotherapy control comparator was aspirin alone, used in 13 trial arm comparisons enrolling 13,647 patients. Clopidogrel alone and dipyridamole alone were used as the monotherapy comparator in 2 trials each. The most common dual therapy regimen tested was clopidogrel plus aspirin, used in 10 randomized trial comparisons enrolling 12,823 patients. The combination of dipyridamole plus aspirin was evaluated in 6 randomized trial comparisons and cilostazol plus aspirin in 1 trial. The 2 largest trials, CHANCE and POINT, evaluated clopidogrel plus aspirin versus aspirin and together contributed 72% of the data (Wang et al., 2013; Johnston et al., 2018). The comparisons with the greatest number of patients were (1) clopidogrel plus aspirin versus aspirin (9 trials, 12,332 patients, 81% of all patients); (2) dipyridamole plus aspirin versus clopidogrel (1 trial, 1360 patients, 9% of all patients); and (3) dipyridamole plus aspirin versus aspirin (3 trials, 748 patients, 5% of all patients).

Time from Onset to Inclusion or Treatment

Permitted time windows for enrolment were up to 12–24 hours for 5 trial comparisons, up to 48 hours for 3 trial comparisons, and up to 72 hours for 9 trial comparisons. Enrolment windows for the 6 trial comparisons contributing the most patients were: within 12 hours in 1 trial – POINT (Johnston et al., 2018); within 24 hours in 3 trials – FASTER, EARLY, and CHANCE (Kennedy et al., 2007; Dengler et al., 2010; Wang et al., 2013); and within 72 hours in 2 trials – PRoFESS and He and colleagues (Bath et al., 2010; He et al., 2015). Among these trials, actual median or mean onset to enrolment or treatment times included 7.4 hours in POINT, 8.5 hours in FASTER, 13 hours in CHANCE, and 58 hours in PRoFESS.

Cerebral Ischaemia Subtype and Severity at Entry

All trials enrolled only patients with non-cardioembolic cerebral ischaemic events. Among these patients, the risk of haemorrhagic transformation of cerebral infarction from intensified antithrombotic therapy is likely to be less in TIA and minor ischaemic stroke patients who have smaller volumes of injured tissue at risk. In addition, observational studies have suggested that patients with early improvement in their deficits during the first 1–7 days after onset are at increased risk for early recurrent ischaemic stroke (Johnston et al., 2003). For these reasons, several of the trials restricted enrolment based on stroke severity.

Four trial comparisons enrolled patients with ischaemic stroke only, 1 enrolled patients with TIA only, and 12 enrolled both patients with ischaemic stroke and TIA. Eight of the trials focused upon patients with mild deficits only, including 6 with either minor ischaemic stroke or TIA, 1 with minor ischaemic stroke only, and 1 with TIA only. The two largest trials, CHANCE and POINT, both enrolled minor ischaemic stroke patients with NIHSS scores of 3 or less and high-risk transient ischaemic attack patients with ABCD2 scores of 4 or higher.

Scheduled Duration of Trial Treatment and Follow-up

The scheduled duration of study treatment included 7 days (2 trials), 14–21 days (2 trials), 30 days (1 trial), 3 months (4 trials), 6 months (1 trial), and 18–42 months (6 trial comparisons). In the two largest trials, scheduled duration of study treatment was 21 days (CHANCE) and 3 months (POINT).

Follow-up duration for assessment of outcome included: 7 days (2 trials), 14 days (1 trial), 1 month (2 trials), 3 months (5 trials), 6 months (1 trial), and 18–42 months (6 trials). In the two largest trials, follow-up assessment was at 3 months (CHANCE and POINT).

Recurrent Stroke

Data regarding recurrent stroke (including ischaemic, haemorrhagic, and unknown subtypes) were available from 17 trial comparisons enrolling 15,227 patients. Overall, early random allocation to dual rather than mono antiplatelet therapy, short-term or long-term, was associated with a decrease in recurrent stroke, 5.4% versus 7.8% (RR 0.68, 95% CI: 0.61–0.77; $p < 0.00001$) (Figure 9.13). In absolute terms, 24 fewer patients had recurrent stroke for every 1000 patients treated with dual therapy. There was no evidence of heterogeneity of effect across the different tested dual and mono antiplatelet regimens.

Considering only studies that evaluated follow-up through up to 3 months after presentation, trial comparisons were available for 10 trials enrolling 14,019 patients (Figure 9.14). Overall, random allocation to dual rather than mono antiplatelet therapy for up to 3 months was associated with a decrease in recurrent stroke (5.5% versus 8.2%, RR 0.67, 95% CI: 0.60–0.76; $p < 0.00001$). In absolute terms, 27 fewer patients had recurrent stroke for every 1000 patients treated with dual therapy. There was no evidence of heterogeneity of effect across the different tested dual and mono antiplatelet regimens, although the preponderance of patients, 86%, came from trials comparing clopidogrel plus aspirin versus aspirin alone.

Composite of Recurrent Stroke, TIA, Acute Coronary Syndrome, and Death

Data regarding the composite outcome of recurrent stroke, TIA, acute coronary syndrome, and death were available from 11 trials enrolling 13,938 patients (see Figure 9.9). Overall, early random allocation to dual rather than mono antiplatelet therapy, continued short-term or long-term, was associated with a decrease in cerebral or cardiac vascular or fatal events, 7.1% versus 9.8% (RR 0.72, 95% CI: 0.65–0.81; $p < 0.00001$). In absolute terms, 27 fewer patients had recurrent cerebral or cardiac vascular events or death for every 1000 patients treated with dual therapy. There was no evidence of heterogeneity of effect across the different tested dual and mono antiplatelet regimens.

Considering only studies that evaluated follow-up through up to 3 months after presentation, trial comparisons were available for 9 trials enrolling 13,352 patients. Overall, random allocation to dual rather than mono antiplatelet therapy was associated with a decrease in cerebral or cardiac vascular or fatal events, 5.5% versus 8.2% (RR 0.67, 95% CI: 0.60–0.76; $p < 0.00001$) (Figure 9.15).

Major Extraparenchymal Bleeding

Data regarding major bleeding were available from 14 trials enrolling 14,946 patients (see Figure 9.10). Overall, random allocation to dual rather than mono antiplatelet therapy was associated with an increase in major bleeding, 0.6% versus 0.3% (RR 1.86, 95% CI: 1.17–2.9; $p = 0.009$). In absolute terms, 3 more patients had major bleeding events for every 1000 patients treated with dual therapy. There was no evidence of heterogeneity of effect across the different tested dual and mono antiplatelet regimens.

Considering only studies that evaluated follow-up through up to 3 months after presentation, trial comparisons were available for 10 trials enrolling 14,038 patients. Overall, random allocation to dual rather than mono antiplatelet therapy was associated with an increase in major bleeding, 0.6% versus 0.3% (RR 1.84, 95% CI: 1.12–3.02; $p = 0.02$) (Figure 9.16).

Patient Subgroups

Study-level and patient-level meta-analyses of dual versus mono antiplatelet therapy have not yet examined early patient subgroups in substantial detail. However, several suggestive exploratory subgroup analyses have been conducted of the large CHANCE trial comparing clopidogrel plus aspirin versus aspirin alone for the first 21 days in 5170 patients with minor ischaemic stroke or TIA.

CYP2C19 Gene Loss-of-Function Alleles

To exert an antiplatelet effect, clopidogrel requires conversion to an active metabolite by hepatic cytochrome P450 (CYP) isoenzymes, and the efficiency of this conversion may be modified by polymorphisms of the *CYP2C19* gene. Loss-of-function alleles are more

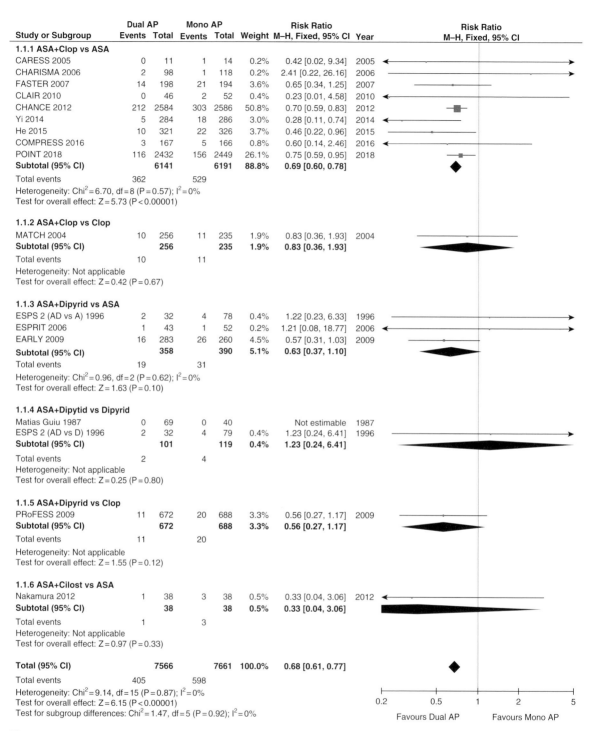

Figure 9.13 *Recurrent stroke (ischaemic, haemorrhagic, or unknown type), early initiation of dual antiplatelet therapy vs early mono antiplatelet therapy*, continued short-term or long-term.

common in Asian individuals. Among 2993 Chinese CHANCE patients who underwent *CYP2C19* genotyping, 59% were carriers of loss-of-function alleles, and

CYP2C19 gene allele status modified the treatment effect of adding clopidogrel to aspirin (Wang et al., 2016). Clopidogrel plus aspirin reduced recurrent

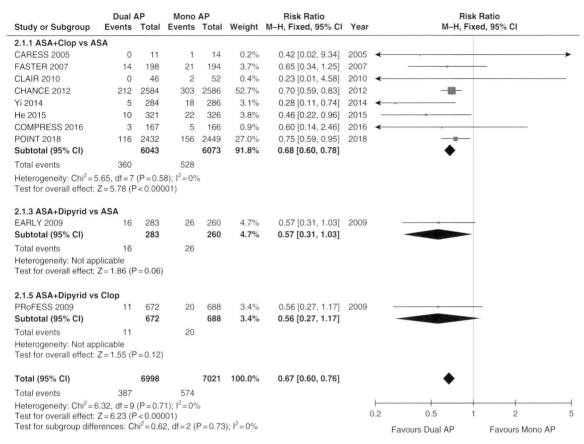

Figure 9.14 *Recurrent stroke (ischaemic, haemorrhagic, or unknown type), early initiation of dual antiplatelet therapy vs early mono antiplatelet therapy,* continued for up to first 3 months.

stroke in non-carriers but not carriers of the loss-of-function alleles ($p = 0.02$ for interaction), with stroke rates among non-carriers of 6.7% versus 12.4% (HR 0.51, 95% CI: 0.35–0.75), and stroke rates among carriers of 9.4% versus 10.8% (HR 0.93, 95% CI: 0.69–1.26).

Large Artery Atherosclerotic Disease with Artery-to-Artery Embolism

Imaging features that exerted a prognostic effect in CHANCE were the presence of large artery intracranial stenosis (ICAS) and acute diffusion magnetic resonance imaging (MRI) infarcts. Among 1,089 CHANCE patients undergoing MRI/MR angiography (MRA) imaging of their presenting event, rates of recurrent ischaemic stroke at 90 days were the following: neither acute infarction nor ICAS – 1.3%; single infarct without ICAS – 6.8%; single infarct with ICAS – 11.9%; and multiple infarcts with ICAS –

18.0% (Pan et al., 2017b). The presence of ICAS did not statistically modify the benefit of clopidogrel plus aspirin versus aspirin alone, HR 0.79 (95% CI: 0.47–1.32) with ICAS versus 1.12 (95% CI: 0.56–2.25) without ICAS, interaction $p = 0.52$ (Liu et al., 2015). However, infarct patterns had a modifying effect on the benefit of clopidogrel plus aspirin versus aspirin alone, with greatest reduction in recurrent stroke among patients with initial multiple infarcts – adjusted HR 0.5 (95% CI: 0.3–0.96), compared with patients with single infarcts – HR 1.1 (95% CI: 0.6–2.0) and patients with no infarcts – HR 1.7 (0.3–11.1), interaction $p = 0.04$ (Jing et al., 2018). Since CHANCE only enrolled patients with non-cardioembolic events, the presence of multiple infarcts likely identifies patients who harbour a highly emboligenic extracranial or intracranial LAA source, and these patients appeared to have a magnified benefit from dual antiplatelet therapy.

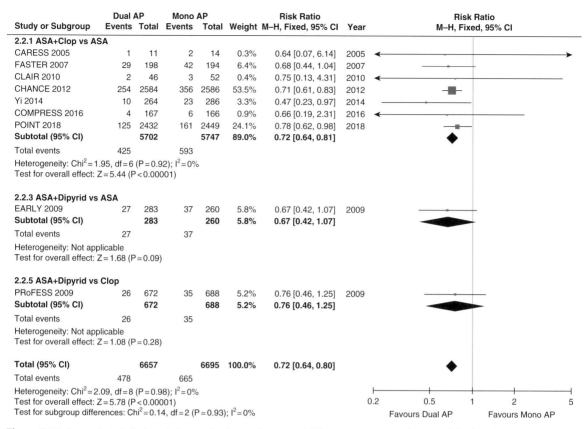

Figure 9.15 *Recurrent stroke (ischaemic, haemorrhagic, or unknown type), TIA, acute coronary syndrome, and death, early initiation of dual antiplatelet therapy vs early mono antiplatelet therapy,* continued for up to first 3 months.

Timing of Beneficial Effects

The ratio of benefit to harm of dual versus mono antiplatelet therapy may vary with time from the index event. The risk of recurrent ischaemic stroke is greatest in the first hours and days after the index ischaemic event, while the thrombotic source remains unstable and collateral growth is still under way. Similarly, the risk of haemorrhagic transformation of cerebral infarction is greatest in the initial hours and days, while endothelial and neural tissues are still freshly injured. However, with minor ischaemic strokes and TIAs, the cerebral haemorrhage risk is relatively low, even in the initial period. In a time course analysis of the CHANCE trial, clopidogrel plus aspirin provided substantial reduction in recurrent ischaemic strokes during the first 10 days of the 21-day treatment course, but from days 11–21 increased major or minor bleeding cases related to dual antiplatelet therapy equalled or exceeded reductions in recurrent ischaemic stroke (Pan et al., 2017a). In the POINT trial, clopidogrel plus aspirin

provided substantial reduction in the primary endpoint of recurrent ischaemic stroke, myocardial infarction, and ischaemic vascular death recurrent ischaemic strokes during the first 20 days of the 90-day treatment course, but from days 21–90 did not confer additional differential benefit (Johnston et al., 2018).

Comparisons of Different Dual Antiplatelet Therapy Regimens

One trial has compared different dual antiplatelet regimens against one another: the PRINCE trial comparing ticagrelor plus aspirin versus clopidogrel plus aspirin (Wang et al., 2018). The trial enrolled 675 Asian patients with non-cardioembolic minor ischaemic stroke (NIHSS score up to 3) or TIA (ABCD2 score ≥4 or relevant large artery stenosis ≥50%) within 24 hours of onset. The mean actual time from onset was 13.9 hours. In the ticagrelor plus aspirin arm, patients received a loading dose of ticagrelor 180 mg

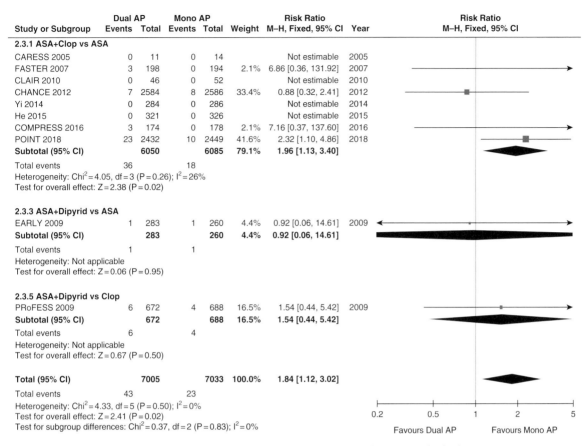

Study or Subgroup	Dual AP Events	Total	Mono AP Events	Total	Weight	Risk Ratio M–H, Fixed, 95% CI	Year
2.3.1 ASA+Clop vs ASA							
CARESS 2005	0	11	0	14		Not estimable	2005
FASTER 2007	3	198	0	194	2.1%	6.86 [0.36, 131.92]	2007
CLAIR 2010	0	46	0	52		Not estimable	2010
CHANCE 2012	7	2584	8	2586	33.4%	0.88 [0.32, 2.41]	2012
Yi 2014	0	284	0	286		Not estimable	2014
He 2015	0	321	0	326		Not estimable	2015
COMPRESS 2016	3	174	0	178	2.1%	7.16 [0.37, 137.60]	2016
POINT 2018	23	2432	10	2449	41.6%	2.32 [1.10, 4.86]	2018
Subtotal (95% CI)		**6050**		**6085**	**79.1%**	**1.96 [1.13, 3.40]**	
Total events	36		18				
Heterogeneity: Chi² = 4.05, df = 3 (P = 0.26); I² = 26%							
Test for overall effect: Z = 2.38 (P = 0.02)							
2.3.3 ASA+Dipyrid vs ASA							
EARLY 2009	1	283	1	260	4.4%	0.92 [0.06, 14.61]	2009
Subtotal (95% CI)		**283**		**260**	**4.4%**	**0.92 [0.06, 14.61]**	
Total events	1		1				
Heterogeneity: Not applicable							
Test for overall effect: Z = 0.06 (P = 0.95)							
2.3.5 ASA+Dipyrid vs Clop							
PRoFESS 2009	6	672	4	688	16.5%	1.54 [0.44, 5.42]	2009
Subtotal (95% CI)		**672**		**688**	**16.5%**	**1.54 [0.44, 5.42]**	
Total events	6		4				
Heterogeneity: Not applicable							
Test for overall effect: Z = 0.67 (P = 0.50)							
Total (95% CI)		**7005**		**7033**	**100.0%**	**1.84 [1.12, 3.02]**	
Total events	43		23				
Heterogeneity: Chi² = 4.33, df = 5 (P = 0.50); I² = 0%							
Test for overall effect: Z = 2.41 (P = 0.02)							
Test for subgroup differences: Chi² = 0.37, df = 2 (P = 0.83); I² = 0%							

Figure 9.16 *Major extraparenchymal haemorrhage, early dual antiplatelet therapy vs early mono antiplatelet therapy.*

and aspirin 100–300 mg, then daily ticagrelor 90 mg and aspirin 100 mg through 21 days, and then ticagrelor 90 mg alone until 3 months. In the clopidogrel plus aspirin arm, patients received a loading dose of clopidogrel 300 mg and aspirin 100–300 mg, then daily clopidogrel 75 mg and aspirin 100 mg through 21 days, and then clopidogrel 75 mg alone until 3 months.

In the trial, directionally favourable effects for combined ticagrelor plus aspirin versus clopidogrel plus aspirin did not reach statistical significance, including reduction in recurrent stroke (6.3% vs 8.8%, HR 0.70, 95% CI: 0.40–1.22) and reduction in the composite of stroke, myocardial infarction, and vascular death (6.5% vs 9.4%, HR 0.68, 95% CI: 0.40–1.18; *p* = 0.17). Though formal interaction testing did not reach statistical significance (interaction *p* = 0.13), there was a suggestion that a differential benefit in stroke reduction may have occurred among the 45% of patients with LAA stroke

mechanisms: LAA (HR 0.45, 95% CI: 0.20–0.96; *p* = 0.04) versus non-LAA (HR 1.10, 95% CI: 0.46–2.63; *p* = 0.84). There were no ticagrelor plus aspirin versus clopidogrel plus aspirin group differences in ICH (0.9% vs 0.6%, HR 1.27, 95% CI: 0.34–4.72), major extracranial haemorrhage (1.5% vs 1.2%, HR 1.27, 95% CI: 0.34–4.72), or all-cause mortality (0.9% vs 0.6%, HR 1.52, 95% CI: 0.25–9.08). However, more minimal bleeding events (19.0% vs 10.6%) and dyspnoea leading to drug discontinuation (4.2% vs 0.0%) did occur in the ticagrelor plus aspirin group.

Comparisons of Triple vs Mono and Dual Antiplatelet Therapy Regimens

One trial has compared a triple antiplatelet regimen against conventional mono and dual antiplatelet therapy options: the TARDIS trial comparing aspirin plus clopidogrel plus dipyridamole against options of clopidogrel alone or combined aspirin plus dipyridamole (Bath et al., 2018). The trial enrolled 3096 patients with either non-cardioembolic ischaemic stroke with limb weakness, dysphasia, or both hemianopia and neuro-imaging confirmed infarction, or with TIA with at least 10 minutes of limb weakness or aphasia. Among the 72% of patients enrolled with ischaemic stroke, the mean entry NIHSS score was 4.0, and across all patients the median time from onset to randomization was 29 hours. The triple antiplatelet regimen was aspirin (300 mg load, then 50–150 mg daily) plus clopidogrel (300 mg load, then 75 mg daily) plus dipyridamole (200 mg extended release twice daily) for 90 days. The same doses were employed in the conventional clopidogrel alone or aspirin plus dipyridamole regimens, which themselves were selected based on local national guidelines and hospital/physician practice.

In the trial, triple antiplatelet therapy compared with conventional antiplatelet therapy did not alter recurrent ischaemic stroke (3.0% vs 3.3%, adjusted HR 0.89, 95% CI: 0.59–1.33). The triple antiplatelet regimen was associated with non-significant increases in ICH (0.9% vs 0.3%, HR 2.77, 95% CI: 0.99–7.75) and major extracranial haemorrhage (1.7% vs 0.8%, HR 1.89, 95% CI: 0.96–3.71). No difference was noted in mortality (1.7% vs 1.8%, HR 0.89, 95% CI: 0.51–1.55).

Comment

Only three single-agent antiplatelet regimens have been tested head-to-head in acute cerebral ischaemia, and all showed comparable net benefits. Compared with aspirin alone, cilostazol alone performed similarly in a trial of moderate sample size and power. Compared with aspirin alone in patients with minor, non-cardioembolic ischaemic stroke and TIA, ticagrelor alone showed signals of a small advantage in reducing progression and recurrence of ischaemic stroke. However, the benefit was modest in absolute terms (8 of every 1000 patients treated), only marginally statistically significant, and offset by small increases in minor bleeding and dyspnoea.

Dual antiplatelet regimens generally show advantages over mono antiplatelet regimens in preventing early stroke recurrence in patients with initial minor, non-cardioembolic ischaemic stroke or TIA. The most well-studied comparison is clopidogrel plus aspirin versus aspirin alone, but dipyridamole plus aspirin, versus aspirin alone or clopidogrel alone, performed

similarly. During the first 3 months after onset, dual antiplatelet therapy started within 72 hours of onset is associated with a moderate reduction in recurrence of all stroke (ischaemic and haemorrhagic), and this benefit is only partially offset by a small risk of major extraparenchymal bleeding. Overall, among 1000 patients treated, 27 fewer will have recurrent stroke (ischaemic or haemorrhagic), though 3 more will have major extraparenchymal bleeding. For the combination of clopidogrel and aspirin, the preponderance, and perhaps all, of the benefit is accrued within the first 10–21 days after onset. In addition, benefit is likely magnified in patients with LAA disease that has generated multiple diffusion MRI infarcts, and may be reduced in patients harbouring *CYP2C19* gene loss-of-function alleles.

The relative advantages and disadvantages of the many combinatorially possible dual and triple antiplatelet regimens have not been yet well interrogated in clinical studies. In one dual versus dual regimen trial, no significant differences were noted, but signals suggested potential greater reduction in recurrent stroke but increase in minor bleeding and dyspnoea with ticagrelor plus aspirin compared with clopidogrel plus aspirin. In one triple regimen trial, the combination of aspirin, clopidogrel, and dipyridamole did not further reduce recurrent ischaemic stroke and was associated with trends toward increased intracranial and extracranial haemorrhage.

Implications for Practice

In patients with early non-cardioembolic minor ischaemic stroke and TIA, dual antiplatelet therapy is beneficial when started within the first 72 hours of onset and continued through 3 weeks.

Clopidogrel plus aspirin, started within 24 hours of onset, is the most well-proven regimen, with clopidogrel given as a 300–600 mg loading dose and 75 mg daily thereafter, and aspirin given at a dose of 50–325 mg daily. In patients known to be poor clopidogrel metabolizers, dipyridamole plus aspirin is a leading alternative option.

In patients who are being treated with intravenous fibrinolytic therapy, antiplatelet therapy should be avoided for the first 24 hours after lytic start, given its known potentiation of bleeding risk (see Chapter 6).

The long-term antithrombotic regimen appropriate for a patient from 3 weeks post-onset forward will depend upon findings from the diagnostic workup regarding ischaemic stroke mechanism (LAA, cardioembolic, small vessel disease, etc.), indications or contraindications arising in other vascular beds, and patient comorbidities. In patients in whom the increased risk of bleeding from dual antiplatelet therapy is outweighed by increased protection against recurrent ischaemic events only during the first 2–3 weeks after an index cerebral ischaemic event, transition to long-term antiplatelet monotherapy is indicated.

Implications for Research

Among patients with minor, non-cardioembolic ischaemic stroke and TIA, some dual combinations of antiplatelet agents that have been understudied merit further investigation. Ticagrelor alone has shown signals of potential benefit compared with aspirin alone in a large trial and added to aspirin versus aspirin alone in a trial of moderate size (Johnston et al., 2016; Wang et al., 2018). The combination of ticagrelor plus aspirin is being further investigated in the THALES trial with an anticipated sample size of 13,000 patients (NCT03354429). The phosphodiesterase inhibitors dipyridamole and cilostazol have also shown preliminary evidence of benefit when added to aspirin in early-presenting patients in completed trials of moderate size, and warrant further study.

It is also desirable to identify optimized early antiplatelet therapy regimens for patients with moderate and severe ischaemic stroke, who have been excluded from the largest trials comparing antiplatelet strategies. While it is reasonable to avoid dual antiplatelet therapy in the first 3–7 days after onset of infarcts of moderate to large volume, given the increased risk of haemorrhagic transformation, trials are warranted of dual versus mono antiplatelet therapy during the 3–21-day time window when the balance of recurrent ischaemia and haemorrhagic risks may again favour more intensive antiplatelet treatment.

In addition, trials focused more closely on specific stroke and pharmacological mechanisms are desirable. The findings from subgroup analyses of several trials that the benefit of dual over mono antiplatelet therapy may be magnified in patients with LAA disease supports further trials to determine whether dual versus mono antiplatelet therapy is beneficial at all for minor ischaemic stroke or TIA due to intrinsic small vessel disease. Further, it might be envisioned that the combination of clopidogrel plus aspirin is particularly advantageous for large artery ischaemia related to highly thrombogenic atherosclerotic lesions, while the combination of phosphodiesterase inhibitors plus aspirin is distinctively beneficial for large artery ischaemia related to LAA lesions that also produce haemodynamic impairment, given their additional vasodilating and collateral-enhancing pharmacological effects. Mechanism assessment by MRI would permit trials to explore tailored dual antiplatelet therapies. Also, the potential benefit of using *CYP2C19* loss-of-function allele genotyping to guide use of clopidogrel versus other agent classes in an initial antiplatelet regimen requires prospective trial testing.

Antiplatelet vs Anticoagulation Therapy

Evidence

In patients with acute cerebral ischaemia early after onset (within 72 h), antiplatelet and arterial-dose anticoagulation therapy have been compared in 5 randomized trials enrolling 10,938 patients (Berge et al., 2002; Wong et al., 2007; Yi et al., 2014). The antiplatelet agent tested in all trials was aspirin. The anticoagulant classes tested were unfractionated heparin, tested in 1 trial comparison enrolling 7284 patients, and low-molecular-weight heparin, tested in 4 trials enrolling 3654 patients.

Permitted time windows for enrolment were within 30 hours in 1 trial and within 48h in 4 trials, and duration of study therapy was for 10 days in 2 trials and 14 days in 3 trials. All trials enrolled only acute ischaemic stroke patients, excluding TIA patients. One trial enrolled a broad range of ischaemic stroke patients (IST, 1997), while 1 enrolled only patients with atrial fibrillation (Berge et al., 2000), 1 enrolled only patients with LAA disease (Wong et al., 2007), 1 enrolled only patients with non-cardioembolic stroke (Yi et al., 2014), and 1 enrolled only patients with moderate-to-severe deficits (Bath et al., 2001).

Death or Dependency

Overall, there was no evidence of a difference in effect between anticoagulants and antiplatelet agents upon death or dependency at final follow-up. Rates of death or dependency with unfractionated heparin versus aspirin were 63.3% versus 62.3% and with low-molecular-weight heparin versus aspirin 46.5% versus 40.1%, with overall RR 1.02, 95% CI: 0.99–1.06; Figure 9.17.

Death

Compared with aspirin, anticoagulation was associated with a non-significantly higher frequency of death by end of follow-up (RR 1.06, 95% CI: 0.98–1.16; Figure 9.18).

Progression or Recurrence of Ischaemic Stroke

There was not an overall effect of anticoagulation versus aspirin on progression or recurrence of ischaemic stroke. There was substantial between-trial heterogeneity for this endpoint (heterogeneity $p < 0.00001$, $I^2 = 86\%$). The heterogeneity was

	Anticoagulant		Antiplatelet			Risk Ratio
Study or Subgroup	Events	Total	Events	Total	Weight	M-H, Fixed, 95% CI
1.1.1 Unfractionated heparin						
IST 1997	1526	2411	2998	4816	73.5%	1.02 [0.98, 1.06]
Subtotal (95% CI)		**2411**		**4816**	**73.5%**	**1.02 [0.98, 1.06]**
Total events	1526		2998			
Heterogeneity: Not applicable						
Test for overall effect: Z = 0.87 (P = 0.39)						
1.1.2 Low molecular-weight heparin						
FISS-tris 2007	28	173	35	180	1.3%	0.83 [0.53, 1.31]
HEAST 2000	148	224	146	225	5.4%	1.02 [0.89, 1.16]
TAIST (hi+med dose) 2001	533	954	279	485	13.6%	1.08 [0.99, 1.18]
Yi 2014	177	683	172	685	6.3%	1.03 [0.86,1.24]
Subtotal (95% CI)		**2034**		**1575**	**26.5%**	**1.04 [0.97, 1.12]**
Total events	946		632			
Heterogeneity: $Chi^2 = 1.66$, df = 3 (P = 0.65); $I^2 = 0\%$						
Test for overall effect: Z = 1.19 (P = 0.23)						
Total (95% CI)		**4445**		**6391**	**100.0%**	**1.02 [0.99, 1.06]**
Total events	2472		3630			
Heterogeneity: $Chi^2 = 2.30$, df = 4 (P = 0.68); $I^2 = 0\%$						
Test for overall effect: Z = 1.39 (P = 0.16)						
Test for subgroup differences: $Chi^2 = 0.43$, df = 1 (P = 0.51), $I^2 = 0\%$						

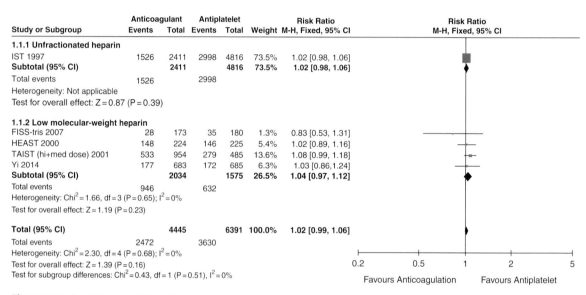

Figure 9.17 *Dependency or death (mRS 3–6 or nearest equivalent) at long-term follow-up, early antiplatelet therapy vs early anticoagulant (arterial-dose) therapy.*

	Anticoagulant		Antiplatelet			Risk Ratio	
Study or Subgroup	Events	Total	Events	Total	Weight	M-H, Fixed, 95% CI	Year
1.2.1 Unfractionated heparin							
IST 1997	549	2411	1018	4816	82.4%	1.08 [0.98, 1.18]	1997
Subtotal (95% CI)		**2411**		**4816**	**82.4%**	**1.08 [0.98, 1.18]**	
Total events	549		1018				
Heterogeneity: Not applicable							
Test for overall effect: Z = 1.59 (P = 0.11)							
1.2.2 Low molecular-weight heparin							
HEAST 2000	40	224	37	225	4.5%	1.09 [0.72, 1.63]	2000
TAIST (hi+med dose) 2001	143	993	73	491	11.9%	1.97 [0.75, 1.26]	2001
FISS-tris 2007	9	179	8	171	1.0%	1.07 [0.42, 2.72]	2007
Yi 2014	2	683	2	685	0.2%	1.00 [0.14, 7.10]	2014
Subtotal (95% CI)		**2079**		**1572**	**17.6%**	1.00 [0.81, 1.24]	
Total events	194		120				
Heterogeneity: $Chi^2 = 0.24$, df = 3 (P = 0.97); $I^2 = 0\%$							
Test for overall effect: Z = 0.05 (P = 0.96)							
Total (95% CI)		**4490**		**6388**	**100.0%**	**1.06 [0.98, 1.16]**	
Total events	743		1138				
Heterogeneity: $Chi^2 = 0.58$, df = 4 (P = 0.96); $I^2 = 0\%$							
Test for overall effect: Z = 1.46 (P = 0.14)							
Test for subgroup differences: $Chi^2 = 0.35$, df = 1 (P = 0.56), $I^2 = 0\%$							

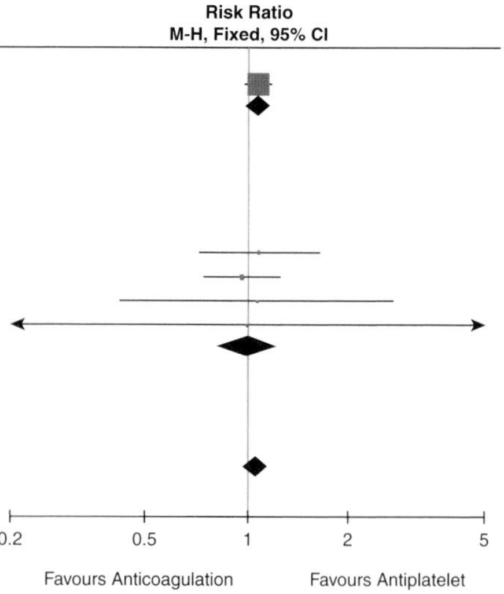

Figure 9.18 *Death at long-term follow-up, early antiplatelet therapy vs early anticoagulant (arterial-dose) therapy.*

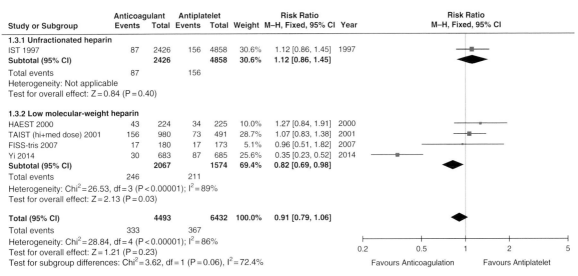

Figure 9.19 *Progression or recurrence of ischaemic stroke, early antiplatelet therapy vs early anticoagulant (arterial-dose) therapy.*

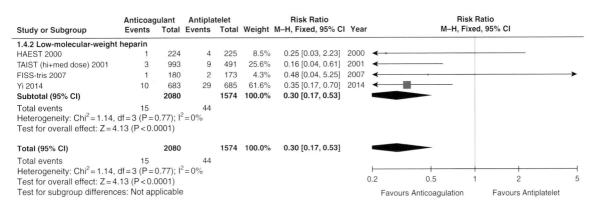

Figure 9.20 *Symptomatic deep vein thrombosis, early antiplatelet therapy vs early anticoagulant (arterial-dose) therapy.*

driven by one open-label trial of low-molecular-weight heparin in patients with non-cardioembolic ischaemic stroke (Yi et al., 2014, heterogeneity *p*). Across all trials, anticoagulation compared with aspirin did not alter the frequency of progression or recurrence of ischaemic stroke (RR 0.91, 95% CI: 0.79–1.06) (Figure 9.19). With exclusion of the outlier trial, remaining trials showed no heterogeneity (heterogeneity *p* = 0.88, I^2 = 0%), and the comparison of anticoagulation versus aspirin showed RR 1.11, 95% CI: 0.94–1.30.

Deep Venous Thrombosis and Pulmonary Embolism

The frequency of deep vein thrombosis was reported in 4 trials enrolling 3654 patients, comparing low-molecular-weight heparin with aspirin. Anticoagulants compared with aspirin were associated with reduced deep vein thrombosis, 0.7% versus 2.8% (RR 0.30, 95% CI: 0.17–0.53; *p* < 0.0001) (Figure 9.20), equivalent to 21 fewer deep venous thrombi per 1000 patients treated. Pulmonary embolism was reported in 5 trials enrolling 10,938 patients, comparing unfractionated heparin or low-molecular-weight heparin with aspirin.

Anticoagulation was associated with non-significantly lower pulmonary embolism (RR 0.67, 95% CI: 0.39–1.18; $p = 0.17$).

Symptomatic Intracranial Haemorrhage

Across the five trials, allocation to anticoagulation rather than aspirin was associated with an increase in SICH (RR 2.68, 95% CI: 1.79–4.01, $p < 0.00001$) (Figure 9.21). In weighted analysis, rates of SICH with anticoagulation versus aspirin were 1.6% versus 0.8%, so that anticoagulation was associated with 8 more symptomatic intracranial haemorrhages per 1000 patients treated.

Major Extracranial Haemorrhage

Collating the five trials, anticoagulation compared with aspirin was associated with an increase in major extraparenchymal haemorrhage (RR 2.01, 95% CI 1.43–2.82) (Figure 9.22). With weighted analysis, rates of major extracranial haemorrhages with

	Anticoagulant		Antiplatelet			Risk Ratio	
Study or Subgroup	Events	Total	Events	Total	Weight	M–H, Fixed, 95% CI	Year
1.6.1 Unfractionated heparin							
IST 1997	43	2426	26	4858	60.4%	3.31 [2.04, 5.38]	1997
Subtotal (95% CI)		**2426**		**4858**	**60.4%**	**3.31 [2.04, 5.38]**	
Total events	43		26				
Heterogeneity: Not applicable							
Test for overall effect: Z = 4.84 (P < 0.00001)							
1.6.2 Low molecular-weight heparin							
HAEST 2000	6	224	4	225	13.9%	1.51 [0.43, 5.27]	2000
TAIST (hi+med dose) 2001	10	993	1	491	4.7%	4.94 [0.63, 38.52]	2001
FISS-tris 2007	1	180	2	173	7.1%	0.48 [0.04, 5.25]	2007
Yi 2014	6	683	4	685	13.9%	1.50 [0.43, 5.31]	2014
Subtotal (95% CI)		**2080**		**1574**	**39.6%**	**1.73 [0.82, 3.65]**	
Total events	23		11				
Heterogeneity: Chi^2 = 2.20, df = 3 (P = 0.53); I^2 = 0%							
Test for overall effect: Z = 1.43 (P = 0.15)							
Total (95% CI)		**4506**		**6432**	**100.0%**	**2.68 [1.79, 4.01]**	
Total events	66		37				
Heterogeneity: Chi^2 = 4.68, df = 4 (P = 0.32); I^2 = 15%							
Test for overall effect: Z = 4.81 (P < 0.00001)							
Test for subgroup differences: Chi^2 = 2.05, df = 1 (P = 0.15); I^2 = 51.3%							

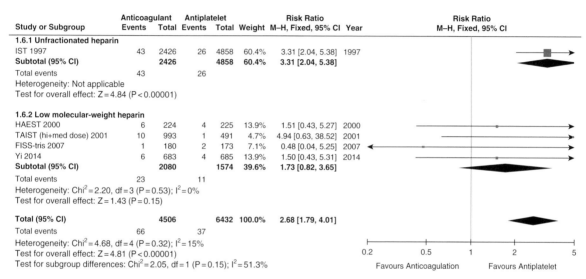

Figure 9.21 *Progression or recurrence of ischaemic stroke, early antiplatelet therapy vs early anticoagulant (arterial-dose) therapy.*

	Anticoagulant		Antiplatelet			Risk Ratio	
Study or Subgroup	Events	Total	Events	Total	Weight	M–H, Fixed, 95% CI	Year
1.7.1 Unfractionated heparin							
IST 1997	33	2426	23	4858	34.2%	2.87 [1.69, 4.88]	1997
Subtotal (95% CI)		**2426**		**4858**	**34.2%**	**2.87 [1.69, 4.88]**	
Total events	33		23				
Heterogeneity: Not applicable							
Test for overall effect: Z = 3.90 (P < 0.0001)							
1.7.2 Low molecular-weight heparin							
HAEST 2000	3	224	0	225	1.1%	7.03 [0.37, 135.34]	2000
TAIST (hi+med dose) 2001	6	993	2	491	6.0%	1.48 [0.30, 7.32]	2001
FISS-tris 2007	25	180	15	173	34.2%	1.60 [0.87, 2.93]	2007
Yi 2014	14	683	11	685	24.5%	1.28 [0.58, 2.79]	2014
Subtotal (95% CI)		**2080**		**1574**	**65.8%**	**1.56 [1.00, 2.45]**	
Total events	48		28				
Heterogeneity: Chi^2 = 1.26, df = 3 (P = 0.74); I^2 = 0%							
Test for overall effect: Z = 1.94 (P = 0.05)							
Total (95% CI)		**4506**		**6432**	**100.0%**	**2.01 [1.43, 2.82]**	
Total events	81		51				
Heterogeneity: Chi^2 = 4.41, df = 4 (P = 0.35); I^2 = 9%							
Test for overall effect: Z = 4.04 (P < 0.0001)							
Test for subgroup differences: Chi^2 = 2.95, df = 1 (P = 0.09), I^2 = 66.2%							

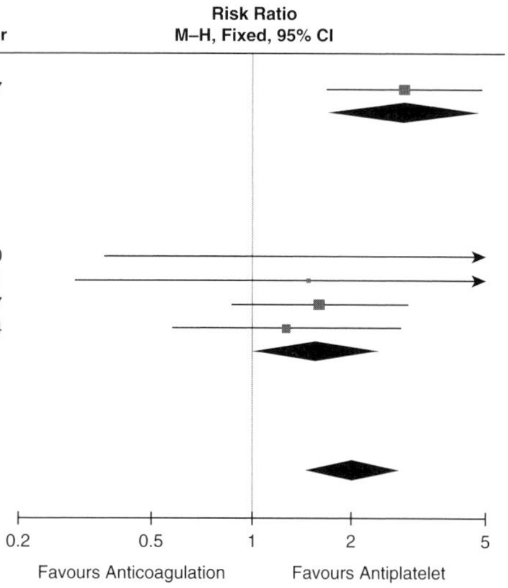

Figure 9.22 *Major extracranial haemorrhage, early antiplatelet therapy vs early anticoagulant (arterial-dose) therapy.*

anticoagulation versus aspirin were 1.7% versus 0.9%, so that anticoagulation was associated with 8 more major extracranial haemorrhages per 1000 patients treated.

Venous Prophylaxis-Dose Anticoagulation Alone vs Antiplatelet Agents Alone

Venous prophylaxis-dose anticoagulation alone versus antiplatelet agents alone among patients with ischaemic stroke largely confirmed by CT imaging has been compared in allocation arms of a single large trial, comparing unfractionated heparin 5000 units subcutaneously twice a day versus aspirin 300 mg orally daily (IST, 1997). Among the 7287 patients enrolled in this trial comparison, low-dose anticoagulation alone was not associated with differences in death or dependency (RR 1.07, 95% CI: 0.95–1.20), recurrent ischaemic stroke (RR 1.00, 95% CI: 0.73–1.38), pulmonary embolism (RR 1.10, 95% CI: 0.59–2.05), SICH (RR 1.23, 95% CI: 0.59–2.57), or major extracranial haemorrhage (RR 0.91, 95% CI: 0.39–2.14), but an unfavourable increase in death did approach statistical significance (RR 1.13, 95% CI: 0.99–1.30).

Comment

Anticoagulants alone offer no net advantage over aspirin in acute ischaemic stroke. At arterial doses, their benefits in reducing deep vein thrombosis are offset by their harms in increasing symptomatic intracranial and extracranial haemorrhages, without an advantage in averting ischaemic stroke progression or recurrence. At venous doses, they tended to be associated with increased mortality.

Antiplatelet Agents Plus Anticoagulant Agents vs Antiplatelet Agents Alone

Evidence

Adding arterial-dose anticoagulation to antiplatelet agents compared with antiplatelet agents alone, was evaluated in the International Stroke Trial, which allocated 2430 patients to aspirin (300 mg daily) plus arterial-dose unfractionated heparin (12,500 units subcutaneous twice daily) and 4858 patients to aspirin alone (300 mg daily) (IST, 1997; Berge et al., 2002).

Aspirin plus high-dose anticoagulation compared with aspirin alone was not associated with differences in death or dependency (62.0% vs 62.3%, RR 1.00, 95% CI: 0.96–1.04), but an unfavourable increase in death did approach statistical significance (23.0% vs 21.1%, RR 1.09, 95% CI: 0.99–1.19). Combined therapy did not significantly alter recurrent ischaemic stroke (2.8% vs 3.2%, RR 0.88, 95% CI: 0.67–1.17), but was associated with reduced pulmonary embolism (0.3% vs 0.7%, RR 0.44, 95% CI: 0.21–0.95). Combined arterial-dose heparin and aspirin versus aspirin alone did increase SICH (1.7% vs 0.5%, RR 3.23, 95% CI: 1.99–5.25) and major extracranial haemorrhage (2.7% vs 0.5%, RR 5.74, 95% CI: 0.3.68–9.20).

Adding venous prophylaxis-dose anticoagulation to antiplatelet agents. All patients were randomized regardless of whether they were ambulatory or non-ambulatory, or had other particular risk factors for venous thrombosis. Aspirin plus low-dose anticoagulation compared with aspirin alone was not associated with differences in death or dependency (62.5% vs 62.3%, RR 1.00, 95% CI: 0.97–1.04) or death (20.8% vs 21.1%, RR 0.98, 95% CI: 0.89–1.08). Combined therapy was associated with reduced recurrent ischaemic stroke (2.1% vs 3.2%, RR 0.64, 95% CI: 0.47–0.88) but not significantly associated with reduced pulmonary embolism (0.5% vs 0.7%, RR 0.72, 95% CI: 0.38–1.36). Combined venous prophylaxis-dose heparin and aspirin versus aspirin alone did not significantly increase SICH (0.78% vs 0.54%, RR 1.46, 95% CI: 0.81–2.63), but an unfavourable increase in major extracranial haemorrhage did approach statistical significance (0.82% vs 0.47%, RR 1.74, 95% CI: 0.96–3.16).

Comment

The combination of venous prophylaxis-dose unfractionated heparin and aspirin, versus aspirin alone, for all patients regardless of stroke mechanism or severity, was associated with a modest beneficial reduction in recurrent ischaemic stroke (11 fewer per 1000 patients treated) that was more marked than an offsetting tendency toward increase in major extracranial haemorrhage (trend towards 3 more per 1000). While no overall alteration in death and dependency or death alone was noted, this favourable profile suggests potential for benefit, meriting further investigation. Selective deployment of combined therapy in patients with particular stroke mechanisms and in patients with ambulatory impairment, increasing the risk of deep vein thrombosis, is a particularly potentially promising strategy. However, the use of intermitted compression boots for mechanical deep vein thrombosis prophylaxis may alter the potential benefits of adding low-dose anticoagulants to aspirin alone.

In contrast, compared with aspirin alone, the combination of arterial-dose unfractionated heparin and aspirin, for all patients regardless of stroke mechanism or severity, was associated with harmful increases in intracranial and extracranial haemorrhage that outweighed the benefit in reducing pulmonary embolism, with an overall trend towards increased mortality. Accordingly, combined high-dose anticoagulation and antiplatelet therapy is not a preferred general strategy in acute ischaemic stroke.

Summary

Aspirin 160–300 mg daily and started within 48 hours of onset of acute ischaemic stroke is associated with a small beneficial reduction in recurrent ischaemic stroke (6 fewer per 1000 patients treated) and pulmonary embolism (1.5 fewer per 1000) that outweighs an associated increased risk of bleeding (2 extra symptomatic intracranial haemorrhages [ICHs] and 4 extra major extracranial haemorrhages). The net impact of these and other effects are that, for every 1000 patients with acute ischaemic stroke who are treated early with aspirin, compared with no aspirin, 22 have reduced disability, including 11 more achieving full recovery.

Only two additional single antiplatelet regimens have been compared head-to-head against aspirin alone in acute cerebral ischaemia. The phosphodiesterase agent cilostazol alone performed similarly to aspirin alone. The glycoprotein (GP) IIa/IIIb receptor antagonist ticagrelor alone compared with aspirin alone, in patients with acute, minor, non-cardioembolic ischaemic stroke and transient ischaemic attack (TIA), showed tendencies towards greater reduction in progression and recurrence of ischaemic stroke but offsetting increases in minor bleeding and dyspnoea, necessitating further study.

Among patients with initial minor, non-cardioembolic ischaemic stroke or TIA, early dual antiplatelet regimens have shown advantages over early single agent regimens. The most well-studied regimen is adding the thienopyridine agent clopidogrel to aspirin, with similar findings in fewer studies for the phosphodiesterase agent dipyridamole added to aspirin. Dual antiplatelet therapy is associated with reduced recurrent strokes of all (ischaemic or haemorrhagic) types (27 fewer per 1000 treated patients), but also with a small increase in major extracranial bleeding (3 more per 1000). Confining dual therapy to the first 3 weeks after the index ischaemic event maximizes the benefit to harm ratio, by limiting treatment to the time period when ischaemic event gains outweigh haemorrhagic harms.

Anticoagulants alone offer no net advantages over antiplatelet drugs alone in acute ischaemic stroke. In addition, arterial-dose anticoagulation added to aspirin, compared with aspirin alone, caused more symptomatic intracranial and major extracranial haemorrhages than pulmonary embolic events averted, and is not a recommended general strategy. However, the combination of venous prophylaxis-dose anticoagulants and aspirin, compared with aspirin alone, was associated with reduced recurrent ischaemic stroke greater than an associated tendency to increased major extracranial haemorrhage, though without alteration in functional outcome or mortality at 3–6 months. This strategy merits further investigation.

References

Abciximab Emergent Stroke Treatment Trial (AbESTT) Investigators. (2005). Emergency administration of abciximab for treatment of patients with acute ischemic stroke. Results of a randomized phase 2 trial. *Stroke*, **36**, 880–90.

Abciximab in Ischemic Stroke (AIST) Investigators. (2000). Abciximab in acute ischemic stroke: a randomized, double-blind, placebo-controlled, dose-escalation study. *Stroke*, **31**, 601–09.

Adams HP Jr, Effron MB, Torner J, Davalos A, Frayne J, Teal P, et al. (2008). Emergency administration of abciximab for treatment of patients with acute ischemic stroke: results of an international phase III trial: Abciximab in Emergency Treatment of Stroke Trial (AbESTT-II). *Stroke*, **39**, 87–99.

Adeoye O, Sucharew H, Khoury J, Vagal A, Schmit PA, Ewing I, et al. (2015). Combined approach to lysis utilizing eptifibatide and recombinant tissue-type plasminogen activator in acute ischemic stroke – full dose regimen stroke trial. *Stroke*, **46**, 2529–33.

Bath PM, Cotton D, Martin RH, Palesch Y, Yusuf S, Sacco R, et al.; PRoFESS Study Group. (2010). Effect of combined aspirin and extended-release dipyridamole versus clopidogrel on functional outcome and recurrence in acute, mild ischemic stroke: PRoFESS subgroup analysis. *Stroke*, **41**, 732–8.

Bath PM, Woodhouse LJ, Appleton JP, Beridze M, Christensen H, Dineen RA, et al.; TARDIS Investigators. (2018). Antiplatelet therapy with aspirin, clopidogrel, and dipyridamole versus clopidogrel alone or aspirin and dipyridamole in patients with acute cerebral ischaemia (TARDIS): a randomized, open-label, phase 3 superiority trial. *Lancet*, **391**, 850–9.

Berge E, Abdelnoor M, Nakstad PH, Sandset PM. (2000). Low molecular-weight heparin versus aspirin in patients with acute ischaemic stroke and atrial fibrillation: a double-blind randomised study. HAEST Study Group. Heparin in Acute Embolic Stroke Trial. *Lancet*, **355**, 1205–10.

Berge E, Sandercock PAG. (2002). Anticoagulants versus antiplatelet agents for acute ischaemic stroke. *Cochrane Database Syst Rev*, 4. CD003242.

CAST (Chinese Acute Stroke Trial) Collaborative Group. (1997). CAST: randomised placebo-controlled trial of early aspirin use in 20,000 patients with acute ischaemic stroke. *Lancet*, **349**, 1641–9.

Chen ZM, Sandercock P, Pan HC, Counsell C, Collins R, Liu LS, et al. (2000). Indications for early aspirin use in acute ischemic stroke: a combined analysis of 40 000 randomized patients from the Chinese Acute Stroke Trial and the international stroke trial. On behalf of the CAST and IST collaborative groups. *Stroke*, **31**, 1240–9.

Ciccone A, Motto C, Abraha I, Cozzolino F, Santilli I. (2014). Glycoprotein IIb-IIIa inhibitors for acute ischaemic stroke. *Cochrane Database Syst Rev*, 3. CD005208. doi:10.1002/14651858.CD005208.pub3.

Ciuffetti G, Aisa G, Mercuri M, Lombardini R, Paltriccia R, Neri C, et al. (1990). Effects of ticlopidine on the neurologic outcome and the hemorheologic pattern in the post acute phase of ischemic stroke: a pilot study. *Angiology*, **41**, 505–11.

Cranston JS, Kaplan BD, Saver JL. (2017). Minimally clinically important difference for safe and simple novel acute ischemic stroke therapies. *Stroke*, **48**, 2946–51.

Dengler R, Diener H-C, Schwartz A, Grond M, Schumacher H, Machnig T, et al.; for the EARLY Investigators. (2010). Early treatment with aspirin plus extended-release dipyridamole for transient ischaemic attack or ischaemic stroke within 24 h of symptom onset (EARLY trial): a randomized, open-label, blinded-endpoint trial. *Lancet Neurol*, **9**, 159–66.

He F, Xia C, Zhang JH, Li XQ, Zhou ZH, Li FP, et al. (2015). Clopidogrel plus aspirin versus aspirin alone for preventing early neurological deterioration in patients with acute ischemic stroke. *J Clin Neurosci*, **22**, 83–6.

International Stroke Trial Collaborative Group. (1997). The International Stroke Trial (IST): a randomised trial of aspirin, subcutaneous heparin, both, or neither among 19435 patients with acute ischaemic stroke. *Lancet*, **349**, 1569–81.

Jing J, Meng X, Zhao X, Liu L, Wang A, Pan Y, et al. (2018). Dual antiplatelet therapy in transient ischemic attack and minor stroke with different infarction patterns: subgroup analysis of the CHANCE randomized clinical trial. *JAMA Neurol*, **75**, 711–19.

Johnston SC, Amarenco P, Albers GW, Denison H, Easton JD, Evans SR, et al; SOCRATES Steering Committee and Investigators. (2016). Ticagrelor versus aspirin in acute stroke or transient ischemic attack. *N Engl J Med*, **375**, 35–43.

Johnston SC, Easton JD, Farrant M, Barsan W, Conwit RA, Elm JJ, et al.; Clinical Research Collaboration, Neurological Emergencies Treatment Trials Network, and the POINT Investigators. (2018). Clopidogrel and aspirin in acute ischemic stroke and high-risk TIA. *N Engl J Med*, **379**, 215–25.

Johnston SC, Leira EC, Hansen MD, Adams HP Jr. (2003). Early recovery after cerebral ischemia risk of subsequent neurological deterioration. *Ann Neurol*, **54**, 439–44.

Kennedy J, Hill MD, Ryckborst KJ, Eliasziw M, Demchuk AM, Buchan AM; FASTER Investigators. (2007). Fast assessment of stroke and transient ischaemic attack to prevent early recurrence (FASTER): a randomised controlled pilot trial. *Lancet Neurol*, **6**, 961–9.

Lee YS, Bae HJ, Kang DW, Lee SH, Yu K, Park JM, et al. (2011). Cilostazol in Acute Ischemic Stroke Treatment (CAIST Trial): a randomized double-blind non-inferiority trial. *Cerebrovasc Dis*, **32**, 65–71.

Liu L, Wong KS, Leng X, Pu Y, Wang Y, Jing J, et al.; CHANCE Investigators. (2015). Dual antiplatelet therapy in stroke and ICAS: subgroup analysis of CHANCE. *Neurology*, **85**, 1154–62.

Multicentre Acute Stroke Trial-Italy (MAST-I) Group. (1995). Randomised controlled trial of streptokinase, aspirin, and combination of both in treatment of acute ischaemic stroke. *Lancet*, **346**, 1509–14.

Pan Y, Jing J, Chen W, Meng X, Li H, Zhao X, Liu L, Wang D, Johnston SC, Wang Y, Wang Y; CHANCE Investigators. (2017a). Risks and benefits of clopidogrel-aspirin in minor stroke or TIA: time course analysis of CHANCE. *Neurology*, **88**, 1906–11.

Pan Y, Meng X, Jing J, Li H, Zhao X, Liu L, et al; CHANCE Investigators. (2017b). Association of multiple infarctions and ICAS with outcomes of minor stroke and TIA. *Neurology*, **88**, 1081–8.

Pancioli AM, Adeoye O, Schmit PA, Khoury J, Levine SR, Tomsick TA, et al.; CLEAR-ER Investigators. (2013). Combined approach to lysis utilizing eptifibatide and recombinant tissue plasminogen activator in acute ischemic stroke-enhanced regimen stroke trial. *Stroke*, **44**, 2381–7.

Rödén-Jüllig Å, Britton M, Malmkvist K, Leijd B. (2003). Aspirin in the prevention of progressing stroke: a randomized controlled study. *J Intern Med*, **254**, 584–90.

Sandercock PAG, Counsell C, Tseng MC, Cecconi E. (2014). Oral antiplatelet therapy for acute ischaemic stroke. *Cochrane Database Syst Rev*, 3. CD000029. doi:10.1002/14651858.CD000029.pub3.

Siebler M, Hennerici MG, Schneider D, von Reutern GM, Seitz RJ, Röther J, et al. (2011). Safety of tirofiban in acute ischemic stroke: the SaTIS trial. *Stroke*, **42**, 2388–92.

Thompson DD, Murray GD, Candelise L, Chen Z, Sandercock PA, Whiteley WN. (2015). Targeting aspirin in acute disabling ischemic stroke: an individual patient data meta-analysis of three large randomized trials. *Int J Stroke*, **10**, 1024–30.

Torgano G, Zecca B, Monzani V, Maestroni A, Rossi P, Cazzaniga M, et al. (2010). Effect of intravenous tirofiban and aspirin in reducing short-term and long-term neurologic deficit in patients with ischemic stroke: a double-blind randomized trial. *Cerebrovasc Dis*, **29**, 275–81.

Wang Y, Meng X, Chen W, Lin Y, Pan Y, Jing J, et al.; PRiNCE Investigators. (2018). Ticagrelor with aspirin on platelet reactivity in acute non-disabling cerebrovascular events (PRINCE) trial – Final analysis. International Stroke Conference. https://professional.heart.org/idc/groups/aha mah-public/@wcm/@sop/@scon/documents/download able/ucm_498791.pdf. Accessed August 2018.

Wang Y, Wang Y, Zhao X, Liu L, Wang D, Wang C, et al.; CHANCE Investigators. (2013). Clopidogrel with aspirin in acute minor stroke or transient ischemic attack. *N Engl J Med*, **369**, 11–19.

Wang Y, Zhao X, Lin J, Li H, Johnston SC, Lin Y, et al.; CHANCE Investigators. (2016). Association between CYP2C19 loss-of-function allele status and efficacy of clopidogrel for risk reduction among patients with minor stroke or transient ischemic attack. *JAMA*, **316**, 70–8.

Wong KS, Chen C, Ng PW, Tsoi TH, Li HL, Fong WC, et al.; FISS-tris Study Investigators. (2007). Low-molecular-weight heparin compared with aspirin for the treatment of acute ischaemic stroke in Asian patients with large artery occlusive disease: a randomised study. *Lancet Neurol*, **6**, 407–13.

Wong KS, Wang Y, Leng X, Mao C, Tang J, Bath PM, et al. (2013). Early dual versus mono antiplatelet therapy for acute non-cardioembolic ischemic stroke or transient ischemic attack: an updated systematic review and meta-analysis. *Circulation*, **128**, 1656–66.

Yang Y, Zhou M, Zhong X, Wang Y, Zhao X, Liu L, et al. (2018). Dual versus mono antiplatelet therapy for acute non-cardioembolic ischaemic stroke or transient ischaemic attack: a systematic review and meta-analysis. *Stroke Vasc Neurol*, **3**, 107–16.

Yi X, Lin J, Wang C, Zhang B, Chi W. (2014). Low-molecular-weight heparin is more effective than aspirin in preventing early neurologic deterioration and improving six-month outcome. *J Stroke Cerebrovasc Dis*, **23**, 1537–44.

Chapter 10

Acute Anticoagulant Therapy for the Treatment of Acute Ischaemic Stroke and Transient Ischaemic Attack

Xinyi Leng
Lawrence K.S. Wong

The purpose of anticoagulation in patients with ischaemic stroke and transient ischaemic attack (TIA) is to prevent recurrent ischaemic stroke and other serious vascular events (by preventing arterial thromboembolism and cardiogenic embolism) and to prevent venous thromboembolism. The current chapter will review evidence of the effects of anticoagulants in the acute phase and in long-term secondary prevention in relatively unselected ischaemic stroke patients, as well as the effects of anticoagulants in the acute phase of ischaemic stroke with atrial fibrillation (AF). For the effects of anticoagulants in long-term secondary prevention of selected stroke patients with cardioembolic risks, please refer to Chapter 18.

Recurrent Stroke

The risk of early recurrence in patients with ischaemic stroke or TIA has been lowered substantially in recent years, due to the development and dissemination into clinical practice of multiple advances in evidence-based treatment strategies. In a large, international observational study of patients with minor ischaemic stroke and TIA, recurrent stroke rates were 2% within 1 week, 3% within 1 month, 4% within 3 months, and 5% within 1 year (Amarenco et al., 2016). However, the risk of early recurrent stroke is much higher in certain subgroups of patients. Among a broad group of acute cerebral ischaemia patients, the hazard for early recurrent stroke was doubled for patients with large artery atherosclerosis as ischaemic mechanism and doubled in patients with multiple acute cerebral infarctions on brain imaging (Amarenco et al., 2016). Similarly, multicentre series have found risks of recurrence by 3 months of up to 15–20% in patients with cervical carotid stenosis (Rothwell, 2008; Johansson and Wester, 2014), and over 10%

in patients with intracranial arterial stenosis (Chimowitz et al., 2011; Liu et al., 2015). In contrast, the risk of recurrence in ischaemic stroke or TIA patients with presumed cardioembolism was reported to be up to 3–7% at 90 days (Ay et al., 2010; Paciaroni et al., 2015).

Theoretically, both anticoagulants and antiplatelet drugs should be at least somewhat effective in reducing recurrent ischaemic strokes that are due to thrombus propagation or recurrent thromboembolism, though not events due to haemodynamic and collateral failure, provided they can be administered safely. Anticoagulants inhibit the formation of predominantly 'red', erythrocyte and fibrin-rich clots in areas of very reduced and stagnant blood flow, such as in cardiac chambers with impaired contractility (e.g. AF, akinetic left ventricle) and in veins (e.g. paralysed leg). Antiplatelet drugs inhibit the formation of predominantly 'white', platelet-rich clots in areas of high shear stress such as in stenotic arteries (e.g. cervical and intracranial large artery atherothrombosis). Because the vascular lesions that cause ischaemic stroke are very heterogeneous, it is unlikely that any one drug or strategy will be dramatically effective in all aetiological subtypes of ischaemic stroke.

Venous Thromboembolism

A few decades ago, without venous thromboembolism prophylaxis, among patients with hemiplegia after stroke, up to 75% would develop deep vein thrombosis (DVT) and up to 20% pulmonary embolism (PE, including fatal PE in 1–2%) (Sherman et al., 2007). In recent trials with mechanical and pharmacological thromboprophylaxis, DVT develops in up to 10% of acute ischaemic stroke patients, but is mostly asymptomatic, and PE occurs in less than 1% of acute ischaemic stroke patients (Sherman et al., 2007; Dennis et al., 2016).

Acute Ischaemic Stroke

Anticoagulation vs Control for Acute Ischaemic Stroke

Evidence

A systematic review identified 24 randomized controlled trials (RCTs) comparing anticoagulant therapy with control in the early treatment (started within 2 weeks of stroke onset) of a total of 23,748 patients with acute ischaemic stroke (Sandercock et al., 2015). One trial enrolled patients within 12 hours of stroke onset, 2 within 24 hours, 10 within 48 hours, and the rest within 14 days. The quality of the trials varied considerably.

The anticoagulants used were standard unfractionated subcutaneous heparin (six trials); standard unfractionated intravenous heparin (two trials); low-molecular-weight heparins (LMWHs) (eight trials: two dalteparin, two nadroparin, one tinzaparin, one fraxiparin, one parnaparin, and one CY 222); subcutaneous heparinoid (two trials: one danaparoid and one mesoglycan); intravenous heparinoid (one danaparoid trial); oral vitamin K antagonists (two trials); and thrombin inhibitors (three trials: two MD805 trials, one argatroban).

Fifteen trials routinely performed a computerized tomography (CT) head scan in all patients to rule out haemorrhage before randomization (Cerebral Embolism Study Group, 1983; Duke et al., 1986; Tazaki et al., 1986; Turpie et al., 1987; Cazzato et al., 1989; Prins et al., 1989; Elias et al., 1990; Sandset et al., 1990; Tazaki, 1992; FISS, 1995; Kwiecinski et al., 1995; Pambianco et al., 1995; Hommel and FISS-bis Investigators Group, 1998; TOAST Investigators, 1998; LaMonte et al., 2004). Three trials performed CT in most patients (Duke et al., 1983; Vissinger, 1995; International Stroke Trial Collaborative Group, 1997). In the International Stroke Trial (IST), 67% of patients were scanned before randomization and 29% after randomization, so that, overall, 96% of patients were scanned. The IST has provided more than 80% of the overall data in this systematic review. It is therefore likely that a small proportion of patients with intracerebral haemorrhage are included in the main analyses of this review, which may have biased the results to mildly underestimate the net beneficial effects in patients with acute cerebral ischaemia.

Death or Dependency at Final Follow-up

Eight RCTs involving a total of 22,125 patients found no evidence that anticoagulants reduced the odds of being dead or dependent at the end of follow-up (more than 1 month after randomization) compared with control (odds ratio [OR]: 0.99, 95% confidence interval [CI]: 0.93–1.04; $I^2 = 47.7\%$) (Figure 10.1).

There was substantial heterogeneity in the analysis of the outcome of death and dependency ($I^2 = 47.7\%$) between studies with different anticoagulant treatment regimens, which was chiefly attributed to the non-significant trends to benefit in studies with LMWH (OR: 0.82, 95% CI: 0.64–1.04) and heparinoid (OR: 0.81, 95% CI: 0.29–2.27), and the non-significant trend to harm in the study with direct thrombin inhibitor (OR: 1.28, 95% CI: 0.62–2.62).

Pre-specified sensitivity analyses showed that the effect of anticoagulants versus control for death and dependency was consistent among studies with low fixed-dose (OR: 1.00, 95% CI: 0.92–1.08), medium fixed-dose (OR: 0.98, 95% CI: 0.91–1.06), or adjusted-dose anticoagulants (OR: 0.95, 95% CI: 0.75–1.20); and also consistent if data from IST were included (OR: 0.99, 95% CI: 0.94–1.05) or excluded (OR: 0.92, 95% CI: 0.78–1.09).

Death at Final Follow-up

Based on 11 trials involving a total of 22,776 patients, there was no evidence that anticoagulant therapy reduced the odds of death from all causes (OR: 1.05, 95% CI: 0.98–1.12; $I^2 = 28.5\%$) at the end of follow-up (more than 1 month after randomization) (Figure 10.2). There was no significant heterogeneity between the included studies with different anticoagulant regimens (Figure 10.2).

Recurrent Stroke

Ischaemic Stroke during the Treatment Period – Eleven trials in 21,605 patients indicated that anticoagulant therapy for acute ischaemic stroke was associated with a statistically significant reduction in recurrent ischaemic stroke (OR: 0.76, 95% CI: 0.65–0.88; $I^2 = 0$), from 3.6% (388/10739) with control to 2.7% (300/10866) with anticoagulants, which translated into a number needed to treat to benefit (NNTB) of 108 (95% CI: 74–266) (Figure 10.3). The majority of the data (95%) were obtained from one trial (IST, 1997).

Symptomatic Haemorrhagic Stroke during the Treatment Period – Sixteen trials in 22,943 patients

Review: Anticoagulants for acute ischaemic stroke
Comparison: 1 Anticoagulant versus control in acute presumed ischaemic stroke
Outcome: 1 Dead or dependent at end of follow up (if > 1 month)

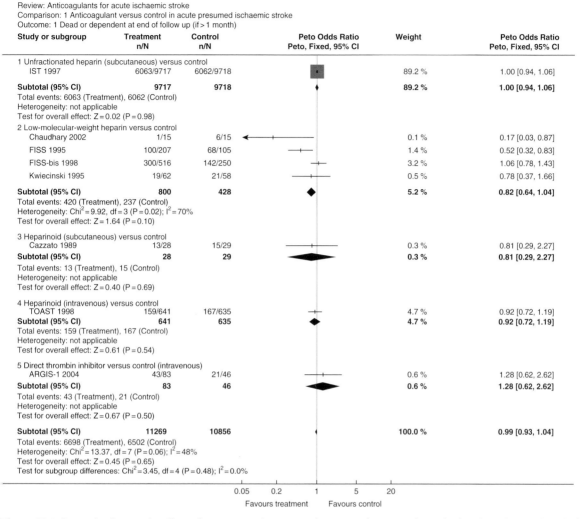

Study or subgroup	Treatment n/N	Control n/N	Peto Odds Ratio Peto, Fixed, 95% CI	Weight	Peto Odds Ratio Peto, Fixed, 95% CI
1 Unfractionated heparin (subcutaneous) versus control					
IST 1997	6063/9717	6062/9718		89.2 %	1.00 [0.94, 1.06]
Subtotal (95% CI)	**9717**	**9718**		**89.2 %**	**1.00 [0.94, 1.06]**
Total events: 6063 (Treatment), 6062 (Control)					
Heterogeneity: not applicable					
Test for overall effect: Z = 0.02 (P = 0.98)					
2 Low-molecular-weight heparin versus control					
Chaudhary 2002	1/15	6/15		0.1 %	0.17 [0.03, 0.87]
FISS 1995	100/207	68/105		1.4 %	0.52 [0.32, 0.83]
FISS-bis 1998	300/516	142/250		3.2 %	1.06 [0.78, 1.43]
Kwiecinski 1995	19/62	21/58		0.5 %	0.78 [0.37, 1.66]
Subtotal (95% CI)	**800**	**428**		**5.2 %**	**0.82 [0.64, 1.04]**
Total events: 420 (Treatment), 237 (Control)					
Heterogeneity: Chi² = 9.92, df = 3 (P = 0.02); I² = 70%					
Test for overall effect: Z = 1.64 (P = 0.10)					
3 Heparinoid (subcutaneous) versus control					
Cazzato 1989	13/28	15/29		0.3 %	0.81 [0.29, 2.27]
Subtotal (95% CI)	**28**	**29**		**0.3 %**	**0.81 [0.29, 2.27]**
Total events: 13 (Treatment), 15 (Control)					
Heterogeneity: not applicable					
Test for overall effect: Z = 0.40 (P = 0.69)					
4 Heparinoid (intravenous) versus control					
TOAST 1998	159/641	167/635		4.7 %	0.92 [0.72, 1.19]
Subtotal (95% CI)	**641**	**635**		**4.7 %**	**0.92 [0.72, 1.19]**
Total events: 159 (Treatment), 167 (Control)					
Heterogeneity: not applicable					
Test for overall effect: Z = 0.61 (P = 0.54)					
5 Direct thrombin inhibitor versus control (intravenous)					
ARGIS-1 2004	43/83	21/46		0.6 %	1.28 [0.62, 2.62]
Subtotal (95% CI)	**83**	**46**		**0.6 %**	**1.28 [0.62, 2.62]**
Total events: 43 (Treatment), 21 (Control)					
Heterogeneity: not applicable					
Test for overall effect: Z = 0.67 (P = 0.50)					
Subtotal (95% CI)	**11269**	**10856**		**100.0 %**	**0.99 [0.93, 1.04]**
Total events: 6698 (Treatment), 6502 (Control)					
Heterogeneity: Chi² = 13.37, df = 7 (P = 0.06); I² = 48%					
Test for overall effect: Z = 0.45 (P = 0.65)					
Test for subgroup differences: Chi² = 3.45, df = 4 (P = 0.48); I² = 0.0%					

0.05   0.2   1   5   20
Favours treatment   Favours control

Figure 10.1 Forest plot showing the effects of *any anticoagulant vs control* in acute ischaemic stroke on *death or dependency at the end of follow-up* (if longer than 1 month).

Reproduced from Sandercock PA, Counsell C, and Kane EJ. (2015). Anticoagulants for acute ischaemic stroke. *Cochrane Database Syst Rev*, 3. CD000024.

indicated that immediate anticoagulant therapy was associated with a statistically significant increase in symptomatic intracranial haemorrhage (ICH) by more than 2-fold (OR: 2.55, 95% CI: 1.95–3.33; $I^2 = 0$), from 0.5% (54/11,242) with control to 1.4% (168/11,701) with various types of anticoagulants, which represented a number needed to treat to harm (NNTH) of 131 (95% CI: 88–213) (Figure 10.4). The majority of the data (76%) were obtained from one trial (IST, 1997).

Indirect comparisons of different types of anticoagulants indicated that there was no significant heterogeneity in the number of excess haemorrhages with different agent classes (see Figure 10.4).

There was a dose-related increase in major ICH in patients treated with anticoagulants in the IST, with an increase in the absolute risk of bleeding from 0.3% to 0.7% to 1.8% for control, low-dose (5000 U bid [twice a day]), and medium-dose (12,500 U bid) subcutaneous unfractionated heparin (UFH), respectively (IST, 1997).

There was possibly bias within the data, since the threshold for rescanning patients with clinical deterioration might be lower, if they were known to be using anticoagulants in trials that were not blinded – for instance, the IST trial. Even in blinded trials, the clinicians could be unblinded if they observed

Review: Anticoagulants for acute ischaemic stroke
Comparison: 1 Anticoagulant versus control in acute presumed ischaemic stroke
Outcome: 3 Dead from all causes at final follow up (if > 1 month)

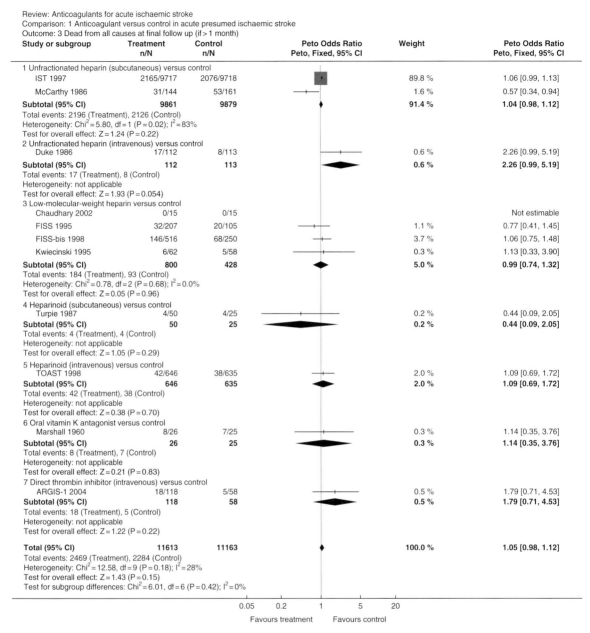

Figure 10.2 Forest plot showing the effects of *any anticoagulant vs control* in acute ischaemic stroke on *death at the end of follow-up*.
Reproduced from Sandercock PA, Counsell C, and Kane EJ. (2015). Anticoagulants for acute ischaemic stroke. *Cochrane Database Syst Rev*, 3. CD000024.

bruising at heparin injection sites. Systematic studies with CT scans before initiation of treatment as well as at the end of the treatment period to detect intracranial haemorrhage in all survivors, and autopsy in all patients who died during the study, may allow unbiased assessment of the effects of anticoagulants on the occurrence of ICH. Five trials in the Cochrane review made a systematic attempt to detect both symptomatic and asymptomatic ICH in this way (Cerebral Embolism Study Group, 1983; Prins et al., 1989; Sandset et al., 1990; FISS, 1995; LaMonte et al., 2004). The numbers of patients and events in these trials was small (symptomatic plus asymptomatic haemorrhages occurring in 20/266

Review: Anticoagulants for acute ischaemic stroke
Comparison: 1 Anticoagulant versus control in acute presumed ischaemic stroke
Outcome: 6 Recurrent ischaemic or unknown stroke during treatment period

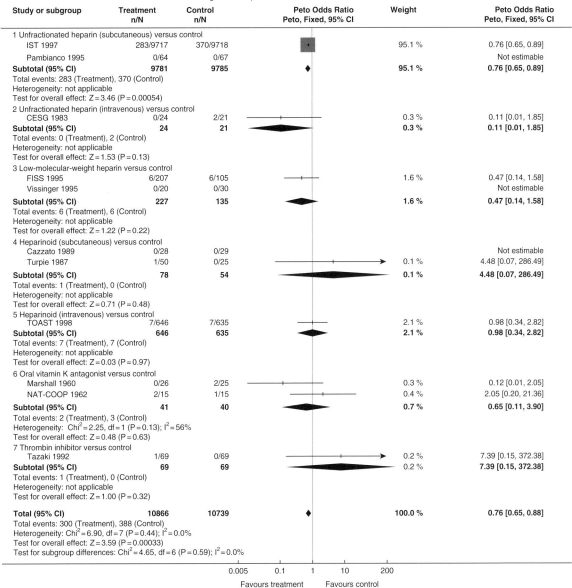

Study or subgroup	Treatment n/N	Control n/N	Peto Odds Ratio Peto, Fixed, 95% CI	Weight	Peto Odds Ratio Peto, Fixed, 95% CI
1 Unfractionated heparin (subcutaneous) versus control					
IST 1997	283/9717	370/9718		95.1 %	0.76 [0.65, 0.89]
Pambianco 1995	0/64	0/67			Not estimable
Subtotal (95% CI)	**9781**	**9785**		**95.1 %**	**0.76 [0.65, 0.89]**
Total events: 283 (Treatment), 370 (Control)					
Heterogeneity: not applicable					
Test for overall effect: Z = 3.46 (P = 0.00054)					
2 Unfractionated heparin (intravenous) versus control					
CESG 1983	0/24	2/21		0.3 %	0.11 [0.01, 1.85]
Subtotal (95% CI)	**24**	**21**		**0.3 %**	**0.11 [0.01, 1.85]**
Total events: 0 (Treatment), 2 (Control)					
Heterogeneity: not applicable					
Test for overall effect: Z = 1.53 (P = 0.13)					
3 Low-molecular-weight heparin versus control					
FISS 1995	6/207	6/105		1.6 %	0.47 [0.14, 1.58]
Vissinger 1995	0/20	0/30			Not estimable
Subtotal (95% CI)	**227**	**135**		**1.6 %**	**0.47 [0.14, 1.58]**
Total events: 6 (Treatment), 6 (Control)					
Heterogeneity: not applicable					
Test for overall effect: Z = 1.22 (P = 0.22)					
4 Heparinoid (subcutaneous) versus control					
Cazzato 1989	0/28	0/29			Not estimable
Turpie 1987	1/50	0/25		0.1 %	4.48 [0.07, 286.49]
Subtotal (95% CI)	**78**	**54**		**0.1 %**	**4.48 [0.07, 286.49]**
Total events: 1 (Treatment), 0 (Control)					
Heterogeneity: not applicable					
Test for overall effect: Z = 0.71 (P = 0.48)					
5 Heparinoid (intravenous) versus control					
TOAST 1998	7/646	7/635		2.1 %	0.98 [0.34, 2.82]
Subtotal (95% CI)	**646**	**635**		**2.1 %**	**0.98 [0.34, 2.82]**
Total events: 7 (Treatment), 7 (Control)					
Heterogeneity: not applicable					
Test for overall effect: Z = 0.03 (P = 0.97)					
6 Oral vitamin K antagonist versus control					
Marshall 1960	0/26	2/25		0.3 %	0.12 [0.01, 2.05]
NAT-COOP 1962	2/15	1/15		0.4 %	2.05 [0.20, 21.36]
Subtotal (95% CI)	**41**	**40**		**0.7 %**	**0.65 [0.11, 3.90]**
Total events: 2 (Treatment), 3 (Control)					
Heterogeneity: Chi² = 2.25, df = 1 (P = 0.13); I² = 56%					
Test for overall effect: Z = 0.48 (P = 0.63)					
7 Thrombin inhibitor versus control					
Tazaki 1992	1/69	0/69		0.2 %	7.39 [0.15, 372.38]
Subtotal (95% CI)	**69**	**69**		**0.2 %**	**7.39 [0.15, 372.38]**
Total events: 1 (Treatment), 0 (Control)					
Heterogeneity: not applicable					
Test for overall effect: Z = 1.00 (P = 0.32)					
Total (95% CI)	**10866**	**10739**		**100.0 %**	**0.76 [0.65, 0.88]**
Total events: 300 (Treatment), 388 (Control)					
Heterogeneity: Chi² = 6.90, df = 7 (P = 0.44); I² = 0.0%					
Test for overall effect: Z = 3.59 (P = 0.00033)					
Test for subgroup differences: Chi² = 4.65, df = 6 (P = 0.59); I² = 0.0%					

0.005   0.1   1   10   200
Favours treatment   Favours control

Figure 10.3 Forest plot showing the effects of *any anticoagulant vs control* in acute ischaemic stroke on *recurrent ischaemic/unknown stroke during the treatment period*.

Reproduced from Sandercock PA, Counsell C, and Kane EJ. (2015). Anticoagulants for acute ischaemic stroke. *Cochrane Database Syst Rev*, 3. CD000024.

[7.5%] patients allocated anticoagulant vs 27/264 [10.2%] patients allocated control). The estimate of risk of 'symptomatic plus asymptomatic' haemorrhage in these few small trials of anticoagulation with control is imprecise and inconclusive (OR: 0.76, 95% CI: 0.38–1.52).

Recurrent Stroke of Any Type during the Treatment Period or Follow-up – Eleven RCTs involving 21,605 patients indicated that anticoagulation was not associated with a net reduction in the odds of the composite of any recurrent ischaemic stroke or any symptomatic intracranial haemorrhage during the treatment period

Review: Anticoagulants for acute ischaemic stroke
Comparison: 1 Anticoagulant versus control in acute presumed ischaemic stroke
Outcome: 7 Symptomatic intracranial haemorrhage during treatment period

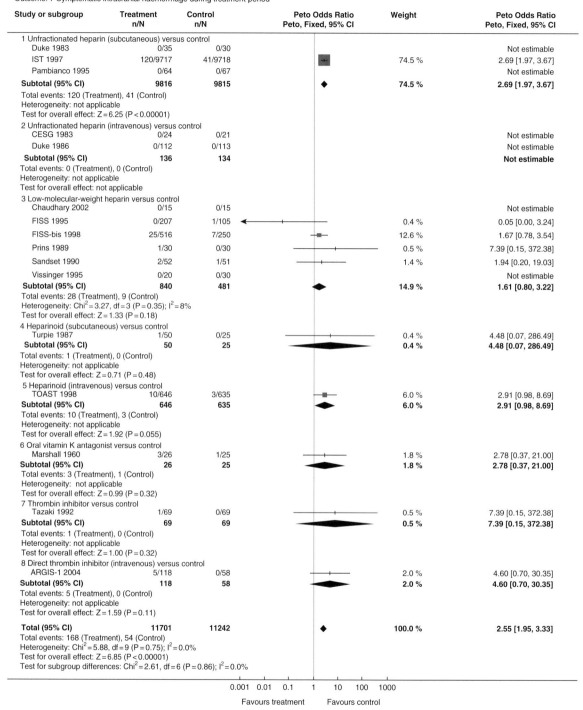

Figure 10.4 Forest plot showing the effects of *any anticoagulant vs control* in acute ischaemic stroke on *symptomatic ICH during the treatment period*.

Reproduced from Sandercock PA, Counsell C, and Kane EJ. (2015). Anticoagulants for acute ischaemic stroke. *Cochrane Database Syst Rev*, 3. CD000024.

Review: Anticoagulants for acute ischaemic stroke
Comparison: 1 Anticoagulant versus control in acute presumed ischaemic stroke
Outcome: 8 Any recurrent stroke or symptomatic intracranial haemorrhage during treatment period or follow up (> 1 month)

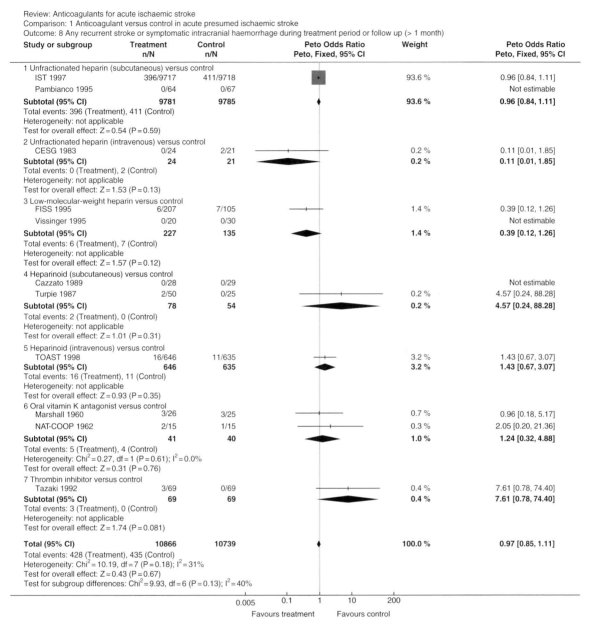

Study or subgroup	Treatment n/N	Control n/N	Peto Odds Ratio Peto, Fixed, 95% CI	Weight	Peto Odds Ratio Peto, Fixed, 95% CI
1 Unfractionated heparin (subcutaneous) versus control					
IST 1997	396/9717	411/9718		93.6 %	0.96 [0.84, 1.11]
Pambianco 1995	0/64	0/67			Not estimable
Subtotal (95% CI)	**9781**	**9785**		**93.6 %**	**0.96 [0.84, 1.11]**
Total events: 396 (Treatment), 411 (Control)					
Heterogeneity: not applicable					
Test for overall effect: Z = 0.54 (P = 0.59)					
2 Unfractionated heparin (intravenous) versus control					
CESG 1983	0/24	2/21		0.2 %	0.11 [0.01, 1.85]
Subtotal (95% CI)	**24**	**21**		**0.2 %**	**0.11 [0.01, 1.85]**
Total events: 0 (Treatment), 2 (Control)					
Heterogeneity: not applicable					
Test for overall effect: Z = 1.53 (P = 0.13)					
3 Low-molecular-weight heparin versus control					
FISS 1995	6/207	7/105		1.4 %	0.39 [0.12, 1.26]
Vissinger 1995	0/20	0/30			Not estimable
Subtotal (95% CI)	**227**	**135**		**1.4 %**	**0.39 [0.12, 1.26]**
Total events: 6 (Treatment), 7 (Control)					
Heterogeneity: not applicable					
Test for overall effect: Z = 1.57 (P = 0.12)					
4 Heparinoid (subcutaneous) versus control					
Cazzato 1989	0/28	0/29			Not estimable
Turpie 1987	2/50	0/25		0.2 %	4.57 [0.24, 88.28]
Subtotal (95% CI)	**78**	**54**		**0.2 %**	**4.57 [0.24, 88.28]**
Total events: 2 (Treatment), 0 (Control)					
Heterogeneity: not applicable					
Test for overall effect: Z = 1.01 (P = 0.31)					
5 Heparinoid (intravenous) versus control					
TOAST 1998	16/646	11/635		3.2 %	1.43 [0.67, 3.07]
Subtotal (95% CI)	**646**	**635**		**3.2 %**	**1.43 [0.67, 3.07]**
Total events: 16 (Treatment), 11 (Control)					
Heterogeneity: not applicable					
Test for overall effect: Z = 0.93 (P = 0.35)					
6 Oral vitamin K antagonist versus control					
Marshall 1960	3/26	3/25		0.7 %	0.96 [0.18, 5.17]
NAT-COOP 1962	2/15	1/15		0.3 %	2.05 [0.20, 21.36]
Subtotal (95% CI)	**41**	**40**		**1.0 %**	**1.24 [0.32, 4.88]**
Total events: 5 (Treatment), 4 (Control)					
Heterogeneity: Chi² = 0.27, df = 1 (P = 0.61); I² = 0.0%					
Test for overall effect: Z = 0.31 (P = 0.76)					
7 Thrombin inhibitor versus control					
Tazaki 1992	3/69	0/69		0.4 %	7.61 [0.78, 74.40]
Subtotal (95% CI)	**69**	**69**		**0.4 %**	**7.61 [0.78, 74.40]**
Total events: 3 (Treatment), 0 (Control)					
Heterogeneity: not applicable					
Test for overall effect: Z = 1.74 (P = 0.081)					
Total (95% CI)	**10866**	**10739**		**100.0 %**	**0.97 [0.85, 1.11]**
Total events: 428 (Treatment), 435 (Control)					
Heterogeneity: Chi² = 10.19, df = 7 (P = 0.18); I² = 31%					
Test for overall effect: Z = 0.43 (P = 0.67)					
Test for subgroup differences: Chi² = 9.93, df = 6 (P = 0.13); I² = 40%					

```
              0.005   0.1    1    10   200
              Favours treatment    Favours control
```

Figure 10.5 Forest plot showing the effects of *any anticoagulant vs control* in acute ischaemic stroke on *recurrent stroke of any type during the treatment period or at the end of follow-up.*

(OR: 0.97, 95% CI: 0.85–1.11; I^2 = 31.3%) (Figure 10.5). The majority of the data (93.6%) were obtained from one trial (IST, 1997). Only three relatively small trials provided data regarding the risk of recurrent stroke of any type at final follow-up, in which there were too few events for reliable analyses.

Major Extracranial Haemorrhage (ECH) during the Treatment Period

Eighteen trials included data from 22,255 randomized patients (93.7% of patients included in the overall review) in whom data on major extracranial haemorrhage (ECH) (defined as bleeding serious enough to cause death or require hospitalization or transfusion) were recorded. Anticoagulation was associated with a significant 3-fold increase in major ECH (OR: 2.99, 95% CI: 2.24–3.99; I^2 = 4%), from 0.4% (42/11,000) with control to 1.3% (143/11,255) with anticoagulation (Figure 10.6), which indicated an NNTH of 128 (95% CI: 85–204).

Deep Vein Thrombosis (DVT) during the Treatment Period

In the meta-analysis combining trials of high-dose and low-dose anticoagulation, 10 RCTs contained data from 916 randomized patients (only 3.9% of patients included in the overall review) in whom the effect of anticoagulants on the occurrence of 'symptomatic or asymptomatic DVT' at the end of the treatment period was sought by (1) I-125 fibrinogen scanning (Sandercock et al., 2015; Pince, 1981; Duke et al., 1983; McCarthy and Turner, 1986; Turpie et al., 1987; Prins et al., 1989; Elias et al., 1990; McCarthy et al., 1977); (2) B mode and Doppler ultrasound (Pambianco et al., 1995); or (3) x-ray contrast venography (Sandset et al., 1990; Vissinger, 1995).

Despite the small numbers of patients studied, anticoagulation was associated with a highly significant reduction in the odds of DVT (OR: 0.21, 95% CI: 0.15–0.29; I^2 = 71.5%), from 44.3% (204/460) with control to 15.1% (69/456) with anticoagulation (Figure 10.7). This result was equivalent to an NNTB of 9 (95% CI: 9–10). However, the majority of DVTs detected were subclinical and asymptomatic.

There was significant heterogeneity in the results of the trials (I^2 = 71.5%). This appeared to be related to three trials that did not show any clear effect of anticoagulation on the odds of DVT (Sandset et al., 1990; Pambianco et al., 1995; Vissinger, 1995), and two trials that did (McCarthy and Turner, 1986; Elias et al., 1990). The three negative trials were the only trials that did not use I-125 fibrinogen scanning. One used ultrasound assessment (Pambianco et al., 1995); the other two used venography (Sandset et al., 1990; Vissinger, 1995). These trials also possessed different features, for instance, in the onset-to-randomization intervals and in the study quality of the concealment.

Symptomatic Pulmonary Embolism (PE) during the Treatment Period

In the meta-analysis combining trials of high-dose and low-dose anticoagulation, 14 RCTs included data from 22,544 patients (95.7% of patients included in the overall review) in which fatal and non-fatal symptomatic PEs were reported, but no trial systematically sought asymptomatic PE by performing ventilation–perfusion scans or computed tomography angiograms (CTAs) in all patients at the end of the treatment period (Sandercock et al., 2015). Anticoagulation was associated with a significant reduction in the odds of symptomatic PE (OR: 0.60, 95% CI: 0.44–0.81; I^2 = 13.7%), from 1.0% (104/11,074) with control to 0.6% (69/11,470) with anticoagulants (Figure 10.8), which translated into an NNTB of 127 (95% CI: 91–268).

Low-dose Prophylactic Anticoagulation – In a later systematic review confined to prophylactic, low-dose anticoagulant regimens, data were available in 14 randomized trials, including 5 trials of UFH, 8 trials of LMWH, and 1 trial of a heparinoid (Dennis et al., 2016). About 90% of the data were contributed by the IST 1 trial of UFH, in which patients were enrolled regardless of mobility status. The occurrence of any (predominantly asymptomatic) DVT was reported in 9 small trials enrolling 605 patients, and was reduced with prophylactic anticoagulation, OR 0.21 ((95% CI: 0.15–0.29). Rates of PE showed heterogeneity of effect by anticoagulation agent class, with less effect in the trial testing UFH regardless of patient mobility. In 7 trials of LMWH enrolling 1090 patients, PE was reduced, 1.3% versus 3.9%, OR 0.34 (95% CI: 0.16–0.71). Rates of symptomatic intracranial haemorrhage and extracranial bleeding were increased with anticoagulation, but nominally less so with LMWH. In 7 trials of LMWH enrolling 970 patients, rates of symptomatic intracranial haemorrhage were 7.7% versus 1.9%, OR 1.36 (95% CI: 0.58–3.18); in 5 LMWH trials enrolling 429 patients, no effect on extracranial bleeding was observed, 0.5% versus 0.5%, OR 1.04 (95% CI: 0.06–16.75). However, although death was not altered across all trials, in 6 LMWH trials enrolling 479 patients, mortality was non-significantly increased, 11.2% versus 6.5%, OR 1.72 (95% CI: 0.92–3.37).

Comment

Interpretation of the Evidence

The data from RCTs indicate that routine immediate anticoagulation (with UFH, LMWH, heparinoid, or a thrombin inhibitor) does not provide any net short- or long-term reduction in death or disability (Table 10.1), in relatively broadly selected patients with acute ischaemic stroke.

Although immediate anticoagulation leads to fewer recurrent ischaemic strokes (OR: 0.76, 95% CI:

Review: Anticoagulants for acute ischaemic stroke
Comparison: 1 Anticoagulant versus control in acute presumed ischaemic stroke
Outcome: 9 Major extracranial haemorrhage during treatment period

Study or subgroup	Treatment n/N	Control n/N	Peto Odds Ratio Peto, Fixed, 95% CI	Weight	Peto Odds Ratio Peto, Fixed, 95% CI
1 Unfractionated heparin (subcutaneous) versus control					
Duke 1983	0/35	0/30			Not estimable
IST 1997	129/9717	37/9718		89.8 %	3.06 [2.25, 4.15]
Pambianco 1995	0/64	0/67			Not estimable
Pince 1981	0/40	0/40			Not estimable
Subtotal (95% CI)	9856	9855		89.8 %	3.06 [2.25, 4.15]
Total events: 129 (Treatment), 37 (Control)					
Heterogeneity: not applicable					
Test for overall effect: Z = 7.17 (P < 0.00001)					
2 Unfractionated heparin (intravenous) versus control					
CESG 1983	0/24	0/21			Not estimable
Subtotal (95% CI)	24	21			Not estimable
Total events: 0 (Treatment), 0 (Control)					
Heterogeneity: not applicable					
Test for overall effect: not applicable					
3 Low-molecular-weight heparin versus control					
Chaudhary 2002	0/15	0/15			Not estimable
Elias 1990	0/15	0/15			Not estimable
FISS 1995	1/207	1/105		1.0 %	0.48 [0.03, 9.05]
Prins 1989	0/30	0/30			Not estimable
Sandset 1990	0/52	0/51			Not estimable
Subtotal (95% CI)	319	216		1.0 %	0.48 [0.03, 9.05]
Total events: 1 (Treatment), 1 (Control)					
Heterogeneity: not applicable					
Test for overall effect: Z = 0.49 (P = 0.62)					
4 Heparinoid (subcutaneous) versus control					
Cazzato 1989	1/28	0/29		0.5 %	7.66 [0.15, 386.16]
Turpie 1987	0/50	0/25			Not estimable
Subtotal (95% CI)	78	54		0.5 %	7.66 [0.15, 386.16]
Total events: 1 (Treatment), 0 (Control)					
Heterogeneity: not applicable					
Test for overall effect: Z = 1.02 (P = 0.31)					
5 Heparinoid (intravenous) versus control					
TOAST 1998	12/646	3/635		8.1 %	3.31 [1.20, 9.15]
Subtotal (95% CI)	646	635		8.1 %	3.31 [1.20, 9.15]
Total events: 12 (Treatment), 13 (Control)					
Heterogeneity: not applicable					
Test for overall effect: Z = 2.30 (P = 0.021)					
6 Oral vitamin K antagonist versus control					
Marshall 1960	0/26	0/25			Not estimable
NAT-COOP 1962	0/15	1/15		0.5 %	0.14 [0.00, 6.82]
Subtotal (95% CI)	41	40		0.5 %	0.14 [0.00, 6.82]
Total events: 0 (Treatment), 1 (Control)					
Heterogeneity: not applicable					
Test for overall effect: Z = 1.00 (P = 0.32)					
7 Thrombin inhibitor versus control					
Tazaki 1986	0/104	0/52			Not estimable
Tazaki 1992	0/69	0/69			Not estimable
Subtotal (95% CI)	173	121			Not estimable
Total events: 0 (Treatment), 0 (Control)					
Heterogeneity: not applicable					
Test for overall effect: not applicable					
8 Direct thrombin inhibitor (intravenous) versus control					
ARGIS-1 2004	0/118	0/58			Not estimable
Subtotal (95% CI)	118	58			Not estimable
Total events: 0 (Treatment), 0 (Control)					
Heterogeneity: not applicable					
Test for overall effect: not applicable					
Total (95% CI)	11255	11000		100.0 %	2.99 [2.24, 3.99]
Total events: 143 (Treatment), 42 (Control)					
Heterogeneity: Chi^2 = 4.17, df = 4 (P = 0.38); I^2 = 4%					
Test for overall effect: Z = 7.41 (P < 0.00001)					
Test for subgroup differences: Chi^2 = 4.17, df = 4 (P = 0.38); I^2 = 4%					

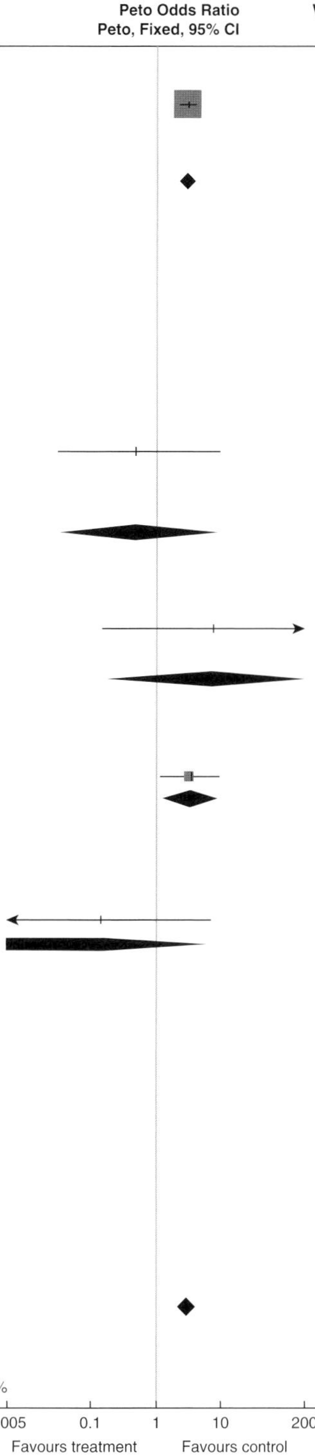

0.005 0.1 1 10 200
Favours treatment   Favours control

Figure 10.6 Forest plot showing the effects of *any anticoagulant vs control* in acute ischaemic stroke on *major extracranial haemorrhage during the treatment period.*

Reproduced from Sandercock PA, Counsell C, and Kane EJ. (2015). Anticoagulants for acute ischaemic stroke. *Cochrane Database Syst Rev*, 3. CD000024.

Review: Anticoagulants for acute ischaemic stroke
Comparison: 1 Anticoagulant versus control in acute presumed ischaemic stroke
Outcome: 4 Deep vein thrombosis during treatment period

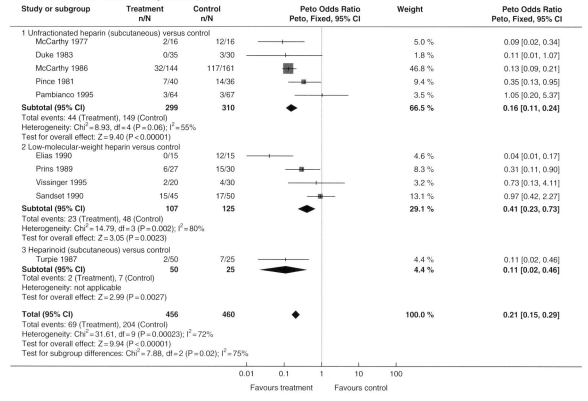

Figure 10.7 Forest plot showing the effects of *any anticoagulant vs control* in acute ischaemic stroke on *DVT during the treatment period*.
Reproduced from Sandercock PA, Counsell C, and Kane EJ. (2015). Anticoagulants for acute ischaemic stroke. *Cochrane Database Syst Rev*, 3. CD000024.

0.65–0.88), with an NNTB of 108 (95% CI: 74–266), it is also associated with a similar-sized increase in the risk of symptomatic ICH (OR: 2.52, 95% CI: 1.95–3.33), with a NNTH of 131 (95% CI: 88–213). The net result is no short- or long-term benefit in terms of preventing recurrent stroke.

Immediate anticoagulation was associated with a highly significant 79% reduction in the odds of DVT during the treatment period (NNTB = 9), similar to that seen with the use of prophylactic heparin in patients undergoing different types of surgery. However, most of these DVT were asymptomatic, and so their detection or prevention is of uncertain clinical relevance. Symptomatic DVT can lead to morbidity (e.g. post-phlebitic leg and varicose ulcers), but neither data specifically on symptomatic DVT nor on these complications of DVT were available from the trials.

The risk of symptomatic PE was reduced significantly with the use of anticoagulants (OR: 0.60, 95%

CI: 0.44–0.81), though the overall risk of symptomatic PE was low, and the absolute benefit small (NNTB = 127). However, there may well have been under-ascertainment of minimally symptomatic PE in all of the trials, since pulmonary emboli were not sought systematically.

Despite the benefit of anticoagulants in preventing asymptomatic DVT and symptomatic PE, such benefit was offset by a similar-sized increase in ECH.

Implications for Practice

The data do not support the routine use of immediate high-dose intravenous or subcutaneous anticoagulants in any form, including LMWHs, heparinoids, and thrombin inhibitors, for relatively unselected patients with acute ischaemic stroke. This is because the benefits of anticoagulant therapies in lowering the risk of arterial and venous thromboembolism are offset by

Review: Anticoagulants for acute ischaemic stroke
Comparison: 1 Anticoagulant versus control in acute presumed ischaemic stroke
Outcome: 5 Symptomatic pulmonary embolism during treatment period

Study or subgroup	Treatment n/N	Control n/N	Peto Odds Ratio Peto, Fixed, 95% CI	Weight	Peto Odds Ratio Peto, Fixed, 95% CI
1 Unfractionated heparin (subcutaneous) versus control					
IST 1997	53/9716	81/9718		79.0 %	0.66 [0.47, 0.92]
Pambianco 1995	2/64	1/67		1.8 %	2.06 [0.21, 20.19]
Pince 1981	1/40	0/40		0.6 %	7.39 [0.15, 372.38]
Subtotal (95% CI)	9820	9825		81.4 %	0.69 [0.49, 0.96]
Total events: 56 (Treatment), 82 (Control)					
Heterogeneity: Chi^2=2.37, df=2 (P=0.31); I^2=16%					
Test for overall effect: Z=2.21 (P=0.027)					
2 Unfractionated heparin (intravenous) versus control					
CESG 1983	0/24	0/21			Not estimable
Subtotal (95% CI)	24	21			Not estimable
Total events: 0 (Treatment), 0 (Control)					
Heterogeneity: not applicable					
Test for overall effect: not applicable					
3 Low-molecular-weight heparin versus control					
Elias 1990	0/15	1/15		0.6 %	0.14 [0.00, 6.82]
FISS 1995	0/207	0/105			Not estimable
FISS-bis 1998	9/516	14/250		11.7 %	0.27 [0.11, 0.65]
Kwiecinski 1995	0/62	2/58		1.2 %	0.12 [0.01, 2.01]
Prins 1989	1/30	2/30		1.7 %	0.50 [0.05, 5.02]
Sandset 1990	2/52	2/51		2.3 %	0.98 [0.13, 7.17]
Vissinger 1995	0/20	0/30			Not estimable
Subtotal (95% CI)	902	539		17.5 %	0.31 [0.15, 0.64]
Total events: 12 (Treatment), 21 (Control)					
Heterogeneity: Chi^2=2.15, df=4 (P=0.71); I^2=0.0%					
Test for overall effect: Z=3.15 (P=0.0016)					
4 Heparinoid (subcutaneous) versus control					
Cazzato 1989	1/28	0/29		0.6 %	7.66 [0.15, 386.16]
Turpie 1987	0/50	0/25			Not estimable
Subtotal (95% CI)	78	54		0.6 %	7.66 [0.15, 386.16]
Total events: 1 (Treatment), 0 (Control)					
Heterogeneity: not applicable					
Test for overall effect: Z=1.02 (P=0.31)					
5 Heparinoid (intravenous) versus control					
TOAST 1998	0/646	1/635		0.6 %	0.13 [0.00, 6.70]
Subtotal (95% CI)	646	635		0.6 %	0.13 [0.00, 6.70]
Total events: 0 (Treatment), 1 (Control)					
Heterogeneity: not applicable					
Test for overall effect: Z=1.01 (P=0.31)					
Total (95% CI)	11470	11074		100.0 %	0.60 [0.44, 0.81]
Total events: 69 (Treatment), 104 (Control)					
Heterogeneity: Chi^2=10.43, df=9 (P=0.32); I^2=14%					
Test for overall effect: Z=3.31 (P=0.00092)					
Test for subgroup differences: Chi^2=5.91, df=3 (P=0.12); I^2=49%					

0.002   0.1   1   10   500
Favours treatment   Favours control

Figure 10.8 Forest plot showing the effects of *any anticoagulant vs control* in acute ischaemic stroke on *symptomatic PE during the treatment period.*

Reproduced from Sandercock PA, Counsell C, and Kane EJ. (2015). Anticoagulants for acute ischaemic stroke. *Cochrane Database Syst Rev*, 3. CD000024.

a similar-sized risk of symptomatic ICH and ECH. For patients at high risk of DVT (e.g. immobile, history of prior venous thromboembolism) and low risk of intracranial haemorrhage (e.g. small infarct less than 3 cm in diameter, no evidence of microhaemorrhages on gradient refocused echo MRI of the brain), low-dose subcutaneous anticoagulation may be worthwhile. Subcutaneous low- molecular-weight heparins likely are mildly more effective than UFH in this setting.

Implications for Research

It is still unclear if certain categories of ischaemic stroke patients may have net benefit from immediate, high-dose anticoagulation therapies over control. However, further large-scale trials comparing immediate

Table 10.1 Summary of the effects of anticoagulation vs control in acute ischaemic stroke

Outcome	OR	95% CI	Absolute risk difference	NNTB or NNTH	95% CI
Death or dependency	0.99	0.93–1.04	NS		
Death	1.05	0.98–1.12	NS		
Recurrent ischaemic stroke	0.76	0.65–0.88	−0.9%	NNTB: 108	74–266
Symptomatic ICH (dose related)	2.55	1.95–3.33	+0.9%	NNTH: 133	88–213
Recurrent stroke of any type	0.97	0.85–1.11	NS		
Major ECH	2.99	2.24–3.99	+0.9%	NNTH: 128	85–204
DVT (most asymptomatic)	0.21	0.15–0.29	−28.1%	NNTB: 9	9–10
Symptomatic PE	0.60	0.44–0.81	−0.4%	NNTB: 127	91–268

CI: confidence interval. NNTB: number needed to treat to benefit. NNTH: number needed to treat to harm. NS: Not significant. ICH: intracranial haemorrhage. ECH: extracranial haemorrhage. DVT: deep vein thrombosis. PE: pulmonary embolism.

anticoagulation as a standalone medical therapy with control in acute ischaemic stroke, even if in a specific aetiological subtype of ischaemic stroke, are unlikely now that intravenous fibrinolysis and endovascular thrombectomy are established treatments of proven value. Future studies could further compare the efficacy and safety of different anticoagulants, including new oral anticoagulants, versus no anticoagulation in select subtypes of ischaemic stroke, such as in the presence of mobile thrombi visualized attached to atherosclerotic plaque or in thin basilar artery occlusion with very slow flow in residual patent basilar segments.

Effective strategies to select patients in whom low-dose prophylactic anticoagulants to prevent DVT and PE will confer net benefit in acute ischaemic stroke require further investigation. However, due to the low rate of symptomatic PE, very large-scale clinical trials are needed to identify the optimal therapy to achieve the most favourable balance of benefit and harm for this particular aim.

LMWHs or Heparinoids vs Standard UFH for Acute Ischaemic Stroke

Evidence

A systematic review identified nine RCTs that directly compared the effects of LMWHs or heparinoids with those of standard UFH in a total of 3137 patients with acute ischaemic stroke (Sandercock and Leong, 2017). Four trials compared a heparinoid (danaparoid) and five trials compared LMWH (enoxaparin, certoparin or unspecified) with standard UFH.

Death during Follow-up

Overall, in 8 trials with 3102 patients, 193 in 1616 (11.9%) allocated LMWH or heparinoids died during the scheduled follow-up period compared with 176 in 1486 (11.8%) of those allocated UFH (OR: 0.98, 95% CI: 0.79–1.23; Figure 10.9). There was no significant heterogeneity among the included studies ($I^2 = 5\%$).

Intracranial Haemorrhage (ICH) during the Treatment Period

In 9 trials of 3137 patients, direct comparisons of the effects of LMWHs or heparinoids with those of UFHs showed no overall statistically significant difference in the rate of ICH during the treatment period (OR: 0.75, 95% CI: 0.46–1.23; $I^2 = 0\%$) (Figure 10.10). However, the analysis of the effects of these anticoagulant regimens on ICH might be biased, since not all patients underwent brain CT scans before randomization and upon occurrence of ICH.

Regarding symptomatic ICH during the treatment period, there was no significant difference between LMWH/heparinoid and UFH (OR: 0.73, 95% CI: 0.35–1.54; $I^2=0\%$). However, the definitions for clinical deterioration in symptomatic ICH varied among the included studies.

Extracranial Haemorrhage during the Treatment Period

Direct comparisons of the effects of LMWH or heparinoid compared with standard UFH show no significant difference in the rate of minor ECH during the treatment period (OR: 0.91, 95% CI: 0.67–1.24; $I^2=0\%$; Figure 10.11). Although there was a significantly higher rate of major ECH in patients treated with LMWH or heparinoid compared with standard UFH

Review: Low-molecular-weight heparins or heparinoids versus standard unfractionated heparin for acute ischaemic stroke
Comparison: 1 LMWH/heparinoid versus standard unfractionated heparin in acute ischaemic stroke
Outcome: 3 Death from all causes during follow up

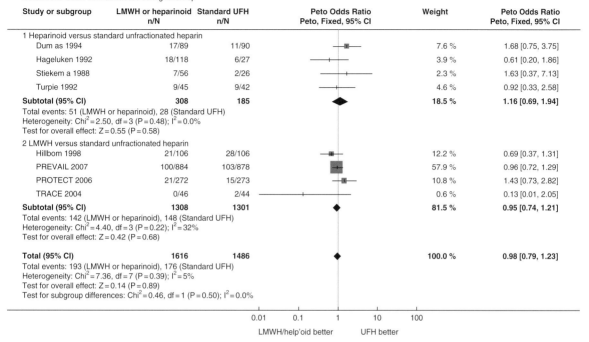

Study or subgroup	LMWH or heparinoid n/N	Standard UFH n/N	Peto Odds Ratio Peto, Fixed, 95% CI	Weight	Peto Odds Ratio Peto, Fixed, 95% CI
1 Heparinoid versus standard unfractionated heparin					
Dum as 1994	17/89	11/90		7.6 %	1.68 [0.75, 3.75]
Hageluken 1992	18/118	6/27		3.9 %	0.61 [0.20, 1.86]
Stiekem a 1988	7/56	2/26		2.3 %	1.63 [0.37, 7.13]
Turpie 1992	9/45	9/42		4.6 %	0.92 [0.33, 2.58]
Subtotal (95% CI)	**308**	**185**		**18.5 %**	**1.16 [0.69, 1.94]**
Total events: 51 (LMWH or heparinoid), 28 (Standard UFH)					
Heterogeneity: Chi² = 2.50, df = 3 (P = 0.48); I² = 0.0%					
Test for overall effect: Z = 0.55 (P = 0.58)					
2 LMWH versus standard unfractionated heparin					
Hillbom 1998	21/106	28/106		12.2 %	0.69 [0.37, 1.31]
PREVAIL 2007	100/884	103/878		57.9 %	0.96 [0.72, 1.29]
PROTECT 2006	21/272	15/273		10.8 %	1.43 [0.73, 2.82]
TRACE 2004	0/46	2/44		0.6 %	0.13 [0.01, 2.05]
Subtotal (95% CI)	**1308**	**1301**		**81.5 %**	**0.95 [0.74, 1.21]**
Total events: 142 (LMWH or heparinoid), 148 (Standard UFH)					
Heterogeneity: Chi² = 4.40, df = 3 (P = 0.22); I² = 32%					
Test for overall effect: Z = 0.42 (P = 0.68)					
Total (95% CI)	**1616**	**1486**		**100.0 %**	**0.98 [0.79, 1.23]**
Total events: 193 (LMWH or heparinoid), 176 (Standard UFH)					
Heterogeneity: Chi² = 7.36, df = 7 (P = 0.39); I² = 5%					
Test for overall effect: Z = 0.14 (P = 0.89)					
Test for subgroup differences: Chi² = 0.46, df = 1 (P = 0.50); I² = 0.0%					

0.01   0.1   1   10   100
LMWH/help'oid better   UFH better

Figure 10.9 Forest plot showing the effects of *LMWH/heparinoid vs standard UFH* in acute ischaemic stroke on *death at the end of follow-up*. Reproduced from Sandercock PAG, Leong TS. (2017). Low-molecular-weight heparins or heparinoids versus standard unfractionated heparin for acute ischaemic stroke. *Cochrane Database Syst Rev*, 4. CD000119.

during the treatment period (OR: 3.79, 95% CI: 1.30–11.06), the extremely small number of the overall major ECH events (n = 14) reported by all the included trials hindered the reliability of such analysis.

Deep Vein Thrombosis (DVT) during the Treatment Period

Seven out of nine trials reported data on the outcome event of DVT. Direct comparisons of the effects of LMWH or heparinoid with those of UFH revealed that 140/1,352 (10.4%) patients allocated LMWH or heparinoid had DVT compared with 206/1,233 (16.7%) of those allocated UFH. This reduction was significant (OR: 0.55, 95% CI: 0.44–0.70), suggesting that LMWH or heparinoid decreases the occurrence of DVT compared with standard UFH (Figure 10.12). There was no significant heterogeneity among included studies (I^2 = 0%), or between subgroups of studies comparing the effects of LMWH versus UFH (OR: 0.56, 95% CI: 0.44–0.73), or heparinoids versus UFH (OR: 0.52, 95% CI: 0.31–0.86; I^2 = 0% for between-subgroup heterogeneity; Figure 10.12).

Low-dose Prophylactic Anticoagulation – A meta-analysis confined to trials comparing low-dose prophylactic anticoagulation with LMWH or heparinoid agents versus UFH identified 7 randomized trials in acute stroke patients (Dennis et al., 2016). Rates of any (predominantly asymptomatic) DVT were reported in 7 trials enrolling 2585 patients, and were reduced with newer agents compared with UFH, OR 0.55 (0.44–0.70). Rates of PE were evaluated in 6 trials enrolling 1250 patients and were not significantly altered, 1.2% versus 2.1%, OR 0.57 (95% CI: 0.23–1.41). Rates of symptomatic intracranial haemorrhage did not differ, but major ECH was more frequent with newer agents than UFH, 0.76% versus 0.14%, OR 3.79 (95% CI: 1.30–11.06).

Comment

Interpretation of the Evidence

These data suggest that LMWH or heparinoids are more effective than UFH for preventing DVT. However, most DVT were asymptomatic, of which the clinical relevance was uncertain, and no substantial agent class advantage

Review: Low-molecular-weight heparins or heparinoids versus standard unfractionated heparin for acute ischaemic stroke
Comparison: 1 LMWH/heparinoid versus standard unfractionated heparin in acute ischaemic stroke
Outcome: 5 Any intracranial haemorrhage/haemorrhagic transformation of the cerebral infarct during treatment period

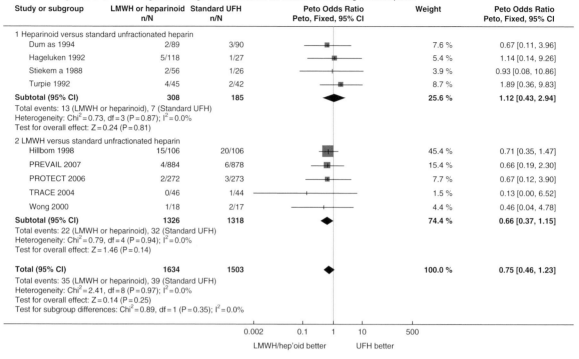

Study or subgroup	LMWH or heparinoid n/N	Standard UFH n/N	Peto Odds Ratio Peto, Fixed, 95% CI	Weight	Peto Odds Ratio Peto, Fixed, 95% CI
1 Heparinoid versus standard unfractionated heparin					
Dum as 1994	2/89	3/90		7.6 %	0.67 [0.11, 3.96]
Hageluken 1992	5/118	1/27		5.4 %	1.14 [0.14, 9.26]
Stiekem a 1988	2/56	1/26		3.9 %	0.93 [0.08, 10.86]
Turpie 1992	4/45	2/42		8.7 %	1.89 [0.36, 9.83]
Subtotal (95% CI)	**308**	**185**		**25.6 %**	**1.12 [0.43, 2.94]**
Total events: 13 (LMWH or heparinoid), 7 (Standard UFH)					
Heterogeneity: Chi² = 0.73, df = 3 (P = 0.87); I² = 0.0%					
Test for overall effect: Z = 0.24 (P = 0.81)					
2 LMWH versus standard unfractionated heparin					
Hillbom 1998	15/106	20/106		45.4 %	0.71 [0.35, 1.47]
PREVAIL 2007	4/884	6/878		15.4 %	0.66 [0.19, 2.30]
PROTECT 2006	2/272	3/273		7.7 %	0.67 [0.12, 3.90]
TRACE 2004	0/46	1/44		1.5 %	0.13 [0.00, 6.52]
Wong 2000	1/18	2/17		4.4 %	0.46 [0.04, 4.78]
Subtotal (95% CI)	**1326**	**1318**		**74.4 %**	**0.66 [0.37, 1.15]**
Total events: 22 (LMWH or heparinoid), 32 (Standard UFH)					
Heterogeneity: Chi² = 0.79, df = 4 (P = 0.94); I² = 0.0%					
Test for overall effect: Z = 1.46 (P = 0.14)					
Total (95% CI)	**1634**	**1503**		**100.0 %**	**0.75 [0.46, 1.23]**
Total events: 35 (LMWH or heparinoid), 39 (Standard UFH)					
Heterogeneity: Chi² = 2.41, df = 8 (P = 0.97); I² = 0.0%					
Test for overall effect: Z = 0.14 (P = 0.25)					
Test for subgroup differences: Chi² = 0.89, df = 1 (P = 0.35); I² = 0.0%					

0.002   0.1   1   10   500
LMWH/hep'oid better   UFH better

Figure 10.10 Forest plot showing the effects of *LMWH/heparinoid vs standard UFH* in acute ischaemic stroke on *any ICH or haemorrhagic transformation during the treatment period.*

Reproduced from Sandercock PAG, Leong TS. (2017). Low-molecular-weight heparins or heparinoids versus standard unfractionated heparin for acute ischaemic stroke. *Cochrane Database Syst Rev*, 4. CD000119.

was seen for clinically relevant major events, including PE, intracerebral and extracerebral haemorrhage and death. Therefore, the systematic reviews did not provide a definite finding of clinically relevant differential benefits and risks of LMWH or heparinoids versus standard UFH in broadly selected acute ischaemic stroke patients.

Implications for Practice

There is no evidence to support the routine use of anticoagulation in broadly selected patients with acute ischaemic stroke because there is no overall net benefit (Sandercock et al., 2015). For the net benefit/harm of LMWH or heparinoids versus standard UFH in unselective acute ischaemic stroke, current evidence does not show clear differences in major clinical outcomes, despite reduced risk of asymptomatic DVT in those treated with LMWH or heparinoids compared with UFH. But in selected acute ischaemic stroke patients at high risk of DVT and PE and at low risk of intracranial haemorrhage, the

use of anticoagulants is reasonable, with LMWH/ heparinoids probably more effective than UFH.

Implications for Research

Further comparison studies of different classes of anticoagulants, including newer oral anticoagulants, in acute ischaemic stroke should not be pursued in broad, unselected acute ischaemic stroke patients, where benefit is not apparent, but is reasonable in certain subgroups of patients. Future studies could further compare the efficacy and safety of high doses of different anticoagulant classes in select subtypes of ischaemic stroke, such as in the presence of mobile thrombi visualized attached to atherosclerotic plaque or in thin basilar artery occlusion with very slow flow in residual patent basilar segments.

Comparisons of different agent classes used at low venous prophylaxis dose would best be conducted in patients with clinical features indicating elevated risk of DVT and PE and low risk of intracerebral haemorrhage.

Review: Low-molecular-weight heparins or heparinoids versus standard unfractionated heparin for acute ischaemic stroke
Comparison: 1 LMWH/heparinoid versus standard unfractionated heparin in acute ischaemic stroke
Outcome: 8 Extracranial haemorrhage during treatment period

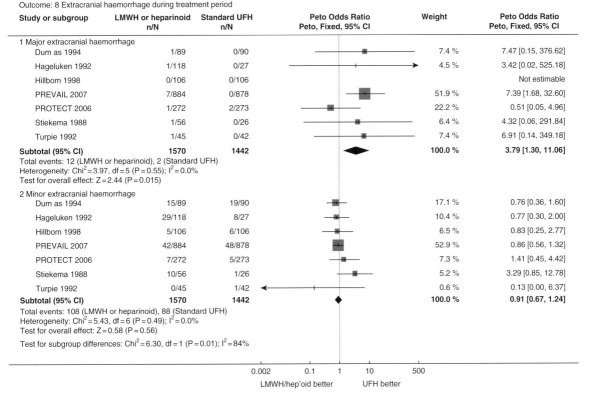

Study or subgroup	LMWH or heparinoid n/N	Standard UFH n/N	Peto Odds Ratio Peto, Fixed, 95% CI	Weight	Peto Odds Ratio Peto, Fixed, 95% CI
1 Major extracranial haemorrhage					
Dum as 1994	1/89	0/90		7.4 %	7.47 [0.15, 376.62]
Hageluken 1992	1/118	0/27		4.5 %	3.42 [0.02, 525.18]
Hillbom 1998	0/106	0/106			Not estimable
PREVAIL 2007	7/884	0/878		51.9 %	7.39 [1.68, 32.60]
PROTECT 2006	1/272	2/273		22.2 %	0.51 [0.05, 4.96]
Stiekema 1988	1/56	0/26		6.4 %	4.32 [0.06, 291.84]
Turpie 1992	1/45	0/42		7.4 %	6.91 [0.14, 349.18]
Subtotal (95% CI)	**1570**	**1442**		**100.0 %**	**3.79 [1.30, 11.06]**

Total events: 12 (LMWH or heparinoid), 2 (Standard UFH)
Heterogeneity: Chi^2 = 3.97, df = 5 (P = 0.55); I^2 = 0.0%
Test for overall effect: Z = 2.44 (P = 0.015)

2 Minor extracranial haemorrhage					
Dum as 1994	15/89	19/90		17.1 %	0.76 [0.36, 1.60]
Hageluken 1992	29/118	8/27		10.4 %	0.77 [0.30, 2.00]
Hillbom 1998	5/106	6/106		6.5 %	0.83 [0.25, 2.77]
PREVAIL 2007	42/884	48/878		52.9 %	0.86 [0.56, 1.32]
PROTECT 2006	7/272	5/273		7.3 %	1.41 [0.45, 4.42]
Stiekema 1988	10/56	1/26		5.2 %	3.29 [0.85, 12.78]
Turpie 1992	0/45	1/42		0.6 %	0.13 [0.00, 6.37]
Subtotal (95% CI)	**1570**	**1442**		**100.0 %**	**0.91 [0.67, 1.24]**

Total events: 108 (LMWH or heparinoid), 88 (Standard UFH)
Heterogeneity: Chi^2 = 5.43, df = 6 (P = 0.49); I^2 = 0.0%
Test for overall effect: Z = 0.58 (P = 0.56)

Test for subgroup differences: Chi^2 = 6.30, df = 1 (P = 0.01); I^2 = 84%

0.002   0.1   1   10   500
LMWH/hep'oid better   UFH better

Figure 10.11 Forest plot showing the effects of *LMWH/heparinoid vs standard UFH* in acute ischaemic stroke on *extracranial haemorrhage during the treatment period*.

Reproduced from Sandercock PAG, Leong TS. (2017). Low-molecular-weight heparins or heparinoids versus standard unfractionated heparin for acute ischaemic stroke. *Cochrane Database Syst Rev*, 4. CD000119.

Anticoagulation for Patients with Acute Ischaemic Stroke Who Are in Atrial Fibrillation (AF)

Patients with acute ischaemic stroke who are in AF have high risk of recurrence in the early phase after stroke onset; for instance, during the first 2 weeks after index stroke, 8% of patients had a recurrent ischaemic stroke despite treatment with dalteparin or aspirin in the Heparin in Acute Embolic Stroke Trial (HAEST) (Berge et al., 2000). However, relatively few data are available for reliable analysis of whether early initiation of anticoagulation improves outcome compared with no antithrombotic therapy or compared with antiplatelet therapy among acute ischaemic stroke patients with AF (Lansberg et al., 2012; Kernan et al., 2014).

Evidence

Initial Anticoagulation vs No Anticoagulation in AF and Stroke

Among 18,451 patients who were randomized within 48 hours of onset of acute ischaemic stroke in the IST to 14 days of treatment with subcutaneous UFH or control, 3169 patients (17%) were in AF, of whom 784 were randomly allocated to high-dose UFH 12,500 units (U) subcutaneously twice daily, 773 to low-dose UFH 5000 U subcutaneously twice daily, and 1612 to no heparin (Saxena et al., 2001). Within each of these groups, half of the patients were randomly assigned to aspirin 300 mg once daily and half to no aspirin.

The proportions of AF patients with further events within 14 days allocated to UFH 12,500 U (n = 784), UFH 5000 U (n = 773), and to no heparin (n = 1,612) groups were: ischaemic stroke, 2.3%, 3.4%, 4.9% (P = 0.001); symptomatic ICH, 2.8%, 1.3%, 0.4% (P < 0.0001);

Review: Low-molecular-weight heparins or heparinoids versus standard unfractionated heparin for acute ischaemic stroke
Comparison: 1 LMWH/heparinoid versus standard unfractionated heparin in acute ischaemic stroke
Outcome: 1 Deep venous thrombosis during treatment period

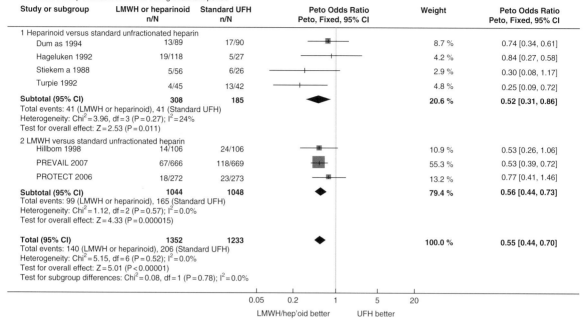

Study or subgroup	LMWH or heparinoid n/N	Standard UFH n/N	Peto Odds Ratio Peto, Fixed, 95% CI	Weight	Peto Odds Ratio Peto, Fixed, 95% CI
1 Heparinoid versus standard unfractionated heparin					
Dum as 1994	13/89	17/90		8.7 %	0.74 [0.34, 0.61]
Hageluken 1992	19/118	5/27		4.2 %	0.84 [0.27, 0.58]
Stiekem a 1988	5/56	6/26		2.9 %	0.30 [0.08, 1.17]
Turpie 1992	4/45	13/42		4.8 %	0.25 [0.09, 0.72]
Subtotal (95% CI)	308	185		20.6 %	0.52 [0.31, 0.86]
Total events: 41 (LMWH or heparinoid), 41 (Standard UFH)					
Heterogeneity: Chi² = 3.96, df = 3 (P = 0.27); I² = 24%					
Test for overall effect: Z = 2.53 (P = 0.011)					
2 LMWH versus standard unfractionated heparin					
Hillbom 1998	14/106	24/106		10.9 %	0.53 [0.26, 1.06]
PREVAIL 2007	67/666	118/669		55.3 %	0.53 [0.39, 0.72]
PROTECT 2006	18/272	23/273		13.2 %	0.77 [0.41, 1.46]
Subtotal (95% CI)	1044	1048		79.4 %	0.56 [0.44, 0.73]
Total events: 99 (LMWH or heparinoid), 165 (Standard UFH)					
Heterogeneity: Chi² = 1.12, df = 2 (P = 0.57); I² = 0.0%					
Test for overall effect: Z = 4.33 (P = 0.000015)					
Total (95% CI)	1352	1233		100.0 %	0.55 [0.44, 0.70]
Total events: 140 (LMWH or heparinoid), 206 (Standard UFH)					
Heterogeneity: Chi² = 5.15, df = 6 (P = 0.52); I² = 0.0%					
Test for overall effect: Z = 5.01 (P < 0.00001)					
Test for subgroup differences: Chi² = 0.08, df = 1 (P = 0.78); I² = 0.0%					

0.05   0.2   1   5   20
LMWH/hep'oid better   UFH better

Figure 10.12 Forest plot showing the effects of *LMWH/heparinoid vs standard UFH* in acute ischaemic stroke on *DVT during the treatment period*.

Reproduced from Sandercock PAG, Leong TS. (2017). Low-molecular-weight heparins or heparinoids versus standard unfractionated heparin for acute ischaemic stroke. *Cochrane Database Syst Rev*, 4. CD000119.

and any stroke or death, 18.8%, 19.4%, 20.7% (P = 0.3), respectively (Table 10.2). No effect of heparin on the proportion of patients dead or dependent at 6 months was apparent (Saxena et al., 2001).

Initial Anticoagulation vs Aspirin in AF and Stroke

The Heparin in Acute Embolic Stroke Trial (HAEST) was a multicentre, randomized double-blind and double-dummy trial comparing the effect of low-molecular-weight heparin versus the effect of aspirin within the acute phase of acute ischaemic stroke with AF (Berge et al., 2000). LMWH (dalteparin 100 U/kg subcutaneously twice a day) was compared with aspirin (160 mg every day), started within 30 hours of stroke onset, for the prevention of recurrent stroke during the first 14 days among 449 patients with acute ischaemic stroke and AF. The frequency of recurrent ischaemic stroke during the first 14 days was 19/244 (8.5%) in dalteparin-allocated patients versus 17/225 (7.5%) in aspirin-allocated patients (OR: 1.13, 95% CI: 0.57–2.24; P = 0.73). There was also no benefit of dalteparin compared with aspirin on secondary events during the first 14 days:

symptomatic cerebral haemorrhage 6/224 versus 4/225; symptomatic and asymptomatic cerebral haemorrhage 26/224 versus 32/225; progression of symptoms within the first 48 hours 24/224 versus 17/225; and death 21/224 versus 16/225. There were no significant differences in functional outcome or death at 14 days or 3 months.

Initial Anticoagulation vs Aspirin or No Antithrombotics in Cardioembolic Stroke

A systematic review of trials of initial anticoagulation in patients with cardioembolic ischaemic stroke identified 7 randomized trials enrolling 4624 patients, among whom 82% had AF and 18% another cardioembolic source (Paciaroni et al., 2007). Randomization was performed within 48 hours of onset, and agents tested were UFH in 3 trials, LMWH in 3 trials, and heparinoid in 1 trial. Control patients received either aspirin or no antithrombotics. Anticoagulants were associated with a non-significant reduction in recurrent stroke within the first 1–2 weeks, 3.0% versus 4.9%, OR 0.68 (95% CI: 0.44–1.06, P = 0.09), but

Table 10.2 Effect of unfractionated heparin in different doses on events within 14 days and outcome at 6 months in patients with atrial fibrillation*

	Heparin 12,500 U (n = 784)	Heparin 5000 U (n = 773)	No heparin (n = 1612)	P for trend
Events within 14 days	(%)	(%)	(%)	
Recurrent ischaemic stroke	2.3	3.4	4.9	0.001
Symptomatic ICH	2.8	1.3	0.4	<0.0001
Recurrent stroke of any type	5.0	4.7	5.3	0.6
Recurrent stroke or death	18.8	19.4	20.7	0.3
Outcome at 6 months	(%)	(%)	(%)	
Dead from any cause	38.9	37.8	39.1	0.8
Dead or dependent	78.1	78.8	78.5	0.8

Source: Reproduced from Saxena R, Lewis S, Berge E, et al. (2001). Risk of early death and recurrent stroke and effect of heparin in 3169 patients with acute ischaemic stroke and atrial fibrillation in the International Stroke Trial. *Stroke*, 32, 2333–7; with permission from Wolters Kluwer Health, Inc.

* Within each of these groups, half of the patients were randomly assigned to aspirin 300 mg once daily.

ICH: intracranial haemorrhage. U: unit.

were also associated with a significant increase in symptomatic intracranial bleeding, 2.5% versus 0.7%, OR 2.89 (95% CI: 1.19–7.01, $P = 0.02$). There was no difference in death or disability at final follow-up, 73.5% vs 73.8%.

Initial Anticoagulation with Non-vitamin-K Oral Anticoagulant (NOAC) vs Warfarin in AF and Stroke

The Triple AXEL trial was a multicentre, randomized trial comparing the effect of the NOAC rivaroxaban with warfarin begun a median 2 days after onset in patients with AF and mild acute ischaemic stroke (Hong et al., 2017). Patients were allocated to treatment strategies for the first 4 weeks of rivaroxaban, 10 mg/day for 5 days followed by 15 or 20 mg/day, or warfarin with a target international normalized ratio of 2.0–3.0. Among 183 randomized patients, median baseline neurological deficit was a National Institutes of Health Stroke Scale (NIHSS) score of 2, and median initial diffusion lesion volume on MRI was 3.5 mL. In both treatment arms, recurrent clinical ischaemic strokes were rare (1 each) and no symptomatic intracranial haemorrhage occurred. On MRI at 4 weeks, no differences for NOAC versus warfarin were seen for new ischaemic lesion, 29.5% versus 35.6%, risk ratio (RR) 0.83 (95% CI: 0.54–1.26; $P = 0.38$) or new intracranial haemorrhage, 31.6% versus 28.7%, RR 1.10 (95% CI: 0.70–1.71; $P = 0.68$).

Timing of Delayed Start of Anticoagulation in AF and Stroke

The risk of haemorrhagic transformation among patients with AF and ischaemic stroke is greatest in the first few hours and days after stroke onset, when the freshly injured brain and neurovasculature have the greatest disruption of blood–brain barrier integrity, and thereafter rapidly declines to a low level (Abdul-Rahim et al., 2015). While the risk of recurrent ischaemic stroke also is highest in the early time period, it then declines to an enduring moderate level. Accordingly, after passage of some time from onset, benefit will outweigh risk, and start of long-term secondary prevention anticoagulation may be initiated.

Several observational studies have explored the best delayed time period at which to initiate anticoagulation in patients with AF and ischaemic stroke (Seiffge et al., 2019). The most broadly generalizable was a multicentre observational study performed in Europe and Asia in which anticoagulation start time was determined by physician discretion in 1029 patients with AF and acute ischaemic stroke (Paciaroni et al., 2015). Overall, 74% of patients were eventually started on anticoagulants, including 44% who received antiplatelet therapy before starting anticoagulation. Anticoagulation agent classes included LMWH alone in 15%, warfarin alone in 37%, NOACs alone in 12%, and LMWH followed by warfarin in 36%. During the first 90 days after onset, 7.6% of patients had recurrent ischaemic stroke, TIA, or systemic embolism; 3.6% had symptomatic intracranial haemorrhage; and 1.4% had major extracerebral haemorrhage. Start of therapeutic anticoagulation between 4 and 14 days after onset was associated with the fewest adverse outcome events, with ischaemic event hazard ratio (HR) 0.43 (95% CI: 0.19–0.97) and haemorrhagic event HR 0.39 (95% CI: 0.12–1.19).

Comment

Immediate anticoagulation upon presentation for all patients with AF and ischaemic stroke is not a recommended policy, as the risks of intracranial and major ECH in the first few days are high and negate the benefits of reduction of early recurrent ischaemic stroke. In contrast, early initiation of oral anticoagulants or LMWH, within 2 weeks of stroke onset but after a short initial delay, is reasonable for acute ischaemic stroke patients with AF (Kernan et al., 2014; Paciaroni et al., 2015). Based on physiological reasoning, it may be reasonable to adjust the timing of initiation of anticoagulation within the first 4–14 days after onset to each patient's individual balance of haemorrhagic and recurrent ischaemic stroke risk. Within this time period, anticoagulation may be initiated earlier in patients with low haemorrhagic risk (small infarct size, absence of cerebral microbleeds or asymptomatic radiological haemorrhagic transformation, normal permeability imaging, well-controlled blood pressure, etc.) and high recurrent ischaemic stroke risk (visualized thrombus in left atrium, asymptomatic microemboli occurring on transcranial Doppler imaging, new silent ischaemic lesions on diffusion MRI, etc.). Anticoagulation may be initiated later in patients in whom the ratio of these risks is reversed. However, such deduction, based on currently available low-quality evidence, might not be reliable. Further studies are warranted to derive and validate algorithms that identify optimal anticoagulation start times for individual patients, maximizing the benefit and reducing the harm of early-initiated anticoagulation therapy in acute ischaemic stroke patients with AF.

Summary

In broad, relatively unselected patients with acute ischaemic stroke, immediate high-dose anticoagulation therapy to avert early stroke progression or recurrence reduces recurrent ischaemic stroke compared with control during the treatment period, but this benefit is offset by an increase in intracranial haemorrhage (ICH) and extracranial haemorrhage (ECH). Immediate antiplatelet therapy has similar efficacy to anticoagulation in averting early stroke progress or recurrence, and is safer when used as an immediate agent in broad, relatively unselected patients in the acute phase of ischaemic stroke (see Chapter 9). In acute ischaemic stroke patients with atrial fibrillation, after start of antiplatelet therapy on presentation, early switchover to anticoagulation therapy 4–14 days after stroke onset is reasonable, but caution should be taken in certain subgroups of patients with high risk of bleeding.

In broad, relatively unselected ischaemic stroke patients, low-dose venous prophylaxis anticoagulation compared with control reduces the occurrence of asymptomatic deep vein thrombosis (DVT) and shows a tendency to reduce pulmonary embolism, but also shows off-setting tendencies to increase ICH and ECH, without conferring a clear net clinical benefit. Low-molecular-weight heparins or heparinoids, compared with unfractionated heparin, appear to further decrease the occurrence of DVT and pulmonary embolism but potentially further increase ICH, but there are too few data to provide reliable information.

References

Abdul-Rahim AH, Fulton RL, Frank B, Tatlisumak T, Paciaroni M, Caso V, et al. (2015). Association of improved outcome in acute ischaemic stroke patients with atrial fibrillation who receive early antithrombotic therapy: analysis from VISTA. *Eur J Neurol*, **22**, 1048–55.

Amarenco P, Lavallée PC, Labreuche J. (2016). One-year risk of stroke after transient ischemic attack or minor ischemic stroke. *N Engl J Med*, **374**, 1533–42.

Ay H, Gungor L, Arsava EM, Rosand J, Vangel M, Benner T, et al. (2010). A score to predict early risk of recurrence after ischemic stroke. *Neurology*, **74**, 128–35.

Berge E, Abdelnoor M, Nakstad PH, Sandset PM on behalf of the Heparin in Acute Embolic Stroke Trial (HAEST) Study Group. (2000). Low molecular-weight heparin versus aspirin in patients with acute ischaemic stroke and atrial fibrillation: a double-blind randomised study. HAEST Study Group. Heparin in Acute Embolic Stroke Trial. *Lancet*, **355**, 1205–10.

Cazzato G, Zorzon M, Mase G, Antonutto L, Iona LG. (1989). Il mesoglicano nelle ischemie cerebrali acute a focolaio [Mesoglycan in the treatment of acute cerebral infarction]. *Rivista di Neurologia*, **59**, 121–6.

Cerebral Embolism Study Group. (1983). Immediate anticoagulation of embolic stroke: a randomized trial. The Cerebral Embolism Study Group. *Stroke*, **14**, 668–76.

Chimowitz MI, Lynn MJ, Derdeyn CP, Derdeyn CP, Turan TN, Fiorella D, et al. (2011). Stenting versus aggressive medical therapy for intracranial arterial stenosis. *N Engl J Med*, **365**, 993–1003

Dennis M, Caso V, Kappelle LJ, Pavlovic A, Sandercock P, for the European Stroke Organisation. (2016). European Stroke Organisation (ESO) guidelines for prophylaxis for venous thromboembolism in immobile patients with acute ischaemic stroke. *Eur Stroke J*, **1**, 6–19.

Duke RJ, Turpie AGG, Bloch RF, Trebilcock RG. (1983). Clinical trial of low-dose subcutaneous heparin for the prevention of stroke progression: natural history of acute partial stroke and stroke-in-evolution. In M Reivich, HI Hurtig, eds., *Cerebrovascular Disease*. New York: Raven Press, pp. 399–405.

Duke RJ, Bloch RF, Turpie AGG, Trebilcock RG, Bayer N. (1986). Intravenous heparin for the prevention of stroke progression in acute partial stable stroke. *Ann Intern Med*, **105**, 825–8.

Elias A, Milandre L, Lagrange G, Aillaud MF, Alonzo B, Toulemonde F, et al. (1990). Prevention of deep venous thrombosis of the leg by a very low molecular weight heparin fraction (CY 222) in patients with hemiplegia following cerebral infarction: a randomized pilot study (30 patients). *Revue de Médecine Interne*, **11**, 95–8.

Hommel M, for the FISS-bis Investigators Group. (1998). Fraxiparine in Ischaemic Stroke Study (FISS bis). *Cerebrovasc Dis*, **8**(Suppl 4), 19.

Hong KS, Kwon SU, Lee SH, Lee JS, Kim YJ, Song TJ, et al. (2017). Rivaroxaban vs warfarin sodium in the ultra-early period after atrial fibrillation-related mild ischemic stroke: a randomized clinical trial. *JAMA Neurol*, **74**, 1206–15.

International Stroke Trial Collaborative Group. (1997). The International Stroke Trial (IST): a randomised trial of aspirin, subcutaneous heparin, both, or neither among 19435 patients with acute ischaemic stroke. *Lancet*, **349**, 1569–81.

Johansson E, Wester P. (2014). Recurrent stroke risk is high after a single cerebrovascular event in patients with symptomatic 50–99% carotid stenosis: a cohort study. *BMC Neurol*, **14**, 23.

Kernan WN, Ovbiagele B, Black HR, Bravata DM, Chimowitz MI, Ezekowitz MD, et al. (2014). Guidelines for the prevention of stroke in patients with stroke and transient ischemic attack: a guideline for healthcare professionals from the American Heart Association/American Stroke Association. *Stroke*, **45**, 2160–2236.

Kwiecinski H, Pniewski J, Kaminska A, Szyluk B. (1995). A randomized trial of fraxiparine in acute ischaemic stroke. *Cerebrovasc Dis*, **5**, 234.

LaMonte MP, Nash ML, Wang DZ, Woolfenden AR, Schulz J, Hursting MJ, et al. (2004). Argatroban anticoagulation in patients with acute ischemic stroke (ARGIS-1). *Stroke*, **35**, 1677–82.

Lansberg MG, O'Donnell MJ, Khatri P, Lang ES, Nguyen-Huynh MN, Schwartz NE, et al. (2012). Antithrombotic and thrombolytic therapy for ischemic stroke: Antithrombotic Therapy and Prevention of Thrombosis, 9th ed: American College of Chest Physicians Evidence-Based Clinical Practice Guidelines. *Chest*, **141**, e601S–636S.

Liu L, Wong KSL, Leng X, Pu Y, Wang Y, Jing J, et al. (2015). Dual antiplatelet therapy in stroke and ICAS Subgroup analysis of CHANCE. *Neurology*, 85, 1154–62.

McCarthy ST, Turner J. (1986). Low-dose subcutaneous heparin in the prevention of deep-vein thrombosis and pulmonary emboli following acute stroke. *Age Ageing*, **15**, 84–8.

McCarthy ST, Turner JJ, Robertson D, Hawkey CJ, Macey DJ. (1997). Low dose heparin as a prophylaxis against deep-vein thrombosis after acute stroke. *Lancet*, **ii**:800–1.

Paciaroni M, Agnelli G, Falocci N, Caso V, Becattini C, Marcheselli S, et al. (2015). Early recurrence and cerebral bleeding in patients with acute ischemic stroke and atrial fibrillation: effect of anticoagulation and its timing: the RAF study. *Stroke*, **46**, 2175–82.

Paciaroni M, Agnelli G, Micheli S, Caso V. (2007). Efficacy and safety of anticoagulant treatment in acute cardioembolic stroke: a meta-analysis of randomized controlled trials. *Stroke*, 38, 423–30.

Pambianco G, Orchard T, Landau P. (1995). Deep vein thrombosis: prevention in stroke patients during rehabilitation. *Arch Phys Med Rehabil*, **76**, 324–30.

Pince J. (1981). *Thromboses veineuses des membres inferieurs et embolies pulmonaires au cours des accidents vasculaires cerebraux. A propos d'un essai comparitif de traitement preventif.* These pour le doctorat d'état en médecine, Toulouse: Université Paul Sabatier.

Prins MH, Gelsema R, Sing AK, van Heerde LR, den Ottolander GJ. (1989). Prophylaxis of deep venous thrombosis with a low-molecular-weight heparin (Kabi 2165/Fragmin) in stroke patients. *Haemostasis*, **19**, 245–50.

Rothwell PM. (2008). Prediction and prevention of stroke in patients with symptomatic carotid stenosis: the high-risk period and the high-risk patient. *Eur J Vasc Endovasc Surg*, **35**, 255–63.

Sandercock PAG, Counsell C, Kane EJ. (2015). Anticoagulants for acute ischaemic stroke. *Cochrane Database Syst Rev*, 3. CD000024.

Sandercock PAG, Leong TS. (2017). Low-molecular-weight heparins or heparinoids versus standard unfractionated heparin for acute ischaemic stroke.

Cochrane Database Syst Rev, 4. CD000119. doi:10.1002/14651858.CD000119.pub4.

Sandset PM, Dahl T, Stiris M, Rostad B, Scheel B, Abildgaard U. (1990). A double-blind and randomized placebo-controlled trial of low molecular weight heparin once daily to prevent deep-vein thrombosis in acute ischemic stroke. *Semin Thromb Hemost*, **16**(Suppl), 25–33.

Saxena R, Lewis S, Berge E, Sandercock PAG, Koudstaal PJ, for the International Stroke Trial Collaborative Group. (2001). Risk of early death and recurrent stroke and effect of heparin in 3169 patients with acute ischemic stroke and atrial fibrillation in the International Stroke Trial. *Stroke*, **32**, 2333–7.

Seiffge DJ, Werring DJ, Paciaroni M, Dawson J, Warach S, Milling TJ, et al. (2019). Timing of anticoagulation after recent ischaemic stroke in patients with atrial fibrillation. *Lancet Neurol*, **18**, 117–26.

Sherman DG, Albers GW, Bladin C, Fieschi C, Gabbai AA, Kase CS, et al. (2007). The efficacy and safety of enoxaparin versus unfractionated heparin for the prevention of venous thromboembolism after acute ischaemic stroke (PREVAIL Study): an open-label randomised comparison. *Lancet*, **369**, 1347–55.

Tazaki Y, Kobayashi S, Togi H, Ohtomo E, Goto F, Araki G, et al. (1986). Therapeutic effect of thrombin inhibitor MD-805 in acute phase of cerebral thrombosis – Phase II double-blinded clinical trial (English translation). *Rinsho to Kenkyu*, 63, 3047–57.

TOAST Investigators. (1998). Low molecular weight heparinoid, ORG 10172 (danaparoid), and outcome after acute ischaemic stroke. *JAMA*, **279**, 1265–72.

Turpie AGG, Levine MN, Hirsh J, Carter CJ, Jay RM, Powers PJ, et al. (1987). Double-blind randomised trial of Org 10172 low-molecular-weight heparinoid in prevention of deep-vein thrombosis in thrombotic stroke. *Lancet*, **1**, 523–6.

Treatment of Brain Oedema

Jeffrey L. Saver
Salvador Cruz-Flores

Rationale

Brain oedema in ischaemic stroke sufficient to cause mass effect and herniation is a complication of large infarcts, which account for up to 15% of patients with anterior circulation infarcts and approximately 20% of patients with cerebellar infarcts (Wijdicks et al., 2014). Cerebral oedema in large infarcts produces additional injury, as regionally expanding oedematous tissues compress and compromise adjacent intact brain tissues and cranial nerves, occlude cerebral arteries at points of herniation leading to cerebral infarcts in other vascular territories, or occlude cerebrospinal fluid (CSF) channels causing hydrocephalus. In ischaemic strokes, oedema in the brain arises through two pathophysiological processes: (1) cytotoxic oedema, increased intracellular fluid due to neuronal energetic failure, and (2) vasogenic oedema, increased extracellular fluid due to blood–brain barrier disruption, with cytotoxic oedema providing the greater contribution.

Microscopic cytotoxic oedema begins to develop within the first minutes after ischaemic stroke onset, when it can be detected on magnetic resonance imaging (MRI) as a decrease in the apparent diffusion coefficient of water. However, macroscopically evident mass effect arising from more advanced cytotoxic oedema and vasogenic oedema develops over a longer time period, typically peaking 3–5 days after ischaemic stroke onset.

The management of substantial brain oedema aims to:

- reduce mass effect;
- prevent secondary injury from herniation;
- resolve hydrocephalus, if present; and
- maintain adequate cerebral perfusion pressure, sufficient to overcome raised intracranial pressure.

Therapies that have been used in practice to treat brain oedema and its complications include:

- elevating head of bed to 20–30 degrees to assist cerebral venous drainage;
- mild fluid restriction to deter brain fluid accumulation (but with potential adverse effect on cerebral perfusion pressure);
- avoiding hypo-osmolar fluids, such as 5% dextrose in water, to prevent osmotic pull of intravascular water into brain tissue;
- administering intravenous crystalloids (hypertonic saline) or colloids (such as mannitol or glycerol) to osmotically draw water out of brain parenchyma;
- avoiding cerebral veno-dilating drugs as they expand the intracranial blood volume within the intravascular compartment;
- hyperventilation, to induce vasoconstriction and reduce the intracranial blood volume within the intravascular compartment;
- hypothermia to reduce intravascular blood volume and stabilize the blood–brain barrier;
- corticosteroids to stabilize the blood–brain barrier and reduce vasogenic oedema;
- glyburide to decrease water flux across neuronal and glial cell membranes and reduce cytotoxic oedema;
- drainage of CSF fluid; and
- surgical decompression.

Some of these diverse therapeutic options have been formally tested in randomized clinical trials, while several have been evaluated only in uncontrolled observational series.

Hyperventilation

Reductions in the partial pressure of carbon dioxide (PCO_2) produce cerebral vasoconstriction and reduced cerebral blood volume. Hyperventilation reducing PCO_2 by 5–10 mm Hg can lower intracranial pressure by 10–40% (Gujjar et al., 1998; Coles et al., 2007). However, this degree of hyperventilation will also reduce cerebral blood flow by 15–30% (Coles et al., 2007), which could aggravate ischaemic brain injury. No randomized trials of hyperventilation for brain oedema in ischaemic stroke have been conducted. Based on its physiological effect profile, hyperventilation, if used at all, likely should be deployed primarily as a temporary measure while preparing surgical interventions to definitively control brain oedema and mass effect.

Corticosteroids

Evidence

Death

A systematic review of eight randomized controlled trial (RCTs) involving 466 patients with early ischaemic stroke revealed that, compared with control, random assignment to corticosteroid treatment within 48 hours of stroke onset did not alter mortality within 1 month (odds ratio [OR]: 0.97, 95% confidence interval [CI]: 0.63–1.47) (Figure 11.1) or within 1 year (OR: 0.87, 95% CI: 0.57–1.34) (Sandercock and Soane, 2011).

Neurological Impairment

Six trials reported neurological impairment outcomes, but used different neurological deficit assessment scales, precluding formal meta-analytic pooling across studies. At the individual study level, four trials reported no difference, one benefit, and one worsening, in neurological impairment with steroid therapy (Sandercock and Soane, 2011).

Adverse Effects

Adverse effects were not systematically reported in most randomized trials of corticosteroids in ischaemic stroke. However, diabetes or hyperglycaemia was reported to be non-significantly nominally more frequent with steroid therapy in four trials.

Comment

Interpretation of the Evidence

The accumulated randomized trial evidence does not indicate a beneficial effect of corticosteroids in patients with early ischaemic stroke on either death or neurological impairment.

Study or subgroup	Treatment n/N	Control n/N	Peto Odds Ratio Peto, Fixed, 95% CI	Weight	Peto Odds Ratio Peto, Fixed, 95% CI
Bauer 1973	5/28	9/26		12.4%	0.42 [0.13, 1.42]
Gupta 1978	2/13	2/17		4.2%	1.35 [0.17, 10.93]
McQueen 1978	12/24	5/24		13.2%	3.49 [1.08, 11.24]
Mulley 1978	42/61	45/57		27.1%	0.60 [0.26, 1.35]
Norris 1976	7/29	5/24		11.0%	1.20 [0.33, 4.33]
Norris 1986	13/54	15/59		25.0%	0.93 [0.40, 2.18]
Ogun 2001	2/5	6/8		3.7%	0.26 [0.03, 2.32]
Patten 1972	1/17	2/20		3.3%	0.58 [0.06, 6.04]
Total (95% CI)	231	235		100.0%	0.87 [0.57, 1.34]

Total events: 84 (Treatment), 89 (Control)

Heterogeneity: Chi^2 = 9.32, df = 7 (P = 0.23); I^2 = 25%

Test for overall effect: Z = 0.62 (P = 0.53)

Test for subgroup differences: Not applicable

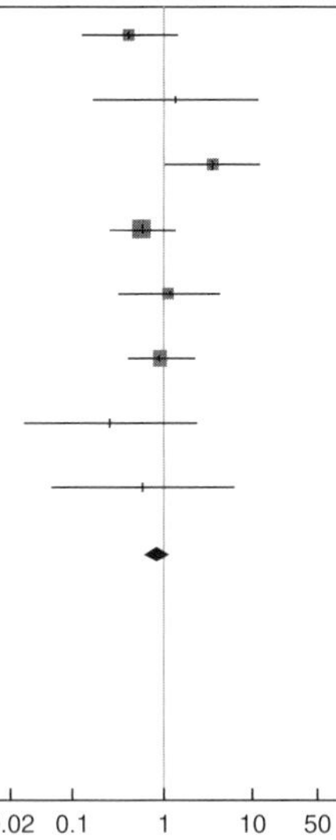

0.02 0.1   1   10 50

Figure 11.1 Forest plot showing the effects of *corticosteroids vs control* in early ischaemic stroke on *death from all causes* during study follow-up. Reproduced from with permission from Sandercock and Soane (2011) and John Wiley & Sons Limited. Copyright Cochrane Library, reproduced with permission.

Implications for Practice

Corticosteroid should not be used in the routine management of brain oedema after acute ischaemic stroke.

Implications for Research

The amount of evidence across all trials is modest, and the great preponderance of studies pre-date the modern era of reperfusion therapy for acute ischaemic stroke. While sufficient data have been accumulated to suggest that corticosteroids are not likely to be a useful broad therapy for all patients with ischaemic stroke, the possibility remains that steroid therapy may be effective for targeted subtypes of patients. Studies may be warranted that are confined to patients with large infarcts and substantial cerebral oedema and that deploy higher doses of corticosteroids (e.g. methylprednisolone 500–1000 mg/day), which may be more effective for vasogenic oedema, and for a shorter duration to avoid potential adverse effects (Davis and Donnan, 2004; Norris, 2004). Also, studies would be of interest in patients with imaging evidence of early blood–brain barrier disruption (e.g. abnormal permeability imaging; Nael et al., 2017), or of early cerebral endothelial injury (e.g. vessel wall enhancement; Renú et al., 2017), identifying patients at increased risk for both vasogenic oedema and haemorrhagic transformation.

Osmotic Agents

Osmotic agents are molecules that do not readily cross the blood–brain barrier, so that their systemic administration yields a higher solute concentration in the blood than in the brain. The resulting osmotic gradient draws free water from brain intracellular and interstitial compartments into the systemic intravascular space. The two main categories of osmatic agents are (1) colloids: large, insoluble molecules, and (2) crystalloids: small, water-soluble molecules (Lewis et al., 2018). For brain oedema, the most well-studied agents are the colloids mannitol and glycerol and the crystalloid hypertonic saline (Fink, 2014).

Mannitol

Mannitol is a colloidal osmotic agent and a free radical scavenger. Mannitol (0.25–0.6 g/kg, e.g. 20–40 g) intravenously over 30 minutes lowers intracranial pressure (ICP). It can be given every 6 hours to a maximum daily dose of 2 g/kg (e.g. about 140 g in a 70 kg person). Mannitol decreases brain oedema by exerting osmotic pressure that draws water out of the brain interstitium.

Evidence

Physiological Effects

In a series of ischaemic stroke patients, mannitol was associated with a shrinking of the volume of the contralateral hemisphere by 8% (Videen et al., 2001), and in another study mannitol was associated with positron emission tomography (PET) scan findings of an increase in cerebral blood flow in peri-infarct regions by 18% ($p = 0.05$) and a trend toward increase in cerebral blood flow in the contralateral hemisphere by 27% ($p = 0.11$) (Diringer et al., 2011). However, mannitol becomes less effective with repeated doses, and delayed 'rebound' increases in ICP can occur as mannitol eventually crosses the blood–brain barrier and enters the cerebral compartment.

Clinical Outcomes

A systematic review identified only one unconfounded RCT in which 77 patients with ischaemic stroke were allocated to mannitol or control (Santambrogio et al., 1978; Bereczki et al., 2007). The mannitol dose was 0.8–0.9 g/kg for 10 days, and the study enrolled both patients with small and those with large ischaemic strokes. The analysed outcomes were the proportion of patients with clinical improvement, clinical stability, and clinical worsening. The outcomes of dependency, death, or adverse effects were not reported. In this small trial, mannitol was not associated with alteration in frequency of improved, unchanged, or worsened patient clinical course as compared with controls. Rates of clinical improvement with mannitol vs control were 33.3% versus 34.1%, risk ratio (RR) 1.02 (95% CI: 0.55–1.91) (Figure 11.2); and rates of clinical worsening were 44.4% versus 43.9%, RR 0.99 (95% CI: 0.60–1.63) (Figure 11.3).

Adverse Effects

The most common complications of mannitol therapy are fluid and electrolyte imbalances, cardiopulmonary oedema, and rebound cerebral oedema. Mannitol also uncommonly causes kidney failure, and hypersensitivity reactions may occur.

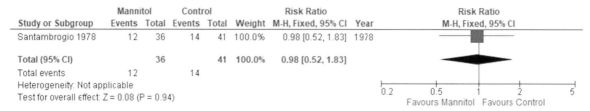

Figure 11.2 Forest plot showing the effects of *mannitol vs control* in early ischaemic stroke on *clinical improvement.*

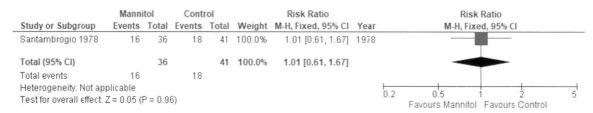

Figure 11.3 Forest plot showing the effects of *mannitol vs control* in early ischaemic stroke on *clinical worsening.*

Comment

Interpretation of the Evidence

There is not enough reliable evidence to determine whether mannitol is effective or ineffective in patients with cerebral oedema due to ischaemic stroke.

Implications for Practice

In the absence of adequate randomized, clinical outcome data to provide definitive guidance, firm recommendations regarding the use of mannitol to treat brain oedema from ischaemic strokes cannot be given. However, based on findings of potentially beneficial physiological effects in ischaemic stroke patients, and larger experience with use of mannitol in neurological conditions, it is reasonable to use mannitol for patients with large hemispheric or cerebellar infarcts, especially as a temporizing measure until a definitive procedural/surgical intervention is delivered, or until patients have crossed the imminent timepoint of expected peak brain swelling.

Implications for Research

The clinical efficacy of mannitol in acute ischaemic stroke has not yet been properly evaluated. Large, placebo-controlled, unconfounded randomized trials of mannitol as bridging, temporizing therapy in patients with sizeable, space-occupying infarcts are desirable.

Glycerol

Glycerol is a polyol compound that acts as a colloidal osmotic agent. In observational series among patients with diverse neurological conditions causing raised ICP, including ischaemic stroke, glycerol reduced ICP and increased indices of cerebral perfusion pressure (Biestro et al., 1997; Treib et al., 1998). Compared with mannitol, glycerol had not only a longer time until achievement of peak effect, but also a longer duration of effect without rebound.

Evidence

A systematic review identified 7 randomized trials, enrolling 601 patients, comparing intravenous glycerol with control, initiated within the first days after onset, in patients with definite or presumed ischaemic stroke (Righetti et al., 2004).

Death

Data regarding death within the scheduled treatment period was available from all 7 trials enrolling 601 patients. Random allocation to glycerol versus control was associated with a reduction in early death, 19.6% versus 25.6% (OR: 0.65, 95% CI: 0.44–0.97; $p = 0.03$). Information on death by end of scheduled follow-up was available from 6 RCTs enrolling 492 patients. Allocation to glycerol versus control was not associated with alteration in death at final follow-up, 36.7%

versus 39.5% (OR: 0.85, 95% CI: 0.59–1.24) (Figure 11.4).

Dependency or Death

Data regarding dependency or death (modified Rankin Scale [mRS] 3–6 or nearest equivalent) at end of follow-up were available from 2 randomized trials enrolling 234 patients with ischaemic stroke. Glycerol compared with control did not show a statistically significant association with dependency or death, 79.5% versus 84.1% (OR: 0.73, 95% CI: 0.37–1.42) (Figure 11.5).

Adverse Effects

Haemolysis was the only relevant adverse effect of glycerol treatment.

Comment

Interpretation of the Evidence

These data indicate a favourable effect of glycerol treatment on short-term survival in patients with definite or presumed ischaemic stroke, though mortality differences did not remain statistically significant at long-term follow-up. Due to the relatively modest total sample size, and the fact that some of the trials were performed in the pre-computed tomography (CT) era and so may have included a few patients with primary haemorrhagic stroke misdiagnosed as ischaemic, the results must be interpreted cautiously. Furthermore, many of the studies included not only patients with large infarcts, but also those with mild-to-moderate infarcts.

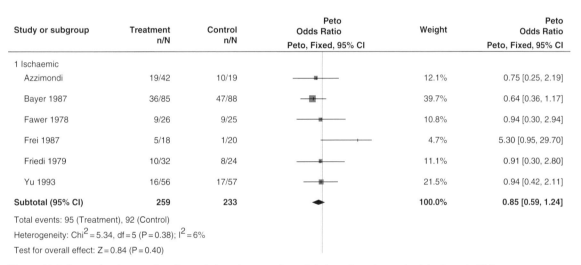

Figure 11.4 Forest plot showing the effects of *glycerol vs control* in early ischaemic stroke on *death by the end of follow-up*.

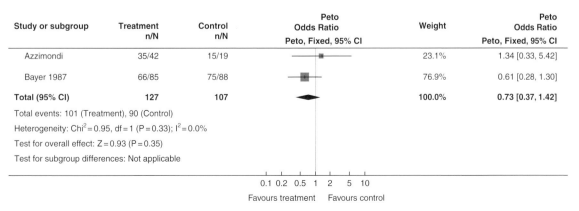

Figure 11.5 Forest plot showing the effects of *glycerol vs control* in early ischaemic stroke on *dependency or death at end of follow-up*.

Implications for Practice

Given the paucity of evidence available regarding effects on functional outcome, and the mixed evidence of potential benefit on mortality, definitive recommendations regarding use of glycerol to treat brain oedema from ischaemic stroke cannot be formulated. Based on findings of potentially beneficial physiological effects and benefit on short-term mortality, it is reasonable to use glycerol in patients with large hemispheric or cerebellar infarcts, especially as a temporizing measure until a definitive procedural/surgical intervention is employed, or until patients cross the imminent timepoint of expected peak brain swelling.

Implications for Research

As glycerol treatment is inexpensive, may be effective, and appears to be safe, it should continue to be tested as a treatment for brain oedema in ischaemic stroke patients, but in much larger RCTs focused upon patients who have clinical and imaging evidence of mass effect, with assessment of long-term functional outcomes as well as survival.

Hypertonic Saline

Hypertonic saline is a crystalloid osmotic agent, producing elevated serum sodium levels that create osmotic pressure drawing water out of brain tissues. Hypertonic saline doses most often studied are a bolus of 23.4% saline for substantial, short-acting effect and a continuous infusion of 3% saline for more modulated, long-lasting effect (Wijdicks et al., 2014; Ong et al., 2015).

Evidence

Physiological Effects

There have been no unconfounded, randomized studies of hypertonic saline confined to patients with ischaemic stroke. In an observational series of 76 transtentorial herniation events among 68 patients with varied neurological conditions (including 8 with ischaemic stroke), bolus therapy with 23.4% hypertonic saline, in tandem with additional medical interventions, was associated with reversal of clinical signs of herniation in 75% of episodes (Koenig et al., 2008). Independent predictors of successful reversal of herniation were an increase in sodium concentration equal to or greater than 5 mmol/L (OR 12.0, 95% CI: 1.6–90.5) and an attained absolute sodium concentration equal to or greater than 145 mmol/L (OR 26.7, 95% CI: 3.6--200.0). In additional studies in patients with diverse neurological causes of raised ICP, including traumatic brain injury, conditions requiring craniotomy, and subarachnoid haemorrhage, hypertonic saline has been shown to reduce ICP, with comparable or slightly greater physiological efficacy compared with mannitol (Li et al., 2015; Pasarikovski et al., 2017; Fang et al., 2018).

Clinical Outcomes

There have been no unconfounded, randomized trials with neurological deficit, disability, or mortality outcomes comparing hypertonic saline with control or with active colloidal osmotic agent therapy in patients with ischaemic stroke.

Adverse Effects

Adverse effects of hypertonic saline are uncommon, but include hyperchloraemic metabolic acidosis, congestive heart failure, acute renal impairment, and seizures (Jeon et al., 2014).

Comment

Interpretation of the Evidence

The absence of any unconfounded randomized trials precludes reliable assessment of whether hypertonic saline is effective or ineffective in patients with cerebral oedema due to ischaemic stroke.

Implications for Practice

In the absence of randomized, clinical outcome data, definite recommendations regarding the use of hypertonic saline to treat brain oedema from ischaemic strokes cannot be advanced. However, based on findings of potentially beneficial physiological effects in ischaemic stroke patients, and larger experience with use of hypertonic saline in other neurological conditions, it is reasonable to use hypertonic saline therapy for patients with large hemispheric or cerebellar infarcts. Using 3% hypertonic saline to counter cerebral salt wasting and maintain euvolaemia while achieving mild hypernatremia with osmotic effects is a reasonable initial strategy in large infarcts. Administration of 23.4% saline bolus in response to signs of progressive herniation or severely elevated ICP also is reasonable as a temporizing measure until a definitive procedural/surgical intervention is delivered.

Implications for Research

The clinical efficacy of hypertonic saline in acute ischaemic stroke has not yet been formally evaluated. Placebo-controlled, unconfounded, randomized trials of hypertonic saline are merited in patients with large hemispheric and cerebellar cerebral infarcts.

Glyburide

In preclinical models, blockade by the sulfonylurea agent glyburide of the inducible sulfonylurea receptor 1 (SUR1)-transient receptor potential melastatin 4 (TRPM4) channel in neurons, astrocytes, and endothelium substantially lessens brain oedema (Simard et al., 2010). Oral glyburide has long been used as an antidiabetic agent, but may not yield predictable blood levels in the critically ill patient, so an intravenous formulation has been developed for potential use as an agent to avert development of substantial brain oedema after large cerebral infarcts (King et al., 2018).

Evidence

One randomized, placebo-controlled, phase 2 trial of intravenous glyburide has been conducted, enrolling patients with large anterior circulation hemispheric infarcts (diffusion MRI infarct volumes 82–300 mL) within 10 hours of onset (Sheth et al., 2016). A total of 86 patients were enrolled and analysed for safety, among whom 77 treated per protocol were analysed for efficacy.

Physiological Outcomes

Allocation to glyburide versus control was associated with reduced growth in midline shift from entry to 72–96 hours, 4.6 versus 8.8 mm, mean difference –4.3 mm (95% CI: –6.3 to –2.4). Differences in growth of ipsilateral hemispheric volume were not statistically significant, 68 versus 78 mL, mean difference –13.4 mL (95% CI: –43.4 to 16.6).

Functional Outcomes

The trial's primary efficacy outcome composite, of avoiding extreme disability (need for continuous care) or death (mRS 5–6) and avoiding decompressive craniectomy, did not differ between glyburide versus control patients (41% versus 39%; OR: 0.87, 95% CI: 0.32–2.32). However, there was a trend for a favourable shift to reduced disability at 3 months across the 7-level mRS, with mean mRS values 4.1 versus 4.6, non-parametric $p = 0.12$.

Death

All-cause mortality by 90 days tended to be less in the glyburide group, 17% versus 36%, hazard ratio (HR) 0.49 (95% CI: 0.21–1.13).

Adverse Effects

In the phase 2 RCT, asymptomatic low blood glucose levels (<3.1 mmol/L) tended to occur more often with glyburide than control, 9% versus 0%, $p = 0.12$, but there were no symptomatic hypoglycaemic events.

Comment

Interpretation of the Evidence

Initial data suggest that glyburide holds promise as a potential agent to minimize the development of brain oedema and herniation in patients with large hemispheric and cerebellar infarcts. Larger, definitive randomized trials are warranted to confirm or disconfirm the initial signals of potential benefit.

Hypothermia

Hypothermia exerts both ICP-lowering and direct neuroprotective effects in preclinical ischaemic stroke models. Reduction in intracranial pressures arises from reduced cerebral blood volume (paralleling reduced metabolic demand), diminished inflammatory injury, and stabilization of the blood–brain barrier (Jeon et al., 2014). In uncontrolled observational series, inducing hypothermia with a target temperature of 32–33°C was associated with reduced mass effect and ICP elevation in patients with large hemispheric infarcts (Schwab et al., 1998, 2001). However, randomized trials of hypothermia in acute ischaemic stroke have focused upon putative neuroprotective effects, by enrolling moderate and large infarct patients very early after onset, rather than upon brain oedema effects, by enrolling only large infarct patients identified as high risk for mass effect and herniation. Given the absence of randomized data, firm recommendations regarding hypothermia for brain oedema management cannot be advanced. Randomized trials targeting patients with large infarcts and elevated risk of herniation risk are desirable.

Cerebrospinal Fluid Drainage

Drainage of CSF via an intra-ventricular catheter can rapidly reduce compartmental shifts due to obstructive hydrocephalus secondary to brain swelling, such as a trapped lateral ventricle exacerbating hemispheric swelling and herniation (Pagani-Estévez et al., 2016), and can also lower overall ICP. In a meta-analysis of observational studies in patients with traumatic brain injury, CSF drainage and hypertonic saline administration were the second-most powerful treatments to lower ICP, after decompressive hemicraniectomy; mean ICP reductions included hemicraniectomy – 19 mm Hg, CSF drainage – 15 mm Hg, hypertonic saline – 15 mm Hg, hypothermia – 10 mm Hg, mannitol – 8 mm Hg, and hyperventilation – 6 mm Hg (Schreckinger and Marion, 2009). However, a cautionary consideration for patients with large cerebellar infarcts is that ventricular drainage above the 4th ventricle can aggravate upward transtentorial cerebellar herniation, by creating a pressure differential with differentially lowered pressure above the obstructed CSF passage. Reverse brain herniation has been reported to occur after as many as 3% of ventriculoperitoneal shunt placements for infratentorial lesions (Raimondi and Tomita, 1981).

Although CSF drainage has not been evaluated in any formal randomized trials in patients with large ischaemic strokes, and so lacks definitive evidence, its use in patients with hydrocephalus complicating large anterior circulation infarcts is reasonably supported by physiological reasoning and observational data. For patients with large cerebellar infarcts and hydrocephalus, the use of CSF drainage in tandem with suboccipital craniectomy is also reasonable, but it is reasonable to restrict its use alone without craniectomy only to subjects with no imaging evidence of early upward herniation.

Surgical Decompression

Rationale

The goal of any surgical approach to the treatment of symptomatic cerebral oedema is to create additional space to accommodate the swelling brain. This can be accomplished by releasing the restriction of the cranial vault and dura or by creating additional space within the cranium by removing non-viable or non-essential brain tissue (Cruz-Flores et al., 2012). For anterior circulation infarcts, external decompression is provided by hemicraniectomy with or without duroplasty. For cerebellar infarcts, external decompression is provided by suboccipital craniectomy. These techniques

may be accompanied by internal decompression via removal of infarcted cerebral tissues ('infarctectomy') and by removal of intact but non-eloquent brain regions. Decompressive craniectomies with relief of mass effect by expanding the cranial vault are the mainstay of surgical interventions. Resection of infarcted and of non-eloquent tissue is added fairly often to suboccipital craniectomy for cerebellar infarcts and added uncommonly to hemicraniectomy for anterior circulation infarcts. These surgical therapies can provide immediate relief from herniation and reduction in raised ICP, but involve risks including secondary cerebral haemorrhage and brain herniation through the craniectomy defect.

Hemicraniectomy

Evidence

Systematic reviews have identified 7 randomized trials enrolling 338 patients with large anterior circulation infarcts and herniation risk and allocating them to hemicraniectomy plus best medical therapy versus best medical therapy alone (Cruz-Flores et al. 2012; Alexander et al., 2016). Three trials focused solely upon younger patients aged 18 to 55 or 60 enrolling 134 patients; 1 trial focused solely upon older patients aged 61 or older, enrolling 109 patients; and the remaining 3 trials enrolled both younger and older patients (n = 95). Patients with nondominant hemisphere infarcts were enrolled more frequently than those with language compromising dominant hemisphere strokes accounting for 59% of the 289 patients enrolled in the 5 trials reporting laterality. Duration from symptom onset to treatment was within 24 hours in 1 trial, between 12 and 36 hours in 1 trial, within 48 hours in 3 trials, and within 96 hours in 2 trials. Follow-up evaluation at 1 year was available from 6 trials, enrolling 93% of the patients, and at 1.5 years from 1 trial enrolling 7%.

Alive and Functionally Independent (mRS 0–2), at 1–1.5 Years

Overall, for all patients, low rates of functional independence at 1–1.5 years were achieved with both hemicraniectomy and medical therapy alone treatment strategies. Random allocation to hemicraniectomy was associated with a nonsignificant trend towards increased functional independence (mRS 0–2) as compared with

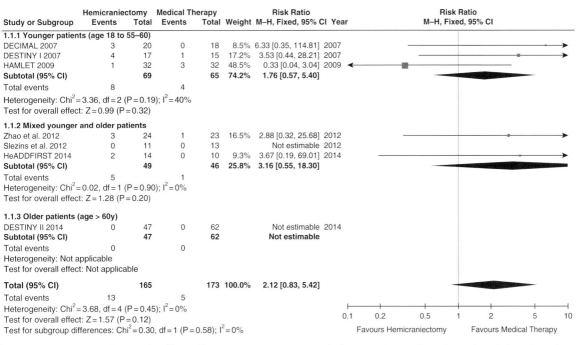

Figure 11.6 Forest plot showing the effects of *hemicraniectomy versus control* in large anterior circulation hemispheric ischaemic stroke on *functional independence (mRS 0–2) at 1–1.5 years.*

medical therapy, 9.1% versus 2.9%, RR: 2.12 (95% CI: 0.83–5.42; $p = 0.12$) (Figure 11.6).

Alive and Capable of Ambulation and Basic Self-care or Better (mRS 0–3), at 1–1.5 Years

Overall, random allocation to hemicraniectomy was associated with an increase in the outcome of being alive and capable of ambulation and basic self-care or better (mRS 0–3) as compared with medical therapy at 1–1.5 years, 26.7% versus 13.9%, RR: 1.74 (95% CI: 1.13–2.67; $p = 0.01$) (Figure 11.7). This represents 128 more patients capable of ambulation and basic self-care or better per 1000 treated with hemicraniectomy compared with control. There was no evidence of heterogeneity of relative treatment effect across individual trials ($I^2 = 0\%$, $p = 0.50$).

Alive and Not Requiring Constant Care or Better (mRS 0–4), at Late Follow-up

Hemicraniectomy in large hemispheric infarct patients was also associated with an increase in the outcome of being alive and not requiring constant care or better (mRS 0–4) at late follow-up, 58.8% hemicraniectomy, 23.7% control; RR: 2.35 (95% CI: 1.76–3.15; $p < 0.00001$) (Figure 11.8). This represents

351 more alive and non–constant care patients per 1000 treated with hemicraniectomy compared with control. There was modest heterogeneity of the relative treatment effect across individual trials ($I^2 = 40\%$, $p = 0.12$).

Death at Late Follow-up

By late follow-up, patients allocated to hemicraniectomy had substantially reduced mortality, 30.3% versus 69.4%, RR: 0.45 (95% CI: 0.35–0.58), $p < 0.00001$, representing 391 fewer deaths per 1000 patients treated with hemicraniectomy compared with control (Figure 11.9). There was mild heterogeneity across individual trials ($I^2 = 14\%$, $p = 0.32$).

Degree of Disability at Long-term Follow-up

Data regarding outcomes across all 7 levels of disability on the mRS are available from 7 trials enrolling 338 patients. Overall, considering the raw combined outcome frequencies across trials, treatment with hemicraniectomy compared with control yielded a lower final level of disability (Mann–Whitney test, $p < 0.00001$) (Figure 11.10). Using the automated algorithmic, min–max joint outcome table method (Saver et al., 2009; Kleinman et al., 2017), mRS

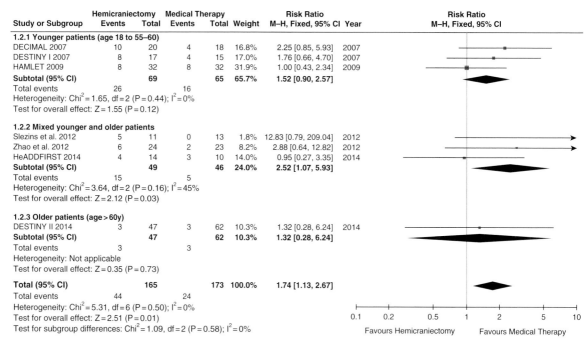

Figure 11.7 Forest plot showing the effects of *hemicraniectomy vs control* in large anterior circulation hemispheric ischaemic stroke on outcome of *being alive and capable of ambulation and basic self-care or better (mRS 0–3) at 1–1.5 years.*

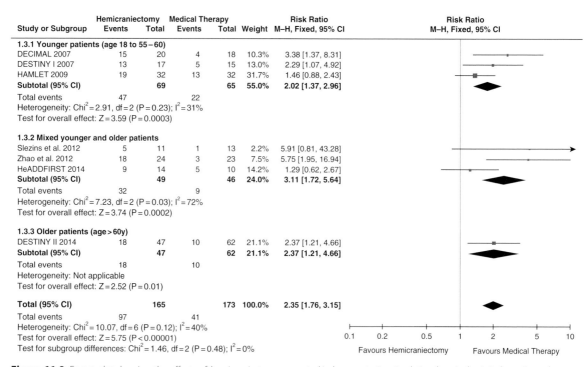

Figure 11.8 Forest plot showing the effects of *hemicraniectomy vs control* in large anterior circulation hemispheric ischaemic stroke on outcome of *being alive and alive and not requiring constant care or better (mRS 0–4) at 1–1.5 years.*

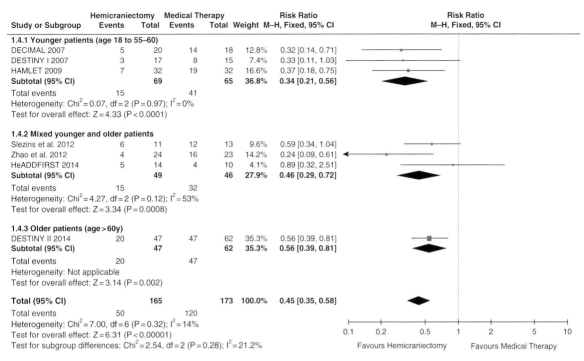

Figure 11.9 Forest plot showing the effects of *hemicraniectomy vs control* in large anterior circulation hemispheric ischaemic stroke on *death by 1–1.5 years.*

outcome distributions indicate that, for every 1000 patients treated with hemicraniectomy, a net of 509 patients will have a lower level of long-term disability as a result. However, the preponderance of benefits was accrued by migration from mortality (391 fewer per 1000) to extreme dependency/needing continuous care (mRS 5: 46 more per 100) and severe dependency/non-ambulatory (mRS 4: 217 more per 1000), with lesser increases in dependency with ambulation (mRS 3: 66 more per 1000), functional independence (mRS 2: 56 more per 1000), and symptoms without disability (mRS 1: 6 more per 1000).

Effect of Age

Randomized trials have shown that older patients with large infarcts benefit from hemicraniectomy to a similar relative degree to younger patients, but with their worse baseline prognosis, their better outcomes are still often ones of severe or extreme disability (see Figures 11.7, 11.8, 11.9, 11.10). In the 4 RCTs with outcomes analysable by age, among the 243 enrolled patients, 55% were up to age 60 and 45% older than age 60. Hemicraniectomy increased survival in both younger patients (78% vs 37%) and older patients (57% vs 24%) (see Figures 11.9, 11.10). In addition,

hemicraniectomy increased the frequency of the outcome of being alive and not requiring constant care or better (mRS 0–4) at late follow-up to similar relative and absolute degrees in both younger patients (70.1% vs 33.3%) and older patients (46.0% vs 13.3%) (see Figures 11.8, 11.10). However, while proportionate increases were similar, absolute increases in favourable outcomes were substantially larger for younger patients for being alive and capable of bodily self-care (mRS 0–3) (younger 39.0% vs 24.0%; older 7.9% vs 4.0%) and for functional independence (younger 14.3% vs 6.7%; older 0% vs 0%) (Figures 11.7, 11.10).

Timing of Hemicraniectomy

Observational series have suggested that outcomes are best if decompressive surgery is performed relatively early during the first 24–36 hours, before substantial, and often irreversible, symptoms from initial stages of herniation have accrued. But early intervention in the absence of definite signs of herniation can result in delivering unnecessary surgical treatment to some patients who were not actually destined for herniation under medical therapy alone. The optimal timepoint at which to pursue hemicraniectomy has been the focus of one RCT, enrolling 46 patients with large

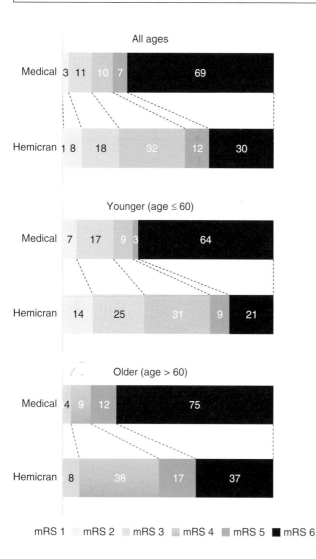

Figure 11.10 *Level of disability at 1–1.5 years, hemicraniectomy (hemicran) versus medical therapy,* pooled cross-trial data.

anterior circulation infarcts (Elsawaf and Galhom, 2018). Patients were enrolled if they: (1) were within 6 hours of presentation; (2) had occlusion of the internal carotid or mainstem middle cerebral artery; and (3) had ischaemic injury volume greater than 145 mL on diffusion MRI. Enrolled patients were randomized to immediate hemicraniectomy versus initial medical management with reactive hemicraniectomy if signs of reduced level of consciousness or uncal herniation developed. Mortality by 6 months was lower with immediate versus delayed craniectomy, 11% versus 52% (RR: 0.20, 95% CI: 0.05–0.79; $p = 0.02$). Functional outcomes were also improved, e.g. alive and capable of ambulation and basic self-care or better (mRS 0–3), 58% versus 26% (RR: 2.23, 95% CI: 1.06–4.70; $p = 0.03$).

Comment

Interpretation of the Evidence

These data indicate that hemicraniectomy is highly effective as a lifesaving procedure in patients with large hemispheric infarcts, but only moderately effective in increasing good functional outcomes and ineffective in increasing excellent outcomes, while being associated with a substantial increase in poor, chronically dependent outcomes.

- In younger individuals up to age 60, hemicraniectomy enables 43 more of 100 treated patients to survive, but only 5 more attain functional independence (mRS 2), 6 more achieve ambulation with dependence (mRS 3), and none achieves freedom from disability (mRS 0–1), while 28 more end up severely or extremely disabled (mRS 4–5).

- The tradeoff is even more challenging in older patients. Among those older than age 60, hemicraniectomy enables 37 more of 100 treated patients to survive, but none achieves freedom from disability (mRS 0–1) or functional independence (mRS 2); perhaps 1 or 2 more achieve ambulation with dependence (mRS 3), but 35 more end up severely or extremely disabled (mRS 4–5).

Implications for Practice

As hemicraniectomy is of proven lifesaving value, but will increase the frequency of severely disabled outcomes more than good functional outcomes, it is critical to educate patients and families regarding the tradeoffs associated with intervention. The patient's perspective on the desirability of treatment is of paramount importance in guiding decision-making, and should be directly elicited if the individual retains communication ability. If the patient cannot currently effectively communicate, his or her perspectives should still play a determinative role if possible, eliciting them based on reports of pre-stroke discussions with family and healthcare providers, and advance directives. As age is strongly associated with prognosis, younger patient age favours a more aggressive therapeutic approach to use of hemicraniectomy. Additional favourable prognostic factors, including excellent pre-stroke function, few medical comorbidities, and non-dominant hemisphere infarction location, also are factors that provide some support for decompressive surgical intervention. Of note, a meta-analysis of studies involving interviews of 382 patients with moderate-to-severe residual physical disability long term after hemicraniectomy found a substantial majority reported worthwhile quality of life (Rahme et al., 2012).

Implications for Research

The optimal timing and patient selection method for hemicraniectomy require further study. The single completed RCT supported early over delayed surgery, but did not use sophisticated monitoring in the initial medical treatment group to identify patients with progressing oedema at an early stage. The best combination of early patient features to use to trigger the decision to proceed to hemicraniectomy, such as imaged initial infarct volume, imaged degree of midline shift, early pace and

trajectory of imaged brain swelling, ICP elevation, and initial mild clinical herniation symptoms, merits clarification by further randomized trials comparing different selection algorithms.

Posterior Fossa Decompression

Physiological reasoning suggests that suboccipital craniectomy with dural expansion, with or without infarct resection, has the potential to be more unequivocally beneficial for large cerebellar infarcts than is hemicraniectomy for anterior circulation infarcts. The smaller size of the posterior fossa cranial vault more tightly restricts how much infarct swelling can accrue before herniation begins. The cerebellum itself has a highly redundant neural architecture, permitting good eventual recovery of function, even after substantial volumetric injury, if damage to surrounding structures can be averted. In addition, the immediately adjacent structures jeopardized by cerebellar herniation are of extreme functional importance: (1) occlusion of the 4th ventricle CSF channel may cause non-communicating hydrocephalus with generalized brain injury and herniation, and (2) direct herniation into the pons, distorting the brainstem, may cause rapidly devastating, often fatal, compromise of brainstem function. Observational series have provided supportive, albeit uncontrolled, evidence of clinical benefit of suboccipital craniectomy. In one multicentre series of 84 patients with massive cerebellar infarction, 40% were treated with surgical craniotomies and 17% with ventricular drainage, and 74% had non-disabled (mRS 0–1) final outcome (Jauss et al., 1999). No randomized trials of suboccipital craniectomy against medical therapy alone have been performed in patients with large cerebellar infarcts. Given the strength of the physiological considerations favouring decompressive surgery, and the available observational evidence of benefit, many investigators lack scientific equipoise. Also, sizeable cerebellar infarcts are uncommon, though not rare, further making RCTs challenging to complete.

On the basis of the available evidence, suboccipital craniectomy with dural expansion appears to be beneficial in patients with massive cerebellar infarctions who are deteriorating neurologically despite maximal medical therapy, conferring both survival and often good final functional capacity (Wijdicks et al., 2014). While randomized trials against medical therapy alone are likely infeasible, the best combination of early patient features to trigger the decision to proceed to suboccipital craniectomy, such as imaged initial infarct volume, imaged degree of downward or upward early herniation, early pace and trajectory of imaged brain swelling, and initial mild clinical herniation symptoms, merits clarification by randomized trials comparing different selection algorithms.

Summary

Among medical therapies, osmotherapy with colloidal agents (mannitol, glycerol) or crystalloid agents (hypertonic saline) is reasonable for patients whose condition is deteriorating due to mass effect and herniation from large anterior circulation hemispheric infarcts or cerebellar infarcts, especially as bridging therapies to more definitive surgical intervention or until the imminent end of the period of maximal post-stroke brain swelling. Hyperventilation and hypothermia may also be reasonable to deploy, though are currently of uncertain benefit and require randomized trial evaluation. The use of corticosteroids is not supported by currently available evidence. Agents that block sulfonylurea receptor-mediated cellular swelling, such as intravenous glyburide, have shown promise but require pivotal trial testing.

Ventriculostomy is useful to treat non-communicating hydrocephalus arising from obstruction of cerebrospinal fluid flow pathways by swollen brain infarcts. But in select large cerebellar infarcts, ventricular drainage in the absence of external decompression has the potential to exacerbate upward herniation of swollen cerebellar tissues, and should be avoided, proceeding instead directly to suboccipital craniectomy along with ventricular drainage.

Decompressive surgery is a potent treatment for brain oedema and mass effect from large cerebral infarcts. Suboccipital craniectomy, often with resection of infarcted tissue, is recommended for massive cerebellar infarcts that may herniate directly into the brainstem, on the basis of powerful physiological and observational evidence, even though randomized controlled trials are lacking.

Hemicraniectomy for brain oedema associated with large anterior circulation hemispheric infarction is a lifesaving measure, but survivors are more often left with severe rather than moderate lifelong disability, especially in individuals older than age 60. Discussions regarding the benefits and drawbacks of hemicraniectomy should be initiated early in individuals with large hemispheric infarcts, eliciting patient and family valuing of potential health outcome states and preferences for or against surgical intervention. If pursued, hemicraniectomy is generally best performed within the first 48 hours of onset and before the development of advanced herniation and neurological deterioration.

References

Alexander P, Heels-Ansdell D, Siemieniuk R, Bhatnagar N, Chang Y, Fei Y, et al. (2016). Hemicraniectomy versus medical treatment with large MCA infarct: a review and meta-analysis. *BMJ Open*, 6(11), e014390. doi:10.1136/bmjopen-2016-014390.

Bereczki D, Liu M, Fernandes do Prado G, Fekete I. (2007). Mannitol for acute stroke. *Cochrane Database Syst Rev*, 3. CD001153. doi:10.1002/14651858.CD001153.pub2.

Biestro A, Alberti R, Galli R, Cancela M, Soca A, Panzardo H, et al. (1997). Osmotherapy for increased intracranial pressure: comparison between mannitol and glycerol. *Acta Neurochir (Wien)*, 139, 725–32.

Coles JP, Fryer TD, Coleman MR, Smielewski P, Gupta AK, Minhas PS, et al. (2007). Hyperventilation following head injury: effect on ischemic burden and cerebral oxidative metabolism. *Crit Care Med*, 35, 568–78.

Cruz-Flores S, Berge E, Whittle IR. (2012). Surgical decompression for cerebral oedema in acute ischaemic stroke. *Cochrane Database Syst Rev*, 1. CD003435. doi:10.1002/14651858.CD003435.pub2.

Davis SM, Donnan GA. (2004). Steroids for stroke: another potential therapy discarded prematurely? *Stroke*, 35, 230–1.

Diringer MN, Scalfani MT, Zazulia AR, Videen TO, Dhar R. (2011). Cerebral hemodynamic and metabolic effects of equi-osmolar doses mannitol and 23.4% saline in patients with edema following large ischemic stroke. *Neurocrit Care*, 14, 11–17.

Elsawaf A, Galhom A. (2018). Decompressive craniotomy for malignant middle cerebral artery infarction: optimal timing and literature review. *World Neurosurg*, 116, e71–e78.

Fang J, Yang Y, Wang W, Liu Y, An T, Zou M, et al. (2018). Comparison of equiosmolar hypertonic saline and mannitol for brain relaxation during craniotomies: a meta-analysis of randomized controlled trials. *Neurosurg Rev*, 41, 945–56.

Fink ME. Osmotherapy for intracranial hypertension: mannitol versus hypertonic saline. *Continuum (Minneap Minn)* 2012, 18, 640–54.

Gujjar AR, Deibert E, Manno EM, Duff S, Diringer MN. (1998). Mechanical ventilation for ischemic stroke and intracerebral hemorrhage: indications, timing, and outcome. *Neurology*, 51, 447–51.

Jauss M, Krieger D, Hornig C, Schramm J, Busse O. (1999). Surgical and medical management of patients with massive cerebellar infarctions: results of the German-Austrian Cerebellar Infarction Study. *J Neurol*, 246, 257–64.

Jeon SB, Koh Y, Choi HA, Lee K. (2014). Critical care for patients with massive ischemic stroke. *J Stroke*, **16**, 146–60.

King ZA, Sheth KN, Kimberly WT, Simard JM. (2018). Profile of intravenous glyburide for the prevention of cerebral edema following large hemispheric infarction: evidence to date. *Drug Des Devel Ther*, **12**, 2539–52.

Kleinman JT, Saver JL, Liebeskind DS, Sharma LK, Gonzalez N, Blanco MB, et al. (2017). DESTINY II joint outcome table analysis: number needed to treat and benefit per hundred. *Neurocrit Care*, **27**, S168.

Koenig MA, Bryan M, Lewin JL 3rd, Mirski MA, Geocadin RG, Stevens RD. (2008). Reversal of transtentorial herniation with hypertonic saline. *Neurology*, **70**, 1023–9.

Lewis SR, Pritchard MW, Evans DJ, Butler AR, Alderson P, Smith AF, et al. (2018). Colloids versus crystalloids for fluid resuscitation in critically ill people. *Cochrane Database Syst Rev*, **8**. CD000567.

Li M, Chen T, Chen SD, Cai J, Hu YH. (2015). Comparison of equimolar doses of mannitol and hypertonic saline for the treatment of elevated intracranial pressure after traumatic brain injury: a systematic review and meta-analysis. *Medicine*, **94**, e736.

Nael K, Knitter JR, Jahan R, Gornbein J, Ajani Z, Feng L, et al. (2017). Multiparametric magnetic resonance imaging for prediction of parenchymal hemorrhage in acute ischemic stroke after reperfusion therapy. *Stroke*, **48**, 664–70.

Norris JW. (2004). Steroids may have a role in stroke therapy. *Stroke*, **35**, 228–9.

Ong CJ, Keyrouz SG, Diringer MN. (2015). The role of osmotic therapy in hemispheric stroke. *Neurocrit Care*, **23**, 285–91.

Pagani-Estévez GL, Couillard P, Lanzino G, Wijdicks EF, Rabinstein AA. (2016). Acutely trapped ventricle: clinical significance and benefit from surgical decompression. *Neurocrit Care*, **24**, 110–17.

Pasarikovski CR, Alotaibi NM, Al-Mufti F, Macdonald RL. (2017). Hypertonic saline for increased intracranial pressure after aneurysmal subarachnoid hemorrhage: a systematic review. *World Neurosurg*, **105**, 1–6.

Rahme R, Zuccarello M, Kleindorfer D, Adeoye OM, Ringer AJ. (2012). Decompressive hemicraniectomy for malignant middle cerebral artery territory infarction: is life worth living? *J Neurosurg*, **117**, 749–54.

Raimondi AJ, Tomita T. (1981). Hydrocephalus and infratentorial tumors. Incidence, clinical picture, and treatment. *J Neurosurg*, **55**, 174–82.

Renú A, Laredo C, Lopez-Rueda A, Llull L, Tudela R, San-Roman L, et al. (2017). Vessel wall enhancement and blood-cerebrospinal fluid barrier disruption after mechanical thrombectomy in acute ischemic stroke. *Stroke*, **48**, 651–7.

Righetti E, Celani MG, Cantisani TA, Sterzi R, Boysen G, Ricci S. (2004). Glycerol for acute stroke. *Cochrane Database Syst Rev*, **2**. CD000096.

Sandercock PAG, Soane T. (2011). Corticosteroids for acute ischaemic stroke. *Cochrane Database Syst Rev*, **2**. CD000065.

Santambrogio S, Martinotti R, Dardella F, Porro F, Randazzo A. (1978). Is there a real treatment for stroke? Clinical and statistical comparison of different treatments in 300 patients. *Stroke*, **9**, 130–2.

Saver JL, Gornbein J, Grotta J, Liebeskind D, Lutsep H, Schwamm L, et al. (2009). Number needed to treat to benefit and to harm for intravenous tissue plasminogen activator therapy in the 3- to 4.5-hour window: joint outcome table analysis of the ECASS 3 trial. *Stroke*, **40**, 2433–2437

Schreckinger M, Marion DW. (2009). Contemporary management of traumatic intracranial hypertension: is there a role for therapeutic hypothermia? *Neurocrit Care*, **11**, 427–36.

Schwab S, Georgiadis D, Berrouschot J, Schellinger PD, Graffagnino C, Mayer SA. (2001). Feasibility and safety of moderate hypothermia after massive hemispheric infarction. *Stroke*, **32**, 2033–5.

Schwab S, Schwarz S, Spranger M, Keller E, Bertram M, Hacke W. (1998). Moderate hypothermia in the treatment of patients with severe middle cerebral artery infarction. *Stroke*, **29**, 2461–6.

Sheth KN, Elm JJ, Molyneaux BJ, Hinson H, Beslow LA, Sze GK, et al. (2016). Safety and efficacy of intravenous glyburide on brain swelling after large hemispheric infarction (GAMES-RP): a randomised, double-blind, placebo-controlled phase 2 trial. *Lancet Neurol*, **15**, 1160–9.

Simard JM, Tsymbalyuk N, Tsymbalyuk O, Ivanova S, Yurovsky V, Gerzanich V. (2010). Glibenclamide is superior to decompressive craniectomy in a rat model of malignant stroke. *Stroke*, **41**, 531–37.

Treib J, Becker SC, Grauer M, Haass A. (1998). Transcranial doppler monitoring of intracranial pressure therapy with mannitol, sorbitol and glycerol in patients with acute stroke. *Eur Neurol*, **40**, 212–19.

Videen TO, Zazulia AR, Manno EM, Derdeyn CP Adams RE, Diringer MN, et al. (2001). Mannitol bolus preferentially shrinks noninfarcted brain in patients with ischemic stroke. *Neurology*, **57**, 2120–2.

Wijdicks EFM, Sheth KN, Carter BS, Greer DM, Kasner SE, Kimberly WT, et al.; on behalf of the American Heart Association Stroke Council. (2014). Recommendations for the management of cerebral and cerebellar infarction with swelling. *Stroke*, **45**, 1222–38.

Neuroprotection for Acute Brain Ischaemia

Nerses Sanossian
Jeffrey L. Saver

Rationale

Normally, cerebral blood flow (CBF) is maintained by cerebral autoregulation at about 50 mL blood/100 g brain/min. In acute ischaemic stroke, a cerebral artery is occluded or there is a reduction in perfusion distal to a severe stenosis, resulting in focal brain ischaemia and infarction. As the regional CBF falls, the regional lack of oxygen and glucose results in a time- and flow-dependent cascade characterized by a fall in energy (adenosine triphosphate [ATP]) production. Neuronal function is affected in two stages. The first threshold is at a blood flow of about 20 mL blood/100 g brain/min, below which neuronal electrical function is compromised, generating clinical deficits, but cellular homeostasis is maintained and recovery remains possible. However, if blood flow falls below the second critical threshold of 10 mL blood/100 g brain/min, an 'ischaemic cascade' of injurious molecular events is triggered (Doyle et al., 2008; Sekerdag et al., 2018). Free radicals are generated. There is excessive release and impaired reuptake of excitatory amino acid (EAA) neurotransmitters such as glutamate, causing overstimulation of neuronal glutamate receptors (excitotoxicity), aerobic mitochondrial metabolism fails, inefficient anaerobic metabolism of glucose takes over, and harmful lactic acidosis evolves. Energy-dependent homoeostatic mechanisms of maintaining cellular ions fail, potassium leaks out of cells, and sodium, water, and calcium enter cells, leading to cytotoxic oedema and calcium-induced mitochondrial failure, respectively. If severe ischaemia (blood flow below 10 mL blood/100 g brain/min) is sustained, irreversible neuronal damage occurs and neuronal cell apoptosis and necrosis ensue.

Preclinical and neuroimaging studies indicate that the untreated penumbra deteriorates over time (Bardutzy et al., 2005; Heiss, 2011). This concept is supported by analyses of reperfusion therapies for acute cerebral ischaemia, which showed greater benefits

of reperfusion by intravenous thrombolysis and by endovascular mechanical thrombectomy with earlier treatment (Emberson et al., 2014; Saver et al., 2016). Just how long ischaemic human brain may survive, and therefore the time window for therapeutic intervention, varies from individual to individual, reflecting degree of CBF compromise, robustness of collateral flow, differential tolerance of grey and white matter to ischaemia, and additional factors. Within the first 3–6 hours after ischaemia onset, nearly all patients still harbour salvageable tissue; from 6 to 24 hours and beyond, a steadily increasing proportion of patients have no remaining tissue at risk, having completed their strokes, but an important, slower progressing subset of patients still possess rescuable tissues.

Neuroprotective treatments are therapies that interrupt the cellular, biochemical, and metabolic processes that lead to brain injury during or after exposure to ischaemia and encompass a wide array of pharmacological and device interventions that block the molecular elaboration of cellular injury in brain tissues exposed to ischaemic stress (Ovbiagele et al., 2003). Neuroprotective treatments may have some mild potential benefits as standalone therapies in settings in which tissues are exposed to permanent ischaemia. However, the settings in which they are likely to exert their greatest benefit are those in which ischaemia will be transient, and neuroprotective interventions can enable ischaemic tissues to tolerate the ischaemic insult until the ischaemia is relieved. A major potential role of neuroprotective therapies is in spontaneous ischaemic stroke, where they can support the ischaemic penumbra until CBF is restored by intravenous thrombolysis and/or endovascular mechanical thrombectomy. They also could be helpful during surgical and endovascular procedures in which the brain is exposed to ischaemia for a delimited period of time.

Although numerous neuroprotective agents have been found beneficial in various preclinical stroke models, successful translation to human stroke patients has been challenging. Over 100 neuroprotective interventions showing signals of effect in preclinical stroke models have been advanced to human clinical trial testing and none was found to be of definite proven benefit (O'Collins et al., 2006; Hong et al., 2011). Several deficiencies in preclinical study and clinical trial designs have been identified as likely contributing to this breakdown in translation (Ovbiagele et al., 2003; O'Collins et al., 2006; Fisher et al., 2009; Lapchak et al., 2013). Preclinical experimental studies have often failed to use robust randomization and blinding techniques to avert bias, started treatments much earlier than achievable in the human clinical setting, and tested agents in young, otherwise healthy rodents and other species rather than older animals with multiple comorbidities. Human clinical trials have often failed to start therapies in the very first minutes and hours after onset, when treatment effect would be maximal, and to confine enrolment to patients likely to have transient rather than permanent ischaemic exposure.

The promise of, and the need for, effective brain cytoprotection remains great, despite past disappointments in neuroprotective development programmes. Reperfusion therapies, which require brain imaging and transport to a treatment-capable centre prior to start, will always have their treatment benefit constrained by the brain injury that accumulates before they can be initiated. For example, in pivotal trials, endovascular mechanical thrombectomy tremendously improves patient outcomes compared with no endovascular intervention, and yet 73% of the patients treated with endovascular therapy still have disabled (modified Rankin Scale [mRS] 2–6) outcomes at 3 months. Neuroprotective agents, many of which are safe and potentially beneficial for haemorrhagic as well as ischaemic stroke, could be started much earlier than reperfusion therapies, in the ambulance or self-administered at home, preserving more brain in a salvageable state until reperfusion can be achieved, potentially substantially magnifying the benefit of CBF restoration. Given the robust signals of benefit of neuroprotection in preclinical focal ischaemic stroke models and the demonstrated benefit of neuroprotection with hypothermia in human global brain ischaemia, there is excellent reason to hope that improved preclinical and clinical study designs will yield clinically useful agents for human stroke.

Among the many classes and individual examples of neuroprotective agents that have been tested in ischaemic stroke, this chapter will review several of the most studied and most promising. A broad mechanistic classification of neuroprotective interventions, with listing of several individual agents, is shown in Table 12.1, and includes: (1) Metabolism Suppressors, (2) Promoters of Genetically Programmed Hypoxia/Injury Tolerance, (3) Free Radical Scavengers and Anti-Oxidants, (4) Promoters of Membrane Repair, (5) Modulators of Excitatory Amino Acids, (6) Modulators of Calcium Influx, (7) Sodium Channel Blockers, (8) Modulators of GABA Inhibition, (9) Nitric Oxide Donors, (10) Modulators of Carnitine + Mitochondrial Function, (11) Anti-Inflammatory, (12) Oxygen Delivery Enhancers, (13) Agents with Multiple Leading Mechanisms, and (14) Uncertain Mechanism.

Hypothermia

Hypothermia is a quintessentially pleiotropic neuroprotective intervention, concurrently inhibiting many of the molecular pathways that elaborate ischaemic injury to neural tissues (Kurisu and Yenari, 2018). Hypothermia decreases the cerebral metabolic rate and metabolic demand, reducing the mismatch between energy supply and energy demand. Hypothermia additionally reduces free radical production, excitotoxicity, apoptosis, and inflammation. Mild (35–36°C), moderate (32–34°C), and profound (<32°C) hypothermia all have protective effects in preclinical models of ischaemic stroke. Achieving profound hypothermia in human patients requires intubation and sedation, to prevent shivering and respiratory compromise. Moderate hypothermia, however, can be achieved in awake patients with concomitant medications to reduce shivering.

Profound hypothermia is already routinely applied to counter the effects of cerebral hypoxia in neurosurgery and open-heart surgery. In cardiac arrest with global brain ischaemia, moderate (32–33°C) hypothermia improves outcome (Arrich et al., 2016). In acute stroke, a high body temperature has been associated with a worse prognosis (Marehbian and Greer, 2017) (see Chapter 5), but it is not known if lowering temperature improves prognosis. Some temperature-lowering agents, like non-steroidal anti-inflammatory drugs, have antiplatelet activity and

Table 12.1 Select categories and examples of neuroprotective agents to protect brain tissue

Category	Agents
Metabolism Suppressors	Hypothermia – profound* Hypothermia – mild–moderate* Transcranial direct current stimulation
Promoters of Genetically Programmed Hypoxia/ Injury Tolerance and Repair	Ischaemic per-conditioning* Ischaemic post-conditioning* Growth factors*
Free Radical Scavengers and Antioxidants	Uric acid* Edaravone* Tirilazad* Disufenton sodium (NXY-059)* Ebselen
Promoters of Membrane Repair	Citicoline*
Modulators of Excitatory Amino Acids	NMDA receptor antagonists* Dextrorphan* Ketamine Xenon Postsynaptic scaffolding proteins* NA-1* AMPA and other receptor antagonists
Modulators of Calcium Influx	Nimodipine* Flunarizine*
Sodium Channel Blockers	Fosphenytoin* Lidocaine
Modulators of GABA Inhibition	Clomethiazole* Diazepam*
Nitric Oxide Donors	Glyceryl trinitrate* L-arginine
Modulators of Carnitine + Mitochondrial Function	Mildronate Coenzyme Q10
Anti-Inflammatory	Enlimomab* Neutrophil inhibitory factor*
Oxygen Delivery Enhancers	Normobaric hyperoxaemia Hyperbaric hyperoxaemia* Aqueous oxygen Trans sodium crocetinate* Haemoglobin-based oxygen carriers*
Multiple Leading Mechanisms	Statins* Minocycline* Magnesium* Albumin* Gangliosides* Melatonin
Uncertain Mechanism	Piracetam*

* Agents receiving focused analysis in this chapter, due to availability in practice, historical importance, and/or current promise.

NMDA: N-methyl-D-aspartate. AMPA: α-amino-3-hydroxy-5-methylisoxazole-4-propionic acid. GABA: gamma-aminobutyric acid.

could increase the risk of bleeding in acute ischaemic and haemorrhagic stroke. Other risks associated with induced hypothermia are mainly sepsis, pneumonia, and coagulopathy.

Evidence

Hypothermia as a neuroprotective intervention for acute ischaemic stroke has largely been evaluated in small randomized trials designed to develop and

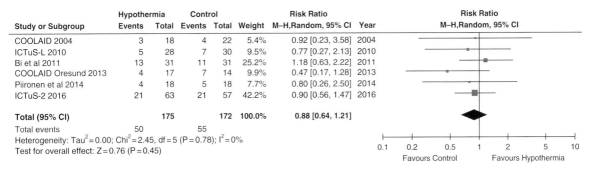

Figure 12.1 Forest plot showing the effects of *hypothermia vs control* for acute ischaemic stroke on *freedom from disability (mRS 0–1) at long-term follow-up.*

validate technically effective regimens for rapid and sustained cooling to targeted temperature and control of shivering, using both surface cooling and indwelling vascular cooling devices. With more recent regimens, rapid attainment and tight maintenance of targeted moderate hypothermia in awake patients has been achieved, and absence of major adverse interaction with intravenous thrombolysis demonstrated. However, in these feasibility and regimen optimization studies, time from onset to enrolment and to time of first achievement of cerebral hypothermia has been prolonged. A meta-analysis of 6 randomized trials enrolling a total of 311 patients does not show a difference in the frequency of disability-free (mRS 0–1) outcome with hypothermia versus control, 25.9% versus 29.6%, risk ratio (RR) 0.88 (95% confidence interval [CI]: 0.64–1.47) (Figure 12.1) (Wan et al., 2014; Lyden et al., 2016).

Hypothermia has also been studied as an antioedema therapy for malignant middle cerebral artery infarction, as reviewed in Chapter 11.

Adverse Effects

Across the 6 randomized trials of hypothermia in human focal ischaemic stroke, mortality did not differ between treated and control groups. An increased risk of pneumonia was observed, 20.0% versus 7.6% (RR 2.65; 95% CI: 1.45–4.83). No differences were found for symptomatic intracerebral haemorrhage (SICH), fatal intracerebral haemorrhage (ICH), deep vein thrombosis (DVT), or atrial fibrillation.

Comment

Human clinical trials have refined device and shivering-control regimens to enable achievement of hypothermia efficiently in awake patients presenting with focal ischaemic stroke. However, there is no evidence from combined analysis of the small randomized controlled trials (RCTs) completed to date that hypothermia improves neurological outcomes in patients with acute ischaemic stroke. In addition, multiple studies have identified increased rates of pneumonia in the hypothermia group. With the advent of endovascular thrombectomy abrogating prolonged ischaemia in many large vessel occlusion patients, hypothermia as a prolonged neuroprotective intervention is no longer a needed therapy. However, hypothermia might play useful roles if it is: (1) initiated as soon as possible after onset, as bridging therapy in the prehospital setting; (2) given after successful reperfusion, to avert reperfusion injury (as in cardiac arrest and global brain ischaemia); or (3) delivered selectively to the cerebrum, via helmet, nasal, or other channels, enabling selective cerebral hypothermia with reduced systemic complications. Future trials evaluating these approaches are desirable.

Ischaemic Conditioning

In ischaemic conditioning, an organ is exposed to one or more brief, non-lethal cycles of ischaemia and reperfusion, activating endogenous cellular protective pathways rendering the target organ more tolerant of prolonged ischaemia. The intermittent ischaemia challenges can occur directly to the target organ; for example, transient ischaemic attacks may render the brain more resistant to subsequent infarction. But the intermittent ischaemia challenges may also be delivered to remote sites, typically simply by intermittent inflation of a blood pressure cuff placed on one or more limbs, with induction of humoral signals that activate hypoxia resistance pathways throughout the body, including the brain (Hess et al., 2015).

In various preclinical models, remote ischaemic conditioning has been found to reduce brain injury when applied before (pre-conditioning), during (per-conditioning), and soon after (post-conditioning) the cerebral ischaemic insult (Wang et al., 2015). Several molecular mechanisms appear to contribute to cerebral ischaemic conditioning, including: (1) increasing antioxidant production and increasing DNA repair capacity; (2) anti-excitotoxic effects by inhibiting glutamate and increasing gamma-aminobutyric acid (GABA) release; (3) anti-inflammatory effects by stimulating Toll-like receptors, which activate proinflammatory pathways; (4) prevention of mitochondrial-dependent cell death pathways; and (5) release of adenosine and activation of adenosine A1 receptors (Narayanan et al., 2013).

Evidence

Two clinical trials have been completed evaluating remote ischaemic per-conditioning (RIPerC) as neuroprotection in the acute ischaemic stroke setting. In a single centre, open-label, blinded outcome observer, prehospital trial in Denmark, 443 patients were randomized and final outcome data were available in 224, with data missingness due to withdrawal of patients without final diagnosis of acute cerebral ischaemia and failure to initially obtain informed consent among patients in the control arm (Hougaard et al., 2014). The intervention arm received 4 inflations of a standard upper limb blood pressure cuff to 200, or 25 mm Hg above the patient's systolic blood pressure, each lasting 5 minutes and separated by 5 minutes of cuff deflation. Among the 133 RIPerC and 91 control patients with final diagnoses of ischaemic stroke or transient ischaemic attack, mixed effects were observed, with a favourable trend in symptom-free outcome (mRS 0), 57% versus 47%, RR 1.21 (95% CI: 0.93–1.57); no difference in disability-free (mRS 0–1) outcome, 72% versus 73%, RR 0.96 (95% CI: 0.81–1.13); and an adverse effect for functional independence (mRS 0–2), 80% versus 88%, RR 0.89 (95% CI: 0.79–0.99).

In a smaller, single centre, sham-controlled, in-hospital trial in Great Britain, 26 patients with ischaemic stroke were randomized to 4 cycles of 5 minutes' inflation in the nonparetic arm, 20 mm Hg above systolic blood pressure in the active group versus 30 mm Hg total in the sham group. The lead tolerability aim of the trial was met, with 12/13 active RIPerC arm patients tolerating and completing the intervention. No difference in disability levels at 3 months was noted, mean mRS for intervention versus control, 2.46 (±1.39) versus 2.69 (±1.79), $p = 0.8$ (England et al., 2017).

Adverse Effects

In the larger Danish trial, patients randomized to rPerC had a higher recall of pain ($p = 0.006$), but not of anxiety, sweating, palpitations, headaches, or nausea. There was no difference in mortality among the acute cerebral ischaemia patients, RIPerC versus control, 4% versus 1%, RR 3.42 (95% CI: 0.41–28.80).

Comments

Remote ischaemic per-conditioning has been shown to be feasible in patients with acute cerebral ischaemia, and without marked adverse effects. Whether further signals to activate hypoxia protection systems generated by remote induced ischaemia in the limbs usefully adds to the signals already being generated directly in the brain during an episode of prolonged cerebral ischaemia remains an open question. Larger trials are needed to definitively assess RIPerC for efficacy in patients experiencing acute cerebral ischaemia, as well as to explore remote ischaemic post-conditioning (RIPostC) to mitigate reperfusion injury and incomplete reperfusion among patients with successful thrombolytic or endovascular thrombectomy reperfusion.

Growth Factors

Growth factors are proteins that regulate the differentiation, survival, and proliferation of neurones, glia, fibroblasts, endothelial cells, and other cell types. Basic fibroblast growth factor (bFGF) promotes neuronal sprouting and proliferation of capillaries and glia during stroke recovery, facilitating neural repair and functional recovery (Paciaroni and Bogousslavsky, 2011). In addition, in stroke models, bFGF initiates a signal transduction cascade, resulting in the expression of cytoprotective genes and their proteins, facilitating cell survival, and reducing infarct volume.

Evidence

Trafermin, a recombinant native form of basic fibroblast growth factor, was studied in 3 double-blind trials in acute ischaemic stroke patients, including 1 dose-escalation trial and 2 pivotal trials. A phase 3 trial in patients within 6 hours of stroke onset in North

America was halted after enrolment of 303 patients on advice of the Data and Safety Monitoring Board (DSMB), due to an increase in adverse neurological events and mortality with active agent. In contrast, a European–Australian phase 3 trial was stopped early for futility, rather than safety, after randomizing 286 patients within 6 hours of stroke onset to 5 or 10 mg of trafermin or placebo intravenously (IV) infused over 24 hours (Paciaroni and Bogousslavsky, 2011). The primary endpoint was favourable outcome at 90 days on a categorized combination of the Barthel and Rankin scales, and did not differ for the 5 mg of trafermin versus placebo (odds ratio [OR]: 1.2, 95% CI: 0.72–2.00, $p = 0.48$) or 10 mg of trafermin versus placebo (OR: 0.74, 95% CI: 0.44–1.22, $p = 0.24$). Mortality rates at 90 days were 17% in the 5 mg group, 24% in the 10 mg group, and 18% in the placebo group. Treatment with trafermin was associated with an increase in leucocytosis and a mean greater decrease in systolic blood pressure (BP) versus placebo of 11 mm Hg in the 5 mg group and 13 mm Hg in the 10 mg group. In a *post hoc* subgroup analysis, patients in the 5 mg group treated more than 5 hours after the onset of symptoms showed an apparent advantage over placebo (OR: 2.1, 95% CI: 1.00–4.41, $p = 0.044$; after age adjustment: OR: 1.9, 95% CI: 0.91–4.13, $p = 0.08$).

Comment

Completed RCTs are modest in size but do not suggest a major neuroprotective effect of bFGF in the acute period of ischaemic stroke. Given its blood pressure lowering effects, which may reduce collateral flow in the acute setting, and its potential for enhancing neuroplasticity in the subacute period, additional studies of bFGF as a subacute neuroreparative agent may be worthwhile.

Free Radical Scavengers and Antioxidants

Free radical, reactive oxygen and nitrogen species are produced by cellular enzymes in settings of oxidative stress, including ischaemia, and damage cellular integrity. Enzymatic and non-enzymatic antioxidant molecules react in one-electron reactions with free radicals to avert oxidative damage (Davis and Pennypacker, 2017).

Uric Acid

Uric acid is the end product of purine degradation in humans and the most abundant antioxidant in the

human body, accounting for up to 60% of plasma antioxidative capacity. Exogenously administered uric acid reduces infarct volume in rodent models of focal cerebral ischaemia (Romanos et al., 2007). In a meta-analysis of 10 observational studies with a total of 8131 acute ischaemic stroke patients, high compared with low serum uric acid level was associated with reduced poor outcomes after acute ischaemic stroke (hazard ratio [HR] = 0.77, 95% CI: 0.68–0.88, $p = 0.0001$) (Wang et al., 2016).

Evidence

Uric acid has been studied in one double-blind, placebo-controlled trial, with 421 ischaemic stroke patients treated with alteplase randomized to 1000 mg intravenous uric acid or placebo over 90 minutes (Chamorro et al., 2014). In the active treatment group, median time from onset to start of alteplase was 140 minutes and from onset to start of uric acid 175 minutes. For the primary 3-month outcome, freedom from disability (mRS 0–1) or continued functional independence if premorbid mRS was 2, a trend to benefit was noted: 39% versus 33%, adjusted RR 1.23 (95% CI: 0.96–1.56), $p = 0.10$). For the secondary endpoint of favourable shift toward reduced disability at 3 months (on a 6-level version of the mRS), a favourable trend was also noted, OR 1.40 (95% CI: 0.99–1.98), $p = 0.06$. The frequency of mortality, symptomatic ICH, and gouty arthritis was similar between the two treatment groups.

Comment

One moderate-sized randomized trial non-significantly suggests that uric acid may be beneficial as a neuroprotective agent in acute ischaemic stroke. Larger randomized trials are warranted to definitively evaluate the potential benefits of acute uric acid therapy.

Edaravone

Edaravone (3-methyl-1-phenyl-2-pyrazolin-5-one) is a broad scavenger of free hydroxyl radicals and peroxynitrite radicals, with evidence in mechanistic studies of protecting neurones, glia, and vascular endothelial cells against oxidative stress.

Evidence

Edaravone has been tested in at least 16 randomized trials for ischaemic stroke, including 10 trials with entire or reported subgroup enrolment within the early post-onset (<48 h) period, enrolling 983 patients

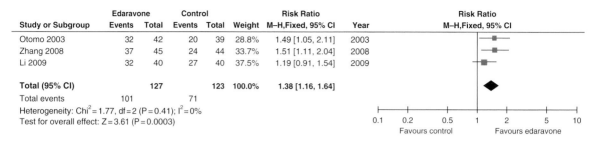

Study or Subgroup	Edaravone Events	Total	Control Events	Total	Weight	Risk Ratio M–H,Fixed, 95% CI	Year
Otomo 2003	32	42	20	39	28.8%	1.49 [1.05, 2.11]	2003
Zhang 2008	37	45	24	44	33.7%	1.51 [1.11, 2.04]	2008
Li 2009	32	40	27	40	37.5%	1.19 [0.91, 1.54]	2009
Total (95% CI)		**127**		**123**	**100.0%**	**1.38 [1.16, 1.64]**	
Total events	101		71				

Heterogeneity: Chi^2 = 1.77, df = 2 (P = 0.41); I^2 = 0%
Test for overall effect: Z = 3.61 (P = 0.0003)

Figure 12.2 Forest plot showing the effects of *edaravone vs control* for acute ischaemic stroke on *functional independence (mRS 0–2 or nearest equivalent)* at long-term follow-up.

(Yang et al., 2015). In these trials, daily edaravone dosage was 60 mg in all, and duration of treatment was median 14 (7–28) days. Adequate protection against bias was not clearly present in the trials, with allocation concealment not clearly described in all trials and double-blind conduct only clearly described in 1 of 10 trials. Among the 3 trials with disability outcome assessment, in 250 patients (127 edaravone, 123 control) edaravone was associated with increased functional independence at long-term follow-up, 79.5% versus 57.7%, RR 1.38 (95% CI: 1.16–1.64), $p = 0.0003$ (Figure 12.2). Among the 8 trials assessing neurological deficit at long-term follow-up on the 100-point European Stroke Scale, in 843 patients (421 edaravone, 422 control), edaravone was associated with reduced neurological deficit, mean difference 7.09 (95% CI: 5.12–9.05), $p < 0.00001$.

Adverse events were analysed across randomized trials for patients with both ischaemic and haemorrhagic stroke. The only signal of a potential adverse event was a trend toward increased mild renal impairment in 3.25% (11/338) versus 1.49% (5/335), RR 1.78 (95% CI: 0.74–4.29), $p = 0.20$.

Comment

Edaravone shows potential promise as a neuroprotective agent for acute ischaemic stroke. However, encouraging efficacy and safety findings among completed trials must be interpreted cautiously, as risk of bias is formally present in all trials reported to date. In addition, the relatively late start and prolonged duration of administration of edaravone in completed trials suggests that completed trials have not closely explored acute neuroprotection for the presenting ischaemic stroke, but rather focused more upon prophylactic neuroprotection against recurrent ischaemic insults and neuroreparative effects. Further trials with rigorous double-blinding and hyperacute treatment start are merited.

Tirilazad

Tirilazad mesylate is a lipid soluble synthetic, non-glucocorticoid, 21-aminosteroid (or lazaroid) that inhibits iron-dependent lipid peroxidation within membranes. However, in 6 randomized trials enrolling 1757 patients with acute ischaemic stroke, tirilazad was associated with increased odds of being dead or disabled at long-term follow-up on the expanded Barthel Index (OR 1.23, 95% CI: 1.01–1.51) and increased odds of infusion site phlebitis (OR 2.81, 95% CI: 2.14–3.69) (Bath et al., 2001). Accordingly, tirilazad has not entered clinical practice and is no longer under active development.

Disufenton Sodium (NXY-059)

Disufenton sodium (NXY-059) is a free-radical trapping agent. Although a first phase 3 trial enrolling 1722 patients had positive results on the primary endpoint of degree of disability at 3 months post-stroke, a second phase 3 trial was non-confirmatory. Pooled, individual participant-level analysis of 5028 patients across both trials found no effect in shifting to a lower disability level, OR 1.02 (95% CI: 0.92–1.13), $p = 0.68$, and no difference in mortality, 16.6% versus 16.4% (Diener et al., 2008). Accordingly, disufenton sodium has not entered clinical practice and is no longer under active development.

Promoters of Membrane Repair

Citicoline

Citicoline (or cytidine-5′-diphosphoholine, CDP-choline) is an intermediate metabolite in membrane phosphatide biosynthesis, normally present in all cells in the body. In preclinical models, exogenously administered citicoline promotes rapid repair of injured cell surface and mitochondrial membranes and maintenance of cell integrity and bioenergetic capacity, downregulates phospholipases to avert apoptotic and necrotic cell death, and reduces free fatty acid release and ensuing generation of injurious free radicals (Saver, 2008).

Evidence

A meta-analysis identified 10 randomized trials of citicoline in ischaemic stroke, enrolling 4420 patients (Secades et al., 2016) The preponderance of trials enrolled patients within 24–48 hours of onset, with 2 trials enrolling 305 patients (7%) having longer enrolment windows of 7–14 days. Few patients in any trial were enrolled in the first few hours of onset; in the largest ICTUS trial, which had a 24-hour enrolment window, the median time from onset to enrolment was 6.7 hours (Dávalos et al., 2012). Across trials, study treatment was administered for up to 10 days to 6 weeks, and doses ranged from 500–2000 mg daily.

Functional Independence

Across the 10 trials, treatment with citicoline was associated with an increased frequency of functional independence (mRS 0–2 or nearest equivalent) at long-term follow-up, 36.4% versus 31.6%, RR (random effect) 1.20 (95% CI: 1.05–1.55), $p = 0.02$ (Figure 12.3). However, substantial heterogeneity was noted, $I^2 = 68\%$, and funnel plot analysis showed some asymmetry suggesting potential publication bias with under-reporting of smaller, nonpositive or less positive trials. The largest and most recent trial, ICTUS, enrolled 2298 patients,

accounting for 52% of all patients in the 10-trial meta-analysis, and had neutral results (Dávalos et al., 2012).

Safety

None of the trials reported any adverse events occurring more frequently in the citicoline than the control groups.

Subgroups

In the large ICTUS trial, enrolling 2298 patients, overall results were neutral on the primary endpoint of recovery at 90 days, measured by a global test combining three measures of success, mRS $\leq$ 1, National Institutes of Health Stroke Scale (NIHSS) $\leq$ 1, and Barthel Index $\geq$ 95, with OR 1.03 (95% CI: 0.86–1.25; $p = 0.36$). However, heterogeneity of effect was noted for 3 of the 5 prespecified subgroups, with signals of greater benefit and less harm among patients over versus under age 70, $p_{\text{interaction}} = 0.001$, patients with less initial deficit severity (NIHSS 8–14 vs 15–22 and 22–42), $p_{\text{interaction}} = 0.02$, and patients ineligible for IV tPA, $p_{\text{interaction}} = 0.04$. Nonetheless, none of the better performing subgroup categories showed nominally significant benefit: age above 70 (OR 1.17, 95% CI: 0.82–1.50); lesser presenting deficit, (NIHSS 8–14, OR 1.08, 95% CI: 0.86–1.35); and IV tissue plasminogen activator (tPA) ineligible (OR 1.11, 95% CI: 0.85–1.46).

Comment

Current randomized trial evidence largely addresses relatively late start and prolonged continued administration of citicoline, and thus evaluates more for potential subacute neuroreparative than acute neuroprotective

Study or Subgroup	Citicoline Events	Total	Control Events	Total	Weight	Risk Ratio M–H,Random, 95% CI	Year	Risk Ratio M–H,Random, 95% CI
Goas 1980	16	31	8	33	5.8%	2.13 [1.06, 4.26]	1980	
Boundouresques 1980	11	23	2	22	1.8%	5.26 [1.31, 21.09]	1980	
Corso 1982	7	17	0	16	0.5%	14.17 [0.87, 229.48]	1982	
Tazaki 1988	68	136	36	136	13.1%	1.89 [1.36, 2.62]	1988	
Citicoline Stroke Study Group Trial 1 1997	80	193	22	64	11.7%	1.21 [0.83, 1.76]	1997	
Citicoline Stroke Study Group Trial 2 - 1999	116	267	50	127	15.2%	1.10 [0.85, 1.42]	1999	
Citicoline 010 Trial - 2000	20	52	19	48	9.0%	0.97 [0.60, 1.59]	2000	
Citicoline Stroke Study Group Trial 3 - 2001	185	452	156	446	17.8%	1.17 [0.99, 1.38]	2001	
Alviarez 2007	13	29	10	30	6.4%	1.34 [0.70, 2.57]	2007	
ICTUS 2012	329	1148	343	1150	18.8%	0.96 [0.85, 1.09]	2012	
Total (95% CI)		**2348**		**2072**	**100.0%**	**1.28 [1.05, 1.55]**		
Total events	845		646					

Heterogeneity: Tau^2 = 0.05; Chi^2 = 27.76, df = 9 (P = 0.001); I^2 = 68%
Test for overall effect: Z = 2.42 (P = 0.02)

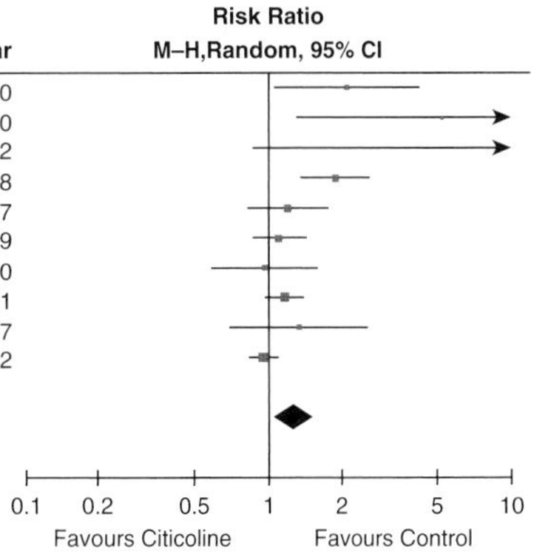

0.1 0.2 0.5 1 2 5 10
Favours Citicoline   Favours Control

Figure 12.3 Forest plot showing the effects of *citicoline vs control* for acute ischaemic stroke *for functional independence (mRS 0–2 or nearest equivalent)* at long-term follow-up.

treatment effects. The trials have demonstrated agent safety but provide mixed indications of potential benefit. Evidence of potential publication bias and neutral results in the largest single trial indicate caution when interpreting the mild favourable effect seen in meta-analytic summary of all trials. Brief administration of citicoline during the first few hours after onset, until reperfusion is achieved, is a strategy not yet explored in human clinical trials of citicoline. The greater signal of potential benefit observed in the large ICTUS trial among patients with older age and moderately severe rather than extremely severe presenting deficits perhaps hints at beneficial neuroreparative effects among patients with less intrinsic neuroplasticity (older age) and more intact brain systems to recruit into recovery pathways (less severe deficits). However, further, larger trials in these patient groups are needed before firm conclusions can be reached regarding potential agent benefit.

Excitatory Amino Acid Antagonists

Focal cerebral ischaemia causes excess release of EAA neurotransmitters, particularly glutamate, from presynaptic vesicles and prevents normal reuptake of glutamate, resulting in very high synaptic concentrations. Glutamate is toxic in neuronal cell culture and *in vivo*. It acts at post-synaptic receptors, notably the N-methyl-D-aspartate (NMDA) receptor complex (to promote entry of calcium and sodium into neurones) and the α-amino-3-hydroxy-5-methylisoxazole-4-propionic acid (AMPA) receptor (to promote principally sodium entry). Resultant cellular depolarization and calcium overload activate intracellular second messenger systems with consequent cell death.

In preclinical models of stroke, antagonists of glutamate release or of postsynaptic glutamate receptors substantially reduce the volume of histological neuronal infarction and improve functional recovery, even when administered up to several hours after the onset of ischaemia (Muir and Lees, 2003). Drugs that modulate EAA toxicity (EAA antagonists) encompass a diversity of pharmacological agents and a number of potential mechanisms of action, including principally inhibition of glutamate release, NMDA receptor antagonism, and AMPA receptor antagonism. The NMDA receptor itself has several modulatory sites that are amenable to pharmacological modification. However, despite multiple supportive studies in preclinical models and advance of many EAA antagonists into human clinical trials, no agent has yet been proven beneficial in acute ischaemic stroke. This section

will briefly survey early studied molecular agents and then provide further details on agents of more recent interest.

Evidence

A systematic review analysed RCTs of EAA antagonists and related agents in acute stroke completed by 2001 (Muir and Lees, 2003). Restricting consideration to agents that had EAA antagonism as their leading or co-leading mechanism, there were 33 completed RCTs evaluating 13 agents. Eight agents were 8 NMDA receptor antagonists, 2 AMPA receptor antagonists, 2 agents that were both sodium channel blockers (reducing glutamate release) and also active calcium channel or cyclic guanosine-3′,5′-monophosphate (cGMP) nitric oxide pathway inhibitors, and 1 agent that was both an NMDA receptor antagonist and a sodium channel inhibitor. Time to treatment averaged under 5 hours in many trials, although only a minority of patients were treated in 3 hours or less after stroke onset.

Death or Dependency

A total of 23 randomized trials testing 10 agents and enrolling 9762 patients provided data on death or dependency at long-term follow-up (Figure 12.4). Random allocation to an EAA antagonist was associated with no significant effect on death or dependency at final follow-up compared with control (53.1% vs 51.7%, OR 1.06; 95% CI: 0.98–1.15). There was moderate heterogeneity across agents, $I^2 = 44\%$.

Death

Random allocation to an EAA antagonist was associated with no significant effect on death at final follow-up compared with control (20.7% vs 19.6%, OR 1.02, 95% CI: 0.92–1.12) (Figure 12.5). There was only mild heterogeneity across study agents, $I^2 = 20\%$.

Comment

None of the surge of EAA agents that entered human clinical trial testing in the period from 1993–2003 was found beneficial. In hindsight, in addition to the several weaknesses in preclinical and clinical study designs recognized at the time (Ovbiagele et al., 2003; O'Collins et al., 2006; Lapchak et al., 2013), another likely major factor was the absence at that time of highly effective reperfusion therapy with which the agents might be combined. EAA antagonists, and most other neuroprotective agents, have

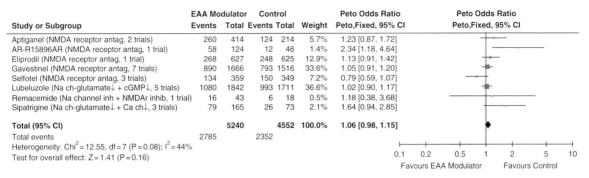

Study or Subgroup	EAA Modulator Events	Total	Control Events	Total	Weight	Peto Odds Ratio Peto,Fixed, 95% CI
Aptiganel (NMDA receptor antag, 2 trials)	260	414	124	214	5.7%	1.23 [0.87, 1.72]
AR-R15896AR (NMDA receptor antag, 1 trial)	58	124	12	46	1.4%	2.34 [1.18, 4.64]
Eliprodil (NMDA receptor antag, 1 trial)	268	627	248	625	12.9%	1.13 [0.91, 1.42]
Gavestinel (NMDA receptor antag, 7 trials)	890	1666	793	1516	33.6%	1.05 [0.91, 1.20]
Selfotel (NMDA receptor antag, 3 trials)	134	359	150	349	7.2%	0.79 [0.59, 1.07]
Lubeluzole (Na ch-glutamate↓ + cGMP↓, 5 trials)	1080	1842	993	1711	36.6%	1.02 [0.90, 1.17]
Remacemide (Na channel inh + NMDAr inhib, 1 trial)	16	43	6	18	0.5%	1.18 [0.38, 3.68]
Sipatrigine (Na ch-glutamate↓ + Ca ch↓, 3 trials)	79	165	26	73	2.1%	1.64 [0.94, 2.85]
Total (95% CI)		**5240**		**4552**	**100.0%**	**1.06 [0.98, 1.15]**
Total events	2785		2352			

Heterogeneity: Chi² = 12.55, df = 7 (P = 0.08); I² = 44%
Test for overall effect: Z = 1.41 (P = 0.16)

Figure 12.4 Forest plot showing the effects of *excitatory amino acid inhibitors vs control* for acute ischaemic stroke on *death or dependency* at long-term follow-up in RCTs reported between 1984 and 2001 (primarily 1995–2001).

Reproduced from Muir and Lees (2003), with permission from John Wiley & Sons Limited. Copyright Cochrane Library.

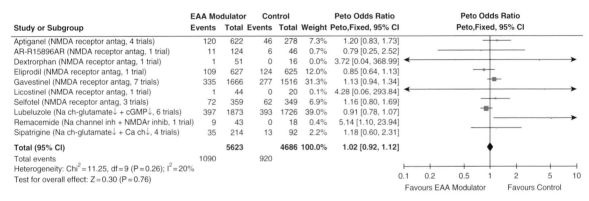

Study or Subgroup	EAA Modulator Events	Total	Control Events	Total	Weight	Peto Odds Ratio Peto,Fixed, 95% CI
Aptiganel (NMDA receptor antag, 4 trials)	120	622	46	278	7.3%	1.20 [0.83, 1.73]
AR-R15896AR (NMDA receptor antag, 1 trial)	11	124	6	46	0.7%	0.79 [0.25, 2.52]
Dextrorphan (NMDA receptor antag, 1 trial)	1	51	0	16	0.0%	3.72 [0.04, 368.99]
Eliprodil (NMDA receptor antag, 1 trial)	109	627	124	625	12.0%	0.85 [0.64, 1.13]
Gavestinel (NMDA receptor antag, 7 trials)	335	1666	277	1516	31.3%	1.13 [0.94, 1.34]
Licostinel (NMDA receptor antag, 1 trial)	1	44	0	20	0.1%	4.28 [0.06, 293.84]
Selfotel (NMDA receptor antag, 3 trials)	72	359	62	349	6.9%	1.16 [0.80, 1.69]
Lubeluzole (Na ch-glutamate↓ + cGMP↓, 6 trials)	397	1873	393	1726	39.0%	0.91 [0.78, 1.07]
Remacemide (Na channel inh + NMDAr inhib, 1 trial)	9	43	0	18	0.4%	5.14 [1.10, 23.94]
Sipatrigine (Na ch-glutamate↓ + Ca ch↓, 4 trials)	35	214	13	92	2.2%	1.18 [0.60, 2.31]
Total (95% CI)		**5623**		**4686**	**100.0%**	**1.02 [0.92, 1.12]**
Total events	1090		920			

Heterogeneity: Chi² = 11.25, df = 9 (P = 0.26); I² = 20%
Test for overall effect: Z = 0.30 (P = 0.76)

Figure 12.5 Forest plot showing the effects of *excitatory amino acid inhibitors vs control* for acute ischaemic stroke on *death* at long-term follow-up in RCTs reported between 1984 and 2001 (primarily 1995–2001).

Reproduced from Muir and Lees (2003), with permission from John Wiley & Sons Limited. Copyright Cochrane Library.

mechanisms of action that slow the pace of ischaemic injury, but that do not reduce its final extent if the ischaemic stress is not eventually relieved. Accordingly, chances of success are likely limited when EAAs are tested as standalone or post-reperfusion treatment therapies, rather than as early bridging therapies followed by reperfusion interventions.

NA-1

NA-1 is a cell-permeant eicosapeptide that perturbs the protein–protein interactions of PSD-95, a postsynaptic scaffolding protein that links NMDA glutamate receptors to neurotoxic signalling pathways, including neuronal nitric oxide synthase, a free radical generator. NA-1 reduced infarct size in rodent and primate ischaemic stroke models.

Evidence

In a phase 2, proof-of-concept trial undertaken to determine whether NA-1 could reduce MRI biomarker evidence of ischaemic injury in humans, 185 patients undergoing non-urgent endovascular repair of unruptured or ruptured aneurysms were randomized to an intravenous bolus of NA-1 or placebo started immediately after completion of the endovascular treatment (Hill et al., 2012). Delaying agent start modelled the post-onset rather than pre-onset initiation of therapy that would be achievable in spontaneous ischaemic stroke patients. None of the primary endpoints reached statistical significance after adjustment for multiplicity, but favourable trends were noted. The number of new diffusion magnetic resonance imaging (MRI) ischaemic lesions after the endovascular procedure was numerically lower in NA-1 versus placebo patients, mean 4.1 versus 7.3, nominal adjusted RR 0.53 (95% CI: 0.38–0.74), and the total volume of new diffusion MRI ischaemic lesions was numerically smaller, median 0.06 versus 0.12 mL, nominal adjusted $p = 0.12$. No difference was noted in the frequency of excellent neurological outcome (NIHSS 0–1) at 30 days, occurring in 89–94% of patients in both treatment groups, with, after adjustment for prognostic features, RR 1.0 (95% CI: 0.9–1.1). No adverse events occurred more frequently in the NA-1 compared with the placebo group.

Comment

Based on the signals of potential efficacy in reducing endovascular procedure-related, subclinical ischaemic brain injury in a phase 2, proof-of-concept trial, and the absence of evidence of any major safety concerns, NA-1 warrants testing in pivotal ischaemic stroke trials. Two trials are under way: the FRONTIER trial (NCT02315443), testing prehospital administration in a broad group of hyperacute suspected stroke patients, and the ESCAPE NA-1 trial (NCT02930018), testing administration in the Emergency Department among patients with acute ischaemic stroke due to large vessel occlusions bound for endovascular mechanical thrombectomy.

Calcium Channel Antagonists

Massive calcium influx into ischaemic brain cells is a final common pathway leading to cell death, and agents that reduce calcium overload lower infarct volumes in preclinical stroke models (Doyle et al., 2008; Sekerdag et al., 2018). Furthermore, the calcium channel agent nimodipine was shown to be effective in decreasing the occurrence of death and disability after aneurysmal and traumatic subarachnoid haemorrhage (SAH) in humans, likely at least in part by conferring neuronal protection against ischaemic injury arising from delayed cerebral vasospasm (see Chapter 14). Nimodipine and other calcium antagonists can act as neuroprotective drugs by diminishing the influx of calcium ions through the voltage-sensitive calcium channels.

Evidence

A systematic review identified 34 RCTs evaluating 6 calcium antagonist agents in 7731 patients predominantly with ischaemic stroke (but some with haemorrhagic stroke and some with no imaging to confirm stroke subtype), with nimodipine being the most predominantly studied agent (Zhang et al., 2012). The trials more closely evaluated calcium channel antagonism in the subacute rather than acute period. Entry windows were typically up to 24–72 hours post-onset; onset time in some trials may have been the time symptoms were first observed rather than time last known well; the study agent typically was continued for 3–21 days; and the first dose was often given orally, resulting in delayed peak serum levels.

Death or Dependency

Data regarding death or dependency at the end of follow-up were available from 22 RCTs evaluating 3 calcium antagonist agents in 6684 patients. The most common agent studied was nimodipine, evaluated in 19 of the trials and 91% (6093/6684) of the patients. Overall, a possible small detrimental effect of calcium antagonists was noted, 46.6% versus 41.5% (RR 1.05; 95% CI: 0.98–1.13; $p = 0.16$) (Figure 12.6). There was no evidence of heterogeneity by agent ($I^2 = 0$%) but mild heterogeneity by individual trial was noted ($I^2 = 29$%).

Death

Data regarding mortality at the end of follow-up were available for 31 RCTs evaluating 6 calcium antagonist agents in 7483 patients. The most common agent studied was nimodipine, evaluated in 24 of the trials and 6312 (84%) of the patients. Among 7483 participants randomized in 31 RCTs, no difference was found for death at the end of follow-up, 21.7% versus 20.4% (RR 1.07; 95% CI: 0.98–1.17, $p = 0.12$). There was no evidence of heterogeneity by treatment agent ($I^2 = 4$%) or by individual trial ($I^2 = 0$%).

Recurrent Stroke

Among the 9 RCTs which reported stroke recurrences among 2460 patients, there was no difference in the proportion of recurrent strokes between calcium antagonists and placebo (2.8% vs 3.0%, RR 0.93; 95% CI: 0.56–1.54, $p = 0.78$).

Adverse Events

In 3 trials reporting salient data, mean systolic blood pressure during or at the end of active treatment was on average 2 mm Hg lower in active than control groups. In 6 trials in which episodes of hypotension sufficient to stop treatment were mentioned, there was a non-significant trend for an increase in hypotensive episodes among patients allocated calcium antagonists compared with control (1.8% vs 1.2%, RR 1.43, 95% CI: 0.61–3.38).

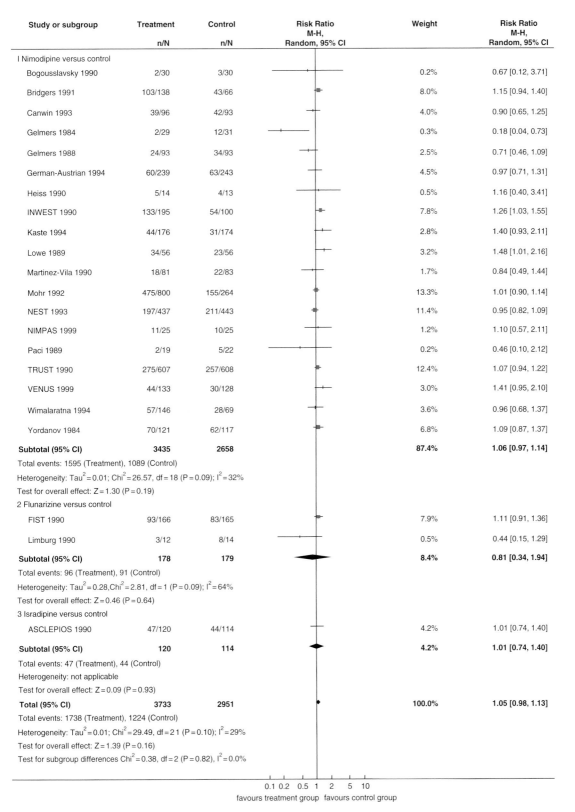

Figure 12.6 Forest plot showing the effects of *calcium antagonists vs control* for acute ischaemic stroke *on death at long-term follow-up*. Reproduced from Zhang et al. (2012), with permission from John Wiley & Sons Limited. Copyright Cochrane Library.

Subgroup Analyses By Dose

Four trials directly compared one dose of nimodipine with another and also reported data on death or dependency at late follow-up. Two contrasted different oral doses, including one trial with 800 participants comparing 60 mg, 120 mg, and 240 mg oral nimodipine daily and one trial with 146 participants comparing 120 mg and 240 mg oral nimodipine daily. No outcome differences were noted across the three dose tiers. Two trials with 333 participants compared an infusion of 1 mg/h and 2 mg/h intravenous nimodipine. The lower dose was associated with less death or dependency at long-term follow-up, 63.8% versus 77.6%, RR 0.82 (95% CI: 0.71–0.95).

By Time of Start of Treatment

Data regarding time of agent start were available for multiple trials only for the time threshold of before or after 12 hours after onset. Across 18 trials, 1879 participants had treatment start within 12 hours and 4071 had treatment start more than 12 hours after onset. Between these two time windows, there was no evidence of heterogeneity of the nonpositive effect on death or dependency at end of follow-up ($p_{interaction} < 0.40$).

Two trials provided specific information regarding treatment started within 6 hours of onset, but both had interpretation difficulty arising from higher potential for bias, active controls, or atypical treatment processes. One single-centre, single-investigator, placebo-controlled trial randomized 93 ischaemic stroke patients to IV nimodipine 2.5 mg/h versus oral nimodipine 30 mg 4 times daily, started within 6 hours of onset (mean 4.8 hours after onset) and continued for 10 days (Chandra, 1995). Among the ischaemic stroke patients, on day 3, the mean neurological deficit score on the Matthew Scale was better (higher), 89 versus 70, but standard deviation and p-values were not provided, and rater blinding from potential unmasking by initial blood pressure effects was not described. One multi-centre, placebo-controlled trial randomized 261 final diagnosis ischaemic stroke patients to oral nimodipine 30 mg 4 times daily or placebo, started within 6 hours of onset and continued for 10 days (Horn et al., 2001). The study agent was commonly started 'prehospital' in a general practitioner's office. Severe dependency or death at 3 months (mRS 4–6) occurred in 32% of nimodipine versus 27% of placebo patients, RR 1.2 (95% CI: 0.9–1.6). The interpretation of this finding is limited by the nonstandard start of nimodipine outside of a continuously monitored setting ahead of any correction for hypovolaemia, the oral agent start with relatively slow attainment of peak blood levels, and the prolonged ongoing study agent administration in the subacute period potentially counteracting effects in the acute period.

Publication Status

There was a trend toward difference in outcomes reported between the 4 unpublished versus 18 published trials, $p_{subgroup\ differences} = 0.20$, with unpublished trials tending to show more of an adverse effect on death or dependency at late follow-up, RR 1.14 versus 1.03.

Comment

Current randomized trial evidence largely addresses relatively late start and prolonged continued administration of calcium channel antagonists, and does not support the use of this treatment strategy in clinical practice. The trials collectively did not demonstrate benefit and suggested potential harm. Hypotensive effects of some calcium channel antagonists may reduce cerebral perfusion pressure, potentially offsetting acute neuroprotective effects by diminishing collateral flow both acutely, when the initial infarct is still evolving, and subacutely, when cerebral oedema and raised intracranial pressure may produce a second period of sensitivity to reduced cerebral perfusion pressure. Brief administration of calcium antagonists during the first hours after onset only, with close control of blood pressure to avert hypotensive effects, until reperfusion is achieved, is a strategy not yet explored in human clinical trials of narrowly targeted calcium channel antagonists. Accordingly, a neuroprotective benefit of this agent class has not yet been well interrogated by randomized trials, although the completed RCTs largely performed in later time windows are certainly not encouraging.

Gamma-Aminobutyric Acid Agonists

Gamma-aminobutyric acid (GABA) is the principal inhibitory cerebral neurotransmitter, and potentiation of GABA activity causes hyperpolarization of neuronal membranes, mitigating the excitotoxic effects of glutamate, including ligand and voltage-gated calcium influx. Two GABA receptor agonists have been studied in clinical trials for acute ischaemic stroke: clomethiazole and diazepam. Clomethiazole has been shown to reduce ischaemia-induced cerebral damage and clinically relevant behavioural abnormalities in rodents and primates at plasma concentrations of 3.5–19 μmol/L (Lyden et al., 2002). Diazepam has been shown to reduce size of injury in focally induced ischaemia in rodent models (Aerden et al., 2004).

Evidence

Functional Independence

A meta-analysis of 4 clinical trials of GABA agonists enrolled 3526 patients, including 3 trials (CLASS, CLASS-I, and CLASS-T) of clomethiazole randomizing 2646 patients within 12 hours of onset and 1 trial of diazepam (EGASIS) randomizing 880 patients within 12 hours of onset (Figure 12.7) (Liu and Wang, 2014). Overall, across all 4 trials, treatment with GABA agonists did not alter the frequency of functional independence at long-term follow-up, 50.7% versus 50.6%, RR 1.00 (95% CI: 0.93–1.08). There was moderate

heterogeneity between drug agent subgroups, I^2 = 55%. Across the 3 trials of clomethiazole, functional independence with long-term follow-up with clomethiazole versus control occurred with RR 0.98 (95% CI: 0.91–1.05), while in the diazepam trial functional independence with diazepam versus control occurred with RR 1.10 (95% CI: 0.96–1.27).

Adverse Events

Across two trials of clomethiazole enrolling 2527 patients, a substantially higher frequency of somnolence occurred with clomethiazole than control, 51.7% versus 11.3% (RR 4.56, 95% CI: 3.50–5.95). In addition, a higher frequency of rhinitis was noted, 13.0% versus 2.5% (RR 4.75, 95% CI: 2.67–8.46).

Comment

Current randomized trial evidence largely addresses the relatively late start of GABA agonists, and does not support the use of this treatment strategy in

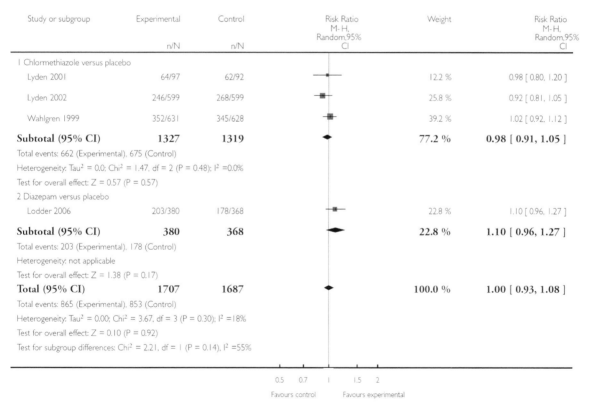

Figure 12.7 Forest plot showing the effects of *GABA agonists vs control* for acute ischaemic stroke *for functional independence (mRS 0–2 or nearest equivalent) at long-term follow-up.*

Reproduced from Liu and Wang (2014), with permission from John Wiley & Sons Limited. Copyright Cochrane Library.

clinical practice. The trials collectively did not demonstrate benefit and a high rate of induced somnolence was noted, complicating patient management. Brief administration of GABA agonists during the first hours after onset only, until reperfusion is achieved, is a strategy not yet explored in human clinical trials. Accordingly, a neuroprotective benefit of this agent class has not yet been well interrogated by randomized trials, although the completed RCTs largely performed in later time windows are certainly not encouraging.

Nitric Oxide Donors

Nitric oxide (NO) is a soluble gas formed from a reaction of L-arginine and oxygen, catalysed by 3 isoforms of nitric oxide synthase (NOS): (1) eNOS, present within endothelial cells, (2) nNOS, present within neurones, and (3) iNOS, present in macrophages, astrocytes, microglia, and vascular smooth muscle cells (Garry et al., 2015). Nitric oxide exerts multiple effects potentially beneficial in acute ischaemic stroke, including vasodilatory, neuromodulatory, anti-inflammatory, and antiplatelet (Bath et al., 2016). While nNOS- and iNOS-derived NO are detrimental in preclinical ischaemic stroke models, eNOS-derived NO is neuroprotective. The nitric oxide donor glyceryl trinitrate (GTN, nitroglycerin) has been tested in human ischaemic stroke trials.

Evidence

Five randomized trials have evaluated transdermal GTN in 3502 ischaemic stroke patients, predominantly at a dose of 5 mg per day (Figure 12.8) (Bath et al., 2017). Four trials, enrolling 3472 ischaemic stroke patients, permitted treatment start in the acute to subacute stage, up to 48 hours to 5 days after onset, while 1 trial, enrolling 30 acute cerebral ischaemia patients, evaluated early initiation in the prehospital ambulance setting, within 4 hours of onset. In all trials, study agent was continued for several days.

Death or Dependency

Overall, among 3502 ischaemic stroke patients, GTN did not alter the frequency of death and dependency at long-term follow-up (mRS 3–6) (OR 0.97, 95% CI: 0.62–1.53).

Death

GTN was associated with a non-significant trend towards reduced death by end of trial (OR 0.85, 95% CI: 0.69–1.05).

Adverse Effects

Consistent with GTN's known blood pressure lowering effects, systolic blood pressure was lower in GTN versus no GTN ischaemic stroke patients when first assessed after start of therapy, by mean 7.05 ± 1.46 mm Hg (Bath et al., 2017), and in 4197 mixed ischaemic and haemorrhagic stroke patients (83% ischaemic), GTN was associated with hypotension deemed by treating physicians as needing medical intervention, 2.7% versus 0.7% (OR 3.66, 95% CI: 2.06–6.51) (Bath et al., 2016). However, xenon computed tomography (CT) and transcranial Doppler studies have indicated that CBF remains relatively preserved in healthy subjects when GTN is administered, as GTN's cerebral vasodilatory effects, reducing vascular resistance, counterbalance systemic hypotensive effects (Willmot et al., 2006). In addition, in mixed ischaemic and haemorrhagic stroke patients, GTN was associated with increased headache, 18.2% versus 8.4% (OR 2.42, 95% CI: 1.99–2.95).

Time from Onset Subgroups

In an individual participant-level data meta-analysis of 4197 mixed ischaemic and haemorrhagic stroke patients (83% ischaemic), the effect of GTN on death or dependency at long-term outcome was modified by time from onset to first dose, $p_{interaction} = 0.01$. Among the 233/3502 (6.7%) ischaemic stroke patients enrolled within 6 hours of onset, GTN was associated with a shift to more favourable long-term disability outcomes over all 7 mRS levels, common odds ratio (cOR) 0.55 (95% CI: 0.34–0.89; $p = 0.01$).

Comment

Transdermal GTN has largely been evaluated in the subacute stroke period and has not shown benefit in this time period. However, available data from 2 randomized trials with enrolments within the first 6 hours after onset suggest potential benefit when given acutely, despite systemic blood pressure lowering and headache adverse effects. Further trials in the hyperacute and acute periods after ischaemic stroke onset are warranted to confirm or disconfirm benefit of this easily administered agent.

Anti-inflammatory Agents

Ischaemic stress and injury trigger a powerful inflammatory tissue reaction that can further extend cerebral tissue damage. In preclinical models, anti-

Review: Nitric oxide donors (nitrates), L-arginine, or nitric oxide synthase inhibitors for acute stroke
Comparison: 1 Glyceryl trinitrate (GTN) compared with no GTN for acute stroke
Outcome: 3 Death or dependency (mRS>2), end of trial, by time to randomization

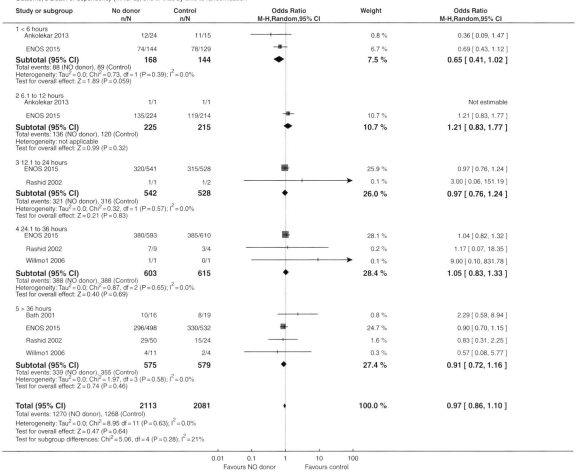

Figure 12.8 Forest plot showing the effects of *glyceryl trinitrate vs control* for acute ischaemic stroke *for death or dependency (mRS 3–6) at long-term follow-up,* by time from onset to enrolment, among 4197 mixed ischaemic and haemorrhagic stroke patients (83% ischaemic). Reproduced from Bath et al. (2017), with permission from the authors and John Wiley & Sons Limited. Copyright Cochrane Library.

inflammatory agents variably reduce final infarct volume. As inflammation is a later-occurring mechanism of injury, the time window may be more prolonged for start of anti-inflammatory agents, compared with other neuroprotective agents, to reduce cerebral ischaemic injury. However, compared with necrotic, apoptotic, and other injury pathways triggered early after ischaemia onset, inflammation appears responsible for only a very small proportion of the cerebral tissue damage in acute ischaemic stroke, limiting its potential for major impact upon clinical course (Heiss et al., 1999). Anti-inflammatory agents investigated in large, human randomized trials include two agents

that block leucocyte adhesion to the endothelial wall and trafficking into the brain parenchyma: enlimomab, an antibody that blocks intercellular adhesion molecule-1; and neutrophil inhibitory factor, a recombinant glycoprotein that blocks an integrin binding site.

Evidence

In a trial enrolling 625 individuals with ischaemic stroke, patients were randomly allocated to enlimomab or placebo begun within 6 hours of onset and continued for 5 days (Enlimomab Acute Stroke Trial Investigators, 2001). Enlimomab was associated with increased death or dependency (mRS

3–6) at 3 months, 45.8% versus 36.1%, $p = 0.02$, and a trend towards increased mortality, 22.2 versus 16.2%, $p = 0.07$. Adverse events more common in enlimomab patients included fever, 51% versus 27%, infection, 56% versus 42%, and aseptic meningitis, 1.9% versus 0%. Neutrophil inhibitory factor was evaluated in an adaptive phase 2, dose–response-finding proof-of-concept study that was stopped for futility after enrolment of 966 patients within 6 hours of ischaemic stroke onset because of no favourable effect of the treatment on the primary outcome measure – a change from baseline to day 90 on the Scandinavian Stroke Scale (Krams et al., 2003). No increased frequency of serious adverse effects was noted.

Comment

Available data do not support the use of anti-inflammatory therapy for acute ischaemic stroke. In addition, immunomodulatory therapies that increase fever with hyperthermia and infectious complications have the potential to worsen rather than improve outcome.

Oxygen Delivery Enhancers

Loss of oxygen supply and conversion from efficient aerobic to inefficient anaerobic energy metabolism is a cardinal feature of cerebral ischaemia. Accordingly, delivery of increased oxygen to hypoxic brain tissues is potentially beneficial in acute ischaemic stroke. Conversely, delivery of oxygen alone without the full complement of energy pathway molecular species in whole human blood also has the potential to have deleterious effect, by increasing oxidative stress through the production of oxygen free-radical species.

Methods to increase oxygen delivery to ischaemic tissues include increasing supplemental gaseous oxygen delivered under atmospheric pressure (normobaric hyperoxaemia) and elevated barometric pressure (hyperbaric hyperoxaemia), intra-arterial delivery of aqueous oxygen, and administration of molecules that enhance oxygen trafficking to cerebral tissues. Modified haemoglobin molecules with increased oxygen-carrying capacity can enhance oxygen delivery to ischaemic tissues. Trans-sodium crocetinate (TSC), a carotenoid derivative, increases the diffusion of oxygen through blood plasma to hypoxic tissues by altering the molecular arrangement of the water molecules, and has been shown to reduce brain infarct size in rodent stroke models (Wang et al., 2014).

Evidence

Normobaric hyperoxaemia is addressed in Chapter 5, and aqueous oxygen and TSC have not yet completed human ischaemic stroke trials.

Hyperbaric oxygen has been evaluated for acute (<48 h of onset) ischaemic stroke in 2 randomized trials, enrolling 77 patients (Bennett et al., 2014). Treatment start was an average of 12–24 hours after onset in both trials. Hyperbaric oxygen therapy (HBOT) did not modify disability or mortality outcomes. In one trial, for HBOT versus control, 6-month disability levels (mRS) were mean mRS 2.6 versus 3.2, difference –0.6 (95% CI: –1.4–0.2). In the other, disability-free (mRS 0–1) 3-month outcome with HBOT versus control was 29.4% versus 56.3%, RR 0.67 (95% CI: 0.27–1.69).

Diaspirin cross-linked haemoglobin, a cell-free, haemoglobin-based, oxygen-carrying solution, was tested at 4 dose tiers, administered over 72 hours, in a saline-controlled trial among 85 patients (40 active agent, 45 control) with ischaemic stroke within 18 hours of onset (Saxena et al., 1999). There was evidence of harm, with functional independence (mRS 0–2) at 3 months achieved in 15% of actively treated versus 49% of control patients, RR 0.31 (95% CI: 0.14–0.68; $p = 0.004$). The diaspirin cross-linked haemoglobin had a marked hypertensive effect, increased mean arterial pressure by 21 mm Hg, and also elevated levels of endothelin-1, a cerebral vasoconstrictor.

Comments

Hyperbaric oxygen therapy has only been minimally trialed in acute ischaemic stroke, so is of uncertain value, and faces substantial practical challenges as an acute neuroprotective intervention given the standard care need to manage many acute patients in catheterization suites, imaging suites, intensive care units, and other settings outside of hyperbaric chambers. Diaspirin cross-linked haemoglobin showed unfavourable effects, likely in part due to off-target effects in raising blood pressure and vasoconstriction; evaluation of more recently developed haemoglobin-based, cell-free oxygen carriers without these adverse effects is desirable (Dhar et al., 2017).

Multiple Leading Mechanisms

Some pharmacological and device interventions exert pleiotropic effects in acute cerebral ischaemia, blocking simultaneously several different molecular pathways that mediate tissue injury in ischaemic environments.

Given the complex, manifold process web of the ischaemic cascade, it seems likely that pleiotropic agents that block multiple rather than only single cell-death pathways, or combinations of single mechanism agents, will be more effective in conferring cytoprotection.

Statins

Statins (HMG CoA-reductases) are a group of lipid-lowering agents that are competitive inhibitors of the enzyme 3-hydroxy-3-methyl-glutaryl-CoA (HMG-CoA) that are of established benefit in the long-term prevention of ischaemic stroke of atherosclerotic origin. Statins may be of benefit in the subacute period after stroke onset through their lead, cholesterol-lowering effect, by stabilizing active atherosclerotic plaque lesions and reducing the frequency of early recurrent ischaemic stroke or myocardial infarction in the first days and weeks after an index event. But statins also exert multiple additional effects that may confer benefit in acute ischaemic stroke, including: inhibition of leucocyte adhesion and inflammatory transcription factors, reducing inflammation; up-regulation of endothelial nitric oxide synthase, bone marrow-derived progenitor endothelial cells, and vascular endothelial growth factor, augmenting CBF; pro-thrombolytic and antiplatelet effects, facilitating reperfusion and deterring thrombus propagation; and promotion of neurogenesis and synaptogenesis, enhancing neural repair (Yaghi and Elkind, 2016). In animal models, the neuroprotective and neuroregenerative effects of statins continue to escalate as doses increase to substantially higher than those used clinically for cholesterol-lowering for long-term prevention.

Evidence

Functional Outcomes

Early statin therapy initiated within the first 48 hours has been investigated in at least 8 RCTs enrolling 1055 patients, with full-length publications in English reporting clinical outcomes. Data on disability-free (mRS 0–1) outcome at late follow-up were available from 3 trials in 402 patients with statin start within 12–24 hours of onset and therapy continued for 7–90 days (Muscari et al., 2011; Montaner et al., 2016; Yoshimura et al., 2017). Disability-free outcome in statin versus control occurred in 51.0% versus 46.0%, RR 1.11, 95% CI: 0.91–1.34 (Figure 12.9). However, moderate heterogeneity across the three trials was present, $I^2 = 43\%$. Data on functional independence (mRS 0–2) at late follow-up were available from 3 trials enrolling 426 patients with statin start within 12–24 hours and therapy continued for 3 to 90 days (Blanco et al., 2007; Montaner et al., 2016; Yoshimura et al., 2017). One of the trials only enrolled patients who had been taking statins pre-stroke, randomizing them to discontinuation or continuation for the first 3 days. Functional independence was attained in 69.2% versus 64.6%, RR 1.06 (95% CI: 0.93–1.21) (Figure 12.10). There was mild heterogeneity across trials, $I^2 = 29\%$.

Recurrent Stroke

Recurrent stroke (ischaemic or haemorrhagic) was evaluated in 2 trials with statin start within 24 hours of onset and therapy continued for 7 days (Kennedy et al., 2007; Yoshimura et al., 2017). Among 649 patients (330 statin, 319 control), recurrent stroke among statin vs control patients occurred in 9.7% versus 6.3%, RR 1.55 (95% CI: 0.90–2.65) (Figure 12.11). Among the 51 recurrent strokes, 47 (92%) were ischaemic.

Additional Clinical Efficacy Outcomes

The most comprehensive clinical endpoints explored in the remaining three RCTs not included in the above analyses were: mean NIHSS at 30 days (1 trial, 40 patients), mean Barthel Index at 90 days (1 trial, 55 patients), and mean mRS at 90 days (1 trial, 56 patients). No statistically significant differences were noted.

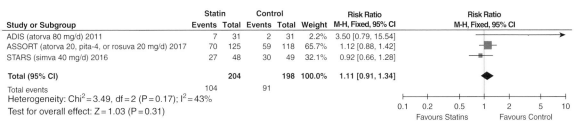

Figure 12.9 Forest plot showing the effects of *statins vs control* for acute ischaemic stroke on *freedom from disability (mRS 0–1) at long-term follow-up*.

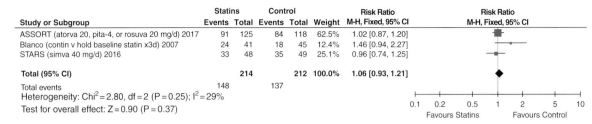

Figure 12.10 Forest plot showing the effects of *statins vs control* for acute ischaemic stroke on *functional independence (mRS 0–2)* at long-term follow-up.

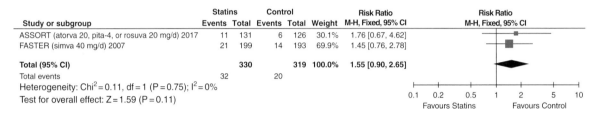

Figure 12.11 Forest plot showing the effects of *statins vs control* for acute ischaemic stroke on *recurrent stroke (ischaemic or haemorrhagic) in* first 3 months.

Subgroup: Statin Withdrawal

While the majority of patients enrolled in RCTs were statin-naïve at study start, two trials provided data specifically on the subset of patients taking statins at stroke onset and then randomized to continuing or initially holding statin therapy. These trials provided contrasting findings. In the one trial confined to 86 statin-at-onset patients, continuing statin therapy was associated with a trend toward more functional independence at long-term follow-up (RR 1.46, 95% CI: 0.94–2.27) (Blanco et al., 2007). However, in another trial, among a subset of 52 statin-at-onset participants, no major shift to lower disability at long-term follow-up was noted (cOR 0.94, 95% CI: 0.35–2.53) (Yoshimura et al., 2017).

Comment

Current randomized trial data do not provide evidence of benefit of early statin therapy on early stroke recurrence or functional outcome. However, the randomized evidence collectively is of only modest size and is primarily regarding low to moderate doses of statin therapy. Further trials are needed of high-potency statin agents administered at the top of the conventional dose range, as well as of statins given hyperacutely at doses that exceed those used for conventional cholesterol lowering and correlate with the greatest neuroprotective and neuroreparative effects of statins in preclinical stroke models.

In addition, from a practical management perspective, long-term treatment with high-dose statins is indicated for patients with ischaemic stroke of large or small artery atherosclerotic origin, and patient adherence to statin therapy is likely to be enhanced if the agent is started within the first days of index stroke, during the 'teachable moment' when patient readiness to adopt new prevention practices may be greatest.

Minocycline

Minocycline is a tetracycline antibiotic that, in addition to its anti-microbial properties, has free radical scavenger, anti-apoptosis, and anti-inflammatory effects in the nervous system. Highly lipophilic, minocycline crosses the blood–brain barrier efficiently and has been shown to reduce cerebral infarct volume in preclinical ischaemic stroke models (Kohler et al., 2013).

Evidence

Functional Independence

Minocycline has been tested in at least 2 unconfounded, open-label trials in acute ischaemic stroke patients reporting broad final functional outcome endpoint in 246 randomized patients. (One additional unconfounded trial reported average neurological deficit score outcomes in 53 patients.) In both these trials, patients were enrolled up to 24 hours after onset, study agent was given for 2.5 or 5 days, and dosage was 200 mg daily. Of note, this dosage is in the low end of the range, up to 10 mg/kg, found to be generally well-tolerated in a formal dose-escalation trial in acute ischaemic stroke patients (Fagan et al., 2010). Overall, across the 2 trials, minocycline was associated with an increased frequency of functional independence (mRS 0–2) at long-term follow-up, 79.3% versus 55.2% (RR 1.44, 95% CI: 1.19–1.73). However, there was substantial heterogeneity between the trials, $p_{(heterogeneity)} < 0.0001$, with the relative risk of functional independence point estimates being 1.94 in one trial and 0.90 in the other. Across both trials, no adverse effects of minocycline were noted. In one trial, minocycline was associated with a reduced frequency of urinary tract infection (14.6% vs 0%, $p = 0.12$), consistent with its antibiotic effects.

Comments

Insufficient data from reliable RCTs exist to recommend use of minocycline as a neuroprotective agent in acute ischaemic stroke. Current randomized trial evidence largely addresses relatively late start of minocycline, and modest size and substantial heterogeneity of the available studies limit conclusions regarding effect in this time window. Further trials are warranted to explore the neuroprotective effects of minocycline for acute ischaemic stroke, including in the hyperacute period and at higher dosages that preliminarily appear well tolerated.

Magnesium

Magnesium is an abundant mineral in the human body. Raising serum magnesium levels can have several potentially neuroprotective effects, including blocking voltage-gated calcium channels, inhibiting presynaptic release of excitatory neurotransmitters, noncompetitively blocking the NMDA receptor, presynaptically potentiating adenosine, suppressing cortical spreading depression and anoxic depolarizations, antagonizing endothelin-1 and other vasoconstrictors, and relaxing vascular smooth muscle, resulting in vasodilation of large and small vascular beds and increased CBF. Magnesium has been shown to reduce cerebral infarct size in several acute ischaemic stroke preclinical models.

Evidence

Six randomized trials have evaluated magnesium sulfate in 4248 acute and subacute stroke patients. All enrolled both ischaemic and haemorrhagic stroke patients, but predominantly ischaemic patients. Four small trials enrolling patients up to 12–24 hours after onset were followed by two pivotal trials: IMAGES, with efficacy data available for 2386 patients (89.6% ischaemic), and FAST-MAG, with efficacy data available for 1700 patients (73.2% ischaemic) (IMAGES Investigators, 2004; Saver et al., 2015). IMAGES enrolled patients up to 12 hours after onset, while FAST-MAG enrolled patients in the prehospital setting hyperacutely, within 2 hours of onset. Both IMAGES and FAST-MAG tested dosing of 4 g bolus over 15 minutes followed by maintenance infusion of 16 g over 24 hours.

Death and Disability

Considering all patients from the first 5 trials and only acute cerebral ischaemia patients from FAST-MAG, data on death or disability (mRS 2–6 or nearest equivalent) at long-term follow-up were available for 4247 patients predominantly with acute brain ischaemia (Figure 12.12). Magnesium did not alter the frequency of death or disability (67.3% vs 69.1%, RR 0.98, 95% CI: 0.94–1.02). In addition, a nonsignificant trend towards increased mortality at long-term follow-up was present (15.4% vs 13.3%, RR 1.14, 95% CI: 0.98–1.32).

Adverse Events

Magnesium sulfate mildly lowered systolic blood pressure during the period of infusion, by mean 4 mm Hg in IMAGES and 3 mm Hg in FAST-MAG. In FAST-MAG, symptomatic haemorrhagic transformation of ischaemic stroke was non-significantly less frequent with magnesium, 2.1% vs 3.3% (OR 0.62, 95% CI: 0.34–1.14). No adverse events occurred with greater frequency in the magnesium sulfate groups.

Prehospital Treatment Start

As the first prehospital pivotal trial of neuroprotective agent administration, the FAST-MAG trial demonstrated the feasibility of hyperacute treatment start. The median time from last known well to start of study agent was 45 minutes (IQR 35–62) and infusion was started within the first 60 minutes after onset in 74% of patients. Among acute cerebral ischaemia patients, potential neuroprotective agent start

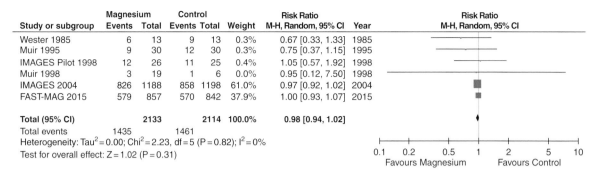

Figure 12.12 Forest plot showing the effects of *magnesium sulfate vs control* for acute ischaemic stroke on *functional independence (mRS 0–2) at long-term follow-up.*

preceded start of intravenous tissue plasminogen activator reperfusion treatment in 447 of the 1245 acute cerebral ischaemia patients (35.9%), by a median of 92 minutes (interquartile range [IQR] 74–117). With paramedic use of the Los Angeles Prehospital Stroke Screen and real-time cellphone patient interview by physician-investigators, the enrolment of stroke-mimic patients was kept to below 4% of the study population.

Comment

Magnesium sulfate did not show evidence of reducing death or disability in acute or subacute ischaemic stroke, and is not recommended for use in routine clinical practice. Mild blood pressure lowering effects and slow trafficking of magnesium across the blood–brain barrier may constrain the benefit attainable with this agent. The FAST-MAG trial has demonstrated the feasibility of hyperacute administration of neuroprotective agents, within the 'golden hour' immediately following stroke onset, when penumbra volume is greatest, and well in advance of reperfusion therapies, potentially enabling larger volumes of salvageable tissue to persist until restoration of CBF.

Albumin

Albumin exerts multiple potentially beneficial effects in preclinical ischaemic stroke systems, including antioxidant effects, binding of transition metals, improvement of tissue perfusion, reversal of microvascular blood-element aggregation and sludging, reduction of brain oedema, normalization of brain water homeostasis, and provision of essential fatty acids (Belayev et al., 2001). Albumin was tested in 2 randomized trials in ischaemic stroke within 5 hours of onset. In a pooled, individual participant data

analysis of these trials, among 1229 randomized patients, functional independence (mRS 0–2) at long-term follow-up was not altered by albumin versus control (52.6% vs 53.4%, RR 0.99, 95% CI: 0.89–1.10) (Martin et al., 2016). In safety analysis, among 1252 patients, an increase in congestive heart failure was seen (RR 7.76, 95% CI: 3.87–15.57), though generally readily addressed with fluid management and diuretic treatment. Overall, mortality was not significantly changed by albumin versus control (15.5% vs 11.5%, RR 1.26, 95% CI: 0.88–1.80). Based on these findings, albumin does not appear to confer benefit when given early after ischaemic stroke onset.

Gangliosides

Gangliosides are glycosphingolipids localized to the outer leaflet of the plasma membrane of vertebrate cells, and are enriched in neuronal membranes, particularly at synapses. Gangliosides in preclinical models have been shown to have neuronotrophic anti-excitotoxic and anti-inflammatory activity, and to facilitate survival and repair of neuronal tissue after ischaemic stress.

Evidence

A systematic review of 13 placebo-controlled, randomized trials of purified monosialoganglioside GM1 in 2265 patients with acute and subacute (within 15 days) ischaemic stroke revealed that allocation to a ganglioside was associated with a non-significant reduction in the odds of death at the end of follow-up (15–180 days) of 9% (95% CI: −13%–27%) (Candelise and Ciccone, 2001). Among the 3 trials that also recorded disability as an outcome measure, random allocation to treatment with gangliosides was not associated with any improvement in Barthel Index (BI) score (weighted mean difference 2.1; 95% CI: –4.8–8.9). In 2 trials, 8 patients exposed to gangliosides experienced adverse effects that led to discontinuation of ganglioside treatment; 7 had skin reactions and one developed Guillain–Barré syndrome.

Comment

There is not enough evidence to conclude that gangliosides are beneficial in acute stroke. Caution is warranted because of reports of sporadic cases of Guillain–Barré syndrome after ganglioside therapy.

Uncertain Mechanism

Piracetam

Piracetam is an agent with neuroprotective effects in ischaemic stroke models that are of uncertain mechanism. Piracetam is a cyclic derivative of the inhibitory neurotransmitter GABA, but does not act through GABA pathways. Piracetam modulates multiple neurotransmitter systems (cholinergic, serotoninergic, noradrenergic, and glutamatergic), increases red blood cell deformability, and reduces platelet aggregability. It has been suggested these diverse influences might arise from a fundamental effect of increasing cell membrane fluidity.

Evidence

A systematic review identified 3 randomized trials comparing piracetam with control in 1002 patients with acute and subacute (within 12 h to 3 days) ischaemic stroke, with active treatment consisting of intravenous piracetam for 4 to 14 days, followed by oral piracetam up to 8 weeks (Ricci et al., 2012). Data regarding death or dependency at 3 months were available from the largest of the 3 trials, PASS, which enrolled 927 patients and found no alteration (OR 1.01, 95% CI: 0.7–1.32). Across all 3 trials, piracetam was associated with a statistically non-significant increase in death at 1 month (OR 1.32, 95% CI: 0.96–1.82). However, the preponderance (93%) of the data came from the PASS trial, which had a potential imbalance in entry stroke severity. In entry-severity-adjusted analysis of the PASS population, there was no correlation between the treatment group and mortality. No adverse effects more frequent in piracetam patients were reported.

Comment

Current randomized trial evidence is limited in magnitude; it largely addresses relatively late start of piracetam and does not support the use of this treatment strategy in clinical practice. Administration of piracetam during the first hours after onset, until reperfusion is achieved, is a strategy not yet explored in human clinical trials. Accordingly, a neuroprotective benefit of this agent has not yet been well interrogated by randomized trials.

Summary

Interpretation of the Evidence
More than 20,000 patients have participated in clinical trials of more than 100 neuroprotective therapies and, despite this enormous effort, none of the studies has provided convincing evidence of a clinically and statistically significant benefit, although some therapies, like glyceryl trinitrate, uric acid, edaravone, and hypothermia, appear promising. Many agents were studied primarily in the subacute period after ischaemic stroke onset, and so never genuinely probed for acute neuroprotective effects. Some of these agents, or agent classes, may merit further testing in hyperacute time windows, if their potential benefits are revalidated in up-to-date preclinical model systems. Others, like magnesium and albumin, have been adequately enough tested in early time windows to reliably exclude a substantial treatment benefit.

Implications for Practice
There is no current role for neuroprotective drugs in acute stroke management because no agent has yet been found to have significant clinical benefits. Further use of any of these agents should occur only in the context of formal clinical trials.

Implications for research
Several improvements to neuroprotective agent development programmes have been identified to increase the rigor of preclinical agent qualification and the likelihood of success of human clinical trials. Preclinical experimental studies should use stringent randomization and blinding techniques to mitigate observer bias, assess treatments in time periods achievable in the human clinical setting, test agents in older animals with comorbidities, and require robust and reproducible benefit magnitudes to advance to

human testing. Human clinical trials should start agents hyperacutely, in the very first minutes and hours after onset, when treatment effect would be maximal, target enrolment of patients likely to have transient rather than permanent ischaemic exposure, and use factorial and platform trial designs that would permit efficient testing of combinations of agents able to block multiple ischaemic injury-mediating pathways concurrently, including both anti-necrotic and anti-apoptotic interventions. Cytoprotection should be the goal, with development of agents or agent combinations that are not just neuroprotective, but gliaprotective and endothelioprotective as well. For agents that allow cells to endure ischaemic stress, human clinical trial testing should deliver study agents as bridging therapies on the way to definitive reperfusion therapy, including prehospital initiation, initiation immediately upon brain imaging in patients destined for endovascular intervention, and initiation at outside hospitals in patients undergoing transfer to a neurothrombectomy centre. In addition, for agents with mechanisms of action likely to be specifically beneficial in mitigating reperfusion injury, treatment start before or concurrent with reperfusion, including intra-arterial administration via catheter immediately after endovascular thrombectomy, should be pursued.

References

Aerden LA, Kessels FA, Rutten BP, Lodder J, Steinbusch HW. (2004). Diazepam reduces brain lesion size in a photothrombotic model of focal ischemia in rats. *Neurosci Lett*, **367**(1), 76–8.

Arrich J, Holzer M, Havel C, Müllner M, Herkner H. (2016). Hypothermia for neuroprotection in adults after cardiopulmonary resuscitation. *Cochrane Database Syst Rev*, **2**. CD004128. doi:10.1002/14651858.CD004128.pub4.

Bardutzky J, Shen Q, Henninger N, Bouley J, Duong TQ, Fisher M. (2005). Perfusion and diffusion imaging in acute focal cerebral ischemia: temporal vs. spatial resolution. *Brain Res*, **1043**, 155–62.

Bath PM, Iddenden R, Bath FJ, Orgogozo JM; Tirilazad International Steering Committee. (2001). Tirilazad for acute ischaemic stroke. *Cochrane Database Syst Rev*, **4**. CD002087.

Bath PMW, Krishnan K, Appleton JP. (2017). Nitric oxide donors (nitrates), L-arginine, or nitric oxide synthase inhibitors for acute stroke. *Cochrane Database Syst Rev*, **4**. CD000398. doi:10.1002/14651858.CD000398.pub2.

Bath PM, Woodhouse L, Krishnan K, Anderson C, Berge E, Ford GA, et al. (2016). Effect of treatment delay, stroke type, and thrombolysis on the effect of glyceryl trinitrate, a nitric oxide donor, on outcome after acute stroke: a systematic review and meta-analysis of individual patients from randomised trials. *Stroke Res Treat*, 9706720. doi:10.1155/2016/9706720.

Belayev L, Liu Y, Zhao W, Busto R, Ginsberg MD. (2001). Human albumin therapy of acute ischemic stroke: marked neuroprotective efficacy at moderate doses and with a broad therapeutic window. *Stroke*, **32**, 553–60.

Bennett MH, Weibel S, Wasiak J, Schnabel A, French C, Kranke P. (2014). Hyperbaric oxygen therapy for acute ischaemic stroke. *Cochrane Database Syst Rev*, **11**. CD004954. doi:10.1002/14651858.CD004954.pub3.

Blanco M, Nombela F, Castellanos M, Rodriguez-Yanez M, Garcia-Gil M, Leira R, et al. (2007). Statin treatment withdrawal in ischemic stroke: a controlled randomized study. *Neurology*, **69**, 904–10.

Candelise L, Ciccone A. (2001). Gangliosides for acute ischaemic stroke. *Cochrane Database Syst Rev*, **4**. CD000094.

Chamorro A, Amaro S, Castellanos M, Segura T, Arenillas J, Marti-Fabregas J, et al. (2014). Safety and efficacy of uric acid in patients with acute stroke (URICO-ICTUS): a randomised, double-blind phase 2b/3 trial. *Lancet Neurol*, **13**(5), 453–60.

Chandra B. (1995). A new form of management of stroke. *J Stroke Cerebrovasc Dis*, **5**, 241–3.

Dávalos A, Alvarez-Sabin J, Castillo J, Diez-Teieder E, Ferro J, Martinez-Vila E, et al. (2012). Citicoline in the treatment of acute ischaemic stroke: an international, randomized, multicenter, placebo-controlled study (ICTUS) trial. *Lancet*, **380**(9839), 349–57.

Davis SM, Pennypacker KR. (2017). Targeting antioxidant enzyme expression as a therapeutic strategy for ischemic stroke. *Neurochem Int*, **107**, 23–32.

Dhar R, Misra H, Diringer MN. (2017). SANGUINATE™ (pegylated carboxyhemoglobin bovine) improves cerebral blood flow to vulnerable brain regions at risk of delayed cerebral ischemia after subarachnoid hemorrhage. *Neurocrit Care*, **27**, 341–9.

Diener, HC, Lees KR, Lyden P, Grotta J, Davalos A, Davis SM, et al. (2008). NXY-059 for the treatment of acute stroke: pooled analysis of the SAINT I and II trials. *Stroke*, **39**, 1751–58.

Doyle KP, Simon RP, Stenzel-Poore MP. (2008). Mechanisms of ischemic brain damage. *Neuropharmacology*, **55**, 310–18.

Emberson J, Lees KR, Lyden P, Blackwell L, Albers G, Bluhmki E, et al.; Stroke Thrombolysis Trialists' Collaborative Group. (2014). Effect of treatment delay, age, and stroke severity on the effects of intravenous thrombolysis with alteplase for acute ischaemic stroke: a meta-analysis of individual patient data from randomised trials. *Lancet*, **384**, 1929–35.

England TJ, Hedstrom A, O'Sullivan S, Donnelly R, Barrett DA, Sarmad S, et al. (2017). RECAST (Remote

Ischemic Conditioning After Stroke Trial): a pilot randomized placebo controlled phase II trial in acute ischemic stroke. *Stroke*, **48**, 1412–1415.

Enlimomab Acute Stroke Trial Investigators. (2001). Use of anti-ICAM-1 therapy in ischemic stroke: results of the Enlimomab Acute Stroke Trial. *Neurology*, **57**, 1428–34.

Fagan SC, Waller JL, Nichols FT, Edwards DJ, Pettigrew LC, Clark WM, et al. (2010). Minocycline to improve neurologic outcome in stroke (MINOS): a dose-finding study. *Stroke*, **41**(10), 2283–7.

Fisher M, Feuerstein G, Howells DW, Hurn PD, Kent TA, Savitz SI, et al; STAIR Group. (2009). Update of the stroke therapy academic industry roundtable preclinical recommendations. *Stroke*, **40**, 2244–50.

Garry PS, Ezra M, Rowland MJ, Westbrook J, Pattinson KT. (2015). The role of the nitric oxide pathway in brain injury and its treatment – from bench to bedside. *Exp Neurol*, **263**, 235–43.

Hess DC, Blauenfeldt RA, Andersen G, Hougaard KD, Hoda MN, Ding Y, Ji X. (2015). Remote ischaemic conditioning – a new paradigm of self-protection in the brain. *Nat Rev Neurol*, **11**, 698–710.

Heiss WD. (2011). The ischemic penumbra: correlates in imaging and implications for treatment of ischemic stroke. *Cerebrovasc Dis*, **32**, 307–20.

Heiss WD, Thiel A, Grond M, Graf R. (1999). Which targets are relevant for therapy of acute ischemic stroke? *Stroke*, **30**, 1486–9.

Hill M, Martin RH, Mikulis D, Wong JH, Silver FL, Terbrugge KG, et al. (2012). Safety and efficacy of NA-1 in patients with iatrogenic stroke after endovascular aneurysm repair (ENACT): a phase 2, randomised, double-blind, placebo-controlled trial. *Lancet Neurol*, **11**, 942–50.

Hong K-S, Lee M, Lee SH, Hao Q, Liebeskind D, Saver JL. (2011). Acute stroke trials in the 1st decade of the 21st century. *Stroke*, **42**, e314.

Horn J, De Haan RJ, Vermeulen M, Limburg M. (2001). Very Early Nimodipine Use in Stroke (VENUS): a randomized, double-blind, placebo-controlled trial. *Stroke*, **32**, 461–5.

Hougaard KD, Hjort N, Zeidler D, Sorensen L, Norgaard A, Hansen TM, et al. (2014). Remote ischemic perconditioning as an adjunct therapy to thrombolysis in patients with acute ischemic stroke. *Stroke*, **45**, 159–167.

Intravenous Magnesium Efficacy in Stroke (IMAGES) Study Investigators. (2004). Magnesium for acute stroke (Intravenous Magnesium Efficacy in Stroke trial): randomised controlled trial. *Lancet*, **363**, 439–45.

Kennedy J, Hill MD, Ryckborst KJ, Eliasziw M, Demchuk AM, Buchan AM; FASTER Investigators. (2007). Fast assessment of stroke and transient ischaemic attack to prevent early recurrence (FASTER): a randomised controlled pilot trial. *Lancet Neurol*, **6**, 961–69.

Kohler E, Prentice DA, Bates TR, Hankey GJ, Claxton A, van Heerden J, et al. (2013). Intravenous minocycline in acute stroke: a randomized, controlled pilot study and meta-analysis. *Stoke*, **44**, 2493–9.

Krams M, Lees KR, Hacke W, Grieve AP, Orgogozo JM, Ford GA; ASTIN Study Investigators. (2003). Acute Stroke Therapy by Inhibition of Neutrophils (ASTIN): an adaptive dose-response study of UK-279,276 in acute ischemic stroke. *Stroke*, **34**, 2543–8.

Kurisu K, Yenari MA. (2018). Therapeutic hypothermia for ischemic stroke; pathophysiology and future promise. *Neuropharmacology*, **134**(Pt B), 302-9. pii: S0028-3908(17)30392-1. doi:10.1016/j.neuropharm.2017.08.025.

Lapchak PA, Zhang JH, Noble-Haeusslein LJ. (2013). RIGOR guidelines: escalating STAIR and STEPS for effective translational research. *Transl Stroke Res*, 4, 279–85.

Liu J, Wang L-N. (2014). Gamma aminobutyric acid (GABA) receptor agonists for acute stroke. *Cochrane Database Syst Rev*, 8. CD009622. doi:10.1002/14651858. CD009622.pub3.

Lyden P, Hemmen T, Grotta J, Rapp K, Ernstrom K, Rzesiewicz, T, et al. (2016). Results of the ICTuS 2 Trial (Intravascular Cooling in the Treatment of Stroke 2). *Stroke*, **47**, 2888–95.

Lyden P, Shuaib A, Ng K, Levin K, Atkinson RP, Rajput A, et al.; CLASS-I/H/T Investigators. (2002). Clomethiazole Acute Stroke Study in ischemic stroke (CLASS-I): final results. *Stroke*, **33**(1), 122–8.

Marehbian J, Greer DM. (2017). Normothermia and stroke. *Curr Treat Options Neurol*, **19**, 4. doi:10.1007/s11940-017-0437-6.

Martin RH, Yeatts SD, Hill MD, Moy CS, Ginsberg MD, Palesch YY, ALIAS Parts 1 and 2 and NETT investigators. (2016). ALIAS (Albumin in Acute Ischemic Stroke) trials: analysis of the combined data from parts 1 and 2. *Stroke*, **47**, 2355–9.

Montaner J, Bustamante J, García-Matas S, Martinez-Zabaleta M, Jimenez C, de la Torre J, et al. (2016). Combination of thrombolysis and statins in acute stroke is safe: results of the STARS Randomized Trial. *Stroke*, **47**, 2870–3.

Muir KW, Lees KR. (2003). Excitatory amino acid antagonists for acute stroke. *Cochrane Database Syst Rev*, 3, CD001244.

Muscari A, Puddu GM, Santoro N, Serafini C, Cenni A, Rossi V, et al. (2011). The Atorvastatin During Ischemic Stroke Study: a pilot randomized controlled trial. *Clin Neuropharm*, **34**, 141–7.

Narayanan S, Dave K, Perez-Pinzon M. (2013). Ischemic preconditioning and clinical scenarios. *Curr Opin Neurol*, 26, 1–7.

O'Collins VE, Macleod MR, Donnan GA, Horky LL, van der Worp BH, Howells DW. (2006). 1,026 experimental treatments in acute stroke. *Ann Neurol*, **59**, 467–77.

Ovbiagele B, Kidwell CS, Starkman S, Saver JL. (2003). Potential role of neuroprotective agents in the treatment of patients with acute ischemic stroke. *Curr Treat Options Neurol*, 5, 367–75.

Paciaroni M, Bogousslavsky J. (2011). Trafermin for stroke recovery: is it time for another randomized clinical trial? *Expert Opin Biol Ther*, 11, 1533–41.

Ricci S, Celani MG, Cantisani TA, Righetti E. (2012). Piracetam for acute ischaemic stroke. *Cochrane Database Syst Rev*, 9. CD000419. doi:10.1002/14651858.CD000419.pub3.

Romanos E, Planas AM, Amaro S, Chamorro A. (2007). Uric acid reduces brain damage and improves the benefits of rt-PA in a rat model of thromboembolic stroke. *J Cereb Blood Flow Metab*, 27, 14–20.

Saxena R, Wijnhoud AD, Carton H, Hacke W, Kaste M, Przybelski RJ, et al. (1999). Controlled safety study of a hemoglobin-based oxygen carrier, DCLHb, in acute ischemic stroke. *Stroke*, 30, 993–6.

Saver JL. (2008). Citicoline: update on a promising and widely available agent for neuroprotection and neurorepair. *Rev Neurol Dis*, 5, 167–77.

Saver JL Goyal M, van der Lugt A, Menon BK, Majoie CB, Dippel DW, et al. (2016). Time to treatment with endovascular thrombectomy and outcomes from ischemic stroke: a meta-analysis. *JAMA*, 316, 1279–88.

Saver JL, Starkman S., Eckstein M, Stratton SJ, Pratt FD, Hamilton S, et al. (2015). Prehospital use of magnesium sulfate as neuroprotection in acute stroke. *N Engl J Med*, 372, 528–36.

Secades JJ, Alvarez-Sabín J, Castillo J, Diez-Tejedor E, Martinez-Vila E, Rios J, et al. (2016). Citicoline for acute ischemic stroke: a systematic review and formal meta-analysis of randomized, double-blind, and placebo-controlled trials. *J Stroke Cerebrovasc Dis*, 25,1984–96.

Sekerdag E, Solaroglu I, Gursoy-Ozdemir Y. (2018). Cell death mechanisms in stroke and novel molecular and cellular treatment options. *Curr Neuropharmacol*, 16(9), 1396–1415. doi:10.2174/1570159X16666180321100439.

Wan YH, Nie C, Wang HL, Huang CY. (2014). Therapeutic hypothermia (different depths, durations, and rewarming speeds) for acute ischemic stroke: a meta-analysis. *J Stroke Cerebrovasc Dis*, 23, 2736–47

Wang Y, Reis C, Applegate R 2nd, Stier G, Martin R, Zhang JH. (2015). Ischemic conditioning-induced endogenous brain protection: applications pre-, per- or post-stroke. *Exper Neurol*, 272, 26–40.

Wang Y, Yoshimura R, Manabe H, Schretter C, Clarke R, Cai Y, et al. (2014). Trans-sodium crocetinate improves outcomes in rodent models of occlusive and hemorrhagic stroke. *Brain Res*, 1583, 245–54.

Wang Z, Lin Y, Liu Y, Chen Y, Wang B, Li C, et al. (2016). Serum uric acid levels and outcomes after acute ischemic stroke. *Mol Neurobiol*, 53, 1753–9.

Willmot M, Ghadami A, Whysall B, Clarke W, Wardlaw J, Bath PM. (2006). Transdermal glyceryl trinitrate lowers blood pressure and maintains cerebral blood flow in recent stroke. *Hypertension*, 47, 1209–15.

Yaghi S, Elkind MSV. (2016). Lipid control and beyond: current and future indications for statin therapy in stroke. *Curr Treat Options Cardio Med*, 18, 27. doi:10.1007/s11936-016-0448-8.

Yang J, Cui C, Li J, Zhang C, Zhang J, Liu M. (2015). Edaravone for acute stroke: Meta-analyses of data from randomized controlled trials. *Devel Neurorehab*, 18, 330–5.

Yoshimura S, Uchida K, Daimon T, Takashima R, Kimura K, Morimoto T; ASSORT Trial Investigator. (2017). Randomized controlled trial of early versus delayed statin therapy in patients with acute ischemic stroke: ASSORT Trial. *Stroke*, 48, 3057–63.

Zhang J, Yang J, Zhang C, Jiang X, Zhou H, Liu M. (2012). Calcium antagonists for acute ischemic stroke. *Cochrane Database Syst Rev*, 5. CD001928. doi:10.1002/14651858.CD001928.pub2.

Chapter

13

Acute Treatment of Intracerebral Haemorrhage

Tom Moullaali
Rustam Al-Shahi Salman
Craig Anderson

Acute non-traumatic intracerebral haemorrhage (ICH) is the most common manifestation of haemorrhagic stroke, which occurs as an isolated haematoma within the brain or extends directly (or indirectly) internally into the ventricular system or externally across the meninges (Figure 13.1). In general, ICH accounts for approximately 10% of strokes, but the proportion is much greater (20–50%) in particular racial-ethnic groups, including Asians, Blacks, and Hispanics, with leading risk factors of older age, male sex, hypertension, poorer socio-economic status, and colder environmental temperature (Feigin et al., 2009; Poon et al., 2015). As haemorrhagic forms of stroke have greater severity than acute ischaemic stroke, the adverse outcomes are disproportionately higher: 49% of all deaths and ~42% (47 million) of all 'disability-adjusted life years lost' due to stroke worldwide each year (Feigin et al., 2015).

There are several reasons why prevention should be the priority of management for ICH, including poor prognosis and limited acute treatments, with case fatality not dramatically changing over recent decades (van Asch et al., 2010; Poon et al., 2014); and, apart from age, the most important risk factor – high blood pressure (BP) – can be effectively modified (O'Donnell et al., 2010). Since two-thirds of incident ICH occurs in people aged ≥75 years in high-income countries (Samarasekera et al., 2015), the burden is likely to rise further as the populations age and primary prevention strategies remain inadequate.

General Management

ICH is a critical illness requiring rapid assessment and management, as patients are often unstable, have altered level of consciousness, and may rapidly deteriorate. An assessment of clinical severity and certain imaging features (i.e. site, volume, and presence of intraventricular haemorrhage [IVH]) of the haematoma are useful in triaging patients for intensive

monitoring, respiratory support, and surgical intervention. Early use of palliative care plans have been shown to adversely influence outcome (Parry-Jones et al., 2016) and should be used cautiously. An active management plan is recommended unless there are clear clinical (e.g. massive ICH with deep coma), comorbid (e.g. advanced dementia or malignancy), or patient autonomy (e.g. advance directive) circumstances to suggest otherwise. Active care allows time to review the rapidity of any progression, for potential complications (e.g. seizures and dehydration) to be resolved, and for family members to adjust to the crisis and receive counselling relevant to their cultural, religious, and personal beliefs. Active care includes monitoring and timely intervention for neurological deterioration and adverse events, which is ideally organized in an intensive care or high dependency unit, where there is a high nurse:patient ratio of care and expertise. Well-organized, acute stroke unit care benefits patients with ICH to the same extent as those with acute ischaemic stroke (Langhorne et al., 2013) by directing effective management according to the type and severity of neurological impairment.

Noncontrast computed tomography (CT) and brain magnetic resonance imaging (MRI) are appropriate initial investigations to diagnose ICH. CT is generally more readily available, but is less useful in establishing any underlying structural cause, which should be suspected when the haematoma is in a lobar or an atypical deep location; when there is a disproportionate amount of subarachnoid haemorrhage or perihaematomal oedema; and in younger patients without a history of hypertension or illicit drug use as predisposing factors. The initial brain imaging may identify the likely cause, such as tumours, large vascular malformations, or underlying infarctions with haemorrhagic transformation. CT or MRI angiography should be the next step to further screen

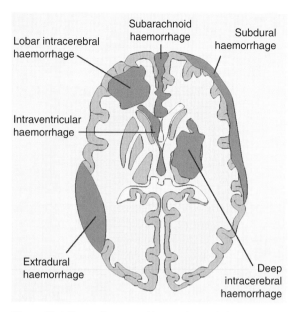

Subarachnoid haemorrhage

Subdural haemorrhage

Lobar intracerebral haemorrhage

Intraventricular haemorrhage

Extradural haemorrhage

Deep intracerebral haemorrhage

Figure 13.1 Types of intracranial haemorrhage (Al-Shahi Salman et al., 2009).

for any underlying vascular anomaly, such as an intracranial aneurysm, arteriovenous malformation, or cavernous angioma; acquired arteriopathies, such as vasculitis or moyamoya disease; reversible vasoconstriction syndrome; cerebral venous sinus thrombosis; and other causes. Catheter cerebral angiography is required where prior investigations identify a potential macrovascular abnormality; suspicion remains high despite negative screening tests (macrovascular abnormalities can go undetected by CT and MR [van Asch et al., 2015]); or interventional treatment is being considered.

Although early mobilization of patients is generally considered beneficial for maintaining muscle strength and to reduce risks associated with immobility, particularly venous thromboembolism, very early and intensive mobilization is not indicated in ICH patients. A large multicentre randomized trial compared very early (median start 18.5 hours after onset), high intensity mobilization with conventional early (median start 22.4 hours after onset), standard intensity mobilization, and found that standard early mobilization was associated with improved outcomes, particularly in those with ICH (AVERT Trial Collaboration Group, 2015). Although elevating the head of patients with large ICH may reduce intracranial pressure, one large randomized trial showed no benefits (or harms) of positioning the patient to be sitting up versus lying flat after acute ICH (Anderson et al., 2017a).

Therapeutic Targets in the Pathophysiology of Acute Intracerebral Haemorrhage

The manifestations of ICH depend on the location of the initial site/tract of haemorrhage and subsequent mass effect from the expanding haematoma on adjacent structures (see Box 13.1). Haematoma expansion

---

BOX 13.1 Manifestations of ICH with Prognostic Significance

- Loss of consciousness at presentation (Glasgow Coma Scale, GCS)
- Progressive neurological deterioration (National Institutes of Health Stroke Scale, NIHSS)
- Location of haematoma
  - internal capsule – damage to motor tracts
  - basal ganglia/thalamus – risk of IVH
  - brainstem/cerebellum – greater risk from mass effect
- Haematoma features
  - volume – more blood, worse outcome
  - volume increase – ongoing bleeding, worse outcome
  - morphology – irregular borders and heterogeneous consistency (e.g. swirl[1] sign) indicate active bleeding
  - spot sign[2] – positivity on CT angiography indicates active bleeding
- Presence of IVH – worse outcome
- Hypertensive response – higher systolic BP, worse outcome
- Hyperglycaemia – higher serum glucose, worse outcome
- Older age – the older brain (with cerebral atrophy) can accommodate greater mass effect from the ICH, but elders have reduced brain/physiological reserve, greater comorbidities, and higher risk of cardiovascular complications

---

[1] Swirl sign describes the appearance of a mixture of hyper- and hypo-attenuation within the ICH lesion on brain imaging, reflecting active bleeding on a background of older haematoma.

[2] Spot sign describes the appearance of one or more discrete foci of hyperattenuation within the ICH lesion on post-contrast imaging, reflecting active bleeding point(s) where contrast has extravasated.

or 'growth' occurs in most patients with ICH: its recognition depends in part on the velocity of growth and in part on the time intervals from symptom onset to initial, and subsequent, brain imaging. Haematoma growth immediately after haemorrhage onset occurs in all patients and contributes to prehospital and early post-arrival neurological deterioration, which occurs in 31% of ICH patients (Shkirkova et al., 2018). Continued radiological haematoma growth between initial post-arrival brain imaging and follow-up imaging affects a fifth of patients with acute ICH, is more common in patients arriving earlier after onset, taking antiplatelet or anticoagulant agents, and with larger haematoma volumes on initial imaging, and is associated with a poor outcome (Davis et al., 2006; Al-Shahi Salman et al., 2018). When ICH is related to anticoagulation therapy, haematoma growth often continues over a more protracted time period. In addition to contributing to local pressure and midline shift, haematoma growth can track into the ventricular system (IVH), causing hydrocephalus, further mass effect, increased intracranial pressure (ICP), and reduced cerebral perfusion. Whether or not ICH growth occurs, any extravasation of blood into the brain parenchyma promotes perihaematomal oedema, initially from infiltration of blood plasma and later from neurotoxicity related to haemoglobin breakdown products causing inflammation (Xi et al., 2006; Yu et al., 2017), and greater oedema worsens prognosis (Yang et al., 2015). Each of the phases of the pathophysiology of ICH influences the degree and rate of recovery and potential therapeutic targets (Poon et al., 2014; Specogna et al., 2014).

Criteria for Selecting Evidence for This Chapter

In this chapter we will outline available treatments for acute ICH, rationale for their use, level of supporting evidence for efficacy and safety, and implications for practice and research. A hierarchical approach has been taken in the selection of Level 1 or 2 of evidence for recommendations; a lower level of evidence is based on expert consensus and summarized in current guidelines (Steiner et al., 2014; Hemphill et al., 2015).

Organized Stroke Unit Care

Rationale

Stroke units provide an integrated package of supportive care potentially beneficial for ICH, including active management of physiological variables relating to fluid balance, pyrexia, oxygenation, and glycaemia; early mobilization out of bed; skilled nursing; and multidisciplinary rehabilitation.

Evidence

A formal meta-analysis identified 8 randomized controlled trials (RCTs) specifically reporting outcomes in 483 enrolled patients with ICH. Among ICH patients, stroke unit care reduced death or dependency, 46.8% vs 74.2%, risk ratio (RR) 0.79 (95% confidence interval [CI]: 0.61–1.00) (Figure 13.2). There was evidence of heterogeneity across trials ($I^2 = 62\%$), but this appeared to arise from bidirectional scatter among small sample size trials without evidence of biasing of the effect estimate. Stroke unit care reduced all-cause mortality, 24.4% vs 50.0%, RR 0.73 (95% CI: 0.54–0.97), without evidence of trial heterogeneity ($I^2 = 21\%$).

Implications for Practice

Patients with ICH should be managed in dedicated stroke units or neurocritical care units that actively monitor and manage physiological variables relating to fluid balance, body temperature, and oxygenation; pursue early mobilization out of bed; have skilled, stroke-knowledgeable nursing; and deliver multidisciplinary rehabilitation.

Surgery

Rationale

Neurosurgery has the potential to improve outcomes from acute ICH through:

- evacuation of the haematoma to reduce early mass effect and elevated intracranial pressure (ICP), and later haematoma-related neurotoxicity, via craniectomy, craniotomy, or minimally invasive approaches (e.g. endoscopic suction or catheter-based drainage)

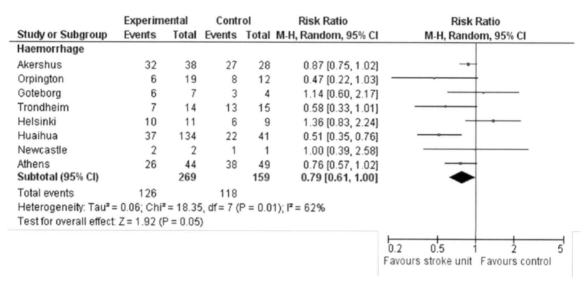

Figure 13.2 Effect of *stroke unit vs general medical ward management* of acute ICH on *death or dependency* at end of scheduled follow-up months (Langhorne et al., 2013).

- placement of an external ventricular drain (EVD) to reduce ICP by clearing IVH with/without local administration of lytic agent.

This section considers both open craniotomy and a variety of minimally invasive neurosurgical approaches to haematoma evacuation. The potential physiological benefits of each approach towards clearance of ICH (± IVH) in relieving mass effect are counterbalanced by the risks of anaesthesia, particularly in an older multi-morbid patient group (Lovelock et al., 2007; Samarasekera et al., 2015); damage to healthy brain tissue trespassed upon to access the haematoma cavity; and post-operative complications (e.g. re-bleeding, infection, thromboembolism). Accordingly, evidence-based analysis and individual case clinical judgement are required. Importantly, it is desirable that improved survival does not solely result in more patients alive but severely disabled, with poor physical function and quality of life.

Evidence

Surgical Evacuation of Supratentorial ICH

The latest Cochrane systematic review included 10 RCTs with a total of 2059 patients randomized to surgery with medical management versus medical management alone (Prasad et al., 2008). Patients undergoing surgery received either craniotomy (open surgery) or stereotactic/endoscopic (catheter-guided) haematoma evacuation. Among 9 trials enrolling 1996 patients contributing to this outcome, surgery combined with medical therapy compared with medical therapy alone reduced death or dependence, 63.1% vs 70.6%, odds ratio (OR) 0.71 (95% CI: 0.58–0.88; $p = 0.001$). No significant heterogeneity of effect across trials was noted ($I^2 = 25\%$). Among all 10 trials, surgery combined with medical therapy compared with medical therapy alone reduced mortality, 27.0% vs 33.6%, OR 0.74 (95% CI: 0.61–0.90; $p = 0.003$). For the mortality outcome, moderate heterogeneity across trials was observed ($I^2 = 49\%$), due at least in part to enhanced mortality benefit in some trials of stereotactic or endoscopic surgery compared with open craniotomy.

A subsequent meta-analysis additionally incorporating later reported trials included 15 RCTs enrolling 3366 patients (Mendelow et al., 2013). In this further analysis, surgery combined with medical therapy compared with medical therapy alone reduced death or unfavourable functional outcome, 59.3% vs 66.5%, OR 0.74 (95% CI: 0.64–0.86). However, there was substantial heterogeneity of effects across trials ($I^2 = 67\%$), heterogeneity p value = 0.0002), and both of the two largest trials, STICH 1 and STICH 2, were individually non-positive and had point estimates for treatment effect less than the aggregate, raising concerns regarding risk of bias of the included RCTs, in addition to uncertainties arising from heterogeneous designs, participants, interventions, and comparators.

Minimally Invasive Surgery

In the Cochrane review, data on the effect of surgery by type of surgical procedure were available from 8 RCTs enrolling 1335 patients, including 566 (42.4%) enrolled in trials of stereotactic or endoscopic surgery plus medical therapy versus medical therapy alone, and 769 (57.6%) enrolled in trials of open craniotomy plus medical therapy versus medical therapy alone (Prasad et al., 2008). A non-significantly greater benefit with minimally invasive surgery than with open craniotomy was noted. For stereotactic or endoscopic surgery plus medical therapy compared with medical therapy alone, rates of death or dependence were 62.3% vs 71.0%, OR 0.66 (95% CI: 0.46–0.95); for open craniotomy plus medical therapy compared with medical therapy alone, 74.9% vs 78.4%, OR 0.82 (95% CI: 0.59–1.15) (Figure 13.3).

A distinctive minimally invasive surgical technique for evacuation of deep ICH is aspiration via catheter assisted by the instillation of fibrinolytic drugs into the haematoma cavity to dissolve the clot for enhanced clearance. The Minimally Invasive Surgery plus recombinant Tissue plasminogen activator (rt-PA) for ICH Evacuation (MISTIE) phase 2 RCT compared imaged-guided catheter placement with local rt-PA administration (0.3 mg or 1.0 mg, every 8 hours for up to 9 doses) added to standard medical care compared to standard medical care alone in 96 randomly allocated patients (Hanley et al., 2019). Patients were enrolled with ICH of at least 20 millilitres (mL) in volume that had been stable in size for at least 6 hours. Haematoma volume at end of treatment, typically around day 4, was reduced in the aspiration group, 20 mL vs 41 mL, $p < 0.0001$, and there was a nonsignificant increase in the rate of being

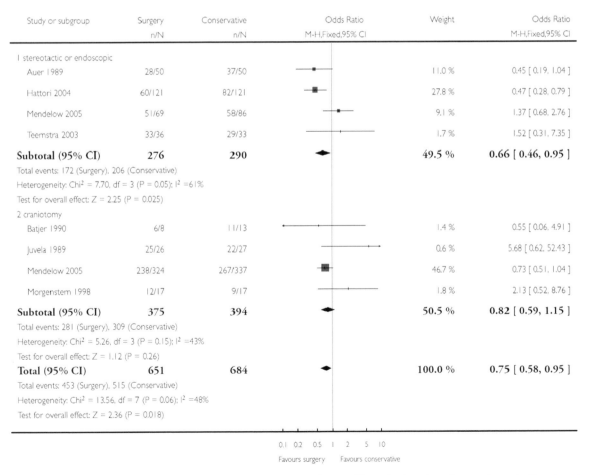

Figure 13.3 Comparison of *surgery type vs conservative management* of acute ICH on *death or dependency at 6 months* (Prasad et al., 2008).

capable of bodily self-care or better (modified Rankin Scale [mRS] 0–3) at 6 months, 33% vs 21%, hazard ratio (HR) 1.32 (95% CI: 0.62–2.82). No significant differences were noted in the lead safety outcomes of 30-day case fatality, 7-day procedure-related case fatality, 72-hour symptomatic bleeding, and 30-day brain infections, although asymptomatic haemorrhages were more common in the surgical group. These results provided support for the phase 3, MISTIE III trial that randomly assigned 506 ICH patients to catheter placement with local administration of 1.0 mg rt-PA every 8 hours for up to 9 doses or standard medical care. Fibrinolytic-assisted catheter aspiration was associated with lower mortality at 1 year (20% vs 27%, HR 0.67, $p = 0.04$), but also with nominally increased severely disabled outcomes (mRS 4–5: 42% vs 38%), with resulting no net significant effect on the primary outcome of ambulatory and capable of bodily self-care or better (mRS 0–3), 45% vs 41%, $p = 0.33$.

Additionally, the MISTIE investigators reported results of a parallel pilot RCT, the Intraoperative Stereotactic Computed Tomography-Guided Endoscopic Surgery (ICES) for Brain Haemorrhage study, that tested the safety and efficacy of image-guided endoscopic haematoma evacuation via a burr hole (Vespa et al., 2016). The investigators compared 14 patients receiving the endoscopic intervention with 42 patients receiving medical care only, with the medical care group comprised of both patients randomized to medical therapy within ICES and patients randomized to medical therapy in MISTIE II. On average, the procedure achieved an immediate reduction in haemorrhage volume of 68%, and a non-significantly higher proportion of patients who received surgical intervention made a good functional recovery (mRS score 0–3) at 180 and 365 days (42.9% vs 23.7%).

Surgical Evacuation of Infratentorial ICH

There have been no RCTs of surgical management of infratentorial ICH. A systematic review of observational studies included 792 patients with primary cerebellar haemorrhage: the overall case fatality was 31%, and surgery (with or without ventriculostomy) was non-significantly associated with a lower case fatality compared to conservative management (29% vs 33%) (Witsch et al., 2013).

Decompressive Hemicraniectomy

A 2017 systematic review and meta-analysis of decompressive hemicraniectomy for spontaneous supratentorial ICH identified one small RCT (n = 40) and 227

cases from 7 observational studies (Yao et al., 2017). Outcomes of hemicraniectomy with or without haematoma evacuation were compared with outcomes of haematoma evacuation alone in the randomized trial and 6 of the 7 non-randomized observational studies, and with medical therapy alone in the remaining non-randomized observational study. Decompressive craniectomy compared with haematoma evacuation or medical therapy alone was associated with reduced frequency of poor outcome (Glasgow Outcome Scale [GOS] score 1–3, or mRS score 4–5), RR 0.91 (95% CI: 0.84–0.99). This result was heavily influenced by the single RCT (Moussa and Khedr, 2017).

Decompressive craniectomy was also associated with reduced mortality, RR 0.67 (95% CI: 0.53–0.85), which was more stable when subjected to sensitivity analyses but the authors were cautious in their interpretation from being unable to adjust for confounding factors. There was no excess of re-bleeding or hydrocephalus among decompressive craniectomy patients.

A multi-centre RCT, the Swiss trial of decompressive craniectomy versus best medical treatment of spontaneous supratentorial intracerebral haemorrhage (SWITCH) (NCT02258919), is currently ongoing with the aim of recruiting 300 patients to compare decompressive craniectomy with best medical management.

EVD Insertion

While no randomized trials have assessed use versus non-use of EVD in ICH, physiological reasoning and observational series provide support. In non-communicating hydrocephalus, the insertion of an EVD in a trapped ventricle and performance of cerebrospinal fluid (CSF) drainage will relieve local pressure; in communicating hydrocephalus, EVD placement and CSF drainage will reduce generalized intracranial pressure. In patients with IVH with or without ICH, a retrospective, single-centre case series of 183 patients noted that EVDs were placed in 37%. EVD placement was an independent predictor of reduced mortality (OR 0.31, 95% CI: 0.10–0.94) and discharge alive and capable of bodily self-care (mRS 0–3) (OR 15.7, 95% CI: 1.83–134.2) (Herrick et al., 2014). In a multicentre analysis of 563 patients with ICH with or without IVH, EVDs were placed in 25%. In propensity score adjusted analysis, EVD placement was associated with improved outcomes among ICH patients who also had IVH, with increased frequency of functional independence (mRS 0–2) at discharge (OR 8.43, 95% CI: 2.39–29.79) and a non-significant reduction in mortality at 30 days (OR 0.60, 95% CI: 0.34–1.05) (Lovasik et al., 2016).

Fibrinolytic Therapy for Intraventricular Haemorrhage

Haemorrhages that are solely or predominantly intraventricular do not produce focal mass effect but can result in damaging hydrocephalus, including non-communicating (obstructive) hydrocephalus due to formation of large clots that plug a particular ventricular conduit and communicating (non-obstructive) hydrocephalus due to diffuse injury by blood degradation products to arachnoid granulations. A systematic review and meta-analysis of 8 small RCTs, 3 prospective cohorts, and 12 retrospective cohorts including 418 patients with ICH and IVH receiving intraventricular fibrinolysis versus 367 controls found that intraventricular fibrinolysis was associated with a lower case fatality (RR 0.55, 95% CI: 0.42–0.71), though benefit did not reach statistical significance in analyses confined to RCTs alone (RR 0.60, 95% CI: 0.35–1.01) (Khan et al., 2014). Intraventricular fibrinolysis was associated with increased good functional outcome (RR 1.66, 95% CI: 1.27–2.19), though not with statistical significance when analyzing only RCTs (RR 1.57, 95% CI: 0.89–2.80). Intraventricular instillation of fibrinolytics was not associated with increased risks of re-haemorrhage or hydrocephalus and was associated with reduced shunt dependence.

More recently, the Clot Lysis: Evaluating Accelerated Resolution of intraventricular haemorrhage phase 3 (CLEAR III) RCT enrolled 500 patients with IVH causing third or fourth ventricle obstruction and no more than 30 mL of accompanying supratentorial ICH (Hanley et al., 2017). All patients received clot removal via EVD, and were randomly allocated to 1 mg doses of rt-PA or placebo saline via EVD, up to a maximum of 12 doses, 8 hours apart. The primary outcome of capable of bodily self-care or better (mRS 0–3) at 180 days was similar in both groups, 48% vs 45%, RR 1.06 (95% CI: 0.88–1.28; $p = 0.55$). The alteplase group had reduced mortality through 180 days, 18% vs 29%, HR 0.60 (95% CI: 0.41–0.86; $p = 0.006$), but also a higher rate of severe disability (mRS 5), 17% vs 9%, RR 1.99 (95% CI: 1.22–3.26; $p = 0.007$). Symptomatic bleeding was similar between groups, and there were fewer cases of ventriculitis in the treatment group.

One RCT has evaluated lumbar drains as an add-on therapy to intraventricular fibrinolysis (IVF) for patients with severe IVH. The placement of lumbar drains may help restore physiological CSF circulation and prevent permanent shunt dependency. Among 30 randomized patients, lumbar drain placement reduced permanent shunt placement, 0% vs 43% ($p = 0.007$) (Staykov et al., 2017).

Interpretation of the Evidence

In view of the lack of clear benefit in individual large RCTs of surgical evacuation and heterogeneity across trials in meta-analyses, early surgery is not clearly beneficial as a treatment strategy for broad, relatively unselected groups of patients with ICH. Minimally invasive endoscopic and stereotactic approaches hold promise, and the results of further RCTs of these interventions and decompressive craniectomy as an adjunctive or alternative surgical manoeuvre are awaited (see below for list of ongoing trials).

Implications for Clinical Practice

At present, based on the available trials and observational series, for patients with supratentorial ICH, guidelines do not recommend early surgical intervention as a broad intervention for individuals who are clinically stable, but do recognize surgical treatment as of potential benefit in select circumstances (Steiner et al., 2014; Hemphill et al., 2015). European guidelines (Steiner et al., 2014) suggest surgical intervention may be of value for patients with a GCS score of 9–12. US guidelines recognize haematoma evacuation as having the potential to reduce mortality, but to increase severe disability, for patients experiencing neurological deterioration. Decompressive hemicraniectomy is also recognized as potentially life-saving, but with increased disability, for patients with coma, large haematomas with midline shift, or elevated intracranial pressure refractory to medical management (Hemphill et al., 2015).

For infratentorial haemorrhage, in the absence of RCT data, the most recent American Heart Association (AHA)/American Stroke Association (ASA) guidelines endorse early neurosurgical removal of haematoma in patients with cerebellar haemorrhage who are deteriorating neurologically, have brainstem compression, or have hydrocephalus, and emphasize that initial management with an EVD alone is insufficient (Hemphill et al., 2015). Evacuation of brainstem haemorrhage is considered harmful and is not recommended.

AHA/ASA guidelines recommend that insertion of an EVD should be considered for the monitoring and management of raised ICP in patients with a GCS score of ≤8, those with evidence of transtentorial herniation, and those with significant IVH or hydrocephalus.

Implications for Research

Current interest is centred on minimally invasive surgery and decompressive craniectomy. Ongoing RCTs include:

1. Minimally invasive surgery versus craniotomy in patients with supratentorial hypertensive intracerebral haemorrhage (MISICH) (NCT02811614)
2. Minimally invasive endoscopic surgery vs medical management in supratentorial intraparenchymal haemorrhage (INVEST) (Fiorella, 2016)
3. Minimally invasive surgery treatment for patients with spontaneous supratentorial intracerebral haemorrhage (MISTICH) (ChiCTR-TRC-12002026)
4. Decompressive hemicraniectomy in intracerebral haemorrhage (SWITCH) (NCT02258919)
5. Decompressive craniectomy combined with haematoma removal to treat ICH (CARICH) (NCT02135783).

Haemostatic Drugs

Rationale

Active ongoing bleeding, causing continued haematoma growth with additional tissue destruction and mass effect, is a mediator of poor outcome in acute ICH. The presence of the CT-angiography spot sign on early imaging, indicating ongoing bleeding, is associated with a 2.4-fold increase in mortality at 3 months (Demchuk et al., 2012). The rationale for using haemostatic drugs is to achieve early resolution of bleeding and attenuate haematoma growth. Several haemostatic therapies have been tested in acute ICH patients:

- Blood coagulation factors
  o Recombinant (activated) factor VII (rFVIIa) – generates thrombin by binding to tissue factor and activated platelets at sites of tissue injury
  o Fresh frozen plasma (FFP) and prothrombin complex concentrate (PCC) – replenishes clotting factors antagonized by warfarin/Coumadin
  o Cryoprecipitate – corrects hypofibrinogenaemia associated with rtPA-related ICH

- Antifibrinolytic drugs
  o Tranexamic acid – competitively inhibits activation of plasminogen to plasmin
- Platelet transfusion
  o Provides functioning platelets to treat antiplatelet therapy-related ICH

Evidence

A Cochrane systematic review identified 12 RCTs enrolling 1732 patients (1150 treated vs 582 controls or active comparators) (Al-Shahi Salman et al., 2018).

Antifibrinolytic Drugs

Three small RCTs of intravenous antifibrinolytic drugs (tranexamic acid in two and aminocaproic acid in the other) enrolled 57 patients (33 active, 24 control). Active antifibrinolytic therapy was associated with a non-significant reduction in ICH growth (RR 0.76, 95% CI: 0.56–1.05). However, antifibrinolytic therapy was also associated with non-significant increases in death or dependency (RR 1.25, 95% CI: 0.57–2.75), death (RR 1.16, 95% CI: 0.31–4.39), and any serious adverse events (SAEs) (RR 1.50, 95% CI: 0.39–5.83) and thromboembolic SAEs (RR 1.59, 95% CI: 0.07–35.15). More recently, the Tranexamic acid for Intracerebral Haemorrhage (TICH-2) RCT randomized 2325 ICH patients within 8 hours of onset to intravenous (IV) tranexamic acid, 1 g loading dose followed by another 1 g infused over 8 hours, or to matching placebo. On the primary outcome of global disability distribution over all 7 levels of the mRS at 3 months, IV tranexamic acid showed a non-significant shift to reduced disability, adjusted common odds ratio (acOR) 0.88 (95% CI: 0.76–1.03; $p = 0.11$). Although there were fewer early deaths by day 7 with IV tranexamic acid (aOR 0.73) deaths by 3 months were not lower (aHR 0.92, 95% CI: 0.77–1.10). No increase in venous or arterial thromboembolism was noted.

Blood Clotting Factors

A recent meta-analysis identified 7 RCTs, enrolling 1480 patients, that have tested blood clotting factors (predominantly rFVIIa) versus placebo/open control (Al-Shahi Salman et al., 2018). Treatment with blood clotting factors was associated with a non-significant reduction in death or incapacity for body self-care (mRS 4–6) in 6 trials that included 1390 patients, RR

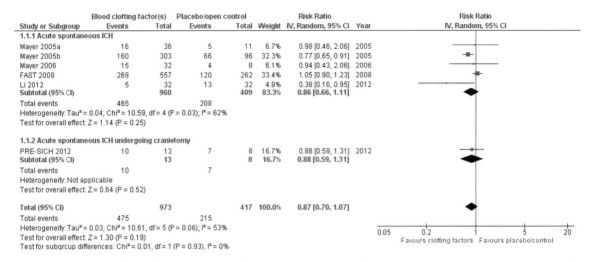

Figure 13.4 The effect of *blood clotting factors versus placebo/open control* for acute ICH not associated with anticoagulant use, *on death or incapacity for body self-care (modified Rankin Scale score 4–6) at day 90* (Al-Shahi Salman et al., 2018).

0.87 (95% CI: 0.70–1.07) (Figure 13.4). Blood clotting factors were also associated with non-significant reductions in death (7 trials, 1480 patients: RR 0.75, 95% CI: 0.51–1.09), all SAEs (2 trials, 81 patients: RR 0.81 95% CI: 0.30–2.22), and ICH growth (3 trials, 151 patients: RR 0.74, 95% CI: 0.36–1.48), but a nonsignificant increase in thromboembolic SAEs (5 trials, 1398 patients: RR 1.24, 95% CI: 0.80–1.91).

Two additional trials have presented pooled preliminary results, both testing rFVIIa in acute ICH patients showing the CT-angiography spot sign indicating ongoing bleeding and higher risk for haematoma expansion. Patients within 6.5 hours of onset were randomized to 80 mg rFVIIa or placebo. Among 69 randomized patients, haematoma expansion did not differ between the treatment arms. In the rFVIIa group, median volume evolution was from 16 mL at baseline to 22 mL at 24 hours, and in the placebo group from 20 mL at baseline to 29 mL at 24 hours, $p = 0.9$. Long-term functional outcomes and mortality also did not differ between the two treatment groups (Jeffrey, 2017).

Vitamin K Antagonist-Associated ICH

The systematic review identified 1 small RCT (n = 13) that evaluated FFP against FFP with factor IX complex concentrate in patients with warfarin-related ICH and showed the addition of factor IX complex concentrate accelerated correction of the international normalized ratio (INR); however, this was not associated with a difference in the underpowered analysis of neurological outcomes (Boulis et al., 1999).

Also of relevance is the INR Normalization in Coumadin Associated Intracerebral Hemorrhage (INCH) RCT, which randomized patients with intracranial haemorrhage to four-factor prothrombin complex concentrate (PCC) versus fresh frozen plasma (Steiner et al., 2016). Among 50 randomized patients, the predominant haemorrhagic subtype was ICH, present in 88%, while the remaining 12% had subdural haematomas. PCC was superior to FFP on the primary endpoint of normalizing the international normalized ratio (INR <1.2) within 3 hours, 67% vs 9%, OR 30.6 (95% CI: 4.7–197.9; $p = 0.0003$), and reduced the amount of haematoma growth at 24 hours, 8.3 vs 22.1 mL ($p = 0.02$). There was also a non-significant reduction in mortality by 3 months in the PCC group (19% vs 35%, $p = 0.14$), but no increase in being alive and capable of bodily self-care or better (mRS 0–3) at 3 months (37% vs 39%, $p = 0.47$).

ICH Associated with Other Anticoagulants

There are no RCTs confined to ICH patients testing specific antidotes to other anticoagulants. Treatment is based on studies in broader groups of patients with major bleeding or planned surgery at diverse organ sites, often including a small subset with ICH, for example in studies of recently developed antidotes for non-vitamin-K oral anticoagulants (NOACs). In the single arm RE-VERSE AD trial studying idarucizumab to reverse the direct thrombin inhibitor dabigatran, ICH accounted for 53/301 (18%) of patients enrolled with life-threatening bleeding (Pollack et al., 2017). Idarucizumab normalized coagulation parameters within 10–30 minutes in more than 95% of patients. Thrombotic events occurred in 4.7% of patients by day 30. In the single arm, ANNEXA-4 trial studying andexanet alfa to reverse any of the four factor Xa inhibitors (apixaban, rivaroxaban, edoxaban, or enoxaparin), ICH accounted for 14/67 (21%) of patients enrolled with life-threatening bleeding (Connolly, 2016). Within 15–30 minutes, andexanet alfa reduced anti-factor Xa activity by a relative 86%–93%. Thrombotic events occurred in 18% of patients by day 30.

Antiplatelet-Related ICH

The Platelet Transfusion in Cerebral Hemorrhage (PATCH) RCT recruited 190 patients with ICH while on antiplatelet therapy and with normal platelet counts (Baharoglu et al., 2016): 97 were randomized to receive a platelet transfusion as soon as possible (within 6 hours of ICH onset and 90 minutes of the diagnostic scan) and 93 received standard care. Allocation to the platelet transfusion group was associated with a shift towards greater disability across all 7 levels of the mRS at 3 months, adjusted common OR 2.05 (95% CI: 1.18–3.56) (Figure 13.5). Patients treated with platelet transfusion tended to be more likely to have an SAE during the hospital stay, 42% vs 29%, OR 1.79 (95% CI: 0.98–3.27), including nominally more brain oedema and intraventricular extension SAEs. Reflecting the small sample size, the treatment groups had some imbalances in baseline prognostic features, including numerically larger ICHs >30 mL in the platelet transfusion group. Nonetheless, the results suggest no benefit and even potential harm from routine use of platelet transfusion in ICH patients taking antiplatelet agents.

Symptomatic ICH Following Thrombolysis for Acute Ischaemic Stroke

Thrombolysis with rt-PA for acute ischaemic stroke is associated with a 3–5% risk of major symptomatic ICH (sICH). However, there are no RCTs to guide management of this uncommon but potentially deadly complication. In 2015, a multicentre retrospective analysis of the treatment of thrombolysis-related ICH reported time to treatment, treatment modality, and clinical outcomes that included haematoma growth and in-hospital mortality (Yaghi et al., 2015). Of 3894 acute ischaemic stroke patients treated with thrombolysis, 128 (3.3%) had a symptomatic ICH. Overall, 49/128 (38%) received one or more haemostatic or surgical therapies, with the most common being cryoprecipitate in 40 (31%), platelet transfusion in 37 (29%), FFP in 26 (20%), and surgical haematoma evacuation or decompressive craniectomy in 18 (15%). Infrequent agents were vitamin K, PCC, aminocaproic acid, and rFVIIa. Median time from sICH diagnosis to treatment was 112 minutes. In-hospital mortality was 52% and was non-significantly lower in patients who received any form of treatment, 41% vs 59% (p = 0.11). Haematoma growth was more common in patients with severe hypofibrinogenaemia, 36% vs 25% (p = 0.01), lending support for the use of cryoprecipitate.

Interpretation of the Evidence

The available evidence does not support the routine use of haemostatic therapies after spontaneous ICH unrelated to antithrombotic drug use. Platelet transfusion seems harmful for ICH associated with antiplatelet drug use. For vitamin K antagonist-associated ICH, four-factor PCC seems superior to FFP for rapid INR reversal and averting haematoma expansion, but whether this translates into improved clinical

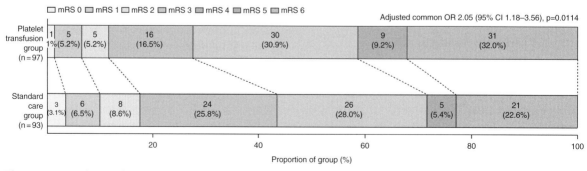

Figure 13.5 Distribution of mRS scores at 3 months in PATCH trial (Baharoglu et al., 2016).

outcomes has not been established. Reversal therapies for other anticoagulant agents are not supported by trials focused solely upon patients with ICH, but have some support from trials in patients with life-threatening bleeding of diverse types, among whom ICH patients constituted about one-fifth the study population.

Implications for Clinical Practice

Clinicians should not routinely use haemostatic therapies where there is no evidence of coagulopathy or anticoagulant use.

For ICH patients who are taking anticoagulation, a prompt assessment of type, last dose, and a coagulation screen are vital in the initial assessment. Immediate cessation of the anticoagulant followed by swift administration of a specific antidote or coagulation factors is recommended with guidance from a haematologist. Based on national guidelines drawing upon the evidence here reviewed (Steiner et al., 2014; Hemphill et al., 2015; Frontera et al., 2016) as well as subsequent trial data (Connolly, 2016; Pollack et al., 2017), recommended approaches include the following:

1. Unfractionated heparin (UHF): use protamine at a dose of 1 mg for every 100 units of UFH given in the previous 2–3 hours (maximum single dose 50 mg), repeat bloods for activated partial thromboplastin time (aPTT), and, if prolonged, give a repeat protamine dose of 0.5 mg per 100 units of UFH.

2. Low-molecular-weight heparin (LMWH): for enoxaparin, give 1 mg of protamine per 1 mg of enoxaparin if the dose was given within 8 hours; if the dose was given within 8–12 hours, then the protamine dose can be halved. Beyond 12 hours, no treatment is recommended. For other LMWH formulations, use 1 mg of protamine per 100 anti-Xa units administered in the past 3–5 half-lives of the drug. In renal insufficiency or ongoing bleeding, use half the dose of protamine and consider rFVIIa, if protamine is contraindicated.

3. Pentasaccharides (e.g. fondaparinux): administer PCC (20 units/kg) or rFVII (90 micrograms/kg) if the former contraindicated. Protamine is not recommended.

4. Direct factor Xa inhibitors (e.g. rivaroxaban, apixaban): establish the timing of last dose. If within 48 hours (or longer if renal or hepatic impairment), administer andexanet alfa if available. If not available, give four-factor PCC. Also, if last dose was within 2 hours, consider activated charcoal for intubated patients.

5. Direct thrombin inhibitors (e.g. dabigatran): if the last dose was within 48 hours and there is no renal failure, administer idarucizumab to reverse dabigatran; where idarucizumab in unavailable, give PCC at a dose of 50 units/kg. If renal failure is present, consider reversal beyond this time, and re-dose if there is ongoing bleeding. Also, if last dose was within 2 hours, consider activated charcoal for intubated patients. Haemodialysis has a role where there is renal insufficiency and idarucizamab is unavailable, or when pharmacological therapy has been ineffective.

For patients with ICH after intravenous rt-PA, immediately discontinue rt-PA and administer cryoprecipitate (or tranexamic acid, if the former is contraindicated) as soon as possible (Frontera et al., 2016). Fibrinogen levels should be re-checked after administration of a reversal agent, and further cryoprecipitate given if serum levels remain low.

Implications for Research

As ICH growth is most pronounced in the first minutes after onset, haemostatic therapy may show a more favourable benefit to risk profile if initiated more quickly. Trials of treatment start confined to within the first 1–2 hours of onset, both in early-hospital-arriving patients and in patients treated in Mobile Stroke Units, hold promise. Trials are also needed to determine which patients with NOAC-related ICH would most benefit from early start of specific reversal agents such as idarucizumab and andexanet alfa. Using the CT spot sign to identify expansion-prone ICH patients for haemostatic therapy merits additional investigation, and trials are under way testing tranexamic acid in this setting, including TRAIGE (NCT02625948) and STOP-AUST (NCT01702636).

Acute Blood Pressure Lowering

Rationale

Blood pressure (BP) elevation is extremely common in ICH patients, present in 75% upon initial presentation (Qureshi et al., 2007), and in more than 90% during the initial hospital course (Asdaghi, 2007). Chronic hypertension is the leading risk factor for

ICH – population attributable risk analysis indicates that chronic hypertension is responsible for 73% of all ICH cases (O'Donnell et al., 2010). The association of elevated BP and incident ICH is the strongest of all the serious cardiovascular events (Rapsomaniki et al., 2014). Chronic hypertension is a risk factor for cerebral small vessel disease (Khan et al., 2007), where persistently raised intraluminal arterial pressure damages the endothelium lining small vessel walls and leads to the formation of microaneurysms at the bifurcation of arterioles (Xi et al., 2006). Moreover, a further increase in systolic BP (SBP) above usual levels often occurs in the weeks and months leading up to ICH (Fischer et al., 2014), suggesting that higher systolic peaks and greater BP variability act as triggers of ICH.

Early after the onset of ICH, impairment of cerebral autoregulation, of vascular tone, activation of neuroendocrine axes that increase BP, and psychological distress contribute to an acute hypertensive response (Manning and Robinson, 2015), which occurs in most patients (Shi et al., 2017). Elevated systolic BP (>140 mm Hg) is associated with haematoma expansion (Brott et al., 1997), neurological deterioration, death, and disability (Willmot et al., 2004). Thus, it seems reasonable to suppose that early lowering of BP might improve outcomes, through attenuation of haematoma growth, reduction in brain oedema, and other mechanisms (Anderson et al., 2008; Arima et al., 2012). However, blood pressure lowering may also precipitate ischaemic injury in brain regions with more advanced occlusive small vessel disease, potentially worsening outcome (Menon et al., 2012; Buletko et al., 2018). Accordingly, blood pressure management strategies are an important domain of clinical trial exploration.

Evidence

Systematic reviews have identified 6 RCTs enrolling 4412 patients comparing early higher and lower intensity BP reduction regimens for hypertensive patients with acute ICH (Anderson et al., 2008; Koch et al., 2008; Anderson et al., 2013; Butcher et al., 2013; Qureshi et al., 2016; Boulouis et al., 2017; Gong et al., 2017; Lattanzi, 2017; Shi et al., 2017). The trials differed in the intensities of targeted and achieved blood pressures in the more intensive and less intensive treatment groups, and in using a single drug regimen or pragmatic selection by physicians among many antihypertensive agents. In all trials, the control group received active blood pressure management, generally targeting

SBP <180. There have been no trials in which the control group is treated by a policy of completely avoiding antihypertensive therapy.

Considering all more versus less intensive regimens together, higher intensity blood pressure lowering was associated with a non-significant reduction in death or dependency (5 trials, 4276 patients: 52.6% vs 55.2%, OR 0.91, 95% CI: 0.81–1.03; $p = 0.14$), without alteration in mortality (5 trials, 4336 patients: 10.8% vs 11.0%, OR 0.98, 95% CI: 0.81–1.19) (Shi et al., 2017). More intensive blood pressure lowering was associated with reduced substantial haematoma growth at 24 hours (5 trials, 2301 patients: 21.6% vs 25.1%, RR 0.86, 95% CI: 0.74–1.00) (Lattanzi, 2017). There were no differences in the rates of hypotension (RR 1.56, 95% CI: 0.61–4.00) or acute coronary events (RR 1.13, 95% CI: 0.45–2.85), but more renal adverse events occurred in more intensively treated patients in the 2 trials providing data (1404 patients: 3.4% vs 1.6%, OR 2.18, 95% CI: 1.08–4.41) (Lattanzi, 2017).

However, based on achieved blood pressures, trial regimens can be seen to have tested 3, not 2, general treatment strategies: mild, moderate, and high intensity blood pressure lowering (Anderson et al., 2017b). During the first 24 hours of treatment, moderate vs mild intensity blood pressure lowering was tested in 3 (INTERACT1, INTERACT2, and ICH ADAPT) and high vs moderate intensity blood pressure lowering was tested in 1 (ATACH-II), reflecting the more uniform and potent intravenous calcium channel blocker regimen used in ATACH-II. Achieved SBPs in the less intensive control group in ATACH-II were actually equal to or lower than the achieved SBPs in the more intensive intervention group in the other trials. For example, at 1 hour, mean SBPs in the two arms of ATACH-II were 133 mm Hg vs 146 mm Hg, while in INTERACT 2 they were 150 mm Hg vs 164 mm Hg; similarly, at 6 hours, mean SBPs in the two arms of ATACH-II were 120 mm Hg vs 141 mm Hg, while in INTERACT they were 139 mm Hg vs 153 mm Hg. Considering just the 3 trials effectively testing moderate versus mild blood pressure lowering, moderate intensity blood pressure lowering was associated with reduced death or dependency (3260 patients: 51.5% vs 55.1%, OR 0.87, 95% CI: 0.76–0.99; $p = 0.04$), but without effect on mortality (3 trials, 3269 patients: 12.0% vs 12.1%, OR 0.99, 95% CI: 0.81–1.20) (Figure 13.6). In contrast, in ATACH-II, no additional benefit of high intensity over moderate intensity blood pressure lowering was noted.

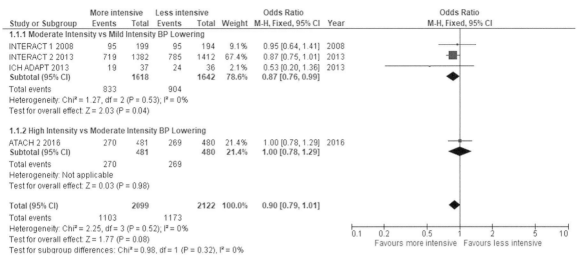

Figure 13.6 The effect of *mild, moderate, and high intensity blood pressure lowering* for acute ICH, on *death or dependency (modified Rankin Scale score 3–6)* (courtesy JL Saver).

Interpretation of the Evidence

Given variable results among individual trials and borderline statistical effects on some endpoints in study-level meta-analyses, caution is warranted in interpreting the results of blood pressure lowering trials for ICH. Moderate BP lowering to a systolic target less than 140 mm Hg within 6 hours of ICH onset is reasonably feasible and apparently safe, and appears to improve functional outcome.

Major differences in patient characteristics and BP management between the two largest trials of BP lowering – INTERACT2 and ATACH-II – are important to note, as they likely account for the differences in efficacy and safety outcomes. First, ATACH-II used almost exclusively intravenous nicardipine, whereas INTERACT2 used a variety of intravenous and oral agents according to their local availability. Second, all ATACH-II patients had a systolic BP >180 mm Hg at presentation, which was an inclusion criterion, whereas a systolic BP >180 mm Hg was present in only half of INTERACT2 participants, reflecting the wider systolic BP inclusion range of 150 to 220 mm Hg. Third, in the more intensive treatment group, ATACH-II used a lower cut-off for the cessation of BP lowering treatment than INTERACT2 (<110 mm Hg vs <130 mm Hg, respectively), and resultant more extreme reductions in BP may have negated potential benefits, as seen in a post-hoc analysis of INTERACT2 where poor outcomes were observed in those with a mean achieved BP <130 mm Hg over 24 hours post-randomization compared with those with a mean achieved BP of 130–139 mm Hg (Arima et al., 2015).

Implications for Clinicians

For ICH patients presenting with systolic blood pressure between 150 and 220 mm Hg and without contraindication to acute BP treatment, acute lowering of SBP to a target of ≤140 mm Hg is reasonable, given evidence of its general safety and potential benefit in improving 90-day functional outcome. However, more intensive lowering of SBP to 110–130 mm Hg in the acute stage should generally be avoided, as evidence beyond this threshold is limited.

Implications for Research

Study-level meta-analyses of aggregate data from acute BP lowering RCTs are limited in their ability to explore how individual patient characteristics may modify the effects of more intensive BP lowering, and do not account for differences in early BP control. An individual patient data meta-analysis would therefore be desirable to identify features of patients who may distinctively benefit from or be harmed by more intensive antihypertensive therapy.

As ICH growth is most pronounced in the first minutes after onset, blood pressure lowering therapy may show a more favourable benefit-to-risk profile if initiated more quickly. Trials of BP lowering initiated within the first 1–2 hours of ICH onset, both in early-hospital-arriving patients and in patients treated in Mobile Stroke Units, are desirable, such as the Rapid Intervention with Glyceryl trinitrate in Hypertensive stroke Trial (RIGHT 2) (ISRCTN26986053).

Trials exploring BP reduction in tandem with haemostatic therapy or surgical therapy are desirable, such as the Perioperative Antihypertensive Treatment in Patients With Spontaneous Intracerebral Haemorrhage (PATICH) (ChiCTR-INR-17011475).

In addition, explanatory trials are desirable to clarify whether more aggressive blood pressure lowering does or does not increase remote ischaemic injury in small vessel territories, and, if so, if clinical and imaging markers can identify risk-prone patients. A trial probing the impact of hypertensive therapies on physiological markers of ischaemic injury on MRI is the Intracerebral Haemorrhage Acutely Decreasing Arterial Pressure Trial (ICH ADAPT 2) (NCT02281838).

Medical Therapies to Reduce Mass Effect and Intracranial Pressure

Rationale

Acute intraparenchymal haemorrhages can produce mass effect and transtentorial herniation through several mechanisms, including haematoma growth, accumulating vasogenic oedema, and non-communicating (obstructive) hydrocephalus. While surgical evacuation or decompression is needed for definitive management of large lesions, medical therapies may be helpful as temporizing treatments.

Evidence

Hyperventilation

As hyperventilation sufficient to cause hypocapnia (partial pressure of carbon dioxide [pCO_2]: 4–4.5 kilopascals [kPa] [normal 4.7 to 6.0 kPa; or 35 to 45 mmHg]) causes cerebral vasoconstriction, it will reduce the volume of the intravascular compartment in the cranium, reducing intracranial pressure and potentially providing additional space to accommodate focal mass effect in ICH patients. However, vasoconstriction raises risk of cerebral ischaemia. There are no RCT data on the safety and efficacy of hyperventilation in acute ICH. Based on its physiological effect profile, hyperventilation, if used at all, likely should be deployed primarily as a temporary measure while preparing surgical interventions to definitively address the source of growing mass effect.

Osmotic Agents

Osmotic agents are molecules that do not readily cross the blood–brain barrier, so that their systemic administration yields a higher solute concentration in the blood than in the brain. The resulting osmotic gradient draws free water from brain intracellular and interstitial compartments into the systemic intravascular space. The two main categories of osmotic agents are (1) colloids – large, insoluble molecules – and (2) crystalloids – small, water-soluble molecules (Lewis et al., 2018). For brain mass lesions, the most well-studied agents are the colloids mannitol and glycerol and the crystalloid hypertonic saline.

Mannitol

Mannitol is an osmotic agent that reduces brain oedema and brain volume by producing an osmotic gradient between the cerebral extracellular space and plasma, thereby drawing away water into the circulation. It may also trigger cerebral vasoconstriction when there is intact autoregulation (Shawkat et al., 2012). However, mannitol becomes less effective with repeated doses, and delayed 'rebound' increases in ICP can occur as mannitol eventually crosses the blood–brain barrier and enters the cerebral compartment.

A systematic review identified 2 RCTs in which a total of 149 ICH patients were allocated to mannitol or control (Bereczki et al., 2008). The mannitol regimen in the larger trial (86% of patients) was 100 mL of 20% mannitol every 4 hours for 5 days; in the smaller trial, it was a one-time dose of 100 mL of 20% mannitol. Only the larger trial evaluated death or disability as an outcome, and rates with mannitol versus control were: 60% vs 54%, OR 1.28 (95% CI: 0.64–2.56). Both trials evaluated case fatality, and rates with mannitol versus control were: 22% vs 22%, OR 1.03 (95% CI: 0.47–2.25).

Glycerol

Glycerol is a polyol compound that acts as a colloidal osmotic agent. Compared with mannitol, glycerol had a longer time until achievement of peak effect, but also a longer duration of effect without rebound. A systematic review identified 2 randomized trials, enrolling 224 patients, comparing intravenous glycerol with control, initiated within the first days after onset in patients with definite or presumed ICH (Righetti, 2002). Random allocation to glycerol vs control was not associated with a change in mortality, 28% vs 30%, OR 0.86 (95% CI: 0.48–1.53).

Hypertonic Saline

Hypertonic saline is a crystalloid osmotic agent, producing elevated serum sodium levels that create osmotic pressure drawing water out of brain tissues. Hypertonic saline doses most often studied are a bolus of 23.4% saline for substantial, short-acting effect and a continuous infusion of 3% saline of more modulated, long-lasting effect (Wijdicks et al., 2014; Ong et al., 2015).

There have been no unconfounded, randomized studies of hypertonic saline confined to patients with ICH. In an observational series of 76 transtentorial herniation events among 68 patients with varied neurological conditions, including 29 (43%) with ICH, bolus therapy with 23.4% hypertonic saline, in tandem with additional medical interventions, was associated with reversal of clinical signs of herniation in 75% of episodes (Koenig et al., 2008). Independent predictors of successful reversal of herniation were an increase in sodium concentration of ≥5 mmol/L (OR 12.0, 95% CI: 1.6–90.5) and an attained absolute sodium concentration ≥145 mmol/L (OR 26.7, 95% CI: 3.6–200.0).

Corticosteroids

Corticosteroids stabilize the blood–brain barrier and reduce vasogenic oedema. A systematic review identified 5 RCTs enrolling 206 patients with ICH to glucocorticoids or control. Corticosteroid therapy did not alter death at end of follow-up, 59% vs 53%, RR 1.09 (95% CI: 0.87–1.35, Figure 13.7) and did not alter combined death or severe disability (3 trials, 146 patients: 84% vs 88%, RR 0.95, 95% CI: 0.83–1.09). A subsequent RCT of 200 patients reported higher mortality in the corticosteroid group (Sharafadinzadeh et al., 2008), but methodological concerns and inconsistences in data reporting were noted for this study (Steiner et al., 2014).

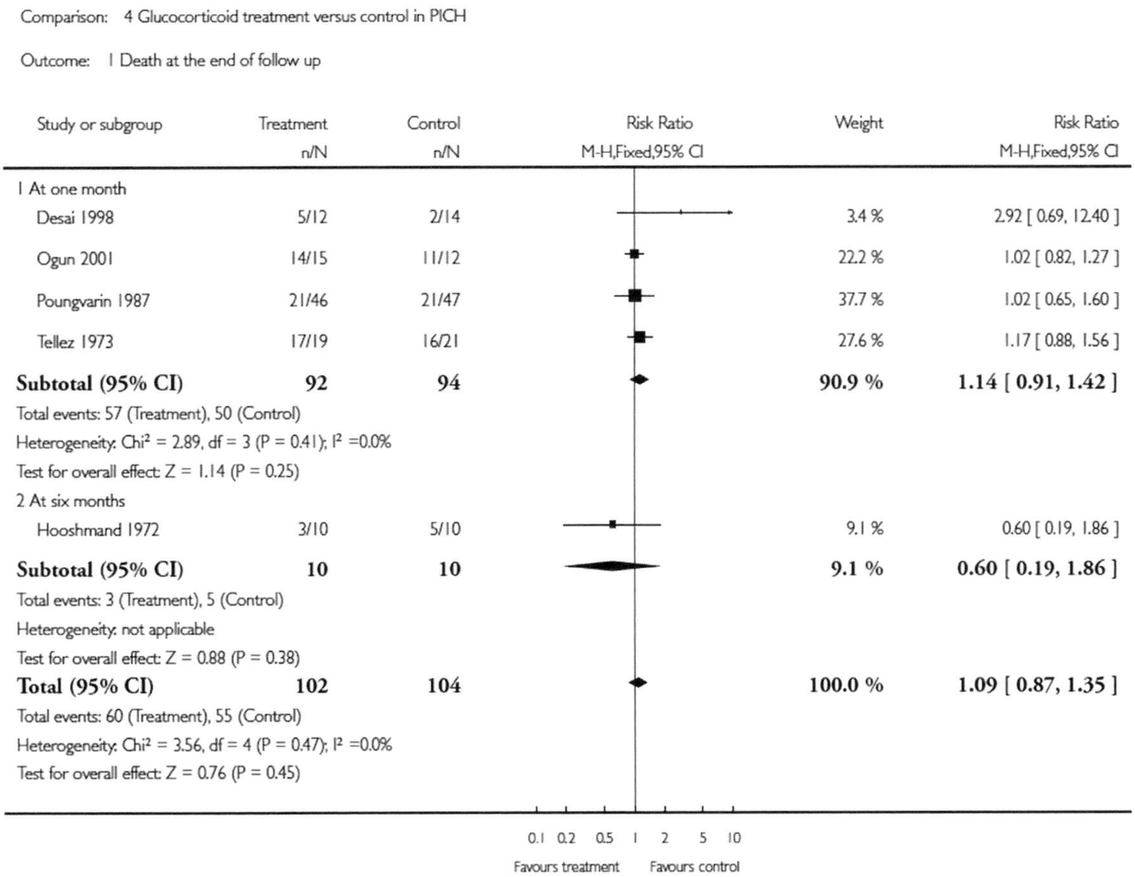

Comparison: 4 Glucocorticoid treatment versus control in PICH

Outcome: 1 Death at the end of follow up

Study or subgroup	Treatment n/N	Control n/N	Risk Ratio M-H,Fixed,95% CI	Weight	Risk Ratio M-H,Fixed,95% CI
1 At one month					
Desai 1998	5/12	2/14		3.4 %	2.92 [0.69, 12.40]
Ogun 2001	14/15	11/12		22.2 %	1.02 [0.82, 1.27]
Poungvarin 1987	21/46	21/47		37.7 %	1.02 [0.65, 1.60]
Tellez 1973	17/19	16/21		27.6 %	1.17 [0.88, 1.56]
Subtotal (95% CI)	**92**	**94**		**90.9 %**	**1.14 [0.91, 1.42]**
Total events: 57 (Treatment), 50 (Control)					
Heterogeneity: Chi² = 2.89, df = 3 (P = 0.41); I² =0.0%					
Test for overall effect: Z = 1.14 (P = 0.25)					
2 At six months					
Hooshmand 1972	3/10	5/10		9.1 %	0.60 [0.19, 1.86]
Subtotal (95% CI)	**10**	**10**		**9.1 %**	**0.60 [0.19, 1.86]**
Total events: 3 (Treatment), 5 (Control)					
Heterogeneity: not applicable					
Test for overall effect: Z = 0.88 (P = 0.38)					
Total (95% CI)	**102**	**104**		**100.0 %**	**1.09 [0.87, 1.35]**
Total events: 60 (Treatment), 55 (Control)					
Heterogeneity: Chi² = 3.56, df = 4 (P = 0.47); I² =0.0%					
Test for overall effect: Z = 0.76 (P = 0.45)					

0.1 0.2 0.5 1 2 5 10

Favours treatment   Favours control

Figure 13.7 The effect of *corticosteroids* versus control of acute ICH not associated with anticoagulant use, on *death at end of follow-up* (Feigin et al., 2005).

Interpretation of the Evidence

There is very limited evidence to guide use of medical therapies to reduce mass effect and ICP after acute ICH.

Implications for Clinicians

As all medical interventions to reduce mass effect and ICP after acute ICH have potential serious adverse effects and lack evidence of general benefit, they should not be employed routinely. However, in patients with imminent herniation, brief, emergent use of hyperventilation and of hypertonic saline or colloidal osmotic agents is reasonable as a temporizing measure until a definitive procedural/surgical intervention is delivered.

Neuroprotective and Anti-Inflammatory Agents

Iron Chelation

Haemoglobin degradation products resulting from haemolysis after ICH include the iron-containing haem. Iron can injure neural cells by generating highly reactive toxic hydroxyl radicals leading to oxidative stress and cell death, activating lipid peroxidation, and exacerbating excitotoxicity (Selim, 2009). The time course for haemoglobin haemolysis and toxicity after ICH is the first 2 to 3 days after onset. The iron chelator deferoxamine mesylate confers neuroprotection after brain haemorrhage in animal models by reducing brain oedema and neuronal death (Nakamura et al., 2004; Gu et al., 2009), an effect attributed to the ability of deferoxamine to form a stable complex with iron and alter regulatory genes that control cellular vulnerability and associated oxidative stress (Selim, 2009).

Three completed RCTs have compared deferoxamine to placebo. The first was stopped prematurely after enrolment of 42 patients, due to an increased frequency of acute respiratory distress syndrome in the deferoxamine group (seen in 5 patients) (Selim, 2013). A successor study was relaunched using a lower deferoxamine dose (32 mg/kg/day for 3 days instead of 62 mg/kg/day for 5 days) with a randomized, placebo-controlled, futility trial design (Selim, 2019). Deferoxamine was safe at the lower dose, but futile on the primary outcome of 'good clinical outcome' on the mRS at 3 and 6 months. A third RCT randomized 42 ICH patients to treatment with deferoxamine 62 mg/kg/day for 3 days or control (Yu et al., 2015). Rates of death or dependency (mRS 3–6) at 1 month did not differ between the deferoxamine and control groups, 43% vs 33% ($p = 0.53$). Serially assessed oedema volumes were lower in the deferoxamine compared with control group – for example, on day 4, the ratio of oedema volume to haematoma volume was 0.57 in deferoxamine group vs 0.99 in the control group ($p = 0.001$).

Other Neuroprotective and Anti-Inflammatory Agents

Multiple additional agents with potentially neuroprotective or anti-inflammatory effects have been tested in ICH patients. The goal of most trials has been to develop beneficial agents for ICH, although some have merely sought to demonstrate that agents being developed to treat acute ischaemic stroke were safe in ICH, permitting treatment to start in advance of brain imaging. Agents tested have included: GABA modulators (clomethiazole and diazepam) (Lyden et al., 2000; Lodder et al., 2006); glycine antagonists (gavestinel) (Haley et al., 2005); free radical scavengers (NXY-059) (Lyden et al., 2007); anti-inflammatory agents (celecoxib, xueshuantong) (Gao et al., 2012; Lee et al., 2013); neurotrophic and membrane repair agents (granulocyte colony-stimulating factor, citicoline) (Iranmanesh and Vakilian, 2008; England et al., 2016); nitric oxide donors (glyceryl trinitrate) (Krishnan et al., 2016); and agents with pleiotropic effects (minocycline, magnesium) (Kohler et al., 2013; Saver et al., 2015). None of the trials showed definite benefit on final functional outcomes in ICH patients.

Interpretation of the Evidence

There is insufficient evidence to support the use of neuroprotective and anti-inflammatory drugs in the management of acute ICH.

Implications for Clinicians

Use of any neuroprotective and anti-inflammatory drugs is not recommended for the management of ICH.

Implications for Research

Ongoing research aims to uncover novel targets and agents for anti-inflammatory effects on ICH. The potential increasing use of catheter aspiration of haematomas makes direct instillation of neuroprotective and anti-inflammatory agents into the haematoma cavity for high penetration into perihaematomal tissues an attractive delivery option for exploration in future neuroprotective trials.

Summary

Intracerebral haemorrhage (ICH) requires prompt clinical diagnosis and radiological confirmation. The following management strategies are recommended on the basis of best available evidence:

1. A combination of clinical and radiological features is useful in determining prognosis, monitoring progression, identifying any underlying structural cause, and evaluating suitability for surgical intervention. Care in a specialized stroke unit or neurointensive care unit improves outcome.

2. Surgical haematoma evacuation should be pursued as soon as possible for patients with cerebellar haemorrhage who are deteriorating neurologically, have hydrocephalus, or have brainstem compression. Early surgery is not recommended for stable patients with supratentorial haemorrhages, but haematoma evacuation may be considered as a life-saving measure in patients with coma, large haematoma with mass effect, or intraventricular haemorrhage (IVH). Minimally invasive surgery in stable patients is of unproven benefit.

3. Clinicians should not routinely use haemostatic therapies where there is no evidence of coagulopathy or anticoagulant use. Randomized controlled trials (RCTs) targeting patients with active bleeding ('spot sign' on computed tomography [CT] angiography) are ongoing. In cases of coagulopathy-related ICH, early corrective measures should be taken with haematology consultation.

4. Early moderate intensity blood pressure (BP) lowering to a systolic BP target of 140 mm Hg is reasonable, in view of its general safety and potential to improve functional outcomes.

5. Medical therapies to reduce mass effect and intracranial pressure should not be used routinely, but hyperventilation and treatment with hypertonic saline or colloidal osmotic agents is reasonable in patients with imminent herniation as a bridge to definitive neurosurgical intervention.

6. Corticosteroids should be avoided in ICH. Novel neuroprotective approaches hold promise and are being evaluated in ongoing RCTs.

References

Al-Shahi Salman R, Frantzias J, Lee RJ, Lyden PD, Battey TWK, Ayres AM, at al. (2018) Absolute risk and predictors of the growth of acute spontaneous intracerebral hemorrhage: a systematic review and meta-analysis of individual patient data. *Lancet Neurol*, 17, 885–94.

Al-Shahi Salman R, Labovitz DL, Stapf C. (2009). Spontaneous intracerebral hemorrhage. *BMJ*, 339, b2586.

Al-Shahi Salman R, Law ZK, Bath PM, Steiner T, Sprigg N. (2018). Hemostatic therapies for acute spontaneous intracerebral hemorrhage. *Cochrane Database Syst Rev*, 4. CD005951. doi:10.1002/14651858.CD005951.pub4.

Anderson C, Heeley E, Huang Y, Wang J, Stapf C, Delcourt C, et al. (2013). Rapid blood-pressure lowering in patients with acute intracerebral hemorrhage. *N Engl J Med*, 368(25), 2355–65.

Anderson CS, Huang Y, Wang JG, Arima H, Neal B, Peng B, et al. (2008). Intensive blood pressure reduction in acute cerebral hemorrhage trial (INTERACT): a randomised pilot trial. *Lancet Neurol*, 7(5), 391–9.

Anderson CS, Arima H, Lavados P, Billot L, Hackett ML, Olavarria VV, et al. (2017a). Cluster-randomized, crossover trial of head positioning in acute stroke. *New Engl J Med*, 376(25), 2437–47.

Anderson CS, Selim MH, Molina CA, Qureshi AI. (2017b). Intensive blood pressure lowering in intracerebral hemorrhage. *Stroke*, 48, 2034–7.

Arima H, Heeley E, Delcourt C, Hirakawa Y, Wang X, Woodward M, et al. (2015). Optimal achieved blood pressure in acute intracerebral hemorrhage: INTERACT2. *Neurology*, 84(5), 464–71.

Arima H, Huang Y, Wang JG, Heeley E, Delcourt C, Parsons M, et al. (2012). Earlier blood pressure-lowering and greater attenuation of hematoma growth in acute intracerebral hemorrhage: INTERACT pilot phase. *Stroke*, 43(8), 2236–8.

Asdaghi, N, Manawadu D, Butcher K. (2007) Therapeutic management of acute intracerebral hemorrhage. *Expert Opin Pharmacother*, 8, 3097–116

AVERT Trial Collaboration Group. (2015). Efficacy and safety of very early mobilisation within 24 h of stroke onset (AVERT): a randomised controlled trial. *Lancet*, 386(9988), 46–55.

Baharoglu MI, Cordonnier C, Al-Shahi Salman R, de Gans K, Koopman MM, Brand A, et al. (2016). Platelet transfusion versus standard care after acute stroke due to spontaneous cerebral hemorrhage associated with antiplatelet therapy (PATCH): a randomised, open-label, phase 3 trial. *Lancet*, 387(10038), 2605–13.

Bereczki D, Liu M, Do Prado, GF, Fekete I. (2008) Mannitol for acute stroke. *Stroke*, 39(2), 512–13.

Boulis NM, Bobek MP, Schmaier A, Hoff JT. (1999). Use of factor IX complex in warfarin-related intracranial hemorrhage. *Neurosurgery*, 45(5), 1113–19.

Boulouis G, Morott A, Goldstein JN, Charidimou A. (2017). Intensive blood pressure lowering in patients with acute intracerebral hemorrhage: clinical outcomes and hemorrhage expansion. Systematic review and meta-analysis of randomised trials. *J Neurol Neurosurg Psychiatry*, **88**(4), 339–45.

Brott T, Broderick J, Kothari R, Barsan W, Tomsick T, Sauerbeck L, Spilker J, et al. (1997). Early hemorrhage growth in patients with intracerebral hemorrhage. *Stroke*, **28**(1), 1–5.

Buletko AB, Thacker T, Cho SM, Mathew J, Thompson NR, Organek N, et al. (2018). Cerebral ischemia and deterioration with lower blood pressure target in intracerebral hemorrhage. *Neurology*, **91**, e1058-e1066.

Butcher KS, Jeerakathil T, Hill M, Demchuk AM, Dowlatshahi D, Coutts SB, et al. (2013). The intracerebral hemorrhage acutely decreasing arterial pressure trial. *Stroke*, **44**(3), 620–6.

Connolly SJ, Milling TJ Jr, Eikelboom JW, Gibson CM, Curnutte JT, Gold A, et al. (2016). Andexanet alfa for acute major bleeding associated with factor Xa inhibitors. *New Engl J Med*, **375**, 1131–41.

Davis SM, Broderick J, Hennerici M, Brun NC, Diringer MN, Mayer SA, et al. (2006). Hematoma growth is a determinant of mortality and poor outcome after intracerebral hemorrhage. *Neurology*, **66**(8), 1175–81.

Demchuk AM, Dowlatshahi D, Rodriguez-Luna D, Molina CA, Glas YS, Dzialowski I, et al. (2012). Prediction of hematoma growth and outcome in patients with intracerebral hemorrhage using the CT-angiography spot sign (PREDICT): a prospective observational study. *Lancet Neurol*, **11**(4), 307–14.

England TJ, Sprigg N, Alasheev AM, Belkin AA, Kumar A, Prasad K, et al. (2016). Granulocyte-colony stimulating factor (G-CSF) for stroke: An individual patient data meta-analysis. *Sci Rep*, **6**, 36567.

Feigin VL, Anderson N, Rinkel, GJE, Algra A, van Gijn J, Bennett D. (2005). Corticosteroids for aneurysmal subarachnoid hemorrhage and primary intracerebral hemorrhage. *Cochrane Database Syst Rev*, 3. CD004583. doi:10.1002/14651858.CD004583.pub2.

Feigin VL, Krishnamurthi RV, Parmar P, Norrving B, Mensah GA, Bennett DA, et al. (2015). Update on the global burden of ischemic and hemorrhagic stroke in 1990–2013: the GBD 2013 study. *Neuroepidemiology*, **45**(3), 161–176.

Feigin VL, Lawes CM, Bennett DA, Barker-Collo SL, Parag V. (2009). Worldwide stroke incidence and early case fatality reported in 56 population-based studies: a systematic review. *Lancet Neurol*, **8**(4), 355–69.

Fiorella D, Arthur AS, Mocco JD. (2016). O-027 The INVEST trial: a randomized, controlled trial to investigate the safety and efficacy of image-guided minimally invasive endoscopic surgery with Apollo vs best medical management for supratentorial intracerebral hemorrhage. *J NeuroInterv Surg*, **8**, A18

Fischer U, Cooney MT, Bull LM, Silver LE, Chalmers J, Anderson CS, et al. (2014). Acute post-stroke blood pressure relative to premorbid levels in intracerebral hemorrhage versus major ischemic stroke: A population-based study. *Lancet Neurol*, **13**(4), 374–84.

Frontera JA, LewinJJ 3rd, Rabinstein AA, Aisiku IP, Alexandrov AW, Cook AM, et al. (2016). Guideline for reversal of antithrombotics in intracranial hemorrhage. *Neurocrit Care*, **24**(1), 6–46.

Gao L, Zhao H, Liu Q, Song J, Xu C, Liu P, et al. (2012). Improvement of hematoma absorption and neurological function in patients with acute intracerebral hemorrhage treated with Xueshuantong. *J Neurolog Sci*, **323**(1–2), 236–40.

Gong S, Lin C, Zhang D, Kong X, Chen J, Wang C, et al. (2017). Effects of intensive blood pressure reduction on acute intracerebral hemorrhage: a systematic review and meta-analysis. *Sci Rep*, **7**(1), 10694.

Gu Y, Hua Y, Keep RF, Morgenstern LB, Xi G. (2009). Deferoxamine reduces intracerebral hematoma-induced iron accumulation and neuronal death in piglets. *Stroke*, **40**(6), 2241–3.

Haley EC, Thompson JLP, Levin B, Davis S, Lees KR, Pittman JG, et al. (2005). Gavestinel does not improve outcome after acute intracerebral hemorrhage: An analysis from the GAIN International and GAIN Americas studies. *Stroke*, **36**(5), 1006–10.

Hanley DF, Lane K, McBee N, Ziai W, Tuhrim S, Lees KR, et al. (2017). Thrombolytic removal of intraventricular hemorrhage in treatment of severe stroke: results of the randomised, multicentre, multiregion, placebo-controlled CLEAR III trial. *Lancet*, **389**(10069), 603–11.

Hanley DF, Thompson RE, Rosenblum M, Yenokyan G, Lane K, McBee N, et al. (2019). Efficacy and safety of minimally invasive surgery with thrombolysis in intracerebral haemorrhage evacuation (MISTIE III): a randomised, controlled, open-label, blinded end-point phase 3 trial. *Lancet*, **393**(10175), 1021–32.

Hemphill JC, Greenberg SM, Anderson CS, Becker K, Bendok BR, Cushman M, et al. (2015). Guidelines for the management of spontaneous intracerebral hemorrhage. *Stroke*, **46**(7), 2032–60.

Herrick DB, Ullman N, Nekoovaght-Tak S, Hanley DF, Awad I, LeDroux S, et al. (2014). Determinants of external ventricular drain placement and associated outcomes in patients with spontaneous intraventricular hemorrhage. *Neurocrit Care*, **21**(3), 426–34.

Iranmanesh F, Vakilian A. (2008). Efficiency of citicoline in increasing muscular strength of patients with nontraumatic cerebral hemorrhage: a double-blind randomized clinical trial. *J Stroke Cerebrovasc Dis*, **17**(3), 153–5.

Jeffrey S. (2017). No benefit of hemostatic therapy in patients with "spot sign" ICH. Medscape Neurology (news article). https://www.medscape.com/viewarticle/877707#vp_2 (accessed Dec 2018).

Khan NR, Tsivgoulis G, Lee SL, Jones GM, Green CS, Katsanos AH, et al. (2014). Fibrinolysis for intraventricular hemorrhage: an updated meta-analysis and systematic review of the literature. *Stroke*, **45**(9), 2662–9.

Khan U, Porteous L, Hassan A, Markus HS. (2007). Risk factor profile of cerebral small vessel disease and its subtypes. *J Neurol Neurosurg Psychiatry*, **78**(7), 702–6.

Koch S, Romano JG, Forteza AM, Otero CM, Rabinstein AA. (2008) Rapid blood pressure reduction in acute intracerebral hemorrhage: feasibility and safety. *Neurocrit Care*, **8**(3), 316–21.

Koenig MA, Bryan M, Lewin JL 3rd, Mirski MA, Geocadin RG, Stevens RD. (2008). Reversal of transtentorial herniation with hypertonic saline. *Neurology*, **70**, 1023–9.

Kohler E, Prentice DA, Bates TR, Hankey GJ, Claxton A, van Heerden J, et al. (2013). Intravenous minocycline in acute stroke: a randomized, controlled pilot study and meta-analysis. *Stroke*, **44**(9), 2493–9.

Krishnan K, Scutt P, Woodhouse L, Adami A, Becker JL, Berge E, et al. (2016). Glyceryl trinitrate for acute intracerebral hemorrhage: results from the Efficacy of Nitric Oxide in Stroke (ENOS) trial, a subgroup analysis. *Stroke*, **47**, 44–52.

Langhorne P, Fearon P, Ronning OM, Kaste M, Palomaki H, Vemmos K, et al. (2013). Stroke unit care benefits patients with intracerebral hemorrhage: Systematic review and meta-analysis. *Stroke*, **44**(11), 3044–9.

Lattanzi S, Cagnetti C, Provinciali L, Silvestrini M. (2017). How should we lower blood pressure after cerebral hemorrhage? A systematic review and meta-analysis. *Cerebrovasc Dis*, **43**(5–6), 207–13.

Lee SH, Park HK, Ryu WS, Lee JS, Bae HJ, Han MK, et al. (2013). Effects of celecoxib on hematoma and edema volumes in primary intracerebral hemorrhage: a multicenter randomized controlled trial. *Eur J Neurol*, **20**(8), 1161–9.

Lewis SR, Pritchard MW, Evans DJ, Butler AR, Alderson P, Smith AF, et al. (2018). Colloids versus crystalloids for fluid resuscitation in critically ill people. *Cochrane Database Syst Rev*, 8. CD000567.

Lodder J, van Raa, L, Hilton A, Hardy E, Kessels A; EGASIS Study Group. (2006). Diazepam to improve acute stroke outcome: results of the early GABA-Ergic activation study in stroke trial. a randomized double-blind placebo-controlled trial. *Cerebrovasc Dis*, **21**(1–2), 120–7.

Lovasik BP, McCracken DJ, McCracken CE, McDougal ME, Frerich JM, Samuels OB, et al. (2016). The effect of external ventricular drain use in intracerebral hemorrhage. *World Neurosurg*, **94**, 309–18.

Lovelock C, Molyneux A, Rothwell P. (2007). Change in incidence and etiology of intracerebral hemorrhage in Oxfordshire, UK, between 1981 and 2006: a population-based study. *Lancet Neurol*, **6**(6), 487–93.

Lyden PD, Shuaib A, Lees KR, Davalos A, Davis SM, Diener HC, et al. (2007). Safety and tolerability of NXY-059 for acute intracerebral hemorrhage: the CHANT trial. *Stroke*, **38**(8), 2262–9.

Lyden PD, Shuaib A, Ng K, Atkinson R. (2000) The clomethiazole acute stroke study in hemorrhagic stroke (CLASS-H): final results. *J Stroke Cerebrovasc Dis*, 9(6), 268–75.

Manning LS, Robinson TG. (2015). New insights into blood pressure control for intracerebral hemorrhage. *Front Neurol Neurosci*, **37**, 35–50.

Mendelow AD, Gregson BA, Rowan EN, Murray GD, Gholkar A, Mitchell PM; STICH II Investigators. (2013). Early surgery versus initial conservative treatment in patients with spontaneous supratentorial lobar intracerebral hematomas (STICH II): a randomised trial. *Lancet*, **382**(9890), 397–408.

Menon RS, Burgess RE, Wing JJ, Gibbons MC, Shara NM, Fernandez S, et al. (2012). Predictors of highly prevalent brain ischemia in intracerebral hemorrhage. *Ann Neurol*, **71**, 199–205.

Moussa WMM, Khedr W. (2017). Decompressive craniectomy and expansive duraplasty with evacuation of hypertensive intracerebral hematoma, a randomized controlled trial. *Neurosurg Rev*, **40**(1), 115–27.

Nakamura T, Keep RF, Hua Y, Schallert T, Hoff JT, Xi G. (2004). Deferoxamine-induced attenuation of brain edema and neurological deficits in a rat model of intracerebral hemorrhage. *J Neurosurg*, **100**(4), 672–8.

O'Donnell MJ, Xavier D, Liu L, Zhang H, Chin SL, Rao-Melacini P, et al. (2010). Risk factors for ischemic and intracerebral hemorrhagic stroke in 22 countries (the INTERSTROKE study): a case-control study. *Lancet*, **376**(9735), 112–23.

Ong CJ, Keyrouz SG, Diringer MN. (2015). The role of osmotic therapy in hemispheric stroke. *Neurocrit Care*, **23**, 285–91.

Parry-Jones AR, Paley L, Bray BD, Hoffman AM, James M, Cloud GC, et al. (2016). Care-limiting decisions in acute stroke and association with survival: Analyses of UK national quality register data. *Int J Stroke*, **11**(3), 321–31.

Pollack CV Jr, Reilly PA, van Ryn J, Eikelboom JW, Glund S, Bernstein RA, et al. (2017). Idarucizumab for dabigatran reversal – full cohort analysis. *N Engl J Med*, **377**, 431–41.

Poon MT, Bell SM, Al-Shahi Salman R. (2015). Epidemiology of intracerebral hemorrhage. *Front Neurol Neurosci*, **37**, 1–12.

Poon MTC, Fonville AF, Al-Shahi Salman R. (2014). Long-term prognosis after intracerebral hemorrhage: systematic review and meta-analysis. *J Neurol Neurosurg Psychiatry*, **85** (6), 660–7.

Prasad K, Mendelow AD, Gregson B. (2008). Surgery for primary supratentorial intracerebral haemorrhage. *Cochrane Database Syst Rev*, 4. CD000200.

Qureshi AI, Ezzeddine MA, Nasar A, Suri MF, Kirmani JF, Husseing HM, et al. (2007). Prevalence of elevated blood pressure in 563,704 adult patients with stroke presenting to the ED in the United States. *Am J Emerg Med*, **25**, 32–8.

Qureshi AI, Palesch YY, Barsan WG, Hanley DF, Hsu CY, Martin RL, et al. (2016). Intensive blood-pressure lowering in patients with acute cerebral hemorrhage. *N Engl J Med*, **375**(11), 1033–43.

Rapsomaniki E, Timmis A, George J, Pujades-Rodriguez M, Shah AD, Denaxas S, et al. (2014). Blood pressure and incidence of twelve cardiovascular diseases: lifetime risks, healthy life-years lost, and age-specific associations in 1·25 million people. *Lancet*, **383**(9932), 1899–1911.

Righetti E, Celani MG, Cantisani TA, Sterzi R, Boysen G, Ricci S. (2002). Glycerol for acute stroke: a Cochrane systematic review. *J Neurol*, **249**(4), 445–51.

Samarasekera N, Fonville A, Lerpiniere C, Farrall AJ, Wardlaw JM, White PM, et al. (2015). Influence of intracerebral hemorrhage location on incidence, characteristics, and outcome: population-based study. *Stroke*, **46**(2), 361–8.

Saver JL, Starkman S, Eckstein M, Stratton SJ, Pratt FD, Hamilton S, et al. (2015). Prehospital use of magnesium sulfate as neuroprotection in acute stroke. *N Engl J Med*, **372** (6), 528–36.

Selim M. (2009). Deferoxamine mesylate: A new hope for intracerebral hemorrhage: from bench to clinical trials. *Stroke*, **40**(3 Suppl), S90–1.

Selim, M. (2013). iDEF: Intracerebral Hemorrhage Deferoxamine Trial. https://www.nihstrokenet.org/docs/default-source/default-document-library/idef_060314.pdf?sfvrsn=2 (accessed Dec 2018).

Selim M, Foster LD, Moy CS, Xi G, Hill MD, Morgenstern LB, et al. (2019). Deferoxamine mesylate in patients with intracerebral haemorrhage (i-DEF): a multicentre, randomised, placebo-controlled, double-blind phase 2 trial. *Lancet Neurol*, **18**, 428–38.

Sharafadinzadeh N, Baghebanian SM, Pipelzadeh M, Moravej Ale Ali A, Ghanavati P. (2008). Effects of dexamethasone in primary intracerebral hemorrhage in the South West of Iran. *Pakistan J Med Sci*, **24**(4), 502–505.

Shawkat H, Westwood, M-M, Mortimer, A. (2012). Mannitol: a review of its clinical uses. *Continuing Educ Anaesth Crit Care Pain*, **12**(2), 82–5.

Shi L, Xu S, Zheng J, Xu J, Zhang J. (2017). Blood pressure management for acute intracerebral hemorrhage: a meta-analysis. *Sci Rep*, **7**(1), 14345.

Shkirkova K, Saver JL, Starkman S, Wong G, Weng J, Hamilton S, et al. (2018). Frequency, predictors, and outcomes of prehospital and early postarrival neurological deterioration in acute stroke: exploratory analysis of the FAST-MAG randomized clinical trial. *JAMA Neurol*, **75**, 1364–74.

Specogna AV, Turin TC, Patten SB, Hill MD. (2014). Factors associated with early deterioration after spontaneous intracerebral hemorrhage: a systematic review and meta-analysis. *PLoS ONE*, **9**(5), e96743.

Staykov D, Kuramatsu JB, Bardutzky J, Volbers B, Gerner ST, Kloska SP, et al. (2017). Efficacy and safety of combined intraventricular fibrinolysis with lumbar drainage for prevention of permanent shunt dependency after intracerebral hemorrhage with severe ventricular involvement: A randomized trial and individual patient data meta-analysis. *Ann Neurol*, **81**(1), 93–103.

Steiner T, Al-Shahi Salman R, Beer R. Christensen H, Cordonnier C, Csiba L, et al. (2014). European Stroke Organisation (ESO) guidelines for the management of spontaneous intracerebral hemorrhage. *Int J Stroke*, **9**(7), 840–55.

Steiner T, Poli S, Griebe M, Husing J, Haida J, Freiberger A, et al. (2016) Fresh frozen plasma versus prothrombin complex concentrate in patients with intracranial hemorrhage related to vitamin K antagonists (INCH): A randomised trial. *Lancet Neurol*, **15**(6), 566–73.

van Asch CJ, Luitse MJ, Rinkel GJ, van der Tweel I, Algra A, Klijn CJ. (2010). Incidence, case fatality, and functional outcome of intracerebral hemorrhage over time, according to age, sex, and ethnic origin: a systematic review and meta-analysis. *Lancet Neurol*, **9**(2), 167–76.

van Asch CJJ, Velthuis BK, Rinkel GJE, Algra A, de Kort GA, Witkamp TD, et al. (2015). Diagnostic yield and accuracy of CT angiography, MR angiography, and digital subtraction angiography for detection of macrovascular causes of intracerebral hemorrhage: Prospective, multicentre cohort study. *BMJ*, **351**.

Vespa P, Hanley D, Betz J, Hoffer A, Engh J, Carter R, et al. (2016). ICES (Intraoperative Stereotactic Computed Tomography-Guided Endoscopic Surgery) for brain hemorrhage: a multicenter randomized controlled trial. *Stroke*, **47**(11), 2749–55.

Wijdicks EFM, Sheth KN, Carter BS, Greer DM, Kasner SE, Kimberly WT, et al.; American Heart Association Stroke Council. (2014). Recommendations for the management of cerebral and cerebellar infarction with swelling. *Stroke*, **45**, 1222–38.

Willmot M, Leonardi-Bee J, Bath PMW. (2004). High blood pressure in acute stroke and subsequent outcome a systematic review. *Hypertension*, **43** (1), 18–24.

Witsch J, Neugebauer H, Zweckberger K, Jüttler E. (2013). Primary cerebellar hemorrhage: complications, treatment and outcome. *Clin Neurol Neurosurg*, **115**(7), 863–869.

Xi G, Keep RF, Hoff JT. (2006). Mechanisms of brain injury after intracerebral hemorrhage. *Lancet Neurol*, **5**(1), 53–63.

Yaghi S, Boehme AK, Dibu J, Leon Guerrero CR, Ali S, Martin-Schild S, et al. (2015). Treatment and outcome of thrombolysis-related hemorrhage: a multicenter retrospective study. *JAMA Neurol*, **72**, 1451–7.

Yang J, Arima H, Wu G, Heeley E, DelcourtC, Zhou J, et al. (2015). Prognostic significance of perihematomal edema in acute intracerebral hemorrhage: pooled analysis from the intensive blood pressure reduction in acute cerebral hemorrhage trial studies. *Stroke*, **46**(4), 1009–13.

Yao Z, Ma L, You C, He M. (2017). Decompressive craniectomy for spontaneous intracerebral hemorrhage: a systematic review and meta-analysis. *World Neurosurg*, **110**, 121–8.

Yu Y, Zhao,W, Zhu C, Kong Z, Xu Y, Liu G, et al. (2015). The clinical effect of deferoxamine mesylate on edema after intracerebral hemorrhage. *PLoS ONE*, **10**(4), e0122371.

Yu Z, Ma L, Zheng J, You C. (2017). Prognostic role of perihematomal edema in intracerebral hemorrhage: a systematic review. *Turk Neurosurg*, doi:10.5137/1019-5149.JTN.19659-16.0. Epub ahead of print.

Acute Treatment of Subarachnoid Haemorrhage

Sherri A. Braksick
Alejandro A. Rabinstein

In patients with subarachnoid haemorrhage (SAH), the initial presentation to the Emergency Department can be very dramatic, with a thunderclap headache (i.e. maximal at onset) followed by sudden unresponsiveness or seizure. In other patients, the presentation may be milder, and clinicians must remain vigilant to recognize subtle clinical presentations. With advances in the quality of computed tomography (CT) scanning, the great majority of cases of aneurysmal SAH are easily identified with this modality. In cases with a clinical history that suggests aneurysmal SAH but negative CT scans, further diagnostic studies may be necessary to determine whether a haemorrhage has occurred.

Following the diagnosis of aneurysmal SAH, the patient must be carefully monitored for multiple early and late complications, and the aneurysm must be definitively secured to prevent re-rupture and clinical worsening.

Over time, the outcomes of patients with SAH have improved, with an overall decrease in mortality (Nieuwkamp et al., 2009). Predictors of good functional outcome in SAH patients include low World Federation of Neurological Surgeons (WFNS) grade, absence of intraparenchymal haemorrhage, absence of delayed infarction, and no requirement for blood transfusion (Pegoli et al., 2015). High-grade initial WFNS score, increased circulating neutrophils, poor haemodynamic status, significant radiographic neurological injury, systemic inflammatory response syndrome, and cardiac dysfunction have been shown to be predictive of a poor clinical outcome (van der Bilt et al., 2009; Tam et al., 2010; Ibrahim et al., 2014). In patients who survive the protracted clinical course and complications associated with aneurysmal SAH, many have good functional outcomes, but cognitive impairment may persist beyond the subacute clinical period (Raya and Diringer, 2014).

Diagnosis

Evidence

A multicentre cohort study evaluating all patients who presented to an Emergency Department with a thunderclap headache (defined as headache peaking within 1 hour of onset) found that 7.7% (240/3132) had a final diagnosis of SAH. CT of the head performed within 6 hours of symptom onset was 100% sensitive and specific for SAH. This required image interpretation by an experienced radiologist, as four false negative readings by physicians in other specialties and trainees were later corrected. Beyond 6 hours, CT performance decreased, with sensitivity 86%, specificity 100% (Perry et al., 2011).

Magnetic resonance imaging (MRI) is more sensitive than CT for the detection of SAH. In one study evaluating detection of SAH present in 146 subarachnoid regions in 25 patients, CT detected 75% of involved regions. In contrast, fluid-attenuated inversion recovery (FLAIR) MRI detected 87%, susceptibility-weighted MRI detected 88%, and combined FLAIR and susceptibility-weighted imaging (SWI) detected 100% (Verma et al., 2013).

When a lumbar puncture is performed and blood is found in the cerebrospinal fluid (CSF), careful analysis of the CSF is needed to differentiate between traumatic tap and aneurysmal haemorrhage as the source. In a multicentre, observational study evaluating CSF findings in alert patients presenting with headache and in whom lumbar puncture was performed after negative CT scans, or in advance of CT imaging at the treating physician's discretion, 36.9% (641/1739) had a bloody tap, but only 0.9% (15/1739) had a final diagnosis of SAH. The combination of $<2000 \times 10^6$ red blood cells/L and absence of xanthochromia excluded SAH (negative predictive value 100%: 95% CI: 99.2–100%), while presence of either or both of these features increased the likelihood of SAH (positive predictive value 21.4%, 95% CI: 12.9–33.2%) (Perry et al., 2015).

The usefulness of xanthochromia alone as a CSF finding in CT-negative patients has varied in different studies. In one single-centre study, patients presenting within 14 days of onset of a thunderclap headache with negative CT scan underwent subsequent CSF analysis. All patients who had evidence of xanthochromia underwent 4-vessel catheter angiography to evaluate for evidence of aneurysm. Among 152 patients, 12% had xanthochromia on visual CSF inspection; and of those, 72% were diagnosed with aneurysmal SAH. Accordingly, for presence of aneurysmal SAH, xanthochromia in CT-negative patients had sensitivity of 93% and specificity of 95% (Dupont et al., 2008). However, in the Ottawa multicentre study of 1739 patients presenting within 14 days of headache onset, xanthochromia had lower sensitivity (47%), though higher specificity (99%) (Perry et al., 2015).

Studies have sought to identify prediction rules that would indicate patients presenting with headache who do not require CT imaging in order to reduce radiation exposure and care costs. However, given the importance of not missing an underlying aneurysm, imaging selection scales are weighted to ensure 100% sensitivity, resulting in relatively low specificity. For example, in a multicentre cohort of 2131 patients, a clinical decision rule, the Ottawa SAH Rule, was derived, which indicated imaging for any patients with age ≥40 years, witnessed loss of consciousness or onset during exertion, neck pain or stiffness, thunderclap onset (pain peaking at onset of headache), or limited neck flexion to predict the presence of SAH. This rule had 100% sensitivity but only 15.3% specificity for the recognition of SAH (Perry et al., 2013). In a validation cohort, this rule had retrospectively retained sensitivity of 100%, and specificity dropped further to 7.6%.

Comment

The data suggest that in patients presenting with acute onset, rapidly peaking headache where clinical suspicion for SAH is high, the initial evaluation should include a non-contrast CT scan of the head. If the CT scan is unrevealing, MRI of the head with gradient echo or SWI could be considered; however, a negative result still requires spinal fluid evaluation to investigate for SAH. Lumbar puncture should evaluate for red blood cells and xanthochromia. As xanthochromia can take hours to develop, ensuring several hours (e.g. 4–6 h) have passed since headache onset before evaluating the spinal fluid may be reasonable. Once an SAH is identified, noninvasive and catheter digital subtraction angiography is necessary for identification and possible management of an identified symptomatic aneurysm.

General Management of Subarachnoid Haemorrhage

Headache

Evidence

There is very limited research on best analgesic regimens for headache in patients with acute SAH. A small retrospective analysis of 53 patients who received gabapentin after SAH found few adverse effects; however, the efficacy was uncertain, as these patients were also receiving other analgesic medications (Dhakal et al., 2015).

Comment

In patients with SAH, sedating medications that may confound serial neurological examinations should be avoided. Opioid medications have adverse effects, including sedation, constipation, and decrease in central respiratory drive, and, in SAH patients, the latter can cause a rise in carbon dioxide with resulting cerebral vasodilation and increased intracranial pressure. Therefore, opioid medications should be avoided if possible. As bleeding risks are an especial concern in patients with SAH, non-steroidal anti-inflammatory agents, which adversely affect platelet aggregation, are typically avoided. For those who have suffered a seizure, analgesic medications such as tramadol, which can further lower the seizure threshold, should be used with caution.

In general, for SAH patients, acetaminophen and judicious use of tramadol and low-dose codeine may be helpful in managing pain without confounding a neurological examination or causing significant risk of increasing intracranial pressure.

Coughing and Straining

Evidence

Valsalva manoeuvres, as during coughing or straining at urinary or bowel movements, produce a brief surge in arterial blood pressure that may increase risk of re-rupture in unsecured aneurysms. In a study of 456 patients whose activities at onset of aneurysmal rupture were known, 13% were engaged in micturition or defaecation (Matsuda et al., 2007).

Comment

It is reasonable to take measures to prevent Valsalva manoeuvres in patients in whom a ruptured aneurysm is not yet secured. Stool softeners should be prescribed routinely. Patients are placed at bed rest and instructed to avoid lifting objects. Antiemetics should be used promptly if nausea develops.

Initial Blood Pressure Management Prior to Securing Aneurysm

Evidence

Elevated blood pressure is a risk factor for early rebleeding in the first 24 hours after initial aneurysmal rupture. In a study of 273 SAH patients, 14% had rebleeding in the ambulance or at the referring hospital before admission arrival to a comprehensive centre. Elevated systolic blood pressure (SBP) (>160 mm Hg) was associated with rebleeding, odds ratio (OR) 3.1 (95% confidence interval [CI]: 1.5–6.8) (Ohkuma et al., 2001).

Whether active blood pressure control reduces rebleeding has not been studied in a randomized trial in the modern management era. In the American Cooperative Study, conducted between 1963 and 1970, 1005 patients with ruptured aneurysms were randomized between four treatment modalities: one arm consisted of drug-induced lowering of the blood pressure, another of bed rest alone, and the other two arms were surgical: carotid ligation and intracranial surgery. In the intention-to-treat analysis, antihypertensive drugs compared with bed rest alone failed to reduce the rate of rebleeding (Torner et al., 1981). However, this study was performed in the pre-CT era, so diagnosis of rebleeding may not have been fully accurate, and the duration of delay before securing the aneurysm was prolonged.

Some nonrandomized studies have tested how well particular continuous intravenous antihypertensive regimens can attain target blood pressures in acute SAH patients awaiting early surgical or endovascular aneurysm treatment. For example, a single arm study analysed 28 acute SAH patients prior to aneurysm securement who had not achieved goal blood pressures with intravenous labetalol or hydralazine. Addition of intravenous nicardipine was effective at lowering blood pressure, decreasing mean SBP from 177 mm Hg at admission and 156 mm Hg with initial agents to 143 mm Hg. Failure to achieve target blood pressure occurred in 4%, hypotension occurred in 11%, and there were no episodes of rebleeding (Varelas et al., 2010).

Comment

In the acute setting, prior to intervention on a ruptured intracranial aneurysm, it is reasonable to control blood pressure to <160 mm Hg to deter early re-rupture. This can be accomplished with small doses of labetalol or hydralazine. In patients with refractory hypertension, continuous infusion of calcium channel blocking agents such as nicardipine or clevidipine can be a reasonable option. Despite theoretical concerns that sodium nitroprusside could increase intracranial pressure due to its potent vasodilatory effect, this effect is rare in practice. Sodium nitroprusside can be useful for the most recalcitrant cases of acute hypertension, though it is prudent to reserve its use for such cases.

After the aneurysm is secured, hypertension should generally not be treated in the absence of signs of heart failure or extremely high pressures reaching the range that could produce hypertensive encephalopathy. Permissive hypertension is especially advisable in patients deemed to be at high risk of delayed cerebral ischaemia (DCI).

Fluids and Electrolytes

Hypotonic solutions (including lactated Ringer's solution) should be avoided in patients with SAH to avoid worsening of brain oedema. Electrolyte imbalances are not uncommon upon presentation. Particular attention should be paid to hypomagnesaemia, which is prevalent and can increase the risk of cardiac arrhythmias. Avoiding intravascular volume depletion should be a priority, especially within the period of maximal risk of DCI (days 3–10), but inducing prophylactic hypervolaemia is not beneficial and can in fact be detrimental (Lennihan et al., 2000; Martini et al., 2012; Kissoon et al., 2015).

For all patients hospitalized with an aneurysmal SAH, careful fluid monitoring requires placement of a urinary catheter. Patients should be hydrated with isotonic or hypertonic solutions. Intravascular volume depletion should be avoided, but without trying to induce hypervolaemia. Additionally, regular monitoring of electrolytes, particularly sodium, allows for early recognition of delayed complications, namely, cerebral salt wasting (CSW) and the syndrome of inappropriate antidiuretic hormone (SIADH).

Hyponatraemia

Patients who present with SAH are at risk for multiple medical complications, and hyponatraemia is one of the most common. Prompt recognition and treatment are necessary to prevent additional complications.

Evidence

The cause of hyponatraemia in SAH patients had previously been attributed to SIADH (Doczi et al., 1981). However, a prospective evaluation of 21 consecutive patients with SAH found that hyponatraemia developed in 9 of 21 patients between post-bleed days 3 and 9, and evaluation of fluid status in those patients identified a decreased plasma volume with a preceding negative sodium balance, indicative of CSW (Wijdicks et al., 1985).

Subsequently, a prospective study of 208 SAH patients identified an incidence of hyponatraemia of 34%, and of these patients, 24% developed DCI compared with 12% of SAH patients who did not have hyponatraemia (Hasan et al., 1990).

A systematic review completed in 2011 identified seven articles evaluating management options for patients with hyponatraemia and SAH, due to either SIADH or CSW. The authors concluded that maintaining a normal volume status and correcting sodium to normal levels was beneficial. Early treatment with mineralocorticoids improved excess sodium loss and serum sodium levels. Most studies evaluated either fludrocortisone or hydrocortisone, with a better side effect profile being seen in patients receiving fludrocortisone. While the use of hypertonic saline improved laboratory values, the clinical benefit was uncertain and, likewise, use of albumin had an unclear clinical benefit. The use of vasopressin antagonists could not be recommended in SAH patients, as these medications had not been studied in this population, and the benefit of the medication compared with the potential harm of inducing hypovolaemia is unknown (Rabinstein and Bruder, 2011).

Clinical Applications

Hyponatraemia in SAH patients is common and primarily due to CSW, although SIADH can occur as well. Maintenance of normovolaemia and correction of sodium to normal levels are recommended. For patients with CSW, mineralocorticoid agents such as fludrocortisone can improve the degree of natriuresis. Maintenance of appropriate volume can be effectively achieved with either isotonic or hypertonic crystalloid fluids. The use of albumin is safe, but the clinical benefit is unclear.

Anaemia

It is common for patients with SAH to present with or develop anaemia during their hospitalization. Anaemia is typically multifactorial.

Evidence

Lower haemoglobin levels have also been associated with an increased risk of an unfavourable functional outcome, especially in patients who have vasospasm (Smith et al., 2004; Wartenberg, et al., 2006; Kramer et al., 2008; Stein et al., 2015). However, red blood cell transfusion (RBCT) has also been consistently associated with worse outcomes and more systemic complications in several retrospective studies (Kramer et al., 2008; Levine et al., 2010; Festic et al., 2013; Pegoli et al., 2015). An extensive review in 2011 included 27 studies evaluating the safety and clinical benefit of RBCT in patients with aneurysmal SAH. Overall, the authors concluded that RBCT might improve some aspects of brain physiology, but is associated with increased risk of medical complications, vasospasm, and poor functional outcomes. Yet, it is unclear if RBCT is responsible for worse clinical outcomes or simply a marker of disease severity (Le Roux, 2011).

Prospective data are very scarce. A small pilot study of 44 patients randomized to a haemoglobin goal of 10 g/dL or 11.5 g/dL found that severity of physical deficits and levels of independence at 14 days, 28 days, or 3 months were not significantly different between the groups (Naidech et al., 2010). Of note, the two haemoglobin targets evaluated in this pilot study would be considered too high by many clinicians.

Fever Management

Evidence

The presence of fever has been shown to negatively impact functional outcomes in SAH and has also been associated with cerebral vasospasm (Oliveira-Filho et al., 2001; Rabinstein and Sandhu, 2007). In a large observational study of 584 consecutive patients with aneurysmal SAH, fever occurred in 48% (Kramer et al., 2017). Fever burden was an independent predictor of poor outcome, OR 1.14 - per day of fever, 95% CI: 1.06–1.22; $p = 0.0006$. In aneurysmal SAH, it is not uncommon for an underlying infectious or systemic inflammatory source to be absent, indicating a likely central cause of fever secondary to neurological injury. In the large observational study, fever without an identified infectious source occurred in 55% of patients (Kramer et al., 2017).

No randomized trial has evaluated induced normothermia in patients with SAH. One case–control study matched 40 consecutive febrile SAH patients treated with a surface-cooling device during the first 14 days after SAH to 80 prior febrile SAH patients managed with conventional fever control, matched by age, Hunt and Hess grade, and SAH severity (Badjatia et al., 2010). On average, over the 2-week treatment period, temperatures were 0.9°C above normal in the conventional treatment group versus 0.2°C above normal in the induced normothermia group, $p < 0.001$. Although patients with induced normothermia had increased rates of cardiac dysrhythmia and hyperglycaemia, induced normothermia was associated with a reduction in poor outcomes at 1 year, OR 0.2, 95% CI: 0.1–0.6, $p = 0.004$.

One small randomized trial evaluated mild therapeutic hypothermia (targeted temperature 34.5°C) or conventional management in 22 poor-grade SAH patients (Choi et al., 2017). Non-significantly fewer patients in the hypothermia group had symptomatic vasospasm (18% vs 36%), delayed cerebral infarction (36% vs 46%), and mortality at 1 month (0% vs 36%).

Clinical Applications

Temperature should be closely monitored and fever should be treated. Central fever is common in neurological patients, but must be a diagnosis of exclusion. Careful evaluation for infection (including ventriculitis/meningitis in patients with a ventricular or lumbar drain), deep vein thrombosis (DVT) or pulmonary embolism, and drug fever must be completed prior to making this diagnosis. For fever occurring between days 3 and 14 after aneurysmal rupture, cerebral vasospasm should also be considered. Management of fever begins with proper identification and treatment of the underlying cause, but also the fever itself should be treated, even if deemed central. Given the known association of fever with poor outcome, a goal of normothermia is reasonable. Various methods, including antipyretic medications, surface or intravascular temperature-modulating devices, and/or cold saline infusions are commonly utilized. There is insufficient evidence at present to support the routine implementation of targeted temperature management to normothermic or hypothermic targets, but further studies are warranted (Madden et al., 2017).

Venous Thromboembolism Prophylaxis

Evidence

Deep vein thrombosis is not as common after SAH as is ischaemic stroke, likely because the patients are restless, less often have leg paralysis, are more aggressively hydrated, and are young. Among 15,968 SAH admissions for aneurysmal SAH in the US Nationwide Inpatient Sample, symptomatic DVTs were documented in 3.5% and pulmonary embolism in 1.2% (Kshettry et al., 2014). Asymptomatic DVTs, found on screening lower extremity Doppler ultrasound, occur more frequently and are reported in 3–24% of patients (Mack et al., 2008; Ray et al., 2009).

In patients with acute SAH, there are limited data regarding the timing of initiation of venous thromboembolism (VTE) chemoprophylaxis. A meta-analysis analysed 18 randomized trials and 12 cohort studies of mechanical and pharmacological prophylaxis in patients undergoing a wide variety of neurosurgical procedures, but few of the patients had SAH and the preponderance of patients were treated with open craniotomy procedures rather than minimally invasive endovascular procedures (Collen et al., 2008). Both low-molecular-weight heparin (LMWH) and intermittent compression devices (ICDs) were effective in reducing DVT (LMWH: risk ratio [RR] 0.60, 95% CI: 0.44–0.81; ICD: RR 0.41, 95% CI: 0.21–0.78). There was no statistical difference in intracranial haemorrhage rates between LMWH and nonpharmacological methods (RR 1.97, 95% CI: 0.64–6.09), though combined intracranial haemorrhage and minor bleeding were higher with pharmacological therapy.

Clinical Applications

For patients admitted with SAH, given the likelihood of limited mobility during the hospital course, VTE prophylaxis should be prescribed. Prior to securing the ruptured aneurysm, ICDs should be used. After the aneurysm is secured (at least 24 hours after the intervention), and if the clinical situation allows, pharmacological prophylaxis may be added (Nyquist et al., 2016). Special consideration and discussion with the neurosurgery team are needed prior to initiation of pharmacological prophylaxis in patients with CSF diversion using an external ventricular drain (EVD) or lumbar drain (LD), and in those where a major surgical procedure (e.g. clipping, haematoma evacuation) was required.

There are no prospective data demonstrating that screening with serial Doppler ultrasounds is cost-effective or beneficial in patients with SAH. Because some of these patients may be unable to receive pharmacological prophylaxis for a prolonged time and have limited mobility, screening ultrasound examinations may be reasonable in certain cases, particularly in patients with poor-grade SAH who may have a higher likelihood of developing a DVT.

Antiepileptic Medications

Evidence

The prophylactic use of antiepileptic medications is controversial. Seizures in the first few weeks after aneurysmal rupture occur in about 10% of patients, and most occur soon after the initial haemorrhage (O'Connor et al., 2014; Panczykowski et al., 2016). Intracranial haematoma and intracranial surgery likely increase the risk. A recent survey of several US medical centres regarding the use of prophylactic antiepileptic drugs (AEDs) in SAH found that 68% of respondents prescribe prophylactic AEDs (Dewan and Mocco, 2015). This practice may not be safe, at least if phenytoin is the drug chosen. Phenytoin use has been associated with worse functional and cognitive outcomes in aneurysmal SAH (Naidech et al., 2005) and it can accelerate the liver metabolism of nimodipine, likely making it less effective (Tartara et al., 1991).

While no randomized trials have included a treatment arm in which use of prophylactic AEDs was completely avoided, one small, single-centre trial randomized 84 patients to a brief (3-day) course of levetiracetam versus an extended (until hospital discharge) course of levetiracetam (Human et al., 2018). Although in-hospital seizures occurred non-significantly more often in the brief than extended prophylaxis group (9% vs 2%, $p = 0.2$), good functional outcome (modified Rankin Scale [mRS] 0–2) was more frequent in the brief treatment group (83% vs 61%, $p = 0.04$). Seizures were more likely to occur

among patients with entry CT evidence of early brain injury (adjusted OR 12.5, 95% CI: 1.2–122; $p = 0.03$).

Clinical Applications

There is no clear evidence that routine use of prophylactic AEDs is beneficial in SAH patients without a history of seizures. If prophylaxis is started, a brief, 3-day period of treatment may be preferred for most patients, avoiding phenytoin and using a medication with few side effects (including less sedation) and limited drug-to-drug interactions, such as levetiracetam. A longer course of prophylaxis may be considered in patients at increased seizure risk due to early brain injury on imaging.

Acute Complications of Subarachnoid Haemorrhage

Patients who experience an SAH are at risk for multiple complications, both in the acute and subacute settings. Clinicians must be mindful of the likely causes of decompensation, and react urgently to stabilize the patient and manage each potential complication.

In the acute post-bleed phase, patients may experience re-rupture and rebleeding, hydrocephalus due to occluded arachnoid granulations or obstruction of foramina, and cardiopulmonary failure.

Aneurysmal Rebleeding

Rebleeding is a known early complication of aneurysmal SAH and typically occurs in the first 24–72 hours after the initial haemorrhage. The clinical presentation of rebleeding can be dramatic, with acute coma or sudden death occurring in some patients. The incidence of rebleeding after SAH has been estimated at 6% within 24 hours (van Donkelaar et al., 2015). The mainstay of treatment after rebleeding is urgent stabilization and definitive management of the aneurysm, with either endovascular or open surgical approaches. Hypertension may contribute to aneurysmal rupture; early blood pressure management has been discussed in a previous section.

Antifbrinolytic Drug Therapy

Rebleeding after SAH is thought to originate from dissolution of the clot at the site of the ruptured aneurysm by natural fibrinolytic activity in the CSF

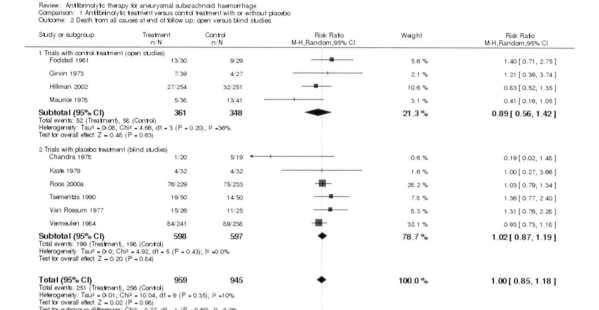

Review: Antifibrinolytic therapy for aneurysmal subarachnoid haemorrhage
Comparison: 1 Antifibrinolytic treatment versus control treatment with or without placebo
Outcome: 2 Death from all causes at end of follow up: open versus blind studies

Figure 14.1 Forest plot showing the effects of *antifibrinolytic therapy vs control* in acute SAH on *death* at end of follow-up. Reproduced from Baharoglu et al. (2013), with permission from the authors and John Wiley & Sons Limited. Copyright Cochrane Library, with permission.

after the SAH. Antifibrinolytic drugs cross the blood–brain barrier rapidly after SAH and reduce fibrinolytic activity. The two most commonly tested drugs have been tranexamic acid and ε-aminocaproic acid. Both agents are structurally similar to lysine and block the lysine sites by which plasminogen molecules bind to fibrin, thereby inhibiting fibrinolysis. Antifibrinolytic drugs potentially have a role in aneurysmal SAH in preventing rebleeding during the period between the initial aneurysm rupture and definitive structural treatment of the aneurysm by clipping or coiling. Most studies of antifibrinolytic agents were performed in an era when there was often a long delay between initial rupture and surgical or endovascular aneurysm treatment, rather than the current practice of proceeding rapidly to definitive aneurysm management.

Evidence

A systematic review for the Cochrane Library identified 10 randomized trials evaluating the effect of antifibrinolytic therapy in a total of 1904 patients with aneurysmal SAH (Baharoglu et al., 2013). For death, data were available from all 10 trials and 1904 patients,

and random allocation to antifibrinolytic therapy was not associated with altered mortality, OR 1.00, 95% CI: 0.85–1.18; $p = 0.98$ (Figure 14.1). For poor outcome (severe disability, vegetative state, or death), data were available from 3 trials and 1546 patients. Random assignment to antifibrinolytic treatment did not change the poor outcome rate, OR 1.02, 95% CI: 0.91–1.15 (Figure 14.2). With regard to rebleeding, all 10 trials and 1904 patients provided data. Treatment with antifibrinolytic therapy did reduce rebleeding rates, 12.7% versus 22.3%, OR 0.65, 95% CI: 0.44–0.97; $p = 0.035$ (Figure 14.3). However, a countervailing effect was seen for occurrence of cerebral ischaemia, for which 6 trials provided data on 1671 patients. Antifibrinolytic therapy increased cerebral ischaemia, 25.6% versus 20.3%, OR 1.41, 95% CI: 1.04–1.91; $p = 0.03$ (Figure 14.4). As prolonged administration of an antifibrinolytic drug increases the incidence of delayed ischaemic infarctions, thus offsetting the early benefit from prevention of rebleeding, a brief duration of antifibrinolytic administration is of interest.

Only 1 of the randomized trials evaluated brief duration therapy, assessing tranexamic acid 1 g IV

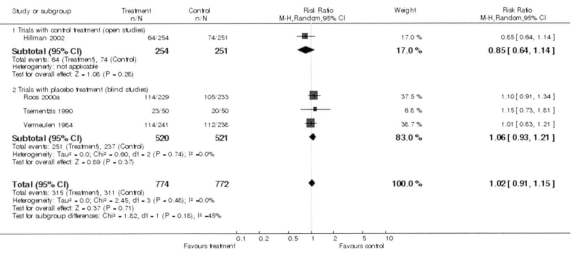

Figure 14.2 Forest plot showing the effects of *antifibrinolytic therapy vs control* in acute SAH on *poor outcome* at end of follow-up. Reproduced from Baharoglu et al. (2013), with permission from the authors and John Wiley & Sons Limited. Copyright Cochrane Library, with permission.

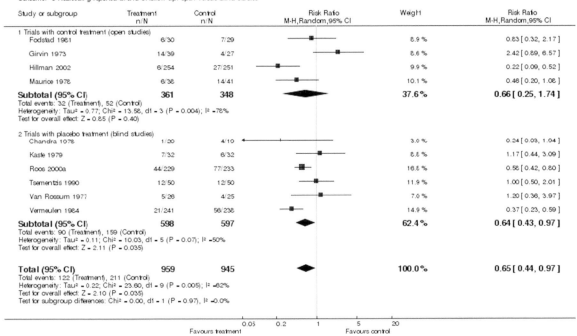

Figure 14.3 Forest plot showing the effects of *antifibrinolytic therapy vs control* in acute SAH on *rebleeding* at end of follow-up. Reproduced from Baharoglu et al. (2013), with permission from the authors and John Wiley & Sons Limited. Copyright Cochrane Library, with permission.

Review: Antifibrinolytic therapy for aneurysmal subarachnoid haemorrhage
Comparison: 1 Antifibrinolytic treatment versus control treatment with or without placebo
Outcome: 6 Cerebral ischaemia reported at end of follow-up: open versus blind studies

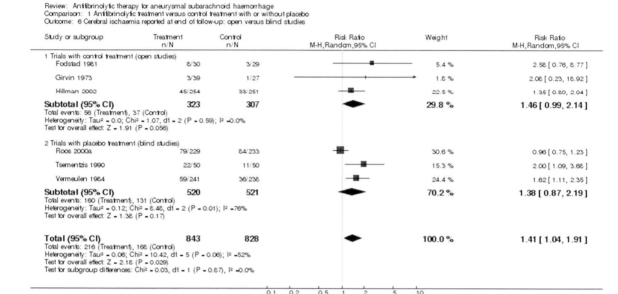

Study or subgroup	Treatment n/N	Control n/N	Risk Ratio M-H,Random,95% CI	Weight	Risk Ratio M-H,Random,95% CI
1 Trials with control treatment (open studies)					
Fodstad 1981	8/30	3/29		5.4 %	2.58 [0.76, 8.77]
Girvin 1973	3/39	1/27		1.8 %	2.08 [0.23, 18.92]
Hillman 2002	45/254	33/251		22.5 %	1.35 [0.80, 2.04]
Subtotal (95% CI)	323	307		29.8 %	1.46 [0.99, 2.14]

Total events: 56 (Treatment), 37 (Control)
Heterogeneity: Tau² = 0.0; Chi² = 1.07, df = 2 (P = 0.59); I² =0.0%
Test for overall effect: Z = 1.91 (P = 0.056)

2 Trials with placebo treatment (blind studies)					
Roos 2000a	79/229	84/233		30.6 %	0.96 [0.75, 1.23]
Tsementzis 1990	22/50	11/50		15.3 %	2.00 [1.09, 3.68]
Vermeulen 1984	59/241	36/238		24.4 %	1.62 [1.11, 2.35]
Subtotal (95% CI)	520	521		70.2 %	1.38 [0.87, 2.19]

Total events: 160 (Treatment), 131 (Control)
Heterogeneity: Tau² = 0.12; Chi² = 8.48, df = 2 (P = 0.01); I² =76%
Test for overall effect: Z = 1.38 (P = 0.17)

Total (95% CI)	843	828		100.0 %	1.41 [1.04, 1.91]

Total events: 216 (Treatment), 168 (Control)
Heterogeneity: Tau² = 0.06; Chi² = 10.42, df = 5 (P = 0.06); I² =52%
Test for overall effect: Z = 2.18 (P = 0.029)
Test for subgroup differences: Chi² = 0.03, df = 1 (P = 0.87), I² =0.0%

0.1   0.2   0.5   1   2   5   10
Favours treatment   Favours control

Figure 14.4 Forest plot showing the effects of *antifibrinolytic therapy vs control* in acute SAH on *cerebral ischaemia* at end of follow-up. Reproduced from Baharoglu et al. (2013), with permission from the authors and John Wiley & Sons Limited. Copyright Cochrane Library, with permission.

every 6 hours until the aneurysm was secured or for not more than 72 hours (Hillman et al., 2002). Among 505 randomized patients, antifibrinolytic therapy reduced rebleeding (OR 0.22, 95% CI: 0.09–0.52; p = 0.0006) with a statistically non-significant offsetting increase in cerebral ischaemia (OR 1.35, 95% CI: 0.89–2.04; p = 0.16). Net effects did not reach statistical significance for final poor outcome (OR 0.85, 95% CI: 0.64–1.14, p = 0.28) or mortality (OR 0.83, 95% CI: 0.52–1.35; p = 0.46).

Clinical Applications

The use of antifibrinolytic agents may reduce the incidence of aneurysmal rebleeding in the acute setting. It is reasonable, in the absence of contraindications, to treat patients with an antifibrinolytic medication (we use tranexamic acid 1 g IV every 6 hours) for the first 72 hours after the haemorrhage or until the aneurysm is secured, whichever occurs first (Connolly et al., 2012). Initiation of antifibrinolytic may increase cerebral ischaemia complications associated with cerebral vasospasm and increases the risk of systemic thrombosis, so these medications should be avoided in patients who have entered the high-risk period of SAH-associated vasospasm (postbleed days 4–14) and in those who have an increased thrombotic risk.

Hydrocephalus

Hydrocephalus is a known complication of SAH, and can present shortly after the initial haemorrhage. It can be communicating (due to blood products blocking CSF absorption at the arachnoid granulations) or non-communicating (from foraminal obstruction). The incidence of hydrocephalus within 72 hours of haemorrhage is 15–20%, and common symptoms include depressed level of consciousness, downward eye deviation, and bradycardia (Yamada et al., 2015; Tso et al., 2016; Chen et al., 2017). The major modern methods of initial hydrocephalus management are EVD and LD, and the leading long-term management technique is ventriculoperitoneal shunting (VPS), with lamina terminalis fenestration used less often. Hydrocephalus is associated with worse functional outcome, and CSF diversion may not be effective in improving prognosis if not started early (Dupont and Rabinstein, 2013).

Evidence

For patients with SAH-associated hydrocephalus, no large, randomized controlled trials have been completed comparing initial treatment strategies. Based on observational series, and the devastating course of untreated hydrocephalus, placement of an EVD is the mainstay of initial therapy. Of note, placement of an EVD is associated with a higher risk of rebleeding, but whether this relationship is causal or reflects bias by indication is uncertain. A systematic review of 16 observational studies with a total of 6804 patients found rebleeding occurred more frequently in patients undergoing EVD, 18.8% versus 6.4%, OR 3.92, p < 0.0001 (Cagnazzo et al., 2017). Pathophysiologically, placement of an EVD might increase rebleeding risk by reducing intracranial pressure, resulting in greater transmural pressure at the aneurysm site. However, the association may reflect confounding by indication, with underlying sicker patient and riskier aneurysm status separately causing more frequent treatment with EVDs and more frequent rebleeding. One small randomized trial enrolling 60 aneurysmal subarachnoid patients with EVDs placed compared continuous CSF drainage with intermittent CSF drainage and found no difference in frequency of vasospasm (65% vs 80%, p = 0.18), independent or better (mRS 0–2) outcomes (32% vs 35%, p = 0.85), or mortality (24% vs 12%, p = 0.24), though nonpatency of EVD occurred more often with continuous drainage (44% vs 12%, p = 0.03) (Olson et al., 2013).

Many patients treated with an EVD will be able to be weaned from ventricular drainage as the subarachnoid blood is reabsorbed. However, an important minority will require placement of a long-term ventriculoperitoneal shunt. Overall, in an analysis of 66 observational studies analysing 41,789 aneurysmal SAH patients, the eventual VPS insertion rate was 12.7% (Tso et al., 2016). Among patients who are initially treated with an EVD, ventriculoperitoneal shunting is pursued in over 30% (Dorai et al., 2003; O'Kelly et al., 2009). One small randomized trial in 81 patients compared rapid (within 24 hours) versus gradual (over 96 hours) weaning of an EVD and found no difference in subsequent requirement for VPS placement, 63% versus 63% (Klopfenstein et al., 2004). Nonetheless, EVD weaning over at least 2–3 days remains common across centres, and the value of this strategy deserves further investigation.

Clinical Applications

CSF diversion in patients with acute symptomatic hydrocephalus after SAH can improve the clinical status rapidly, and this treatment is indispensable in many cases. Removal of CSF can be achieved using lumbar puncture, LD, or an EVD. EVD is the only option when hydrocephalus is non-communicating (typically from obstruction at the aqueduct, thus causing dilation of the third ventricle but not the fourth ventricle). Deferring CSF diversion until after the ruptured aneurysm has been secured is advocated by some, but should only be acceptable if the delay will be short and the patient is not frankly symptomatic from the hydrocephalus.

Ventriculoperitoneal shunting (or, less often, lumboperitoneal shunting) is necessary when attempts at clamping the external drain fail because of recurrent symptoms or intracranial hypertension. Further randomized trials are needed to guide use of intermittent versus continuous EVD drainage and the rate of EVD weaning.

Neurogenic Cardiopulmonary Injury

Patients with acute neurological injury, including SAH, are at risk of developing secondary cardiac injury in the absence of coronary disease, typically referred to as 'stress cardiomyopathy' or Takotsubo cardiomyopathy, mediated by a surge in adrenal circulating catecholamines or direct myocardial sympathetic stimulation by dysfunctional insular cortex. Neurogenic pulmonary oedema can also occur acutely after aneurysmal SAH, though most often combined with a cardiogenic component.

Evidence

Approximately one-third of patients with SAH have elevation of troponin, and this, as well as elevated B-type natriuretic peptide, and Q wave, T wave, and ST segment abnormalities, is associated with death, poor overall outcome, and development of delayed cerebral infarction. Cardiac arrhythmias are also common, occurring in approximately one-third of patients, although life-threatening arrhythmias only occur in a small minority. Pulmonary oedema is associated with poor-grade haemorrhages, elevated serum troponin, and increased mortality (van der Bilt et al., 2009; Bruder and Rabinstein, 2011).

In large series, independent predictors of development of neurogenic stress cardiomyopathy have included higher Hunt and Hess score, older age, and female sex (Tung et al., 2004; Malik et al., 2015).

In the modern era of early aneurysm coiling or clipping, no randomized trial has assessed different therapies for prevention or treatment of neurogenic cardiopulmonary injury. In the preceding treatment era, a trial randomizing 224 aneurysmal SAH patients to prophylactic beta-blockade therapy with propranolol or control for 3 weeks found beta-blocker treatment associated with more frequent non-disabled outcome (72.1% vs 51.6%, $p = 0.003$) and fewer deaths (11.7% vs 22.6%, $p = 0.02$) (Neil-Dwyer et al., 1978; Neil-Dwyer et al., 1985). However, beta-blockers potentially adversely affect cerebral perfusion in the setting of vasospasm and may raise intracranial pressure, and have not been tested in a randomized study in the modern treatment era (Chang et al., 2016).

Clinical Applications

Cardiopulmonary complications are common in SAH patients. Electrolytes should be carefully monitored and adequately replaced to prevent cardiac arrhythmias. Treatment of stress-induced cardiomyopathy is supportive, with anti-hypertensives or diuretics as needed, and occasionally ionotropic agents. However, these treatments should be carefully monitored in patients with SAH, particularly those who are developing or are at high risk of vasospasm, as hypotension or hypovolaemia may precipitate cerebral ischaemia.

Definitive Management of Ruptured Aneurysms

In the first day after hospital admission for the initial SAH, up to 15% of patients experience rebleeding. In patients who survive the first day, the risk of rebleeding without medical or surgical therapy directed at preventing recurrent haemorrhage is 35–40% over the next 4 weeks, and is more or less evenly distributed over those 4 weeks (Hijdra et al., 1987). Between 4 weeks and 6 months after the initial haemorrhage, the risk of rebleeding gradually decreases, from the initial 1–2% per day to a long-term risk of about 3% per year, if the ruptured aneurysm is not therapeutically occluded. Given its high rates of occurrence and morbidity and mortality, averting rebleeding is a dominant therapeutic aim in the management of aneurysmal SAH. The leading techniques for definitive aneurysm occlusion are: (1) endovascular coiling, in which catheter-delivered platinum coils are released to pack the aneurysm and induce thrombosis to completely fill the aneurysm sac; and (2) open surgical clipping, in which a small metallic clip or clips are placed across the neck of the aneurysm, excluding it from the circulation. The endovascular technique

allows for the diagnostic angiogram and the therapeutic coiling to be completed in the same intervention. The differential efficacy and safety of each approach for different aneurysm targets must be considered when determining the ideal treatment for each individual patient.

In addition to whether and how to occlude a ruptured aneurysm, the best time period to do so has been an important focus of study. Performing the occlusion procedure early after aneurysm rupture prevents rebleeding and, with the aneurysm secured, permits more aggressive blood pressure and fluid support to treat vasospasm and avert delayed cerebral infarction. However, it requires the obliterative procedure to take place when the patient is under acute physiological stress.

Timing of Treatment

Evidence

The practice of performing aneurysm occlusion procedures early after initial SAH first became widespread in the era when microsurgical clipping was the main treatment procedure, after the publication of a randomized trial from Finland and a large international observational study. The Finnish study, the only randomized controlled trial (RCT) addressing this topic identified in systematic review, randomized 216 patients with aneurysmal SAH to planned surgery at 3 different time points after SAH: early (0–3 days), intermediate (3–7 days), or late (>7 days) (Ohman and Heiskanen, 1989; Whitfield and Kirkpatrick, 2001). The outcome of death or dependency at 3 months was lower in patients undergoing early- compared with intermediate-period surgery (OR 0.34, 95% CI: 0.12–0.93), and also tended to be lower compared with late-period surgery (OR 0.40, 95% CI: 0.13–1.02).

A similar advantage of early- over intermediate-period surgery was found in the large, observational International Cooperative Study on the Timing of Aneurysm Surgery, a prospective, nonrandomized study of 3521 patients (Kassell et al., 1990). Good recovery rates were higher when surgery was planned to occur in early (0–3 days) or late (15–32 days), compared with intermediate (e.g. 7–10 days) time periods: early 63%, intermediate 56%, late 63%, $p = 0.046$. Among the 722 patients enrolled in the United States, where patients may have had access to more advanced intensive care postoperatively, good recovery rates were highest with early period surgery: early 71%, intermediate 56%, late 63%, $p < 0.05$ (Haley et al., 1992).

The development of endovascular coiling further entrenched early aneurysm obliteration as a widely employed treatment strategy, as coiling, compared with clipping, potentially has less differentially higher intra-procedural risk when performed early after SAH. In the era of coiling, observational studies, but no randomized trials, have investigated whether performing endovascular aneurysm occlusion procedures ultra-early, in the first 24 hours after SAH, is advantageous compared with later time periods. A systematic review identified 8 observational series with a total of 1594 SAH patients (Rawal et al., 2017). Endovascular coiling in the ultra-early period at <1 day was associated with a reduced frequency of poor outcome compared with treatment at >1 day (RR 0.56, 95% CI: 0.45–0.70; $I^2 = 0\%$) but not when compared with treatment at 1–3 days (RR 1.12, 95% CI: 0.58–2.15; $I^2 = 80\%$) (Figure 14.5).

Clinical Applications

A treatment policy of procedural treatment of the ruptured aneurysm in the early, initial 0- to 3-day period following SAH is highly reasonable, though supported preponderantly by observational series rather than randomized trials. Securing the aneurysm early after rupture reduces rebleeding frequency and permits more aggressive vasoactive management to prevent delayed

cerebral infarction from vasospasm. Further compressing the target procedural period to just the first 24 hours after aneurysm rupture, rather than days 1–3, does not consistently provide additional improved outcomes.

Endovascular Coiling vs Surgical Clipping

Evidence

A systematic review identified 4 randomized trials enrolling 2458 participants comparing endovascular coiling and surgical clipping of ruptured aneurysms (Lindgren et al., 2018). Only patients deemed treatable by either modality were enrolled. A preponderance of the patients, 87%, were contributed by one large trial, the International Subarachnoid Aneurysm Trial (ISAT) (Molyneux et al., 2002; Molyneux et al., 2015). The majority of enrolled patients had mild-to-moderate rather than severe-grade SAH, and most aneurysms were located within the anterior circulation. All 4 trials contributed data on outcomes through 1 year. Only ISAT contributed data on long-term outcomes, with follow-up extending to 18 years.

With regard to functional outcomes, allocation to endovascular coiling compared with surgical clipping and reduced death and dependency at 1 year, 24% versus 32% (RR 0.77, 95% CI: 0.67–0.87; $p = 0.00005$) (Figure 14.6). At 10 years, the reduction in death or dependency was sustained (RR 0.81, 95% CI: 0.70–0.92; $p = 0.002$).

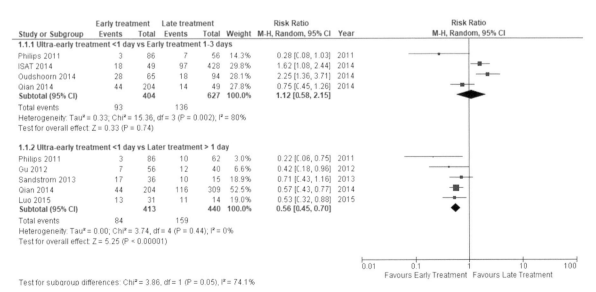

Figure 14.5 Forest plot showing the effects of *ultra-early vs later endovascular coiling* for ruptured cerebral aneurysms on *poor functional outcome* at end of follow-up in non-randomized studies. Figure courtesy of JL Saver, under a Creative Commons 4.0 CC-BY license (JL Saver).

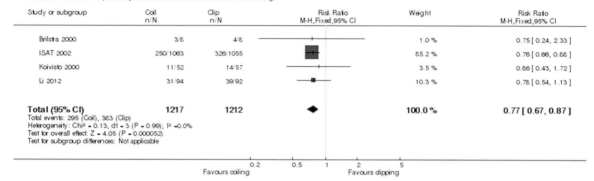

Figure 14.6 Forest plot showing the effects of *endovascular coiling vs surgical clipping* for ruptured cerebral aneurysms on *poor outcome* at 1 year. Reproduced from Lindgren et al. (2018), with permission from the authors and John Wiley & Sons Limited. Copyright Cochrane Library, with permission.

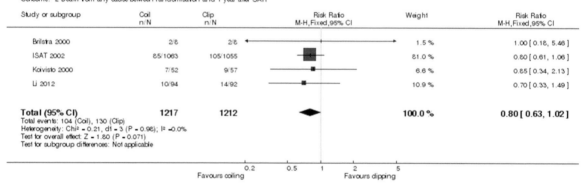

Figure 14.7 Forest plot showing the effects of *endovascular coiling vs surgical clipping* for ruptured cerebral aneurysms on *death* at 1 year. Reproduced from Lindgren et al. (2018), with permission from the authors and John Wiley & Sons Limited. Copyright Cochrane Library, with permission.

For mortality, assignment to endovascular coiling was associated with a non-significant reduction in death at 1 year, 8.5% versus 10.7% (RR 0.80, 95% CI: 0.63–1.02; $p = 0.07$) (Figure 14.7). At 10 years, the reduction in mortality reached nominal statistical significances (RR 0.78, 95% CI: 0.64–0.96; $p = 0.02$).

Data regarding DCI by 2–3 months were available for 2450 patients from the 4 trials. Allocation to endovascular coiling compared with surgical clipping reduced DCI, 23.8% versus 28.5% (RR 0.84, 95% CI: 0.74–0.96; $p = 0.01$) (Figure 14.8).

Data regarding the degree of sustained aneurysm obliteration were available from 3 trials for 1626 patients. At 1 year, non-complete obliteration of the target aneurysm was more frequent with endovascular coiling than with neurosurgical clipping, 33.3% versus 16.4% (RR 2.02, 95% CI: 1.65–2.47; $p < 0.00001$) (Figure 14.9). However, substantial non-complete obliteration (<90% occlusion) was less frequent, and not statistically different, 7.6% versus 5.1% (RR 1.43, 95% CI: 0.93–2.21; $p = 0.11$) (2 trials, 1440 patients).

Rebleeding was evaluated in two time periods: (1) before the aneurysm procedural treatment, and (2) after. Rebleeding could occur differentially after random allocation to the assigned treatment strategy but before the procedure if one takes longer to initiate. Among 3 trials with data on 2272 patients, assignment to endovascular coiling compared with surgical clipping was

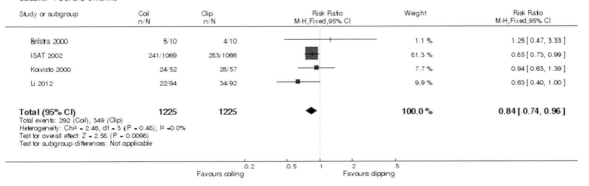

Figure 14.8 Forest plot showing the effects of *endovascular coiling vs surgical clipping* for ruptured cerebral aneurysms on *delayed cerebral infarction*. Reproduced from Lindgren et al. (2018), with permission from the authors and John Wiley & Sons Limited. Copyright Cochrane Library, with permission.

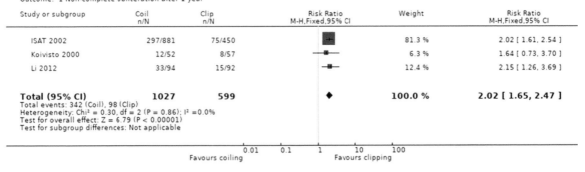

Figure 14.9 Forest plot showing the effects of *endovascular coiling vs surgical clipping* for ruptured cerebral aneurysms on incomplete aneurysm obliteration. Reproduced from Lindgren et al. (2018), with permission from the authors and John Wiley & Sons Limited. Copyright Cochrane Library, with permission.

associated with non-significantly lower pre-procedural rebleeding in 1.7% versus 2.6% (RR 0.64, 95%: 0.37–1.12; p = 0.12). In contrast, post-procedural rebleeding was higher with endovascular coiling than with microsurgical clipping, reflecting greater definitiveness of surgery in permanently excluding the aneurysm from the circulation. Among 4 trials with data on 2458 patients, with endovascular coiling versus surgical clipping, postprocedural rebleeding through 1 year occurred in 2.6% versus 1.4% (RR 1.83, 95% CI: 1.04–3.23; p = 0.04) (Figure 14.10). In long-term follow-up in the ISAT trial, through 10 years, postprocedural

rebleeding occurred in 6.1% versus 2.3% (RR 2.69, 95% CI: 1.50–4.81; p = 0.0009).

One additional controlled trial has been performed, the Barrow-Ruptured Aneurysm Trial (BRAT), which was excluded from the systematic Cochrane review because of design features increasing risk of bias, including alternating rather than random allocation to treatment groups and a high (30%) rate of not receiving allocated therapy. Among 403 patients available for evaluation at 1 year, death or dependency (mRS 3–6) was more frequent with clipping than coiling, 33.7% versus 23.2% (OR 1.68, 95% CI: 1.08–2.61; p = 0.02) (McDougall et al., 2012).

273

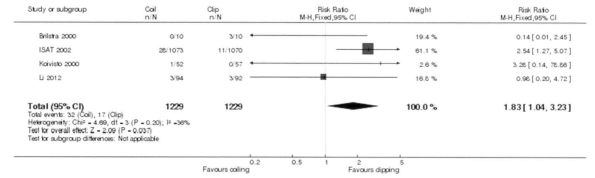

Review: Endovascular coiling versus neurosurgical clipping for people with aneurysmal subarachnoid haemorrhage
Comparison: 4 Rebleeding
Outcome: 2 Rebleed postprocedure up to 1 year

Study or subgroup	Coil n/N	Clip n/N	Risk Ratio M-H,Fixed,95% CI	Weight	Risk Ratio M-H,Fixed,95% CI
Brilstra 2000	0/10	3/10		19.4 %	0.14 [0.01, 2.45]
ISAT 2002	28/1073	11/1070		61.1 %	2.54 [1.27, 5.07]
Koivisto 2000	1/52	0/57		2.6 %	3.28 [0.14, 78.86]
Li 2012	3/94	3/92		16.8 %	0.98 [0.20, 4.72]
Total (95% CI)	**1229**	**1229**		**100.0 %**	**1.83 [1.04, 3.23]**

Total events: 32 (Coil), 17 (Clip)
Heterogeneity: Chi² = 4.69, df = 3 (P = 0.20); I² =36%
Test for overall effect: Z = 2.09 (P = 0.037)
Test for subgroup differences: Not applicable

0.2   0.5   1   2   5
Favours coiling   Favours clipping

Figure 14.10 Forest plot showing the effects of *endovascular coiling vs surgical clipping* for ruptured cerebral aneurysms on *preprocedural rebleeding*. Bottom panel: forest plot showing the effects of *endovascular coiling vs surgical clipping* for ruptured cerebral aneurysms on *postprocedural rebleeding through 1 year*. Reproduced from Lindgren et al. (2018), with permission from the authors and John Wiley & Sons Limited. Copyright Cochrane Library, with permission.

Clinical Applications

Deciding the proper modality for definitive aneurysm securement is complex and the final decision should consider multiple patient and aneurysm characteristics. The decision on how to treat a ruptured aneurysm should be made by multidisciplinary consensus with participation of experts in open surgical and endovascular techniques. Furthermore, these aneurysms should be treated at centres with broad expertise in both modalities and with a specialized neurocritical care unit to optimize the management of the patient before and after the intervention.

Based on the results of randomized trials, coiling should generally be preferred over clipping for the treatment of ruptured aneurysms amenable to both modalities. However, there are aneurysms that will be better treated with an open surgical approach, notably including those located in the middle cerebral artery bifurcation and those associated with an intraparenchymal haematoma that demands evacuation. Aneurysms with arterial branches arising from the sac are also best approached with craniotomy and clipping. In addition, coiling should be preferred in cases under-represented in the randomized trials as they historically were judged more amenable to coiling than clipping, including most posterior circulation aneurysms and for poor-grade patients who have a greater surgical risk.

When the aneurysm is coiled, a repeat angiogram at 6 months should be performed to exclude a recurrence that needs retreatment, even if there is no remnant noted at the time of the initial intervention.

Endovascular and Surgical Treatment of Ruptured Wide-necked Aneurysms

Wide-necked aneurysms are more difficult to obliterate for both endovascular and surgical strategies. The surgical approach requires greater vessel exposure and manipulation and more extensive clip placement. The endovascular approach was initially limited by the risk of coils escaping and embolizing from wide-necked aneurysm sacs, but was made more powerful by the technical developments of: (1) stent-assisted coiling, enabling safer delivery and packing of coils within the aneurysm; and (2) flow diverters, directing blood flow past rather than into the aneurysm sac, promoting thrombosis and closure of the aneurysm.

Evidence

There have been no randomized studies comparing surgical, endovascular coiling, stent-assisted coiling, and flow diverters for treatment of acutely ruptured, wide-necked aneurysms. One systematic review analysed observational series of surgical and endovascular treatment of mixed unruptured, remotely ruptured, and acutely ruptured wide-neck aneurysms, with 43 studies (2749 aneurysms) providing efficacy data and 65 studies (5366 patients) providing safety data (Fiorella et al., 2017).

Complete aneurysm occlusion was achieved in 53% of surgically treated patients and 40% of endovascularly treated patients. However, the endovascular techniques employed were frequently coiling alone.

For stent-assisted coiling, a systematic review identified 17 observational studies reporting outcomes in 339 patients with acutely ruptured, wide-necked aneurysms (Bodily et al., 2011). Complete aneurysm occlusion at the time of initial procedural treatment was attained in 63% (130/207). Crossover to open surgery, usually for failure in stent placement or for intraprocedural aneurysm rupture, was required in 2%. Clinically significant intracranial haemorrhagic complications, potentially related to intra-procedural anticoagulation, occurred in 8% (27/339). Clinically significant thromboembolic events occurred in 6% (16/288). Favourable functional outcomes occurred in 67%, poor functional outcomes in 14%, and death in 19%.

Flow diverters in acutely ruptured intracranial aneurysms were assessed in a systematic review of 20 observational studies reporting 223 patients (Cagnazzo et al., 2018). Immediate angiographic occlusion was obtained in 32% (29/86) and long-term complete/near-complete aneurysm occlusion in 89% (162/189). The treatment-related complication rate was 17.8% (42/223). Aneurysm rebleeding after treatment occurred in 4% (5/223), most often in the first 72 hours after treatment.

Clinical Applications

For patients with acutely ruptured, wide-necked, aneurysms, open surgical clipping will often be the preferred procedural treatment modality. However, when microsurgical clipping or simple coiling is not feasible, stent-assisted coiling and flow diverters can be reasonable options for pursuing aneurysm occlusion.

Subacute and Late Complications of Subarachnoid Haemorrhage

Preventing Vasospasm and Delayed Cerebral Ischaemia

Cerebral ischaemia or infarction due to vasospasm is a complication of SAH that tends to peak around 4–10 days after the SAH. The molecular drivers of vasospasm remain incompletely understood. Vasospasm can occur in multiple arteries and is strongly related to the amount of extravasated blood. The morbidity from cerebral ischaemia can be severe, and multiple interventions have been evaluated for prevention and treatment of DCI and symptomatic vasospasm.

Calcium Channel Antagonists

Calcium channel antagonists have two major modes of action of potential benefit: (1) vasodilatory – they inhibit the contractile properties of smooth-muscle cells, particularly those in the walls of cerebral arteries, potentially leading to vessel reopening; and (2) neuroprotective – they inhibit calcium flux across cell membranes into neurones and glia, an important molecular mediator of cell injury in hypoxic environments (Inzitari and Poggesi, 2005). The use of systemically administered (oral and intravenous) calcium channel blockers to avert vasospasm and DCI is covered in this section. (The use of intra-arterially administered calcium channel blockers to reverse established vasospasm is covered in a later section.)

Evidence

A systematic review for the Cochrane Library identified 13 randomized trials comparing oral or intravenous calcium channel blockers with no calcium channel blockers in patients with aneurysmal SAH (Dorhout Mees et al., 2007a). A total of 2976 patients were randomized to calcium channel blockers or control, and tested agents included: nimodipine (8 trials, 1694 patients), nicardipine (2 trials, 974 patients), AT877 (1 trial, 276 patients), and magnesium (1 trial, 52 patients),

Poor Outcome

Overall, among 9 trials (2589 patients), random allocation to treatment with a calcium antagonist compared with control was associated with a reduction in death or dependency, 24.3% versus 29.6% (RR 0.81, 95% CI: 0.72–0.92; $p = 0.001$) (Figure 14.11). Four of the trials (enrolling 853 patients), specifically tested nimodipine administered orally, the agent and treatment route used most commonly in clinical practice. Oral nimodipine was associated with a reduction in death or dependency, 26.5% versus 40.3% (RR 0.67, 95% CI: 0.55–0.81; $p = 0.00002$).

Death

In 11 trials enrolling 2775 patients, treatment with a calcium antagonist was not associated with

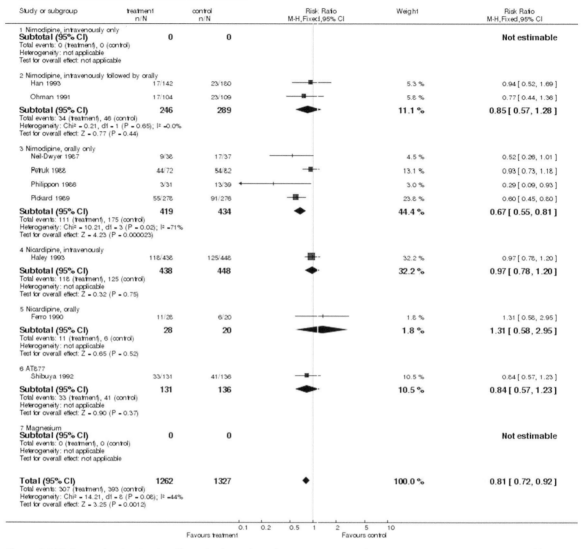

Figure 14.11 Forest plot showing the effects of *calcium channel antagonists vs control* in acute SAH on *poor outcome* at end of follow-up. Reproduced from Dorhout Mees et al. (2007a), with permission from the authors and John Wiley & Sons Limited. Copyright Cochrane Library, with permission.

a statistically significant reduction in death, 14.6% versus 16.8% (RR 0.86, 95% CI: 0.73–1.02; *p* = 0.09) (Figure 14.12). Among 4 trials (899 patients), oral nimodipine effects on mortality also did not reach statistical significance, 18.9% versus 24.0% (RR 0.80, 95% CI: 0.63–1.03; *p* = 0.08).

Delayed Cerebral Ischaemia

Calcium antagonists were associated with a significant reduction in clinical signs of secondary ischaemia (11 trials, 2203 patients): 26.8% versus 40.5% (RR 0.66, 95% CI: 0.59–0.75) (Figure 14.13). In addition, calcium channel blockers reduced the occurrence of

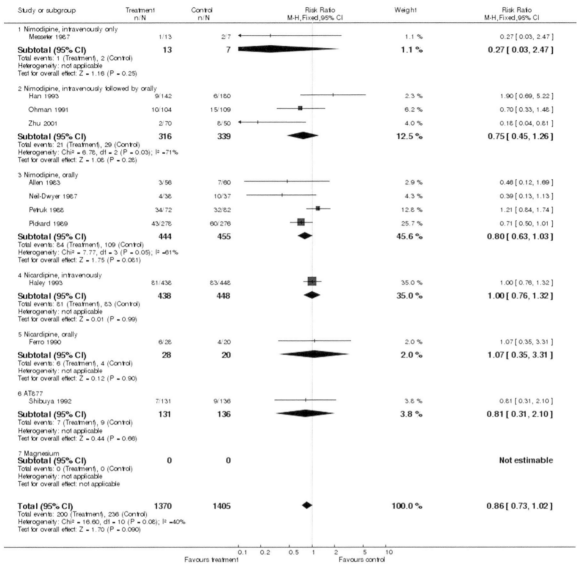

Review: Calcium antagonists for aneurysmal subarachnoid haemorrhage
Comparison: 2 Case fatality
Outcome: 1 Case fatality according to type and route of study medication

Figure 14.12 Forest plot showing the effects of *calcium channel antagonists vs control* in acute SAH on *death* at end of follow-up. Reproduced from Dorhout Mees et al. (2007a), with permission from the authors and John Wiley & Sons Limited. Copyright Cochrane Library, with permission.

cerebral infarction on CT or MRI (8 trials, 1830 patients): 34.0% versus 45.1% (RR 0.78, 95% CI: 0.70–0.87).

Rebleeding

Calcium antagonists were associated with reduced rebleeding (8 trials, 2215 patients), 7.2% versus 9.8% (RR 0.75, 95% CI: 0.57–0.98) (Figure 14.14).

Vasospasm

Vasospasm on angiography as an outcome was assessed in an earlier systematic review, encompassing 5 trials enrolling 687 patients (Feigin et al., 1998). Random allocation to treatment with a calcium channel blocker reduced the occurrence of angiographic vasospasm (RR 0.80, 95% CI: 0.72–0.89). Though point estimates for

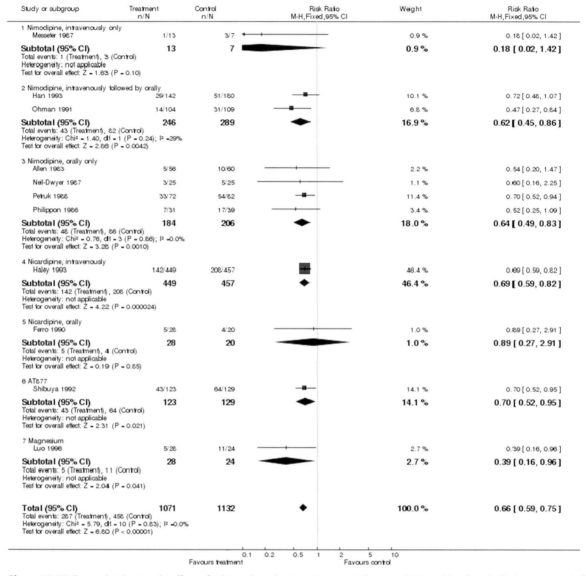

Review: Calcium antagonists for aneurysmal subarachnoid haemorrhage
Comparison: 3 Secondary ischaemia
Outcome: 1 Clinical signs of secondary ischaemia

Figure 14.13 Forest plot showing the effects of *calcium channel antagonists vs control* in acute SAH on *delayed cerebral ischaemia* at end of follow-up. Reproduced from Dorhout Mees et al. (2007a), with permission from the authors and John Wiley & Sons Limited. Copyright Cochrane Library, with permission.

this reduction were lower for nimodipine than for nicardipine or AT877, formal heterogeneity testing did not show a significant difference in this treatment effect across agents.

The available evidence suggests that oral nimodipine may exert benefit upon outcome, not only by vasodilatory effects but also by direct neuroprotective or other mechanisms, given the greater magnitude of the point estimate for improvements in outcome and DCI than for vasospasm. However, the evidence for this differential effect is fragile, and further studies are needed.

Clinical Application

Oral nimodipine (60 mg every 4 hours, continued for 3 weeks) is a standard treatment in patients following aneurysmal SAH. If the patient is unable to swallow,

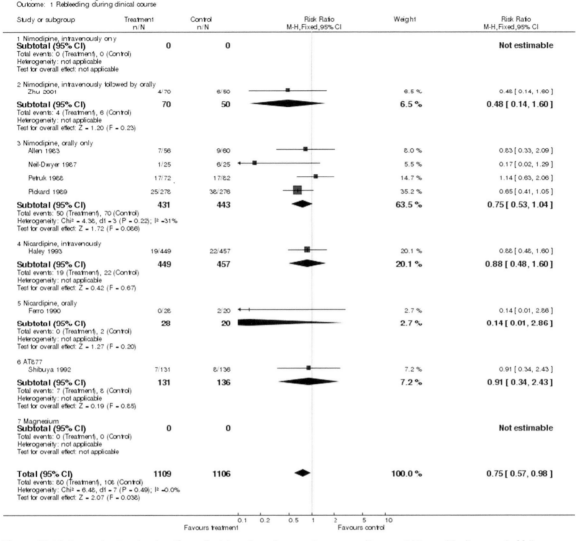

Review: Calcium antagonists for aneurysmal subarachnoid haemorrhage
Comparison: 4 Rebleeding
Outcome: 1 Rebleeding during clinical course

Figure 14.14 Forest plot showing the effects of *calcium channel antagonists vs control* in acute SAH on *rebleeding* at end of follow-up. Reproduced from Dorhout Mees et al. (2007a), with permission from the authors and John Wiley & Sons Limited. Copyright Cochrane Library, with permission.

the tablets should be crushed and washed down a nasogastric tube with normal saline.

Low blood pressure may complicate administration of nimodipine, not only with the intravenous route but also when the drug is given orally. In the presence of hypotension, if no treatable cause such as sepsis or blood loss is identified, nimodipine should be reduced in dosage or, if necessary, discontinued.

Magnesium

Magnesium exerts several effects potentially beneficial in SAH, including acting as an indirect calcium antagonist with vasodilatory and neuro-protective properties. A systematic review identified 10 RCTs assigning 2199 SAH patients to magnesium or control (Reddy et al., 2014). Magnesium generally showed a null effect, including for poor functional outcome (RR 0.93, 95% CI: 0.82–1.06), mortality (RR 0.95, 95% CI: 0.76–1.17), and clinical signs of DCI (RR 0.93, 95% CI: 0.62–1.39), though a reduction was noted in the occurrence of cerebral infarction on brain imaging (RR 0.54, 95% CI: 0.38–0.75).

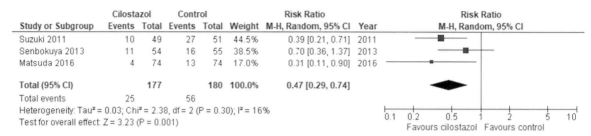

| | Cilostazol | | Control | | | Risk Ratio | | Risk Ratio |
Study or Subgroup	Events	Total	Events	Total	Weight	M-H, Random, 95% CI	Year	M-H, Random, 95% CI
Suzuki 2011	10	49	27	51	44.5%	0.39 [0.21, 0.71]	2011	
Senbokuya 2013	11	54	16	55	38.5%	0.70 [0.36, 1.37]	2013	
Matsuda 2016	4	74	13	74	17.0%	0.31 [0.11, 0.90]	2016	
Total (95% CI)		177		180	100.0%	0.47 [0.29, 0.74]		
Total events	25		56					

Heterogeneity: Tau² = 0.03; Chi² = 2.38, df = 2 (P = 0.30); I² = 16%
Test for overall effect: Z = 3.23 (P = 0.001)

Figure 14.15 Forest plot showing the effects of *cilostazol vs control* in acute SAH on *poor functional outcome* at end of follow-up. Figure courtesy of JL Saver, under a Creative Commons 4.0 CC-BY license (JL Saver).

Statins

Statins in preclinical studies have shown the capacity to improve cerebral endothelial vasomotor function through cholesterol-dependent and cholesterol-independent mechanisms, and also to exert direct neuroprotective effects. A systematic review identified 10 RCTs, enrolling 1214 patients, of statins for aneurysmal SAH (Akhigbe et al., 2017). Agents studied were simvastatin (9 trials) and pravastatin (1 trial). Nine of the trials had modest sample sizes, and one large study with 803 patients, the Simvastatin in Aneurysmal Subarachnoid Hemorrhage (STASH) trial, accounted for 66% of the participants (Kirkpatrick et al., 2014).

Overall, statins were not associated with statistically significant differences in poor functional outcome (OR 0.96, 95% CI: 0.75–1.23) or mortality (OR 0.77, 95% CI: 0.54–1.11). An association with reduced delayed ischaemic neurological deficit was observed (OR 0.72, 95% CI: 0.54–0.97). There was evidence of moderate heterogeneity across trials for the outcomes of delayed ischaemic neurological deficit (I^2 = 43%) and mortality (I^2 = 36%). Imbalanced funnel plots suggested potential publication bias. The results of the largest, most precise trial, STASH, were null for all three outcomes.

Accordingly, current evidence does not support the use of statin agents for the treatment of aneurysmal SAH.

Antiplatelet and Combined Antiplatelet–Vasodilatory Medications

A Cochrane Library systematic review identified 7 trials, enrolling 1385 patients, performed through 2007 evaluating the effectiveness of antiplatelet agents in preventing DCI and improving outcome (Dorhout Mees et al., 2007b). Agents assessed included aspirin (3 trials), OKY-046 (2 trials), dipyridamole (1 trial),

and ticlopidine (1 trial). There were no statistically significant changes in brain ischaemia (RR 0.79, 95% CI: 0.56–1.22), intracranial haemorrhagic complications (RR 1.36, 95% CI: 0.59–3.12), aneurysmal rebleeding (RR 0.98, 95% CI: 0.78–1.38), or mortality (RR 1.01, 95% CI: 0.74–1.37). A trend towards reduced poor outcomes was noted, but did not reach statistical significance (RR 0.79, 95% CI: 0.62–1.01). These data do not support the use of antiplatelet agents without major vasodilatory effects in SAH.

Subsequently, several clinical trials focused on cilostazol, a phosphodiesterase inhibitor with both vasodilatory and antiplatelet effects. A systematic review identified 3 RCTs enrolling 357 patients (Suzuki et al., 2011; Senbokuya et al., 2013; Matsuda et al., 2016; Saber et al., 2018). Random effects meta-analysis of these 3 trials indicates that allocation to cilostazol was associated with reduced systematic vasospasm (RR 0.34, 95% CI: 0.17–0.69), reduced cerebral infarction on imaging (RR 0.47, 95% CI: 0.29–90.74), and reduced poor functional outcome (14.1% vs 31.1%, RR 0.47, 95% CI: 0.29–0.74; p = 0.001) (Figure 14.15). For mortality, 2 trials (209 patients) provided data, and no effect was noted (RR 0.64, 95% CI: 0.15–2.76).

Endothelin Receptor Antagonists

Endothelin is a potent vasoconstrictor upregulated in patients with aneurysmal SAH who develop vasospasm. Endothelin receptor antagonists, like clazosentan, therefore have the potential to avert vasospasm and prevent DCI. A systematic review identified 5 RCTs of endothelin receptor antagonists enrolling 2601 patients, including 4 trials (2181 patients) of clazosentan and 1 trial (420 patients) of TAK-044 (Vergouwen et al., 2012). Allocation to an endothelin receptor antagonist reduced angiographic vasospasm (RR 0.58, 95% CI: 0.48–0.71), but did not reduce new cerebral infarction (RR 1.04, 95% CI: 0.91–1.19) and did not alter rates of poor functional outcome (RR 1.06, 95% CI: 0.93–1.22). The net neutral results likely in part reflected off-target adverse effects of the endothelin receptor antagonists, which included pulmonary oedema due to fluid retention, anaemia, and hypotension.

Haemodynamic Augmentation

Induced hypertension and hypervolaemia have the potential to prevent or minimize DCI in patients with vasospasm by augmenting cerebral blood flow, through both vasospastic arteries and collateral vessels.

Evidence

Three small controlled clinical trials have evaluated haemodynamic augmentation therapy started routinely after securing of the ruptured aneurysm, before the development of vasospasm. The first two trials were collated in a systematic review in the Cochrane Library (Rinkel et al., 2004). Interventions assessed were volume expansion with 5% albumin (1 trial, 84 patients), and combined high-volume saline and colloids and anaemia induction to haematocrit of 0.30–0.35 (1 trial, 32 patients). In combined analysis, no statistically significant effects were seen for poor functional outcome (RR 1.0, 95% CI: 0.45–2.22), death (RR 0.75, 95% CI: 0.18–3.20), DCI signs (RR 1.08, 95% CI: 0.54–2.16), or cerebral infarct on brain imaging (RR 1.75, 95% CI: 0.55–5.53). The third trial used a 2-way factorial design to allocate 20 patients: (1) to normovolaemia versus hypervolaemia (achieved with high-volume intravenous fluids targeting central venous pressure higher than 8 mm Hg); and (2) to normotension (target SBP 120–140) versus hypertension (target BP 140–160, achieved with inotropes and vasopressors) (Togashi et al., 2015). There were no statistically significant differences in any analysed clinical endpoint.

Recognizing that prophylactic use of haemodynamic augmentation exposes patients not destined to develop symptomatic vasospasm to the adverse cardiopulmonary side effects of hyperdynamic intervention, one small randomized trial (42 patients) evaluated more selective deployment only among patients early after onset of symptoms of DCI (Gathier et al., 2018). Patients within 3 hours of onset of DCI symptoms were randomized to induced hypertension or no induced hypertension. In the active arm patients, hypertension was induced with fluids and noradrenaline over a central venous line, raising pressure until improvement of neurological deficits, occurrence of a complication, a maximum mean arterial pressure of 130 mm Hg, or SBP of 230 mm Hg. Although early neurological improvement within 24 hours tended to occur more frequently in the induced hypertension group, 52% versus 30%, poor outcome (mRS 4–6) at 3 months was non-significantly more frequent in the induced hypertension group, 57% versus 40%, RR 1.4 (95% CI: 0.7–2.7). Serious adverse events tended to occur more frequently in the induced hypertension group, RR 2.1 (95% CI: 0.9–5.0).

Clinical Applications

Haemodynamic augmentation became a widespread therapy largely on the basis of physiological studies and observational series. Concerningly, though their sample sizes are too small to provide definitive findings, the few randomized trials completed to date have not been supportive of a net beneficial effect. Though augmenting blood pressure may initially reverse ischaemic deficits, prolonged hyperdynamic therapy may provoke cardiac dysrhythmias, cardiac ischaemia, pulmonary oedema, and electrolyte and acid–base disorders. The available evidence supports national guideline recommendations that, prior to development of DCI, euvolaemia should be maintained and induced hypertension avoided (Connolly et al., 2012; Cho et al., 2018). Among patients who develop DCI, induced hypertension likely can provide early reversal of deficits in some patients, but is of uncertain long-term benefit and, if pursued, should be used cautiously, with strict monitoring of cardiopulmonary status.

Tirilazad

Tirilazad is a non-glucocorticoid 21-aminosteroid with neuroprotective properties in preclinical models of cerebral ischaemia. A systematic review in the Cochrane Library identified 5 RCTs comprising a total of 3821 patients comparing tirilazad against placebo or open control (Zhang et al., 2010). Although fewer patients developed DCI in the tirilazad group than in the control group (OR 0.80, 95% CI: 0.69–0.93), there were no differences in long-term poor functional outcome (OR 1.04, 95% CI: 0.90–1.21) or death (OR 1.04, 95% CI: 0.90–1.21). These data do not support use of tirilazad in routine care.

Additional Pharmacological Agents

Additional pharmacological agents from different therapeutic categories studied in single randomized clinical trials in SAH have included (1) neuroprotective agents: omega-3 fatty acids (Yoneda et al., 2014); (2) combined neuroprotective and intravascular volume agents: albumin (Suarez et al., 2012; Suarez et al., 2015); and (3) anti-inflammatory agents: high-dose methylprednisolone (Gomis et al., 2010) and meloxicam (Ghodsi et al., 2015). There is insufficient evidence from these studies to support use of these agents in routine practice.

Subarachnoid Blood Clearance by Lumbar Drains

While drainage of CSF via EVDs relieves hydrocephalus, it does not promote clearance of extravasated blood in the basal cisterns, and may even promote clot stasis and more prolonged exposure of basal arteries to vasospasm-promoting blood products. A systematic review identified 3 RCTs enrolling 377 patients assessing external lumbar CSF drainage versus control (Alcalá-Cerra et al., 2016). Across all 3 trials, patients allocated to lumbar drainage had reduced clinical deterioration caused by DCI (RR 0.49, 95% CI: 0.36–0.66). For final clinical outcomes, point estimates were directionally favourable but did not reach statistical significance: disability (0.40, 95% CI: 0.04–3.91) and mortality (RR 0.56, 95% CI: 0.19–1.66). These initial results are promising, and more trials are merited to determine net therapeutic benefit and explore different duration and rates of CSF diversion (Panni et al., 2017).

Endovascular Intervention for Symptomatic Vasospasm

Endovascular intervention is recommended when symptomatic vasospasm is refractory to medical therapy (Diringer et al., 2011; Connolly et al., 2012; Cho et al., 2018). Options include transluminal balloon angioplasty (TBA) for vasospasm affecting proximal arterial segments (supraclinoid internal carotid arteries, M1 segments of the middle cerebral arteries, A1 segments of the anterior cerebral arteries, basilar artery, and sometimes P1 segments of the posterior cerebral arteries) and selective intra-arterial infusion of vasodilators (verapamil, nicardipine, or nimodipine) for the same arteries plus more distal or diffuse vasospasm. Balloon angioplasty to expand arterial segments has more long-lasting effects than intra-arterial pharmacotherapy. Both techniques can be combined.

Balloon Angioplasty and Intra-arterial Administration of Vasodilator Drugs

The only randomized trial of endovascular balloon angioplasty assessed the strategy of prophylactic angioplasty before development of vasospasm, randomizing 170 patients with Fisher grade III SAH to prophylactic TBA within 96 hours of aneurysm rupture or to conventional management (Zwienenberg-Lee et al., 2008). Allocation to TBA was associated with reduced need for later rescue endovascular angioplasty or intra-arterial infusions (26% vs 12%, p = 0.03). However, delayed ischaemic neurological deficits were not statistically reduced (24% vs 32%, p = 0.30), nor were final poor functional outcome rates (51% vs 57%, p = 0.73). Mortality rates did not differ (21% vs 19%), although 4 patients in the prophylactic TBA group experienced intraprocedural vascular perforation, fatal in 3 (Zwienenberg-Lee et al., 2008).

Only observational series have assessed the strategy of using transluminal balloon angioplasty to directly dilate and treat spastic arteries in patients with symptomatic vasospasm refractory to medical therapy. A systematic review identified 3 observational series (total 346 patients) reporting active treatment and comparable untreated cohorts (Boulouis et al., 2017). Use of TBA in refractory vasospasm patients was associated with a reduction in poor functional outcomes, RR 0.68 (95% CI: 0.57–0.80).

Intra-arterial Administration of Vasodilator Drugs

Intra-arterial delivery of vasodilator drugs into spastic arteries can induce vasorelaxation and improve cerebral blood flow. Intra-arterial administration of pharmacological vasodilators to reverse vasospasm has not been tested in randomized clinical trials. A meta-analysis of observational series identified 55 studies reporting 1571 patients (Venkatraman et al., 2018). The most common intra-arterial agents delivered were nimodipine (14 studies), papaverine (12 studies), and nicardipine (7 studies), with the remaining studies investigating fasudil, verapamil, milrinone, and combinations of these agents. Immediate angiographic vasodilation was reported to occur in 89% of treated arteries and neurological deficit improvement to occur in 57% of patients.

The largest cohort of patients treated with endovascular interventions for vasospasm following SAH was reported from a nationwide registry in Japan (Hayashi et al., 2014). A total of 645 treatment sessions was recorded in 480 patients, with use of intra-arterial vasodilator drugs in 78% (495/645) and transluminal angioplasty in 22% (140/645). After start of neurological dysfunction, treatment was initiated within 0–3 hours in 39.8%, 3–6 hours in 30.1%, and more than 6 hours in 30.1%. Radiological improvement in vasospasm was reported in 96.6% of treatment sessions and early neurological improvement in 64.7%. Treatment-related complications occurred in 3.1% (20 cases), including intracranial haemorrhage in 0.9% and cerebral ischaemia in 0.8%.

Clinical Application

The use of endovascular therapy for patients with vasospasm refractory to medical therapy is reasonable, though formal RCTs to validate this treatment approach are desirable. Transluminal balloon angioplasty may be preferable for proximal, easily navigated arteries, as it provides more durable vasodilation. Intra-arterial vasodilator pharmacotherapy may be of distinctive benefit when vasospasm affects more distal parts of the vasculature, beyond safe access or addressability by angioplasty. Effects of intra-arterial vasodilator pharmacological agents are time-limited, and multiple, repeated treatments may be necessary. Systemic hypotension and other adverse effects can occur and require close monitoring.

Summary

Aneurysmal subarachnoid haemorrhage (SAH) is a very severe disease, and the post-haemorrhage period is fraught with potential complications that must be recognized and treated early to provide the best chance for favourable outcome. While the diagnosis of SAH is clear in many cases based on the clinical history and initial computed tomography scan, some patients will require further evaluation of the cerebrospinal fluid (CSF). Patients with aneurysmal SAH should be managed by a team of nurses and physicians with neurocritical care, neuroendovascular, and neurosurgical expertise, preferably in a dedicated neurosciences intensive care unit.

Early complications that may be encountered include aneurysmal rebleeding, hydrocephalus, and neurogenic cardiopulmonary injury. In the subacute phase, delayed cerebral ischaemia and hyponatraemia are more commonly seen. If recognized early, these complications can be ameliorated with appropriate management strategies.

For definitive management of a ruptured aneurysm, endovascular coiling is preferable when feasible, but in some cases surgical clipping may be necessary based on patient or aneurysmal characteristics, and when SAH is accompanied by intraparenchymal haemorrhage that may necessitate emergent clot evacuation. Treatment of symptomatic hydrocephalus with CSF diversion is also crucial to maximize the chances of good recovery.

With optimal multidisciplinary management, aneurysmal SAH is no longer a sentence to death or permanent disability. Many patients can return to their previous level of function only weeks after the aneurysm rupture. Still, most treatments in SAH are based on insufficient evidence, and more collaborative research from the bench to the bedside is necessary to continue improving the prognosis of these patients.

References

Akhigbe T, Zolnourian A, Bulters D. (2017). Cholesterol-reducing agents for treatment of aneurysmal subarachnoid hemorrhage: systematic review and meta-analysis of randomized controlled trials. *World Neurosurg*, **101**, 476–85.

Alcalá-Cerra G, Paternina-Caicedo Á, Díaz-Becerra C, Moscote-Salazar LR, Gutiérrez-Paternina JJ, Niño-Hernández LM; en representación del Grupo de Investigación en Ciencias de la Salud y Neurociencias (CISNEURO). (2016). External lumbar cerebrospinal fluid drainage in patients with aneurysmal subarachnoid hemorrhage: a systematic review and meta-analysis of controlled trials. *Neurologia*, **31**(7), 431–44.

Badjatia N, Fernandez L, Schmidt JM, Lee K, Claassen J, Connolly ES, Mayer SA. (2010). Impact of induced normothermia on outcome after subarachnoid hemorrhage: a case-control study. *Neurosurgery*, **66**(4), 696–700.

Baharoglu MI, Germans MR, Rinkel GJ, Algra A, Vermeulen M, van Gijn J, et al. (2013). Antifibrinolytic therapy for aneurysmal subarachnoid haemorrhage. *Cochrane Database Syst Rev*, 8. CD001245.

Bodily KD, Cloft HJ, Lanzino G, Fiorella DJ, White PM, Kallmes DF. (2011). Stent-assisted coiling in acutely ruptured intracranial aneurysms: a qualitative, systematic review of the literature. *AJNR Am J Neuroradiol*, **32**(7), 1232–6.

Boulouis G, Labeyrie MA, Raymond J, Rodriguez-Régent C, Lukaszewicz AC, Bresson D, et al. (2017). Treatment of cerebral vasospasm following aneurysmal subarachnoid haemorrhage: a systematic review and meta-analysis. *Eur Radiol*, **27**(8), 3333–42.

Bruder N, Rabinstein A. (2011). Cardiovascular and pulmonary complications of aneurysmal subarachnoid hemorrhage. *Neurocrit Care*, **15**(2), 257–69.

Cagnazzo F, di Carlo DT, Cappucci M, Lefevre PH, Costalat V, Perrini P. (2018). Acutely ruptured intracranial aneurysms treated with flow-diverter stents: a systematic review and meta-analysis. *AJNR Am J Neuroradiol*, **39**(9), 1669–75.

Cagnazzo F, Gambacciani C, Morganti R, Perrini P. (2017). Aneurysm rebleeding after placement of external ventricular drainage: a systematic review and meta-analysis. *Acta Neurochir (Wien)*, **159**(4), 695–704.

Chang MM, Raval RN, Southerland JJ, Adewumi DA, Bahjri KA, Samuel RK, et al. (2016). Beta blockade and clinical outcomes in aneurysmal subarachnoid hemorrhage. *Open Neurol J*, **30**(10), 155–63.

Chen S, Luo J, Reis C, Manaenko A, Zhang J. (2017). Hydrocephalus after subarachnoid hemorrhage: pathophysiology, diagnosis, and treatment. *Biomed Res Int*, **2017**, 8584753.

Cho WS, Kim JE Park SQ, Ko JK, Kim DW, Park JC, et al. (2018). Korean Clinical Practice Guidelines for aneurysmal subarachnoid hemorrhage. *J Korean Neurosurg Soc*, **61**(2), 127–66.

Choi W, Kwon SC, Lee WJ, Weon YC, Choi B, Lee H, et al. (2017). Feasibility and safety of mild therapeutic hypothermia in poor-grade subarachnoid hemorrhage: prospective pilot study. *J Korean Med Sci*, **32**(8), 1337–44.

Collen JF, Jackson JL, Shorr AF, Moores LK. (2008). Prevention of venous thromboembolism in neurosurgery: a metaanalysis. *Chest*, **134**(2), 237–49.

Connolly ES, Jr, Rabinstein AA, Carhuapoma JR Derdeyn CP, Dion J, Higashida RT, et al. (2012). Guidelines for the management of aneurysmal subarachnoid hemorrhage: a guideline for healthcare professionals from the American Heart Association/American Stroke Association. *Stroke*, **43**(6), 1711–37.

Dewan MC, Mocco J. (2015). Current practice regarding seizure prophylaxis in aneurysmal subarachnoid hemorrhage across academic centers. *J Neurointerv Surg*, **7**(2), 146–9.

Dhakal LP, Hodge DO, Nagal J, Mayes M, Richie A, Ng LK, et al. (2015). Safety and tolerability of gabapentin for aneurysmal subarachnoid hemorrhage (SAH) headache and meningismus. *Neurocrit Care*, **22**(3), 414–21.

Diringer MN, Bleck TP, Claude Hemphill J 3rd, Menon D, Shutter L, Vespa P, et al.; Neurocritical Care Society. (2011). Critical care management of patients following aneurysmal subarachnoid hemorrhage: recommendations from the Neurocritical Care Society's Multidisciplinary Consensus Conference. *Neurocrit Care*, **15**, 211–40.

Doczi T, Bende J, Huszka E, Kiss J. (1981). Syndrome of inappropriate secretion of antidiuretic hormone after subarachnoid hemorrhage. *Neurosurgery*, **9**(4), 394–7.

Dorai Z, Hynan LS, Kopitnik TA, Samson D. (2003). Factors related to hydrocephalus after aneurysmal subarachnoid hemorrhage. *Neurosurgery*, **52**(4), 763–9; discussion 769–771.

Dorhout Mees SM, Rinkel GJ, Feigin VL, Algra A, van den Bergh WM, Vermeulen M, et al. (2007a). Calcium antagonists for aneurysmal subarachnoid haemorrhage. *Cochrane Database Syst Rev*, 3. CD000277.

Dorhout Mees SM, van den Bergh WM, Algra A, Rinkel GJ. (2007b). Antiplatelet therapy for aneurysmal subarachnoid haemorrhage. *Cochrane Database Syst Rev*, 4. CD006184.

Dupont S, Rabinstein AA. (2013). Extent of acute hydrocephalus after subarachnoid hemorrhage as a risk factor for poor functional outcome. *Neurol Res*, **35**(2), 107–110.

Dupont SA, Wijdicks EF, Manno EM, Rabinstein AA. (2008). Thunderclap headache and normal computed tomographic results: value of cerebrospinal fluid analysis. *Mayo Clin Proc*, **83**(12), 1326–31.

Feigin VF, Rinkel GJE, Algra A, Vermeulen M, van Gijn J. (1998). Calcium antagonists in patients with aneurysmal subarachnoid hemorrhage: a systematic review. *Neurology*, **50**, 876–83.

Festic E, Rabinstein AA, Freeman WD, Mauricio EA, Robinson MT, Mandrekar J, et al. (2013). Blood transfusion is an important predictor of hospital mortality among patients with aneurysmal subarachnoid hemorrhage. *Neurocrit Care*, **18**(2), 209–15.

Fiorella D, Arthur AS, Chiacchierini R, Emery E, Molyneux A, Pierot L. (2017). How safe and effective are existing treatments for wide-necked bifurcation aneurysms? Literature-based objective performance criteria for safety and effectiveness. *Neurointerv Surg*, **9**(12), 1197–1201.

Gathier CS, van den Bergh WM, van der Jagt M, Verweij BH, Dankbaar JW, Müller MC, et al.; HIMALAIA Study Group. (2018). Induced hypertension for delayed cerebral ischemia after aneurysmal subarachnoid hemorrhage: a randomized clinical trial. *Stroke*, **49**(1), 76–83.

Ghodsi SM, Mohebbi N, Naderi S, Anbarloie M, Aoude A, Habibi Pasdar SS. (2015). Comparative efficacy of meloxicam and placebo in vasospasm of patients with subarachnoid hemorrhage. *Iran J Pharm Res*, **14**(1), 125–30.

Gomis P, Graftieaux JP, Sercombe R, Hettler D, Scherpereel B, Rousseaux P. (2010). Randomized, double-blind, placebo-controlled, pilot trial of high-dose methylprednisolone in aneurysmal subarachnoid hemorrhage. *J Neurosurg*, **112**(3), 681–8.

Haley EC Jr, Kassell NF, Torner JC. (1992). The International Cooperative Study on the Timing of Aneurysm Surgery. The North American experience. *Stroke*, **23**(2), 205–14.

Hasan D, Wijdicks EF, Vermeulen M. (1990). Hyponatremia is associated with cerebral ischemia in patients with aneurysmal subarachnoid hemorrhage. *Ann Neurol*, **27**(1), 106–08.

Hayashi K, Hirao T, Sakai N, Nagata I; JR-NET2 Study Group. (2014). Current status of endovascular treatment for vasospasm following subarachnoid hemorrhage: analysis of JR-NET2. *Neurol Med Chir (Tokyo)*, **54**(2), 107–12.

Hijdra A, Vermeulen M, van Gijn J, van Crevel H. (1987). Rerupture of intracranial aneurysms: a clinicoanatomic study. *J Neurosurg*, **67**(1), 29–33.

Hillman J, Fridriksson S, Nilsson O, Yu Z, Saveland H, Jakobsson KE. (2002). Immediate administration of tranexamic acid and reduced incidence of early rebleeding after aneurysmal subarachnoid hemorrhage: a prospective randomized study. *J Neurosurg*, **97**(4), 771–8.

Human T, Diringer MN, Allen M, Zipfel GJ, Chicoine M, Dacey R, et al. (2018). Randomized trial of brief versus extended seizure prophylaxis after aneurysmal subarachnoid hemorrhage. *Neurocrit Care*, **28**, 169–74.

Ibrahim GM, Morgan BR, Macdonald RL. (2014). Patient phenotypes associated with outcomes after aneurysmal subarachnoid hemorrhage: a principal component analysis. *Stroke*, **45**(3):, 670–6.

Inzitari D, Poggesi A. (2005). Calcium channel blockers and stroke. *Aging Clin Exp Res*, **17**(4 Suppl), 16–30.

Kassell NF, Torner JC, Haley EC Jr, Adams HP. (1990). The International Cooperative Study on the Timing of Aneurysm Surgery. Part 2: surgical results. *J Neurosurg*, **73** (1), 37–47.

Kirkpatrick PJ, Turner CL, Smith C, Hutchinson PJ, Murray GD; STASH Collaborators. (2014). Simvastatin in aneurysmal subarachnoid haemorrhage (STASH): a multicentre randomised phase 3 trial. *Lancet Neurol*, **13** (7), 666–75.

Kissoon NR., Mandrekar JN, Fugate JE, Lanzino G, Wijdicks EF, Rabinstein AA. (2015). Positive fluid balance is associated with poor outcomes in subarachnoid hemorrhage. *J Stroke and Cerebrovasc Dis*, **24**(10), 2245–51. Epub 8/19/2015.

Klopfenstein JD, Kim LJ, Feiz-Erfan I, Hott JS, Goslar P, Zabramski JM, et al. (2004). Comparison of rapid and gradual weaning from external ventricular drainage in patients with aneurysmal subarachnoid hemorrhage: a prospective randomized trial. *J Neurosurg*, **100**(2), 225–9.

Kramer AH, Gurka MJ, Nathan B, Dumont AS, Kassell NF, Bleck TP. (2008). Complications associated with anemia and blood transfusion in patients with aneurysmal subarachnoid hemorrhage. *Crit Care Med*, **36**(7), 2070–5.

Kramer CL, Pegoli M, Mandrekar J, Lanzino G, Rabinstein AA. (2017). Refining the association of fever with functional outcome in aneurysmal subarachnoid hemorrhage. *Neurocrit Care*, **26**(1), 41–7. doi:10.1007/ s12028–016–0281–7.

Kshettry VR, Rosenbaum BP, Seicean A, Kelly ML, Schiltz NK, Weil RJ. (2014). Incidence and risk factors associated with in-hospital venous thromboembolism after aneurysmal subarachnoid hemorrhage. *J Clin Neurosci.*, **21** (2), 282–6.

Le Roux PD. (2011). Anemia and transfusion after subarachnoid hemorrhage. *Neurocrit Care*, **15**(2), 342–53.

Lennihan L, Mayer SA, Fink ME, Beckford A, Paik MC, Zhang H, et al. (2000). Effect of hypervolemic therapy on cerebral blood flow after subarachnoid hemorrhage: a randomized controlled trial. *Stroke*, **31**(2), 383–91.

Levine J, Kofke A, Cen L, Chen Z, Faerber J, Elliott JP, et al. (2010). Red blood cell transfusion is associated with infection and extracerebral complications after subarachnoid hemorrhage. *Neurosurgery*, **66**(2), 312–18; discussion 318.

Lindgren A, Vergouwen MD, van der Schaaf I, Algra A, Wermer M, Clarke MJ, Rinkel GJ. (2018). Endovascular coiling versus neurosurgical clipping for people with aneurysmal subarachnoid haemorrhage. *Cochrane Database Syst Rev*, 8. CD003085. doi:10.1002/14651858.CD003085. pub3.

Mack WJ, Ducruet AF, Hickman ZL, Kalyvas JT, Cleveland JR, Mocco J, et al. (2008). Doppler ultrasonography screening of poor-grade subarachnoid hemorrhage patients increases the diagnosis of deep venous thrombosis. *Neurol Res*, **30**(9), 889–92.

Madden LK, Hill M, May TL, Human T, Guanci MM, Jacobi J, et al. (2017).The implementation of targeted temperature management: an evidence-based guideline from the Neurocritical Care Society. *Neurocrit Care*, **27**(3), 468–87. doi:10.1007/s12028–017–0469–5.

Malik AN, Gross BA, Rosalind Lai PM, Moses ZB, Du R. (2015). Neurogenic stress cardiomyopathy after aneurysmal subarachnoid hemorrhage. *World Neurosurg*, **83**(6), 880–5

Martini RP, Deem S, Brown M, Souter MJ, Yanez ND, Daniel S, et al. (2012). The association between fluid balance and outcomes after subarachnoid hemorrhage. *NeurocritCare*, **17**(2), 191–8.

Matsuda M, Watanabe K, Saito A, Matsumura K, Ichikawa M. (2007). Circumstances, activities, and events precipitating aneurysmal subarachnoid hemorrhage. *J Stroke Cerebrovasc Dis*, **16**(1), 25–9.

Matsuda N, Naraoka M, Ohkuma H, Shimamura N, Ito K, Asano K, et al. (2016). Effect of cilostazol on cerebral vasospasm and outcome in patients with aneurysmal subarachnoid hemorrhage: a randomized, double-blind, placebo-controlled trial. *Cerebrovasc Dis*, **42**(1–2), 97–105.

McDougall CG, Spetzler RF, Zabramski JM, Partovi S, Hills NK, Nakaji P, et al. (2012). The Barrow Ruptured Aneurysm Trial. *J Neurosurg*, **116**(1), 135–44.

Molyneux AJ, Birks J, Clarke A, Sneade M, Kerr, RSC. (2015). The durability of endovascular coiling versus neurosurgical clipping of ruptured cerebral aneurysms: 18 year follow-up of the UK cohort of the International Subarachnoid Aneurysm Trial (ISAT). *Lancet*, **385**(9969), 691–7.

Molyneux A, Kerr R, Stratton I, Sandercock P, Clarke M, Shrimpton J, Holman R; International Subarachnoid

Aneurysm Trial (ISAT) Collaborative Group. (2002). International Subarachnoid Aneurysm Trial (ISAT) of neurosurgical clipping versus endovascular coiling in 2143 patients with ruptured intracranial aneurysms: a randomised trial. *Lancet*, **360**, 1267–74.

Naidech AM, Kreiter KT., Janjua N, Ostapkovich N, Parra A, Commichau C, et al. (2005). Phenytoin exposure is associated with functional and cognitive disability after subarachnoid hemorrhage. *Stroke*, **36**(3), 583–7.

Naidech AM, Shaibani A, Garg RK, Duran IM, Liebling SM, Bassin SL, et al. (2010). Prospective, randomized trial of higher goal hemoglobin after subarachnoid hemorrhage. *Neurocritl Care*, **13**(3), 313–20.

Neil-Dwyer G, Walter P, Cruickshank JM. (1985). Beta-blockade benefits patients following a subarachnoid haemorrhage. *Eur J Clin Pharmacol*, **28** Suppl., 25–29.

Neil-Dwyer G, Walter P, Cruickshank JM, Doshi B, O'Gorman P. (1978). Effect of propranolol and phentolamine on myocardial necrosis after subarachnoid haemorrhage. *Br Med J*, **2**(6143), 990–2.

Nieuwkamp DJ, Setz LE, Algra A, Linn FH, de Rooij NK, Rinkel GJ. (2009). Changes in case fatality of aneurysmal subarachnoid haemorrhage over time, according to age, sex, and region: a meta-analysis. *Lancet Neurol*, **8**(7), 635–42.

Nyquist P, Bautista C, Jichici D, Burns J, Chhangani S, DeFilippis M, et al. (2016). Prophylaxis of venous thrombosis in neurocritical care patients: an evidence-based guideline: a statement for healthcare professionals from the Neurocritical Care Society. *Neurocrit Care*, **24**(1), 47–60.

O'Connor KL, Westover MB, Phillips MT, Iftimia NA, Buckley DA, Ogilvy CS, et al. (2014). High risk for seizures following subarachnoid hemorrhage regardless of referral bias. *Neurocrit Care*, **21**, 476–82.

O'Kelly CJ, Kulkarni AV, Austin PC, Urbach D, Wallace MC. (2009). Shunt-dependent hydrocephalus after aneurysmal subarachnoid hemorrhage: incidence, predictors, and revision rates. Clinical article. *J Neurosurg*, **111**(5), 1029–35.

Ohkuma H. Tsurutani H, Suzuki S. (2001). Incidence and significance of early aneurysmal rebleeding before neurosurgical or neurological management. *Stroke*, **32**(5), 1176–80.

Ohman J, Heiskanen O. (1989). Timing of operation for ruptured supratentorial aneurysms: a prospective randomized study. *J Neurosurg*, **70**(1), 55–60.

Oliveira-Filho J, Ezzeddine MA, Segal AZ, Buonanno FS, Chang Y, Ogilvy CS, et al. (2001). Fever in subarachnoid hemorrhage: relationship to vasospasm and outcome. *Neurology*, **56**(10), 1299–1304.

Olson DM, Zomorodi M, Britz GW, Zomorodi AR, Amato A, Graffagnino C. (2013). Continuous cerebral spinal fluid drainage associated with complications in patients admitted with subarachnoid hemorrhage. *J Neurosurg*, **119**(4), 974–80.

Panczykowski D, Pease M, Zhao Y, Weiner G, Ares W, Crago E, et al. (2016). Prophylactic antiepileptics and seizure incidence following subarachnoid hemorrhage: a propensity score-matched analysis. *Stroke*, **47**, 1754–60.

Panni P, Fugate JE, Rabinstein AA, Lanzino G. (2017). Lumbar drainage and delayed cerebral ischemia in aneurysmal subarachnoid hemorrhage: a systematic review. *J Neurosurg Sci*, **61**(6), 665–72.

Pegoli M, Mandrekar J, Rabinstein AA, Lanzino G. (2015). Predictors of excellent functional outcome in aneurysmal subarachnoid hemorrhage. *J Neurosurg*, **122**(2), 414–18.

Perry JJ, Alyahya B, Sivilotti ML, Bullard MJ, Emond M, Sutherland J, et al. (2015). Differentiation between traumatic tap and aneurysmal subarachnoid hemorrhage: prospective cohort study. *BMJ*, **350**, h568.

Perry JJ, Stiell IG, Sivilotti ML, Bullard MJ, Symington C, Worster A, et al. (2011). Sensitivity of computed tomography performed within six hours of onset of headache for diagnosis of subarachnoid haemorrhage: prospective cohort study. *BMJ*, **343**, d4277.

Perry JJ, Stiell IG, Sivilotti ML, Bullard MJ, Hohl CM, Sutherland J, et al. (2013). Clinical decision rules to rule out subarachnoid hemorrhage for acute headache. *JAMA*, **310**(12), 1248–55.

Rabinstein AA, Bruder N. (2011). Management of hyponatremia and volume contraction. *Neurocrit Care*, **15**(2), 354–60.

Rabinstein AA, Sandhu K. (2007). Non-infectious fever in the neurological intensive care unit: incidence, causes and predictors. *J Neurol Neurosurg Psychiatry*, **78**(11), 1278–80.

Rawal S, Alcaide-Leon P, Macdonald RL, Rinkel GJ, Victor JC, Krings T, et al. (2017). Meta-analysis of timing of endovascular aneurysm treatment in subarachnoid haemorrhage: inconsistent results of early treatment within 1 day. *J Neurol Neurosurg Psychiatry*, **88**(3), 241–8.

Ray WZ, Strom RG, Blackburn SL, Ashley WW, Sicard GA, Rich KM. (2009). Incidence of deep venous thrombosis after subarachnoid hemorrhage. *J Neurosurg*, **110**(5), 1010–14.

Raya AK, Diringer MN. (2014). Treatment of subarachnoid hemorrhage. *Crit Care Clin*, **30**(4), 719–33.

Reddy D, Fallah A, Petropoulos JA, Farrokhyar F, Macdonald RL, Jichici D. (2014). Prophylactic magnesium sulfate for aneurysmal subarachnoid hemorrhage: a systematic review and meta-analysis. *Neurocrit Care*, **21**(2), 356–64.

Rinkel GJ, Feigin VL, Algra A, van Gijn J. (2004). Circulatory volume expansion therapy for aneurysmal subarachnoid haemorrhage. *Cochrane Database Syst Rev*, 4. CD000483.

Saber H, Desai A, Palla M, Mohamed W, Seraji-Bozorgzad N, Ibrahim M (2018). Efficacy of cilostazol in prevention of delayed cerebral ischemia after aneurysmal subarachnoid hemorrhage: a meta-analysis. *J Stroke Cerebrovasc Dis*, 27 (11), 2979–85.

Senbokuya N, Kinouchi H, Kanemaru K, Ohashi Y, Fukamachi A, Yagi S, et al. (2013). Effects of cilostazol on cerebral vasospasm after aneurysmal subarachnoid hemorrhage: a multicenter prospective, randomized, open-label blinded end point trial. *J Neurosurg*, 118(1), 121–30.

Smith MJ, Le Roux PD, Elliott JP, Winn HR. (2004). Blood transfusion and increased risk for vasospasm and poor outcome after subarachnoid hemorrhage. *J Eurosurg*, 101 (1), 1–7.

Stein, M., Brokmeier L., Herrmann J., Scharbrodt W, Schreiber V, Bender M, et al. (2015). Mean hemoglobin concentration after acute subarachnoid hemorrhage and the relation to outcome, mortality, vasospasm, and brain infarction. *J Clin Neurosci*, 22(3), 530–4.

Suarez JI, Martin RH, Calvillo E, Bershad EM, Venkatasubba Rao CP. (2015). Effect of human albumin on TCD vasospasm, DCI, and cerebral infarction in subarachnoid hemorrhage: the ALISAH study. *Acta Neurochir. Suppl*, 120, 287–90.

Suarez JI, Martin RH, Calvillo E, Dillon C, Bershad EM, Macdonald RL, et al. (2012). The Albumin in Subarachnoid Hemorrhage (ALISAH) multicenter pilot clinical trial: safety and neurologic outcomes. *Stroke*, 43(3), 683–90.

Suzuki S, Sayama T, Nakamura T, Nishimura H, Ohta M, Inoue T, et al. (2011). Cilostazol improves outcome after subarachnoid hemorrhage: a preliminary report. *Cerebrovasc Dis*, 32(1), 89–93.

Tam AK, Ilodigwe D, Mocco J, Mayer S, Kassell N, Ruefenacht D, et al. (2010). Impact of systemic inflammatory response syndrome on vasospasm, cerebral infarction, and outcome after subarachnoid hemorrhage: exploratory analysis of CONSCIOUS-1 database. *Neurocrit Care*, 13(2), 182–9.

Tartara A, Galimberti CA, Manni R, Parietti L, Zucca C, Baasch H, et al. (1991). Differential effects of valproic acid and enzyme-inducing anticonvulsants on nimodipine pharmacokinetics in epileptic patients. *Br J Clin Pharmacol*, 32(3), 335–40.

Togashi K, Joffe AM, Sekhar L, Kim L, Lam A, Yanez D, et al. (2015). Randomized pilot trial of intensive management of blood pressure or volume expansion in subarachnoid hemorrhage (IMPROVES). *Neurosurgery*, 76 (2), 125–34; discussion 134–125; quiz 135.

Torner JC, Nibbelink DW, Burmeister LF. (1981). Statistical comparison of end results of a randomised treatment study. In AL Sahs, DW Nibbelink, JC Torner, eds., *Aneurysmal Subarachnoid Haemorrhage. Report of the Cooperative Study*. Baltimore: Urban & Schwarzenberg, pp. 249–75.

Tso MK, Ibrahim GM, Macdonald RL. (2016). Predictors of shunt-dependent hydrocephalus following aneurysmal subarachnoid hemorrhage. *World Neurosurg*, 86, 226–32.

Tung P, Kopelnik A, Banki N, Ong K, Ko N, Lawton MT, et al. (2004). Predictors of neurocardiogenic injury after subarachnoid hemorrhage. *Stroke*, 35(2), 548–51.

van der Bilt IA, Hasan D, Vandertop, WP, Wilde AA, Algra A, Visser FC, et al. (2009). Impact of cardiac complications on outcome after aneurysmal subarachnoid hemorrhage: a meta-analysis. *Neurology*, 72(7), 635–42.

van Donkelaar CE, Bakker NA, Veeger NJ, Uyttenboogaart M, Metzemaekers JD, Luijckx GJ, et al. (2015). Predictive factors for rebleeding after aneurysmal subarachnoid hemorrhage: rebleeding aneurysmal subarachnoid hemorrhage study. *Stroke*, 46(8), 2100–06. Epub 6/13/2015.

Varelas PN, Abdelhak T, Wellwood J, Shah I, Hacein-Bey L, Schultz L, et al. (2010). Nicardipine infusion for blood pressure control in patients with subarachnoid hemorrhage. *Neurocrit Care*, 13(2), 190–8.

Venkatraman A, Khawaja AM, Gupta S, Hardas S, Deveikis JP, Harrigan MR, Kumar G. (2018). Intra-arterial vasodilators for vasospasm following aneurysmal subarachnoid hemorrhage: a meta-analysis. *J Neurointerv Surg*, 10(4), 380–7.

Vergouwen MD, Algra A, Rinkel GJ. (2012). Endothelin receptor antagonists for aneurysmal subarachnoid hemorrhage: a systematic review and meta-analysis update. *Stroke*, 43(10), 2671–6.

Verma RK, Kottke R, Andereggen L, Weisstanner C, Zubler C, Gralla J, et al. (2013). Detecting subarachnoid hemorrhage: comparison of combined FLAIR/SWI versus CT. *Eur J Radiol*, 82 1539–45.

Wartenberg KE, Schmidt JM, Claassen J, Temes RE, Frontera JA, Ostapkovich N, et al. (2006). Impact of medical complications on outcome after subarachnoid hemorrhage. *Crit Care Med*, 34(3), 617–23; quiz 624.

Whitfield PC, Kirkpatrick PJ. (2001). Timing of surgery for aneurysmal subarachnoid haemorrhage. *Cochrane Database Syst Rev*, 2. CD001697.

Wijdicks EF, Vermeulen M, ten Haaf JA, Hijdra A, Bakker Wh, van Gijn J. (1985). Volume depletion and natriuresis in patients with a ruptured intracranial aneurysm. *Ann Neurol*, 18(2): 211–16.

Yamada S, Ishikawa M, Yamamoto K, Ino T, Kimura T, Kobayashi S. (2015). Aneurysm location and clipping versus coiling for development of secondary normal-pressure hydrocephalus after aneurysmal subarachnoid hemorrhage: Japanese Stroke DataBank. *J Neurosurg*, **123**(6), 1555–61.

Yoneda H, Shirao S, Nakagawara J, Ogasawara K, Tominaga T, Suzuki M. (2014). A prospective, multicenter, randomized study of the efficacy of eicosapentaenoic acid for cerebral vasospasm: the EVAS study. *World Neurosurg*, **81**(2), 309–15.

Zhang S, Wang L, Liu M, Wu B. (2010). Tirilazad for aneurysmal subarachnoid haemorrhage. *Cochrane Database Syst Rev*, 2. CD006778.

Zwienenberg-Lee M, Hartman J, Rudisill N, Madden LK, Smith K, Eskridge J, et al. (2008). Effect of prophylactic transluminal balloon angioplasty on cerebral vasospasm and outcome in patients with Fisher grade III subarachnoid hemorrhage: results of a phase II multicenter, randomized, clinical trial. *Stroke*, **39**(6): 1759–65.

Chapter 15

Prevention of Stroke by Lowering Blood Pressure

Meng Lee

Jeffrey L. Saver

Bruce Ovbiagele

By the year 1990, it was established that there is a direct log-linear relationship between usual blood pressure levels and risk of any stroke (MacMahon et al., 1990). Moreover, it was shown to be a causal relationship when a systematic review of randomized clinical trials demonstrated that lowering BP in hypertensive individuals significantly reduced the risk of first-ever stroke (Collins et al., 1990). Subsequently, additional clinical trials extended these findings to show that blood pressure reduction among individuals with elevated pressure prevented recurrent stroke (Liu et al., 2009).

More recently, blood pressure lowering among individuals with blood pressures in a range then designated as 'pre-hypertensive', systolic blood pressure (SBP) 130–139 mm Hg or diastolic blood pressure (DBP) 80–89 mm Hg, was also shown to reduce stroke occurrence (Lee et al., 2011; Sipahi et al., 2012; Huang et al., 2014). The benefit of detecting and treating blood pressures in lower ranges led to redefinition of high blood pressure, with normal being less than 120/80; elevated being SBP between 120–129 and DBP less than 80; stage 1 hypertension being SBP between 130 and 139 or DBP between 80 and 89; stage 2 hypertension being SBP being 140–180 or DBP 90–120; hypertensive crisis being SBP above 180 or DBP above 120 (Whelton et al., 2018).

Though a risk factor for both cerebral and coronary ischaemia, hypertension has a heightened association with cerebrovascular compared with cardiovascular events. Modest reductions in blood pressure by about 10 mm Hg systolic and 5 mm Hg diastolic reduced the relative risk (RR) of stroke by about 41% and the RR of coronary heart disease by about 22% within a few years of beginning the treatment (Blood Pressure Lowering Treatment Trialists' Collaboration, 2003; Law et al., 2009).

However, despite tremendous advances in our understanding and ability to prevent stroke through treatment of elevated blood pressure, concerns linger about whether a differential approach is warranted for lowering blood pressure in patients with known cerebrovascular disease, and especially those with significant occlusive cerebrovascular disease, because doing so may compromise cerebral perfusion and perhaps even increase the rate of recurrent ischaemic stroke due to haemodynamic insufficiency (Boan et al., 2014).

Evidence

Broad Patient Populations

A systematic review collated 123 randomized controlled trials (RCTs), enrolling 613,815 patients, of blood pressure lowering performed in diverse populations, including cerebrovascular primary prevention (patients without a history of stroke or transient ischaemic attack [TIA]), vascular primary prevention (patients without a history of symptomatic cardiac, cerebral, or peripheral events), cerebrovascular secondary prevention (patients who have already had had one or more strokes/TIAs), and vascular secondary prevention (patients who have had one or more symptomatic vascular events in any circulatory bed) (Ettehad et al., 2016). For the occurrence of stroke, in 54 RCTs enrolling 265,323 individuals, every 10 mm Hg reduction in SBP significantly reduced the risk of stroke occurrence (RR 0.73, 95% confidence interval [CI]: 0.68–0.77). In addition, blood pressure lowering also reduced coronary heart disease (RR 0.83, 95% CI: 0.78–0.88), heart failure (RR 0.72, 95% CI: 0.67–0.78), the composite of all major cardiovascular disease events (RR 0.80, 95% CI: 0.77–0.83), and all-cause mortality (RR 0.87, 95% CI: 0.84–0.91).

The same meta-analysis also investigated the relative effectiveness of the five main classes of antihypertensive drugs: angiotensin-converting enzyme (ACE) inhibitors, angiotensin-receptor blockers (ARB), beta-blockers, calcium channel blockers, and diuretics (Ettehad et al., 2016). Two class differences were noted in averting stroke. Compared with pooled effects of the other drug classes, calcium channel blockers were superior for stroke prevention (RR 0.90, 95% CI: 0.85–0.95) and beta-blockers were inferior for stroke prevention (RR 1.24, 95% CI: 1.14–1.35). In contrast, all classes performed comparably in averting myocardial infarcts. The reduced effectiveness of beta-blockers may reflect off-target effects promoting dyslipidaemia, glucose intolerance, and atrial fibrillation (Sardana et al., 2017; Whelton et al., 2018).

Primary Stroke Prevention

For patients without a history of symptomatic cardiovascular disease, a systematic review of 8 large RCTs showed that every 10 mm Hg reduction in SBP significantly reduced *first-ever* stroke (RR 0.75, 95% CI: 0.63–0.89). Blood pressure reduction also reduced first-ever heart failure (RR 0.77, 95% CI: 0.59–1.00) and all-cause mortality (RR 0.84, 95% CI: 0.75–0.93), though not first-ever coronary artery events (RR 0.85, 95% CI: 0.55–1.32) (Ettehad et al., 2016). Another systematic review specifically evaluated blood pressure lowering therapy in primary prevention patients who had mildly elevated blood pressure at entry (SBP 140–159 or DBP of 90–99), pooling individual participant level data from 14,906 patients enrolled in 10 trials (Sundstrom et al., 2015). Though the average reduction in blood pressure was modest, at 3.6 mm Hg systolic and 2.4 mm Hg diastolic, the risk of *first-ever* stroke was reduced importantly (RR 0.72, 95% CI: 0.55–0.92), with projected effects in a primary care cohort of reducing first-ever stroke events over 5 years from occurring in 4.2% to 3.0% of patients

Among primary prevention patients with an indication for blood pressure lowering, failure to prescribe is common and failure to adhere to antihypertensive therapy is associated with increased stroke rates. A UK study showed that among 7008 patients presenting with a first-ever stroke or TIA, 25% had not been prescribed blood pressure lowering agents despite have a clinical indication for antihypertensive therapy (Turner et al., 2016). Moreover, in a Korean study of 33,748 hypertensive patients, those with poor antihypertensive medication adherence had elevated rates of fatal cerebral

haemorrhage (hazard ratio [HR] 2.19, 95% CI: 1.28–3.77) and fatal cerebral infarction (HR 1.92, 95% CI: 1.25–2.96) (Kim et al., 2016).

Recent investigations have explored the relative benefits and risks of intensive blood pressure lowering to levels beyond the prior conventional target of SBP at or below 140 mm Hg. Among individuals with starting blood pressures in the 130–139 range and who have prediabetes, diabetes, or subclinical renal impairment (but not symptomatic cardiovascular disease), systematic reviews of trials testing lowering SBP to below 130 mm Hg have found suggestions of additional benefit (Lee et al., 2012; Brunstrom and Carlberg, 2018). Among 11 trials enrolling 62,751 patients, there was a non-significant trend towards reduced stroke incidence (RR 0.85, 95% CI: 0.68–1.06) (Brunstrom and Carlberg, 2018). Among individuals with starting SBPs over a broader range, 130–180 mm Hg, two large RCTs compared the strategies of blood pressure lowering to an aggressive <120 mm Hg target versus a standard <140 mm Hg target, in patients with diabetes (ACCORD Study Group et al, 2010) and without diabetes (SPRINT Research Group et al., 2015). Combined analysis of the 14,094 patients from the two trials showed that allocation to aggressive blood pressure lowering targets was associated with fewer incident strokes (RR 0.75, 95% CI: 0.58–0.97) (Perkovic and Rodgers, 2015) (Figure 15.1). In addition, in the SPRINT trial, over a median 5-year follow-up, allocation to intensive blood pressure treatment to a SBP goal of <120 mm Hg was associated with reduced mild cognitive impairment (14.6 vs 18.3 cases per 1000 person-years; HR 0.81, 95% CI: 0.69–0.94) and a trend towards reduced dementia (7.2 vs 8.6 cases per 1000 person-years; HR 0.83, 95% CI: 0.67–1.04) (SPRINT MIND Investigators, 2019).

Implications for Practice

This evidence supports a tailored, primary prevention approach to blood pressure reduction across the range of presenting levels of SBP to prevent first stroke and other cardiovascular events (Whelton et al., 2018). Individuals with elevated blood pressure within the normal range (SBP 120–129 and DBP < 80) may be treated with nonpharmacological management, including healthy diet, weight loss, physical activity, and moderate alcohol intake. Individuals with stage 1 hypertension (SBP 130–139 or DBP 80–89) who have no major risk factors for cardiovascular disease may also be treated with nonpharmacological management; those

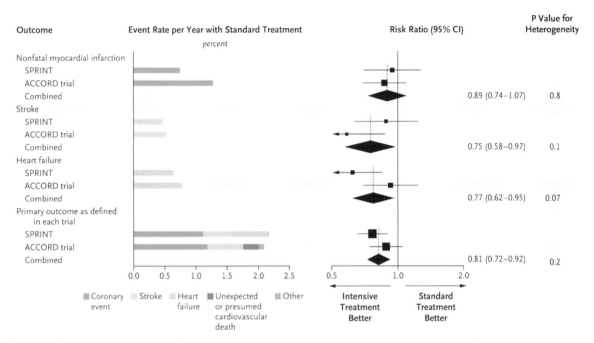

Figure 15.1 Forest plots showing the effects on outcome of blood pressure lowering to an *intensive target of <120 mm Hg vs a less-intensive target of <140 mm Hg*, among patients with vascular risk factors but no history of stroke, TIA, or symptomatic vascular disease. Adapted from Perkovic et al. (2015).

with stage 1 hypertension with age, diabetes, tobacco, cholesterol, or other risk factors placing them at a 10-year risk of cardiovascular events of 10% or more are best also treated with start of single-agent pharmacological antihypertensive therapy. Individuals with stage 2 hypertension (SBP ≥ 140 or DBP ≥ 90) should be treated with a combination of nonpharmacological management plus antihypertensive drug therapy, using 2 agents of different pharmacological classes. When pharmacological therapy is indicated, consideration should be given to including a calcium channel antagonist and to avoiding a beta-blocker to maximize stroke reduction.

Secondary Stroke Prevention

A systematic review in the Cochrane Library identified 11 RCTs enrolling 38,742 participants assessing long-term blood pressure lowering to prevent recurrent stroke and major cardiovascular events after an initial stroke or TIA (Zonneveld et al., 2018). Eight of the trials (35,110 participants) compared antihypertensive therapy with no antihypertensive therapy and three of the trials (3632 participants) compared different SBP targets.

Recurrent Stroke

Among 35,110 patients with prior stroke or TIA who were randomized in eight RCTs to pharmacological blood pressure lowering or control, the frequency of recurrent stroke was reduced (8.7% versus 10.1%, RR 0.81, 95% CI: 0.70–0.93) (Figure 15.2).

With regard to potential modification of treatment effect by the subtype of the index stroke, data were available from one trial with 5854 participants (PROGRESS, 2001). Antihypertensive therapy showed consistent effects across qualifying event types: TIA – RR 0.77; ischaemic stroke – RR 0.76; haemorrhagic stroke – RR 0.59; $I^2 = 0\%$.

Stratified analysis by baseline SBP levels was available from three trials (6656 participants). Pharmacological antihypertensive therapy demonstrated a mild graded increase in relative degree of stroke reduction with higher SBP levels at trial entry: SBP ≥160 – RR 0.65; SBP 140–159 – RR 0.71; SBP 120–139 – RR 0.86; SBP <120 – RR 1.01 (Figure 15.3).

There was evidence of differential efficacy among tested antihypertensive agent classes in reducing recurrent stroke (subgroup heterogeneity $I^2 = 72\%$, $p = 0.01$).

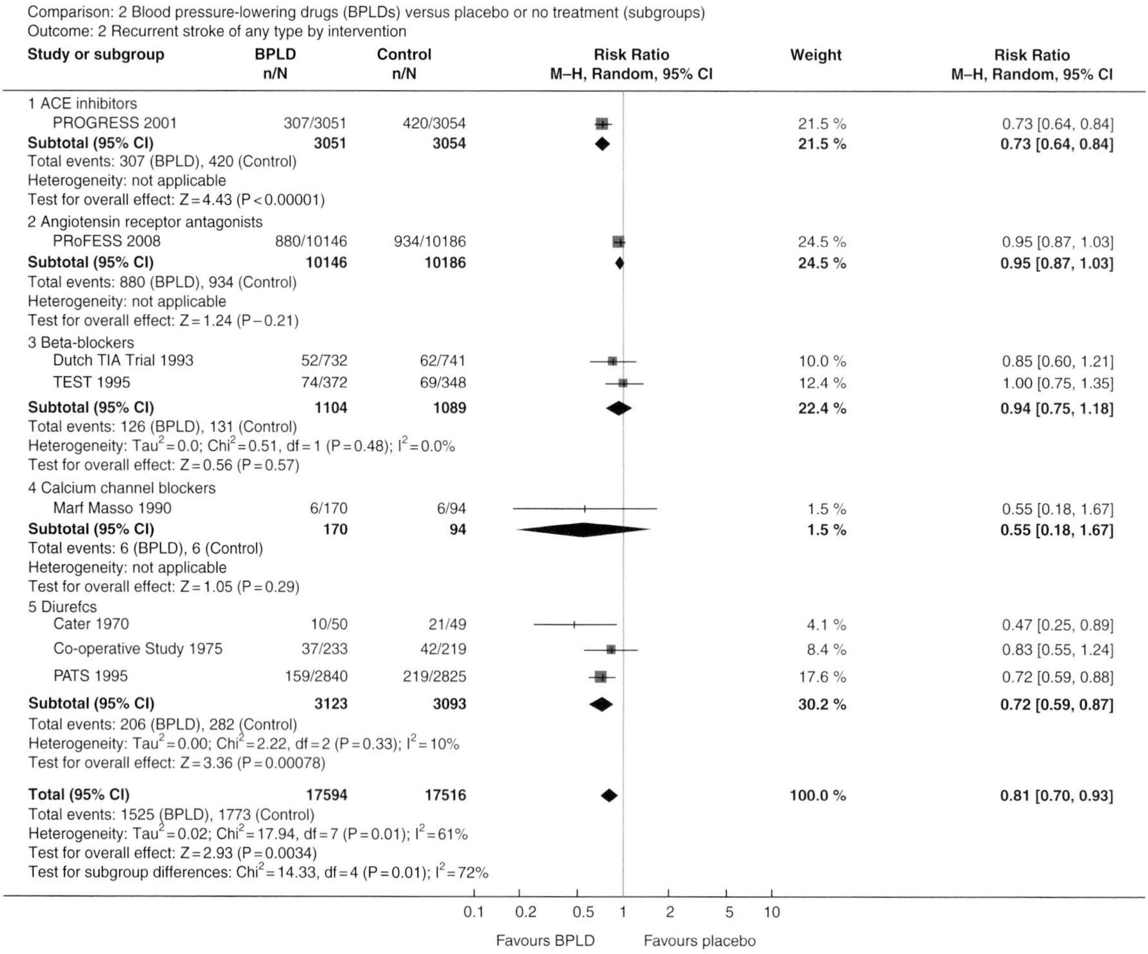

Comparison: 2 Blood pressure-lowering drugs (BPLDs) versus placebo or no treatment (subgroups)
Outcome: 2 Recurrent stroke of any type by intervention

Study or subgroup	BPLD n/N	Control n/N	Risk Ratio M–H, Random, 95% CI	Weight	Risk Ratio M–H, Random, 95% CI
1 ACE inhibitors					
PROGRESS 2001	307/3051	420/3054		21.5 %	0.73 [0.64, 0.84]
Subtotal (95% CI)	3051	3054		21.5 %	0.73 [0.64, 0.84]
Total events: 307 (BPLD), 420 (Control)					
Heterogeneity: not applicable					
Test for overall effect: Z = 4.43 (P < 0.00001)					
2 Angiotensin receptor antagonists					
PRoFESS 2008	880/10146	934/10186		24.5 %	0.95 [0.87, 1.03]
Subtotal (95% CI)	10146	10186		24.5 %	0.95 [0.87, 1.03]
Total events: 880 (BPLD), 934 (Control)					
Heterogeneity: not applicable					
Test for overall effect: Z = 1.24 (P – 0.21)					
3 Beta-blockers					
Dutch TIA Trial 1993	52/732	62/741		10.0 %	0.85 [0.60, 1.21]
TEST 1995	74/372	69/348		12.4 %	1.00 [0.75, 1.35]
Subtotal (95% CI)	1104	1089		22.4 %	0.94 [0.75, 1.18]
Total events: 126 (BPLD), 131 (Control)					
Heterogeneity: Tau^2 = 0.0; Chi^2 = 0.51, df = 1 (P = 0.48); I^2 = 0.0%					
Test for overall effect: Z = 0.56 (P = 0.57)					
4 Calcium channel blockers					
Marf Masso 1990	6/170	6/94		1.5 %	0.55 [0.18, 1.67]
Subtotal (95% CI)	170	94		1.5 %	0.55 [0.18, 1.67]
Total events: 6 (BPLD), 6 (Control)					
Heterogeneity: not applicable					
Test for overall effect: Z = 1.05 (P = 0.29)					
5 Diurefcs					
Cater 1970	10/50	21/49		4.1 %	0.47 [0.25, 0.89]
Co-operative Study 1975	37/233	42/219		8.4 %	0.83 [0.55, 1.24]
PATS 1995	159/2840	219/2825		17.6 %	0.72 [0.59, 0.88]
Subtotal (95% CI)	3123	3093		30.2 %	0.72 [0.59, 0.87]
Total events: 206 (BPLD), 282 (Control)					
Heterogeneity: Tau^2 = 0.00; Chi^2 = 2.22, df = 2 (P = 0.33); I^2 = 10%					
Test for overall effect: Z = 3.36 (P = 0.00078)					
Total (95% CI)	17594	17516		100.0 %	0.81 [0.70, 0.93]
Total events: 1525 (BPLD), 1773 (Control)					
Heterogeneity: Tau^2 = 0.02; Chi^2 = 17.94, df = 7 (P = 0.01); I^2 = 61%					
Test for overall effect: Z = 2.93 (P = 0.0034)					
Test for subgroup differences: Chi^2 = 14.33, df = 4 (P = 0.01); I^2 = 72%					

0.1 0.2 0.5 1 2 5 10
Favours BPLD   Favours placebo

Figure 15.2 Forest plot showing the effects of *antihypertensive drugs vs control* for patients with an index stroke or TIA on *recurrent stroke,* by *pharmacological agent class.*

Reproduced from Zonneveld et al. (2018), with permission from the authors and John Wiley & Sons Limited. Copyright Cochrane Library, with permission.

Reductions in recurrent stroke were greater for diuretics – RR 0.72, ACE inhibitors – RR 0.73, and calcium channel blockers – RR 0.55; and less for beta-blockers – RR 0.94 and angiotensin receptor blockers – RR 0.95 (Figure 15.2). However, these differences across trials could be confounded by other factors, such as differences in enrolled populations, magnitude of attained blood pressure reduction, and permitted concomitant antihypertensive therapies. Also, the calcium channel antagonist estimate came from one small trial, so was highly imprecise (95% CI: 0.18–1.67).

Myocardial Infarction

In six RCTs enrolling 34,747 patients with prior stroke or TIA, the frequency of myocardial infarction

(MI) among patients randomized to active antihypertensive agents, compared with control, was 1.9% versus 2.1%, RR 0.90, 95% CI: 0.72–1.11 (Figure 15.4). A contributor to the non-positive result was the lower risk for MI than for recurrent stroke among patients with a first cerebral ischaemic event, affording less scope for an intervention to alter outcomes. In control groups, rates of recurrent stroke (10.1%) were 5-fold higher than rates of MI (2.1%).

Major Vascular Events (stroke, MI, or vascular death)

For the composite outcome of major vascular events (nonfatal stroke, nonfatal MI, or vascular death), among 28,630 participants from four RCTs, occurrences associated with allocation to active

Comparison: 2 Blood pressure-lowering drugs (BPLDs) versus placebo or no treatment (subgroups)
Outcome: 1 Recurrent stroke of any type by baseline systolic blood pressure (SBP)

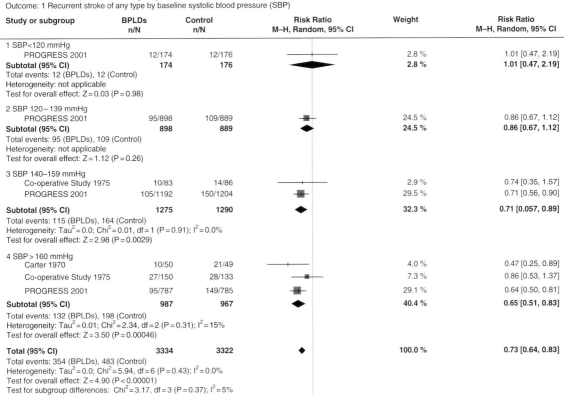

Study or subgroup	BPLDs n/N	Control n/N	Risk Ratio M–H, Random, 95% CI	Weight	Risk Ratio M–H, Random, 95% CI
1 SBP<120 mmHg					
PROGRESS 2001	12/174	12/176		2.8 %	1.01 [0.47, 2.19]
Subtotal (95% CI)	**174**	**176**		**2.8 %**	**1.01 [0.47, 2.19]**
Total events: 12 (BPLDs), 12 (Control)					
Heterogeneity: not applicable					
Test for overall effect: Z = 0.03 (P = 0.98)					
2 SBP 120–139 mmHg					
PROGRESS 2001	95/898	109/889		24.5 %	0.86 [0.67, 1.12]
Subtotal (95% CI)	**898**	**889**		**24.5 %**	**0.86 [0.67, 1.12]**
Total events: 95 (BPLDs), 109 (Control)					
Heterogeneity: not applicable					
Test for overall effect: Z = 1.12 (P = 0.26)					
3 SBP 140–159 mmHg					
Co-operative Study 1975	10/83	14/86		2.9 %	0.74 [0.35, 1.57]
PROGRESS 2001	105/1192	150/1204		29.5 %	0.71 [0.56, 0.90]
Subtotal (95% CI)	**1275**	**1290**		**32.3 %**	**0.71 [0.057, 0.89]**
Total events: 115 (BPLDs), 164 (Control)					
Heterogeneity: Tau² = 0.0; Chi² = 0.01, df = 1 (P = 0.91); I² = 0.0%					
Test for overall effect: Z = 2.98 (P = 0.0029)					
4 SBP > 160 mmHg					
Carter 1970	10/50	21/49		4.0 %	0.47 [0.25, 0.89]
Co-operative Study 1975	27/150	28/133		7.3 %	0.86 [0.53, 1.37]
PROGRESS 2001	95/787	149/785		29.1 %	0.64 [0.50, 0.81]
Subtotal (95% CI)	**987**	**967**		**40.4 %**	**0.65 [0.51, 0.83]**
Total events: 132 (BPLDs), 198 (Control)					
Heterogeneity: Tau² = 0.01; Chi² = 2.34, df = 2 (P = 0.31); I² = 15%					
Test for overall effect: Z = 3.50 (P = 0.00046)					
Total (95% CI)	**3334**	**3322**		**100.0 %**	**0.73 [0.64, 0.83]**
Total events: 354 (BPLDs), 483 (Control)					
Heterogeneity: Tau² = 0.0; Chi² = 5.94, df = 6 (P = 0.43); I² = 0.0%					
Test for overall effect: Z = 4.90 (P < 0.00001)					
Test for subgroup differences: Chi² = 3.17, df = 3 (P = 0.37); I² = 5%					

0.1 0.2 0.5 1 2 5 10
Favours BPLDs   Favours placebo

Figure 15.3 Forest plot showing the effects of *antihypertensive drugs vs control* for patients with an index stroke or TIA on *recurrent stroke,* by *baseline systolic blood pressure.*

Reproduced from Zonneveld et al. (2018), with permission from the authors and John Wiley & Sons Limited. Copyright Cochrane Library, with permission.

antihypertensive therapy versus control therapy were 13.6% versus 15.1%, RR 0.90, 95% CI: 0.78–1.04. However, there was significant heterogeneity among trials ($I^2 = 75\%$, heterogeneity $p = 0.01$), which appeared to be related to agent classes tested. Major vascular events were reduced in the trial testing ACE inhibitors with or without diuretics (RR 0.76, 95% CI: 0.68–0.85), but not in trials testing beta-blockers (RRs 1.03 and 0.99) or ARBs (RR 0.94).

Blood Pressure Treatment Intensity

Among the three RCTs in the Cochrane review comparing more intensive versus less intensive blood pressure lowering among patients with an index stroke or TIA, one trial (529 patients) compared targets of SBP <130 versus <140, one trial (83 patients) compared targets of SBP <125 versus <140, and one trial (3020 patients) compared targets

of SBP <130 versus SBP 130–149 (Zonneveld et al., 2018). Overall, allocation to more intensive blood pressure targets was associated with a borderline significant reduction in recurrent stroke (6.6% vs 8.4%, RR 0.80, 95% CI: 0.63–1.00; $p = 0.052$). Less strong signals were seen for other outcomes, including MI (RR 0.90, 95% CI: 0.58–1.38), and combined stroke, MI, or vascular death (RR 0.58, 95% CI: 0.23–1.46) (Figure 15.5).

Implications for Practice

After a stroke or TIA, long-term blood pressure lowering is an essential component of secondary prevention and will reduce recurrent stroke by about one-fifth. Beneficial effects on MI or all-cause mortality have not been established, but averting stroke is sufficient reason for therapy to proceed.

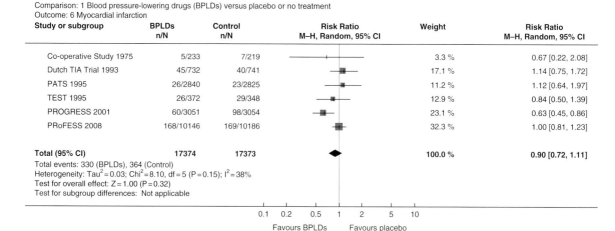

Figure 15.4 Forest plot showing the effects of *antihypertensive drugs vs control* for patients with an index stroke or TIA on *myocardial infarction*.

Reproduced from Zonneveld et al. (2018), with permission from the authors and John Wiley & Sons Limited. Copyright Cochrane Library, with permission.

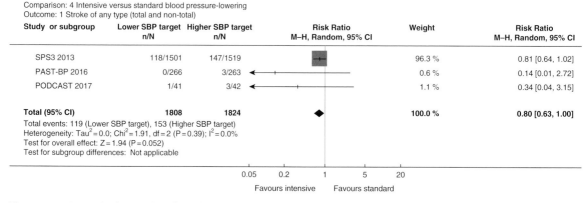

Figure 15.5 Forest plot showing the effects of *more intensive vs less intensive blood pressure lowering* for patients with an index stroke or TIA on *recurrent stroke*.

Reproduced from Zonneveld et al. (2018), with permission from the authors and John Wiley & Sons Limited. Copyright Cochrane Library, with permission.

In ischaemic stroke and TIA patients, antihypertensive therapy start should generally wait until after the first 24 hours after stroke onset. Lowering blood pressure while penumbral tissue is still salvageable could reduce cerebral perfusion and worsen outcome, due to impaired cerebral autoregulation in the ischaemic area. Trials have shown that antihypertensive agents may be safely be started or resumed between 24 and 72 hours after onset in most patients (Chapter 5).

Thereafter, treatment should be introduced slowly and gently in all patients with elevated blood pressures, irrespective of pathological stroke type, age, sex, and race-ethnicity. A blood pressure of less than 130/80 is a reasonable eventual goal (Whelton et al., 2018). All patients should receive non-pharmacological blood pressure lowering therapy and those with blood pressure ≥140/90 should receive antihypertensive agents. It is reasonable to initiate treatment with an ACE inhibitor, a thiazide diuretic, or both, as these classes have the strongest evidence in the secondary prevention setting. Drugs from other classes, such as calcium channel blockers or angiotensin receptor blockers, can then be added if blood pressure remains high. Beta-blockers are not a preferred option for secondary stroke prevention, but can be useful if they already are firmly required by another indication. However, the decision of which drugs should be used lies with the preferences of the responsible clinician and patient, and they are influenced by the presence of other diseases for which certain drug classes are specifically indicated (e.g. ACE inhibitors or ARBs in heart failure) or contraindicated (e.g. the avoidance of ACE inhibitors and ARBs in renal artery stenosis and beta-receptor antagonists in asthma).

Although RCTs for secondary stroke prevention usually followed patients for only up to 5 years, it is reasonable to maintain lifelong antihypertensive therapy for patients with prior stroke.

They are also greater for preventing recurrent stroke than for preventing MI, in both primary and secondary prevention.

The degree of reduction in blood pressure more greatly influences the degree of reduction in stroke and other vascular events than does the agent classes of pharmacological drugs used. Arriving at a highly effective, well-tolerated regimen is therefore a key long-term goal. Nonetheless, unless otherwise indicated, beta-blockers are not a preferred agent, as they show less efficacy for stroke prevention in both primary and secondary prevention settings. Calcium channel antagonists may be preferred agents for primary stroke prevention, as some evidence supports their stronger efficacy. In secondary prevention after first stroke or TIA, calcium channel antagonists have been understudied, and angiotensin-converting enzyme inhibitors and thiazide diuretics may be preferred on the basis of their more robust evidence base.

Summary

For hypertensive patients without prior stroke, transient ischaemic attack (TIA), or other symptomatic vascular disease, anti-hypertensive therapy, which reduces systolic blood pressure (SBP) modestly by 10 mm Hg, is associated with significant reductions in the relative risk of stroke (by about one-quarter) and of combined stroke, myocardial infarction (MI), and vascular death (by about one-fifth). Combined pharmacological and non-pharmacological therapy to lower blood pressure is indicated in all individuals with SBP >140 or diastolic blood pressure (DBP) >90, and in individuals with SBP 130–139 or DBP 80–89 who have additional vascular risk factors. Non-pharmacological blood pressure lowering is indicated in individuals with SBP 130–139 or DBP 80–89 without important additional vascular risk factors.

For hypertensive patients with prior stroke or TIA, antihypertensive therapy is associated with significant reductions in the relative risks of recurrent stroke and combined stroke, MI, and vascular death, regardless of patient age, race-ethnicity, and pathological stroke subtype. A goal blood pressure less than 130/80 is reasonable. For ischaemic stroke and TIA, treatment may be gradually started as early as 24–72 hours after onset of the index stroke.

The absolute benefits of antihypertensive therapy are greater with greater reductions in blood pressure.

References

ACCORD Study Group et al. (2010). Effects of intensive blood-pressure control in type 2 diabetes mellitus. *N Engl J Med*, **362**, 1575–85.

Blood Pressure Lowering Treatment Trialists' Collaboration. (2003). Effects of different blood-pressure-lowering regimens on major cardiovascular events: results of prospectively-designed overviews of randomised trials. *Lancet*, **362**, 1527–35.

Boan AD, Lackland DT, Ovbiagele B. (2014). Lowering of blood pressure for recurrent stroke prevention. *Stroke*, **45**, 2506–13.

Brunström M, Carlberg B. (2018). Association of blood pressure lowering with mortality and cardiovascular disease across blood pressure levels: a systematic review and meta-analysis. *JAMA Intern Med*, **178**(1), 28–36.

Collins R, Peto R, MacMahon S, Hebert P, Fiebach NH, Eberlein KA, et al. (1990). Blood pressure, stroke, and coronary heart disease. Part 2, short-term reductions in blood pressure: overview of randomised drug trials in their epidemiological context. *Lancet*, **335**(8693), 827–38.

Ettehad D, Emdin CA, Kiran A, Anderson SG, Callender T, Emberson J, et al. (2016). Blood pressure lowering for prevention of cardiovascular disease and death: a systematic review and meta-analysis. *Lancet*, **387**(10022), 957–67.

Huang Y, Cai X, Li Y, Su L, Mai W, Wang S, et al. (2014). Prehypertension and the risk of stroke: a meta-analysis. *Neurology*, **82**, 1153–61.

Kim S, Shin DW, Yun JM, Hwang Y, Park SK, Ko YJ, et al. (2016). Medication adherence and the risk of cardiovascular mortality and hospitalization among patients with newly prescribed antihypertensive medications. *Hypertension*, **67**, 506–12.

Law MR, Morris JK, Wald NJ. (2009). Use of blood pressure lowering drugs in the prevention of cardiovascular disease: meta-analysis of 147 randomised trials in the context of expectations from prospective epidemiological studies. *BMJ*, **338**, b1665. doi:10.1136/bmj.b1665.

Lee M, Saver JL, Chang B, Chang KH, Hao Q, Ovbiagele B, et al. (2011). Presence of baseline prehypertension and risk of incident stroke: a meta-analysis. *Neurology*, **77**, 1330–1337.

Lee M, Saver JL, Hong K-S, Hao Q, Ovbiagele B. (2012). Does achieving an intensive versus usual blood pressure level prevent stroke? *Ann Neurol*, **71**, 133–140.

Liu L, Wang Z, Gong L, Zhang Y, Thhijs L, Staessen JA, et al. (2009). Blood pressure reduction for the secondary prevention of stroke: a Chinese trial and a systematic review of the literature. *Hypertens Res*, **32**, 1032–40.

MacMahon S, Peto R, Cutler J. (1990). Blood pressure, stroke, and coronary heart disease. Part 1, prolonged differences in blood pressure: prospective observational studies corrected for the regression dilution bias. *Lancet*, **335**, 765–74.

Perkovic V, Rodgers A. (2015). Redefining blood-pressure targets – SPRINT starts the marathon. *N Engl J Med*, **373**, 2175–8.

PROGRESS Collaborative Group. (2001). Randomised trial of a perindopril-based blood-pressure-lowering regimen among 6,105 individuals with previous stroke or transient ischaemic attack. *Lancet*, **358**, 1033–41.

Sardana M, Syed AA, Hashmath Z, Phan TS, Koppula MR, Kewan U, et al. (2017). Beta-blocker use is associated with impaired left atrial function in hypertension. *J Am Heart Assoc*, **6**. doi:10.1161/JAHA.116.005163.

Sipahi I, Swaminathan A, Natesan V, Debanne SM, Simon DI, Fang JC. (2012). Effect of antihypertensive therapy on incident stroke in cohorts with prehypertensive blood pressure levels: a meta-analysis of randomized controlled trials. *Stroke*, **43**, 432–40.

SPRINT MIND Investigators for the SPRINT Research Group. (2019). Effect of intensive vs standard blood pressure control on probable dementia: a randomized clinical trial. *JAMA*, **322**, 169–70.

SPRINT Research Group et al. (2015). A randomized trial of intensive versus standard blood-pressure control. *N Engl J Med*, **373**, 2103–16.

Sundstrom J, Arima H, Jackson, R, Turnbull F, Rahimi K, Chalmers J, et al. (2015). Effects of blood pressure reduction in mild hypertension: a systematic review and meta-analysis. *Ann Intern Med*, **162**, 184–91.

Turner GM, Calvert M, Feltham MG, Ryan R, Fitzmaurice D, Cheng KK, et al. (2016). Under-prescribing of prevention drugs and primary prevention of stroke and transient ischaemic attack in UK general practice: a retrospective analysis. *PLoS Med*, **13**, e1002169.

Whelton PK, Carey RM, Aronow WS, Casey DE Jr, Collins KJ, Dennison Himmelfarb C, et al. (2018). 2017 ACC/AHA/AAPA/ABC/ACPM/AGS/APhA/ASH/ASPC/NMA/PCNA Guideline for the Prevention, Detection, Evaluation, and Management of High Blood Pressure in Adults: a report of the American College of Cardiology/American Heart Association Task Force on Clinical Practice Guidelines. *Hypertension*, **71**(6), e13–e115.

Zonneveld TP, Richard E, Vergouwen MD, Nederkoorn PJ, de Haan R, Roos YB, et al. (2018). Blood pressure-lowering treatment for preventing recurrent stroke, major vascular events, and dementia in patients with a history of stroke or transient ischaemic attack. *Cochrane Database Syst Rev*, 7. CD007858. doi:10.1002/14651858.CD007858.pub2.

Prevention of Stroke by Lowering Blood Cholesterol Concentrations

Maurizio Paciaroni

Blood Cholesterol and Risk of Stroke

A Review of Observational Epidemiological Studies

All Stroke

Whether increased serum cholesterol levels are risk factors for stroke remains controversial. A systematic review of 45 observational studies over 16 years including around 450,000 individuals reported no significant correlation between total plasma cholesterol and any stroke (after adjusting for age, gender, ethnicity, blood pressure, and history of cardiac disease), suggesting that cholesterol is not a risk factor for stroke (Prospective Studies Collaboration, 1995). Furthermore, a meta-analysis of individual data from 61 prospective studies, most of which were carried out in the USA and Europe, reported no independent positive association between total cholesterol and ischaemic or total stroke mortality (Lewington et al., 2007). Finally, a review of 14 Japanese cohort studies, including subject pools ranging from 1621 to 19,219 (mean follow-up period ranged from 7.6 to 32 years), reported no association between hypercholesterolaemia and total stroke (Tanaka and Tomonori, 2012).

Even though an association between total cholesterol and all strokes has not been confirmed, it could be that total cholesterol and all stroke dilutes associations between cholesterol and pathological subtypes of stroke and between cholesterol fractions and pathological and aetiological subtypes of stroke.

Subtypes of Stroke

A weak (positive) association between increasing plasma cholesterol concentrations and increasing risk of ischaemic stroke has been reported, which is partially offset by a weaker (negative) association between decreasing plasma cholesterol concentrations and an increasing risk of haemorrhagic stroke in both Western and Asiatic populations (Nagasawa et al., 2012; Zhang et al., 2012; Wang et al., 2013).

Fractions of Cholesterol

Low-density Lipoprotein-cholesterol

Increasing low-density lipoprotein-cholesterol (LDL-C) concentrations of 1.03 mmol/L (40 mg/dL) have been associated independently with a 14% (95% confidence interval [CI]: 0–26%) increase in the odds of ischaemic stroke or transient ischaemic attack (TIA) (Koran-Morag et al., 2002).

High-density Lipoprotein-cholesterol

A significant, independent (negative) association between decreasing plasma high-density lipoprotein (HDL) concentrations and increasing risk of ischaemic stroke has been identified in several studies (Leppala et al., 1999; Koran-Morag et al., 2002; Pikula et al., 2015; Orozco-Beltran et al., 2017).

Total Cholesterol/HDL-cholesterol Concentration Ratio

A significant, independent, positive association has been reported between the ratio of total cholesterol/HDL-C concentrations and ischaemic stroke (Simons et al., 2001).

Apolipoproteins

Apolipoproteins make up the protein moiety of lipoproteins, with apolipoprotein B (apo B) being found mainly in LDL and apolipoprotein A1 (apo A1) in HDL. The assessment of apo B and apo A1 levels provides information on the total number of atherogenic (apo B) and antiatherogenic (apo A1) particles.

A study has suggested that apo B and the ratio of apo B/apo A1 are better predictors of ischaemic stroke than total cholesterol, LDL-C or HDL-C (hazard ratio [HR] 2.27; 95% CI: 1.14–4.50 and HR 2.86; 95% CI:

1.37–5.88, respectively) (Bhatia et al., 2004). Additionally, a collaborative analysis of 79,036 individuals reported that lipoprotein-associated phospholipase A_2 (Lp-PLA$_2$) activity and mass are associated with the risk of ischaemic stroke (Lp-PLA$_2$ Studies Collaboration, 2010).

Aetiological Subtypes of Ischaemic Stroke

Increasing LDL-C concentrations have been associated independently with a 68% (95% CI: 23–230%) increase in odds of ischaemic stroke, due to large artery atherothrombosis (Koran-Morag et al., 2002). Also lacunar stroke, but not cardioembolic types, is associated with an increase in LDL-C levels (Imamura et al., 2009; Bezerra et al., 2012).

Type of Cholesterol Lowering Intervention and Stroke Prevention

A Systematic Review of Randomized Controlled Trials

A systematic review and meta-analysis of 58 randomized controlled trials (RCTs) investigating cholesterol lowering by any means reported that lowering the concentration of LDL-C by 1.0 mmol/L decreased the risk of all stroke by 10%, and lowering cholesterol by 1.8 mmol/L decreased the risk of stroke by 17% (95% CI: 9–25%) and the risk of coronary events by 61% (95% CI: 51–71%) (Law et al., 2003).

Non-pharmacological (e.g. diets) and non-statin lipid-lowering interventions are less effective in reducing plasma cholesterol concentrations, compared with statins (3-hydroxy-3-methylglutaryl coenzyme A [HMG-CoA] reductase inhibitors). In fact, the mean reduction in cholesterol concentrations among trials of non-statin interventions were reported to be half as great when compared with trials of statin drugs (Di Mascio et al., 2000). Indeed, a significant decrease in stroke incidence has only been observed in trials on statin drugs.

Non-pharmacological Interventions to Lower Plasma Lipid Concentrations

Among the five trials to date investigating the benefit of non-pharmacological interventions in lowering plasma lipid concentrations (diet, ileal bypass, LDL apheresis) in 2198 patients (1102 in intervention group and 1096 in control group), total cholesterol was reduced by 14.5% (standard deviation [SD]: 3.7) the odds of stroke was reduced by 28% (95%CI: -17% to +56%), from 3.6% (40/1096) in the control group to 2.6% (29/1102) in the intervention group P for heterogeneity 0.7 (Di Mascio et al., 2000).

In a meta-regression analysis including 26,969 participants treated with non-statin therapies that act via upregulation of LDL receptor expression to reduce LDL-C (diet, bile acid sequestrants, ileal bypass, and ezetimibe), the risk ratio (RR) for major vascular events (a composite of cardiovascular death, acute myocardial infarction [MI] or other acute coronary syndrome, coronary revascularization, or stroke) per 1 mmol/L reduction in LDL-C level was 0.77 (95% CI: 0.75–0.79; $P = 0.01$). No significant heterogeneity was seen (Silverman et al., 2016).

Reduction of saturated fat intake is known to reduce serum cholesterol levels, therein reducing the risk of MI, while the benefits on stroke are less clear (any stroke, RR 1.00; 95% CI: 0.89–1.12; 8 trials with 50,952 participants) (Hopper et al., 2015).

Non-statin Lipid-lowering Drugs

Primary Prevention Trials

Among the 12 trials of non-statin lipid-lowering drugs (clofibrate, niacin, colestipol, cholestyramine, gemfibrozil, probucol) in 27,519 patients (12,143 in intervention group, 15,376 in control group) published before 1998, total cholesterol was reported to be reduced by 12.6% (SD: 5.9) and stroke reduced by 21%; 1.76% (270/15,376) with control and 1.39% (169/12,143) with intervention (Di Mascio et al., 2000).

Since 1998, the Veterans Affairs High-Density Lipoprotein Cholesterol Intervention Trial (VAHIT) has reported that, compared with placebo, men with ischaemic heart disease allocated to gemfibrozil 1200 mg for 5 years, experienced no change in LDL-C levels (2.87 mmol/L), an increase in HDL levels by 6% (0.82–0.85 mmol/L), a reduction in triglyceride levels by 31% (1.81–1.25 mmol/L), and a reduction in the incidence of stroke (as designated by the investigators), from 6.9% (88/1267) to 5.1% (64/1264); relative risk reduction (RRR): 27% (95% CI: 1–47, $P = 0.04$) (Rubins et al., 1999). However, the rate of stroke (a secondary outcome event in this trial), as confirmed by the blinded adjudication committee of three neurologists, was not significantly different: 6% (76/1267) for patients allocated placebo versus 4.6%

(58/1264) for patients allocated gemfibrozil; RRR: 24% (95% CI: −7% to +45%, *P* = 0.1). Furthermore, the BIP trial reported that patients with known coronary heart disease (CHD) allocated to bezafibrate, compared with placebo, had a 6.5% reduction (3.82 to 3.6 mmol/L) in LDL-C levels, a fall in triglyceride levels of 21% (1.63 to 1.29 mmol/L), an increase in HDL levels of 18% (0.89 to 1.03 mmol/L), but no significant difference in the rate of all stroke (placebo: 5.0% [77/1542], bezafibrate: 4.6% [72/1548]; RRR: 7% [95% CI: −27% to +32%, *P* = 0.66]), or ischaemic stroke (placebo: 4.5% [69/1542], bezafibrate: 3.8% [59/1548]; RRR: 15% [95% CI: −20% to +39%, *P* = 0.36]) (BIP Study Group, 2000).

Three classes of agents targeted at increasing HDL levels included in a meta-analysis (niacin, fibrates, and cholesteryl ester transfer protein [CETP] inhibitors), were not associated with a significantly reduced risk of stroke in both the pre-statin era and the present era (HPS2-THRIVE Collaborative Group, 2014; Keene et al., 2014). A meta-analysis that included 39,195 participants concluded that niacin does not reduce overall mortality (RR 1.05; 95% CI: 0.97–1.12) and the number of fatal or non-fatal strokes (RR 0.93; 95% CI: 0.74–1.22). Participants randomized to niacin were more likely to discontinue treatment due to side effects than participants randomized to control group (RR 2.17; 95% CI: 1.70–2.77) (Schandelmaier et al., 2017). A randomized trial involving 30,449 adults with atherosclerotic vascular disease (6781 with history of cerebrovascular atherosclerotic disease), who were receiving intensive atorvastatin therapy and who had a mean LDL-C level of 61 mg/dL, showed that the primary outcome (composite of coronary death, MI, or coronary revascularization) occurred in significantly fewer patients in the anacetrapib (a CE inhibitor) group than in the placebo group (RR 0.91; 95% CI: 0.85–0.97; *P* = 0.004). There were no significant between-group differences in the risk of death, cancer, or other serious adverse events. However, the risk of presumed ischaemic stroke (secondary endpoint) was similar between the two groups (RR 0.99; 95% CI: 0.87–1.12) (HPS3/TIMI55–REVEAL Collaborative Group, 2017).

Trials have compared ezetimibe, a lipid-lowering agent that inhibits intestinal absorption of dietary cholesterol plus a lipid-lowering drug, with ezetimibe; reporting a non-significant impact in reducing the incidence of stroke (RR 0.65; 95% CI: 0.08–4.59). Furthermore, ezetimibe plus simvastatin versus simvastatin alone was not associated with a reduction in stroke (RR 2.38; 95% CI: 0.46–12.35) (Battaggia et al., 2015). Conversely, a meta-analysis including 7 trials, enrolling 31,048 patients, reported that ezetimibe versus placebo or ezetimibe plus another hypolipidaemic agent versus the same hypolipidaemic drug alone significantly reduced the risk of any stroke by 16.0% (RR 0.840, 95% CI: 0.744–0.949; *P* = 0.005), without any effect on all-cause and cardiovascular mortalities (RR 1.003, 95% CI: 0.954–1.055; *P* = 0.908; RR 0.958, 95% CI: 0.879–1.044; *P* = 0.330; respectively) as well as the risk of new cancer (RR 1.040, 95% CI: 0.965–1.120; *P* = 0.303) (Savarese et al., 2015). Another meta-analysis including 23,499 participants showed that adding ezetimibe to statins probably reduces the risk of non-fatal MI (RR 0.88; 95% CI: 0.81–0.95) and non-fatal stroke (RR 0.83; 95% CI: 0.71–0.97), but trials reporting all-cause mortality used ezetimibe with statins or fenofibrate found they have no effect on this outcome (RR 0.98; 95% CI: 0.91–1.05) (Zhan et al., 2018).

Secondary Prevention Trials

Until 1998, there were 25 secondary prevention trials including 33,000 patients (14,979 in the intervention group, 18,237 in the control group) (Di Mascio et al., 2000). Total cholesterol was reduced by 18.1% (SD: 6.6), and the odds of stroke was reduced by 20% (95% CI: 9–29%), from 3.53% (643/18,237) in the control group to 2.86% (428/14,979) in the intervention group (Di Mascio et al., 2000).

A later systematic review of lipid-lowering interventions for preventing stroke recurrence reported that among 627 patients with a history of stroke or TIA randomized in two trials (Acheson and Hutchinson, 1972; The Veterans Administration Cooperative Study Group, 1973) to clofibrate (n = 315) or control (n = 312), the odds of a recurrent stroke were non-significantly increased among patients allocated to clofibrate (14.4% control, 19.0% clofibrate; odds ratio [OR] 1.48, 95% CI: 0.94–2.30) (Manktelow et al., 2002; Wang et al., 2015).

Statin Drugs

Numerous statin trials, including patients with known CHD and primary prevention trials including high-risk populations, have declared a decrease in stroke incidence in patients treated with statins (Paciaroni et al., 2007). The Stroke Prevention by Aggressive Reduction of Cholesterol Levels (SPARCL) study evidenced the positive effects of statin therapy also in the secondary prevention of cerebrovascular diseases (SPARCL Investigators, 2006).

Primary Prevention Trials

Statins and Their Benefits in Stroke Prevention for Both CHD and High-risk Vascular Disease Patients (mainly diabetic and hypertensive patients without CHD)

The Cholesterol Treatment Trialists' Collaborators reported on the results of a prospective meta-analysis examining data from 90,056 individuals in 14 randomized trials on the benefits from statin use (Cholesterol Treatment Trialists' [CTT] Collaboration, 2005): 42,131 (47%) had pre-existing CHD, 21,575 (24%) were women, 18,686 (21%) had a history of diabetes, and 49,689 (55%) had a history of hypertension. Regarding cerebrovascular events, data were available for a total of 2,957 first-ever strokes after randomization. Overall, 2282 strokes were reported among 65,138 patients in the 9 trials that collected information on stroke type: 204 (9%) haemorrhagic, 1565 (69%) ischaemic, and 513 (22%) unknown type. A significant 17% proportional reduction in the incidence of first stroke of any type (1340 [3.0%] was reported in the statin group versus 1617 [3.7%] for the control group: RR 0.83, 95% CI: 0.78–0.88; $P < 0.0001$) per 1 mmol/L LDL-C reduction. This overall reduction in stroke was associated with highly significant 19% proportional reduction (RR 0.81, 99% CI: 0.74–0.89; $P < 0.0001$) in stroke not attributed to haemorrhage (i.e. presumed ischaemic) per 1 mmol/L LDL-C reduction, and no apparent difference in haemorrhagic stroke. The total reduction in presumed ischaemic stroke was associated with a significant 22% proportional reduction in confirmed ischaemic stroke (RR 0.78, 99% CI: 0.70–0.87; $P < 0.0001$) per 1 mmol/L LDL-C reduction and a 12% proportional reduction in stroke of unknown type (RR 0.88, 99% CI: 0.7–1.02; $P = 0.03$). There was no significant reduction in stroke during the first year after randomization (RR 0.96, 99% CI: 0.79–1.17; $P = 0.6$), yet there were significant reductions ranging from 20–25% over the 3 subsequent years, and thereafter favourable trends were recorded. During an average 5-year treatment period, the reduction in the overall incidence of stroke was roughly one-sixth for each 1 mmol/L LDL-C decrease, predicting 8/1000 fewer subjects would have any stroke in the pre-existing CHD disease group at baseline, compared with 5/1000 fewer subjects with no such history.

The beneficial effect of statins in stroke prevention for high-risk patients, with or without CHD, has been confirmed also by other meta-analyses. In a Cochrane review including 18 randomized control trials (19 trial arms; 56,934 subjects; 14 trials recruited patients with specific conditions such as elevated lipid levels, diabetes, hypertension, and microalbuminuria), all-cause mortality was reduced by statins (OR 0.86, 95% CI: 0.79–0.94), as was combined fatal and non-fatal stroke (RR 0.78, 95% CI: 0.68–0.89) (Taylor et al., 2013). Another meta-analysis of randomized trials on statins, in combination with other preventive strategies, included 165,792 subjects, reporting that each 1 mmol/L (39 mg/dL) decrease in LDL-C equated to a reduction in relative risk for stroke of 21.1% (95% CI: 6.3–33.5; $P = 0.009$) (Amarenco and Labreuche, 2009).

In men and women at an equivalent risk of cardiovascular disease, statin therapy is of similar effectiveness for the prevention of major vascular events (Cholesterol Treatment Trialists' [CTT] Collaboration, 2015).

Benefit of Statins in Stroke Prevention for Patients at Low Risk of Vascular Disease

A meta-analysis including data from 22 trials on statin use versus controls (n = 134,537 subjects; mean LDL-C difference 1.08 mmol/L; median follow-up 4.8 years) and 5 trials of higher-dose versus lower-dose statin use ($n = 39,612$ subjects, difference 0.51 mmol/L; 5.1 years) reported that for stroke, the reduction in risk for subjects with 5-year risk of major vascular events lower than 10% (RR per 1 mmol/L LDL-C reduction 0.76, 99% CI: 0.61–0.95; $P = 0.0012$) was also similar to that seen in higher-risk categories (trend $P = 0.3$) (Cholesterol Treatment Trialists' [CTT] Collaboration, 2012).

In a meta-analysis of 8 RCTs ($n = 25,952$) comparing any statins with placebo or usual care for primary prevention of CVD in subjects aged 65 years or older, statins significantly reduced the risks of composite major adverse cardiovascular events (RR 0.82, 95% CI: 0.74–0.92), nonfatal MI (0.75, 95% CI: 0.59–0.94), and total MI (0.74, 95% CI: 0.61–0.90). Treatment effects of statins were statistically insignificant in fatal MI (0.43, 95% CI: 0.09–2.01), stroke (fatal: 0.76, 95% CI: 0.24–2.45; nonfatal: 0.76, 95% CI: 0.53–1.11; total: 0.85, 95% CI: 0.68–1.06) and all-cause mortality (0.96, 95% CI: 0.88–1.04) (Teng et al., 2015).

Secondary Prevention Trials

Among 821 patients with a history of stroke or TIA (and CHD), who were randomized in the CARE and LIPID trials (Plehn et al., 1999; White et al., 2000) to pravastatin (n = 436) or placebo (n = 385), the odds of a recurrent stroke were reduced by 33% (95% CI: –1% to +56%) from 15.1% (placebo) to 10.6% (pravastatin) (Manktelow et al., 2002). Patients with a history of only stroke had similar results.

Among the 3289 subjects in the HPS trial with a history of symptomatic ischaemic cerebrovascular disease a mean of 4.3 (standard error [SE]: 0.1) years previously, 1820 had a past history of stroke only and 1460 had a past history of CHD and stroke. For these 1820 with previous stroke only, allocation to simvastatin was associated with a significant reduction in major vascular events: 23.6% (placebo) to 18.7% (simvastatin). This resulted in an RRR of 21% (95% CI: 5–34%, $P < 0.001$), and an absolute risk reduction (ARR) of 49 major vascular events (4.9%) per 1000 stroke patients allocated to simvastatin over 5 years. Among the 1460 subjects with known CHD and a past history of stroke, allocation to simvastatin was associated with a similar reduction in any major vascular event: 37.4% (placebo) to 32.4% (simvastatin) that resulted in an RRR of 14% (95% CI: 0.5–25%), and an ARR of 5% over 5 years.

A retrospective subgroup analysis of HPS data suggested that in subjects with a history of cerebrovascular disease, simvastatin did not reduce the overall rate of recurrent stroke compared with placebo (simvastatin: 10.3%, placebo: 10.4%; RR: 0.98, 95% CI: 0.79–1.22), in contrast to other high-risk subjects who had a highly significant reduction in stroke (simvastatin: 3.2%, placebo: 4.8%; heterogeneity $P = 0.002$). Those with a history of cerebrovascular disease who were assigned to simvastatin had a 19% (SE: 12, $P = 0.1$) reduction in the RR of ischaemic stroke (simvastatin: 6.1%, placebo: 7.5%) but a nearly 2-fold increase in RR for haemorrhagic stroke (placebo: 0.7%, simvastatin: 1.3%). This latter result was in contrast with other high-risk subjects who had a non-significantly lower risk of haemorrhagic stroke (heterogeneity $P = 0.03$).

The SPARCL study was the first to investigate the effects of statins on the risk of cerebrovascular events in patients without a history of CHD. This double-blind, randomized, placebo-controlled, multicentre trial examined the effect of aggressive atorvastatin therapy (80 mg/day) on specified cerebrovascular endpoints. Patients were eligible for the study if they had had a previous TIA or stroke and an LDL level between 100 mg/dL (2.58 mmol/L) and 190 mg/dL (4.91 mmol/L), without any evidence of CHD. The primary clinical endpoint was the time to first occurrence of a fatal or nonfatal stroke. In this study, 4731 patients who had had a stroke or TIA within the past 6 months were randomized. After 6 years of follow-up, 265 patients in the atorvastatin group had a fatal or nonfatal stroke compared with 311 in the control group. This resulted in a 16% risk reduction in time to first occurrence of stroke for atorvastatin (adjusted hazard ratio 0.84, 95% CI: 0.71–0.99; number needed to treat 46). For the secondary endpoint of time to stroke or TIA, a 23% risk reduction was reported (HR 0.77, 95% CI: 0.67–0.88) with 375 events in the atorvastatin group and 476 in controls. Moreover, there was a 35% reduction in coronary events (HR 0.65, 95% CI: 0.49–0.87) (SPARCL Investigators, 2006). The treatment effect did not differ between men and women, in individuals aged younger than 65 years and those older than 65 years, in those with carotid stenosis at entry compared with those with no carotid stenosis, in patients with diabetes compared with those without, and across ischaemic stroke subtype at entry.

In Figure 16.1, the forest plot shows the effect of statins compared with controls, in patients with and without a history of either stroke or TIA, on the incidence of subsequent stroke (fatal and not-fatal) of any pathological type. In the secondary prevention of non-cardioembolic stroke, a significant reduction in LDL-C levels due to statin use significantly reduced the risks of recurrent stroke (RR 0.84, 0.71–0.99, $P = 0.03$) and major cardiovascular events (0.80, 0.69–0.92, $P = 0.002$) (Amarenco and Labreuche, 2009).

Is Statin Treatment Safe?

There is no strong evidence that statins increase the overall incidence of cancer (OR 1.02, 95% CI: 0.97–1.07) at any particular site, or cancer death (OR 1.01, 95% CI: 0.93–1.09) (Dale et al., 2006). Regarding other side effects, the occurrence of myopathy with currently available statins has been reported (Thompson et al., 2003; Bays, 2006; Peto and Collins, 2018). Myopathy (defined as muscle pain or weakness with large increases in creatine kinase levels) is rare and most muscle-related symptoms are not myopathy. The frequency of muscle-related symptoms recorded in randomized trials depends on whether such symptoms

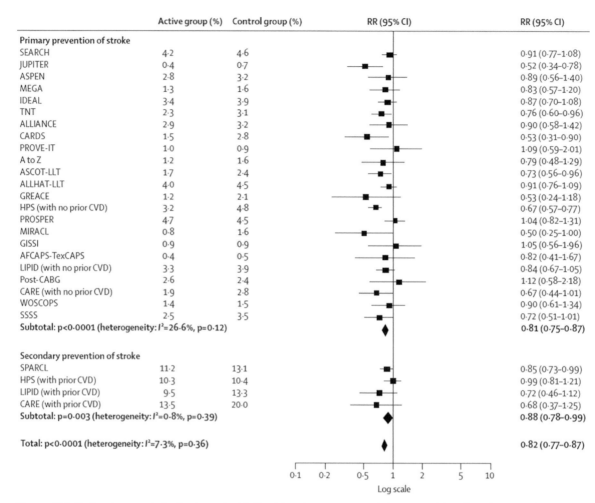

	Active group (%)	Control group (%)	RR (95% CI)	RR (95% CI)
Primary prevention of stroke				
SEARCH	4·2	4·6		0·91 (0·77–1·08)
JUPITER	0·4	0·7		0·52 (0·34–0·78)
ASPEN	2·8	3·2		0·89 (0·56–1·40)
MEGA	1·3	1·6		0·83 (0·57–1·20)
IDEAL	3·4	3·9		0·87 (0·70–1·08)
TNT	2·3	3·1		0·76 (0·60–0·96)
ALLIANCE	2·9	3·2		0·90 (0·58–1·42)
CARDS	1·5	2·8		0·53 (0·31–0·90)
PROVE-IT	1·0	0·9		1·09 (0·59–2·01)
A to Z	1·2	1·6		0·79 (0·48–1·29)
ASCOT-LLT	1·7	2·4		0·73 (0·56–0·96)
ALLHAT-LLT	4·0	4·5		0·91 (0·76–1·09)
GREACE	1·2	2·1		0·53 (0·24–1·18)
HPS (with no prior CVD)	3·2	4·8		0·67 (0·57–0·77)
PROSPER	4·7	4·5		1·04 (0·82–1·31)
MIRACL	0·8	1·6		0·50 (0·25–1·00)
GISSI	0·9	0·9		1·05 (0·56–1·96)
AFCAPS-TexCAPS	0·4	0·5		0·82 (0·41–1·67)
LIPID (with no prior CVD)	3·3	3·9		0·84 (0·67–1·05)
Post-CABG	2·6	2·4		1·12 (0·58–2·18)
CARE (with no prior CVD)	1·9	2·8		0·67 (0·44–1·01)
WOSCOPS	1·4	1·5		0·90 (0·61–1·34)
SSSS	2·5	3·5		0·72 (0·51–1·01)
Subtotal: p<0·0001 (heterogeneity: I²=26·6%, p=0·12)				**0·81 (0·75–0·87)**
Secondary prevention of stroke				
SPARCL	11·2	13·1		0·85 (0·73–0·99)
HPS (with prior CVD)	10·3	10·4		0·99 (0·81–1·21)
LIPID (with prior CVD)	9·5	13·3		0·72 (0·46–1·12)
CARE (with prior CVD)	13·5	20·0		0·68 (0·37–1·25)
Subtotal: p=0·003 (heterogeneity: I²=0·8%, p=0·39)				**0·88 (0·78–0·99)**
Total: p<0·0001 (heterogeneity: I²=7·3%, p=0·36)				**0·82 (0·77–0·87)**

Figure 16.1 Updated meta-analysis of major statin trials (24 trials with 165,792 patients) that assessed the effect of statins on fatal and non-fatal stroke.

(Amarenco and Labruche, 2009; with permission of Elsevier.)

were systematically sought and on the questions asked. However, although the rates differ between the trials, the proportions reporting these symptoms within each of these trials were similar among patients assigned statin or placebo (Peto and Collins, 2018).

In meta-analyses of the available results from the randomized trials, standard statin dose regimens were associated with a proportional increase of about 10% in reported diabetes and more intensive statin regimens with about a 10% further increase (Sattar et al., 2010; Preiss et al., 2011), but the cardiovascular benefits of statin therapy are substantial despite any increase in diabetes-related morbidity (Collins et al., 2016). The underlying incidence of new-onset diabetes in the primary prevention trials was about 1%

per year (Sattar et al., 2010), so the absolute excess with statin therapy was about 10–20 per 10,000 per year, with this range reflecting the intensity of the statin regimen (Collins et al., 2016).

Several studies have suggested that low cholesterol is a risk factor for intracerebral haemorrhage, whereas other studies have claimed that high cholesterol is protective against intracerebral haemorrhage. For this, lipid-lowering drugs may increase the risk of cerebral haemorrhage. To this regard, SPARCL evidenced an association between statin use and a higher incidence of haemorrhagic stroke. Specifically, of the 88 patients who had at least one intracerebral haemorrhage, 55 were assigned to atorvastatin and 33 to placebo. The RR related to intracerebral haemorrhage increased by 66% for the atorvastatin group. Nonetheless, the overall benefit in terms of stroke risk reduction was significant despite an increase in intracerebral haemorrhage in the same group. Secondary analyses of the SPARCL study have been conducted to address the implications of statin therapy on patients having intracerebral haemorrhage during the trial. A preliminary exploratory analysis has suggested that brain haemorrhage is not related to a major lowering of LDL-C levels.

Likewise, HPS reported a similar observation in a subset of 3200 patients having stroke before randomization: a 91% relative increase in the risk of haemorrhagic stroke for patients assigned to statin treatment.

A meta-analysis including 91,588 subjects in the active group and 91,215 in the control group evidenced no significant difference in the incidence of intracerebral haemorrhage observed in the active treatment group versus controls (OR 1.08; 95% CI: 0.88–1.32; $P = 0.47$). Moreover, intracerebral haemorrhage risk was not related to the degree of LDL reduction or achieved LDL-C (McKinney and Kostis, 2012).

The above results suggest that statins have a good overall safety profile. Yet, we need to further investigate their safety in patients with prior cerebral haemorrhage and if they have a role in causing brain haemorrhage in secondary prevention of stroke.

What Is the Ideal LDL-C Level?

In a meta-analysis of data compiled on 170,000 subjects from 26 randomized trials, the size of the proportional reduction in major vascular events was reported to be directly proportional to the absolute LDL reduction achieved, with further benefit coming from more intensive statin therapy, even if LDL-C was already lower than 2.0 mmol/L. Each 1 mmol/L reduction reduced the risk of occlusive vascular events by about a fifth, irrespective of baseline cholesterol concentration, suggesting that a 2–3 mmol/L reduction would reduce risk by 40–50% (Cholesterol Treatment Trialists' [CTT] Collaboration, 2010). Furthermore, a meta-analysis that included randomized trials of LDL-C lowering with data in populations starting with LDL-C levels averaging 1.8 mmol/L (70 mg/dL) or less found a consistent relative risk reduction in major vascular events (RR 0.79 per 1 mmol/L reduction; 95% CI: 0.71–0.87; $P < 0.001$) achieving levels as low as a median of 0.5 mmol/L (21 mg/dL) with no observed offsetting adverse effects (Sabatine et al., 2018).

These findings suggest that physicians need to prescribe statins in patients at high risk of occlusive vascular events to further reduce LDL-C as much as possible in order to lower the incidence of vascular events. Regarding different types of statins, atorvastatin and rosuvastatin decrease blood total cholesterol and LDL-C in a linear dose-related manner over the commonly prescribed dose range (10–80 mg for atorvastatin and 10–40 mg for rosuvastatin). Based on an informal comparison, rosuvastatin is more than 3-fold more potent than atorvastatin (Adams et al., 2014, 2015).

What Is the Optimal Duration for Statin Treatment?

Prolonged follow-up in the HPS reported that a reduction of about a quarter in vascular mortality and morbidity – produced by an average 1 mmol/L reduction in LDL-C with 5 years of statin therapy – persisted largely unchanged during the subsequent 6 years. Moreover, no adverse effects on particular causes of non-vascular mortality or major morbidity (including site-specific cancers) emerged during the 11 year follow-up (Heart Protection Study Collaborative Group, 2011).

These findings support prompt initiation and long-term statin treatment for patients at increased risk of vascular events. In clinical practice, statins are underused, and poor patient adherence to a medication regimen can affect the success of lipid-lowering treatment. A meta-analysis demonstrates that intensification of patient care interventions (e.g. electronic reminders, pharmacist-led interventions, healthcare professional education of patients) improves short-term (OR 1.93, 95% CI: 1.29–2.88) and long-term (OR 2.87, 95% CI: 1.91–4.29) medication adherence, as well as total cholesterol and LDL-C levels (van Driel et al., 2016).

Inhibition of Pro-protein Convertase Subtilisin/kexin Type 9 (PCSK9)

Inhibition of pro-protein convertase subtilisin/kexin type 9 (PCSK9), a novel therapeutic agent for the treatment of hypercholesterolaemia, has been studied for its LDL-C lowering effects. A meta-analysis reported that both evolocumab and alirocumab were safe and well-tolerated, and both antibodies substantially reduced LDL-C levels by over 50%, increased the HDL-C levels, and resulted in favourable changes in other lipids (Zhang et al., 2015).

A meta-analysis included 20 studies with data on 67,237 participants: 12 trials randomized participants to alirocumab, 3 trials to bococizumab, 1 to RG7652, and 4 to evolocumab. Compared with placebo, PCSK9 inhibitors decreased LDL-C by 53.86% (95% CI: 58.64–49.08) at 24 weeks; compared with ezetimibe, PCSK9 inhibitors decreased LDL-C by 30.20% (95% CI: 34.18–26.23); and compared with ezetimibe and statins, PCSK9 inhibitors decreased LDL-C by 39.20% (95% CI: 56.15–22.26). Compared with placebo, PCSK9 inhibitors decreased the risk of cardiovascular events, with a risk difference of 0.91% (OR 0.86, 95% CI: 0.80–0.92). Compared with ezetimibe and statins, PCSK9 inhibitors appeared to have a stronger protective effect on cardiovascular risk, although with considerable uncertainty (OR 0.45, 95% CI: 0.27–0.75). No data were available for the ezetimibe-only comparison. Compared with placebo, PCSK9 inhibitors probably had little or no effect on mortality (OR 1.02, 95% CI: 0.91–1.14). Compared with placebo, PCSK9 inhibitors increased the risk of any adverse events (OR 1.08, 95% CI: 1.04–1.12). Similar effects were observed for the comparison of ezetimibe and statins (OR 1.18, 95% CI: 1.05–1.34). Clinical event data were unavailable for the ezetimibe-only comparison (Schmidt et al., 2017).

In the randomized FOURIER trial, inhibition of PCSK9 with subcutaneous injections of evolocumab, on a background of statin therapy, lowered LDL-C levels to a median of 30 mg per decilitre (0.78 mmol per litre) and reduced the risk of cardiovascular events. Overall, 19% of patients in the FOURIER study had a prior history of non-haemorrhagic stroke (n = 5337). In this subgroup analysis, stroke patients treated with evolocumab experienced a 56% mean reduction in LDL-C levels, compared with placebo (median LDL-C level of 29 mg/dL for patients on evolocumab versus median LDL-C of 89 mg/dL for placebo; $P < 0.001$). In this same subgroup analysis, the hazard ratio associated with evolocumab compared with placebo for the composite primary endpoint, which included hospitalization for unstable angina, coronary revascularization, heart attack, stroke, or cardiovascular death, was 0.85 (95% CI: 0.72–1.00; $P = 0.047$). Moreover, there were no significant differences in the overall rate of adverse events. (Sabatine et al., 2017).

Comments

Interpretation of the Evidence and Implications for Clinicians

Whether increased serum cholesterol levels are a risk factor for stroke remains controversial. However, several clinical trials have reported that statins significantly reduce stroke risk in vascular disease patients, including patients with prior stroke. It is not known, however, whether these findings are associated only with the cholesterol reduction effect of statins or to other effects, including those of a pleiotropic nature, such as improved endothelial function, decreased platelet aggregability, and reduced vascular inflammation.

Large-scale evidence from RCTs demonstrates clearly that, after a somewhat smaller risk reduction in the first year of treatment, statin therapy reduces the risk of major vascular events in many different types of patients (lower and higher risk, women and men, older and younger) during each subsequent year by about one-quarter for each mmol/L reduction in LDL-C (Collins et al., 2016).

In the secondary prevention of non-cardioembolic stroke, a reduction of LDL-C by statins was also reported to significantly reduce the relative risk of recurrent stroke by about 16%.

The use of statins has never been reported to increase the risk of haemorrhagic stroke in primary prevention or cancer. Yet, statins need to be further investigated in secondary prevention of stroke for their possible association in triggering cerebral bleedings.

Implications for Research

The benefit–risk ratio of statin therapy in symptomatic cerebrovascular disease patients could be improved if high-risk haemorrhage patients were better identified (e.g. presence of leucoaraiosis, cerebral microbleeds on MRI, multi-lacunes, and additional clinical features such as hypertension and alcohol abuse) for those for whom treatment is not suited or pursued at lower doses.

Another issue is whether statins are effective for secondary prevention of stroke in the subgroups excluded from the SPARCL study: very elderly, cardioembolic stroke, disabling stroke, and uncontrolled hypertension patients. Furthermore, trial results suggest that physicians need to prescribe statins in high-risk patients to reduce LDL-C as much as possible in order to lower the risk of vascular events. The Treat Stroke to Target trial recently reported that after an atherosclerotic ischaemic stroke or TIA, patients who were treated to a target LDL-C level of less than 70 mg/dL had a lower risk of subsequent cardiovascular events than those who had a target of 90 mg/dL to 110 mg/dL. Specifically, the composite primary endpoint (stroke, myocardial infarction, or vascular death) occurred in 8.5% of the lower target group and in 10.9% in the higher target group (adjusted HR 0.78; 95% CI 0.61–0.98, p=0.04). The incidence of intracranial haemorrhage and newly diagnosed diabetes did not differ significantly between the two groups (Amarenco et al. 2020).

As for inhibitors of PCSK9, it has been reported that they may reduce the overall rate of cardiovascular events. However, studies with long-term follow-up are needed, especially to further investigate them in patients with history of either stroke or TIA.

Summary

Although higher plasma cholesterol concentrations have not been reported to be associated with increased stroke risk, a lowering of the concentrations has been reported to decrease this risk.

This decrease can be achieved with statins, which are well-tolerated, provided they are not given to patients with active liver or muscle diseases.

Statin treatment in addition to a healthy lifestyle is recommended for the primary prevention of ischaemic stroke in patients with pre-existing coronary heart disease or other high-risk conditions such as diabetes and hypertension.

Statins with intensive lipid-lowering effects are recommended for their positive influence on reducing the risks of stroke and cardiovascular events for patients with prior ischaemic stroke or transient ischaemic attack (TIA) presumed to be of non-cardioembolic origin, even with an low-density lipoprotein-cholesterol (LDL-C) LDL-C level ≤100 mg/dL, with or without evidence of other clinical atherosclerotic cardiovascular diseases. The Treat Stroke to Target trial reported that among patients with an ischaemic stroke or TIA and evidence of atherosclerosis, those assigned a target LDL cholesterol level of less than 70 mg per decilitre with the use of statins and, if required, ezetimibe had a lower risk of a composite end point of major

cardiovascular events than those assigned to a target range of 90 mg to 110 mg per decilitre.

Despite the good safety profile of statins to date, further studies are needed to investigate their safety in patients with prior cerebral haemorrhage and whether they have a role in causing brain haemorrhage in secondary prevention of stroke.

The use of inhibitors of PCSK9 is advised as add-on therapy to statins for patients with a high cardiac risk not able to achieve an optimal LDL-C level. Nonetheless, future studies with long-term follow-up are needed to further investigate the efficacy and safety of this therapy in patients with history of stroke or TIA.

References

Acheson J, Hutchinson EC. (1972). Controlled trial of clofibrate in cerebral vascular disease. *Atherosclerosis*, **15**, 177–83.

Adams SP, Sekhon SS, Wright JM. (2014). Lipid-lowering efficacy of rosuvastatin. *Cochrane Database Syst Rev*, 11. CD010254.

Adams SP, Tsang M, Wright JM. (2015). Lipid-lowering efficacy of atorvastatin. *Cochrane Database Syst Rev*, 3. CD008226

Amarenco P, Kim JS, Labreuche J, et al. (2020). A comparison of two LDL cholesterol targets after ischemic stroke. *N Engl J Med*, **382**, 9–19.

Amarenco P, Labreuche J. (2009). Lipid management in the prevention of stroke: review and updated meta-analysis of statins for stroke prevention. *Lancet Neurol*, **8**, 453–63.

Battaggia A, Donzelli A, Font M, Molteni D, Galvano A. (2015). Clinical efficacy and safety of ezetimibe on major cardiovascular endpoints: systematic review and meta-analysis of randomized controlled trials. *PLoS ONE*, **10**, e0124587.

Bays H. (2006). Statin safety: an overview and assessment of the data – 2005. *Am J Cardiol*, **97**(suppl), 6 C–26 C.

Bezerra DC, Sharrett AR, Matsushita K, Gottesman RF, Shibata D, Mosley TH Jr, et al. (2012). Risk factors for lacunar subtype in the atherosclerosis risk in Communities (ARIC) Study. *Neurology*, **78**, 102–108.

Bhatia M, Howard SC, Clarke TG, Murphy MFG, Rothwell PM. (2004). Apo-lipoproteins predict ischaemic stroke in patients with a previous transient ischaemic attack. Presented at the World Stroke Congress, Vancouver, Canada.

Cholesterol Treatment Trialists' (CTT) Collaboration. (2005). Efficacy and safety of cholesterol lowering treatment: prospective meta-analysis of data from 90,056 participants in 14 randomised trials of statins. *Lancet*, **366**, 1267–78.

Cholesterol Treatment Trialists' (CTT) Collaboration. (2010). Efficacy and safety of more intensive lowering of LDL cholesterol: a meta-analysis of data from 170,000 participants in 26 randomized trials. *Lancet*, **376**, 1670–81.

Cholesterol Treatment Trialists' (CTT) Collaboration. (2012). The effect of lowering LDL-cholesterol with statin therapy in people at low risk of vascular disese: meta-analysis of individual data from 27 randomised trials. *Lancet*, **380**, 581–90.

Cholesterol Treatment Trialists' (CTT) Collaboration. (2015). Efficacy and safety of LDL-lowering therapy among men and women: meta-analysis of individual data from 174,000 participants in 27 randomised studies. *Lancet*, **385**, 1397–1405.

Collins R, Reith C, Emberson J, Armitage J, Baigent C, Blackwell L, et al. (2016). Interpretation of the evidence for the efficacy and safety of statin therapy. *Lancet*, **388**(10059), 2532–61.

Dale KM, Coleman CI, Henyan NN, Kluger J, White CM. (2006). Statins and cancer risk. *JAMA*, **295**, 74–80.

Di Mascio R, Marchioli R, Tognoni G. (2000). Cholesterol reduction and stroke occurrence: an overview of randomised clinical trials. *Cerebrovasc Dis*, **10**, 85–92.

Heart Protection Study Collaborative Group. (2011). Effects on 11-year mortality and morbidity of lowering LDL cholesterol with simvastatin for about 5 years in 20,536 high-risk individuals: a randomized controlled trial. *Lancet*, **578**, 2013–20.

Hopper L, Martin N, Abpelhamid A, Davey Smith G. (2015). Reduced in saturated fat intake for cardiovascular disease. *Cochrane Database Syst Rev*, 6. CD011737.

HPS2-THRIVE Collaborative Group. (2014). Effects of extended-release niacin with laropiprant in high-risk patients. *N Engl J Med*, **371**, 203–12.

HPS3/TIMI55–REVEAL Collaborative Group. (2017). Effects of anacetrapib in patients with atherosclerotic vascular disease. *N Engl J Med*, **377**(13), 1217–27

Imamura T, Doi Y, Arima H, Yonemoto K, Hata J, Kubo M, et al. (2009). LDL-cholesterol and the development of stroke subtypes and coronary heart disease in a general Japanese population. *Stroke*, **40**, 382–8.

Keene D, Price C, Shun-Shin MJ, Francis DP. (2014). Effect on cardiovascular risk of high density lipoprotein targeted drug treatment niacin, fibrates, and CEPT inhibitors: meta-analysis of randomized controlled trials including 117,411 patients. *BMJ*, **349**, 1–14.

Koren-Morag N, Tanne D, Graff E, Goldbourt U, for the Bezafibrate Infarction Prevention Study Group. (2002). Low- and high-density lipoprotein cholesterol and ischemic cerebrovascular disease. The Bezafibrate Infarction Prevention Registry. *Arch Int Med*, **162**, 993–9.

Law MR, Wald NJ, Rudnicka AR. (2003). Quantifying effect of statins on low density lipoprotein cholesterol, ischaemic

heart disease and stroke: systematic review and meta-analysis. *BMJ*, **326**, 1423–9.

Leppala JM, Virtamo J, Fogelholm R, Albanes D, Heinonen OP. (1999). Different risk factors for different stroke subtypes. *Stroke*, **30**, 2535–40.

Lewington S, Whitelock G, Clarke R, Sherliker P, Emberson J, Halsey J, et al. (2007). Blood cholesterol and vascular mortality by age, sex, and blood pressure: a meta-analysis of individual data from 61 prospective studies with 55,000 vascular deaths. *Lancet*, **370**, 1829–39.

Lp-PLA$_2$ Studies Collaboration. (2010). Lipoprotein-associated phospholipase A$_2$ and risk of coronary disease, stroke and mortality: collaborative analysis of 32 prospective studies. *Lancet*, **375**, 1536–44.

Manktelow B, Gillies C, Potter JF. (2002). Interventions in the management of serum lipids for preventing stroke recurrence. *Cochrane Database Syst Rev*, 3. CD002091. doi:10.1002/14651858.CD002091.

McKinney JS, Kostis WJ. (2012). Statin therapy and risk of intracerebral hemorrhage. A meta-analysis of 31 randomized controlled trials. *Stroke*, **43**, 2149–56.

Nagasawa S, Okamura T, Iso H, Tamakoshi A, Yarada M, Watanabe M, et al. (2012). Relation between serum total cholesterol level and cardiovascular disease stratified by sex and age group: a pooled analysis of 65,594 individuals from cohort studies in Japan. *J Am Heart Assoc*, 1, e001974.

Orozco-Beltran D, Gil-Guillen VF, Redon J, Martin-Moreno JM, Pallares-Carratala V, Navarro-Perez J, et al.; ESCARVAL Study Group. (2017). Lipid profile, cardiovascular disease and mortality in a Mediterranean high-risk population: the ESCARVAL-RISK study. *PLoS One*, **12**(10), e0186196.

Paciaroni M, Hennerici M, Agnelli G, Bogousslavsky J. (2007). Statins and stroke prevention. *Cerebrovasc Dis*, **24**, 170–82.

Peto R, Collins R. (2018). Trust the blinded randomized evidence that statin therapy rarely causes symptomatic side effects. *Circulation*, **138**(15), 1499–1501.

Pikula A, Belser AS, Wang J, Himali JJ, Kelly-Haynes M, Kase CS, et al. (2015). Lipid and lipoprotein measurement and the risk of ischemic vascular events. *Framingham Study. Neurology*, **84**, 472–9.

Plehn JF, Davis BR, Sacks FM, Rouleau JL, Pfeffer MA, Bernstein V, et al. (1999). Reduction of stroke incidence after myocardial infarction with pravastatin: the Cholesterol and Recurrent Events (CARE) study. The CARE Investigators. *Circulation*, **99**, 216–23.

Preiss D, Seshasai SR, Welsh P, Murphy SA, Ho JE, Waters DD, et al. (2011). Risk of incident diabetes with intensive-dose compared with moderate-dose statin therapy: a meta-analysis. *JAMA*, **305**, 2556–64.

Prospective Studies Collaboration. (1995). Cholesterol, diastolic blood pressure, and stroke: 13,000 strokes in 450,000 people in 45 prospective cohorts. *Lancet*, **346**, 1647–53.

Sabatine MS, Giugliano RP, Keech AC, Honarpour N, Wiviott SD, Murphy SA, et al.; FOURIER Steering Committee and Investigators. (2017). Evolocumab and clinical outcomes in patients with cardiovascular disease. *N Engl J Med*, **376**(18), 1713–22.

Sabatine MS, Wiviott SD, Im K, Murphy SA, Giugliano RP. (2018). Efficacy and safety of further lowering of low-density lipoprotein cholesterol in patients starting with very low levels: a meta-analysis. *JAMA Cardiol*, **3**(9), 823–8.

Sattar N, Preiss D, Murray HM, Welsh P, Buckley BM, de Craen AJ, et al. (2010). Statins and risk of incident diabetes: a collaborative meta-analysis of randomized statin trials. *Lancet*, **375**, 735–42.

Savarese G, De Ferrari GM, Rosano GM, Perrone-Filardi P. (2015). Safety and efficacy of ezetimibe: a meta-analysis. *Int J Cardiol*, **10**(201), 247–52.

Schandelmaier S, Briel M, Saccilotto R, Olu KK, Arpagaus A, Hemkens LG, et al. (2017). Niacin for primary and secondary prevention of cardiovascular events. *Cochrane Database Syst Rev*, 6. CD009744.

Silverman MG, Ference BA, Im K, Wiviott SD, Giugliano RP, Grundy SM, et al. (2016). Association between lowering ldl-c and cardiovascular risk reduction among different therapeutic interventions: a systematic review and meta-analysis. *JAMA*, **316**(12), 1289–97.

Simons LA, Simons J, Friedlander Y, McCallum J. (2001). Cholesterol and other lipids predict CHD and ischaemic stroke in the elderly, but only in those below 70 years. *Atherosclerosis*, **159**, 201–08.

SPARCL Investigators. (2006). High-dose atorvastatin after stroke or transient ischemic attack. *N Engl J Med*, **355**, 549–59.

Tanaka T, Tomonori O. (2012). Blood cholesterol level and risk of stroke in Community-based or Worksite cohort studies: a review of Japanese Cohort Studies in the past 20 years. *Keio J Med*, **81**, 79–88.

Taylor F, Huffman MD, Macedo AF, Moore TH, Burke M, Davey Smith G, et al. (2013). Statins for the primary prevention of cardiovascular disease. *Cochrane Database Syst Rev*, 1. CD004816.

Teng M, Lin L, Zhao YJ, Khoo AL, Davis BR, Yong QW. (2015). Statins for primary prevention of cardiovascular disease in elderly patients: systematic review and meta-analysis. *Drugs Aging*, **32**(8), 649–61.

Thompson PD, Clarkson P, Karas RH. (2003). Statin associated myopathy. *JAMA*, **289**, 1681–90.

van Driel ML, Morledge MD, Ulep R, Shaffer JP, Davies P, Deichmann R. (2016). Interventions to improve adherence to lipid-lowering medication. *Cochrane Database Syst Rev*, 12. CD004371.

Veterans Administration Cooperative Study Group. (1973). The treatment of cerebrovascular disease with Clofibrate. Final report of the Veterans Administration Cooperative Study of Atherosclerosis, Neurology Section. *Stroke*, **4**, 684–93.

Wang D, Liu B, Tao W, Hao Z, Liu M. (2015). Fibrates for secondary prevention of cardiovascular disease and stroke. *Cochrane Database Syst Rev*, 10. CD009580.

Wang X, Dong Y, Qi X, Huang C, Hou L. (2013). Cholesterol levels and risk of hemorrhagic stroke. A systematic review and meta-analysis. *Stroke*, **44**, 1833–9.

White HD, Simes RJ, Anderson NE, Hankey GJ, Watson JDG, Hunt D, et al. (2000). Pravastatin therapy and the risk of stroke. *N Engl J Med*, **343**, 317–26.

Zhan S, Tang M, Liu F, Xia P, Shu M, Wu X. (2018). Ezetimibe for the prevention of cardiovascular disease and all-cause mortality events. *Cochrane Database Syst Rev*, 11. CD012502.

Zhang XL, Zhu QQ, Zhu L, Chen JZ, Chen QH, Li GN, et al. (2015). Safety and efficacy of anti-PCSK9 antibodies: a meta-analysis of 25 randomized, controlled trials. *BMC Med*, **13**, 123. doi:10.1186/s12916.

Zhang Y, Tuomilehto J, Jousilahti P, Wang Y, Antikainen R, Hu G. (2012). Total and high-density lipoprotein cholesterol and stroke risk. *Stroke*, **4**, 1768–74.

Prevention of Stroke by Modification of Additional Vascular and Lifestyle Risk Factors

Amytis Towfighi
Jeffrey L. Saver

Diabetes Mellitus and Glucose Intolerance

Evidence

Risk Factors for Stroke

Diabetes prevalence is increasing in low-, middle-, and high-income countries, affecting 451 million people worldwide (Whiting et al., 2011), and is a well-established risk factor for ischaemic stroke. The extent to which diabetes affects stroke risk varies by age, sex, and race. In the Greater Cincinnati/Northern Kentucky Stroke Study, the risk ratio for ischaemic stroke in patients younger than 65 years of age was 5.2 (95% confidence interval [CI]: 3.6–6.9) for black people compared with 12.0 (95% CI: 8.8–15.2) for white. Among those 65 years or older, the risk ratio was 2.1 (95% CI: 1.5–2.7) for black people and 2.7 (95% CI: 2.1–3.4) for white (Khoury et al., 2013). A systematic review of 64 cohort studies representing 775,385 individuals and 12,539 strokes revealed that the pooled maximum adjusted risk ratio (RR) of stroke associated with diabetes was 2.28 (95% CI: 1.93–2.69) in women and 1.83 (95% CI: 1.60–2.08) in men. Compared with men with diabetes, women with diabetes had a 27% greater RR for stroke when baseline differences in other major cardiovascular risk factors were taken into account, RR 1.27 (95% CI: 1.10–1.46) (Peters et al., 2014). In the INTERSTROKE case–control study of 26,919 participants from 32 countries, among 10 common vascular risk factors, diabetes contributed to 7.5% (95% CI: 5.0–11.1%) of all ischaemic strokes (population attributable risk) (O'Donnell et al., 2016). Diabetes is also an independent risk factor for stroke recurrence: in a meta-analysis of 18 studies involving 43,899 participants with prior stroke, the increased hazard of recurrent

stroke associated with diabetes was hazard ratio (HR) 1.45 (95% CI: 1.32–1.59) (Shou et al., 2015).

Pre-diabetes is also associated with greater stroke risk. A meta-analysis of 15 prospective cohort studies including 760,925 participants revealed that when pre-diabetes was defined as fasting glucose 110–125 mg/dL (5 studies), the adjusted relative risk for stroke was 1.21 (95% CI: 1.02–1.44; $p = 0.03$) (Lee et al., 2012).

The prevalence of diabetes among stroke survivors in the United States has been increasing. Data from the United States Nationwide Inpatient Sample revealed that from 1997 to 2006, the absolute number of acute ischaemic stroke hospitalizations declined by 17%; however, the absolute number of acute ischaemic stroke hospitalizations with comorbid diabetes rose by 27% (from 97,577 [20%] to 124,244 [(30%]). Factors independently associated with higher odds of diabetes in acute ischaemic stroke patients were black or 'other' (versus white) race, congestive heart failure, peripheral vascular disease, and history of myocardial infarction, renal disease, or hypertension (Towfighi et al., 2012).

Effective Strategies to Reduce the Risk of Stroke in Diabetics

Effective strategies to reduce the risk of stroke in diabetics include:

1. Preventing or delaying the onset of diabetes of patients with prediabetes. A meta-analysis of randomized controlled trials (RCTs) found that diet, exercise, and pharmacological interventions reduced diabetes onset (RR 0.83, 95% CI: 0.80–0.86), and reduced fatal and nonfatal strokes (RR 0.76, 95% CI: 0.58–0.99) (Hopper et al., 2011).

2. Preventing atherogenesis by optimally controlling risk factors such as high blood pressure (Emdin et al., 2015), high blood cholesterol (Cholesterol Treatment Trialists, et al., 2008; Sabatine et al.,

2017), high blood glucose (Brunstrom and Carlberg, 2016), and smoking (Pan et al., 2015).

3. Preventing atherothrombosis, should an atherosclerotic plaque become eroded or rupture, with optimal antiplatelet therapy (Antithrombotic Trialists, 2002; Antithrombotic Trialists et al., 2009).

4. Recanalizing a cervical carotid artery with atherosclerotic stenosis that is moderate–severe and symptomatic or severe and asymptomatic by means of carotid stenting or endarterectomy (Rothwell et al., 2003; Moresoli et al., 2017).

Blood Glucose Control

Randomized trials have shown that more intensive treatment of hyperglycaemia results in fewer microvascular complications (retinopathy and renal damage) of diabetes type 2, but has limited impact upon macrovascular complications (Marso et al., 2010; Zoungas et al., 2017). A meta-analysis of 4 RCTs including 27,544 patients revealed that those randomized to intensive glucose control did not have a reduction in stroke risk compared with those with conventional glucose control; however, there was a 14% reduction in non-fatal myocardial infarction (odds ratio [OR] 0.86, 95% CI: 0.77–0.97) (Marso et al., 2010).

Blood Pressure Control in Diabetics

A meta-analysis of 40 RCTs of blood pressure (BP) lowering among 100,354 participants with diabetes revealed a lower risk of stroke (RR 0.73, 95% CI: 0.64–0.83; absolute risk reduction [ARR] 4.06, 95% CI: 2.53–5.40) (Emdin et al., 2015). While benefits of blood pressure lowering in diabetic patients with systolic blood pressure (SBP) >140 mm Hg are present for all major cardiovascular and stroke endpoints, differential benefits and harms accrue with blood pressure lowering therapy for patients with SBP <140 mm Hg. Using lower targets, such as SBP <130 mm Hg, tends to further reduce stroke events, but tends to increase cardiovascular mortality. In a meta-analysis of 49 trials of blood pressure lowering enrolling 73,738 diabetic patients, among patients whose baseline SBP was <140 mm Hg before randomization to more aggressive antihypertensive therapy, stroke events had RR of 0.81 (95% CI: 0.53–1.22) but cardiovascular mortality had RR of 1.15 (95% CI: 1.00–1.32 (Brunstrom and Carlberg, 2016). Similarly, regardless of entry SBP level, among patients during trial conduct whose attained SBP on more aggressive antihypertensive therapy was <130 mm Hg, stroke events had RR of 0.65

(95% CI: 0.42–0.99) but cardiovascular mortality had RR of 1.26 (95% CI: 0.89–1.77).

Cholesterol Lowering in Diabetics

Diet and pharmacological cholesterol-lowering have both shown evidence of benefit in reducing stroke risk in patients with prediabetes and diabetes. It is important to note that statins are associated with a small increase in diabetes incidence; in a meta-analysis of 13 trials enrolling 91,140 nondiabetic patients, statins increased diabetes onset, OR 1.09 (95% CI: 1.02–1.17) (Sattar et al., 2010). However, the absolute effect was small, an increase of 0.49% over 5 years of therapy, and is outweighed by the benefit in averting cardiovascular and neurovascular events. In a meta-analysis of 14 trials enrolling 90,056 patients, statins substantially reduced major vascular events and stroke among both diabetics and nondiabetics (Cholesterol Treatment Trialists et al., 2008). In diabetics, the effect on major vascular events was RR 0.79 (95% CI: 0.72–0.86), with an absolute reduction of 4.2% over 5 years; the effect on strokes was RR 0.83 (95% CI: 0.77–0.88), with an absolute reduction of 1.2% over 5 years. Pro-protein convertase subtilisin/kexin type 9 (PCSK9) inhibitors added to statin therapy in diabetic patients further reduce the frequency of major vascular events, including stroke. In the FOURIER trial, among 11,031 patients with diabetes, allocation to a PCSK9 inhibitor reduced the composite of cardiovascular death, myocardial infarction, and stroke, HR 0.82 (95% CI: 0.72–0.93), with a homogeneous effect on the component stroke endpoint, HR 0.79 (95% CI: 0.62–1.01) (Sabatine et al., 2017).

Comment

Early detection of diabetes and prediabetes, followed by careful control of glycaemia and atherosclerotic vascular risk factors to optimal levels are likely to reduce stroke and other major vascular events (Fox et al., 2015). In diabetics, rigorous long-term control of blood pressure and blood cholesterol is essential to reduce stroke risk. Control of blood glucose levels to a moderate target, glycosylated haemoglobin ≤7%, also is likely to reduce future stroke incidence; more aggressive control to intensified targets, though beneficial for retinal and renal health, is not likely to confer substantial additional reduction of incident stroke.

Hormone Replacement Therapy

Evidence

Although prothrombotic, oestrogen has other effects that potentially could reduce vascular events, including improving lipid profiles, enhancing endothelial function, and improving insulin sensitivity. Large observational studies suggested that, among postmenopausal women, hormone replacement therapy (HRT) was associated with reduced frequency of stroke and other vascular events. However, RCT data indicate that the use of oestrogen plus progestin, as well as oestrogen alone, increases stroke risk in postmenopausal, generally healthy women and provides no protection for postmenopausal women with established coronary heart disease (CHD) and recent stroke or transient ischaemic attack (TIA). One systematic review of 28 RCTs assessing the effect of HRT on subsequent risk of stroke in a total of 39,769 subjects showed that random assignment to HRT was associated with a significant increase in total stroke (OR 1.29, 95% CI: 1.13–1.47), non-fatal stroke (OR 1.23, 95% CI: 1.06–1.44), stroke leading to death or disability (OR 1.56, 95% CI: 1.11–2.20), and ischaemic stroke (OR 1.29, 95% CI: 1.06–1.56). HRT was not associated with haemorrhagic stroke (OR 1.07, 95% CI: 0.65–1.75) (Bath and Gray, 2005).

It appears that the timing of HRT initiation may play a critical role in the effect of HRT. Another meta-analysis of 19 trials enrolling 40,410 post-menopausal women examined the timing of HRT start, finding a beneficial effect on coronary disease events when HRT was started less than 10 years after menopause onset, but not later. However, there was no heterogeneity for the increased risk of stroke in both time frames: within 10 years of menopause, RR 1.37, 95% CI: 0.89–2.34, versus more than 10 years after menopause, RR 1.21, 95% CI: 1.06–1.38 (Boardman et al., 2015) (Figure 17.1) Venous thromboembolism was also increased in both time frames.

Comment

There is reasonably strong evidence from RCTs that HRT increases the risk of stroke in postmenopausal women with or without a history of vascular disease. Therefore, long-term oestrogen or oestrogen plus progestin is not indicated as a long-term stroke prevention therapy. However, the risks of HRT are small in absolute terms for short duration therapy. Accordingly, HRT remains a suitable option for women with bothersome menopausal symptoms, but they should understand that there are some risks involved and should regularly re-assess their need for treatment with their clinician. It is prudent to use the lowest effective dose for the shortest period.

Hormonal Contraceptive Use

Evidence

There have been no large RCTs of oral, transdermal, or vaginal hormonal contraceptive use versus non-hormonal barrier methods, so high-level evidence is lacking. But there is a large body of evidence from observational studies, though these are prone to bias and confounding, as highlighted in Chapter 2. When initial observational studies indicated increased risk of stroke, myocardial infarction, and venous thrombosis with early oestrogen and combined oestrogen and progestin contraceptives, later generation agents were developed with lower oral oestrogen doses, progestin-only formulations, and different variants of hormonal molecules, seeking to reduce thrombotic risk. Oestrogen doses declined from 50 µg (first generation) to 20–35 µg (second and later generations).

Several meta-analyses of cohort and case–control studies have shown that oral contraceptive (OC) therapy increases the risk of ischaemic stroke by 1.5- to 3.0-fold, with a lesser but still significant risk associated with later generation agents. A meta-analysis of 16 case–control and cohort studies between 1960 and 1999 estimated a 2.75-fold increased odds (95% CI: 2.24–3.38) of stroke associated with OC use (Gillum et al., 2000). A second meta-analysis of 20 studies published between 1970 and 2000 found no increased risk of stroke in the cohort studies but an increased risk with OC use in case-control studies (OR 2.13, 95% CI: 1.59–2.86) (Chan et al., 2004). Only 2 of the 4 cohort studies reported strokes by subtype, and risk was increased for ischaemic but not haemorrhagic strokes. A more recent meta-analysis of 18 case–control and cohort studies between 1970 and 2014 found an overall increased risk of first-ever ischaemic stroke, OR 2.47 (95% CI: 2.04–2.99). The risk of ischaemic stroke among current OCP users declined with decreasing oestrogen dose: oestrogen doses of ≥50 µg had OR 3.28 (95% CI: 2.49–4.32); 30–40 µg had OR 1.75 (95% CI: 1.61–1.89), and 20 µg had OR 1.56 (95% CI: 1.36–1.79) (Xu et al., 2015) A similar oestrogen dose-related pattern was seen in a meta-analysis evaluating the composite outcome of stroke or myocardial infarction (Roach et al., 2015)(Figure 17.2).

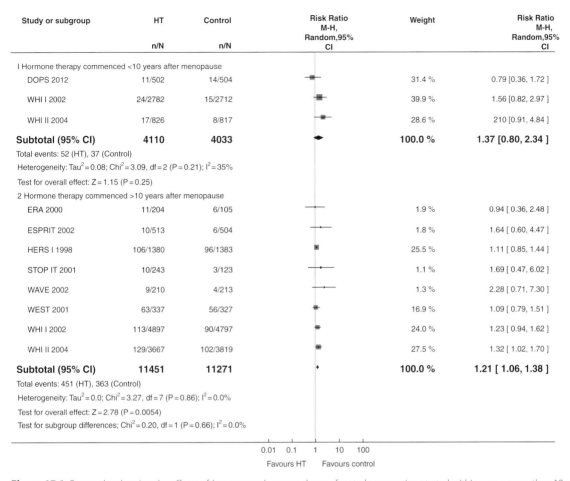

Study or subgroup	HT	Control	Risk Ratio M-H, Random,95% CI	Weight	Risk Ratio M-H, Random,95% CI
	n/N	n/N			
1 Hormone therapy commenced <10 years after menopause					
DOPS 2012	11/502	14/504		31.4 %	0.79 [0.36, 1.72]
WHI I 2002	24/2782	15/2712		39.9 %	1.56 [0.82, 2.97]
WHI II 2004	17/826	8/817		28.6 %	210 [0.91, 4.84]
Subtotal (95% CI)	**4110**	**4033**		**100.0 %**	**1.37 [0.80, 2.34]**
Total events: 52 (HT), 37 (Control)					
Heterogeneity: Tau^2=0.08; Chi^2=3.09, df=2 (P=0.21); I^2=35%					
Test for overall effect: Z=1.15 (P=0.25)					
2 Hormone therapy commenced >10 years after menopause					
ERA 2000	11/204	6/105		1.9 %	0.94 [0.36, 2.48]
ESPRIT 2002	10/513	6/504		1.8 %	1.64 [0.60, 4.47]
HERS I 1998	106/1380	96/1383		25.5 %	1.11 [0.85, 1.44]
STOP IT 2001	10/243	3/123		1.1 %	1.69 [0.47, 6.02]
WAVE 2002	9/210	4/213		1.3 %	2.28 [0.71, 7.30]
WEST 2001	63/337	56/327		16.9 %	1.09 [0.79, 1.51]
WHI I 2002	113/4897	90/4797		24.0 %	1.23 [0.94, 1.62]
WHI II 2004	129/3667	102/3819		27.5 %	1.32 [1.02, 1.70]
Subtotal (95% CI)	**11451**	**11271**		**100.0 %**	**1.21 [1.06, 1.38]**
Total events: 451 (HT), 363 (Control)					
Heterogeneity: Tau^2=0.0; Chi^2=3.27, df=7 (P=0.86); I^2=0.0%					
Test for overall effect: Z=2.78 (P=0.0054)					
Test for subgroup differences: Chi^2=0.20, df=1 (P=0.66); I^2=0.0%					

```
          0.01  0.1   1   10   100
          Favours HT    Favours control
```

Figure 17.1 Forest plot showing the effects of *hormone replacement therapy* for *stroke prevention,* started within versus more than 10 years after menopause, among 22,722 patients.
Reproduced from Boardman et al. (2015), with permission from the authors and John Wiley & Sons Limited. Copyright Cochrane Library.

The risk of ischaemic stroke was not increased with progestin-only agents, OR 0.99 (95% CI: 0.71–1.37).

Risk factors for stroke on hormonal contraceptives include older age, cigarette smoking, hypertension, migraine headaches, obesity, and hypercholesterolaemia (Chang et al., 1999; Kemmeren et al., 2002; Xu et al., 2015). In addition, an increased risk of stroke was seen in those with heterozygosity for factor V Leiden (OR 11.2, 95% CI: 4.2–29.0), the methyltetrahydrofolate reductase (MTHFR) 677TT mutation (OR 5.4, 95% CI: 2.4–12.0), β2 glycoprotein-1 antibodies (OR 2.3, 95% CI: 1.4–3.7), lupus anticoagulant (OR 43.1, 95% CI: 12.2–152.0), and von Willebrand factor levels >90th percentile (OR 11.4, 95% CI: 5.2–25.3) (Chang et al., 1999; Kemmeren et al., 2002). Although there is an increased risk of thromboembolism in women with these hypercoagulable states, the absolute risk is low; therefore, routine screening is not recommended. Selective screening based on prior personal or family history of venous thromboembolism is more cost-effective than universal screening in women who initiate OC (Wu et al., 2006).

Comment

The available evidence suggests that oestrogen-containing hormonal contraceptives are a risk factor for ischaemic but not haemorrhagic stroke. The risk of ischaemic stroke increases with higher doses of oestrogen. With lower dose agents, the relative risk is about 1.75-fold, equivalent to a small absolute increase in risk from about 3.5 to about 6.1 per 100,000 women per year (Nightingale and Farmer, 2004). Of note, this risk is low compared with the absolute stroke risk of pregnancy, 34.2 per 100,000 deliveries (James et al. 2005).

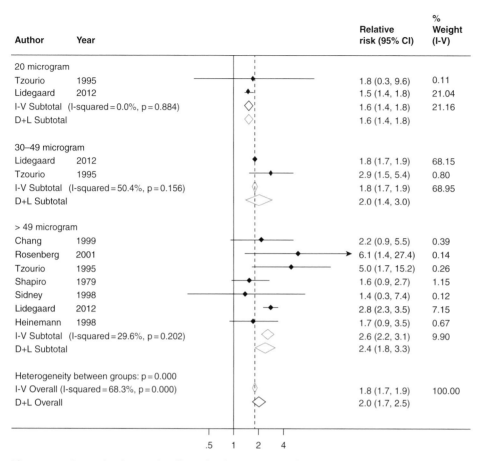

Figure 17.2 Forest plot showing the effects of *oral contraceptives of three oestrogen dose levels* on the composite of *myocardial infarction and stroke*.

Reproduced from Roach et al. (2015), with permission from John Wiley & Sons Limited. Copyright Cochrane Library.

Avoidance of oestrogen-containing contraceptives should be considered in women with additional risk factors, including older age, cigarette smoking, hypertension, migraine headaches, obesity, hypercholesterolaemia, and prior thromboembolic events. Progestin-only contraceptives do not appear to have increased stroke risk, and are a potential contraceptive option, as are barrier methods, for patients with risk factors for stroke on oestrogen-containing agents.

Tobacco Smoking

Evidence

Tobacco Smoking as a Risk Factor for Stroke

Observational studies suggest that tobacco smoking is a causal risk factor for ischaemic stroke and subarachnoid haemorrhage because the association is independent of other risk factors, consistent among different studies, dose-related, strong, and biologically plausible (Woodward et al., 2005; Bhat et al., 2008; Shah and Cole, 2010). A meta-analysis of 81 prospective cohort studies that included 3,980,359 individuals and 42,401 strokes revealed that smoking was an independent risk factor for stroke in both sexes (Peters et al., 2013). The risk of stroke associated with current smoking was RR 1.83 (95% CI: 1.58–2.12) for women and RR 1.67 (95% CI: 1.49–1.88) for men. The risk associated with being a former smoker versus never having smoked was RR 1.17 (95% CI: 1.12–1.22) for women and RR 1.08 (95% CI: 1.03–1.13) for men. Compared with never-smokers, the beneficial effects of quitting smoking among former smokers on stroke risk were similar between the sexes (RR 1.10, 95% CI: 0.99–1.22). In the INTERSTROKE international case–control study, among 10 common vascular risk factors, current smoking contributed to 15.1% (95% CI: 12.8–17.8%) of all ischaemic strokes (population attributable risk) (O'Donnell et al., 2016).

Secondhand Tobacco Smoke as a Risk Factor for Stroke

Exposure to secondhand tobacco smoke, also termed passive smoking or environmental tobacco smoke, increases the risk of stroke by approximately 1.25-fold, with a dose–response relationship (Lee and Forey, 2006; Oono et al., 2011). Data from the REasons for Geographic And Racial Differences in Stroke (REGARDS) study showed that the risk of stroke was increased among nonsmokers exposed to secondhand smoke in the prior year, HR 1.30 (95% CI: 1.02–1.67) (Malek et al., 2015). Analysis of participants in the US National Health and Nutrition Examination Surveys found a dose-dependent relationship between secondhand smoke exposure and all-cause mortality after stroke, with 10-year cumulative mortality rates of 39.0%, 40.7%, 58.3%, and 65.4% across increasing nicotinine quartiles (trend $p = 0.02$) (Lin et al., 2016).

Tobacco Smoking Cessation

There have been no RCTs wherein people have been randomized to 'continue smoking' or 'stop smoking', and observed for the risk of first-ever or recurrent stroke. And there likely never will be, as it would now be considered unethical given the strength of the observational evidence of the adverse health effects of smoking. Evidence from observational studies, however, suggests that quitting smoking is associated with a decreased risk of stroke, with risk declining to a substantially lower level 2–4 years after cessation (Kawachi et al., 1993; Peters et al., 2013; Epstein et al., 2017).

Health Provider Advice to Quit Tobacco Smoking

A systematic review identified 42 randomized trials, enrolling 31,000 smokers, of smoking cessation advice from a medical practitioner, in which abstinence was assessed at least 6 months after advice was first provided (Stead et al., 2013). In some trials, participants were identified as at risk for specified diseases (lung disease, diabetes, ischaemic heart disease), but most were from unselected populations. The most common setting for delivery of advice was primary care. Combined data from 28 RCTs showed that advice versus no advice (or usual care) increased the rate of quitting (8.0% vs 4.8%, RR 1.76, 95% CI: 1.58–1.96).

Among 15 trials comparing intensive versus minimal advice, an advantage of intensive advice was seen, RR 1.37 (95% CI: 1.20–1.56). Direct comparison RCTs also indicated greater efficacy of repeating advice at follow-up visits compared with advice at a single visit, RR 1.52 (95% CI: 1.08–2.14).

Nicotine Replacement Therapy

Gum, Patches, Nasal Spray, Tablets/Lozenges

A systematic review identified 150 randomized trials, including 117 enrolling over 50,000 patients in which nicotine replacement therapy (NRT) was compared with placebo or no treatment, and 28 which compared different doses or combinations of NRT (Stead et al., 2012). Allocation to NRT compared with control increased achievement of abstinence from smoking (17.3% vs 10.3%, RR 1.60, 95% CI: 1.53 to 1.68). The RR for different forms of NRT were: 1.49 (95% CI: 1.40–1.60) for gum; 1.64 (95% CI: 1.52–1.78) for patches; 1.90 (95% CI: 1.36–2.67) for inhalators; 2.02 (95% CI: 1.49–2.73) for nasal spray; and 1.95 (95% CI: 1.61–2.36) for nicotine sublingual tablets/lozenges. The effects of NRT were largely independent of the duration of therapy, intensity of behavioural support provided, or the setting in which the NRT was offered. In highly dependent smokers, there was a dose-related benefit of 4 mg gum compared with 2 mg gum (RR 1.85, 95% CI: 1.36–2.50), but weaker evidence of a benefit from higher doses of patch. Combining a nicotine patch with a rapid delivery form of NRT was more effective than a single type of NRT (RR 1.34, 95% CI: 1.18–1.51). Adverse effects of NRT include skin irritation from patches and irritation to the inside of the mouth from gum and tablets. There was no evidence that NRT increased the risk of myocardial infarction.

Electronic Cigarettes (vaping)

Electronic cigarettes (ECs) are electronic devices that heat a liquid – usually comprising propylene glycol and glycerol, with or without nicotine and flavours, stored in disposable or refillable cartridges or a reservoir – into an aerosol for inhalation. While concern exists about potential long-term effects of EC use, they may provide some benefit in reducing tobacco exposure among smokers. In a systematic meta-analysis, among 662 patients in 2 RCTs comparing ECs with nicotine versus ECs without nicotine, smokers allocated to ECs with nicotine were more likely to have abstained from smoking for at least 6 months (RR 2.29, 95% CI: 1.05–4.96) (McRobbie et al., 2014).

Nicotine Receptor Partial Agonist Therapy

The addictive properties of nicotine arise mainly from agonistic action at neuronal nicotinic acetylcholine receptors, stimulating release of brain mesolimbic dopamine. Pharmacological nicotine receptor partial agonists produce a moderate, sustained release of dopamine, counteracting both withdrawal symptoms from tobacco abstinence and reward from tobacco re-use. The most extensively tested agent is varenicline. A systematic meta-analysis of 31 trials of varenicline enrolling 13,891 patients found that tobacco abstinence was increased by both standard-dose varenicline (RR 2.24, 95% CI: 2.06–2.43; 27 trials, 12,625 people) and lower- or variable-dose varenicline (RR 2.08, 95% CI: 1.56–2.78; 4 trials, 1266 people) (Cahill et al., 2016). Although uncontrolled observational studies raised concerns, large subsequent randomized trials found that varenicline did not increase rates of agitation, suicidal behaviour, or cardiovascular events (Anthenelli et al., 2016; Cahill et al., 2016; Eisenberg et al., 2016; Benowitz et al., 2018).

Antidepressants for Tobacco Cessation

Bupropion is an aminoketone with dopaminergic and adrenergic actions, and an antagonist at the nicotinic acetylcholinergic receptor. Bupropion may aid smoking cessation by blocking nicotine effects, by relieving withdrawal, by reducing depressed mood, and by substituting for noradrenergic effects of nicotine. In a systematic meta-analysis of 44 RCTs enrolling 13,728 patients, bupropion increased long-term smoking cessation (RR 1.62, 95% CI: 1.49–1.76) (Hughes et al., 2014). Adverse effects with bupropion include insomnia, dry mouth, nausea, and, rarely (0.1%), seizures. Nortriptyline, a tricyclic with noradrenergic activity, may aid smoking cessation by reducing depressed mood and by substituting for noradrenergic effects of nicotine. In the same meta-analysis, among 6 RCTs enrolling 975 patients, nortriptyline increased long-term tobacco cessation (RR 2.03, 95% CI: 1.48–2.78) (Hughes et al., 2014). Adverse effects with nortriptyline at the relatively low doses (75–150 mg daily) used for smoking cessation include dry mouth, drowsiness, constipation, and, rarely, seizures.

Comparisons of Single and Combined Interventions

A systematic network meta-analysis of 267 RCTs of pharmacological interventions for smoking cessation in 101,804 smokers compared each therapy with the others and with placebo, both directly and indirectly (Cahill et al., 2013). The most effective single therapy was varenicline, which yielded predicted higher cessation rates than either NRT (OR 1.57, 95% credible interval [CredI]: 1.29–1.91) or bupropion (OR 1.59, 95% CredI: 1.29–1.96), while bupropion and NRT were equally effective (OR 0.99, 95% CredI: 0.86–1.13) (Figure 17.3). However, varenicline was not more effective than combined rapid delivery plus patch NRT (OR 1.06, 95% CredI: 0.75–1.48). Neither nortriptyline nor bupropion added to NRT increased quitting rates compared with NRT alone.

A meta-analysis of 47 trials enrolling more than 18,000 smokers found that adding more intensive behavioural support to pharmacotherapy, compared to pharmacotherapy with minimal behavioural support, mildly further increased tobacco cessation rates (RR 1.17, 95% CI: 1.11–1.24) (Stead et al., 2015).

Tobacco Cessation Interventions Specifically in Stroke Patients

Few RCTs of tobacco cessation interventions have been conducted specifically in stroke patients. A systematic review identified 4 RCTs enrolling a total of 354 stroke survivors (Edjoc et al., 2012). Different trials evaluated: (1) providing advice to patients and general practitioners on NRT for smoking cessation (1 trial); (2) stroke nurse specialist patient counselling (2 trials); and (3) NRT plus smoking cessation counselling. Though underpowered, the effect observed in these small trials was directionally homogeneous with the benefit observed in the much larger set of trials in primary prevention and mixed vascular disease populations: tobacco abstinence rates after allocation to an active smoking cessation intervention versus control were 23.9% versus 20.8% (RR 1.15, 95% CI: 0.78–1.70).

Comment

All persons who use tobacco in any form (cigarettes, pipes, cigars, chewing tobacco), in both primary and secondary stroke prevention settings, should be advised to stop. The risks of subsequent stroke decline substantially within 2–5 years of stopping.

Simple advice from a healthcare provider is modestly effective (and highly cost-effective) in facilitating smoking cessation. Repeated and sustained advice and behavioural support programmes are more effective than one-time counselling.

In addition, pharmacological therapies, including NRT (gum, transdermal patch, nasal spray, inhaler, or sublingual tablets), varenicline, or

Comparison		Odds ratio (95% credible interval)	No. of studies (direct comparisons)
NRT vs Placebo		1.84 (1.71 , 1.99)	119
Burpropion vs Placebo		1.82 (1.6 , 2.06)	36
Varenicline vs Placebo		2.88 (2.4 , 3.47)	15
Bupropion vs NRT		0.99 (0.86 , 1.13)	9
Varenicline vs NRT		1.57 (1.29 , 1.91)	0
Varenicline vs Bupropion		1.59 (1.29 , 1.96)	3

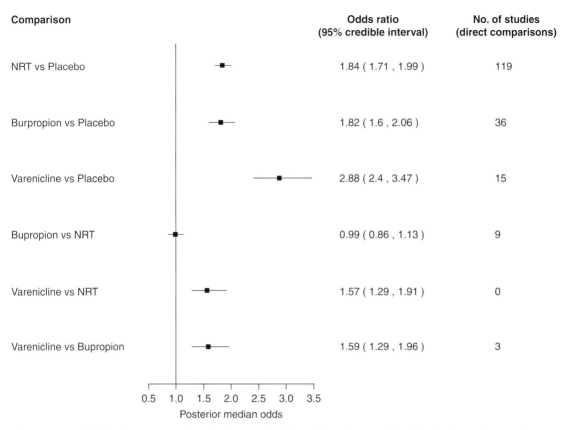

Figure 17.3 Probability of treatment ranking plot showing the effects of *three pharmacological therapies for smoking cessation.*
Reproduced from Cahill et al. (2013), with permission from John Wiley & Sons Limited. Copyright Cochrane Library.

bupropion, are effective for increasing smoking cessation rates in the short and long term. They increase quit rates by 1.5-fold to 2.25-fold. Among the pharmacological agents, the most effective approaches appear to be: (1) varenicline, and (2) combined NRT using fast-acting delivery systems plus a slower-release patch. Among NRT options, for patients who are particularly nicotine dependent, higher-dose, 4 mg gum is more effective than lower dose. In less highly dependent smokers, the different NRT preparations are comparable in efficacy, but nicotine patches offer greater convenience and minimal need for instruction. Inhalers and nasal sprays may be useful in patients with particularly severe nicotine craving, and combined patches and fast-acting forms of NRT are more effective than either alone. Bupropion is associated with a very low rate of seizure, and so is relatively contra-indicated in patients with a seizure history. Combining NRT with either varenicline or bupropion does not enhance cessation.

Combining counselling and behavioural interventions with drug treatments mildly increases cessation rates over drug therapy alone, and is recommended.

The role of ECs (vaping) with nicotine in tobacco cessation is at present uncertain. While associated with increased short-term smoking abstinence in 2 modest-sized RCTs, their long-term safety has not yet been fully established, and, more than other NRT methods, they may perpetuate behaviours and cultural triggers associated with smoking, potentially increasing risk of late relapse (Bhatnagar et al., 2014). They may be an option in patients who have been refractory to other tobacco abstinence interventions.

It is also reasonable to advise patients with stroke or TIA to avoid environmental smoke exposures (Kernan et al., 2014). Encouraging smoking partners and family members of patients to quit smoking may reduce the patient exposure to environmental tobacco smoke and reduce the risk of stroke or other serious vascular events for all family members.

Alcohol

Evidence

Risk Factor for Stroke

A meta-analysis of 27 prospective cohort studies reporting data on over 1.4 million individuals found that alcohol intake had a U-shaped curve relationship with ischaemic stroke and a J-shaped curve relationship with haemorrhagic stroke (Larsson et al., 2016). For ischaemic stroke, compared with no alcohol consumption, risk was reduced with light alcohol intake (less than 1 drink/day, RR 0.90, 95% CI: 0.85–0.95) and moderate alcohol intake (1–2 drinks/day, RR 0.92, 95% CI: 0.87–0.97), and increased with high alcohol intake (between 2 and 4 drinks/day, RR 1.08, 95% CI: 1.01–1.15) and heavy alcohol intake (more than 4 drinks/day, RR 1.14, 95% CI: 1.02–1.28). For intracerebral haemorrhage, compared with no alcohol consumption, risk was unchanged with light-to-moderate alcohol intake (<1 to 2 drinks/day, RR 0.95, 95% CI: 0.84–1.07) and increased with high-to-heavy alcohol intake (>2 drinks/day, RR 1.45, 95% CI: 1.18–1.78). Similarly, for subarachnoid haemorrhage, compared with no alcohol consumption, risk was unchanged with light-to-moderate alcohol intake (<1 to 2 drinks/day, RR 1.16, 95% CI: 0.98–1.37) and increased with high-to-heavy alcohol intake (>2 drinks/day, RR 1.57, 95% CI: 1.18–2.09). In the INTERSTROKE international case–control study, among 10 common vascular risk factors, high or heavy alcohol intake contributed to 4.6% (95% CI: 2.0–10.0%) of all ischaemic strokes and 9.8% (95% CI: 6.4–14.8%) of all haemorrhagic strokes (population attributable risk) (O'Donnell et al., 2016).

Among 428 nationally representative US stroke survivors, a healthy lifestyle, including light-to-moderate alcohol consumption (up to 2 drinks per day for men and up to 1 drink per day for nonpregnant women), was associated with reduced mortality after stroke (Towfighi et al., 2012).

The protective effect of light-to-moderate alcohol consumption for ischaemic stroke may be related to antithrombotic and favourable lipid effects of alcohol (Mukamal et al., 2005; Brien et al., 2011). Heavy alcohol use likely increases the risk of haemorrhagic stroke in part by antithrombotic effects, and the risk of both haemorrhagic and ischaemic stroke by increasing the risk of hypertension, atrial fibrillation, cardiomyopathy, and diabetes (Baliunas et al., 2009; Kodama et al., 2011; Briasoulis et al., 2012).

Treatments for Alcohol Dependence

Behavioural

In a meta-analysis of brief (<1 hour) motivational counselling interventions in heavy alcohol drinkers, among 8 RCTs enrolling over 2500 heavy drinkers, those who received brief motivational interventions were close to two times more likely to decrease and moderate their drinking compared with those who received no intervention (OR 1.95, 95% CI: 1.66–2.30) (Wilk et al., 1997). A more recent meta-analysis of 73 controlled studies of brief, single-session interventions in heavy-drinking college students reduced alcohol use by 0.18 of the standard deviation of baseline use (95% CI: 0.12–0.24) (Samson and Tanner-Smith, 2015). Insufficient unconfounded trials of 12-step programmes and other longer interventions are available to assess their effectiveness (Ferri et al., 2006).

Pharmacological

A systematic network meta-analysis of several pharmacological therapies analysed 122 RCTs and 1 cohort study (Jonas et al., 2014). In 16 trials enrolling 4847 patients, acamprosate reduced the absolute rate of return to any drinking by 9% (95% CI: 4–14%); in 7 trials, acamprosate did not modify the risk of return to heavy drinking, absolute risk reduction 1% (95% CI: –3–4%). In 16 trials enrolling 2347 patients, naltrexone at moderate 50 mg oral dose reduced the absolute rate of return to any drinking by 5% (95% CI: 0.2–10%); in 19 trials, naltrexone at moderate 50 mg dose reduced the rate of return to heavy drinking by 9% (95% CI: 4–13%). In 2 trials enrolling 492 patients, disulfiram did not statistically modify the rate of return to any drinking, ARR 4% (95% CI: –3 to 11%).

Comment

Reducing heavy alcohol intake is advisable, as it is associated with increased ischaemic and haemorrhagic stroke in observational studies. Brief counselling interventions, pharmacological therapy with acamprosate, and pharmacological therapy with naltrexone are effective interventions to increase abstinence among heavy drinkers. Light to moderate amounts of alcohol consumption (up to 2 drinks per day for men and up to 1 drink per day for nonpregnant women) are not associated with increased stroke risk and may even help prevent ischaemic stroke. Light to moderate drinkers may be counselled to continue with moderate intake; however, given the risk of addiction, nondrinkers should not be counselled to start drinking (Kernan et al., 2014).

Physical Activity

Evidence

Physical Activity and Risk of Stroke

A systematic review of 9 prospective cohort studies following more than 390,000 participants typically for 12 years found a dose–response relationship between weekly physical activity and stroke incidence, with the greatest gain occurring with the transition from complete inactivity to at least low activity (Wahid et al., 2016). Compared with inactivity, stroke occurrence was lower with low physical activity (0.1–11.5 hours per week) by RR 0.85 (95% CI: 0.80–0.91); medium physical activity (11.5–29.5 hours per week) by RR 0.81 (95% CI: 0.74–0.89), and high physical activity (more than 29.5 hours per week) by RR 0.76 (95% CI: 0.68–0.85). In the INTERSTROKE international case–control study, among 10 common vascular risk factors, physical inactivity contributed to 33.4% (95% CI: 24.2–44.0%) of all ischaemic strokes and 34.6% (95% CI: 21.3–50.7%) of all haemorrhagic strokes (population attributable risk) (O'Donnell et al., 2016).

The mechanisms by which physical activity might reduce stroke risk include lowering body weight, blood pressure, blood viscosity, fibrinogen concentrations, and platelet aggregability; enhancing fibrinolysis; and improving lipid profiles and endothelial function (Billinger et al., 2014). Individuals who have had a stroke often have reduced physical activity due to motor and other deficits, potentially predisposing them to heightened risk of recurrent stroke and cardiovascular disease.

Physical activity and exercise programmes after stroke and TIA have been found to improve vascular risk factor profiles. A systematic review of 14 RCTs in 720 stroke and TIA patients of exercise with or without additional lifestyle interventions found reductions in SBP, mean difference (MD) −5.32 mm Hg, 95% CI: −9.46 to −1.18, fasting glucose, MD −0.11 mmol/L, 95% CI: −0.17 to −0.06, and fasting insulin, MD −17.14 pmol/L, 95% CI: −32.90 to −1.38, $P = 0.03$, and increases in high-density lipoprotein cholesterol, MD 0.10 mmol/L, 95% CI: 0.03–0.18 (D'Isabella et al.,

2017). Similar effects were seen when analysis was confined to the 9 RCTs in which exercise was the only intervention. However, insufficient long-term trials have been performed to determine whether these favourable effects on vascular risk factors translate into actual reduced recurrent stroke and cardiovascular events.

The optimal time to resume physical activity after stroke remains unknown. In the AVERT trial, among 2104 stroke patients randomized to very early and frequent mobilization, commencing within 24 hours, or usual care, patients randomized to usual care had more frequent functional independence (modified Rankin Scale [mRS] 0–2) outcome at 3 months, 50% versus 46% (OR 1.37, 95% CI: 1.11–1.69) (Avert Trial Collaboration Group, 2015). They found a consistent pattern of improved odds of favourable outcome in efficacy and safety outcomes with increased daily frequency of out-of-bed sessions (OR 1.13, 95% CI: 1.09–1.18; $p < 0.001$), keeping time to first mobilization and mobilization amount constant. On the other hand, increased amount (minutes per day) of mobilization reduced the odds of a good outcome (OR 0.94, 95% CI: 0.91 to 0.97, $p < 0.001$) (Bernhardt et al., 2016).

Comment

Based on available, largely observational evidence, regular physical activity to improve aerobic capacity is likely to reduce stroke risk. American Heart/Stroke Association guideline recommendations for primary prevention of stroke have suggested at least 40 minutes of moderate- to vigorous-intensity activity 3–4 times per week (Meschia et al., 2014). Among individuals who have already had a stroke or TIA, based on short-term trials evaluating modification of risk factors rather than actual stroke and other vascular events in the long-term, regular physical activity also appears likely to reduce risk of recurrent stroke and cardiovascular events. While highly vigorous activity within the first 24 hours of stroke onset should be avoided, eventually at least three to four 40-minute sessions per week of moderate- to vigorous-intensity aerobic physical exercise in stroke patients able to engage in physical activity appears desirable (Kernan et al., 2014). In addition to potential reduction in recurrent stroke risk by aerobic exercise, stroke patient engagement in regular strength, flexibility, and coordination-building physical activities may bring other benefits, including greater recovery of post-stroke motor deficits and decreased fall risk (Billinger et al., 2014).

Obesity

Evidence

Risk Factor for Stroke

In a systematic review of 25 prospective cohort studies with over 2.27 million participants experiencing over 30,700 stroke events over an average follow-up of 17.5 years, higher body mass index (BMI) was associated with increased risk of ischaemic and haemorrhagic stroke (Strazzullo et al., 2010). Overweight was defined as BMI 25–29.9 kg/m^2 in Western countries and 23–27.5 kg/m^2 in Asian countries, and obesity defined as BMI ≥30 kg/m^2 in Western countries and >27.5 kg/m^2 in Asian countries. For ischaemic stroke, compared with normal weight, incidence was increased in overweight individuals, RR 1.22 (95% CI: 1.05–1.41) and obese individuals, RR 1.64 (95% CI: 1.36–1.99). For haemorrhagic stroke, incidence was not increased for overweight individuals, RR 1.01 (95% CI: 0.88–1.17) but tended to be increased for obese individuals, RR 1.24 (95% CI: 0.99–1.54) Considering only young adults, aged 18–50, a meta-analysis of eight cohort studies found that for overweight individuals the pooled adjusted RR of stroke was 1.36 (95% CI: 1.28–1.44), and for obese individuals it was 1.81 (95% CI: 1.45–2.25) (Guo et al., 2016).

Abdominal obesity, reflecting visceral adipose tissue, compared with general obesity, reflecting also subcutaneous fat, has been more closely related to metabolic dysfunctions, inflammatory cytokines, and lipid profiles predisposing to vascular events. In a meta-analysis of 15 prospective cohort studies of over 405,000 participants experiencing over 11,700 stroke events, ischaemic strokes were associated with abdominal obesity, assessed as higher waist circumference, RR 1.41 (95% CI: 1.21–1.56), waist-to-hip ratio, RR 1.35 (95% CI: 1.21–1.50), and waist-to-height ratio, RR 1.55 (95% CI: 1.37–1.76) (Zhong et al., 2016). In contrast, haemorrhagic strokes were not increased with abdominal adiposity. In the INTERSTROKE international case–control study, among 10 common vascular risk factors, abdominal obesity contributed to 20.4% (95% CI: 13.3–25.3%) of all ischaemic strokes and 13.1% (95% CI: 6.4–25.1%) of all haemorrhagic strokes (population attributable risk) (O'Donnell et al., 2016).

Within the general framework of increased stroke incidence with higher body weight, nuances include:

1. Metabolically healthy obesity (MHO): Within the obese population, a subgroup has been identified who may not be at increased risk of cardiovascular events, as they do not display the typical metabolic disorders associated with obesity. Metabolically healthy obesity has been defined as obese individuals who do not have insulin resistance, lipid disorders, or hypertension, and occurs in 10–25% of the obese population (Roberson et al., 2014). In a prospective cohort study of 354,000 Korean adults experiencing 4884 strokes over a mean 7.4 years, compared with metabolically healthy normal weight individuals, stroke incidence was not increased in metabolically healthy obese individuals, HR 1.09 (95% CI: 0.89–1.33), but was increased in metabolically unhealthy obese individuals, HR 4.90 (95% CI: 4.42–5.42) (Lee et al., 2018).

2. The effects of below normal weight: Several studies have suggested a U-shaped relation between body weight and stroke, with below normal body weight associated with increased incidence in addition to above normal (Chen et al., 2013).

3. The 'obesity paradox' and recurrent stroke events: In contrast to the increasing incidence of first stroke with increasing BMI in the general population, a paradoxical reduction of recurrent stroke incidence with increasing BMI has been suggested by several studies in patients with index first strokes. In a qualitative review, 10 of 12 studies (total 162,921 stroke patients) reported reduced mortality rates post-stroke among stroke patients with higher BMI values, and 7 of 9 studies (total 92,718 stroke patients) reported a favourable effect of excess body weight on functional outcomes and avoidance of recurrent vascular events (Oesch et al., 2017). A formal, quantitative meta-analysis of 5 studies including 54,372 first stroke patients suggested a similar pattern; compared with normal weight patients, overweight patients had RR for recurrent stroke of 0.96 (95% CI: 0.90–1.04; $p = 0.32$) and obese patients had RR 0.89 (95% CI: 0.77–1.02; $p = 0.096$) (Huang et al., 2016). These paradoxically more favourable outcomes in post-stroke patients may simply be an artefact of survival-to-event bias (unfit overweight patients may die more often before having a stroke) (Towfighi and Ovbiagele, 2009), but also could reflect greater metabolic reserve against post-stroke catabolism and anti-inflammatory endocrine effects of adipose tissue (Oesch et al., 2017).

Interventions to Reduce Weight

General obesity-related health risks can be substantially reduced with weight loss of as little as 5% of body weight (Jensen et al., 2014), and a number of interventions have been found to be effective for weight loss and weight-loss maintenance, with some specifically evaluated for effect on stroke.

Behaviour, Physical Activity, and Dietary Interventions to Reduce Weight

Behaviour-change interventions targeting diet and physical activity are effective in facilitating clinically meaningful weight loss of 3 to 5 kg at 12 months (Greaves et al., 2011). In a systematic meta-analysis of 47 randomized trials, group-based diet and/or physical activity interventions reduced weight compared with control, mean difference (MD) 3.44 kg (95% CI: 2.85–4.23) at 1 year and 2.56 kg (95% CI: 1.33–3.79) at 2 years (Borek et al., 2018). In a meta-analysis of 48 RCTs enrolling 7286 individuals, compared with no diet intervention, the largest weight loss was associated with low-carbohydrate diets, 7.25 kg (95% CredI: 5.33–9.25) at 1 year, and low-fat diets, 7.27 kg (95% CredI: 5.26–9.34 kg) at 1 year (Johnston et al., 2014).

Drugs to Reduce Weight

Currently available drug therapies to reduce weight include orlistat, sibutramine, combined phentermine/topiramate rimonabant, liraglutide, lorcaserin, metformin, and combined naltrexone/bupropion. In a meta-analysis of RCTs of pharmacological weight loss agents in hypertensive patients, compared with placebo, orlistat (4 trials, 2080 patents) reduced weight by MD 3.73 kg (95% CI: 2.80–4.65) and also diastolic blood pressure (DBP) by MD 1.9 mm Hg (95% CI: 0.9–3.0); in contrast, sibutramine (4 trials, 574 patients) reduced weight by MD 3.74 kg (95% CI: 2.64–4.84), but increased DBP by MD 3.2 mm Hg (95% CI: 1.4–4.9) (Siebenhofer et al., 2016).

Gastric Balloons and Bariatric Surgery for Weight Loss

In a systematic network meta-analysis of 15 RCTs, 13 versus control and 2 comparisons of different devices, compared with control, fluid-filled balloons reduced total body weight at 6 months by 5.78% (95% CI: 4.11–7.46) and gas-filled balloons reduced total body weight by 3.58% (95% CI: 0.94–6.22) (Bazerbachi et al., 2018).

In patients with extreme obesity, bariatric surgery is the most effective means to achieve durable weight loss. In one systematic analysis, in 37 RCTs and 127 observational studies enrolling 161,756 patients, mean age 45 and BMI 46 kg/m^2, BMI reduction at 5 years post-surgery was 12–17 kg/m^2 (Chang et al., 2014). Peri-operative (<30 day) mortality was 0.08%, the complication rate was 17% (95% CI: 11%–23%), and reoperation rate was 7% (95% CI: 3%–12%).

In a systematic meta-analysis of 14 randomized trials and controlled cohort studies with 29,208 surgical patients and 166,200 nonsurgical controls, mean age 48, 70% female, follow-up 2.0–14.7 years, bariatric surgery reduced all-cause mortality, OR 0.48, 95% CI: 0.35–0.64, and, in 4 studies examining neurovascular outcome, reduced stroke, OR 0.49, 95% CI: 0.32–0.75 (Kwok et al., 2014).

Comment

Observational studies suggest that elevated BMI confers stroke risk, in part by increasing hypertension, hyperlipidaemia, and diabetes, but also via an additional, independent, incremental contribution to stroke frequency.

For individuals with extreme obesity, bariatric surgery and gastric balloon placement procedures substantially reduce weight; have favourable effects on vascular risk factors including blood pressure, diabetes, and cholesterol; and have suggestive evidence of reducing long-term stroke clinical events. Though associated with peri-procedural complications and need for repeat interventions, these procedures are of value for the severely obese patients at high vascular risk.

For patients with more moderate obesity, group-based diet and/or physical activity interventions reduce weight modestly, including both low-carbohydrate and low-fat diet regimens. While it has not been shown in RCTs that the resulting modest BMI lowering prevents stroke, it is reasonable to adopt reduction of BMI in overweight individuals as a strategy to reduce the risk of stroke and other serious vascular events.

Among pharmacological agents for weight reduction, orlistat has shown the most consistent favourable short-term effect on both weight and blood pressure reduction, but long-term trials are needed to determine whether these changes result in reduced stroke clinical events and are sufficient to offset potential side effects like loose stool.

Diet

Dietary intake varies among individuals not only by total calories consumed, but also by the proportions of different classes of nutrient molecules and different food groups contributing to the caloric total. Studies of diet and prevention of stroke and cardiovascular disease may be divided into investigations that focus more narrowly on risk and interventions at the level of individual nutrient classes or individual food groups and investigations that focus more broadly on risk and interventions at the level of broad dietary patterns with several concurrent alterations in nutrient and individual food group intake.

Dietary Intake of Nutrients

Evidence
Overview

Large-scale observational studies have evaluated the epidemiological relation of dietary intake of multiple nutrients (Table 17.1) and food groups (Table 17.2) with first and recurrent stroke. In meta-analyses of prospective cohort studies, nutrients likely associated with a reduced incidence of stroke included: mono-unsaturated fat, omega-3 polyunsaturated fat, fibre, dietary potassium, and dietary magnesium.

Nutrients associated or likely associated with increased incidence of stroke included: total carbohydrate, carbohydrate-linked glycaemic load, and dietary sodium. Nutrients with less reliable point estimates suggesting potential unfavourable effect on stroke risk included trans fat.

Nutrients associated with a neutral effect on stroke risk include saturated fat.

Additional systematic meta-analyses have evaluated the effect in controlled clinical trials of long-term dietary alterations or supplementary administration of particular dietary nutrients in pill form (Table 17.3). In combined RCTs, interventions associated with reduced stroke incidence were the Mediterranean Diet and supplemental administration of included B vitamins, particularly folic acid (vitamin B9).

Interventions associated with neutral effect on subsequent stroke included reducing dietary intake of saturated fatty acids and supplemental administration of omega-3 polyunsaturated fatty acids, vitamin D, and the antioxidant nutrients vitamin E, vitamin C, beta-carotene, and selenium.

Dietary Macromolecules: Fats and Carbohydrates

Evidence

Risk Factor for Stroke

Of the four types of dietary macromolecules (lipids, carbohydrates, proteins, and nucleic acids), two have been linked by some studies to stroke risk: lipids (fats) and carbohydrates (carbs). The lipid composition of atherosclerotic plaques and their relation with higher serum levels of certain lipid molecules historically cast concern on dietary fat. Carbohydrates may mediate risk by raising serum insulin and glucose, reducing catabolism of body fat to meet energy demands.

Among dietary lipids, important subclasses include: (1) trans fats, which can increase serum low-density lipoprotein (LDL) level, be pro-inflammatory, and enhance insulin resistance; (2) saturated fats, which can increase serum LDL; and (3) mono- and polyunsaturated fats, which can lower serum LDL. In meta-analyses of prospective cohort studies, dietary intake of trans and saturated fats has had a neutral association with subsequent stroke, while dietary mono- and polyunsaturated fats have been associated with reduced stroke incidence (see Table 17.3). In a meta-analysis of 11 prospective cohorts with 339,000 participants experiencing 6226 stroke events, comparing highest versus lowest dietary consumption groups, monounsaturated fat was associated with decreased stroke occurrence, RR 0.83 (95% CI: 0.71–0.97) (Schwingshackl and Hoffmann, 2014). In a different meta-analysis, of 8 prospective cohort studies following 242,076 participants who experienced 5238 stroke events, comparing highest versus lowest dietary consumption groups, polyunsaturated omega-3 fatty acids from seafood sources were associated with decreased stroke occurrence, RR 0.83 (95% CI: 0.71–0.97) (Larsson et al., 2012).

For carbohydrates, a meta-analysis of 7 prospective cohort studies enrolling 225,205 participants who experienced 3046 strokes, higher dietary carbohydrate-related glycaemic index trends towards association with incident stroke, RR 1.10 (95% CI: 0.99–1.21), and in a smaller set of 179,348 individuals, the relation of total dietary carbohydrate and stroke occurrence was 1.12 (95% CI: 0.93, 1.35) (Cai et al., 2015).

Table 17.1 Meta-analyses of relation of dietary nutrients to stroke incidence

Nutrient	Studies	Subjects	Events	Unit	RR (95% CI)	Citation
Carbohydrates						
Total carbohydrate	4 PCs	179,348	1851	high vs low	1.12 (0.93, 1.35)	(Cai et al., 2015)
Glycaemic index	7 PCs	225,205	3046	high vs low	1.10 (0.99, 1.21)	(Cai et al., 2015)
Glycaemic load	6 PCs	222,308	2951	high vs low	1.19 (1.05, 1.36)	(Cai et al., 2015)
Fats						
Saturated fat	12 PCs	332,864	6226	high vs low	1.03 (0.91, 1.16)	(de Souza et al., 2015)
Trans fat	3 PCs	190,284	1905	high vs low	1.07 (0.88, 1.28)	(de Souza et al., 2015)
Monounsaturated fat	10 PCs	314,511	5827	high vs low	0.86 (0.74, 1.00)	(Schwingshackl and Hoffmann, 2014)
Polyunsaturated fat – omega-3	14 PCs	514,483	9065	high vs low	0.87 (0.79, 0.95)	(Cheng et al., 2015)
Fibre						
Fibre	8 PCs	324,641	9836	7 g/d	0.93 (0.88, 0.98)	(Threapleton et al., 2013)
Ions						
Sodium	12 PCs, 3 CCs	225,693	8135	high vs low	1.34 (1.19, 1.51)	(Li et al., 2012)
Potassium	16 PCs	639,440	19,522	high vs low	0.87 (0.80, 0.94)	(Vinceti et al. 2016)
Calcium	10 PCs	371 495	10 408	high vs low	0.96 (0.89, 1.04)	(Tian et al. 2015)
Magnesium	14 PCs	692,930	15,160	high vs low	0.88 (0.82, 0.95)	(Fang et al. 2016)

PC: Prospective cohort study. CC: Case–control study.

Table 17.2 Meta-analyses of relation of food groups to stroke incidence

Food or beverage	Studies	Subjects	Events	Unit	RR (95% CI)	Meta-analysis
Fruits	16 PCs	964,142	46,203	2 serving/d (200 g/d)	0.82 (0.74, 0.90)	(Aune et al., 2017)
Vegetables	13 PCs	441,670	14,973	2 serving/d (200 g/d)	0.87 (0.79, 0.96)	(Aune et al., 2017)
Legumes	6 PCs	254,628	6690	4 servings/wk (400 g)	0.98 (0.84, 1.14)	(Afshin et al., 2014)
Nuts	11 PCs	396,768	9272	1 servings/d (28 g)	0.93 (0.83, 1.05)	(Aune et al., 2016a)
Whole grains	6 PCs	245,012	2337	5.6 servings/d (90 g/d)	0.88 (0.75, 1.03)	(Aune et al., 2016b)
Olive oil	2 PCs, 1 RCT	38,673	–	2 tbsp/d (25 g/d)	0.76 (0.67–0.86)	(Martinez-Gonzalez et al., 2014)
Fish	8 PCs	394,958	16,890	≥5 vs 1 serving/wk	0.88 (0.81, 0.96)	(Chowdhury et al., 2012)
Red meat – processed	17 PCs	2,079,236	21,730	1 serving/d (50 g)	1.14 (1.05, 1.24)	(Yang et al., 2016)
Total dairy	9 PCs	336,188	12,043	1.1 servings/d (200 g)	0.99 (0.96, 1.02)	(de Goede et al., 2016)
Milk	14 PCs	603,920	25,269	0.8 servings/d (200 g)	0.93 (0.88, 0.98)	(de Goede et al., 2016)
Cheese	7 PCs	272,368	11,126	0.9 servings/d (40 g)	0.97 (0.94, 1.01)	(de Goede et al., 2016)
Butter	3 PCs	47,227	2230	0.7 servings/d (10 g)	1.00 (0.99, 1.01)	(de Goede et al., 2016)
Eggs	9 PCs	436,088	13,645	≥7 eggs vs <1 egg/wk	0.91 (0.85, 0.98)	(Xu et al., 2019)
Chocolate	7 PCs	231,128	–	highest vs lowest	0.84 (0.78–0.90)	(Yuan et al., 2017)
Sugar-sweetened drinks	3 PCs	235,701	–	high vs low	1.10 (0.97–1.25)	(Narain et al., 2016)
Coffee	17 PCs	1,283,685	12,030	3.5 vs 0 cups/d	0.80 (0.75, 0.86)	(Ding et al., 2014)
Tea	8 PCs	307,968	11,329	3 servings/d (3 cups)	0.82 (0.73, 0.92)	(Zhang et al., 2015)

PC: Prospective cohort study. RCT: Randomized clinical trial.

Table 17.3 Meta-analyses of randomized trials of dietary interventions and stroke

Intervention	RCTs	RR	95% CI	Meta-analysis
Diet				
Mediterranean	3	0.66	0.48–0.92	(Liyanage et al., 2016)
Nutrient				
Reduced saturated fat intake	8	1.00	0.89–1.12	(Hooper et al., 2015)
Supplements				
Vitamin B9 (folic acid)	22	0.89	0.84–0.96	(Zhao et al., 2017)
Vitamin D	12	1.09	0.92–1.30	(Ford et al., 2014)
Omega-3 PUFAs	10	1.03	0.93–1.13	(Aung et al., 2018)
Antioxidant – Vitamin C	4	0.98	0.88–1.09	(Myung et al., 2013)
Antioxidant – Vitamin E	12	1.00	0.93–1.09	(Myung et al., 2013)
Antioxidant – beta-carotene	2	0.98	0.89–1.07	(Myung et al., 2013)
Antioxidant – Selenium	1	1.09	0.68–1.72	(Myung et al., 2013)

PUFAs: polyunsaturated fatty acids.

Low-fat Diet Interventions

In a meta-analysis of 13 RCTs enrolling 53,300 participants of whom 4337 had a subsequent cardiovascular event, allocation to diets targeting lower saturated fat intake by reducing or modifying dietary fat was associated with fewer incident cardiovascular events (RR 0.86, 95% CI: 0.72–0.96) (Hooper et al., 2015). However, for stroke alone, in 8 trials enrolling 50,952 participants, diets to lower saturated fats did not reduce event rates (RR 1.00, 95% CI: 0.89–1.12).

Administration of omega-3 as a supplementary pill, unaccompanied by other polyunsaturated fats, was evaluated in a meta-analysis of 10 RCTs enrolling 77,917 individuals who subsequently had 1713 stroke events. Omega-3 supplements did not reduce stroke incidence, RR 1.03 (95% CI: 0.93–1.13) (Aung et al., 2018).

Low-carbohydrate Diet Interventions

In a meta-analysis of 17 trials in 1141 obese patients, a low-carbohydrate diet was associated with reduced weight by 7.04 kg (95% CI: 6.88–7.20), reduced abdominal circumference by 5.74 cm (95% CI: 5.41–6.07), lower SBP by 4.81 mm Hg (95% CI: 4.29–5.33), lower glycated haemoglobin by 0.21% (95% CI: 0.18–0.24), lower plasma insulin by 2.24 microIU/mL (95% CI: 1.82–2.65), and increased high-density lipoprotein (HDL) cholesterol by 1.73 mg/dL (95% CI: 1.44–2.01), though there was no change in LDL cholesterol (Santos et al., 2012).

Low-carb vs Low-fat Diet Interventions

In a systematic meta-analysis of 17 trials enrolling 1797 patients comparing low-fat with low-carbohydrate diets, the low-carbohydrate diet was associated with greater reduction in weight by 2.0 kg (95% CI: 0.9–3.1) and in SBP, 4.4 mm Hg (95% CI: 1.5–7.2), and a greater increase in HDL cholesterol, by 5.1 mg/dL (95% CI: 3.5–6.7), but also a greater increase in LDL cholesterol, by 8.6 mg/dL (95% CI: 3.6–13.7) (Sackner-Bernstein et al., 2015). The resulting changes in atherosclerotic risk factor profiles lowered the expected vascular event rate more greatly for low-carbohydrate patients; for example, for white patients with high (4.89%) risk of cardiovascular events, the expected event rate was lowered to 4.03% with low-carb diet versus 4.49% with low-fat, mean difference 0.44% (95% CI: 0.06–0.83).

Comment

Large-scale observational data suggest that dietary saturated fat intake is likely not a major risk factor for stroke, though it may be a risk factor for coronary artery disease. Consistent with these epidemiological observations, randomized trials of diets lowering intake of saturated fat have failed to demonstrate a reduction in stroke events, despite indications of potential modest benefit for CHD. Accordingly, narrowly focused, low-saturated-fat diets are not a supported recommendation for stroke-prevention-focused patient care. In contrast, dietary unsaturated fat consumption, of both mono- and polyunsaturated fats, is associated with reduced inci-dence of both neurovascular and cardiovascular disease events. Randomized trials of diets focused solely upon increasing unsaturated fat intake with stroke outcomes have not been performed, but it appears reasonable to include increased intake of unsaturated fat in diet regi-mens aiming to reduce stroke risk. Conversely, admin-istration of the polyunsaturated fatty acid omega-3 as a supplement in isolated pill form is not beneficial for reducing future stroke, suggesting the benefits of unsa-turated fat intake are not conveyed by the omega 3 fatty acid subtype alone.

The large prospective cohort studies also indicate that higher dietary carbohydrate intake is likely a risk factor for stroke. Trials of low-carbohydrate diets completed to date have generally had relatively short follow-up periods and so have not been able to address whether there is benefit for actual stroke events. Trials do show that low-carbohydrate diets cause potentially beneficial alterations in weight, blood pres-sure, insulin, and HDL cholesterol, though slightly adverse change in LDL cholesterol, with a cumulative effect profile that appears more likely than low-fat diets to favourably reduce subsequent stroke. However, long-term trials assessing actual incident stroke rates are needed before a definite recommendation regarding the role of narrowly focused low-carbohydrate diets in stroke prevention can be advanced.

Dietary Intake of B Vitamins

Evidence

Risk Factor for Stroke

Homocysteine, an amino acid generated in the inter-mediate metabolism of the essential amino acid cysteine, exerts several potential stroke-risk-enhancing actions, including pro-atherosclerotic, prothrombotic, and vaso-constrictive effects. Large prospective cohort studies have found that elevated plasma homocysteine is an independent predictor of future stroke. A meta-analysis of 9 prospective cohort studies with 13,284 participants, comparing the highest versus lowest quar-tile of homocysteine levels, had increased frequency of first ischaemic strokes of RR 1.69 (95% CI: 1.29–2.20) and of recurrent strokes, RR 1.76 (95% CI: 1.37–2.24) (He et al., 2014). A causal role of homocysteine is further supported by Mendelian randomization studies analys-ing the gene encoding methylenetetrahydrofolate reduc-tase (MTHFR), an enzyme in homocysteine

metabolism, as an instrumental variable. A meta-analyses of genetic epidemiological studies found that, compared with individuals homozygous for the more common allele (CC), individuals homozygous for the MTHFR polymorphism (TT) had both higher plasma homocysteine concentration, mean difference 1.93 $\mu mol/L$ (95% CI: 1.38–2.47) and increased incidence of stroke, OR 1.26 (95% CI: 1.14–1.40) (Qin et al., 2016).

B-vitamin Supplementation Intervention

Vitamins B_9 (folic acid), B_6 (pyridoxine), and B_{12} (coba-lamin) are cofactors of enzymes involved in homocys-teine metabolism and lower plasma homocysteine levels when administered as supplements. Folic acid has the most potent effect, reducing homocysteine by 20–25%. In systematic meta-analyses, homocysteine-lowering therapy with folic acid, often accompanied by vitamin B_6 and vitamin B_{12}, has been associated with reduced occurrence of stroke (Figure 17.4) (Marti-Carvajal et al., 2017; Zhao et al., 2017). Among 22 trials enrolling 82,723 patients, stroke rates with and without homocysteine-lowering therapy with folic acid were 3.8% versus 4.2%, RR 0.89 (95% CI: 0.84–0.96) (Zhao et al., 2017). The effect was greater in regions without governmental poli-cies requiring low-level folic acid fortification of food to deter spina bifida (11 trials, 49,957 patients, RR 0.85, 95% CI: 0.77–0.94) compared with the effect in regions with concomitant, society-wide folic acid fortification (7 trials, 14,655 patients, RR 1.05, 95% CI: 0.90–1.23) (Zhao et al., 2017). A subsequent larger meta-analysis, confined to countries without fortification, of 13 RCTs enrolling 65,812 patients, also found folic acid supple-mentation was associated with decreased stroke inci-dence (RR 0.85, 95% CI: 0.77–0.95) (Hsu et al., 2018).

Vitamin B_{12} is available in pill form complexed with different molecules, including cyanide (cyanoco-balamin) or a methyl group (methylcobalamin). Although quite low, the levels of thiocyanate that accumulate in patients with renal impairment when the cyanocobalamin formulation is used may be suffi-cient to counteract folic acid benefit, by promoting LDL oxidation and impairing endothelial function. In a meta-analysis of 9 folic acid RCTs enrolling 31,872 individuals, patients with impaired renal function exposed to high-dose cyanocobalamin did not have reduced stroke, RR 1.04 (95% CI: 0.84–1.27), but patients with both normal renal function and nonex-posure to high-dose cyanocobalamin had reduced stroke occurrence, RR 0.78 (95% CI: 0.67–0.90), $p_{(interaction)} = 03$ (Spence et al., 2017).

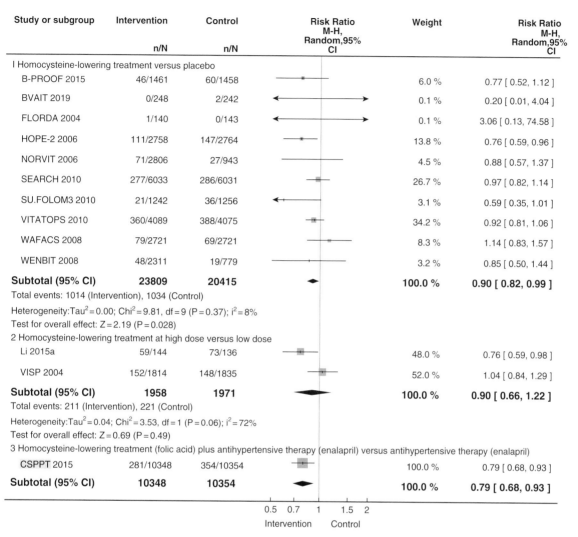

Figure 17.4 Forest plot showing the effects of *folic acid, B₆, and B₁₂ homocysteine-lowering therapy* for *stroke prevention*, among a total of 68,853 patients.

Reproduced from Marti-Carvajal et al. (2017), with permission from John Wiley & Sons Limited. Copyright Cochrane Library.

Comment

The now substantial randomized clinical trial literature suggests that homocysteine-lowering therapy with supplemental folic acid (vitamin B_9), often accompanied by vitamin B_6 and vitamin B^{12}, mildly reduces the risk of first or recurrent stroke. Folic acid supplementation of bread and other foods, undertaken at the societal level to reduce spina bifida, likely also confers benefit at the population level in reducing stroke incidence. In regions in which folic acid food fortification has not been implemented by governmental action, administration of folic acid, accompanied by low levels of vitamins B_6 and B_{12}, to individual patients in pill form likely reduces subsequent stroke risk. In regions with implementation of folic acid food fortification, supplemental, pill-form folic acid has not been shown to confer additional stroke prevention benefit. Further clinical trials are desirable to explore the possibility that, even in regions with folic acid food fortification, additional administration of a nuanced regimen of folic acid supplements accompanied by low-dose vitamin B_{12} in methylcobalamin form, rather than cyanocobalamin form, may be beneficial, especially in patients with normal renal function.

Dietary Intake of Antioxidants

Evidence

Laboratory evidence suggests that oxidative modification of LDL cholesterol may be an important stage in the formation and rupture of atherosclerotic plaques. A number of dietary constituents have antioxidant properties, such as certain minerals (e.g. selenium, copper, zinc, manganese), vitamins (A, C, and E), provitamins (beta-carotene), and flavonoids, and low dietary intake of several was associated with stroke incidence in observational studies.

However, meta-analyses of randomized trials have not found a benefit of vitamin C, selenium, vitamin E, or beta-carotene in reducing stroke (see Table 17.3). Moreover, in a meta-analysis of 57 trials enrolling 244,056 participants, antioxidant supplements tended to be associated with increased all-cause mortality, 11.7% versus 10.2%, random effect model RR 1.02 (95% CI: 0.98–1.05), fixed-effect model RR 1.03 (95% CI: 1.01–1.05) (Bjelakovic et al., 2012).

Comment

Sufficient large randomized trials have now been performed to definitively disconfirm the hypotheses generated by observational studies that antioxidant nutrient supplements would reduce the risk of stroke. Moreover, the studies suggest an actual overall harmful effect of chronic antioxidant supplements in mildly increasing all-cause mortality, potentially due in part to providing protection to nascent neoplastic cells against immune system clearance in part mediated by targeted oxidative injury against highly metabolically active cells. Accordingly, at present, use of oxidative nutrient supplements is not recommended to prevent incident stroke.

The disjunction between observational data and randomized trials with regard to the effects of antioxidant molecules highlights the importance of not relying on data from observational studies to establish causality, because bias cannot be entirely eliminated in prospective cohort studies. 'Healthy cohort' bias is a particularly common source of confounding, in which non-causal associations arise since healthier, more well-to-do patients are both more likely to be aware of, afford, and pursue a particular health practice due to their baseline healthier state, and also less likely to have stroke due to their baseline healthier state. RCTs are needed to demonstrate causality, as only random allocation fully controls for known and unknown covariates that may influence stroke occurrence.

Dietary Intake of D Vitamins

Evidence

Risk Factor for Stroke

Physiological studies suggest several mechanisms by which low vitamin D levels might increase vascular event risk, including promoting endothelial dysfunction, reducing myocyte contractility via diminished calcium flux, and increasing chronic inflammation. However, observational studies have not reliably shown a relation between dietary vitamin D intake and stroke, and a meta-analysis of 12 randomized trials enrolling 11,841 individuals failed to show a reduction in stroke occurrence with use of supplemental vitamin D, RR 1.09 (95% CI: 0.92–1.30) (Ford et al., 2014)(see Table 17.3).

Comment

Dietary intake of vitamin D has not been consistently associated with stroke risk in observational studies, and randomized trials of vitamin D supplements have not found benefit in reducing stroke incidence. Accordingly, routine vitamin D supplementation is not indicated in stroke prevention regimens.

Dietary Intake of Salt (sodium chloride)

Evidence

Risk of Stroke

There is a clear relationship between sodium chloride salt intake and hypertension, the leading modifiable risk factor for stroke. In a meta-analysis of 12 prospective cohort and 3 case–control studies, with 225,693 participants (follow-up 3.5–19 years) and over 8135 stroke events, higher salt intake was associated with greater stroke incidence, RR 1.23 (95% CI: 1.06–1.43) (Li et al., 2012).

Low-salt Diet Intervention

A systematic meta-analysis of 6 RCTs enrolling 5762 individuals found that advice and salt substitution,

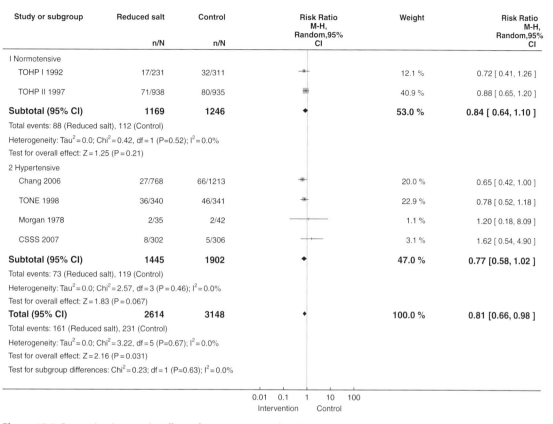

Study or subgroup	Reduced salt	Control	Risk Ratio M-H, Random,95% CI	Weight	Risk Ratio M-H, Random,95% CI
	n/N	n/N			
1 Normotensive					
TOHP I 1992	17/231	32/311		12.1 %	0.72 [0.41, 1.26]
TOHP II 1997	71/938	80/935		40.9 %	0.88 [0.65, 1.20]
Subtotal (95% CI)	**1169**	**1246**		**53.0 %**	**0.84 [0.64, 1.10]**
Total events: 88 (Reduced salt), 112 (Control)					
Heterogeneity: Tau^2=0.0; Chi^2=0.42, df=1 (P=0.52); I^2=0.0%					
Test for overall effect: Z=1.25 (P=0.21)					
2 Hypertensive					
Chang 2006	27/768	66/1213		20.0 %	0.65 [0.42, 1.00]
TONE 1998	36/340	46/341		22.9 %	0.78 [0.52, 1.18]
Morgan 1978	2/35	2/42		1.1 %	1.20 [0.18, 8.09]
CSSS 2007	8/302	5/306		3.1 %	1.62 [0.54, 4.90]
Subtotal (95% CI)	**1445**	**1902**		**47.0 %**	**0.77 [0.58, 1.02]**
Total events: 73 (Reduced salt), 119 (Control)					
Heterogeneity: Tau^2=0.0; Chi^2=2.57, df=3 (P=0.46); I^2=0.0%					
Test for overall effect: Z=1.83 (P=0.067)					
Total (95% CI)	**2614**	**3148**		**100.0 %**	**0.81 [0.66, 0.98]**
Total events: 161 (Reduced salt), 231 (Control)					
Heterogeneity: Tau^2=0.0; Chi^2=3.22, df=5 (P=0.67); I^2=0.0%					
Test for overall effect: Z=2.16 (P=0.031)					
Test for subgroup differences: Chi^2=0.23; df=1 (P=0.63); I^2=0.0%					

0.01   0.1   1   10   100
Intervention   Control

Figure 17.5 Forest plot showing the effects of *interventions to reduce dietary salt* on *combined cardiovascular and stroke events.* Reproduced from Adler et al. (2014), with permission from John Wiley & Sons Limited. Copyright Cochrane Library.

aimed at lowering dietary salt, tended to reduce cardiovascular disease events, including stroke, both in participants normotensive at baseline, 0.84, 95% CI: 0.64–1.10 (2 trials, 2415 individuals) and in participants hypertensive at baseline, 0.77, 95% CI: 0.58–1.02 (4 trials, 3347 individuals) (Adler et al., 2014) (Figure 17.5). Stroke events were not analysed as a separate endpoint. Advice to reduce salt tended to be associated with reduced SBP in normotensives, mean difference (MD) –1.15 mm Hg, 95% CI: –2.32 to 0.02, and was associated with reduced SBP in hypertensives, MD –4.14 mm Hg, 95% CI: –5.84 to –2.43.

Comment

Adding sodium chloride salt to food appears to be a risk factor for stroke, particularly haemorrhagic stroke. Salt reduction has been shown in randomized clinical trials to reduce BP to a modest degree. The 1–6 mm Hg reductions in SBP are sufficient to be projected to reduce long-term stroke risk to a small but worthwhile degree in individual patients, and to have a substantial impact at the population level. Although long-term randomized trials confirming actual benefit in stroke reduction have not been conducted, it is reasonable to advise patients to lower salt intake. The American Heart Association guidelines recommend that those with a history of stroke or TIA reduce their sodium intake to <2.4 g/day. Further reduction to <1.5 g/day is also reasonable and is associated with even greater blood pressure reduction (Kernan et al., 2014). Sustained reduction in dietary salt intake may help people on antihypertensive drugs to reduce the number and dose of their medications while maintaining adequate control of blood pressure.

Dietary Intake of Potassium

Evidence

Potassium is an essential mineral that can counteract sodium and lower blood pressure levels. In a meta-analysis of 12 prospective studies following 333,250 participants who had 10,659 stroke events, greater intake of dietary potassium was associated with reduced stroke incidence, RR 0.80 (95% CI: 0.72–0.90) (D'Elia et al., 2014).

Comment

The inverse epidemiological association of dietary potassium intake and stroke frequency provides some support for the use of potassium chloride salts as a table and recipe substitute for sodium chloride salt. Long-term randomized trials of potassium chloride salt substitution as an isolated intervention are desirable to confirm or disconfirm benefit in reducing neurovascular events.

Magnesium

Evidence

Magnesium is an essential mineral and cofactor for more than 300 enzymatic reactions in the human body (Adebamowo et al., 2015). Higher dietary magnesium intake has been associated with effects that could reduce stroke risk, including lowering blood pressure and improving endothelial function. In a meta-analysis of 14 prospective cohort studies of 692,930 individuals having 15,160 stroke events, higher dietary magnesium was associated with a lower incidence of stroke, RR 0.88 (95% CI: 0.82–0.95) (Fang et al., 2016).

Comment

Increased dietary magnesium intake is associated with reduced stroke risk in observational studies, but RCTs of extended duration and sample size of magnesium sulfate or magnesium chloride dietary supplements have not been performed to confirm or disconfirm the hypothesis that daily 'Slow-Mag' supplements would reduce stroke risk. At present, correction of low serum magnesium levels to normal range is reasonable, but chronic daily supplemental magnesium to achieve high normal or supra-normal magnesium levels has insufficient supportive data to endorse as a standard practice.

Food Groups

Evidence

Overview

Large-scale studies have evaluated the epidemiological relation of dietary intake of diverse food (and drink) categories with stroke incidence. As shown in Table 17.2, in meta-analyses of prospective cohort studies, food groups associated with reduced incidence of stroke included: fruits, vegetables, nuts and seeds, fish, eggs, coffee, and tea. Food groups likely associated with reduced stroke incidence included cheese, and food groups with less reliable point estimates suggesting potential favourable effect on stroke risk included whole grains. Conversely, food groups associated with increased occurrence of stroke included both processed and unprocessed red meat. Food groups associated with a neutral effect on stroke risk included legumes and butter.

The directionality of these associations of diverse food groups with stroke risk largely accord with long-standing expectation, but for eggs (9 studies, 436,088 individuals, RR 0.91, 95% CI: 0.85–0.98) and coffee (22 studies, RR 0.80, 95% CI: 0.75–0.86) the actual observed protective associations are at variance with some prior conventional assumptions. Several potential mediators of the observed protective association have been postulated. For eggs, body LDL cholesterol levels chiefly reflect liver production of LDL, not dietary intake; eggs are rich in cholesterol but low in saturated or trans fat, so stimulate little hepatic LDL production. Coffee is a complex chemical mixture with hundreds of compounds, including several with beneficial vascular system effects, including the minerals potassium and magnesium and cholesterol-lowering niacin and its precursor trigonelline. It also remains possible that the apparent protective association of dietary intake of these food groups with stroke occurrence is a non-causal relationship, arising from confounding by covarying third variables, such as socioeconomic status. Being well-off may enable individuals both to have a lower risk of stroke and to afford to purchase more of these food categories, leading to a non-causal, inverse association between the foods and stroke events.

Dietary Patterns

Evidence

Risk of Stroke

A wide variety of diets have been developed that focus broadly upon dietary patterns at the level of broad food groups, rather than more narrowly upon intake of particular nutrients. Dietary patterns have been strongly associated with stroke risk in epidemiological studies. In the INTERSTROKE case–control study of 26,919 participants from 32 countries, among 10 common vascular risk factors, diet quality, as assessed with the food group-based Alternative Healthy Eating Index, contributed to 22.4% (95% CI: 17.0–29.0) of all ischaemic strokes and 24.5% (95% CI: 16.5–34.8) of all haemorrhagic strokes (population attributable risk) (O'Donnell et al., 2016). In prospective cohort studies, reduced stroke incidence has been associated with greater adherence to several different recommended dietary patterns, including the Mediterranean Diet, the DASH Diet, the Nordic Diet, the Healthy Eating Index, and the Alternative Healthy Eating Index (Hankey, 2017; Schwingshackl et al., 2018).

Dietary Pattern Interventions: Mediterranean Diet and DASH Diet

The two food-group-pattern diets that have the strongest randomized trial evidence for favourable effect on stroke risk are the Mediterranean Diet and the DASH Diet (Table 17.4). The Mediterranean Diet was first conceptualized in the 1960s, based on the eating patterns of long-lived people on the Mediterranean coast, including Greece, Italy, and Spain. The Dietary Approaches to Stop Hypertension (DASH) Diet was originally developed in the 1990s by the US National Institutes of Health specifically to reduce blood pressure, but also had, and has been further modified to increase, additional elements to promote overall vascular health.

The Mediterranean Diet and the DASH Diet share several core features. Both diets increase intake of fruit and vegetables, whole grains, legumes, and nuts, and reduce intake of red meat, sweets, and sugary drinks. Consequently, both diets increase intake of unsaturated fats and fibre and both reduce intake of carbohydrates and saturated fats. Beyond these predominant commonalities, the diets differ in some respects. The Mediterranean Diet is higher in intake of olive oil, seafood, and red wine. The DASH Diet reduces sodium intake explicitly, has more dairy (non-fat or low-fat) intake, and is higher in red meat.

In short-term studies, a meta-analysis of 3 randomized trials found that the Mediterranean Diet was associated with blood pressure reduction, SBP mean difference –3.02 mm Hg (95% CI: –3.47 to –2.58) (Ndanuko et al., 2016). In long-term studies with vascular event outcomes, a meta-analysis of 2 high-quality randomized trials enrolling 8052 participants found that allocation to the Mediterranean Diet was associated with reduced stroke occurrence, 1.2% versus 2.2%, RR 0.66 (95% CI: 0.48–0.92) (Liyanage et al., 2016). In addition, the Mediterranean Diet was

Table 17.4 Mediterranean and DASH Diets*

Mediterranean Diet		DASH Diet	
Food Group	Recommendation	Food Group	Servings
Whole grains Vegetables Fruits Nuts Seeds Beans Olive Oil Legumes	Base every meal on these foods	Whole grains	7 to 8 daily
		Vegetables	4 to 5 daily
		Fruits	4 to 5 daily
		Nuts Seeds Beans (dry)	4 to 5 per week
Fish, seafood	Eat at least twice a week	Fish Poultry Lean red meats	≤2 daily
Poultry Eggs Yogurt Cheese	Eat moderate portions daily to weekly	Dairy, low-fat or nonfat	2 to 3 daily
Wine	Drink in moderation	Fats and oils	2 to 3 daily
Red meats Sweets	Eat less often than other foods	Sweets	5 per week

* Based in part on reference: Harvard Women's Health Watch (2015).

Table 17.5 Optimal lifestyle to prevent stroke

Goal/Metric	Ideal
Physical activity	≥150 min/wk moderate or ≥75 min/wk vigorous intensity
Body weight and waist-to-hip ratio	<25 kg/m^2, minimize intra-abdominal/visceral obesity
Diet	Mediterranean Diet (or DASH Diet)
Alcohol	≤1 drink/d for women and ≤2 drinks/d for men
Fasting plasma glucose	<100 mg/dL
Smoking	Avoid
Long-term oestrogen hormone replacement	Avoid

associated with reduction in all vascular events (RR 0.69, 95% CI: 0.55–0.86) and a trend towards reduction in coronary events (RR 0.73, 95% CI: 0.51–1.05).

In short-term studies, a meta-analysis of 11 randomized trials found that the DASH Diet was associated with blood pressure reduction, SBP mean difference –4.90 mm Hg (95% CI: –6.22 to –3.58) (Ndanuko et al., 2016). Long-term RCTs with vascular event outcomes have not been reported for the DASH Diet.

Comment

The Mediterranean Diet reduces vascular risk factors and reduces stroke events. It is a recommended diet for stroke prevention. The DASH Diet, which in some ways is an Americanized version of the Mediterranean Diet, also reduces vascular risk factors, but has not yet been validated in long-term trials as reducing stroke events. It is a reasonable alternative diet for stroke prevention for individuals not able to adhere to the Mediterranean Diet.

Summary

For a few risk factors reviewed in this chapter, there is evidence from randomized controlled trials (RCTs) to guide clinical practice: adhering to a Mediterranean Diet pattern, avoiding long-term oestrogen hormone replacement, and treating severe obesity with gastric balloons or bariatric surgery reduce stroke risk. In addition, while there is no reliable evidence from RCTs that quitting smoking, controlling blood glucose, losing weight in moderately obese individuals, exercising regularly, abandoning heavy

alcohol consumption, and improving diet (less salt and more unsaturated fats) via other approaches reduces the risk of recurrent stroke, such evidence is very difficult to obtain, and observational studies suggest these changes probably do all help to reduce the stroke risk.

It therefore is appropriate for individuals to endeavour to reduce their risk of stroke and other serious vascular events by the modifications to their lifestyle as listed in Table 17.5, in part based on the American Heart Association Life's Simple 7 ideal goals (Lloyd-Jones et al., 2010). The potential beneficial effects of these measures in reducing stroke risk are likely largely mediated by their effects on well-established risk factors such as blood pressure, cholesterol, diabetes, and coagulation status, but may also be conferred in part through other effects.

In order to achieve these lifestyle changes, both the individual and the community must share responsibility. Governments have a responsibility to improve public education, access to healthy foods, and built environments with pedestrian, bicycle, and exercise infrastructure; to responsibly work with the food, tobacco, and alcohol industries; and to legislate and impose taxes against hazardous lifestyle behaviours (e.g. smoking, alcohol, and perhaps salt or sugar in foods). Continued cultural change is also required among individuals and communities to further incorporate regular physical activity, a healthy diet, and minimal exposure to smoking into everyday life.

References

Aburto NJ, Ziolkovska A, Hooper L, Elliott P, Cappuccio FP, Meerpohl JJ. (2013). Effect of lower sodium intake on health: systematic review and meta-analyses. *BMJ*, **346**, f1326.

Adebamowo SN, Spiegelman D, Willett WC, Rexrode KM. (2015). Association between intakes of magnesium, potassium, and calcium and risk of stroke: 2 cohorts of US women and updated meta-analyses. *Am J Clin Nutr*, **101**(6), 1269–77.

Adler AJ, Taylor F, Martin N, Gottlieb S, Taylor RS, Ebrahim S. (2014). Reduced dietary salt for the prevention of cardiovascular disease. *Cochrane Database Syst Rev*, 12. CD009217.

Afshin A, Micha R, Khatibzadeh S, Mozaffarian D. (2014). Consumption of nuts and legumes and risk of incident ischemic heart disease, stroke, and diabetes: a systematic review and meta-analysis. *Am J Clin Nutr*, **100**(1), 278–88.

Anthenelli RM, Benowitz NL, West R, St Aubin L, McRae T, Lawrence D, et al. (2016). Neuropsychiatric safety and efficacy of varenicline, bupropion, and nicotine patch in smokers with and without psychiatric disorders (EAGLES): a double-blind, randomised, placebo-controlled clinical trial. *Lancet*, **387**(10037), 2507–20.

Antithrombotic Trialists, C. (2002). Collaborative meta-analysis of randomised trials of antiplatelet therapy for prevention of death, myocardial infarction, and stroke in high risk patients. *BMJ*, **324**(7329), 71–86.

Antithrombotic Trialists Collaboration, Baigent C Blackwell L, Collins R, Emberson J, Godwin J, Peto R, et al. (2009). Aspirin in the primary and secondary prevention of vascular disease: collaborative meta-analysis of individual participant data from randomised trials. *Lancet*, **373**(9678), 1849–60.

Aune D, Giovannucci E, Boffetta P, Fadnes LT, Keum N, Norat, T, et al. (2017). Fruit and vegetable intake and the risk of cardiovascular disease, total cancer and all-cause mortality-a systematic review and dose-response meta-analysis of prospective studies. *Int J Epidemiol*, **46**(3), 1029–56.

Aune D, Keum N, Giovannucci E, Fadnes LT, Boffetta P, Greenwood DC, et al. (2016a). Nut consumption and risk of cardiovascular disease, total cancer, all-cause and cause-specific mortality: a systematic review and dose-response meta-analysis of prospective studies. *BMC Med*, **14**(1), 207.

Aune D, Keum N, Giovannucci E, Fadnes LT, Boffetta P, Greenwood, DC, et al. (2016b). Whole grain consumption and risk of cardiovascular disease, cancer, and all cause and cause specific mortality: systematic review and dose-response meta-analysis of prospective studies. *BMJ*, **353**, i2716.

Aung T, Halsey J, Kromhout D, Gerstein HC, Marchioli R, Tavazzi L, et al., and Omega-3 Treatment Trialists. (2018). Associations of omega-3 fatty acid supplement use with cardiovascular disease risks: meta-analysis of 10 trials involving 77917 individuals. *JAMA Cardiol*, **3**(3), 225–34.

Avert Trial Collaboration Group. (2015). Efficacy and safety of very early mobilisation within 24 h of stroke onset (AVERT): a randomised controlled trial. *Lancet*, **386**(9988), 46–55.

Baliunas DO, Taylor BJ, Irving H, Roerecke, Patra J, Mohapatra S, et al. (2009). Alcohol as a risk factor for type 2 diabetes: A systematic review and meta-analysis. *Diabetes Care*, **32**(11), 2123–32.

Bath PM, Gray LJ. (2005). Association between hormone replacement therapy and subsequent stroke: a meta-analysis. *BMJ*, **330**(7487), 342.

Bazerbachi F, Haffar S, Sawas T, Vargas EJ, Kaur RJ, Wang Z, et al. (2018). Fluid-filled versus gas-filled intragastric balloons as obesity interventions: a network meta-analysis of randomized trials. *Obes Surg*, **28**(9), 2617–25.

Benowitz NL, Pipe A, West R, Hays JT, Tonstad S, McRae, T, et al. (2018). Cardiovascular safety of varenicline, bupropion, and nicotine patch in smokers: a randomized clinical trial. *JAMA Intern Med*, **178**(5), 622–31.

Bernhardt J, Churilov L, Ellery F, Collier J, Chamberlain J, Langhorne, P, et al., and A. C. Group (2016). Prespecified dose-response analysis for A Very Early Rehabilitation Trial (AVERT). *Neurology*, **86**(23), 2138–45.

Bhat VM, Cole JW, Sorkin JD, Wozniak MA, Malarcher AM, Giles WH, et al. (2008). Dose-response relationship between cigarette smoking and risk of ischemic stroke in young women. *Stroke*, **39**(9), 2439–43.

Bhatnagar A, Whitsel LP, Ribisl KM, Bullen C, Chaloupka F, Piano MR, et al.; American Heart Association Advocacy Coordinating Committee, Council on Cardiovascular and Stroke Nursing, Council on Clinical Cardiology, and Council on Quality of Care and Outcomes Research. (2014). Electronic cigarettes: a policy statement from the American Heart Association. *Circulation*, **130**(16), 1418–36.

Billinger SA, Arena R, Bernhardt J, Eng JJ, Franklin BA, Johnson, CM, et al.; American Heart Association Stroke Council; Council on Cardiovascular and Stroke Nursing; Council on Lifestyle and Cardiometabolic Health; Council on Epidemiology and Prevention; Council on Clinical Cardiology. (2014). Physical activity and exercise recommendations for stroke survivors: a statement for healthcare professionals from the American Heart Association/American Stroke Association. *Stroke*, **45**(8), 2532–53.

Bjelakovic, G, Nikolova D, Gluud LL, Simonetti RG, Gluud C. (2012). Antioxidant supplements for prevention of mortality in healthy participants and patients with various diseases. *Cochrane Database Syst Rev*, 3. CD007176.

Boardman HM, Hartley L, Eisinga A, Main C, Roque i Figuls M, Bonfill Cosp X, et al. (2015). Hormone therapy for preventing cardiovascular disease in post-menopausal women. *Cochrane Database Syst Rev*, 3. CD002229.

Borek AJ, Abraham C, Greaves CJ, Tarrant M. (2018). Group-based diet and physical activity weight-loss interventions: a systematic review and meta-analysis of randomised controlled trials. *Appl Psychol Health Well Being*, **10**(1), 62–86.

Briasoulis A, Agarwal V, Messerli FH. (2012). Alcohol consumption and the risk of hypertension in men and women: a systematic review and meta-analysis. *J Clin Hypertens (Greenwich)*, **14**(11), 792–8.

Brien SE, Ronksley PE, Turner BJ Mukamal KJ, Ghali, WA. (2011). Effect of alcohol consumption on biological markers associated with risk of coronary heart disease: systematic review and meta-analysis of interventional studies. *BMJ*, **342**, d636.

Brunstrom M, Carlberg B. (2016). Effect of antihypertensive treatment at different blood pressure levels in patients with diabetes mellitus: systematic review and meta-analyses. *BMJ*, **352**, i717.

Cahill K, Lindson-Hawley N, Thomas KH, Fanshawe TR, Lancaster T. (2016). Nicotine receptor partial agonists for smoking cessation. *Cochrane Database Syst Rev*, 5. CD006103.

Cahill K, Stevens S, Perera R, Lancaster T. (2013). Pharmacological interventions for smoking cessation: an overview and network meta-analysis. *Cochrane Database Syst Rev*, 5. CD009329.

Cai X, Wang C, Wang S, Cao G, Jin C, Yu J, et al. (2015). Carbohydrate intake, glycemic index, glycemic load, and stroke: a meta-analysis of prospective cohort studies. *Asia Pac J Public Health*, **27**(5), 486–96.

Chan WS., Ray J, Wai EK, Ginsburg S, Hannah ME, Corey PN, et al. (2004). Risk of stroke in women exposed to low-dose oral contraceptives: a critical evaluation of the evidence. *Arch Intern Med*, **164**(7), 741–7.

Chang CL, Donaghy M, Poulter N. (1999). Migraine and stroke in young women: case-control study. The World Health Organization Collaborative Study of Cardiovascular Disease and Steroid Hormone Contraception. *BMJ*, **318** (7175), 13–18.

Chang SH, Stoll CR, Song J, Varela JE, Eagon CJ, Colditz GA. (2014). The effectiveness and risks of bariatric surgery: an updated systematic review and meta-analysis, 2003–2012. *JAMA Surg*, **149**(3), 275–87.

Chen Y, Copeland WK, Vedanthan R, Grant E, Lee JE, Gu, D, et al. (2013). Association between body mass index and cardiovascular disease mortality in east Asians and south Asians: pooled analysis of prospective data from the Asia Cohort Consortium. *BMJ*, **347**, f5446.

Cheng P, Huang W, Bai W, Wu Y, Yu J, Zhu, X, et al. (2015). BMI affects the relationship between long chain n-3 polyunsaturated fatty acid intake and stroke risk: a meta-analysis. *Sci Rep*, **5**, 14161.

Cholesterol Treatment Trialists, Kearney PM, Blackwell L, Collins R, Keech A, Simes J, Peto, R, et al. (2008). Efficacy of cholesterol-lowering therapy in 18,686 people with diabetes in 14 randomised trials of statins: a meta-analysis. *Lancet*, **371**(9607), 117–25.

Chowdhury R, Stevens S, Gorman D, Pan A, Warnakula S, Chowdhury S, et al. (2012). Association between fish consumption, long chain omega 3 fatty acids, and risk of cerebrovascular disease: systematic review and meta-analysis. *BMJ*, **345**, e6698.

D'Elia L, Iannotta C, Sabino P, Ippolito R. (2014). Potassium-rich diet and risk of stroke: updated meta-analysis. *Nutr Metab Cardiovasc Dis*, **24**(6), 585–7.

D'Isabella NT, Shkredova DA, Richardson JA, Tang A. (2017). Effects of exercise on cardiovascular risk factors following stroke or transient ischemic attack: a systematic review and meta-analysis. *Clin Rehabil*, **31**(12), 1561–72.

de Goede J, Soedamah-Muthu SS, Pan, A Gijsbers L, Geleijnse JM. (2016). Dairy consumption and risk of stroke: a systematic review and updated dose-response meta-analysis of prospective cohort studies. *J Am Heart Assoc*, **5**(5):e002787. doi: 10.1161/JAHA.115.002787 May 20;5(5):e002787. doi: 10.1161/JAHA.115.002787.

de Souza RJ, Mente, A, Maroleanu, A, Cozma, AI, Ha, V, Kishibe, T, et al. (2015). Intake of saturated and trans unsaturated fatty acids and risk of all cause mortality, cardiovascular disease, and type 2 diabetes: systematic review and meta-analysis of observational studies. *BMJ*, **351**, h3978.

Ding M, Bhupathiraj SN, Satija A, van Dam RM, Hu FU. (2014). Long-term coffee consumption and risk of cardiovascular disease: a systematic review and a dose-response meta-analysis of prospective cohort studies. *Circulation*, **129**(6), 643–59.

Edjoc RK, Reid RD, Sharma M. (2012). The effectiveness of smoking cessation interventions in smokers with cerebrovascular disease: a systematic review. *BMJ Open*, **2**(6), e002022.

Eisenberg MJ, Windle SB, Roy N, Old W, Grondin FR, Bata I, et al., and EVITA investigators. (2016). Varenicline for smoking cessation in hospitalized patients with acute coronary syndrome. *Circulation*, **133**(1), 21–30.

Emdin CA, Rahimi K, Neal B, Callender T, Perkovic V, Patel A. (2015). Blood pressure lowering in type 2 diabetes: a systematic review and meta-analysis. *JAMA*, **313**(6), 603–15.

Epstein KA, Viscoli CM, Spence JD, Young LH, Inzucchi SE, Gorman M, et al, and I. T. Investigators. (2017). Smoking cessation and outcome after ischemic stroke or TIA. *Neurology*, **89**(16), 1723–9.

Fang X, Wang K, Han D, He X, Wei J, Zhao L, et al. (2016). Dietary magnesium intake and the risk of cardiovascular disease, type 2 diabetes, and all-cause mortality: a dose-response meta-analysis of prospective cohort studies. *BMC Med*, **14**(1), 210.

Ferri M, Amato L, Davoli M. (2006). Alcoholics Anonymous and other 12-step programmes for alcohol dependence. *Cochrane Database Syst Rev*, 3. CD005032.

Ford JA, MacLennan GS, Avenell A, Bolland M, Grey A, Witham M, et al. (2014). Cardiovascular disease and vitamin D supplementation: trial analysis, systematic review, and meta-analysis. *Am J Clin Nutr*, **100**(3), 746–55.

Fox CS, Golden SH, Anderson C, Bray GA, Burke LE, de Boer IH, et al.; American Heart Association Diabetes Committee of the Council on Lifestyle and Cardiometabolic Health; Council on Clinical Cardiology, Council on Cardiovascular and Stroke Nursing, Council on Cardiovascular Surgery and Anesthesia, Council on Quality of Care and Outcomes Research; American Diabetes Association. (2015). Update on prevention of cardiovascular disease in adults with type 2 diabetes mellitus in light of recent evidence: a scientific statement from the American Heart Association and the American Diabetes Association. *Circulation*, **132**(8), 691–718.

Gillum LA, Mamidipudi SK, Johnston SC. (2000). Ischemic stroke risk with oral contraceptives: a meta-analysis. *JAMA*, **284**(1), 72–8.

Greaves CJ, Sheppard KE, Abraham C, Hardeman W, Roden M, Evans, PH, et al., I. S. Group (2011). Systematic review of reviews of intervention components associated with increased effectiveness in dietary and physical activity interventions. *BMC Public Health*, **11**, 119.

Guo Y, Yue XJ, Li HH, Song ZX, Yan HQ, Zhang, P, et al. (2016). Overweight and obesity in young adulthood and the risk of stroke: a meta-analysis. *J Stroke Cerebrovasc Dis*, **25** (12), 2995–3004.

Hankey GJ. (2017). The role of nutrition in the risk and burden of stroke: an update of the evidence. *Stroke*, **48**(11), 3168–74.

Harvard Women's Health Watch (2015). DASH or Mediterranean: which diet is better for you? *Harvard Women's Health Watch*, **14**(9), 4.

He Y, Li Y, Chen Y, Feng L, Nie Z. (2014). Homocysteine level and risk of different stroke types: a meta-analysis of prospective observational studies. *Nutr Metab Cardiovasc Dis*, **24**(11), 1158–65.

Hooper L, Martin N, Abdelhamid A., Davey Smith G. (2015). Reduction in saturated fat intake for cardiovascular disease. *Cochrane Database Syst Rev*, 6. CD011737.

Hopper I, Billah B, Skiba M, Krum H. (2011). Prevention of diabetes and reduction in major cardiovascular events in studies of subjects with prediabetes: meta-analysis of randomised controlled clinical trials. *Eur J Cardiovasc Prev Rehabil*, **18**(6), 813–23.

Hsu, CY, Chiu SW, Hong KS, Saver JL, Wu YL, Lee JD, et al. (2018). Folic acid in stroke prevention in countries without mandatory folic acid food fortification: a meta-analysis of randomized controlled trials. *J Stroke*, **20**(1), 99–109.

Huang K, Liu F, Han X, Huang C, Huang J, Gu D, et al. (2016). Association of BMI with total mortality and recurrent stroke among stroke patients: A meta-analysis of cohort studies. *Atherosclerosis*, **253**(10), 94–101.

Hughes JR, Stead LF, J. Hartmann-Boyce J, Cahill K, Lancaster T. (2014). Antidepressants for smoking cessation. *Cochrane Database Syst Rev*, 1. CD000031.

James AH, Bushnell CD, Jamison MG, Myers ER. (2005). Incidence and risk factors for stroke in pregnancy and the puerperium. *Obstet Gynecol*, **106**(3), 509–16.

Jensen MD, Ryan DH, Apovian CM, Ard JD Comuzzie AG, Donato, KA, et al., American College of Cardiology/American Heart Association Task Force on Practice Guidelines; Obesity Society. (2014). 2013 AHA/ACC/TOS guideline for the management of overweight and obesity in adults: a report of the American College of Cardiology/American Heart Association Task Force on Practice Guidelines and The Obesity Society. *J Am Coll Cardiol* **63**(25 Pt B): 2985–3023.

Johnston BC, Kanters S, Bandayrel K, Wu P, Naji F, Siemieniuk RA, et al. (2014). Comparison of weight loss among named diet programs in overweight and obese adults: a meta-analysis. *JAMA*, **312**(9), 923–933.

Jonas DE, Amick HR, Feltner C, Bobashev G, Thomas K, Wines R, et al. (2014). Pharmacotherapy for adults with alcohol use disorders in outpatient settings: a systematic review and meta-analysis. *JAMA*, **311**(18), 1889–1900.

Kawachi I, Colditz GA, Stampfer MJ, Willett WC, Manson JE, Rosner B, et al. (1993). Smoking cessation and decreased risk of stroke in women. *JAMA*, **269**(2), 232–6.

Kemmeren JM, Tanis BC, van den Bosch MA, Bollen EL, Helmerhorst FM, van der Graaf Y, et al. (2002). Risk of Arterial Thrombosis in Relation to Oral Contraceptives (RATIO) study: oral contraceptives and the risk of ischemic stroke. *Stroke*, **33**(5), 1202–08.

Kernan WN, Ovbiagele B, Black HR, Bravata, DM, Chimowitz, MI, Ezekowitz, MD, et al. (2014). Guidelines for the prevention of stroke in patients with stroke and transient ischemic attack: a guideline for healthcare professionals from the American Heart Association/American Stroke Association. *Stroke*, **45**(7), 2160–2236.

Khoury JC, Kleindorfer D, Alwell K, Moomaw CJ, Woo D, Adeoye O, et al. (2013). Diabetes mellitus: a risk factor for ischemic stroke in a large biracial population. *Stroke*, **44**(6), 1500–04.

Kodama S, Saito K, Tanaka, S, Horikawa C, Saito A, Heianza Y, et al. (2011). Alcohol consumption and risk of atrial fibrillation: a meta-analysis. *J Am Coll Cardiol*, **57**(4), 427–36.

Kwok CS, Pradhan A, Khan MA, Anderson SG, Keavney BD, Myint PK, et al. (2014). Bariatric surgery and its impact on cardiovascular disease and mortality: a systematic review and meta-analysis. *Int J Cardiol*, **173**(1), 20–8.

Larsson SC, Wallin A, Wolk A, Markus HS. (2016). Differing association of alcohol consumption with different stroke types: a systematic review and meta-analysis. *BMC Med*, **14**(1), 178.

Lee HJ, Choi EK, Lee SH, Kim YJ, Han D, Oh S. (2018). Risk of ischemic stroke in metabolically healthy obesity: a nationwide population-based study. *PLoS One*, **13**(3), e0195210.

Lee M, Saver JL, Hong KS, Song S, Chang KH, Ovbiagele B. (2012). Effect of pre-diabetes on future risk of stroke: meta-analysis. *BMJ*, **344**, e3564.

Lee PN, Forey BA. (2006). Environmental tobacco smoke exposure and risk of stroke in nonsmokers: a review with meta-analysis. *J Stroke Cerebrovasc Dis*, **15**(5), 190–201.

Li XY, Cai XL, Bian PD, Hu LR. (2012). High salt intake and stroke: meta-analysis of the epidemiologic evidence. *CNS Neurosci Ther*, **18**(8), 691–701.

Lin MP, Ovbiagele, B, Markovic D, Towfighi A. (2016). Association of secondhand smoke with stroke outcomes. *Stroke*, **47**(11), 2828–35.

Liyanage T, Ninomiya T, Wang A, Neal B, Jun M, Wong, MG, et al. (2016). Effects of the Mediterranean Diet on cardiovascular outcomes – a systematic review and meta-analysis. *PLoS One*, **11**(8), e0159252.

Lloyd-Jones DM, Hong Y, Labarthe D, Mozaffarian D, Appel LJ, Van Horn L, et al. (2010). Defining and setting national goals for cardiovascular health promotion and disease reduction: the American Heart Association's strategic Impact Goal through 2020 and beyond. *Circulation*, **121**(4), 586–613.

Malek AM, Cushman, M, Lackland, DT, Howard G, McClure LA. (2015). Secondhand smoke exposure and stroke: the Reasons for Geographic and Racial Differences in Stroke (REGARDS) Study. *Am J Prev Med*, **49**(6), e89–97.

Marso SP, Kennedy KF, House JA, McGuire DK. (2010). The effect of intensive glucose control on all-cause and cardiovascular mortality, myocardial infarction and stroke in persons with type 2 diabetes mellitus: a systematic review and meta-analysis. *Diab Vasc Dis Res*, **7**(2), 119–30.

Marti-Carvajal AJ, Sola I, Lathyris D, Dayer M. (2017). Homocysteine-lowering interventions for preventing cardiovascular events. *Cochrane Database Syst Rev*, 8. CD006612.

Martinez-Gonzalez MA, Dominguez LJ, Delgado-Rodriguez M. (2014). Olive oil consumption and risk of CHD and/or stroke: a meta-analysis of case-control, cohort and intervention studies. *Br J Nutr*, **112**(2), 248–59.

McRobbie H, Bullen C, Hartmann-Boyce J, Hajek P. (2014). Electronic cigarettes for smoking cessation and reduction. *Cochrane Database Syst Rev*, 12. CD010216.

Meschia JF, Bushnell C, Boden-Albala B, Braun LT, Bravata DM, Chaturvedi S, et al.; American Heart Association Stroke Council; Council on Cardiovascular and Stroke Nursing; Council on Clinical Cardiology; Council on Functional Genomics and Translational Biology; Council on Hypertension. (2014). Guidelines for the primary prevention of stroke: a statement for healthcare professionals from the American Heart Association/American Stroke Association. *Stroke*, **45**(12), 3754–3832.

Moresoli P, Habib B, Reynier P, Secrest MH, Eisenberg MJ, Filion KB. (2017). Carotid stenting versus endarterectomy for asymptomatic carotid artery stenosis: a systematic review and meta-analysis. *Stroke*, **48**(8), 2150–7.

Mukamal KJ, Massaro JM, Ault KA, Mittleman MA, Sutherland PA, Lipinska I, (2005). Alcohol consumption and platelet activation and aggregation among women and men: the Framingham Offspring Study. *Alcohol Clin Exp Res*, **29**(10), 1906–12.

Myung SK, Ju W, Cho B, Oh SW, Park SM, Koo, BK, Park BJ, and Korean Meta-Analysis Study Group. (2013). Efficacy of vitamin and antioxidant supplements in prevention of cardiovascular disease: systematic review and meta-analysis of randomised controlled trials. *BMJ*, **346**, f10.

Narain A, Kwok CS, Mamas MA. (2016). Soft drinks and sweetened beverages and the risk of cardiovascular disease and mortality: a systematic review and meta-analysis. *Int J Clin Pract*, **70**(10), 791–805.

Ndanuko RN, Tapsell, LC, Charlton, KE, Neale EP, Batterham MJ. (2016). Dietary patterns and blood pressure in adults: a systematic review and meta-analysis of randomized controlled trials. *Adv Nutr*, **7**(1), 76–89.

Nightingale AL, Farmer RD. (2004). Ischemic stroke in young women: a nested case-control study using the UK General Practice Research Database. *Stroke*, **35**(7), 1574–8.

O'Donnell MJ, Chin SL, Rangarajan S, Xavier D, Liu L, Zhang H, et al.; and INTERSTROKE Investigators. (2016). Global and regional effects of potentially modifiable risk factors associated with acute stroke in 32 countries (INTERSTROKE): a case-control study. *Lancet*, **388** (10046), 761–75.

Oesch L, Tatlisumak T, Arnold M, Sarikaya H. (2017). Obesity paradox in stroke – myth or reality? A systematic review. *PLoS One*, **12**(3), e0171334.

Oono IP, Mackay DF, Pell JP. (2011). Meta-analysis of the association between secondhand smoke exposure and stroke. *J Public Health (Oxf)*, **33**(4), 496–502.

Pan A, Wang Y, Talaei M, Hu FB. (2015). Relation of smoking with total mortality and cardiovascular events among patients with diabetes mellitus: a meta-analysis and systematic review. *Circulation*, **132**(19), 1795–1804.

Peters SA, Huxley RR, Woodward M. (2013). Smoking as a risk factor for stroke in women compared with men: a systematic review and meta-analysis of 81 cohorts, including 3,980,359 individuals and 42,401 strokes. *Stroke*, **44**(10), 2821–8.

Peters SA, Huxley RR, Woodward M. (2014). Diabetes as a risk factor for stroke in women compared with men: a systematic review and meta-analysis of 64 cohorts, including 775,385 individuals and 12,539 strokes. *Lancet*, **383**(9933), 1973–80.

Qin X, Li J, Spence JD, Zhang Y, Li Y, Wang, X, et al. (2016). Folic acid therapy reduces the first stroke risk associated with hypercholesterolemia among hypertensive patients. *Stroke*, **47**(11), 2805–12.

Roach RE, Helmerhorst FM, Lijfering WM, Stijnen T, Algra A, Dekkers OM. (2015). Combined oral contraceptives: the risk of myocardial infarction and ischemic stroke. *Cochrane Database Syst Rev*, 8. CD011054.

Roberson LL, Aneni EC, Maziak W, Agatston A, Feldman T, Rouseff M, et al. (2014). Beyond BMI: the metabolically healthy obese phenotype & its association with clinical/subclinical cardiovascular disease and all-cause mortality – a systematic review. *BMC Public Health*, **14**, 14.

Rothwell PM, Eliasziw M, Gutnikov SA, Fox AJ, Taylor DW, Mayberg MR, et al. (2003). Analysis of pooled data from the randomised controlled trials of endarterectomy for symptomatic carotid stenosis. *Lancet*, **361**(9352), 107–16.

Sabatine MS, Leiter LA, Wiviott SD, Giugliano RP, Deedwania P, De Ferrari GM, et al. (2017). Cardiovascular safety and efficacy of the PCSK9 inhibitor evolocumab in patients with and without diabetes and the effect of evolocumab on glycaemia and risk of new-onset diabetes: a prespecified analysis of the FOURIER randomised controlled trial. *Lancet Diabetes Endocrinol*, **5**(12), 941–50.

Sackner-Bernstein J, Kanter D, Kaul S. (2015). Dietary intervention for overweight and obese adults: comparison of low-carbohydrate and low-fat diets. a meta-analysis. *PLoS One*, **10**(10), e0139817.

Samson JE, Tanner-Smith EE. (2015). Single-session alcohol interventions for heavy drinking college students: a systematic review and meta-analysis. *J Stud Alcohol Drugs*, **76**(4), 530–43.

Santos FL, Esteves SS, da Costa Pereira A, Yancy WS Jr, Nunes JP. (2012). Systematic review and meta-analysis of clinical trials of the effects of low carbohydrate diets on cardiovascular risk factors. *Obes Rev*, **13**(11), 1048–66.

Sattar N, Preiss D, Murray HM, Welsh P, Buckley BM, de Craen AJ, et al. (2010). Statins and risk of incident diabetes: a collaborative meta-analysis of randomised statin trials. *Lancet*, **375**(9716), 735–42.

Schwingshackl L, Bogensberger B, Hoffmann G. (2018). Diet quality as assessed by the Healthy Eating Index, Alternate Healthy Eating Index, Dietary Approaches to Stop Hypertension Score, and Health Outcomes: an updated systematic review and meta-analysis of cohort studies. *J Acad Nutr Diet*, **118**(1), 74–100 e111.

Schwingshackl L, Hoffmann G. (2014). Monounsaturated fatty acids, olive oil and health status: a systematic review and meta-analysis of cohort studies. *Lipids Health Dis*, **13**, 154.

Shah RS, Cole JW. (2010). Smoking and stroke: the more you smoke the more you stroke. *Expert Rev Cardiovasc Ther*, **8**(7), 917–32.

Shou J, Zhou L, Zhu S, Zhang X. (2015). Diabetes is an independent risk factor for stroke recurrence in stroke patients: a meta-analysis. *J Stroke Cerebrovasc Dis*, **24**(9), 1961–8.

Siebenhofer A, Jeitler K, Horvath K, Berghold A, Posch N, Meschik J, et al. (2016). Long-term effects of weight-reducing drugs in people with hypertension. *Cochrane Database Syst Rev*, 3. CD007654.

Spence JD, Yi Q, Hankey GJ. (2017). B vitamins in stroke prevention: time to reconsider. *Lancet Neurol*, **16**(9), 750–60.

Stead LF, Buitrago D, Preciado N, Sanchez G, Hartmann-Boyce J, Lancaster T. (2013). Physician advice for smoking cessation. *Cochrane Database Syst Rev*, 5. CD000165.

Stead LF, Koilpillai P, Lancaster T. (2015). Additional behavioural support as an adjunct to pharmacotherapy for smoking cessation. *Cochrane Database Syst Rev*, 10. CD009670.

Stead LF, Perera R, Bullen C, Mant D, Hartmann-Boyce J, Cahill K, et al. (2012). Nicotine replacement therapy for smoking cessation. *Cochrane Database Syst Rev*, 11. CD000146.

Strazzullo P, D'Elia L, Cairella G, Garbagnati F, Cappuccio FP, Scalfi L. (2010). Excess body weight and incidence of stroke: meta-analysis of prospective studies with 2 million participants. *Stroke*, **41**(5): e418–26.

Threapleton DE, Greenwood DC, Evans CE, Cleghorn CL, Nykjaer C, Woodhead C, et al. (2013). Dietary fiber intake and risk of first stroke: a systematic review and meta-analysis. *Stroke*, **44**(5), 1360–8.

Tian DY, Tian J, Shi CH, Song B, Wu J, Ji Y, et al. (2015). Calcium intake and the risk of stroke: an up-dated meta-analysis of prospective studies. *Asia Pac J Clin Nutr*, **24**(2), 245–52.

Towfighi A, Markovic D, Ovbiagele B. (2012a). Current national patterns of comorbid diabetes among acute ischemic stroke patients. *Cerebrovasc Dis*, **33**(5), 411–18.

Towfighi A, Markovic D, Ovbiagele B. (2012b). Impact of a healthy lifestyle on all-cause and cardiovascular mortality after stroke in the USA. *J Neurol Neurosurg Psychiatry*, **83**(2), 146–151.

Towfighi A, Ovbiagele B. (2009). The impact of body mass index on mortality after stroke. *Stroke*, **40**(8), 2704–08.

Vinceti M, Filippini T, Crippa A, de Sesmaisons A, Wise LA, Orsini N. (2016). Meta-analysis of potassium intake and the risk of stroke. *J Am Heart Assoc*, **5**(10), e004210.

Wahid A, Manek N, Nichols M, Kelly P, Foster C, Webster, P, et al. (2016). Quantifying the association between physical activity and cardiovascular disease and diabetes: a systematic review and meta-analysis. *J Am Heart Assoc*, **5**(9).

Whiting DR, Guariguata L, Weil C, Shaw J. (2011). IDF diabetes atlas: global estimates of the prevalence of diabetes for 2011 and 2030. *Diabetes Res Clin Pract*, **94**(3), 311–21.

Wilk AI, Jensen NM, Havighurst TC. (1997). Meta-analysis of randomized control trials addressing brief interventions in heavy alcohol drinkers. *J Gen Intern Med*, **12**(5), 274–83.

Woodward M, Lam TH, Barzi F, Patel A, Gu D, Rodgers A, et al., and Asia Pacific Cohort Studies Collaboration. (2005). Smoking, quitting, and the risk of cardiovascular disease among women and men in the Asia-Pacific region. *Int J Epidemiol*, **34**(5), 1036–45.

Wu O, Robertson L, Twaddle S, Lowe GD, Clark P, Greaves M, et al. (2006). Screening for thrombophilia in high-risk situations: systematic review and cost-effectiveness analysis. The Thrombosis: Risk and Economic Assessment of Thrombophilia Screening (TREATS) study. *Health Technol Assess*, **10**(11), 1–110.

Xu L, Lam TH, Jiang CQ, Zhang WS, Zhu F, Jin, YL, et al. (2019). Egg consumption and the risk of cardiovascular disease and all-cause mortality: Guangzhou Biobank Cohort Study and meta-analyses. *Eur J Nutr*, **58**(2), 785–96.

Xu Z, Li Y, Tang S, Huang X, Chen T. (2015). Current use of oral contraceptives and the risk of first-ever ischemic stroke: a meta-analysis of observational studies. *Thromb Res*, **136**(1), 52–60.

Yang C, Pan L, Sun C, Xi Y, Wang L, Li D. (2016). Red meat consumption and the risk of stroke: a dose-response meta-analysis of prospective cohort studies. *J Stroke Cerebrovasc Dis*, **25**(5), 1177–86.

Yuan S, Li X, Jin Y, Lu J. (2017). Chocolate consumption and risk of coronary heart disease, stroke, and diabetes: a meta-analysis of prospective studies. *Nutrients*, **9**(7):688. doi: 10.3390/nu9070688.

Zhang C, Qin YY, Wei X, Yu FF, Zhou YH, He J. (2015). Tea consumption and risk of cardiovascular outcomes and total mortality: a systematic review and meta-analysis of prospective observational studies. *Eur J Epidemiol*, **30**(2), 103–13.

Zhao M, Wu G, Li Y, Wang X, Hou FF, Xu X, et al. (2017). Meta-analysis of folic acid efficacy trials in stroke prevention: insight into effect modifiers. *Neurology*, **88**(19), 1830–8.

Zhong CK, Zhong XY, Xu T, Zhang YH. (2016). Measures of abdominal adiposity and risk of stroke: a dose-response meta-analysis of prospective studies. *Biomed Environ Sci*, **29**(1), 12–23.

Zoungas S, Arima H, Gerstein HC, Holman RR, Woodward M, Reaven P, et al.; Collaborators on Trials of Lowering Glucose. (2017). Effects of intensive glucose control on microvascular outcomes in patients with type 2 diabetes: a meta-analysis of individual participant data from randomised controlled trials. *Lancet Diabetes Endocrinol*, **5**(6), 431–7.

Chapter 18

Drugs, Devices, and Procedural Therapies to Prevent Recurrent Cardiogenic Embolic Stroke

Graeme J. Hankey

It has traditionally been considered that about 20% of first-ever and recurrent ischaemic strokes are due to embolism from the heart. However, recent population-based studies, such as the 2009–2010 Adelaide Stroke Incidence Study, suggest that embolism from the heart is now the major cause of ischaemic stroke, accounting for 42% (95% confidence interval [CI]: 36–49%) of all ischaemic strokes in this community (Leyden et al., 2013).

The major cardiac sources of embolism are the left atrium and left atrial appendage (particularly atrial fibrillation [AF]), the left ventricle (myocardial infarction [MI], cardiomyopathy), the mitral and aortic valves (mitral stenosis, infective endocarditis), and the venous system and right atrium via a patent foramen ovale (paradoxical embolism).

This chapter will review the evidence for antithrombotic therapies, left atrial appendage occlusive devices, antibiotics, and percutaneous closure of a patent foramen ovale (PFO) to prevent recurrent ischaemic stroke due to embolism from the heart.

Atrial Fibrillation

Atrial fibrillation is a major causal risk factor for embolic ischaemic stroke. It is conducive to thrombogenesis in the left atrium and left atrial appendage because it predisposes to each of Virchow's classic triad: endothelial/endocardial damage or dysfunction, stasis of blood, and hypercoagulability of blood (Goldberger et al., 2015).

Diagnosis and Detection

Screening High-risk, Asymptomatic Populations

In view of the known association of AF with stroke, and the evidence that anticoagulation can prevent up to 80% of strokes in patients with clinical nonvalvular AF, it is attractive to hypothesize that screening high-risk, asymptomatic populations with electrocardiography (ECG) should identify patients with AF for whom anticoagulation can be initiated and thromboembolic complications such as ischaemic stroke prevented.

However, the US Preventive Services Task Force (USPSTF) has recently highlighted that, although ongoing studies are evaluating this hypothesis, there is no current evidence to support it. (US Preventive Services Task Force et al., 2018). Accordingly, the task force concludes that the current evidence is insufficient to assess the balance of benefits and harms of screening for AF with ECG.

This recommendation statement of the USPSTF is based on a recent evidence report and systematic review for the USPSTF, which concluded that although screening with ECG can detect previously unknown cases of AF, it has not been shown to detect more cases than screening focused on pulse palpation (Jonas et al., 2018). Furthermore, although treatments for AF reduce the risk of stroke and all-cause mortality, they increase the risk of bleeding. Trials have not assessed whether treatment of screen-detected asymptomatic older adults results in better health outcomes than treatment after detection by usual care or after symptoms develop.

Screening Patients with Stroke and Transient Ischaemic Attack

Observational Studies

A systematic review and random effects meta-analysis of 50 studies of the yield of cardiac monitoring for diagnosing new AF after stroke or transient ischaemic attack (TIA) in a total of 11,658 patients reported that the overall proportion of patients diagnosed with AF after stroke was

- 7.7% (95% CI: 5.0–10.8) by admission electrocardiogram (ECG) in the emergency room (phase 1);
- 5.1% (3.8–6.5) by serial ECG in hospital, continuous inpatient ECG monitoring,

337

continuous inpatient cardiac telemetry, and in-hospital Holter monitoring (phase 2);

- 10.7% (5.6–17.2) by ambulatory Holter (phase 3); and
- 16.9% (13.0–21.2) by mobile cardiac outpatient telemetry, external loop recording, and implantable loop recording (phase 4) (Sposato et al., 2015).

The overall AF detection yield after all phases of sequential cardiac monitoring was 23.7% (95% CI: 17.2–31.0) (Sposato et al., 2015).

An analysis of individual patient data from three prospective studies of 1556 patients with stroke suggests that the AS5F score (Age: 0.76 points per year, Stroke severity National Institutes of Health Stroke Scale [NIHSS] <5 = 9 points, NIHSS >5 = 21 points) may be useful for selecting ischaemic stroke patients for prolonged ECG monitoring (to detect paroxysmal AF) (Uphaus et al., 2019). This score awaits external validation in independent data sets.

Clinical Trials

In the EMBRACE trial, noninvasive ambulatory ECG monitoring for 30 days in 572 patients with a recent cryptogenic stroke or TIA who were >55 years of age significantly improved the detection of AF by a factor of more than 5 (16.1% vs 3.2%, absolute difference 12.9%, 95% CI: 8.0–17.6%) as compared with the standard practice of short-duration 24-hour ECG monitoring. Noninvasive ambulatory ECG monitoring for 30 days also nearly doubled the rate of anticoagulant treatment at 90 days after randomization compared with the short-duration 24-hour ECG monitoring (18.6% vs 11.1%, absolute difference 7.5%, 95% CI: 1.6–13.3) (Gladstone et al., 2014).

In the CRYSTAL AF study, long-term monitoring with an insertable cardiac monitor (ICM) was more effective than conventional follow-up (control) for detecting AF at 6 months in 441 patients >40 years of age with cryptogenic stroke (<90 days ago) and no evidence of AF during >24 hours prior ECG monitoring (19 [8.9%] patients ICM vs 3 [1.4%] control; hazard ratio [HR] 6.4; 95% CI: 1.9–21.7; p < 0.001) (Sanna et al., 2014).

Interpretation

Atrial fibrillation might be newly detected in nearly a quarter of patients with stroke or TIA by sequentially combining cardiac monitoring methods.

Implications for Practice

It is recommended that for patients with acute ischaemic stroke or TIA and no apparent cause, prolonged rhythm monitoring ($\approx$30 days) for AF is reasonable within 6 months of the event (Kernan et al., 2014).

Risk Stratification

Predictors of Stroke and Systemic Embolism in Patients with AF

For patients with AF, the main predictors of an increased risk of stroke are those comprising the $CHADS_2$ and CHA_2DS_2-VASc scores (Tables 18.1 and 18.2) and the age, biomarkers (N-terminal fragment B-type natriuretic peptide [NT-proBNP] and cardiac troponin high sensitivity [cTn-hs]), and clinical history (prior stroke or TIA) (ABC) score (Lip et al., 2010; Olesen et al., 2011; Hijazi et al., 2016a; Borre et al., 2018; Chen et al., 2019). However, these scores demonstrate only mediocre predictive values with C statistics ranging from 0.55 to 0.64.

Additional clinical predictors of stroke in anticoagulated patients with AF include vitamin K antagonist (VKA)-naive status (for VKA-experienced patients, risk ratio [RR] 0.85, 95% CI: 0.74–0.97), moderate

Table 18.1 Definitions and scores for $CHADS_2$ and CHA_2DS_2-VASc stratification methods for identifying patients with atrial fibrillation at risk of stroke

Item	$CHADS_2$ Score	CHA_2DS_2-VASc Score
Congestive heart failure	1	1
Hypertension	1	1
Age ≥75 years	1	2
Diabetes mellitus	1	1
Stroke, transient ischaemic attack, or thromboembolism	2	2
Vascular disease (previous MI, PAD, or aortic plaque)		1
Age 65–74 years		1
Sex category (female sex)		1
Maximum score	*6*	*9*

LV: left ventricular. MI: myocardial infarction. PAD: peripheral artery disease.

Table 18.2 Prevalence and stroke rate at 1 year of CHADS$_2$ and CHA$_2$DS$_2$-VASc scores in 73,538 patients with non-valvular atrial fibrillation (Olesen et al., 2011)

	CHADS$_2$		CHA$_2$DS$_2$-VASc	
	Prevalence (%)	Stroke rate at 1 year, % (95% CI)	Prevalence %	Stroke rate at 1 year, (95% CI)
0	22%	1.7% (1.5–1.9)	8%	0.8% (0.6–1.0)
1	31%	4.7% (4.4–5.1)	12%	2.0% (1.7–2.4)
2	23%	7.3% (6.9–7.8)	18%	3.7% (3.3–4.1)
3	15%	15.5% (14.6–16.3)	23%	5.9% (5.5–6.3)
4	7%	21.5% (20.0–23.2)	19%	9.3% (8.7–9.9)
5	2%	19.7% (16.9–22.9)	12%	15.3% (14.3–16.2)
6	0.2%	22.4% (14.6–34.3)	6%	19.7% (18.2–21.4)
7			2%	21.5% (18.7–24.6)
8			0.4%	22.4% (16.3–30.8)
9			0.1%	23.6% (10.6–52.6)

All patients in this study were discharged from a hospital in Denmark between 1997 and 2006 with non-valvular atrial fibrillation, were not anticoagulated, and were followed up for 1 year. CHA$_2$DS$_2$-VASc scores: 0 = no antithrombotic therapy recommended. 1 = antithrombotic therapy with oral anticoagulation or antiplatelet therapy recommended (preferably oral anticoagulation). ≥ 2 = oral anticoagulation recommended (Olesen et al., 2011).

renal impairment (1.54, 1.30–1.81), severe renal impairment (2.22, 1.85–2.66), previous aspirin use (1.19, 1.04–1.37), and Asian race (1.70, 1.42–2.03). (Albertsen et al., 2013).

Additional electrocardiographic predictors of ischaemic stroke in non-anticoagulated people with AF, independent of CHA$_2$DS$_2$-VASc variables, include an abnormal P-wave axis (Maheshwari et al., 2019).

Echocardiographic predictors of incident and recurrent stroke include echocardiographic evidence of stasis in the left atrium (spontaneous echo contrast ['smoke'] or diminished left atrial appendage (LAA) flow velocities [specifically peak LAA emptying velocity <0.2 m/s]), large LA dimension/volume, and LAA geometry; one study reported that patients with chicken wing morphology of the LAA were associated with a lower risk of stroke or TIA compared to other LAA morphologies, such as the cactus, cauliflower, and windsock morphology (odds ratio [OR] 0.21, 95% CI: 0.05–0.91) (Di Biase et al., 2012; Goldberger et al., 2015).

An advantage of the CHA$_2$DS$_2$-VASc score over the CHADS$_2$ score is that it helps identify very low-risk patients in whom anticoagulation may be associated with a net disadvantage (Friberg et al., 2012).

A limitation of the CHADS$_2$ and CHA$_2$DS2-VASc scores is that high scores are associated with increased risks of stroke and systemic embolism and also of bleeding and death (Oldgren et al., 2011). This association exists because many of the predictors of ischaemic stroke that contribute to the CHADS$_2$ and CHA$_2$DS$_2$-VASc scores (see Table 18.1) are also predictors of major bleeding that comprise the HAS-BLED score (Table 18.3). One study showed that, of the so-called shared predictors, older age and previous stroke or TIA were more closely associated with ischaemic stroke than with intracerebral haemorrhage, whereas a history of hypertension, diabetes mellitus, renal impairment, and alcohol intake was not more strongly associated with either ischaemic or haemorrhagic stroke (McGrath et al., 2012).

Predictors of Major Bleeding

The main predictors of an increased risk of major bleeding while taking oral anticoagulants are those comprising the HAS-BLED score (Tables 18.3 and 18.4) and ABC bleeding score (Age, Biomarkers [haemoglobin, cTn-hs, and GDF-15 or cystatin C/CKD-EPI] and Clinical history of previous bleeding]) (Pisters et al., 2010; Hijazi et al., 2016b; Borre et al., 2018).

Table 18.3 Definitions and scores for the HAS-BLED stratification method for identifying patients with atrial fibrillation at risk of major bleeding with oral anticoagulation

HAS-BLED score	
Hypertension (uncontrolled, systolic blood pressure ≥160 mm Hg)	1
Abnormal renal[†] or liver[††] function (1 point each)	1 or 2
Stroke (previous history)	1
Bleeding history or predisposition (anaemia)	1
Labile INR (if on warfarin, time in the therapeutic range <60%)	1
Elderly (age >65 years)	1
Drugs (antiplatelet or NSAID)[†††] or excess alcohol[††††] (1 point each)	1 or 2
Maximum score	*9*

† Abnormal renal function is classified as the presence of chronic dialysis, renal transplantation, or serum creatinine ≥200 micromol/L.

†† Abnormal liver function is defined as chronic hepatic disease (e.g. cirrhosis) or biochemical evidence of significant hepatic derangement (bilirubin >2 times the upper limit of normal, in association with aspartate aminotransferase, alanine aminotransferase, or alkaline phosphatase >3 times the upper limit normal).

††† Drugs = concomitant use of antiplatelet or non-steroidal anti-inflammatory drugs (NSAIDs).

†††† Excess Alcohol = ≥8 units/week.

INR: international normalized ratio.

Table 18.4 The risk of major bleeding within 1 year according to the HAS-BLED score in 3071 patients with non-valvular atrial fibrillation enrolled in the Euro Heart Survey (Pisters et al., 2010)

HAS-BLED score	Patients, n	Bleeds, n	Bleeds per 100 patient-years
0	798	9	1.13
1	1286	13	1.02
2	744	14	1.88
3	187	7	3.74
4	46	4	8.7
5	8	1	12.5
6	2	0	0
7	0	..	..
8	0		..
9	0	..	..
Any score	3071	48	1.56

Patients in the survey were followed up for 1 year. 48 patients had a major bleed at an overall rate of 1.56 per 100 patient-years. A HAS-BLED score of ≥3 indicates a major bleeding risk of about 3.7 per 100 patient-years, and means that caution is warranted in the prescription of oral anticoagulation, and treatment of modifiable risk factors for bleeding (e.g. hypertension, abnormal renal and liver function, drugs, and alcohol) and regular review are recommended.

Predictors of Intracranial Haemorrhage in Anticoagulated Patients with AF

ROCKET AF Trial Cohort

In the Rivaroxaban Once Daily, Oral, Direct Factor Xa Inhibition Compared With Vitamin K Antagonism for Prevention of Stroke and Embolism Trial in Atrial Fibrillation (ROCKET AF) trial cohort of 14,264 patients with AF who were anticoagulated with rivaroxaban or warfarin, 172 patients (1.2%) experienced 175 intracranial haemorrhage (ICH) events at a rate of 0.67% per year during 1.94 years (median) of follow-up (Hankey et al., 2014).

The significant, independent predictors of ICH were race (Asian: HR, 2.02; 95% CI: 1.39–2.94; black: HR, 3.25; 95% CI: 1.43–7.41), age (1.35; 1.13–1.63 per 10-year increase), reduced serum albumin (1.39; 1.12–1.73 per 0.5 g/dL decrease), reduced platelet count below 210×10^9/L (1.08; 1.02–1.13 per 10×10^9/L decrease), previous stroke or TIA (1.42; 1.02–1.96), and increased diastolic blood pressure (1.17; 1.01–1.36 per 10 mm Hg increase).

Predictors of a reduced risk of ICH were randomization to rivaroxaban (0.60; 0.44–0.82) and history of congestive heart failure (0.65; 0.47–0.89). The ability of the model to discriminate individuals with and without ICH was good (C-index, 0.69; 95% CI: 0.64–0.73).

Table 18.5 shows the platelets, albumin, no CHF, warfarin, age, race, diastolic blood pressure, stroke (PANWARDS) nomogram for predicting absolute risk of ICH in the ROCKET AF cohort of 14,000 anticoagulated patients with AF, which is based on the independent, significant prognostic factors for ICH and the strength of their association with risk of ICH.

Table 18.6 shows the predicted probabilities of ICH at 2.5 years according to the score derived from the variables within the PANWARDS nomogram.

Other Cohorts – The ROCKET AF cohort did not measure or analyse all potential risk factors for ICH in anticoagulated AF patients, such as imaging features of leucoaraiosis and cerebral microbleeds, which could be incorporated in ICH risk scores (SPIRIT Trial Investigators, 1997; Wilson et al., 2018).

The CROMIS-2 observational study of 1490 patients with AF and recent acute ischaemic stroke or TIA, treated with a VKA or direct oral

Table 18.5 PANWARDS nomogram for predicting risk of intracranial haemorrhage

Variable	Points
Platelets, × 10⁹/L	
<125	11
125–149	8
150–174	5
175–199	3
≥200	0
Albumin, g/dL	
<3.0	18
3.0–3.49	14
3.5–3.99	9
4.0–4.49	5
≥4.5	0
No history of CHF	6
Warfarin instead of rivaroxaban	7
Age, years	
<55	0
55–64	4
65–74	8
75–84	13
≥85	17
Race	
Black	18
Asian	9
White or other	0
Diastolic blood pressure, mm Hg	
<50	0
50–69	4
70–89	9
90–109	13
≥110	17
Stroke or TIA in past	5

CHF: congestive heart failure. PANWARDS: platelets, albumin, no CHF, warfarin, age, race, diastolic blood pressure, stroke. TIA: transient ischaemic attack.

Table 18.6 Predicted probabilities of intracranial haemorrhage (ICH) at 2.5 years according to total score on PANWARDS nomogram (Table 18.5)

Total score	n	Probability of ICH at 2.5 years
10	20	0.002
15	161	0.003
20	679	0.004
25	1465	0.006
30	2185	0.008
35	3001	0.012
40	2788	0.017
45	1889	0.025
50	994	0.035
55	406	0.049
60	166	0.070
65	62	0.098
70	12	0.137
75	4	0.190

n, number of patients

Rivaroxaban Once Daily, Oral, Direct Factor Xa Inhibition Compared with Vitamin K Antagonism for Prevention of Stroke and Embolism Trial in Atrial Fibrillation (ROCKET AF) cohort with PANWARDS score. ICH: intracranial haemorrhage. PANWARDS: platelets, albumin, no congestive heart failure, warfarin, age, race, diastolic blood pressure, stroke.

Compared with the HAS-BLED score alone (C-index 0.41, 95% CI: 0.29–0.53), prediction models which included cerebral microbleeds and HAS-BLED (0.66, 0.53–0.80) and cerebral microbleeds, diabetes, anticoagulant type, and HAS-BLED (0.74, 0.60–0.88) predicted symptomatic ICH significantly better (difference in C-index 0.25, 95% CI: 0.07–0.43, $p = 0.0065$; and 0.33, 0.14–0.51, $p = 0.00059$, respectively) (Wilson et al., 2018).

Long-term Prevention of Recurrent Cardiogenic Ischaemic Stroke

Aspirin vs Control

TIA and Ischaemic Stroke Patients

Recurrent Stroke – The European Atrial Fibrillation Trial found that aspirin is not significantly more effective than control for preventing recurrent stroke in patients with ischaemic stroke or TIA with AF (HR

anticoagulant, and followed up for a mean period of 850 days (standard deviation [SD] 373) reported that the rate of symptomatic ICH in patients with cerebral microbleeds was 9.8 per 1000 patient-years (95% CI: 4.0–20.3) compared with 2.6 per 1000 patient-years (95% CI: 1.1–5.4) in those without cerebral microbleeds (adjusted HR: 3.67, 95% CI: 1.27–10.60) (Wilson et al., 2018).

0.83, 95% CI: 0.65–1.05) (European Atrial Fibrillation Trial Study Group, 1993).

Interpretation

The result from this single secondary prevention trial in patients with prior stroke or TIA is consistent with the results of several primary prevention trials which also found that aspirin is not significantly more effective than placebo in preventing (first-ever) stroke in people with AF (RR 0.81, 95% CI: 0.65–1.01) (Hart et al., 2007).

Implications for Practice

Aspirin is not recommended for the secondary prevention of recurrent stroke in patients with AF and previous ischaemic stroke or TIA.

Clopidogrel Plus Aspirin vs Aspirin
Atrial Fibrillation Patients

The ACTIVE-A trial randomized 7554 patients with AF for whom VKA therapy was considered unsuitable (physician's judgement that VKA was inappropriate, 50%; specific risk of bleeding, 23%; patient's preference not to take VKA, 27%) to 75 mg clopidogrel once daily plus aspirin. Patients were followed up for a median of 3.6 years after randomization. Only 892 (13%) patients in this trial had a previous stroke or TIA (ACTIVE Investigators, 2009; Connolly et al., 2011a).

Major Vascular Events – Dual antiplatelet therapy (75 mg clopidogrel once daily plus aspirin) was associated with a marginal but statistically significant reduction in the primary outcome of stroke, MI, non-central nervous system (CNS) systemic embolism, or death from vascular causes, after a median of 3.6 years of follow-up, compared with placebo plus aspirin (6.8% per year clopidogrel plus aspirin vs 7.6% per year aspirin; RR 0.89 [95% CI: 0.81–0.98]) (ACTIVE Investigators, 2009).

Stroke – The combination of clopidogrel and aspirin was more effective than aspirin alone in preventing stroke (2.4% per year, clopidogrel plus aspirin, vs 3.3% per year, aspirin; RR 0.72, 95% CI: 0.62–0.83).

Major Bleeding – Major bleeding was greater among patients assigned clopidogrel plus aspirin versus those on aspirin alone (2.0% vs 1.3% per year; RR 1.57 [1.29–1.92]).

Interpretation

The ACTIVE-A trial data suggest that treating 1000 patients with AF for 1 year with clopidogrel plus aspirin prevents eight major vascular events (including two fatal and three disabling strokes) and causes seven major haemorrhages (one fatal) compared with aspirin alone.

Implications for Practice

For ischaemic stroke or TIA, AF, and being unable to take oral anticoagulants, the use of the combination of clopidogrel and aspirin therapy might be reasonable (Class IIb; Level of Evidence B) (Kernan et al., 2014).

Anticoagulation (warfarin) vs Control
TIA and Ischaemic Stroke Patients

Two randomized trials have compared oral anticoagulation versus control (no treatment) or placebo in a total of 485 patients with non-valvular AF and previous TIA or minor ischaemic stroke (Saxena and Koudstaal, 2004a).

Recurrent Stroke – For patients with AF and prior stroke or TIA, long-term adjusted-dose warfarin (international normalized ratio [INR]: 2.5–4.0) over about 2 years reduced the risk of recurrent stroke by two-thirds, compared with no antithrombotic therapy (8.9% warfarin vs 22.6% control, OR 0.36, 95% CI: 0.22–0.58) (Figure 18.1) (European Atrial Fibrillation Trial Study Group, 1993; Saxena and Koudstaal, 2004a)

Bleeding – Anticoagulation (INR 2.5 to 4.0 in the European Atrial Fibrillation Trial, 1993) significantly increased major extracranial bleeding complications compared with control (2.8% per year [oral anticoagulants] vs 0.7% per year [control]; OR 4.32, 95% CI: 1.55–12.1, absolute excess 2.1% per year) (Figure 18.2), but there was no association with any excess of intracranial bleeds compared to control in the two trials (OR 0.13, 95% CI: 0.00–6.49) (European Atrial Fibrillation Trial Study Group, 1993; Saxena and Koudstaal, 2004a).

The lack of excess intracranial bleeding with warfarin is most likely explained by the inclusion of highly selected patients in the historical European Atrial Fibrillation trial and low statistical power to reliably identify or exclude a modest but clinically significant increase in risk.

Interpretation

The results of the two studies indicate that in patients with nonrheumatic atrial fibrillation (NRAF) and a recent TIA or minor ischaemic

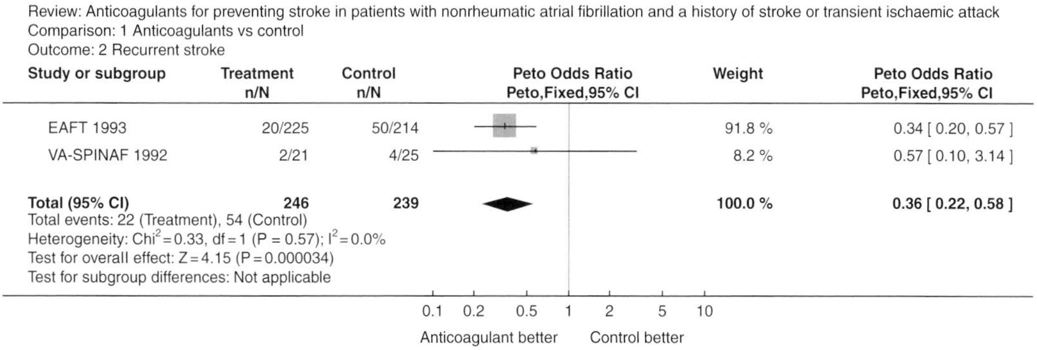

Review: Anticoagulants for preventing stroke in patients with nonrheumatic atrial fibrillation and a history of stroke or transient ischaemic attack
Comparison: 1 Anticoagulants vs control
Outcome: 2 Recurrent stroke

Study or subgroup	Treatment n/N	Control n/N	Peto Odds Ratio Peto,Fixed,95% CI	Weight	Peto Odds Ratio Peto,Fixed,95% CI
EAFT 1993	20/225	50/214		91.8 %	0.34 [0.20, 0.57]
VA-SPINAF 1992	2/21	4/25		8.2 %	0.57 [0.10, 3.14]
Total (95% CI)	**246**	**239**		**100.0 %**	**0.36 [0.22, 0.58]**

Total events: 22 (Treatment), 54 (Control)
Heterogeneity: Chi^2 = 0.33, df = 1 (P = 0.57); I^2 = 0.0%
Test for overall effect: Z = 4.15 (P = 0.000034)
Test for subgroup differences: Not applicable

0.1 0.2 0.5 1 2 5 10
Anticoagulant better   Control better

Figure 18.1 Forest plot showing the effects of *oral anticoagulants vs control* in patients with nonrheumatic atrial fibrillation (NRAF) and a history of stroke or TIA on *recurrent stroke* at the end of follow-up.

Reproduced from Saxena and Koudstaal (2004a), with permission from the authors and John Wiley & Sons Limited. Copyright Cochrane Library, reproduced with permission.

Review: Anticoagulants for preventing stroke in patients with nonrheumatic atrial fibrillation and a history of stroke or transient ischaemic attack
Comparison: 1 Anticoagulants vs control
Outcome: 4 Major extracranial bleed

Study or subgroup	Treatment n/N	Control n/N	Peto Odds Ratio Peto,Fixed,95% CI	Weight	Peto Odds Ratio Peto,Fixed,95% CI
EAFT 1993	13/225	2/214		100.0 %	4.32 [1.55, 12.10]
Total (95% CI)	**225**	**214**		**100.0 %**	**4.32 [1.55, 12.10]**

Total events: 13 (Treatment), 2 (Control)
Heterogeneity: not applicable
Test for overall effect: Z = 2.79 (P = 0.0053)
Test for subgroup differences: Not applicable

0.1 0.2 0.5 1 2 5 10
Anticoagulant better   Control better

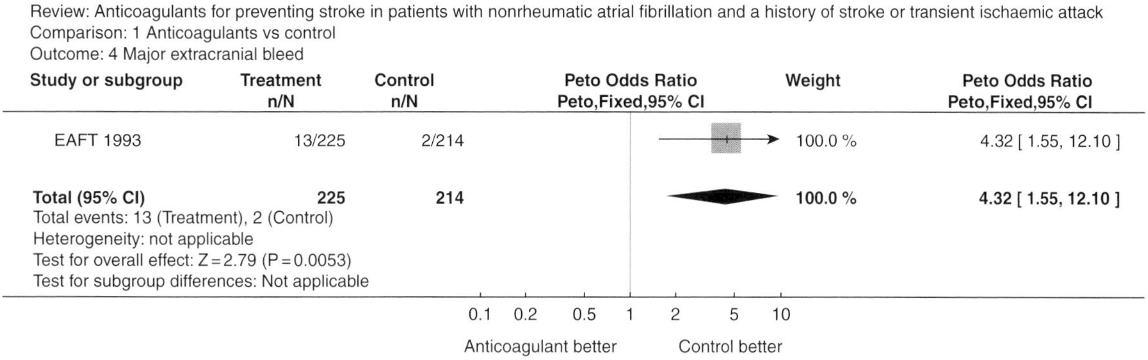

Figure 18.2 Forest plot showing the effects of *oral anticoagulants vs control* in patients with NRAF and a history of stroke or TIA on *major extracranial haemorrhages* at the end of follow-up.

Reproduced from Saxena and Koudstaal (2004a), with permission from the authors and John Wiley & Sons Limited. Copyright Cochrane Library, reproduced with permission.

stroke, oral anticoagulant treatment decreases the odds of recurrent stroke (disabling and non-disabling) by two-thirds, from about 12% per year (control) to 4% per year (oral anticoagulants; absolute risk reduction [ARR] 8% per year) and almost halves the odds of serious vascular events.

Although there was a 4-fold increase in serious bleeding complications, the absolute excess of 2.1% per year did not negate the absolute benefit in preventing recurrent stroke (8% per year).

Implications for Practice

These results indicate that anticoagulants should be prescribed to patients with NRAF and a recent TIA or minor ischaemic stroke, unless there is a major contraindication.

The target value for the INR should be set between 2.0 and 3.0 for safe and effective stroke prevention.

Timing of Anticoagulation after Stroke – There remains uncertainty about the ideal timing of initiating anticoagulant therapy after an acute cardioembolic stroke due to non-valvular AF (Ng and Whiteley, 2017; Seiffge et al., 2019).

Oral anticoagulation is generally started (or restarted) after about 2 weeks have elapsed because the risks of haemorrhagic transformation of the fresh brain infarct in the first 2 weeks may offset any benefits of earlier anticoagulation in reducing recurrent embolic ischaemic stroke. Patients with small ischaemic strokes, controlled blood pressure, and perhaps no evidence of microbleeding on gradient echo or susceptibility-weighted magnetic resonance imaging (MRI) sequences might be considered for earlier initiation of anticoagulant therapy, within the first week or so of ischaemic stroke, if they are at high risk of recurrent stroke. Hence, it is generally recommended that oral anticoagulation be initiated after the first 1–2 weeks of stroke onset. Patients with no residual brain infarction, such as those with TIA, should be safe to start anticoagulation immediately.

Peri-procedural Bridging Anticoagulation with Low-molecular-weight Heparin – The Bridging Anticoagulation in Patients who Require Temporary Interruption of Warfarin Therapy for an Elective Invasive Procedure or Surgery (BRIDGE) was a randomized, double-blind, placebo-controlled trial which showed that in 1884 patients with AF who stopped warfarin therapy 5 days before an elective operation or other elective invasive procedure (and which was resumed within 24 hours after the procedure), random assignment to bridging anticoagulation therapy with low-molecular-weight heparin (100 International Units [IU] of dalteparin per kilogram of body weight) or matching placebo administered subcutaneously twice daily, from 3 days before the procedure until 24 hours before the procedure and then for 5 to 10 days after the procedure, forgoing bridging anticoagulation was noninferior to perioperative bridging with low-molecular-weight heparin for the prevention of arterial thromboembolism and decreased the risk of major bleeding (Douketis et al., 2015).

The incidence of arterial thromboembolism (stroke, systemic embolism, or TIA) at 30 days after the procedure was 0.4% in the no-bridging group and 0.3% in the bridging group (risk difference, 0.1 %, 95% CI: −0.6–0.8; *p* = 0.01 for noninferiority). However, the incidence of major bleeding was 1.3% in the no-bridging group and 3.2% in the bridging group (relative risk, 0.41, 95% CI: 0.20–0.78; *p* = 0.005 for superiority) (Douketis et al., 2015).

Anticoagulation (warfarin) vs Single Antiplatelet Therapy

TIA and Ischaemic Stroke Patients

Two randomized trials have compared oral anticoagulation versus single antiplatelet therapy in a total of 1371 patients with non-valvular AF and previous TIA or minor ischaemic stroke (Saxena and Koudstaal, 2004a).

The European Atrial Fibrillation Trial (EAFT) randomized 455 patients with AF and recent (<3 months) TIA or minor ischaemic stroke to receive either anticoagulants (INR 2.5 to 4.0) or aspirin (300 mg/day) for a mean follow-up period of 2.3 years.

The Studio Italiano Fibrillazione Atriale (SIFA) trial randomized 916 AF patients within 15 days of prior TIA or minor ischaemic stroke to anticoagulation (INR 2.0 to 3.5) or indobufen (a reversible platelet cyclooxygenase inhibitor, 100 or 200 mg bid) for a follow-up period of 1 year.

Stroke – Adjusted-dose warfarin reduced the risk of recurrent stroke by about half (OR 0.49, 95% CI: 0.33–0.72) compared with antiplatelet therapy (European Atrial Fibrillation Trial Study Group, 1993; Saxena and Koudstaal, 2004b) (Figure 18.3).

This proportional reduction is consistent with the effect of adjusted-dose warfarin compared with

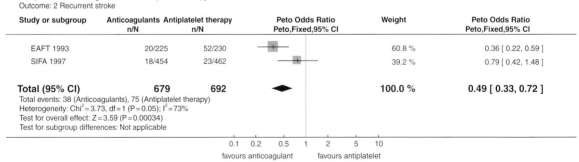

Figure 18.3 Forest plot showing the effects of *oral anticoagulants vs antiplatelet therapy* in patients with NRAF and a history of stroke or TIA on *recurrent stroke* at the end of follow-up.

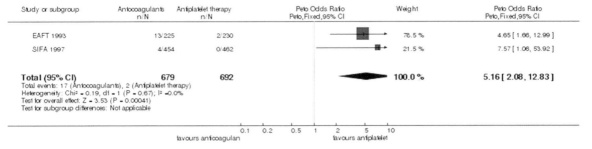

Figure 18.4 Forest plot showing the effects of *oral anticoagulants vs antiplatelet therapy* in patients with *NRAF and a history of stroke or TIA* on *major extracranial bleeding* at the end of follow-up.

antiplatelet therapy in the prevention of first-ever stroke (RR 0.61 [0.48–0.78]) (Hart et al., 2007).

Serious Vascular Events – Anticoagulants were also significantly more effective than antiplatelet therapy in reducing the odds of all vascular events by about one-third (OR 0.67, 95% CI: 0.50–0.91).

Bleeding – Adjusted-dose warfarin increased major extracranial bleeding by several-fold compared with antiplatelet therapy (OR 5.2, 95% CI: 2.1–12.8) but the absolute difference observed in the trials was small (2.8% per year [oral anticoagulants] vs 0.9% per year [antiplatelet therapy] in EAFT and 0.9% per year [oral anticoagulants] vs 0% [antiplatelet therapy] in SIFA) (European Atrial Fibrillation Trial Study Group, 1993; Saxena and Koudstaal, 2004b) (Figure 18.4).

Warfarin did not cause a significant increase of intracranial bleeds versus antiplatelet therapy (OR 1.99, 95% CI: 0.40–9.88).

Anticoagulation (warfarin) vs Dual Antiplatelet Therapy

TIA and Ischaemic Stroke Patients

For individuals with AF and previous stroke or TIA, adjusted-dose warfarin was significantly more effective for prevention of stroke than the combination of clopidogrel plus aspirin (2.99% per year with warfarin vs 6.22% with clopidogrel plus aspirin; RR 0.47, 95% CI: 0.25–0.81) in the ACTIVE-W trial (Healey et al., 2008).

The benefit of oral anticoagulant over antiplatelet therapy in AF depended on the quality of INR control achieved by centres and countries as measured by time in therapeutic range (Connolly et al., 2008).

For patients enrolled in the ACTIVE-W trial with $CHADS_2 > 1$, major bleeding occurred at a rate of 2.63% per year on clopidogrel plus aspirin and 2.75% per year on oral anticoagulation (RR 0.97, 95% CI: 0.69–1.35; $p = 0.84$). The relative risk of major bleeding with clopidogrel plus aspirin, compared with oral anticoagulation was not significantly different between patients with high and low $CHADS_2$ scores (p for interaction = 0.15); however, the absolute risk of major bleeding on oral anticoagulation was significantly lower among patients with $CHADS_2 = 1$ compared to $CHADS_2 > 1$ (RR 0.49, 95% CI: 0.30–0.79; $p = 0.0003$).

Interpretation

Anticoagulant therapy is more effective than single or dual antiplatelet therapy (DAPT) for the prevention of stroke in people with NRAF and recent non-disabling stroke or TIA.

Anticoagulation Plus Dual Antiplatelet Therapy vs Anticoagulation Plus Single Antiplatelet Therapy

Patients with ischaemic stroke/TIA and AF often have coexisting atherosclerotic vascular disease because hypertension and ischaemic heart disease are common causes of both AF and ischaemic stroke/TIA.

Traditionally, it has been considered that anticoagulation prevents the formation of fibrin-rich thrombus (so-called red clot) in areas of stasis of blood flow, such as the LAA associated with AF, whereas antiplatelet treatment prevents the formation of the platelet-rich thrombus (so-called white clot) in areas of high shear stress and endothelial injury associated with arterial

345

vascular disease. Hence, for patients with AF who present with unstable vascular disease manifested by an acute coronary syndrome, or who are undergoing vascular injury by means of percutaneous coronary or carotid intervention or stenting, the combination of aspirin plus clopidogrel is usually prescribed, at least in the short term (to prevent arterial thrombosis), in addition to prophylactic anticoagulation (to prevent left atrial thrombosis).

However, the WOEST trial reported that among 573 anticoagulated patients with AF who had an acute coronary syndrome or underwent percutaneous coronary stent (drug eluting stent or bare metal stent) implantation, dual treatment with clopidogrel 75 mg daily plus oral anticoagulation (INR as originally indicated) caused less bleeding than triple therapy with clopidogrel 75 mg daily plus aspirin 80–100 mg daily plus oral anticoagulation (INR as originally indicated) (19.4% dual vs 44.4% triple; HR 0.36, 95% CI: 0.26–0.50) without increasing thrombotic events or the composite of death, MI, target vessel revascularization, stroke, or stent thrombosis (11.3% dual vs 17.7% triple; HR 0.60, 95% CI: 0.34–0.94) (DeWilde et al., 2013).

In view of the increased risk of bleeding with standard anticoagulation with a VKA plus DAPT with a P2Y12 inhibitor and aspirin in patients with AF undergoing percutaneous coronary intervention (PCI) with placement of stents, the PIONEER AF-PCI trial aimed to determine the effectiveness and safety of anticoagulation with a non-vitamin K antagonist oral anticoagulant (NOAC) (rivaroxaban) plus either one or two antiplatelet agents are (Gibson et al., 2016; Chi et al., 2018).

A total of 2124 participants with nonvalvular AF who had undergone PCI with stenting were randomly assigned to receive, in a 1:1:1 ratio, low-dose rivaroxaban (15 mg once daily) plus a P2Y12 inhibitor for 12 months (group 1); very-low-dose rivaroxaban (2.5 mg twice daily) plus DAPT for 1, 6, or 12 months (group 2); or standard therapy with a dose-adjusted VKA (once daily) plus DAPT for 1, 6, or 12 months (group 3).

The rates of clinically significant bleeding (the primary safety outcome) were lower in the two groups receiving rivaroxaban than in the group receiving standard therapy (16.8% in group 1, 18.0% in group 2, and 26.7% in group 3; hazard ratio for group 1 vs group 3, 0.59; 95% CI: 0.47–0.76; $p < 0.001$; hazard ratio for group 2 vs group 3, 0.63; 95% CI: 0.50–0.80; $p < 0.001$). The rates of death from cardiovascular causes, MI, or stroke were similar in the three groups

(Kaplan–Meier estimates, 6.5% in group 1, 5.6% in group 2, and 6.0% in group 3; p-values for all comparisons were non-significant).

The RE-DUAL PCI trial randomly assigned 2725 patients with AF who had undergone PCI to triple therapy with warfarin plus a P2Y12 inhibitor (clopidogrel or ticagrelor) and aspirin (for 1 to 3 months) (triple-therapy group) or dual therapy with dabigatran (110 mg or 150 mg twice daily) plus a P2Y12 inhibitor (clopidogrel or ticagrelor) and no aspirin (110 mg and 150 mg dual-therapy groups). Outside the USA, elderly patients (≥80 years of age; ≥70 years of age in Japan) were randomly assigned to the 110 mg dual-therapy group or the triple-therapy group (Cannon et al., 2017).

The incidence of a major or clinically relevant non-major bleeding event (the primary endpoint) was 15.4% in the 110 mg dual-therapy group as compared with 26.9% in the triple-therapy group (HR 0.52; 95% CI: 0.42–0.63; $p < 0.001$ for noninferiority; $p < 0.001$ for superiority) and 20.2% in the 150 mg dual-therapy group as compared with 25.7% in the corresponding triple-therapy group, which did not include elderly patients outside the USA (HR 0.72; 95% CI: 0.58–0.88; $p < 0.001$ for noninferiority). The incidence of the composite efficacy endpoint was 13.7% in the two dual-therapy groups combined as compared with 13.4% in the triple-therapy group (HR 1.04; 95% CI: 0.84–1.29; $p = 0.005$ for noninferiority). The rate of serious adverse events did not differ significantly among the groups.

Interpretation of the Evidence

For patients with AF who have stable vascular disease, there is no reliable evidence that adding aspirin or clopidogrel, or both, to oral anticoagulation is safe and effective compared with anticoagulation alone.

For patients with AF who have unstable vascular disease, the WOEST trial suggests that adding aspirin to the combination of clopidogrel and effective anticoagulation may not prevent more ischaemic events yet may increase bleeding. The PIONEER AF PCI trial suggests that for patients with AF undergoing PCI, the administration of either low-dose rivaroxaban plus a P2Y12 inhibitor for 12 months or very-low-dose rivaroxaban plus DAPT for 1, 6, or 12 months is associated with a lower rate of clinically significant bleeding, and similar efficacy rates to standard therapy with a VKA plus DAPT for 1, 6, or 12 months. The RE-DUAL PCI trial suggests that for patients with AF who have undergone PCI, the risk of bleeding is lower among those who received dual therapy with

igatran and a P2Y12 inhibitor than among those
received triple therapy with warfarin, a P2Y12
ibitor, and aspirin. Dual therapy was also nonin-
or to triple therapy with respect to the risk of
mboembolic events.

A bivariate analysis that simultaneously
racterized both risk and benefit demonstrated that
roxaban-based and dabigatran-based regimens
e both favourable over VKA plus DAPT among
ents with AF undergoing PCI (Chi et al., 2018).

ication for Practice

comitant antiplatelet and anticoagulant therapy is
recommended in patients with AF and ischaemic
ke/TIA unless there is a specific indication, such
a mechanical heart valve (see below), or a recent
te coronary syndrome, or coronary stent, in which
e the anticoagulant should probably be a NOAC
er than VKA.

itations of Warfarin

pite the effectiveness and affordability of vitamin
ntagonists such as warfarin for the prevention of
irrent ischaemic stroke in patients with AF, these
gs have several limitations.

Warfarin has a slow onset of action and initially
uires variable dose adjustments that may be due, in
t, to genetic variability of vitamin K epoxide reduc-
complex 1 (which is involved in γ-carboxylation

of vitamin K-dependent clotting factors) and cytochrome P450 enzymes, such as CYP2C9 (which are
involved in the metabolism of warfarin).

Fluctuations in dietary intake of vitamin K and
alcohol, and several drug–drug interactions, further
contribute to inter-individual and intra-individual
variability in anticoagulant effects of warfarin.

Consequently, despite close monitoring of coagulation to maintain the INR in the therapeutic range (INR
2.0–3.0), this ratio is frequently outside the therapeutic
range, limiting the effectiveness of warfarin in up to 60%
of patients with AF, and increasing the risk of bleeding
(if INR too high) or thromboembolism (if INR too low).

These limitations have prompted the development
and assessment of several alternative antithrombotic
strategies.

Non-vitamin K Antagonist Oral Anticoagulants (NOACs) vs Warfarin

Pharmacology of the NOACs

The NOACs are target-specific, direct anticoagulants
which target thrombin (dabigatran etexilate) or factor
Xa (rivaroxaban, apixaban, and edoxaban)
(Heidbuchel et al., 2017; Steffel et al., 2018).

The pharmacological characteristics of the
NOACs are summarized in Table 18.7.

Dabigatran Etexilate – Dabigatran etexilate is a
prodrug of dabigatran that directly inhibits thrombin.

able 18.7 Pharmacological properties of non-vitamin K antagonist oral anticoagulants (NOACs)

eature	Dabigatran	Rivaroxaban	Apixaban	Edoxaban
arget	Thrombin	Factor Xa	Factor Xa	Factor Xa
osing	150 mg or 110 mg twice daily	15 or 20 mg once daily	2.5 or 5 mg twice daily	30 or 60 mg once daily
me to peak plasma oncentration	2 h	3 h	3 h	3 h
alf-life*	12–14 h	7–13 h	10–14 h	9–11 h
enal excretion	80%	33% (66%)	25%	35%
lonitoring	No	No	No	No
nteractions	P-gp†	CYP450 3A4‡ P-gp†	CYP450 3A4 ‡ P-gp†	CYP450 3A4‡ P-gp†
dverse effects	Dyspepsia, Bleeding	Bleeding	Bleeding	Bleeding

In patients with normal renal function.

P-glycoprotein inhibitors include azole antifungals (e.g. ketoconazole, itraconazole, voriconazole, posaconazole) and protease inhibitors (e.g. ritonavir).

Cytochrome P450 isoenzyme inhibitors include azole antifungals, protease inhibitors (e.g. atazanavir), and macrolide antibiotics (e.g. clarithromycin).

Thrombin has a pivotal role in blood coagulation by converting fibrinogen to fibrin; activating factors V, VIII, and XI; and activating platelets. Absorption from the gut depends on an acid environment, achieved with tartaric acid pellets coated with dabigatran etexilate. Despite this, bioavailability is only 6–7%. After oral administration, dabigatran etexilate is converted rapidly to dabigatran by hepatic and plasma esterases, and peak plasma concentrations are reached within 2 hours. Dabigatran is predominantly (80%) cleared by the kidneys. The drug half-life is 12–14 hours in patients with normal renal function, 18 hours if creatinine clearance is 30–50 mL/min, and more than 24 hours if creatinine clearance is less than 30 mL/min.

Dabigatran etexilate is a substrate for the P-glycoprotein transporter. P-glycoprotein is an efflux transporter that extrudes hydrophobic substances, such as toxins, out of cells into the gut, bile, and urine, and out of the brain and other organs. Since P-glycoproteins block absorption from the gut, co-administration of potent P-glycoprotein inhibitors (e.g. ketoconazole), which increase plasma concentrations of dabigatran, and co-administration of potent P-glycoprotein inducers (e.g. rifampicin), which reduce plasma concentrations of dabigatran, are contraindicated.

Rivaroxaban – Rivaroxaban is a direct-acting factor Xa inhibitor with a half-life of 7–13 hours. The 20 mg dose has a bioavailability of about 66% in the fasted state and the 10 mg dose has a bioavailability of about 80–100%; co-administration with food increases the bioavailability. A third of rivaroxaban is excreted unchanged via the kidneys and the remainder is broken down via CYP3A4-dependent and CYP3A4-independent pathways in the liver and excreted as inactive metabolites in the urine (half) and faeces (half). Rivaroxaban is also a substrate for P-glycoprotein. Co-administration of potent inhibitors of both P-glycoprotein and CYP3A4 (e.g. ketoconazole) results in higher drug concentrations and is contraindicated.

Apixaban – Apixaban is a direct-acting factor Xa inhibitor with similar pharmacological properties to those of rivaroxaban. It is partly broken down via CYP3A4 and excreted via several pathways. A quarter is excreted via the kidneys and the half-life is about 12 hours. Co-administration of potent P-glycoprotein and CYP3A4 inhibitors is contraindicated because it can lead to apixaban toxicity with increased risk of bleeding.

Edoxaban – Edoxaban is an oral, reversible, di factor Xa inhibitor with a linear and predictable p macokinetic profile and 62% oral bioavailability achieves maximum concentrations within 1 2 hours, and 50% is excreted by the kid Pharmacokinetic modelling and simulation s that patients with low body weight, moderate severe renal dysfunction, or concomitant use a potent P-glycoprotein inhibitor should have edoxaban dose reduced by 50%.

Advantages of the NOACs

Advantages of the NOACs include a rapid o of action; low propensity for interactions food, alcohol, and drugs; and administration fixed doses with a predictable anticoagulant ef that makes routine coagulation monitoring necessary.

Despite concerns that measurement of drug c centration or anticoagulant activity might be nee to prevent excessively low or high drug concen tions, which may significantly increase thromb and bleeding risk, respectively, data from ENGAGE AF-TIMI 48 trial suggest that adjustmen edoxaban dose based on clinical factors alone preve excess drug concentration and the risk of bleeding eve (Ruff et al., 2015). Edoxaban (or placebo-edoxaba warfarin group) doses were halved at randomizatio during the trial if patients had creatinine cleara 30–50 mL/min, body weight 60 kg or less, or c comitant medication with potent P-glycoprot interaction. Although dose reduction decrea mean anti-FXa activity by 25% and 20% in higher-dose and lower-dose regimens, respectiv dose reduction preserved the efficacy of edoxa compared with warfarin (stroke or systemic em lism: higher dose p interaction = 0.85, lower d p interaction = 0.99) and provided even greater sa (major bleeding: higher dose p interaction 0 lower dose p interaction = 0.002).

These findings validate the strategy that tailor of the dose of edoxaban on the basis of clin factors alone (renal function, body weight, conco tant P-glycoprotein transport inhibitor or indu achieves the dual goal of preventing excess d concentrations and helping to optimize an ind dual patient's risk of ischaemic and bleeding eve The results also showed that the therapeutic wind for edoxaban is narrower for major bleeding tha is for thromboembolism.

Disadvantages of the NOACs

Disadvantages include twice daily administration for dabigatran etexilate and apixaban; underdeveloped methods of coagulation monitoring; potential for drug toxicity in patients with renal insufficiency, liver insufficiency, or taking P glycoprotein or CYP3A4 inhibitors; and, until the US Food and Drug Administration (FDA) approved the use of idracuzimab as an antidote to dabigatran in 2015 and andexanet alfa as an antidote to rivaroxaban and apixaban in 2018, the absence of an antidote that is widely accessible and affordable, proven to reverse the anticoagulation effects of the drug, stop bleeding, and reduce death and disability due to bleeding (the latter of which remains to be proven).

Clinical Trials of the Non-vitamin K Antagonist Oral Anticoagulants (NOACs) vs Warfarin

The efficacy and safety of dabigatran, rivaroxaban, apixaban, and edoxaban have been compared with warfarin for stroke prevention in atrial fibrillation in four large, phase 3 clinical trials: RE-LY (Connolly et al., 2009, 2010), ROCKET AF (Patel et al., 2011), ARISTOTLE (Granger et al., 2011), and ENGAGE AF-TIMI (Giugliano et al., 2013; Ruff et al., 2014; Verheugt and Granger, 2015).

Dabigatran vs Warfarin in Patients with Atrial Fibrillation

RE-LY (Randomised Evaluation of Long-term anticoagulant therapY) was a three-armed trial that compared two doses of dabigatran (110 mg twice a day or 150 mg twice a day) with standard dose-adjusted warfarin (target INR 2.0–3.0). Although healthcare providers and patients were blinded to dabigatran dose, warfarin was open label. All outcome events were independently adjudicated by two panel members blinded to treatment allocation.

Patients were excluded if they had poor renal function (creatinine clearance of <30 mL/min), active liver disease, or a stroke within 14 days of randomization, or were considered at high risk for bleeding. Twenty per cent of patients had a history of stroke or TIA. Low-dose aspirin was taken by about a third of all patients.

Stroke or Systemic Embolism – The lower dose of dabigatran etexilate (110 mg twice a day) was non-inferior to warfarin in reducing the rate of stroke or systemic embolism (warfarin 1.71% per year vs dabigatran 110 mg bid: 1.54% per year; RR 0.90, 95% CI: 0.74–1.10, $p < 0.001$ for non-inferiority, $p = 0.30$ for superiority).

The higher dose (150 mg twice a day) was superior to warfarin (warfarin: 1.71% per year vs dabigatran 150 mg bid: 1.11% per year; RR 0.65, 95% CI: 0.52–0.81; $p < 0.001$ for superiority).

The higher dose also significantly reduced the rate of ischaemic stroke compared with warfarin (RR 0.76, 95% CI: 0.59–0.97; $p = 0.03$).

Major Bleeding – The rates of all major haemorrhages were reduced in the lower-dose dabigatran group compared with warfarin (RR 0.80, 95% CI: 0.70–0.93), and roughly equal in the higher-dose dabigatran and warfarin groups (RR 0.93, 95% CI: 0.81–1.07). The exception was major gastrointestinal (GI) haemorrhage, which was increased in the higher-dose dabigatran group versus warfarin (1.56%/yr vs 1.15%/yr, RR 1.48, 95% CI: 1.18–1.85; $p < 0.001$).

Both doses of dabigatran significantly reduced haemorrhagic stroke and intracerebral haemorrhage compared with warfarin. The annual rates of haemorrhagic stroke were 0.12%/yr for the lower dose of dabigatran (HR vs warfarin 0.31, 95% CI: 0.17–0.56), 0.10%/yr for the higher dose (HR vs warfarin 0.26, 95% CI: 0.14–0.49), and 0.38%/yr for warfarin. The case fatality rate of intracerebral haemorrhage, which averaged 52%, was not significantly different in participants assigned dabigatran or warfarin (Hart et al., 2012).

Subsequent secondary analyses have shown that elderly patients (>75 years) had an increased risk of major haemorrhage with dabigatran 150 mg bid versus warfarin, and both doses of dabigatran had a higher risk of extracranial and GI haemorrhage compared with warfarin. However, the rate of ICH remained less with dabigatran than warfarin for all age groups.

Adverse Effects – Dabigatran caused higher rates of dyspepsia than did warfarin (11.8% with dabigatran 110 mg twice a day and 11.3% with dabigatran 150 mg twice a day vs 5.8% with warfarin), presumably related to the tartaric acid content of the dabigatran etexilate capsule.

A numerical increase in MI was reported with both doses of dabigatran compared with warfarin. A meta-analysis of all trials of dabigatran, including RE-LY, suggests that the absolute increase in MI is slight (0.14–0.17% per year), not statistically significant, and outweighed by the reduction in stroke and systemic embolism (0.6% per year).

Dabigatran vs Warfarin in Patients with Atrial Fibrillation and Previous TIA or Ischaemic Stroke

The relative effects of dabigatran versus warfarin in the 3623 patients with previous stroke or TIA were consistent with the effects of dabigatran versus warfarin in the 14,490 patients without previous stroke or TIA for both stroke or systemic embolism and major bleeding (Diener et al., 2010).

Stroke or Systemic Embolism – The rate of stroke or systemic embolism among patients treated with dabigatran 110 mg per day compared with warfarin was consistent among patients with prior stroke or TIA (2.32%/year dabigatran 110 mg vs 2.78%/year warfarin; RR 0.84, 95% CI: 0.58–1.20) and patients without prior stroke or TIA (1.34%/year vs 1.45%/year; RR 0.93, 95% CI: 0.73–1.18; interaction $p = 0.62$).

The rate of stroke or systemic embolism among patients treated with dabigatran 150 mg per day compared with warfarin was consistent among patients with prior stroke or TIA (2.07%/year dabigatran 150 mg vs 2.78%/year warfarin; RR 0.75, 95% CI: 0.52–1.08) and patients without prior stroke or TIA (0.87%/year vs 1.45%/year; RR 0.60, 95% CI: 0.45–0.78; interaction $p = 0.34$).

Major Bleeding – The rate of major bleeding among patients treated with dabigatran 110 mg per day compared with warfarin was consistent among patients with prior stroke or TIA (2.74%/year dabigatran 110 mg vs 4.15%/year warfarin; RR 0.66, 95% CI: 0.48–0.90) and patients without prior stroke or TIA (2.91%/year vs 3.43%/year; RR 0.85, 95% CI: 0.72–0.99; interaction $p = 0.15$).

The rate of major bleeding among patients treated with dabigatran 150 mg per day compared with warfarin was consistent among patients with prior stroke or TIA (4.15%/year dabigatran 150 mg vs 4.15%/year warfarin; RR 1.01, 95% CI: 0.77–1.34) and patients without prior stroke or TIA (3.10%/year vs 3.43%/year; RR 0.91, 95% CI: 0.77–1.06; interaction $p = 0.51$).

Rivaroxaban vs Warfarin in Patients with Atrial Fibrillation

The oral factor Xa inhibitor rivaroxaban was compared with warfarin in ROCKET AF (Rivaroxaban – Once daily oral direct factor Xa inhibition compared with vitamin K antagonism [target INR 2.0–3.0] for prevention of stroke and Embolism Trial in Atrial Fibrillation) (Patel et al., 2011). The study population in ROCKET AF was at high risk of stroke; 55% of patients had a previous stroke or TIA, and 90% had

either a previous stroke or TIA, or three or more risk factors for stroke. Patients were randomly assigned to receive fixed-dose rivaroxaban (20 mg daily, or 15 mg daily in patients with a creatinine clearance of 30–49 mL per minute) or adjusted-dose warfarin (target INR 2.0–3.0).

Stroke or Systemic Embolism – Rivaroxaban was non-inferior to warfarin for the prevention of stroke or systemic embolism in the primary per-protocol, on-treatment analysis (1.71% per year rivaroxaban vs 2.16% per year warfarin, HR: 0.79; 95% CI: 0.66–0.96; $p < 0.001$ for noninferiority), but was not better than warfarin according to the intention-to-treat analysis (2.12% vs 2.42% per year; HR 0.88; 95% CI: 0.74–1.03; $p < 0.001$ for noninferiority; $p = 0.117$ for superiority).

Bleeding – The rates of major and clinically relevant non-major bleeding were similar with rivaroxaban (14.91% per year) and warfarin (14.52% per year; HR 1.03, 95% CI: 0.96–1.11; $p = 0.44$).

However, rivaroxaban was associated with lower rates of intracranial haemorrhage ($p = 0.019$) and fatal bleeding (0.24% per year with rivaroxaban vs 0.48% with warfarin; HR 0.50, 95% CI: 0.31–0.79), but higher rates of major gastrointestinal bleeding (3.15% vs 2.16% per year; $p < 0.001$).

Rivaroxaban vs Warfarin in Patients with Atrial Fibrillation and Previous TIA or Ischaemic Stroke

The relative effects of rivaroxaban versus warfarin in the 7468 patients with previous stroke or TIA were consistent with the effects of rivaroxaban versus warfarin in the 6796 patients without previous stroke or TIA for stroke or systemic embolism (Hankey et al., 2012).

Stroke or Systemic Embolism – The rate of stroke or systemic embolism among patients treated with rivaroxaban compared with warfarin was consistent among the 7468 patients with prior stroke or TIA (2.79%/year rivaroxaban vs 2.96%/year warfarin; HR 0.94, 95% CI: 0.77 to 1.16) and the 6796 patients without prior stroke or TIA (1.44%/year vs 1.88%/year; HR 0.77, 95% CI: 0.58–1.01; interaction $p = 0.23$).

Major Bleeding – The rate of major bleeding among patients treated with rivaroxaban compared with warfarin was also consistent among patients with prior stroke or TIA (3.13%/year rivaroxaban vs 3.22%/year warfarin; HR 0.97, 95% CI: 0.79–1.19) and patients without prior stroke or TIA (4.10%/year vs 3.69%/year; HR 1.11, 95% CI: 0.92–1.34; interaction p = 0.36).

Apixaban vs Warfarin in Patients with Atrial Fibrillation

The ARISTOTLE (Apixaban for Reduction in Stroke and Other Thromboembolic Events in Atrial Fibrillation) trial compared apixaban with warfarin (target INR 2.0–3.0) (Granger et al., 2011). Patients with impaired renal function (serum creatinine >2.5 mg/dL [221 μmol/L] or creatinine clearance <25 mL/min) were excluded. Patients who were elderly (80 years or older), had low body weight (60 kg or lighter), or a serum creatinine of 133 μmol/L (1.5 mg/dL) or greater received a lower dose of apixaban (2.5 mg twice a day) than did other patients (5 mg twice a day).

Stroke or Systemic Embolism – Apixaban was better than warfarin in reducing the rate of stroke or systemic embolism (1.27% per year apixaban vs 1.60% per year warfarin; HR: 0.79, 95% CI: 0.66–0.95; p < 0.001 for noninferiority; p = 0.01 for superiority).

Bleeding – Apixaban was also associated with significantly less major bleeding (2.13% per year apixaban vs 3.09% per year warfarin; HR 0.69, 95% CI: 0.60–0.80; p < 0.001), less ICH (0.33% per year apixaban vs 0.80% per year warfarin; HR 0.42, 95% CI: 0.30–0.58; p < 0.001), and lower mortality (3.52% apixaban vs 3.94% warfarin; HR 0.89, 95% CI: 0.80–0.99; p = 0.047) than warfarin.

The occurrence of gastrointestinal haemorrhage and MI was similar in both groups.

Apixaban vs Warfarin in Patients with Atrial Fibrillation and Previous TIA or Ischaemic Stroke

The relative effects of apixaban versus warfarin in the 3436 patients with previous stroke or TIA in the ARISTOTLE trial were consistent with the effects of apixaban versus warfarin in the 14,765 patients without previous stroke or TIA for stroke or systemic embolism and major bleeding (Diener et al., 2012).

Stroke or Systemic Embolism – The rate of stroke or systemic embolism among patients treated with apixaban compared with warfarin was consistent among the 3436 patients with prior stroke or TIA (2.46%/year apixaban vs 3.24%/year warfarin; HR 0.76, 95% CI: 0.56–1.03) and the 14,765 patients without prior stroke or TIA (1.01%/year vs 1.23%/year; HR 0.82, 95% CI: 0.65–1.03; interaction p = 0.71).

Major Bleeding – The rate of major bleeding among patients treated with apixaban compared with warfarin was also consistent among patients with prior stroke or TIA (2.84%/year apixaban vs 3.91%/year warfarin; HR 0.73, 95% CI: 0.55–0.98) and patients without prior stroke or TIA (1.98%/year vs 2.91%/year; HR 0.68, 95% CI: 0.58–0.80; interaction p = 0.69).

Edoxaban vs Warfarin in Patients with Atrial Fibrillation

The Effective Anticoagulation with Factor Xa Next Generation in Atrial Fibrillation–Thrombolysis in Myocardial Infarction 48 (ENGAGE AF-TIMI 48) trial was a three-group, randomized, double-blind, double-dummy trial comparing two once-daily regimens of edoxaban (higher-dose edoxaban [60 mg once daily], or lower-dose edoxaban [30 mg once daily]) with adjusted dose warfarin (INR 2.0–3.0) in 21,105 patients with moderate-to-high risk of AF (median follow-up, 2.8 years) (Giugliano et al., 2013).

The ENGAGE AF-TIMI 48 trial showed that both once-daily regimens of edoxaban were noninferior to warfarin with respect to the prevention of stroke or systemic embolism and were associated with significantly lower rates of bleeding and death from cardiovascular causes.

Stroke or Systemic Embolism – The annualized rate of stroke or systemic embolism during treatment was 1.50% with warfarin (median time in the therapeutic range, 68.4%), as compared with 1.18% with high-dose edoxaban (HR 0.79; 97.5% CI: 0.63–0.99; p < 0.001 for noninferiority) and 1.61% with low-dose edoxaban (HR 1.07; 97.5% CI: 0.87–1.31; p = 0.005 for noninferiority).

In the intention-to-treat analysis, there was a trend favouring high-dose edoxaban versus warfarin (HR 0.87; 97.5% CI: 0.73–1.04; p = 0.08) and an unfavourable trend with low-dose edoxaban versus warfarin (HR 1.13; 97.5% CI: 0.96–1.34; p = 0.10).

Stroke – Patients randomized to high-dose edoxaban had fewer strokes on-treatment (HR 0.80; 95% CI: 0.65–0.98) than those on warfarin (median time-in-therapeutic range, 68.4%); patients in the low-dose edoxaban group had similar rates (HR 1.10 versus warfarin; 95% CI: 0.91–1.32) (Giugliano et al., 2014).

Rates of ischaemic stroke or TIA were similar with high-dose edoxaban (1.76% per year) and warfarin (1.73% per year; P = 0.81), but more frequent with low-dose edoxaban (2.48% per year; p < 0.001).

Major Bleeding – The annualized rate of major bleeding was 3.43% with warfarin versus 2.75% with high-dose edoxaban (HR 0.80; 95% CI: 0.71–0.91; $p < 0.001$) and 1.61% with low-dose edoxaban (HR 0.47; 95% CI: 0.41–0.55; $p < 0.001$).

Both edoxaban regimens significantly reduced haemorrhagic stroke and other subtypes of intracranial bleeds.

Other Outcome Events – The corresponding annualized rates of death from cardiovascular causes were 3.17% versus 2.74% (HR 0.86; 95% CI: 0.77–0.97; $p = 0.01$), and 2.71% (HR 0.85; 95% CI: 0.76–0.96; $p = 0.008$), and the corresponding rates of the composite of stroke, systemic embolism, or death from cardiovascular causes were 4.43% versus 3.85% (HR 0.87; 95% CI: 0.78–0.96; $p = 0.005$), and 4.23% (HR 0.95; 95% CI: 0.86–1.05; $p = 0.32$).

Meta-analyses of the Four Large Phase III Trials of Warfarin vs One of the Non-vitamin K Antagonist Oral Anticoagulants (NOACs) in Atrial Fibrillation

Atrial Fibrillation Patients

A meta-analysis, using a random effects model, of all 71,683 participants included in the RE-LY, ROCKET AF, ARISTOTLE, and ENGAGE AF-TIMI 48 trials, reported that a total of 42,411 participants received a new oral anticoagulant and 29,272 participants received warfarin (Ruff et al., 2014).

The meta-analysis showed that the NOACs have a favourable risk–benefit profile, with significant reductions in stroke, ICH, and mortality, and with similar major bleeding to warfarin but with increased gastrointestinal bleeding. The relative efficacy and safety of new oral anticoagulants are consistent across a wide range of patients. Updated meta-analyses support these observations (Lowenstern et al., 2018).

Stroke or Systemic Embolism – The NOACs significantly reduced stroke or systemic embolic events by 19% compared with warfarin (RR 0.81, 95% CI: 0.73–0.91; $p < 0.0001$; $I^2 = 47\%$, heterogeneity $p = 0.13$). This was mainly driven by a reduction in haemorrhagic stroke (0.49, 0.38–0.64; $p < 0.0001$). There was no heterogeneity for stroke or systemic embolic events in important clinical subgroups.

Although indirect comparisons suggest that the relative effects of each of the NOACs compared with warfarin were reasonably consistent for stroke and systemic embolism (p-value for heterogeneity = 0.13), indirect comparisons of the NOACs should be interpreted cautiously because the trials had different designs, participants, and interventions (e.g. time in the therapeutic range [TTR] in those assigned warfarin differed between the trials).

Low-dose NOAC regimens showed similar overall reductions in stroke or systemic embolic events compared with warfarin (RR: 1.03, 0.84–1.27; $p = 0.74$), but significantly more ischaemic strokes (RR 1.28, 1.02–1.60; $p = 0.045$).

Major Bleeding – The NOACs were associated with a non-significant trend towards reduced major bleeding events by 14% compared with warfarin, but there was substantial heterogeneity among the trials (RR 0.86, 95% CI: 0.73–1.00; $p = 0.06$; $I^2 = 83\%$, heterogeneity $p = 0.001$). There was a greater relative reduction in major bleeding with NOACs when the centre-based time in the therapeutic range was less than 66% than when it was 66% or more (RR 0.69, 95% CI: 0.59–0.81 vs RR 0.93, 95% CI: 0.76–1.13; p for interaction = 0.022).

Low-dose NOAC regimens showed a trend towards a more favourable bleeding profile compared with warfarin (RR 0.65, 95% CI: 0.43–1.00; $p = 0.05$) (Huang et al., 2018).

Other Outcome Events – The NOACs also significantly reduced all-cause mortality (RR 0.90, 95% CI: 0.85–0.95; $p = 0.0003$) and ICH (RR 0.48, 95% CI: 0.39–0.59; $p < 0.0001$), but increased gastrointestinal bleeding (RR 1.25, 95% CI: 1.01–1.55; $p = 0.04$).

Low-dose new oral anticoagulant regimens showed similar overall rates of stroke or systemic embolic events compared with warfarin (RR 1.03, 0.84–1.27; $p = 0.74$) but significantly more ischaemic strokes (RR 1.28, 1.02–1.60; $p = 0.045$).

Atrial Fibrillation Patients and Previous TIA or Ischaemic Stroke

Stroke or Systemic Embolism – The relative effects of the NOACs versus warfarin in preventing stroke or systemic embolism were consistent among patients with AF and previous TIA or ischaemic stroke (4.94% NOAC vs 5.73% warfarin; RR 0.86; 95% CI: 0.76–0.98) and among patients with AF and no history of previous TIA or ischaemic stroke (2.33% NOAC vs 2.98% warfarin; RR 0.78; 95% CI: 0.66–0.91; interaction $p = 0.30$) (Ruff et al., 2014; Ntaios et al., 2017).

ajor Bleeding – The relative effects of the NOACs vs *rfarin* on major bleeding were consistent among *tients* with AF and previous TIA or ischaemic *oke* (5.71% NOAC vs 6.43% warfarin; RR 0.89, % CI: 0.77–1.02) and among patients with AF and history of previous TIA or ischaemic stroke (5.18% *JAC* vs 6.21% warfarin; RR 0.85; 95% CI: 0.72–ⓐ); interaction *p* = 0.70 (Ruff et al., 2014; Ntaios al., 2017).

ta-analysis of Direct Thrombin Inhibitors versus amin K Antagonists in Atrial Fibrillation

systematic review identified eight randomized *ntrolled* trials (RCTs) comparing DTIs versus *KAs* for prevention of stroke and systemic *abolism* in a total of 27,557 participants with non-*lvular* AF and one or more risk factors for stroke *alazar* et al., 2014).

The DTIs included dabigatran 110 mg twice daily *d* 150 mg twice daily (three studies, 12,355

participants), AZD0837 300 mg once per day (two studies, 233 participants), and ximelagatran 36 mg twice per day (three studies, 3726 participants). The VKA comparator was warfarin (10,287 participants).

The review showed that DTIs were as efficacious as VKAs for the composite outcome of vascular death and ischaemic events, and only the dose of dabigatran 150 mg twice daily was found to be superior to warfarin. DTIs were associated with fewer major haemorrhagic events, including haemorrhagic strokes. Adverse events that led to discontinuation of treatment occurred more frequently with the DTIs. There was no difference in death from all causes.

Vascular Death and Ischaemic Events

The odds of vascular death and ischaemic events were not significantly different between all DTIs and warfarin (OR 0.94, 95% CI: 0.85–1.05) (Figure 18.5).

Review: Direct thrombin inhibitors versus vitamin K antagonists for preventing cerebral or systemic embolism in people with non-valvular atrial fibrillation
Comparison: 1 Efficacy
Outcome: 1 Vascular deaths and ischaemic events

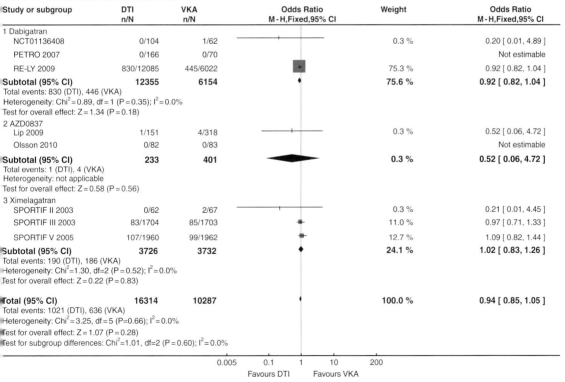

Figure 18.5 Forest plot showing the effects of *direct thrombin inhibitors vs vitamin K antagonists* in patients with *non-valvular atrial fibrillation* * schaemic events and vascular death* at the end of follow-up.

Review: Direct thrombin inhibitors versus vitamin K antagonists for preventing cerebral or systemic embolism in people with non-valvular atrial fibrillation
Comparison: 2 Safety
Outcome: 1 Fatal and non-fatal haemorrhages

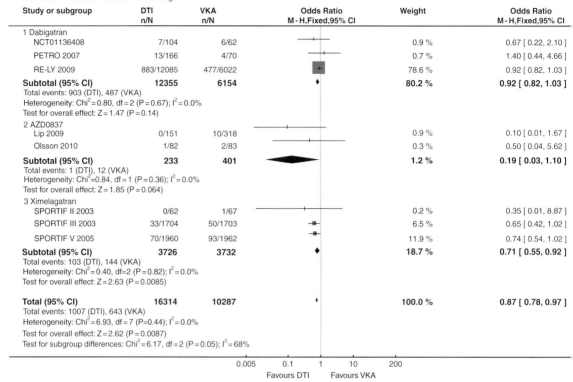

Figure 18.6 Forest plot showing the effects of *direct thrombin inhibitors vs vitamin K antagonists* in patients with *non-valvular atrial fibrilla* on *fatal and non-fatal haemorrhage* at the end of follow-up.

Reproduced from Salazar et al. (2014) with permission from the authors and John Wiley & Sons Limited. Copyright Cochrane Library, reproduced with permission.

Sensitivity analysis by dose of dabigatran on reduction in ischaemic events and vascular mortality indicated that dabigatran 150 mg twice daily was superior to warfarin, although the effect estimate was of borderline statistical significance (OR 0.86, 95% CI: 0.75–0.99). Sensitivity analyses by other factors did not alter the results.

Major Bleeding

Fatal and non-fatal major bleeding events, including haemorrhagic strokes, were less frequent with the DTIs (OR 0.87, 95% CI: 0.78–0.97) (Figure 18.6).

Other Outcome Events

Adverse events that led to discontinuation of treatment were significantly more frequent with the DTIs (OR 2.18, 95% CI: 1.82–2.61). All-cause mortality was similar between DTIs and warfarin (OR 0.91, 95% CI: 0.83–1.01).

Meta-analysis of Factor Xa Inhibitors versus Vitamin K Antagonists in Atrial Fibrillation

Atrial Fibrillation Patients

A systematic review identified 13 RCTs that directly compared the effects of long-term treatment (>4 weeks) with factor Xa inhibitors and a VKA (warfarin) for the prevention of stroke and systemic embolism in 67,688 participants with a confirmed diagnosis of AF (or atrial flutter) (Bruins Slot and Berge, 2018).

The trials directly compared dose-adjusted warfarin, with a target INR of 2.0 to 3.0, with either apixaban, betrixaban, darexaban, edoxaban, idraparinux, idrabiotaparinux, or rivaroxaban. The majority of the included data (approximately 90%) were from apixaban, edoxaban, and rivaroxaban.

Review: Factor Xa inhibitors versus vitamin K antagonists for preventing cerebral or systemic embolism in patients with atrial fibrillation
Comparison: 1 Factor Xa inhibitors versus VKA
Outcome: 1 Stroke and other systemic embolic events

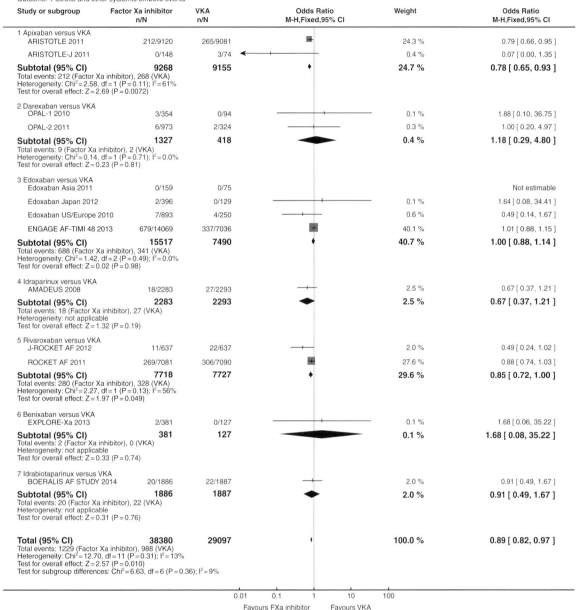

Figure 18.7 Forest plot showing the effects of *factor Xa inhibitors versus vitamin K antagonists* in patients with *non-valvular atrial fibrillation* on *stroke and other systemic embolic events* at the end of follow-up.

Reproduced from Bruins Slot and Berge (2018) with permission from the authors and John Wiley & Sons Limited. Copyright Cochrane Library, reproduced with permission.

The review found that factor Xa inhibitors significantly reduced the number of strokes and systemic embolic events compared with warfarin in patients with AF. The absolute effect of factor Xa inhibitors compared with warfarin treatment was, however, rather small.

Factor Xa inhibitors also reduced the number of ICHs, all-cause deaths, and major bleedings

Review: Factor Xa inhibitors versus vitamin K antagonists for preventing cerebral or systemic embolism in patients with atrial fibrillation
Comparison: 1 Factor Xa inhibitors versus VKA
Outcome: 6 Major bleedings

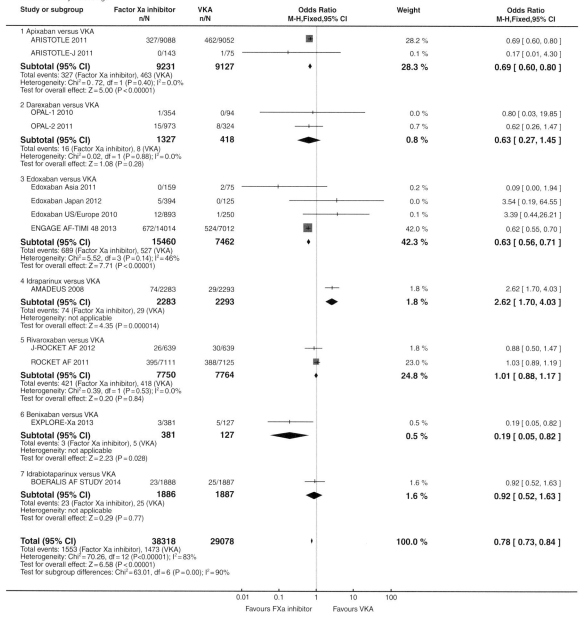

Figure 18.8 Forest plot showing the effects of *factor Xa inhibitors versus vitamin K antagonists* in patients with *non-valvular atrial fibrillation* on *major bleeding events* at the end of follow-up.

Reproduced from Bruins Slot et al. (2013) with permission from the authors and John Wiley & Sons Limited. Copyright Cochrane Library, reproduced with permission.

compared with warfarin, although the evidence for a reduction of major bleedings is less robust.

Stroke and Systemic Embolism – The composite primary efficacy endpoint of all strokes (both ischaemic and

haemorrhagic) and non-central nervous systemic embolic events was reported in all of the included studies.

Treatment with a factor Xa inhibitor significantly decreased the composite of stroke and systemic

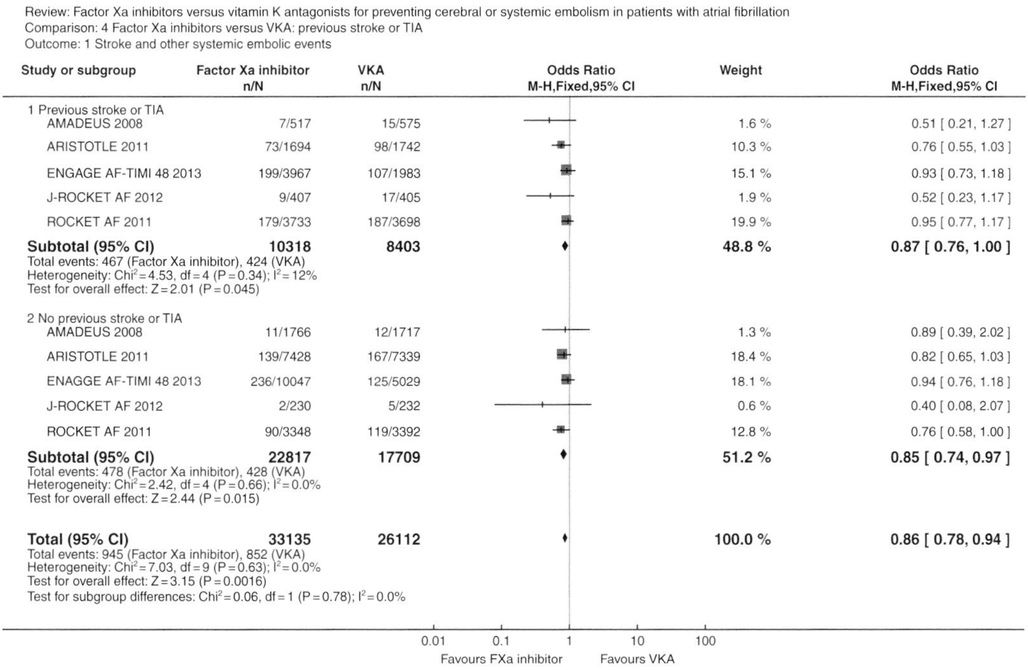

Review: Factor Xa inhibitors versus vitamin K antagonists for preventing cerebral or systemic embolism in patients with atrial fibrillation
Comparison: 4 Factor Xa inhibitors versus VKA: previous stroke or TIA
Outcome: 1 Stroke and other systemic embolic events

Study or subgroup	Factor Xa inhibitor n/N	VKA n/N	Odds Ratio M-H,Fixed,95% CI	Weight	Odds Ratio M-H,Fixed,95% CI
1 Previous stroke or TIA					
AMADEUS 2008	7/517	15/575		1.6 %	0.51 [0.21, 1.27]
ARISTOTLE 2011	73/1694	98/1742		10.3 %	0.76 [0.55, 1.03]
ENGAGE AF-TIMI 48 2013	199/3967	107/1983		15.1 %	0.93 [0.73, 1.18]
J-ROCKET AF 2012	9/407	17/405		1.9 %	0.52 [0.23, 1.17]
ROCKET AF 2011	179/3733	187/3698		19.9 %	0.95 [0.77, 1.17]
Subtotal (95% CI)	**10318**	**8403**		**48.8 %**	**0.87 [0.76, 1.00]**
Total events: 467 (Factor Xa inhibitor), 424 (VKA)					
Heterogeneity: Chi² = 4.53, df = 4 (P = 0.34); I² = 12%					
Test for overall effect: Z = 2.01 (P = 0.045)					
2 No previous stroke or TIA					
AMADEUS 2008	11/1766	12/1717		1.3 %	0.89 [0.39, 2.02]
ARISTOTLE 2011	139/7428	167/7339		18.4 %	0.82 [0.65, 1.03]
ENAGGE AF-TIMI 48 2013	236/10047	125/5029		18.1 %	0.94 [0.76, 1.18]
J-ROCKET AF 2012	2/230	5/232		0.6 %	0.40 [0.08, 2.07]
ROCKET AF 2011	90/3348	119/3392		12.8 %	0.76 [0.58, 1.00]
Subtotal (95% CI)	**22817**	**17709**		**51.2 %**	**0.85 [0.74, 0.97]**
Total events: 478 (Factor Xa inhibitor), 428 (VKA)					
Heterogeneity: Chi² = 2.42, df = 4 (P = 0.66); I² = 0.0%					
Test for overall effect: Z = 2.44 (P = 0.015)					
Total (95% CI)	**33135**	**26112**		**100.0 %**	**0.86 [0.78, 0.94]**
Total events: 945 (Factor Xa inhibitor), 852 (VKA)					
Heterogeneity: Chi² = 7.03, df = 9 (P = 0.63); I² = 0.0%					
Test for overall effect: Z = 3.15 (P = 0.0016)					
Test for subgroup differences: Chi² = 0.06, df = 1 (P = 0.78); I² = 0.0%					

0.01   0.1   1   10   100
Favours FXa inhibitor   Favours VKA

Figure 18.9 Forest plot showing the effects of *factor Xa inhibitors versus vitamin K antagonists* in patients with *non-valvular atrial fibrillation and previous stroke or TIA* on *stroke and other systemic embolic events* at the end of follow-up.

Reproduced from Bruins Slot and Berge (2018) with permission from the authors and John Wiley & Sons Limited. Copyright Cochrane Library, reproduced with permission.

embolic events compared with dose-adjusted warfarin in participants with AF (OR 0.89, 95% CI: 0.82–0.97; 13 studies; 67,477 participants; high-quality evidence) (Figure 18.7).

Major Bleeding – Treatment with a factor Xa inhibitor significantly reduced the number of major bleeding events compared with warfarin (OR 0.78, 95% CI: 0.73–0.84; 13 studies; 67,396 participants; moderate-quality evidence) (Figure 18.8). There was, however, statistically significant and high heterogeneity (I^2 = 83%). When this analysis was repeated using a random-effects model, it did not show a statistically significant decrease in the number of major bleedings (OR 0.88, 95% CI: 0.66–1.17).

A pre-specified sensitivity analysis excluding all open-label studies showed that treatment with a factor Xa inhibitor significantly reduced the number of major bleeding events compared with warfarin (OR 0.75, 95% CI: 0.69–0.81), but high heterogeneity was also observed in this analysis (I^2 = 72%). The same sensitivity analysis using a random-effects

model also showed a statistically significant decrease in the number of major bleedings in participants treated with factor Xa inhibitors (OR 0.76, 95% CI: 0.60–0.96).

Intracranial Haemorrhage – Treatment with a factor Xa inhibitor significantly reduced the risk of ICHs compared with warfarin (OR 0.50, 95% CI: 0.42–0.59; 12 studies; 66,259 participants; high-quality evidence). Moderate, but statistically significant, heterogeneity was present (I^2 = 55%).

The pre-specified sensitivity analysis excluding open-label studies showed that treatment with a factor Xa inhibitor significantly reduced the number of ICHs compared with warfarin (OR 0.47, 95% CI: 0.40–0.56), with low, non-statistically significant heterogeneity (I^2 = 27%).

Death from Any Cause – Treatment with a factor Xa inhibitor significantly reduced the number of all-cause deaths compared with warfarin (OR 0.89, 95% CI: 0.83–0.95; 10 studies; 65,624 participants; moderate-quality evidence).

357

Review: Factor Xa inhibitors versus vitamin K antagonists for preventing cerebral or systemic embolism in patients with atrial fibrillation
Comparison: 4 Factor Xa inhibitors versus VKA: previous stroke or TIA
Outcome: 2 Major bleedings

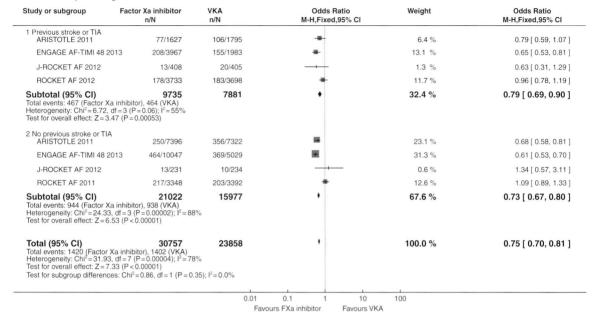

Study or subgroup	Factor Xa inhibitor n/N	VKA n/N	Odds Ratio M-H,Fixed,95% CI	Weight	Odds Ratio M-H,Fixed,95% CI
1 Previous stroke or TIA					
ARISTOTLE 2011	77/1627	106/1795		6.4 %	0.79 [0.59, 1.07]
ENGAGE AF-TIMI 48 2013	208/3967	155/1983		13.1 %	0.65 [0.53, 0.81]
J-ROCKET AF 2012	13/408	20/405		1.3 %	0.63 [0.31, 1.29]
ROCKET AF 2012	178/3733	183/3698		11.7 %	0.96 [0.78, 1.19]
Subtotal (95% CI)	**9735**	**7881**		**32.4 %**	**0.79 [0.69, 0.90]**
Total events: 467 (Factor Xa inhibitor), 464 (VKA) Heterogeneity: Chi²=6.72, df=3 (P=0.06); I²=55% Test for overall effect: Z=3.47 (P=0.00053)					
2 No previous stroke or TIA					
ARISTOTLE 2011	250/7396	356/7322		23.1 %	0.68 [0.58, 0.81]
ENGAGE AF-TIMI 48 2013	464/10047	369/5029		31.3 %	0.61 [0.53, 0.70]
J-ROCKET AF 2012	13/231	10/234		0.6 %	1.34 [0.57, 3.11]
ROCKET AF 2011	217/3348	203/3392		12.6 %	1.09 [0.89, 1.33]
Subtotal (95% CI)	**21022**	**15977**		**67.6 %**	**0.73 [0.67, 0.80]**
Total events: 944 (Factor Xa inhibitor), 938 (VKA) Heterogeneity: Chi²=24.33, df=3 (P=0.00002); I²=88% Test for overall effect: Z=6.53 (P<0.00001)					
Total (95% CI)	**30757**	**23858**		**100.0 %**	**0.75 [0.70, 0.81]**
Total events: 1420 (Factor Xa inhibitor), 1402 (VKA) Heterogeneity: Chi²=31.93, df=7 (P=0.00004); I²=78% Test for overall effect: Z=7.33 (P<0.00001) Test for subgroup differences: Chi²=0.86, df=1 (P=0.35); I²=0.0%					

0.01   0.1   1   10   100
Favours FXa inhibitor   Favours VKA

Figure 18.10 Forest plot showing the effects of *factor Xa inhibitors versus vitamin K antagonists* in patients with *non-valvular atrial fibrillation and previous stroke or TIA* on *major bleeding* at the end of follow-up.

Reproduced from Bruins Slot and Berge (2018) with permission from the authors and John Wiley & Sons Limited. Copyright Cochrane Library, reproduced with permission.

Atrial Fibrillation Patients with Previous Stroke or TIA

Stroke and Systemic Embolism – The risk of stroke and systemic embolic events was significantly lower in people treated with factor Xa inhibitors who had previously suffered a stroke or TIA (OR 0.87, 95% CI: 0.76–1.00), as well as in people who did not have a previous stroke or TIA (OR 0.85, 95% CI: 0.74–0.97), compared with warfarin (Figure 18.9).

Major Bleeding – The number of major bleedings was significantly lower in participants with or without a previous stroke or TIA who received treatment with factor Xa inhibitors compared with warfarin: OR 0.79 (95% CI: 0.69–0.90) and OR 0.73 (95% CI: 0.67–0.80), respectively (Figure 18.10).

Non-vitamin K Antagonist Oral Anticoagulants (NOACs) vs Aspirin

Atrial Fibrillation Patients

The AVERROES (Apixaban Versus Aspirin to Reduce the Risk of Stroke) study compared apixaban (5 mg twice daily) versus aspirin (81–324 mg per day) in patients with AF who were thought to be unsuitable or unwilling to receive a VKA (Connolly et al., 2011b).

The reasons for unsuitability for a VKA varied, but most (>70%) were related to issues with INR monitoring, INR instability, and patient refusal to take vitamin K antagonists.

The AVERROES trial showed that in patients unable or unwilling to take a VKA, apixaban was more effective than aspirin for the prevention of embolic events, but it was also as safe as aspirin for major bleeding and cerebral haemorrhage.

Stroke and Systemic Embolism – The rate of stroke and systemic embolism was significantly lower with apixaban than with aspirin (1.6% per year apixaban vs 3.7% per year aspirin, HR 0.45, 95% CI: 0.32–0.62; *p* < 0.001) (Connolly et al., 2011b).

Major Bleeding – The rates of major bleeding (1.4% per year apixaban vs 1.2% aspirin; HR: 1.13, 95% CI:

,74–1.75; $p = 0.57$), ICH (0.4% per year apixaban vs ,4% per year aspirin; HR: 0.85, 95% CI: 0.38–1.90; $= 0.69$), and gastrointestinal bleeding ($p = 0.71$) ere similar in both groups.

trial Fibrillation Patients with Previous Stroke or TIA

he relative effects of apixaban versus aspirin in the 64 patients with previous stroke or TIA were con- stent with the effects of apixaban versus aspirin in he 4832 patients without previous stroke or TIA Diener et al., 2012).

troke or Systemic Embolism – The rate of stroke or ystemic embolism among 764 patients with previous roke or TIA was 2.39% at one year with apixaban ersus 9.16% at one year with aspirin (HR: 0.29, 0.15) 0.60).

Major Bleeding – The rates of major bleeding mong patients with previous stroke and TIA ere: 4.1% at 1 year apixaban vs 2.89% at 1 year spirin (HR: 1.28, 95% CI: 0.58–2.82; interaction $= 0.73$).

Management of Anticoagulant-associated Bleeding

atients Treated with NOACs

he management of bleeding complications in atients treated with NOACs depends on

) Bleeding factors: nuisance/minor, major non- life threatening, or life-threatening bleeding.

) Patient factors: the time of last NOAC intake, prescribed dosing regimen, renal function, other factors influencing plasma concentrations (including co-medication), and haemostasis (such as concomitant use of antiplatelet drugs) (Steffel et al., 2018).

or nuisance bleeding, management may involve ocal mechanical compression, delaying or withhold- ng intake of 1 dose of the NOAC until the anti- oagulant activity of the NOAC effect wanes as result of spontaneous clearance of the drug (facili- ated by maintaining and/or stimulating diuresis), nd re-starting the NOAC once the bleeding has topped.

Minor bleeding may require treatment of the cause f the bleeding (e.g. proton pump inhibitor [PPI] for astric ulcers, antibiotics for urinary tract infection). pistaxis and gum bleeds can be treated with local nti-fibrinolytics.

Recurrent minor bleeding, despite efforts to treat the cause, should trigger a review of diagnostic investigations seeking an occult source of bleeding and potential effective treatments of any underlying cause. An alternative NOAC with a potentially different bleeding profile may be required also. Any cessation or temporary interruption of the NOAC should be balanced against a subsequently increased thromboembolic risk.

Major and/or life-threatening bleeding requires immediate aggressive management, including the use of specific and non-specific reversal strategies. Initial steps are to do the following:

- Enquire about the exact time of last intake of the NOAC, the dosing regime, and factors influencing plasma concentrations (e.g. chronic kidney disease, p-glycoprotein transport inhibitors or inducers), and haemostasis (e.g. concomitant antiplatelet therapy).
- Stop the anticoagulant.
- Identify and compress the source of bleeding (local haemostatic measures).
- Take blood for routine laboratory coagulation tests (INR, PT, aPTT, fibrinogen) and assays that measure plasma concentrations of NOACs (including the dilute thrombin time [Haemoclot test] for dabigatran and anti-factor Xa assays for rivaroxaban, apixaban, and edoxaban), renal function, and complete blood count, including platelet count, to estimate normalization of haemostasis and the cause and extent of the bleeding:
  - Normal results of dTT/ecarin clotting time (for dabigatran) and anti-Xa activity (for anti-FXa treated patients) usually exclude relevant levels of the anticoagulant. Specific assays allow for the quantification of plasma levels of the anticoagulant (Gosselin et al., 2018).
  - Coagulation tests may be abnormal due to reasons other than the effect of the NOAC, particularly when bleeding is severe.
- Administer fluids (colloids if necessary) to assist diuresis and renal excretion of the drug.
- Consider specific reversal of dabigatran with idarucizumab (a humanized antibody fragment that specifically binds dabigatran, see below)

359

(Eikelboom et al., 2015; Pollack et al., 2017) and of FXa inhibitors (rivaroxaban and apixaban) with andexanet alfa (a recombinant human FXa analogue that competes with FXa to bind FXa inhibitors, see below) (Connolly et al., 2016), or perhaps, if approved in the future, with ciraparantag (PER977), a small synthetic molecule that seems to have more generalized antagonistic effects (Ansell et al., 2014):

- After direct reversal, significant NOAC concentrations may reappear in some patients and contribute to recurrent or continued bleeding (particularly after andexanet alfa, less after idarucizumab administration), underlining the necessity for continued clinical and laboratory monitoring.

• In the absence of specific reversal drugs, consider non-specific support of haemostasis using coagulation factor concentrates, such as 4-factor prothrombin complex concentrate (PCC) (see below).

- Clinical trials and registry data with NOACs have shown that administration of coagulation factors is rarely needed (Healey et al., 2012; Beyer-Westendorf et al., 2014).
- Prothrombin complex concentrates consist of 4-factor concentrates (which contain coagulation factors II, VII, IX, and X) and 3-factor concentrates (which contain II, IX, and X). Four-factor PCCs are available in activated or nonactivated clotting factor formulations.
- Activated PCC (FIEBA) 50 U/kg (with additional 25 U/kg if clinically needed, and up to a maximum of 200 U/kg/day) stimulates thrombin formation and bypasses the anticoagulant effect of thrombin and factor Xa antagonists.
- There is increasing information about the effects of (activated) PCC concentrates in cohorts of NOAC-treated patients with bleeding (Beyer-Westendorf et al., 2014).
- The place of recombinant activated factor VIIa (90 mcg/kg) needs further evaluation. In a recent study, activated PCC and rFVIIa, but not PCC, seemed to reverse, at least partially, some effects of dabigatran on coagulation parameters (Lindahl et al., 2015).

- Fresh frozen plasma is not considered a usef reversal strategy in NOAC-treated patients with bleeding, because any remaining NOAC in the bloodstream inhibit newly administered coagulation factors upon activation.
- Vitamin K and protamine administration ha no role in the management of bleeding unde NOACs, but are useful in the management c bleeding in the presence of NOACs when vitamin K deficiency is suspected or in case concomitant treatment with heparin, respectively.
- Restoring coagulation may not necessarily improve clinical outcome and may have a potential adverse prothrombotic effect.

• Consider red blood cell transfusion if necessary.

• Consider fresh frozen plasma as a plasma expander (not as a reversal agent).

• Consider tranexamic acid (antifibrinolytic) as a adjuvant.

• Consider desmopressin in special cases of coagulopathy or thrombopathy.

• Haemodialysis can be used to remove the two-thirds of circulating dabigatran that is n protein-bound. However, the time to obtain vascular access in patients who are anticoagulated and bleeding might be longer than the half-life of the drug, except in patien with impaired renal function (for whom dialysis might be practical and worthwhile). Dialysis is not effective for the factor Xa inhibitors because these drugs are mostly protein-bound.

Idarucizumab for Direct Reversal of Dabigatran (dire thrombin inhibitor) – Idarucizumab (aDabi-Fab, 655075, UNII-97RWB5S1U6) is a humanize monoclonal antibody fragment [Fab] that bind specifically to dabigatran in a 1:1 molar ratio. has an affinity for dabigatran that is ~350 tim greater than that of thrombin (Eikelboom et a 2015).

In a randomized, placebo-controlled, doubl blind, proof-of-concept phase 1 study of the safet tolerability, and efficacy of increasing doses of idar cizumab for the reversal of anticoagulant effects dabigatran, 47 healthy volunteers (aged 18–45 year with a body mass index of 18.5–29.9 kg/m^2 who ha ceived oral dabigatran etexilate 220 mg twice daily r 3 days and a final dose on day 4 were randomly signed to receive placebo or idarucizumab (1 g, 2 g, 4 g 5-min infusion, or 5 g plus 2.5 g in two 5-min fusions given 1 h apart) about 2 hours after the final bigatran etexilate dose. Idarucizumab was assoated with immediate, complete, and sustained reverl of dabigatran-induced anticoagulation in healthy en, and was well tolerated with no unexpected or nically relevant safety concerns (Glund et al., 2015).

In a prospective cohort study of patients who were ticoagulated with dabigatran and had serious bleedg (group A, n = 51) or who required an urgent ocedure (group B, n = 39), idarucizumab (5 g intranously in two 50 mL boluses of 2.5 g each, less than 5 minutes apart) was safe and completely reversed the ticoagulant effect of dabigatran in 88–98% of tients, and within minutes (Pollack et al., 2015). he median maximum percentage reversal of the ticoagulant effect of dabigatran within 4 hours after e administration of idarucizumab was 100% (95% I: 100–100). Concentrations of unbound dabigatran mained below 20 ng per millilitre at 24 hours in 79% the patients. Among 35 patients in group A with rious bleeding who could be assessed, haemostasis as restored at a median of 11.4 hours. Among 36 tients in group B who underwent a procedure, noral intraoperative haemostasis was reported in 33. ne thrombotic event occurred within 72 hours after arucizumab administration in a patient in whom ticoagulants had not been reinitiated.

In the REVERSE-AD study, idarucizumab was iccessfully used in patients on dabigatran presenting ith major or life-threatening bleeding, or with the ecessity of emergency surgery. Idarucizumab cometely reversed the anticoagulant activity of dabigaan within minutes in almost all patients (Pollack al., 2017).

Idarucizumab (Praxbind) was approved by the US DA in October 2015 for reversal of the anticoagulant fect of the direct thrombin inhibitor dabigatran etexte (Pradaxa) in patients taking dabigatran who have ajor or life-threatening bleeding or need for emergency rgery (Idarucizumab (Praxbind), 2015). A total of 5 g arucizumab is administered intravenously in two bolus oses of 2.5 g no more than 15 minutes apart. Continued inical and laboratory monitoring is recommended, nce a 5 g dose of idarucizumab may not completely eutralize an exceptionally high level of dabigatran (e.g. case of overdose or renal insufficiency). Also, low

levels of dabigatran may reappear after 12–24 hours. After 24 hours, dabigatran can be re-started if clinically indicated and feasible, with normal kinetics.

Andexanet Alfa for Direct Reversal of Apixaban and Rivaroxaban (FXa inhibitors) – Andexanet alfa (coagulation factor Xa [recombinant], inactivated-zhzo) is a modified recombinant inactive form of human factor Xa designed to bind and sequester factor Xa inhibitor molecules with an affinity that is similar to that of native factor Xa, thereby reducing antifactor Xa activity, and reversing the anticoagulant effects of Xa inhibitors rapidly and nearly completely with a 420 mg dose (Lu et al., 2013; Das and Liu, 2015). It therefore acts as a modified decoy of factor Xa, binding to factor Xa inhibitors and neutralizing their anticoagulant effect.

Phase 2 trials and animal studies indicate that andexanet alfa effectively reduces the anti-factor Xa activity of all direct factor Xa antagonists (apixaban, betrixaban, edoxaban, and rivaroxaban) (Sartori and Cosmi, 2018). Andexanet alfa also reduces the antifactor Xa activity of indirect (enoxaparin and fondaparinux) factor Xa inhibitors.

In May 2018, andexanet alfa was approved by the US FDA for urgent reversal of the anticoagulant effect of the direct factor Xa inhibitors apixaban (Eliquis) and rivaroxaban (Xarelto) in patients with life-threatening or uncontrolled bleeding (Heo, 2018). It has not been approved, to date, for reversal of anticoagulation with the direct factor Xa inhibitors edoxaban (Savaysa) or betrixaban (Bevyxxa). Intravenous andexanet alfa is under regulatory review in the EU and is undergoing clinical development in Japan.

Approval of andexanet alfa was based on the results of two randomized, placebo-controlled trials (ANNEXA-A and ANNEXA-R) that showed that andexanet rapidly reduced both the unbound fraction of the plasma level of factor Xa inhibitor and antifactor Xa activity following administration to healthy volunteers 50–75 years old who had received either apixaban or rivaroxaban (Siegal et al., 2015).

In the ANNEXA-A and ANNEXA-R studies, no thromboembolic events occurred among 223 healthy volunteers who received factor Xa inhibitors and were treated with andexanet alfa. In healthy volunteers, infusion reactions were the only adverse events that occurred more often with andexanet alfa than with placebo. No antibodies to factor X or Xa developed in any healthy volunteers, and no neutralizing antibodies against andexanet alfa were detected (Siegal et al., 2015).

In the Andexanet Alfa, a Novel Antidote to the Anticoagulation Effects of Factor Xa Inhibitors (ANNEXA-4), single-group cohort study of 352 patients with acute major bleeding (64% intracranial, 26% gastrointestinal) who had received a factor Xa inhibitor (apixaban, rivaroxaban, or edoxaban) within the previous 18 hours, the administration of a bolus of andexanet over 15–30 minutes (400–800 mg), followed by a 2-hour infusion (480–960 mg), markedly reduced anti–factor Xa activity from baseline, and 82% of patients had excellent or good haemostatic efficacy at 12 hours after the andexanet infusion, with consistent effects across all subgroups (Connolly et al., 2019). At 30 days, 14% of patients died and 10% experienced thrombotic events, most in patients in whom resumption of oral anticoagulation was delayed or not started.

Two dosage regimens of andexanet alfa are recommended, based on the factor Xa inhibitor taken, its dose, and the time since the last factor Xa inhibitor dose.

Patients taking ≤10 mg of rivaroxaban or ≤5 mg of apixaban per dose should receive the low-dose regimen, a 400 mg IV bolus dose of andexanet alfa over 15–30 minutes, followed by a 4 mg/minute continuous infusion over 2 hours.

Patients taking >10 mg of rivaroxaban or >5 mg of apixaban per dose should receive the high-dose regimen, an 800 mg IV bolus dose of andexanet alfa, followed by an 8 mg/minute continuous infusion for up to 120 minutes if their last dose was <8 hours before starting andexanet alfa; if the last dose was ≥8 hours before starting andexanet alfa, the low-dose regimen should be used.

If the dose and/or timing since the last dose of the factor Xa inhibitor is unknown, the high-dose regimen should be used. The optimal dosage of andexanet alfa for patients taking other factor Xa inhibitors has not been established.

PER977 for Direct Reversal of Apixaban, Rivaroxaban, and Dabigatran

PER977 (Perosphere) is a small, synthetic, water-soluble, cationic molecule that binds factor Xa inhibitors, DTIs, and heparin, and has been shown to reverse anticoagulation with each of the NOACs.

A double-blind, placebo-controlled trial involving 80 healthy persons of escalating, single intravenous doses of PER977 (5 to 300 mg) administered alone and after a 60 mg oral dose of edoxaban showed that baseline haemostasis was restored from the anticoagulated state within 10 to 30 minutes after administration of 100 to 300 mg of PER977 and was sustained for 24 hours (Ansell et al., 2014).

Coagulation Factors – As stated above, PCCs and activated PCCs (aPCCs) can facilitate the normalization of coagulation parameters under NOAC treatment (Song et al., 2017) and appear efficacious in supporting haemostasis on observational studies of patients with major bleeding (Majeed et al., 2017). The efficacy on clinical outcomes of PCCs or aPCCs in patients taking NOACs who are actively bleeding has not, however, been firmly established in a RCT. As indicated above, data from the large phase 3 trials demonstrated that outcomes of bleedings under NOACs were similar (if not better) than in the VKA arm with similar treatment used (including PCC/aPCC).

The administration of PCCs or aPCCs can be considered in a patient with life-threatening bleeding if immediate haemostatic support is required, especially in situations where a specific reversal agent is not available.

The choice between PCC and aPCC may depend on their availability and the experience of the treatment centre. Particularly, aPCC induce a strong procoagulant effect and should only be used by physicians experienced in their use.

PCC and aPCC are preferred over recombinant activated factor VIIa (NovoSeven, 90 mg/kg), the latter of which has a pronounced pro-coagulant effect (Warkentin et al., 2012).

Patients Treated with Vitamin K Antagonists (VKAs)

For non-compressible major haemorrhage or emergency surgery, the effects of warfarin can be reversed with PCC or fresh frozen plasma in conjunction with vitamin K. The haemostatic efficacy of PCC in patients with major bleeding who were treated with VKAs was 72% in one study (Sarode et al., 2013).

Four-factor PCC is non-inferior and superior to plasma for rapid INR reversal and effective haemostasis in patients needing VKA reversal for urgent surgical or invasive procedures (Goldstein et al., 2015) or patients with ICH related to vitamin K antagonists and an INR greater than or equal to 1.4 at admission (Steiner et al., 2016).

Vitamin K injection is also recommended as standard treatment, despite insufficient supporting evidence. The aim of the reversal treatment is to obtain an INR lower than 1.4 as soon as possible. INR values should be followed up at 3- to 6-hour intervals for the first 24 hours to detect rebound coagulopathy and further need for reversal if necessary.

Left Atrial Appendage Occlusion

Although the mechanism of thromboembolism in AF is multifactorial, the LAA appears to be the major source of thrombus and is a target for transcatheter interventional therapy with device occlusion or ligation.

For patients with AF who have had a stroke but in whom oral anticoagulation is contraindicated because of risks of bleeding (e.g. previous recurrent intracerebral haemorrhages due to amyloid angiopathy), the LAA can be occluded surgically or non-surgically, such as by endoscopic placement of a device such as the WATCHMAN filter (a self-expanding cage placed in the LAA via a transseptal approach with femoral access) (Reddy et al., 2017; Sahay et al., 2017; Gurol, 2018).

Atrial Fibrillation Patients

All Left Atrial Appendage Occlusion Procedures – A conventional meta-analysis of five RCTs of LAA occlusion versus warfarin for stroke prevention in a total of 1285 patients with AF found no difference between groups for the occurrence of stroke (RR 0.78, 95% CI: 0.47–1.29) but a significant reduction in mortality (5 trials, 1285 patients; RR 0.71, 95% CI: 0.51–0.99) favouring LAA occlusion versus warfarin (Sahay et al., 2017; Hanif et al., 2018).

A network meta-analysis demonstrated a trend towards a reduction in stroke (OR 0.84, 95% CrI: 0.47–1.55) and mortality (OR 0.69, 95% CrI: 0.44–1.10) for LAA occlusion versus warfarin, but no statistically significant effect (Hanif et al., 2018).

Statistical ranking curves placed LAA occlusion as the most efficacious treatment on the outcomes of stroke and mortality when compared with warfarin, aspirin, or placebo.

No significant differences between groups were seen in major bleeding or operative time for surgical trials. The overall quality of the evidence was low as assessed by the Grading of Recommendations Assessment, Development and Evaluation (GRADE) working group.

WATCHMAN Left Atrial Appendage Device – The PROTECT AF (WATCHMAN Left Atrial Appendage System for Embolic Protection in Patients With Atrial Fibrillation) and PREVAIL (Evaluation of the WATCHMAN LAA Closure Device in Patients With Atrial Fibrillation Versus Long Term Warfarin Therapy) trials randomized a total of 1114 patients with AF in a 2:1 ratio to left atrial appendage closure (LAAC) (*n* = 732) or warfarin (*n* = 382), who were followed for 4343 patient-years (Reddy et al., 2017).

Stroke, Systemic Embolism, or Cardiovascular/Unexplained Death – – Rates of the composite endpoint of stroke, systemic embolism, or cardiovascular/unexplained death were similar between groups (2.8 per 100 patient-years device vs 3.4 per 100 patient-years warfarin; HR: 0.82, 95% CI: 0.58–1.17; *p* = 0.27).

Stroke or Systemic Embolism – – Rates of all-stroke/systemic embolism were also similar between groups (1.7 per 100 patient-years device vs 1.8 per 100 patient-years warfarin; HR: 0.96, 95% CI: 0.60–1.54; *p* = 0.87).

Ischaemic Stroke or Systemic Embolism – – The ischaemic stroke/systemic embolism rate was numerically but not significantly higher with LAAC than warfarin (1.6% vs 0.95%, HR 1.71, 95% CI: 0.94–3.11; *p* = 0.80), whereas the rate of haemorrhagic stroke was numerically but not significantly lower with LAAC than warfarin (0.17% vs 0.87%, HR 0.20, 0.07–0.56).

Major Bleeding – – There was no significant different in major bleeding (3.1% vs 3.5%; HR 0.91, 95% CI: 0.64–1.29).

Death – – The rate of all-cause death was lower with LAAC versus warfarin (3.6% vs 4.9%; HR 0.73, 95% CI: 0.54–0.98) (Reddy et al., 2017).

These 5-year outcomes of the PROTECT AF and PREVAIL trials indicate that LAAC with the WATCHMAN device provides stroke prevention in nonvalvular AF comparable to warfarin and reductions in major bleeding and mortality.

A cost-effectiveness analysis of LAAC with the WATCHMAN device compared with warfarin or NOACs for the secondary prevention of stroke in patients with AF suggests that the initial, upfront procedure costs initially make LAAC a higher cost than warfarin and the NOACs, but within 10 years, LAAC is likely to deliver more quality-adjusted life-years and lower total costs than anticoagulation (Reddy et al., 2018).

Atrial Fibrillation and Prior Ischaemic Stroke Patients – **Stroke, Systemic Embolism, and Cardiovascular/ Unexplained Death** – Among patients who had sustained a stroke or TIA prior to enrolment in the PROTECT AF trial, there was a non-significant trend towards a reduction in stroke, systemic embolism, and cardiovascular/unexplained death with the device strategy (82/463 [17.7%] in the device group vs 49/244 [20.1%] in the warfarin group; HR 0.66; 95% CI: 0.30–1.45) (Reddy et al., 2014).

Left Ventricular Thrombus

Large anterior MI accompanied by a left ventricular ejection fraction (LVEF) of <40% and anteroapical wall-motion abnormalities predisposes to stasis of blood in the ventricular cavity, endocardial injury with associated inflammation, and an increased risk of mural thrombus formation in the left ventricle.

Left ventricular mural thrombus arises in about 15% of patients with anterior MI, and 27% of patients with anterior ST-segment elevation MI (STEMI) and LVEF <40%.

The risk of thromboembolization after large MI is uncertain, but appears highest in the first 1 to 2 weeks, declining over 3 months, when residual thrombus becomes organized, fibrotic, and adherent to the LV wall.

The risk of embolization after MI in patients with mural thrombus who are not anticoagulated is about 10–20% at 3 months (Vaitkus and Barnathan, 1993; Kontny et al., 1997).

Recommendations for Practice

- For most patients with ischaemic stroke/TIA in the setting of acute MI and LV thrombus, VKA therapy (target INR, 2.5; range, 2.0–3.0) for 3 months is recommended. Additional antiplatelet therapy may be indicated.
- For patients with ischaemic stroke/TIA in the setting of acute anterior STEMI and anterior apical akinesis or dyskinesis but without LV thrombus, VKA therapy (target INR, 2.5; range, 2.0–3.0) for 3 months may be considered.
- For patients with ischaemic stroke/TIA in the setting of acute MI and LV thrombus or anterior or apical wall-motion abnormalities with LVEF <40% intolerant of VKA therapy, a low-molecular -weight heparin or direct oral anticoagulant for 3 months may be considered.

Cardiomyopathy/Heart Failure

Dilated cardiomyopathy (ischaemic or nonischaemic) predisposes to an increased risk of stroke.

In one study of 2114 patients with sinus rhythm and LVEF ≤35%, the risk of stroke was 1.7% per year (Freudenberger et al., 2007), and in another of 1886 patients with sinus rhythm + LVEF ≤35%, the risk of stroke was similar at 3.9% over 3 years (Mahajan et al., 2010).

Recommendations for Practice

- For patients with ischaemic stroke/TIA, sinus rhythm and dilated cardiomyopathy (LVEF ≤35%), or restrictive cardiomyopathy without left atrial or LV thrombus, the choice between anticoagulation or antiplatelet prescription is uncertain and should be individualized.
- For patients with ischaemic stroke/TIA, sinus rhythm and dilated cardiomyopathy (LVEF ≤35%), restrictive cardiomyopathy, or a mechanical left ventricular assist device (LVAD) in those who are intolerant to VKA therapy because of nonhaemorrhagic adverse events, the effectiveness of dabigatran, rivaroxaban, or apixaban versus VKA therapy for prevention of recurrent stroke is uncertain.
- For patients with ischaemic stroke/TIA, sinus rhythm, and left atrial or LV thrombus, anticoagulation with a VKA is recommended for ≥3 months.
- For patients with ischaemic stroke/TIA in the setting of a mechanical LVAD, anticoagulation with VKA therapy (target INR, 2.5; range, 2.0–3.0) is reasonable in the absence of major contraindications (e.g. active gastrointestinal bleeding).

Valvular Heart Disease (mitral, aortic)

Mitral Stenosis, Regurgitation, and Prolapse; Mitral Annular Calcification and Aortic Valve Disease

Mitral stenosis is usually caused by rheumatic fever.

Streptococcal infection leads to fibrosis of the mitral valve leaflets, which narrows the orifice. The risk of embolic stroke within 6–12 years is 30–65% without anticoagulation, half within the first year. The risk of stroke increases with left atrial enlargement,

F, reduced cardiac output, older age, and a history of rior embolic event (Chandrashekhar et al., 2009).

Antithrombotic therapy has not been examined in rials but there is consensus that "anticoagulation (vitamin K antagonist [VKA] or heparin) is indicated in atients with 1) MS and AF (paroxysmal, persistent, or ermanent), 2) MS and a prior embolic event, or 3) MS nd a left atrial thrombus. (Nishimura et al., 2014).

ecommendations for Practice

For patients with ischaemic stroke or TIA with rheumatic mitral valve disease and AF, long-term VKA therapy, INR target 2.5 (range, 2.0–3.0) is recommended.

For patients with ischaemic stroke or TIA with rheumatic mitral valve disease without AF or another likely cause for their symptoms (e.g. carotid stenosis), long-term VKA therapy, INR target 2.5 (range, 2.0–3.0) may be considered instead of antiplatelet therapy.

For patients with rheumatic mitral valve disease who are prescribed VKA therapy after an ischaemic stroke or TIA, antiplatelet therapy should not be routinely added.

For patients with rheumatic mitral valve disease who have an ischaemic stroke or TIA while being treated with adequate VKA therapy, the addition of an antiplatelet drug might be considered.

- For patients with ischaemic stroke or TIA and native aortic or nonrheumatic mitral valve disease who do not have AF or another indication for anticoagulation, antiplatelet therapy is recommended.

- For patients with ischaemic stroke or TIA and mitral annular calcification who do not have AF or another indication for anticoagulation, antiplatelet therapy is recommended (as it would be without the mitral annular calcification).

- For patients with mitral valve prolapse who have ischaemic stroke or TIAs and who do not have AF or another indication for anticoagulation, antiplatelet therapy is recommended (as it would be without mitral valve prolapse).

Prosthetic Heart Valves (mechanical, bioprosthetic)

Patients with prosthetic heart valves are at increased risk for valve thrombosis and arterial thromboembolism. Oral anticoagulation alone, without or with the addition of antiplatelet drugs, has been used to minimize this risk.

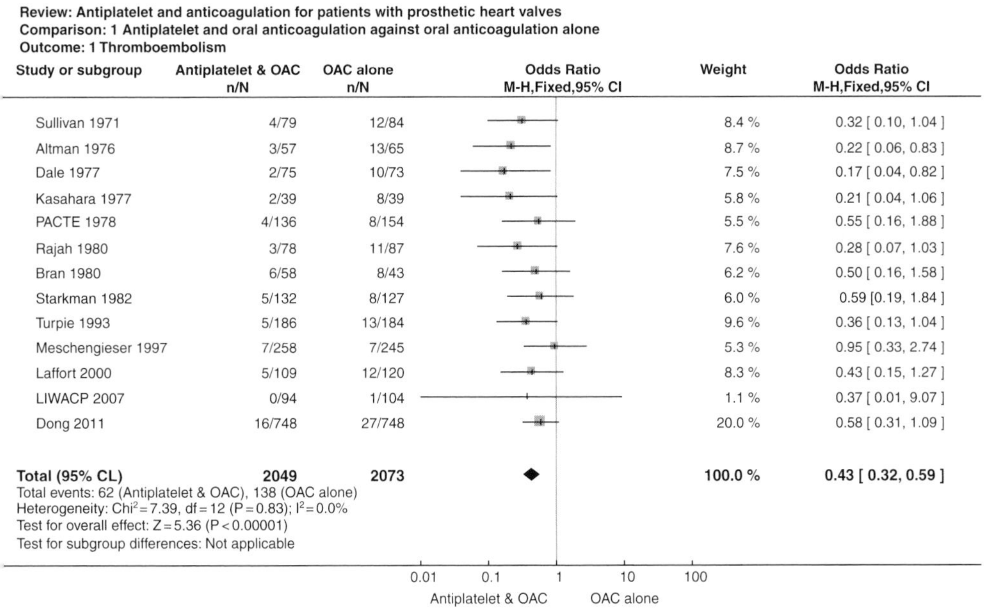

Figure 18.11 Forest plot showing the effects of *antiplatelet + oral anticoagulation (OAC) vs oral anticoagulation alone* in patients with *rosthetic heart valves* on *thromboembolic events* at the end of follow-up.

eproduced from Massel and Little (2013) with permission from the authors and John Wiley & Sons Limited. Copyright Cochrane Library, eproduced with permission.

Review: Antiplatelet and anticoagulation for patients with prosthetic heart valves
Comparison: 1 Antiplatelet and oral anticoagulation against oral anticoagulation alone
Outcome: 3 Major bleeding

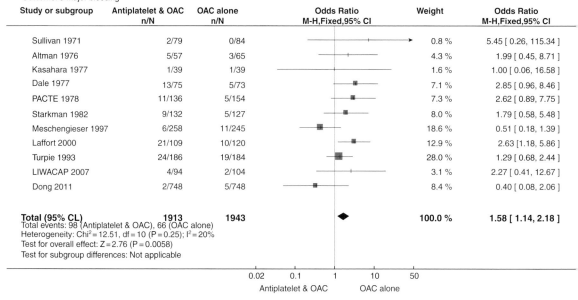

Study or subgroup	Antiplatelet & OAC n/N	OAC alone n/N	Odds Ratio M-H,Fixed,95% CI	Weight	Odds Ratio M-H,Fixed,95% CI
Sullivan 1971	2/79	0/84		0.8 %	5.45 [0.26, 115.34]
Altman 1976	5/57	3/65		4.3 %	1.99 [0.45, 8.71]
Kasahara 1977	1/39	1/39		1.6 %	1.00 [0.06, 16.58]
Dale 1977	13/75	5/73		7.1 %	2.85 [0.96, 8.46]
PACTE 1978	11/136	5/154		7.3 %	2.62 [0.89, 7.75]
Starkman 1982	9/132	5/127		8.0 %	1.79 [0.58, 5.48]
Meschengieser 1997	6/258	11/245		18.6 %	0.51 [0.18, 1.39]
Laffort 2000	21/109	10/120		12.9 %	2.63 [1.18, 5.86]
Turpie 1993	24/186	19/184		28.0 %	1.29 [0.68, 2.44]
LIWACAP 2007	4/94	2/104		3.1 %	2.27 [0.41, 12.67]
Dong 2011	2/748	5/748		8.4 %	0.40 [0.08, 2.06]
Total (95% CL)	**1913**	**1943**		**100.0 %**	**1.58 [1.14, 2.18]**

Total events: 98 (Antiplatelet & OAC), 66 (OAC alone)
Heterogeneity: Chi² = 12.51, df = 10 (P = 0.25); I² = 20%
Test for overall effect: Z = 2.76 (P = 0.0058)
Test for subgroup differences: Not applicable

0.02   0.1   1   10   50
Antiplatelet & OAC   OAC alone

Figure 18.12 Forest plot showing the effects of *antiplatelet + oral anticoagulation (OAC) vs oral anticoagulation alone* in patients with *prosthetic heart valves* on *major bleeding events* at the end of follow-up.

Reproduced from Massel and Little (2013) with permission from the authors and John Wiley & Sons Limited. Copyright Cochrane Library, reproduced with permission.

Oral Anticoagulation (Warfarin) vs Oral Anticoagulation (Warfarin) + Antiplatelet Therapy

Warfarin vs Warfarin + Aspirin

A meta-analysis identified 13 RCTs comparing standard-dose oral anticoagulation with standard-dose oral anticoagulation and antiplatelet therapy in 4122 patients with one or more prosthetic heart valves published between 1971 and 2011 (Massel and Little, 2013). The patients had mechanical prosthetic valves or biological valves and indicators of high risk such as AF or prior thromboembolic events.

In general, the quality of the included trials tended to be low, possibly reflecting the era when the majority of the trials were conducted (1970s and 1980s when trial methodology was less advanced).

Thromboembolic Events – Compared with anticoagulation alone, the addition of an antiplatelet agent reduced the risk of thromboembolic events (odds ratio [OR] 0.43, 95% CI: 0.32–0.59; $p < 0.00001$) (Figure 18.11).

Aspirin and dipyridamole reduced these events similarly.

Mortality – Compared with anticoagulation alone, th[e] addition of an antiplatelet agent reduced the risk of tot[al] mortality (OR 0.57, 95% CI: 0.42–0.78; $p = 0.0004$).

Major Bleeding – The risk of major bleeding wa[s] increased when antiplatelet agents were added t[o] oral anticoagulants (OR 1.58, 95% CI: 1.14–2.18; p 0.006) (Figure 18.12).

There was no evidence of heterogeneity betwee[n] aspirin and dipyridamole, or in the comparison o[f] trials performed before and after 1990, which i[s] around the time when anticoagulation standardiza[-] tion with INR testing was being implemented.

A lower daily dose of aspirin (<100 mg) may b[e] associated with a lower major bleeding risk than highe[r] doses.

Interpretation – Adding antiplatelet therapy, eithe[r] dipyridamole or low-dose aspirin, to oral anticoagula[-] tion decreased the risk of systemic embolism or deat[h] among patients with prosthetic heart valves. The effec[-] tiveness and safety of low-dose aspirin (100 mg daily[)] were similar to higher-dose aspirin and dipyridamol[e.] The risk of major bleeding was increased with antiplate[-] let therapy.

Dabigatran vs Warfarin in Patients with Mechanical Heart Valves

Although dabigatran, an oral direct thrombin inhibitor, is an effective alternative to warfarin for preventing stroke and systemic embolism in patients with AF, has, so far, not proved as effective or safe as adjusted-dose warfarin in patients with mechanical heart valves (Eikelboom et al., 2013).

In a phase 2 dose-validation study, 252 patients who had undergone aortic- or mitral-valve replacement were randomly assigned in a 2:1 ratio to receive either dabigatran or warfarin. The selection of the initial dabigatran dose (150, 220, or 300 mg twice daily) was based on kidney function, and dabigatran doses were subsequently adjusted to obtain a trough plasma level of at least 50 ng per millilitre. The warfarin dose was adjusted to obtain an INR of 2–3 or 2.5–3.5 on the basis of thromboembolic risk. Although the primary endpoint was the trough plasma level of dabigatran, the trial was terminated prematurely (after the enrolment of 252 patients) because of an excess of thromboembolic and bleeding events among patients in the dabigatran group. Ischaemic or unspecified stroke occurred in 9 patients (5%) in the dabigatran group and in no patients in the warfarin group; major bleeding occurred in 7 patients (4%) and 2 patients (2%), respectively. All patients with major bleeding had pericardial bleeding. In the as-treated analysis, dose adjustment or discontinuation of dabigatran was required in 52 of 162 patients (32%).

Interpretation

The use of dabigatran in patients with mechanical heart valves was associated with increased rates of thromboembolic and bleeding complications, as compared with warfarin, thus showing no benefit and an excess risk.

Recommendations for Practice

For patients with a mechanical aortic valve and a history of ischaemic stroke or TIA before its insertion, VKA therapy is recommended with an INR target of 2.5 (range, 2.0–3.0).

For patients with a mechanical mitral valve and a history of ischaemic stroke or TIA before its insertion, VKA therapy is recommended with an INR target of 3.0 (range, 2.5–3.5).

For patients with a mechanical mitral or aortic valve who have a history of ischaemic stroke or TIA before its insertion and who are at low risk for bleeding, the addition of aspirin 75

to 100 mg/day to VKA therapy is recommended.

- For patients with a mechanical heart valve who have an ischaemic stroke or systemic embolism despite adequate antithrombotic therapy, it is reasonable to intensify therapy by increasing the dose of aspirin to 325 mg/day or increasing the target INR, depending on bleeding risk.
- For patients with a bioprosthetic aortic or mitral valve, a history of ischaemic stroke or TIA before its insertion, and no other indication for anticoagulation therapy beyond 3 to 6 months from the valve placement, long-term therapy with aspirin 75 to 100 mg/day is recommended in preference to long-term anticoagulation.
- For patients with a bioprosthetic aortic or mitral valve who have a TIA, ischaemic stroke, or systemic embolism despite adequate antiplatelet therapy, the addition of VKA therapy with an INR target of 2.5 (range, 2.0–3.0) may be considered.

Infective Endocarditis

Infective endocarditis causes ischaemic stroke or TIA in about one-fifth of patients. The cause is embolism of valvular vegetations. Although TIA and stroke may be the initial manifestation, stroke more commonly manifests in patients who are unwell with uncontrolled infection.

Infective endocarditis may also be complicated by haemorrhagic transformation of a brain infarct, sometimes as a consequence of unwise anticoagulation, and intracerebral or subarachnoid haemorrhage due to a pyogenic vasculitis and vessel wall necrosis, or mycotic aneurysm(s) of the distal branches of a cerebral artery. Other non-stroke, neurological complications of infective endocarditis include meningitis; a diffuse encephalopathy, perhaps as a result of showers of small emboli; acute mononeuropathy; rarely, cerebral abscess; discitis; and headache.

Patients with active endocarditis should not be treated with oral anticoagulants because of their high risk of intracerebral haemorrhage; bactericidal antibiotics with or without surgery (radical valve replacement or vegetectomy and valve repair) are the cornerstone of therapy.

The main indications for surgery comprise refractory cardiac failure caused by valvular insufficiency, persistent sepsis caused by a surgically removable focus or a valvular ring or myocardial abscess, and persistent life-threatening embolization (Wang et al., 2018). Surgery for active endocarditis is associated with a mortality rate of 8–16%, and actuarial survival rates of 75–76% at 5 years and 61% at 10 years.

Mycotic aneurysms do not always rupture and tend to resolve with time so that, on balance, cerebral angiography to detect unruptured aneurysms with a view to surgery and surgical repair of any asymptomatic aneurysm are unnecessary.

Recommendations for Medical Therapy

- In patients with (septic) embolic ischaemic or haemorrhagic stroke due to infective endocarditis, appropriate antibiotic therapy should be initiated and continued after blood cultures are obtained with guidance from antibiotic sensitivity data and infectious disease consultants (Nishimura et al., 2014; Baddour et al., 2015). Patients with infective endocarditis on the left side of the heart are typically treated with intravenous antibiotic agents for up to 6 weeks. However, once the patient is in a stable condition, changing to oral antibiotic treatment was noninferior to continued intravenous antibiotic treatment in a recent randomized trial (Iversen et al., 2019).
- In patients with infective endocarditis who are anticoagulated for another indication (e.g. prosthetic heart valve) and who develop central nervous system symptoms compatible with embolism or stroke, the anticoagulation should be discontinued temporarily because of the risks of haemorrhagic transformation of the brain infarct or rupture of a mycotic aneurysm (but antibiotics +/– plans for surgical treatment of the infected heart valve should be continued).

Recommendations for Surgical Therapy

Early valve surgery is **indicated** in the following cases:
- Valve dysfunction resulting in symptoms or signs of heart failure
- Symptoms or signs of heart failure resulting from valve dehiscence, intracardiac fistula, or severe prosthetic valve dysfunction
- Infective endocarditis complicated by heart block, annular or aortic abscess, or destructive penetrating lesions

- Evidence of persistent infection (i.e. persistent bacteraemia or fever lasting >5–7 days and provided that other sites of infection and fever have been excluded) after the start of appropriate antibiotic therapy.

Early valve surgery should be **considered** or a **reasonable** strategy in the following:
- Infective endocarditis caused by fungi or resistant organisms (e.g. vancomycin-resistant enterococci [VRE], multidrug-resistant [MDR] gram-negative bacilli)
- Recurrent emboli and persistent or enlarging vegetations despite appropriate antibiotic therapy
- Severe valvular regurgitation and mobile vegetations >10 mm
- Mobile vegetations >10 mm, particularly when involving the anterior leaflet of the mitral valve and associated with other relative indications for surgery
- Relapsing prosthetic valve infective endocarditis

Patent Foramen Ovale

A PFO is a remnant of embryological development. It is common; echocardiographic and autopsy studies indicate that it fails to close completely after birth in about 25% (19–36%) of the general population and is usually an incidental finding. The size of the defect varies from 1 to 19 mm (mean 4.9 mm), and is much like a flap valve, sealed closed by the higher pressure in the left atrium. However, at times of elevated right atrial pressure, blood may pass from the right atrium into the left atrium and, therefore, into the systemic arterial circulation.

This paradoxical route for venous embolic material to reach the systemic arterial circulation has been recognized by rare autopsy findings of thrombus straddling a PFO in the setting of a fatal stroke. Paradoxical embolism in the context of PFO has also been documented with stroke during pulmonary embolus, cerebral lesions from gas embolism in divers, and cerebral infarction from fat embolism post orthopaedic trauma. However, these clinical settings are often associated with increased pressure in the right heart and therefore predispose to paradoxical embolism. Nevertheless, right-to-left shunting may occur with normal right heart pressures during normal respiration or the Valsalva manoeuvre.

The proposed mechanisms by which a PFO may cause a stroke include not only paradoxical embolization, but also *in situ* thrombosis within the canal of the PFO, associated atrial dysrhythmias and concomitant hypercoagulable states.

Patients with cryptogenic ischaemic stroke or TIA and a PFO have a similar rate of recurrent ischaemic stroke (1.6% per year, 95% CI: 1.1–2.1%) to patients without a PFO (RR 1.1, 95% CI: 0.8–1.5) (Almekhlafi et al., 2009). However, an additional atrial septal aneurysm increases the risk of recurrent stroke (HR for both PFO and atrial septal aneurysm vs neither 4.17, 95% CI: 1.5–11.8) (Mas et al., 2001).

Possible strategies to reduce recurrent stroke from paradoxical embolism include antiplatelet drugs, anticoagulation, surgical PFO closure, and percutaneous closure of the PFO with a device (Saver et al., 2018).

Antithrombotic Therapy

The role of antithrombotic therapy for the prevention of recurrent stroke associated with PFO is uncertain because of the absence of reliable evidence from RCTs.

A recent systematic review identified only three trials which randomly allocated patients with cryptogenic stroke who had PFO confirmed by TOE to long-term anticoagulation versus antiplatelet therapy and reported the outcome of ischaemic stroke (Kasner et al., 2018).

The PFO in Cryptogenic Stroke Study (PICSS) comprised a cohort of 98 patients with cryptogenic stroke who were randomly assigned to receive warfarin or aspirin (Homma et al., 2002). The Patent Foramen Ovale Closure or Anticoagulants versus Antiplatelet Therapy to Prevent Stroke Recurrence (CLOSE) trial comprised a cohort of 361 patients who were randomly allocated to anticoagulation or antiplatelet therapy, with the choice of medication within each category left to the treating physician (336 [93%] of 361 patients on anticoagulation were given vitamin K antagonists) (Mas et al., 2017).

The NAVIGATE ESUS trial randomized 7213 patients with embolic stroke of undetermined source (ESUS) to receive rivaroxaban (n = 3609) or aspirin (n = 3604). Transthoracic echocardiogram (TTE) was done in 6884 patients, transoesophageal echocardiogram (TOE) in 1382, and either TTE or TOE in 7210. PFO was detected in 313 (4.6%) patients by TTE and in 379 (27.4%) by TOE. Recurrent ischaemic stroke occurred at a rate of 3.7 events per

100 person-years among patients with PFO on TTE or TOE, or both, compared with 4.8 events per 100 person-years in those without evidence of PFO (unadjusted hazard ratio [HR] 0.80, 95% CI: 0.51–1.26; $p = 0.33$; adjusted HR 0.84 [after adjustment for age, hypertension, diabetes, coronary disease, and heart failure], 95% CI: 0.53–1.32; $p = 0.44$). Among the 379 patients with PFO in the TOE cohort from NAVIGATE ESUS, there was a trend to a lower rate of recurrent ischaemic stroke among participants allocated anticoagulation (7/182 [3.8%]) versus antiplatelet therapy (12/197 [6.1%] – OR 0.62, 95% CI: 0.24–1.60) (Kasner et al., 2018).

A random-effects meta-analysis of these three studies, in which patients with cryptogenic stroke and PFO were randomly assigned to receive anticoagulant or antiplatelet therapy (NAVIGATE ESUS, PICSS, and CLOSE), yielded a summary odds ratio of 0.48 (95% CI: 0.24–0.96; $p = 0.04$) for recurrent ischaemic stroke in favour of anticoagulation, without evidence of heterogeneity. ($I^2 = 0\%$) (Kasner et al., 2018)

Interpretation

For patients with a cryptogenic ischaemic stroke or TIA and a PFO, the relative efficacy and safety of oral anticoagulation versus antiplatelet therapy is uncertain; anticoagulation might reduce the risk of recurrent stroke by up to half compared with antiplatelet therapy.

Recommendations for Practice

Randomized trials comparing different antithrombotic approaches in patients with cryptogenic stroke and PFO are needed, as are studies to determine whether the source of the thrombus (that embolized to the brain via the PFO) and the presence of an inherited and acquired thrombophilia influence the selection of concurrent anticoagulation or antiplatelet therapy in patients with PFO and cryptogenic ischaemic stroke (Hankey and McQuillan, 2018).

Surgical Closure of the Patent Foramen Ovale

Surgical PFO closure, requiring thoracotomy and cardiopulmonary bypass with their attendant risks, is rarely pursued as a standalone therapy. It may be

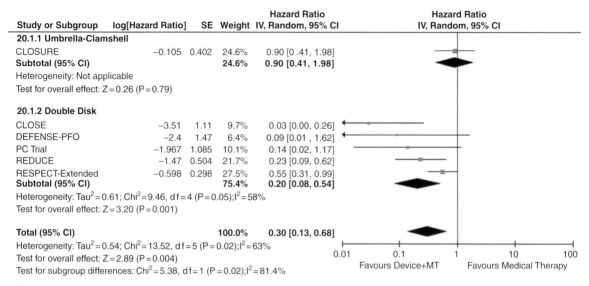

Figure 18.13 Forest plot of trials showing the effects of *PFO closure plus long-term medical antithrombotic (primarily antiplatelet) therapy* vs *medical antithrombotic (antiplatelets or anticoagulants) therapy alone,* in patients with *a patent foramen ovale and a history of cryptogenic stroke or TIA* on *recurrent ischaemic stroke* at the end of follow-up.

Wherever available, data reflect ischaemic stroke defined using the modern tissue-based definition. The forest plot analyses hazard ratio, rather than odds or risk ratio, because of the imbalance in duration of study follow-up between treatment groups in all trials. IV, inverse variance; and MT, medical therapy.

Adapted from Saver et al. (2018).

a useful option when a patient is undergoing cardiac surgery for another indication (Saver et al., 2018). In observational series, open surgical closure had minimal peri-operative mortality, but morbidity included AF, pericardial effusion, post-operative bleeding, infection, and postpericardiotomy syndrome. The annual event rate for recurrent stroke or TIA has ranged from 0% to 9%. Recurrence of cerebral ischaemia may be related to incomplete PFO closure by open surgical treatment, occurring in up to 73% of patients (Schneider and Bauer, 2005).

Percutaneous Closure of the Patent Foramen Ovale

There have now been six RCTs that have compared PFO closure devices with medical management alone, and they provide the first firm evidence to guide treatment selection. Collectively, the trials enrolled 3560 fully reported patients followed for 13,850 patient-years. They differed in several important aspects, including devices tested in the device arm, medications tested in the medication arm, permitted qualifying events, and extent of workup mandated to

exclude competing causes of stroke (Mir et al., 2018; Ntaios et al., 2018; Saver et al., 2018; Turc et al., 2018).

After device placement, there was effective PFO closure (no, or only trace, residual shunting) in 93–96% of patients in double-disk trials and in 87% in the umbrella-clamshell trial.

Recurrent Ischaemic Stroke

A meta-analysis of the 6 RCTs reveals that device closure plus medical therapy (MT), compared with MT alone, reduced the rate of recurrent ischaemic stroke (0.49 [device + medical therapy] vs 1.27 [medical therapy] per 100 patient-years; or 1.96% [device + medical therapy] vs 4.73% [medical therapy] of patients; HR 0.30; 95% CI: 0.13–0.68; $p = 0.004$; Figure 18.13) (Saver et al., 2018).

There was heterogeneity of treatment effect across different device classes (tests for subgroup differences: $I^2 = 81.4\%$; $p = 0.02$), with a greater and significant reduction in recurrent stroke with double-disk devices (HR 0.20, 95% CI: 0.08–0.54; $p = 0.001$) in contrast to an umbrella-clamshell device (HR 0.90, 95% CI: 0.41–1.98; $p = 0.79$).

In the 5 trials of double-disk devices, the recurrent ischaemic stroke rate over 5 years after randomization

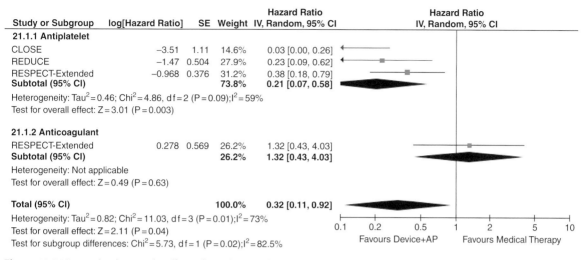

Figure 18.14 Forest plot showing the effects of *PFO closure with predominantly double-disk devices plus long-term medical therapy* vs *medical therapy alone,* in patients with *a patent foramen ovale and a history of cryptogenic stroke or TIA* on *recurrent ischaemic stroke* overall, and in medical therapy antiplatelet and anticoagulant subgroups.
Adapted from Saver et al. (2018).

was 6.0% on medical therapy versus 1.8% with device closure plus long-term antiplatelet therapy. Three patient features were associated or likely associated with magnified reduction in recurrent ischaemic stroke with device therapy: (1) atrial septal aneurysm (ASA) (HR 0.13, 95% CI: 0.03–0.45, ASA; vs HR 0.43, 0.06–3.34, no ASA); (2) larger shunt sizes; and (3) index ischaemic stroke topography not confined to a single, deep, penetrating artery (HR 0.34, 0.29–0.50, superficial or deep and large; vs HR 2.25, 0.41–12.3, small, deep, single perforator) (Saver et al., 2018).

One RCT compared PFO closure versus anticoagulation (353 patients; HR 0.14, 95% CI: 0.00–1.45) and 2 RCTs compared PFO closure versus antiplatelet therapy (1137 patients; HR 0.18, 95% CI: 0.05–0.63; I^2 = 12%).

Medical Therapy Subgroups

Patients randomly allocated to medical therapy in the trials were treated with a mix of antiplatelet agents and anticoagulant agents in 4 of the 6 trials and with antiplatelets alone in 2 trials (Saver et al., 2018).

In contrast, among patients randomly allocated to PFO closure with a device, early concomitant medical antithrombotic therapy was confined to antiplatelet agents alone in 5 of the 6 trials, and early anticoagulation was used in <1% of device-treated patients.

Among the 3 trials which separately reported medical therapy treatment subgroups, there was evidence of heterogeneity of the treatment effect depending on the type of medical antithrombotic therapy (*p* [subgroup difference] = 0.02). Compared with medical antiplatelet therapy alone, device closure plus long-term medical antiplatelet therapy was superior in averting recurrent stroke (HR 0.19, 95% CI: 0.06–0.56; *p* = 0.003). In contrast, in the underpowered comparison of medical therapy with anticoagulants alone versus device closure plus long-term antiplatelet therapy, no benefit of device closure was noted (HR 1.32, 95% CI: 0.43–4.03) (Saver et al., 2018) (Figure 18.14).

Mortality

There was no significant difference in all-cause mortality with PFO closure versus medical treatment (0.18 vs 0.23 per 100 patient-years, respectively; OR 0.73; 95% CI: 0.34–1.56) (Ntaios et al., 2018).

Complications

Immediate, serious, procedure-related complications were infrequent among the 1780 of 1889 patients allocated to the device groups who actually underwent a placement procedure and included access site or retroperitoneal haemorrhage in 1.01%, pericardial tamponade in 0.17%, and cardiac perforation in 0.06% (Saver et al., 2018). Overall, major

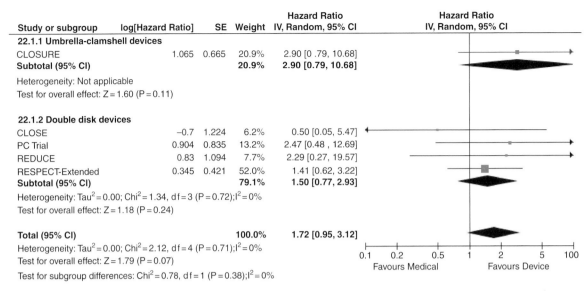

Study or subgroup	log[Hazard Ratio]	SE	Weight	Hazard Ratio IV, Random, 95% CI	Hazard Ratio IV, Random, 95% CI
22.1.1 Umbrella-clamshell devices					
CLOSURE	1.065	0.665	20.9%	2.90 [0 .79, 10.68]	
Subtotal (95% CI)			**20.9%**	**2.90 [0.79, 10.68]**	
Heterogeneity: Not applicable					
Test for overall effect: Z = 1.60 (P = 0.11)					
22.1.2 Double disk devices					
CLOSE	−0.7	1.224	6.2%	0.50 [0.05, 5.47]	
PC Trial	0.904	0.835	13.2%	2.47 [0.48 , 12.69]	
REDUCE	0.83	1.094	7.7%	2.29 [0.27, 19.57]	
RESPECT-Extended	0.345	0.421	52.0%	1.41 [0.62, 3.22]	
Subtotal (95% CI)			**79.1%**	**1.50 [0.77, 2.93]**	
Heterogeneity: Tau^2 = 0.00; Chi^2 = 1.34, d f = 3 (P = 0.72); I^2 = 0%					
Test for overall effect: Z = 1.18 (P = 0.24)					
Total (95% CI)			**100.0%**	**1.72 [0.95, 3.12]**	
Heterogeneity: Tau^2 = 0.00; Chi^2 = 2.12, d f = 4 (P = 0.71); I^2 = 0%					
Test for overall effect: Z = 1.79 (P = 0.07)					
Test for subgroup differences: Chi^2 = 0.78, d f = 1 (P = 0.38); I^2 = 0%					

0.1 0.2 0.5 1 2 5 100
Favours Medical   Favours Device

Figure 18.15 Forest plot showing the effects of *PFO closure plus long-term medical therapy* vs *medical therapy alone,* in patients with *a patent foramen ovale and a history of cryptogenic stroke or TIA* on *atrial fibrillation in the post-procedural period.*
Adapted from Saver et al. (2018).

complications occurred in 2.40% (95% CI: 1.03–4.25; I^2=77%) of procedures (Turc et al., 2018).

The most common complication of device placement was AF, occurring in 3.2% of patients undergoing a device procedure.

Among the 4 double-disk device trials with available data, device placement showed a non-significant increase in annual risk of AF in the post peri-procedural period (30–45 days after randomization or device placement), 0.39% versus 0.26% per year (HR 1.50, 95% CI: 0.77–2.93; p = 0.24) (Figure 18.15).

Most episodes of AF were transient, occurring during the first 4 to 6 weeks after device placement, and associated with first settling of device elements into atrial tissue. The AF resolved in 72% of cases within 45 days (Ntaios et al., 2018; Turc et al., 2018).

Interpretation

The data from RCTs show that PFO closure is superior to antithrombotic therapy for preventing stroke recurrence after cryptogenic stroke in selected patients, despite some limitations of the RCTs, which include a lack of double-blinding in all trials and incomplete follow-up in some trials. Whilst the CLOSURE and CLOSE trials had acceptable losses to follow-up of 1.2% and 0.4%, respectively, the other three major RCTs had losses to follow-up of 10% to 21%. Missing data exceeded

differences in outcome by 11 to 22 times (Powers, 2018).

These data thereby establish a causal role for PFO and paradoxical embolism in the genesis of embolic ischaemic stroke in some patients. The results also endorse the approval by the US FDA of the AMPLATZER PFO occluder for PFO closure to prevent paradoxical embolism in appropriately selected patients.

The annual absolute risk reduction of stroke with PFO closure is low, however, and most of the potentially preventable strokes (in the CLOSE medical group at least) were very mild (Powers, 2018). However, this has to be weighed against a substantial time at risk (at least 5 years) in young and middle-aged patients with PFO and cryptogenic stroke.

PFO closure is also associated with an increased risk of AF.

Implications for Practice and Research

For clinicians, PFO closure is now an additional treatment option to long-term antiplatelet therapy and vascular risk factor control, as appropriate, for lowering the risk of recurrent ischaemic stroke in selected young patients (<60 years) with ischaemic stroke that is most likely attributable to a PFO (Hankey and McQuillan, 2018; Kuijpers et al., 2018).

The first step in selecting patients for PFO closure is to establish a clinical diagnosis of stroke and to confirm that the pathological type is ischaemic by early brain imaging. The next step is to determine the aetiological subtype, or cause, of the ischaemic stroke. This can be difficult because the cause can only be inferred, rather than established, from the site and pattern of the ischaemic brain lesion(s) on brain imaging and circumstantial evidence of a potential cause of cerebral arterial occlusion, such as AF or atherosclerosis in the symptomatic arterial circulation (i.e. a smoking gun). Frequently, more than one potential cause is present. Despite careful evaluation, the cause of ischaemic stroke remains uncertain in about one-quarter (10–40%) of cases and is deemed cryptogenic.

About 35% of patients with cryptogenic stroke have a PFO detected by contrast transoesophageal or transthoracic echocardiography. However, because a PFO is also detected in ≈25% of the general population, any PFO in patients with cryptogenic stroke is more likely to be coincidental than causal. Moreover, any PFO detected among patients with ischaemic stroke with other sources of embolism to the brain (e.g. AF, atherosclerosis) or with nonembolic (e.g. lacunar) ischaemic stroke is even more likely to be coincidental than causal.

Clinical features that increase the probability that a PFO caused the ischaemic stroke are younger age, an embolic pattern of infarction on brain imaging (e.g. cortical infarct), a potential source of embolization (e.g. a venous thrombus or hypercoagulable state), and the absence of risk factors for atherosclerosis (e.g. hypertension, diabetes mellitus, and smoking), no other causes of ischaemic stroke, and a history of prior stroke or TIA.

Transoesophageal echocardiographic factors associated with paradoxical embolism across a PFO include larger size of the PFO on colourflow Doppler, larger right-to-left interatrial shunt as measured by high right-to-left microbubble count following intravenous agitated saline contrast injection, an ASA, and left bowing of an aneurysmal septum (implying higher right atrial than left atrial pressure).

The participants enrolled in the RCTs of PFO closure were carefully selected according to standardized clinical, imaging, and echocardiographic evaluation that increased the probability that paradoxical embolism via a PFO caused the qualifying stroke. Participants were <60 years of age (mean age 45 years) with nonlacunar ischaemic stroke, few vascular risk factors, no alternative demonstrable cause of embolic ischaemic stroke (e.g. atheroma, dissection, or AF), and echocardiographic characteristics of PFO, many with a large right-to-left shunt or ASA. Participants were also treated by experienced cardiologists with complication rates that may not be generalizable. A recent observational study reported serious peri-procedural adverse outcomes or death among 7.0% (95% CI: 5.9–8.2) of 1887 patients undergoing percutaneous transcatheter PFO closure after ischaemic stroke or TIA (Merkler et al., 2017).

The many caveats of selecting appropriate patients for PFO closure emphasize the need for multidisciplinary, personalized evaluation of patients by stroke physicians and cardiologists, perhaps in jointly staffed units or clinics:

- to confirm the accuracy of the clinical, pathological, and aetiological diagnosis of embolic ischaemic stroke that is most likely attributable to PFO;
- to determine the prognosis for recurrent stroke without and with PFO closure added to optimal medical management;
- to determine the potential peri-operative and long-term risks of PFO closure; and
- to engage patients in shared decision-making that incorporates their understanding of the issues and their expectations and values.

Uniform, evidence-based, joint recommendations from professional societies could help facilitate a widespread, multidisciplinary approach to patient care and standardize the indications for financial reimbursement.

Meanwhile, further research is needed to optimize the selection criteria for appropriate and cost-effective PFO closure, to determine the clinical implications of AF related to PFO closure, to reduce the complications and costs associated with PFO closure, to monitor the long-term safety and efficacy of PFO closure in routine clinical practice, to evaluate the optimal antithrombotic regimen that complements PFO closure, and to determine the role of PFO closure in the prevention of recurrent stroke in older patients with cryptogenic TIA or stroke (Kuijpers et al., 2018; Mazzucco et al., 2018).

The population-based Oxford Vascular Study (OXVASC) reported that contrast-enhanced transcranial Doppler (bubble-TCD) to detect probable PFO, as indicated by a right-to-left shunt (RLS), was feasible in most (about 91%) older patients (>60 years) with TIA or non-disabling stroke, and also that the association of a right-to-left shunt with cryptogenic TIA and ischaemic stroke remained at older ages. Compared with those with TIA or stroke of known cause, patients with cryptogenic events had a higher prevalence of RLS overall (OR 1.93, 95% CI: 1.32–2.82; $p = 0.001$), and in those aged older than 60 years (2.06, 1.32–3.23; $p = 0.001$) (Mazzucco et al., 2018).

Pooled data from OXVASC and two previous, smaller studies of bubble-TCD in patients aged 50 years or older also revealed an association between RLS and cryptogenic events (OR 2.35, 95% CI: 1.42–3.90; $p = 0.0009$; p for heterogeneity = 0.15), which was consistent with the equivalent estimate from transoesophageal echocardiography studies (2.20, 1.15–4.22; $p = 0.02$; p for heterogeneity = 0.02). These data suggest that randomized trials of PFO closure in patients with cryptogenic TIA and ischaemic stroke older than 60 years should be feasible and worth undertaking.

Antiphospholipid Syndrome

Antiphospholipid syndrome (APS) is an autoimmune disease characterized by the presence of antiphospholipid (aPL) antibodies that have prothrombotic activity. Antiphospholipid antibodies are associated with an increased risk of pregnancy complications (recurrent miscarriage, premature birth, intrauterine growth retardation) and thrombotic events (both arterial and venous), of which the most common are brain ischaemia (stroke or TIA) and deep vein thrombosis.

The diagnosis of APS is established by the presence of aPL antibodies in two measurements and at least one thrombotic event or pregnancy complication.

A systematic review of nine RCTs that compared any antiplatelet or anticoagulant agents, or their combinations, at any dose and mode of delivery with placebo, no intervention, or other intervention in a total 1044 participants with APS reported insufficient evidence to demonstrate benefit or harm of any regimen (Bala et al., 2018). Studies that are adequately powered and that focus mainly on thrombotic events are needed to draw any firm conclusions on the primary and secondary prevention of thrombotic events in people with antiphospholipid antibodies.

Summary

Recurrent cardiogenic embolism is a major cause of recurrent ischaemic stroke. The cardiac source of embolism is usually the left atrial appendage and atrium due to atrial fibrillation (AF), but other sources include the left ventricle, heart valves, and the venous system or right atrium via a patent foramen ovale (PFO).

Interpretation of Evidence

- Atrial fibrillation may be newly detected in nearly a quarter of patients with stroke or transient ischaemic attack (TIA) by sequentially combining cardiac monitoring methods.
- In patients with non-valvular AF and a recent TIA or minor ischaemic stroke, oral anticoagulant treatment decreases the odds of recurrent stroke by two-thirds compared with no anticoagulation.
- Anticoagulant therapy with a vitamin K antagonist (VKA), such as warfarin, is also more effective than antiplatelet therapy for preventing stroke in people with nonrheumatic atrial fibrillation (NRAF) and recent non-disabling stroke or TIA.
- The four non-vitamin K antagonist anticoagulants (NOACs) that are target-specific direct inhibitors of thrombin (dabigatran etexilate) and factor Xa (rivaroxaban, apixaban, and edoxaban) have a favourable risk–benefit profile compared with warfarin for stroke prevention in AF, with significant reductions in stroke (by about 14%, 95% CI: 2–24), intracranial haemorrhage (by about half), and mortality, and with similar major bleeding as for warfarin, but increased gastrointestinal bleeding.
- The relative efficacy and safety of the NOACs are consistent across a wide range of patients.
- For patients with AF in whom anticoagulation is unsuitable, the combination of clopidogrel and aspirin is more effective than is aspirin alone in preventing stroke (RR 0.72, 95% CI: 0.62–0.83), but causes more major bleeding (RR 1.57, 1.29–1.92). Treating 1000 patients with AF for 1 year with clopidogrel plus aspirin prevents about eight major vascular events (including two fatal and three disabling strokes) and causes seven major haemorrhages (one fatal) compared with aspirin alone.
- Apixaban is superior to aspirin for preventing stroke and systemic embolism among patients with AF who are unable or unwilling to take a vitamin K antagonist, and it is also as safe as aspirin for major bleeding and cerebral haemorrhage.

- For patients taking NOACs who experience severe, potentially fatal bleeding or require urgent surgery, idarucizumab (Praxbind) was approved in 2015 for reversal of the anticoagulant effect of the direct thrombin inhibitor dabigatran etexilate (Pradaxa); and recombinant coagulation factor Xa (andexanet alfa; Andexxa – Portola) was approved in 2018 for urgent reversal of the anticoagulant effect of the direct factor Xa inhibitors apixaban (Eliquis) and rivaroxaban (Xarelto).

- In patients with NVAF, left atrial appendage closure (LAAC) is associated with similar rates of stroke and lower rates of mortality compared to warfarin but the overall quality of the evidence to date is low as assessed by the GRADE working group.

- For ischaemic stroke/TIA, sinus rhythm and dilated cardiomyopathy (left ventricular ejection fraction [LVEF] ≤35%) or restrictive cardiomyopathy without left atrial or LV thrombus, the effectiveness of anticoagulation versus antiplatelet prescription is uncertain.

- For ischaemic stroke/TIA, sinus rhythm and dilated cardiomyopathy (LVEF ≤35%), restrictive cardiomyopathy, or a mechanical left ventricular assist device (LVAD) in patients who are intolerant of VKA therapy because of nonhaemorrhagic adverse events, the effectiveness of dabigatran, rivaroxaban, or apixaban versus VKA therapy for prevention of recurrent stroke is uncertain.

- For patients with prosthetic heart valves, adding antiplatelet therapy, either dipyridamole or low-dose aspirin, to oral anticoagulation decreases the risk of systemic embolism or death. The effectiveness and safety of low-dose aspirin (100 mg daily) appear to be similar to higher-dose aspirin and dipyridamole. The risk of major bleeding is increased with antiplatelet therapy.

- The use of dabigatran in patients with mechanical heart valves is associated with increased rates of thromboembolic and bleeding complications, as compared with warfarin, thus showing no benefit and an excess risk.

- A PFO may be more common in cryptogenic stroke than stroke of known cause, but its presence may not increase the risk of recurrent stroke.

- There are insufficient data to establish whether anticoagulation is equivalent or superior to aspirin for secondary stroke prevention in patients with PFO.

- In patients aged <60 years with a cryptogenic ischaemic stroke after extensive workup for other causes of stroke, and a PFO, closure of the PFO plus long-term medical antithrombotic (primarily antiplatelet) therapy confers an important reduction in ischaemic stroke recurrence compared with long-term antiplatelet therapy alone. It is uncertain whether PFO closure is more effective in preventing recurrent stroke compared with long-term anticoagulation. PFO closure incurs a risk of persistent atrial fibrillation and device-related adverse events. Compared with alternatives, anticoagulation probably increases major bleeding.

Implications for Practice

- Embolism from the heart, particularly the left atrium due to atrial fibrillation, is a major cause of recurrent stroke.

- For patients with acute ischaemic stroke or TIA and no apparent cause, prolonged rhythm monitoring (≈30 days) for AF is reasonable within 6 months of the event (Kernan et al., 2014).

- Patients with TIA and ischaemic stroke who have atrial fibrillation should be treated with anticoagulation, unless there is a major contraindication.

- There remains uncertainty about the ideal timing of initiating anticoagulant therapy, but it is generally recommended that oral anticoagulation be initiated within the first 1–2 weeks of stroke onset, depending on the size of brain infarct(s).

- Warfarin, dabigatran, apixaban, rivaroxaban, and edoxaban are all indicated for preventing recurrent stroke in patients with non-valvular AF, whether paroxysmal or permanent.

- For some patients, the individual's preferences, level of disability, prognosis, and overall clinical status might preclude oral anticoagulation.

- The selection of an anticoagulant agent should be individualized on the basis of renal and hepatic function, potential for drug interactions, patient preference, cost, tolerability, and other clinical characteristics, including time in international normalized ratio (INR) therapeutic range if the patient has been taking warfarin.

- For patients with ischaemic stroke/TIA and AF, thromboprophylaxis with warfarin is indicated in the presence of:
  - Prosthetic heart valve or rheumatic mitral valve disease
  - Poor renal function (estimated creatinine clearance < 25–30 mL/min)
  - P-glycoprotein and CYP3A4 inhibitors (strong) concurrently.
- Warfarin will also remain the anticoagulant of choice for patients who cannot afford the new anticoagulants, and perhaps those who have concerns about compliance with twice-daily doses of dabigatran, apixaban, and edoxaban (e.g. patients taking several medications, and patients who are poorly motivated and forgetful), because the risks of embolic stroke are likely to increase substantially with poor adherence to shorter-acting, new oral anticoagulants.
- If a VKA such as warfarin is prescribed, the target value for the INR should be set between 2.0 and 3.0 for safe and effective stroke prevention.
- For patients with atrial fibrillation who are receiving warfarin and require an elective operation or other elective invasive procedure, the need for bridging anticoagulation during peri-operative interruption of warfarin treatment is uncertain. Warfarin treatment is typically stopped 5 days before an elective procedure to allow its anticoagulant effect to wane; it is resumed after the procedure, when haemostasis is secured, at which point 5 to 10 days of treatment is required to attain therapeutic anticoagulation. During the interruption of warfarin treatment, bridging anticoagulation therapy, typically with low-molecular-weight heparin, can be given to minimize the time that patients do not have an adequate level of anticoagulation, with the intent of minimizing the risk of peri-operative arterial thromboembolism, such as stroke. However, the BRIDGE trial suggests that peri-operative bridging with low-molecular-weight heparin is no more effective than forgoing bridging in preventing arterial thromboembolism, yet it increases the risk of major bleeding (Douketis et al., 2015).
- For patients with ischaemic stroke/TIA and AF, thromboprophylaxis with one of the NOACs is indicated by:

- Previous poor INR control (time in the therapeutic range [TTR]) whilst taking warfarin due to:
  - Genetic polymorphisms affecting warfarin metabolism
  - Drug interactions with warfarin
  - Inadequate access to monitoring, cannot self-monitor
  - Patients unwilling to take warfarin
  - Patient or physician preference for a NOAC.
- If transitioning from warfarin to a NOAC, delay starting the NOAC until the INR is in the lower therapeutic range (e.g. <2.5 or 3.0).
- Monitoring of blood concentrations or anticoagulant activity of the NOACs is not required routinely because:
  - The NOACs demonstrate predictable linear pharmacokinetics with dose-proportional increases in drug exposure and anticoagulation.
  - The therapeutic window of the NOACs is sufficiently wide to allow fixed-dose administration without monitoring.
  - The concept of fixed-dose administration without monitoring proved effective and safe in RE-LY, ROCKET AF, ARISTOTLE, ENGAGE AF-TIMI, and AVERROES trials.
  - The ENGAGE AF-TIMI 48 trial showed that the dose of the NOAC can be tailored based on clinical factors alone (older age, body weight <60 kg, renal dysfunction, concomitant potent P-gp interaction) without the need for a blood test (Ruff et al., 2015).
  - There is currently no standardized, widely and rapidly available test which has proved a therapeutic range that correlates with risk of bleeding and embolic ischaemic events and which adds to clinical risk prediction:
- Because the half-lives and time to anticoagulant activity of NOACs are shorter than for warfarin, bridging therapy is not thought to be necessary with these agents.
- If anticoagulation is complicated by intracerebral haemorrhage, reversal agents should be considered as soon as possible.
  - If the patient is taking a vitamin K antagonist and the INR is ≥1.4 at admission, 4-factor prothrombin complex concentrate is preferable to fresh frozen plasma. Vitamin K injection is also recommended. The aim is to lower the INR below 1.4 as soon as possible. INR values should

be followed up at 3- to 6-hour intervals for the first 24 hours to detect rebound coagulopathy and possible further need for reversal.

- In patients taking NOACs, specific reversal drugs (idarucizumab for dabigatran and andexanet-alfa for factor Xa inhibitors) can be used if available. Otherwise, 4-factor prothrombin complex concentrate can be used.

- Apixaban 2.5 mg twice daily should be considered as an alternative to aspirin in stroke patients with non-valvular atrial fibrillation who are judged unsuitable for vitamin K antagonist therapy if their creatinine clearance is >25 mL per minute.

- Otherwise, for patients with AF and prior ischaemic stroke or TIA who are unable to take oral anticoagulants, the use of the combination of clopidogrel and aspirin therapy might be reasonable.

- For patients with AF who are at high risk of both embolic ischaemic stroke and bleeding, left atrial appendage (LAA) occlusion appears to preserve the benefits of oral anticoagulation therapy for stroke prevention, but the current evidence is of low quality.

- For most patients with ischaemic stroke/TIA in setting of acute myocardial infarction (MI) and LV thrombus, vitamin K antagonist (VKA) therapy (target INR, 2.5; range, 2.0–3.0) for 3 months is recommended. Additional antiplatelet therapy may be indicated.

- For patients with ischaemic stroke/TIA in the setting of acute anterior ST-segment elevation MI (STEMI) and anterior apical akinesis or dyskinesis but without LV thrombus, VKA therapy (target INR, 2.5; range, 2.0–3.0) for 3 months may be considered.

- For ischaemic stroke/TIA, sinus rhythm and dilated cardiomyopathy (LVEF ≤35%) or restrictive cardiomyopathy without left atrial or LV thrombus, the choice between anticoagulation and antiplatelet prescription is uncertain and should be individualized.

- For ischaemic stroke/TIA, sinus rhythm and left atrial or LV thrombus, anticoagulation with a VKA is recommended for ≥3 months.

- For patients with ischaemic stroke/TIA in the setting of a mechanical LVAD, anticoagulation with VKA therapy (target INR, 2.5; range, 2.0–3.0) is reasonable in the absence of major contraindications (e.g. active gastrointestinal bleeding).

- For ischaemic stroke or TIA with rheumatic mitral valve disease and AF, long-term VKA therapy, INR target 2.5 (range, 2.0–3.0) is recommended.

- For ischaemic stroke or TIA with rheumatic mitral valve disease without AF or another likely cause for their symptoms (e.g. carotid stenosis), long-term VKA therapy, INR target 2.5 (range, 2.0–3.0), may be considered instead of antiplatelet therapy.

- For patients with ischaemic stroke or TIA and native aortic or nonrheumatic mitral valve disease who do not have AF or another indication for anti-coagulation, antiplatelet therapy is recommended.

- For patients with ischaemic stroke or TIA and mitral annular calcification who do not have AF or another indication for anticoagulation, antiplatelet therapy is recommended, as it would be without the mitral annular calcification.

- For patients with mitral valve prolapse who have ischaemic stroke or TIAs and who do not have AF or another indication for anticoagulation, antiplatelet therapy is recommended, as it would be without mitral valve prolapse.

- For patients with a mechanical aortic valve and a history of ischaemic stroke or TIA before its insertion, VKA therapy is recommended with an INR target of 2.5 (range, 2.0–3.0).

- For patients with a mechanical mitral valve and a history of ischaemic stroke or TIA before its insertion, VKA therapy is recommended with an INR target of 3.0 (range, 2.5–3.5).

- For patients with a mechanical mitral or aortic valve who have a history of ischaemic stroke or TIA before its insertion and who are at low risk for bleeding, the addition of aspirin 75 to 100 mg/day to VKA therapy is recommended.

- For patients with a bioprosthetic aortic or mitral valve, a history of ischaemic stroke or TIA before its insertion, and no other indication for anticoagulation therapy beyond 3 to 6 months from the valve placement, long-term therapy with aspirin 75 to 100 mg/day is recommended in preference to long-term anticoagulation.

- Patients with active infective endocarditis should not be treated with oral anticoagulants because of their high risk of intracerebral haemorrhage; bactericidal antibiotics (with or without valve surgery) are the mainstay of therapy.

- For patients with a cryptogenic ischaemic stroke or TIA and a PFO, the relative efficacy and safety of oral anticoagulation versus antiplatelet therapy is uncertain.

- For patients under 60 years old with a cryptogenic embolic (non-lacunar) ischaemic stroke or TIA and a PFO, PFO closure plus antiplatelet therapy is recommended (weak) rather than anticoagulant therapy. For patients in whom anticoagulation is contraindicated or declined, a strong recommendation is made for PFO closure plus antiplatelet therapy versus antiplatelet therapy alone. For patients in whom closure is contraindicated or declined, a weak recommendation is made for anticoagulant therapy rather than antiplatelet therapy. Further research may alter the recommendations that involve anticoagulant therapy.

References

ACTIVE Investigators. (2009). Effect of clopidogrel added to aspirin in patients with atrial fibrillation. *N Engl J Med*, **360**, 2066–78.

Albertsen IE, Rasmussen LH, Overvad TF, Graungaard T, Larsen TB, Lip GY. (2013). Risk of stroke or systemic embolism in atrial fibrillation patients treated with warfarin: a systematic review and meta-analysis. *Stroke*, **44**, 1329–36.

Alli OO, Holmes DR Jr. (2015). Left atrial appendage occlusion for stroke prevention. *Curr Probl Cardiol*, **40**, 429–76.

Almekhlafi MA, Wilton SB, Rabi DM, Ghali WA, Lorenzetti DL, Hill MD. (2009). Recurrent cerebral ischemia in medically treated patent foramen ovale: a meta-analysis. *Neurology*, **73**, 89–97.

Ansell JE, Bakhru SH, Laulicht BE, Steiner SS, Grosso M, Brown K, et al. (2014). Use of PER977 to reverse the anticoagulant effect of edoxaban. *N Engl J Med*, **371**, 2141–2

Baddour LM, Wilson WR, Bayer AS, Fowler VG Jr, Tleyjeh IM, Rybak MJ, et al. (2015) Infective endocarditis in adults: diagnosis, antimicrobial therapy, and management of complications: a scientific statement for healthcare professionals from the American Heart Association. *Circulation*, **132**, 1435–86.

Bala MM, Paszek E, Lesniak W, Wloch-Kopec D, Jasinska K, Undas A. (2018) Antiplatelet and anticoagulant agents for primary prevention of thrombosis in individuals with antiphospholipid antibodies. *Cochrane Database Syst Rev*, 7, CD012534.

Beyer-Westendorf J, Forster K, Pannach S, Ebertz F, Gelbricht V, Thieme C, et al. (2014). Rates, management, and outcome of rivaroxaban bleeding in daily care: results from the Dresden NOAC registry. *Blood*, **124**, 955–962.

Borre ED, Goode A, Raitz G, Shah B, Lowenstern A, Chatterjee R, et al. (2018). Predicting thromboembolic and bleeding event risk in patients with non-valvular atrial fibrillation: a systematic review. *Thromb Haemost*, **118**, 2171–87.

Bruins Slot KM, Berge E. (2018). Factor Xa inhibitors versus vitamin K antagonists for preventing cerebral or systemic embolism in patients with atrial fibrillation. *Cochrane Database Syst Rev*, 3, CD008980. doi:10.1002/14651858. CD008980.pub3.

Cannon CP, Bhatt DL, Oldgren J, Lip GYH, Ellis SG, Kimura T, et al.; RE-DUAL PCI Steering Committee and Investigators. (2017). Dual antithrombotic therapy with dabigatran after PCI in atrial fibrillation. *N Engl J Med*, **377**, 1513–24.

Chandrashekhar Y, Westaby S, Narula J. (2009) Mitral stenosis. *Lancet*, **374**, 1271–83.

Chen LY, Norby FL, Chamberlain AM, MacLehose RF, Bengtson LG, Lutsey PL, et al. (2019). CHA_2DS_2-VASc score and stroke prediction in atrial fibrillation in whites, blacks and Hispanics. *Stroke*, **50**, 28–33.

Chi G, Kerneis M, Kalayci A, Liu Y, Mehran R, Bode C, et al (2018). Safety and efficacy of non-vitamin K oral anticoagulant for atrial fibrillation patients after percutaneous coronary intervention: A bivariate analysis of the PIONEER AF-PCI and RE-DUAL PCI trial. *Am Heart J*, **203**,17–24.

Connolly SJ, Pogue J, Eikelboom J, Flaker G, Commerford P, Franzosi MG, et al. (2008). Benefit of oral anticoagulant over antiplatelet therapy in atrial fibrillation depends on the quality of international normalized ratio control achieved by centers and countries as measured by time in therapeutic range. *Circulation*, **118**, 2029–37.

Connolly SJ, Ezekowitz MD, Yusuf S, Eikelboom J, Oldgren J, Parekh A, et al., for the RE-LY Steering Committee and Investigators. (2009). Dabigatran versus warfarin in patients with atrial fibrillation. *N Engl J Med*, **361**, 1139–51.

Connolly SJ, Ezekowitz MD, Yusuf S, Reilly PA, Wallentin L, for the Randomized Evaluation of Long-Term Anticoagulation Therapy Investigators. (2010). Newly identified events in the RE-LY trial (letter to the editor). *N Engl J Med*, **363**, 1875–6.

Connolly SJ, Eikelboom JW, Ng J, Hirsh J, Yusuf S, Pogue J, et al., and the ACTIVE (Atrial Fibrillation Clopidogrel Trial with Irbesartan for Prevention of Vascular Events) Steering Committee and Investigators. (2011a). Net clinical benefit of adding clopidogrel to aspirin therapy in patients with atrial fibrillation for whom vitamin K antagonists are unsuitable. *Ann Intern Med*, **155**, 579–86.

Connolly SJ, Eikelboom J, Joyner C, Diener HC, Hart R, Golitsyn S, et al., and the AVERROES Steering Committee and Investigators. (2011b). Apixaban in patients with atrial fibrillation. *N Engl J Med*, **364**, 806–17.

Connolly SJ, Milling TJ, Eikelboom JW, Gibson CM, Curnutte JT, Gold A, et al., ANNEXA-4 Investigators.

(2016). Andexanet Alfa for acute major bleeding associated with factor Xa inhibitors. *N Engl J Med*, **375**, 1131–41.

Connolly SJ, Crowther M, Eikelboom JW, Gibson CM, Curnutte JT, Lawrence JH, et al; ANNEXA-4 Investigators. (2019). Full study report of Andexanet Alfa for bleeding associated with factor Xa inhibitors. *N Engl J Med*, **380**, 1326–35.

Das A, Liu D. (2015). Novel antidotes for target specific oral anticoagulants. *Exp Hematol Oncol*, **4**, 25.

DeWilde WJ, Oirbans T, Verheugt FW, Kelder JC, De Smet JP, Adriaenssens T, et al.; WOEST Study Investigators. (2013). Use of clopidogrel with or without aspirin in patients taking oral anticoagulant therapy and undergoing percutaneous coronary intervention: an open-label, randomized, controlled trial. *Lancet*, **381**, 1107–15.

Di Biase L, Santangeli P, Anselmino M, Mohanty P, Salvetti I, Gili S, et al. (2012). Does the left atrial appendage morphology correlate with the risk of stroke in patients with atrial fibrillation? Results from a multicenter study. *J Am Coll Cardiol*, **60**, 531–8.

Diener HC, Eikelboom J, Connolly SJ, Joyner CD, Hart RG, Lip GY, et al.; AVERROES Steering Committee and Investigators. (2012). Apixaban versus aspirin in patients with atrial fibrillation and previous stroke or transient ischaemic attack: a predefined subgroup analysis from AVERROES, a randomized trial. *Lancet Neurol*, **11**, 225–31.

Douketis JD, Spyropoulos AC, Kaatz S, Becker RC, Caprini JA, Dunn AS, et al.; BRIDGE Investigators. (2015). Perioperative bridging anticoagulation in patients with atrial fibrillation. *N Engl J Med*, **373**, 823–33.

Eikelboom JW, Connolly SJ, Brueckmann M, Granger CB, Kappetein AP, Mack MJ, et al.; RE-ALIGN Investigators. (2013). Dabigatran versus warfarin in patients with mechanical heart valves. *N Engl J Med*, **369**, 1206–14.

Eikelboom JW, Quinlan DJ, van Ryn J, Weitz JI. (2015). Idarucizumab: the antidote for reversal of dabigatran. *Circulation*, **132**, 2412–22.

European Atrial Fibrillation Trial Study Group. (1993). Secondary prevention in non-rheumatic atrial fibrillation after transient ischemic attack or minor stroke. *Lancet*, **342**, 1255–62.

Freudenberger RS, Hellkamp AS, Halperin JL, Poole J, Anderson J, Johnson G, et al. (2007). Risk of thromboembolism in heart failure: an analysis from the Sudden Cardiac Death in Heart Failure Trial (SCD-HeFT). *Circulation*, **115**, 2637–41.

Friberg L, Rosenqvist M, Lip GY. (2012). Evaluation of risk stratification schemes for ischaemic stroke and bleeding in 182678 patients with atrial fibrillation: the Swedish Atrial Fibrillation cohort study. *Eur Heart J*, **33**, 1500–10.

Gibson CM, Mehran R, Bode C, Halperin J, Verheugt FW, Wildgoose P, et al. (2016). Prevention of bleeding in patients with atrial fibrillation undergoing PCI. *N Engl J Med*, **375**, 2423–34.

Giugliano RP, Ruff CT, Braunwald E, Murphy SA, Wiviott SD, Halperin JL, et al.; ENGAGE AF-TIMI 48 Investigators. (2013). Edoxaban versus warfarin in patients with atrial fibrillation. *N Engl J Med*, **369**, 2093–104.

Giugliano RP, Ruff CT, Rost NS, Silverman S, Wiviott SD, Lowe C, et al.; ENGAGE AF-TIMI 48 Investigators. (2014). Cerebrovascular events in 21 105 patients with atrial fibrillation randomized to edoxaban versus warfarin: Effective Anticoagulation with Factor Xa Next Generation in Atrial Fibrillation-Thrombolysis in Myocardial Infarction 48. *Stroke*, **45**, 2372–8.

Gladstone DJ, Spring M, Dorian P, for the EMBRACE Investigators and Coordinators. (2014). Atrial fibrillation in patients with cryptogenic stroke. *N Engl J Med*, **370**, 2467–77.

Glund S, Stangier J, Schmohl M, Gansser D, Norris S, van Ryn J, et al. (2015). Safety, tolerability, and efficacy of idarucizumab for the reversal of the anticoagulant effect of dabigatran in healthy male volunteers: a randomised, placebo-controlled, double-blind phase 1 trial. *Lancet*, **386**, 680–90.

Goldberger JJ, Arora R, Green D, Greenland P, Lee DC, Lloyd-Jones DM, et al. (2015). Evaluating the atrial myopathy underlying atrial fibrillation: identifying the arrhythmogenic and thrombogenic substrate. *Circulation*, **132**, 278–91.

Goldstein JN, Refaai MA, Milling TJ Jr, Lewis B, Goldberg-Alberts R, Hug BA, et al. (2015). Four-factor prothrombin complex concentrate versus plasma for rapid vitamin K antagonist reversal in patients needing urgent surgical or invasive interventions: a phase 3b, open-label, non-inferiority, randomised trial. *Lancet*, **385**, 2077–87.

Gosselin RC, Adcock DM, Bates SM, Douxfils J, Favaloro EJ, Gouin-Thibault I, et al., International Council for Standardization in Haematology (ICSH). (2018). Recommendations for laboratory measurement of direct oral anticoagulants. *Thromb Haemost*, **118**, 437–50.

Granger CB, Alexander JH, McMurray JJV, Lopes RD, Hylek EM, Hanna M, et al., for the ARISTOTLE Committees and Investigators. (2011). Apixaban versus warfarin in patients with atrial fibrillation. *N Engl J Med*, **365**, 981–92.

Gurol ME. (2018). Nonpharmacological management of atrial fibrillation in patients at high intracranial hemorrhage risk. *Stroke*, **49**, 247–254.

Hankey GJ, Patel MR, Stevens SR, Becker RC, Breithardt G, Carolei A, et al.; ROCKET AF Steering Committee Investigators. (2012). Rivaroxaban compared with warfarin in patients with atrial fibrillation and previous stroke or transient ischaemic attack: a subgroup analysis of ROCKET AF. *Lancet Neurol*, 11, 315-22.

Hankey GJ, McQuillan BM. (2018). Patent foramen ovale closure: the pendulum swings. *Circulation*, **137**, 1991–3.

Hankey GJ, Stevens SR, Piccini JP, Lokhnygina Y, Mahaffey KW, Halperin JL, et al.; ROCKET AF Steering Committee and Investigators. (2014). Intracranial hemorrhage among patients with atrial fibrillation anticoagulated with warfarin or rivaroxaban: the rivaroxaban once daily, oral, direct factor XA inhibition compared with vitamin K antagonism for prevention of stroke and embolism trial in atrial fibrillation. *Stroke*, **45**, 1304–12.

Hanif H, Belley-Cote EP, Alotaibi A, Dvirnik N, Neupane B, Beyene J, et al. (2018). Left atrial appendage occlusion for stroke prevention in patients with atrial fibrillation: a systematic review and network meta-analysis of randomized controlled trials. *J Cardiovasc Surg (Torino)*, **59**, 128–39.

Hart RG, Diener HC, Yang S, Connolly SJ, Wallentin L, Reilly PA, et al. (2012). Intracranial hemorrhage in atrial fibrillation patients during anticoagulation with warfarin or dabigatran: the RE-LY trial. *Stroke*, **43**, 1511–17.

Hart RG, Pearce LA, Aguilar MI. (2007). Meta-analysis: antithrombotic therapy to prevent stroke in patients who have nonvalvular atrial fibrillation. *Ann Intern Med*, **146**, 857–67.

Healey JS, Eikelboom J, Douketis J, Wallentin L, Oldgren J, Yang S, et al. (2012). Periprocedural bleeding and thromboembolic events with dabigatran compared with warfarin: results from the Randomized Evaluation of Long-Term Anticoagulation Therapy (RE-LY) randomized trial. *Circulation*, **126**, 343–8.

Healey JS, Hart RG, Pogue J, Pfeffer MA, Hohnloser SH, De Caterina R, et al. (2008). Risks and benefits of oral anticoagulation compared with clopidogrel plus aspirin in patients with atrial fibrillation according to stroke risk: the atrial fibrillation clopidogrel trial with irbesartan for prevention of vascular events (ACTIVE-W). *Stroke*, **39**, 1482–6.

Heidbuchel H, Verhamme P, Alings M, Antz M, Hacke W, Oldgren J, et al.; European Heart Rhythm Association. (2013). European Heart Rhythm Association Practical Guide on the use of new oral anticoagulants in patients with non-valvular atrial fibrillation. *Europace*, **15**, 625–51.

Heidbuchel H, Verhamme P, Alings M, Antz M, Diener HC, Hacke W, et al.; ESC Scientific Document Group. (2017) Updated European Heart Rhythm Association practical guide on the use of non-vitamin-K antagonist anticoagulants in patients with non-valvular atrial fibrillation: executive summary. *Eur Heart J*, **38**, 2137–49.

Heo YA. (2018). Andexanet alfa: first global approval. *Drugs*, **78**, 1049–55.

Hijazi Z, Lindbäck J, Alexander JH, Hanna M, Held C, Hylek EM, et al., for the ARISTOTLE and STABILITY Investigators. (2016a). The ABC (age, biomarkers, clinical history) stroke risk score: a biomarker-based risk score for predicting stroke in atrial fibrillation. *Eur Heart J*, **37**, 1582–90.

Hijazi Z, Oldgren J, Lindbäck J, Alexander JH, Connolly SJ, Eikelboom JW, et al., for the ARISTOTLE and RE-LY Investigators. (2016b). The novel biomarker-based ABC (age, biomarkers, clinical history)-bleeding risk score for patients with atrial fibrillation: a derivation and validation study. *Lancet*, **387**, 2302–11.

Homma S, Sacco RL, Di Tullio MR, Sciacca RR, Mohr JP; PFO In Cryptogenic Stroke Study (PICSS) Investigators. (2002). Effect of medical treatment in stroke patients with patent foramen ovale: Patent foramen ovale In Cryptogenic Stroke Study. *Circulation*, **105**, 2625–31.

Huang WY, Singer DE, Wu YL, Chiang CE, Weng HH, Lee M, et al. (2018). Association of intracranial haemorrhage risk with non-vitamin K antagonist oral anticoagulant use vs aspirin use. A systematic review and meta-analysis. *JAMA Neurol*, **75**, 1511–18.

Idarucizumab (Praxbind) – an antidote for dabigatran. (2015). *Med Lett Drugs Ther*, **57**, 157–8.

Iversen K, Ihlemann N, Gill SU, Madsen T, Elming H, Jensen KT, et al. (2019). Partial oral versus intravenous antibiotic treatment of endocarditis. *N Engl J Med*, **380**, 415–24.

Jonas DE, Kahwati LC, Yun JDY, Middleton JC, Coker-Schwimmer M, Asher GN. (2018). Screening for atrial fibrillation with electrocardiography: evidence report and systematic review for the US Preventive Services Task Force. *JAMA*, **320**, 485–98.

Kasner SE, Swaminathan B, Lavados P, Sharma M, Muir K, Veltkamp R, et al.; NAVIGATE ESUS Investigators. (2018). Rivaroxaban or aspirin for patent foramen ovale and embolic stroke of undetermined source: a prespecified subgroup analysis from the NAVIGATE ESUS trial. *Lancet Neurol*, **17**, 1053–60.

Kernan WN, Ovbiagele B, Black HR, Bravata DM, Chimowitz MI, Ezekowitz MD, et al. (2014). Guidelines for the prevention of stroke in patients with stroke and transient ischemic attack: a guideline for healthcare professionals from the American Heart Association/American Stroke Association. *Stroke*, **45**, 2160–236.

Kontny F, Dale J, Abildgaard U, Pedersen TR. (1997). Randomized trial of low molecular weight heparin (dalteparin) in prevention of left ventricular thrombus formation and arterial embolism after acute anterior myocardial infarction: the Fragmin in Acute Myocardial Infarction (FRAMI) Study. *J Am Coll Cardiol*, **30**,962–9.

Kuijpers T, Spencer FA, Siemieniuk RAC, Vandvik PO, Otto CM, Lytvyn L, et al. (2018). Patent foramen ovale closure, antiplatelet therapy or anticoagulation therapy alone for management of cryptogenic stroke? A clinical practice guideline. *BMJ*, **362**, k2515.

Leyden JM, Kleinig TJ, Newbury J, Castle S, Cranefield J, Anderson CS, et al. (2013). Adelaide Stroke Incidence Study: declining stroke rates but many preventable cardioembolic strokes. *Stroke*, **44**, 1226–31.

Lindahl TL, Wallstedt M, Gustafsson KM, Persson E, Hillarp A. (2015). More efficient reversal of dabigatran inhibition of coagulation by activated prothrombin complex concentrate or recombinant factor VIIa than by four-factor prothrombin complex concentrate. *Thromb Res*, **135**, 544–7.

Lip GY, Nieuwlaat R, Pisters R, Lane DA, Crijns HJ. (2010). Refining clinical risk stratification for predicting stroke and thromboembolism in AF using a novel risk factor-based approach: the Euro Heart Survey on Atrial Fibrillation. *Chest*, **137**, 263–72.

Lowenstern A, Al-Khatib SM, Sharan L, Chatterjee R, Allen LaPointe NM, Shah B, et al. (2018). Interventions for preventing thromboembolic events in people with atrial fibrillation. A systematic review. *Ann Intern Med*, **169**, 774–87.

Lu G, DeGuzman FR, Hollenbach SJ, Karbarz MJ, Abe K, Lee G, et al. (2013). A specific antidote for reversal of anticoagulation by direct and indirect inhibitors of coagulation factor Xa. *Nat Med*, **19**, 446–51.

Mahajan N, Ganguly J, Simegn M, Bhattacharya P, Shankar L, Madhavan R, et al. (2010). Predictors of stroke in patients with severe systolic dysfunction in sinus rhythm: role of echocardiography. *Int J Cardiol*, **145**, 87–9.

Maheshwari A, Norby FL, Roetker NS, Soliman EZ, Koene RJ, Rooney MR, et al. (2019). Refining predictions of atrial fibrillation-related stroke using the P_2- CHA_2DS_2-VASc score. ARIC and MESA. *Circulation*, **139**,180–91.

Majeed A, Agren A, Holmstrom M, Bruzelius M, Chaireti R, Odeberg J, et al. (2017). Management of rivaroxaban- or apixaban-associated major bleeding with prothrombin complex concentrates: a cohort study. *Blood*, **130**,1706–12

Mas JL, Arquizan C, Lamy C, Zuber M, Cabanes L, Derumeaux G, et al., and the Patent Foramen Ovale and Atrial Septal Aneurysm Study Group. (2001). Recurrent cerebrovascular events associated with patent foramen ovale, atrial septal aneurysm, or both. *N Engl J Med*, **345**, 1740–6.

Mas JL, Derumeaux G, Guillon B, Massardier E, Hosseini H, Mechtouff L, et al., CLOSE Investigators. (2017) Patent foramen ovale closure or anticoagulation vs. antiplatelets after stroke. *N Engl J Med*, **377**, 1011–21.

Massel DR, Little SH. (2013). Antiplatelet and anticoagulation for patients with prosthetic heart valves. *Cochrane Database Syst Rev*, 7, CD003464. doi:10.1002/14651858.CD003464.pub2.

Mazzucco S, Li L, Binney L, Rothwell PM; Oxford Vascular Study Phenotyped Cohort. (2018). Prevalence of patent foramen ovale in cryptogenic transient ischaemic attack and non-disabling stroke at older ages: a population-based study, systematic review, and meta-analysis. *Lancet Neurol*; **17**, 609–17.

McGrath ER, Kapral MK, Fang J, Eikelboom JW, o Conghaile A, Canavan M, et al., and the Investigators of the Registry of the Canadian Stroke Network. (2012). Which risk factors are more associated with ischemic stroke than intracerebral hemorrhage in patients with atrial fibrillation? *Stroke*, **43**, 2048–54.

Merkler AE, Gialdini G, Yaghi S, Okin PM, Iadecola C, Navi BB, Kamel H. (2017). Safety outcomes after percutaneous transcatheter closure of patent foramen ovale. *Stroke*, **48**, 3073–7.

Mir H, Siemieniuk RAC, Ge LC, Foroutan F, Fralick M, Syed T, et al (2018). Patent foramen ovale closure, antiplatelet therapy or anticoagulation in patients with patent foramen ovale and cryptogenic stroke: a systematic review and network meta-analysis incorporating complementary external evidence. *BMJ Open*, **8**, e023761.

Nishimura RA, Otto CM, Bonow RO, Carabello BA, Erwin JP 3rd, Guyton RA, et al. (2014). 2014 AHA/ACC Guideline for the Management of Patients with Valvular Heart Disease: executive summary: a report of the American College of Cardiology/American Heart Association Task Force on Practice Guidelines. *Circulation*, **129**, 2440–92.

Ng KKH, Whiteley W. (2017). Anticoagulation timing for atrial fibrillation in acute ischemic stroke: time to reopen Pandora's box? *JAMA Neurol*, **74**, 1174–5.

Ntaios G, Papavasileiou V, Diener HC, Makaritsis K, Michel P. (2017). Nonvitamin-K-antagonist oral anticoagulants versus warfarin in patients with atrial fibrillation and previous stroke or transient ischemic attack: an updated systematic review and meta-analysis of randomized controlled trials. *Int J Stroke*, **12**, 589–96.

Ntaios G, Papavasileiou V, Sagris D, Makaritsis K, Vemmos K, Steiner T, Michel P. (2018). Closure of patent foramen ovale versus medical therapy in patients with cryptogenic stroke or transient ischemic attack: updated systematic review and meta-analysis. *Stroke*, **49**, 412–18.

Oldgren J, Alings M, Darius H, Diener HC, Eikelboom J, Ezekowitz MD, et al., and the RE-LY Investigators. (2011). Risks for stroke, bleeding, and death in patients with atrial fibrillation receiving dabigatran or warfarin in relation to the CHADS2 score: a subgroup analysis of the RE-LY trial. *Ann Intern Med*, **155**, 660–7.

Olesen JB, Lip GY, Hansen ML, Tolstrup JS, Lindhardsen J, Selmer C, et al. (2011). Validation of risk stratification schemes for predicting stroke and thromboembolism in patients with atrial fibrillation: a nationwide cohort study. *BMJ*, **342**, d124.

Patel MR, Mahaffey KW, Garg J, Pan G, Singer DE, Hacke W, et al., for the ROCKET AF Investigators. (2011). Rivaroxaban versus warfarin in nonvalvular atrial fibrillation. *N Engl J Med*, **365**, 883–91.

Pisters R, Lane DA, Nieuwlaat R, de Vos CB, Crijns HJ, Lip GY. (2010). A novel user-friendly score (HAS-BLED) to assess one-year risk of major bleeding in AF patients: the Euro Heart Survey. *Chest*, **138**, 1093–100.

Pollack CV Jr, Reilly PA, Eikelboom J, Glund S, Verhamme P, Bernstein RA, et al. (2015). Idarucizumab for Dabigatran Reversal. *N Engl J Med*. **373**, 511–20.

Pollack CV Jr, Reilly PA, van Ryn J, Eikelboom JW, Glund S, Bernstein RA, et al. (2017). Idarucizumab for dabigatran reversal – full cohort analysis. *N Engl J Med*, **377**, 431–41.

Powers WJ. (2018) Additional factors in considering patent foramen ovale closure to prevent recurrent ischemic stroke. *JAMA Neurol*, **75**, 895.

Reddy VY, Sievert H, Halperin J, Doshi SK, Buchbinder M, Neuzil P, et al., PROTECT AF Steering Committee and Investigators. (2014). Percutaneous left atrial appendage closure vs warfarin for atrial fibrillation: a randomized clinical trial. *JAMA*, **312**, 1988–98.

Reddy VY, Doshi SK, Kar S, Gibson DN, Price MJ, Huber K, et al.; PREVAIL and PROTECT AF Investigators. (2017). 5-year outcomes after left atrial appendage closure: from the PREVAIL and PROTECT AF trials. *J Am Coll Cardiol*, **70**, 2964–75.

Reddy VY, Akehurst RL, Amorosi SL, Gavaghan MB, Hertz DS, Holmes DR Jr. (2018). Cost-effectiveness of left atrial appendage closure with the WATCHMAN device compared with warfarin or non-vitamin K antagonist oral anticoagulants for secondary prevention in nonvalvular atrial fibrillation. *Stroke*, **49**, 1464–70.

Ruff CT, Giugliano RP, Braunwald E, Hoffman EB, Deenadayalu N, Ezekowitz MD, et al. (2014). Comparison of the efficacy and safety of new oral anticoagulants with warfarin in patients with atrial fibrillation: a meta-analysis of randomised trials. *Lancet*, **383**, 955–62.

Ruff CT, Giugliano RP, Braunwald E, Morrow DA, Murphy SA, Kuder JF, et al. (2015). Association between edoxaban dose, concentration, anti-factor Xa activity, and outcomes: an analysis of data from the randomised, double-blind ENGAGE AF-TIMI 48 trial. *Lancet*, **385**, 2288–95.

Sahay S, Nombela-Franco L, Rodes-Cabau J, Jimenez-Quevedo P, Salinas P, Biagioni C, et al. (2017). Efficacy and safety of left atrial appendage closure versus medical treatment in atrial fibrillation: a network meta-analysis from randomised trials. *Heart*, **103**, 139–47.

Salazar CA, del Aguila D, Cordova EG. (2014). Direct thrombin inhibitors versus vitamin K antagonists for preventing cerebral or systemic embolism in people with non-valvular atrial fibrillation. *Cochrane Database Syst Rev*, 3, CD009893. doi:10.1002/14651858.CD009893.pub2.

Sanna T, Diener HC, Passman RS, Di Lazzaro V, Bernstein RA, Morillo CA, et al., for the CRYSTAL AF Investigators. (2014). Cryptogenic stroke and underlying atrial fibrillation. *N Engl J Med*, **370**, 2478–86.

Sarode R, Milling TJ Jr, Refaai MA, Mangione A, Schneider A, Durn BL, et al. (2013). Efficacy and safety of a 4-factor prothrombin complex concentrate in patients on vitamin K antagonists presenting with major bleeding: a randomized, plasma-controlled, phase IIIb study. *Circulation*, **128**, 1234–43.

Sartori M, Cosmi B. (2018). Andexanet alfa to reverse the anticoagulant activity of factor Xa inhibitors: a review of design, development and potential place in therapy. *J Thromb Thrombolysis*, **45**, 345–52.

Saver JL, Mattle HP, Thaler D. (2018). Patent foramen ovale closure versus medical therapy for cryptogenic ischemic stroke: a topical review. *Stroke*, **49**, 1541–8.

Saxena R, Koudstaal PJ. (2004a). Anticoagulants for preventing stroke in patients with nonrheumatic atrial fibrillation and a history of stroke or transient ischaemic attack. *Cochrane Database Syst Rev*, 2, CD000185.

Saxena R, Koudstaal PJ. (2004b). Anticoagulants versus antiplatelet therapy for preventing stroke in patients with nonrheumatic atrial fibrillation and a history of stroke or transient ischemic attack. *Cochrane Database Syst Rev*, 4, CD000187.

Schneider B, Bauer R. (2005). Is surgical closure of patent foramen ovale the gold standard for treating interatrial shunts? An echocardiographic follow-up study. *J Am Soc Echocardiogr*, **18**, 1385–91.

Seiffge DJ, Werring DJ, Paciaroni M, Dawson J, Warach S, Milling TJ, et al. (2019). Timing of anticoagulation after recent ischaemic stroke in patients with atrial fibrillation. *Lancet Neurol*, **18**, 117–26.

Siegal DM, Curnutte JT, Connolly SJ, Lu G, Conley PB, Wiens BL, et al. (2015). Andexanet alfa for the reversal of factor Xa inhibitor activity. *N Engl J Med*, **373**, 2413–24.

Song Y, Wang Z, Perlstein I, Wang J, LaCreta F, Frost RJA, Frost C. (2017). Reversal of apixaban anticoagulation by four-factor prothrombin complex concentrates in healthy subjects: a randomized three-period crossover study. *J Thromb Haemost*, **15**, 2125–37.

SPIRIT Trial Investigators. (1997). A randomized trial of anticoagulants versus aspirin after cerebral ischemia of presumed arterial origin. The Stroke Prevention in Reversible Ischemia Trial (SPIRIT) Study Group. *Ann Neurol*, **43**, 857–65.

Sposato LA, Cipriano LE, Saposnik G, Ruíz Vargas E, Riccio PM, Hachinski V. (2015). Diagnosis of atrial fibrillation after stroke and transient ischaemic attack: a systematic review and meta-analysis. *Lancet Neurol*, **14**, 377–87.

Steffel J, Verhamme P, Potpara TS, Albaladejo P, Antz M, Desteghe L, et al.; ESC Scientific Document Group. (2018). The 2018 European Heart Rhythm Association Practical Guide on the use of non-vitamin K antagonist oral anticoagulants in patients with atrial fibrillation. *Eur Heart J*, **39**, 1330–93.

Steiner T, Poli S, Griebe M, Husing J, Hajda J, Freiberger A, et al. (2016). Fresh frozen plasma versus prothrombin complex concentrate in patients with intracranial haemorrhage related to vitamin K antagonists (INCH): a randomised trial. *Lancet Neurol*, **15**, 566–73.

Turc G, Calvet D, Guérin P, Sroussi M, Chatellier G, Mas JL; CLOSE Investigators. (2018). Closure, anticoagulation, or antiplatelet therapy for cryptogenic stroke with patent foramen ovale: systematic review of randomized trials, sequential meta-analysis, and new insights from the CLOSE Study. *J Am Heart Assoc*, **7**, pii: e008356.

Uphaus T, Weber-Kruger M, Grond M, Toenges G, Jahn-Eimermacher A, Jauss M, et al. (2019). Development and validation of a score to detect paroxysmal atrial fibrillation. *Neurology*, **92**, e115–e124.

US Preventive Services Task Force, Curry SJ, Krist AH, Owens DK, Barry MJ, Caughey AB, Davidson KW, et al. (2018). Screening for atrial fibrillation with electrocardiography: US Preventive Services Task Force Recommendation Statement. *JAMA*, **320**, 478–84

Vaitkus PT, Barnathan ES. (1993). Embolic potential, prevention and management of mural thrombus complicating anterior myocardial infarction: a meta-analysis. *J Am Coll Cardiol*, **22**, 1004–9.

Verheugt FW, Granger CB. (2015). Oral anticoagulants for stroke prevention in atrial fibrillation: current status, special situations, and unmet needs. *Lancet*, **386**, 303–10.

Wang A, Gaca JG, Chu VH. (2018). Management considerations in infective endocarditis: a review. *JAMA*, **320**, 72–83.

Warkentin TE, Margetts P, Connolly SJ, Lamy A, Ricci C, Eikelboom JW. (2012). Recombinant factor VIIa (rFVIIa) and hemodialysis to manage massive dabigatran-associated postcardiac surgery bleeding. *Blood*, **119**, 2172–4.

Wilson D, Ambler G, Shakeshaft C, Brown MM, Charidimou A, Al-Shahi Salman R, et al.; CROMIS-2 collaborators. (2018). Cerebral microbleeds and intracranial haemorrhage risk in patients anticoagulated for atrial fibrillation after acute ischaemic stroke or transient ischaemic attack (CROMIS-2): a multicentre observational cohort study. *Lancet Neurol*, **17**, 539–47.

Chapter 19

Long-term Antithrombotic Therapy for Large and Small Artery Occlusive Disease

Graeme J. Hankey

Antiplatelet Therapy

Aspirin vs Control

TIA and Ischaemic Stroke Patients

There have been 10 randomized controlled trials (RCTs) of long-term aspirin versus control in about 10,000 patients with previous ischaemic stroke or transient ischaemic attack (TIA) (Antithrombotic Trialists' [ATT] Collaboration et al., 2009).

Major Vascular Events

Long-term aspirin therapy for about 3 years reduced the risk ratio (RR) of serious vascular events (stroke, myocardial infarction (MI), or vascular death) by about 17% (95% confidence interval [CI]: 7–25%) compared with control (6.78%/yr aspirin vs 8.06%/yr control; RR 0.83, 95% CI: 0.75–0.93; absolute risk ratio [ARR] 1.28%/year; $p = 0.001$) (Table 19.1).

This corresponds to an absolute reduction in risk of serious vascular events of about 13/1000 per year (Antithrombotic Trialists' Collaboration, 2009). There was no significant heterogeneity among the 10 trials (chi square 6.3; $p = 0.7$).

Any Recurrent Stroke

Long-term aspirin therapy for about 3 years reduced the RR of any recurrent stroke (ischaemic or haemorrhagic) by about 17% (95% CI: 4–28%) compared with control (3.90%/yr aspirin vs 4.68%/yr control; RR 0.83, 95% CI: 0.72–0.96; ARR 0.78% per year; $p = 0.01$) (see Table 19.1).

This corresponds to an absolute reduction in risk of recurrent stroke of about 8/1000 per year (Antithrombotic Trialists' Collaboration, 2009). There was no significant heterogeneity among the 10 trials (chi square 8.4; $p = 0.5$).

Ischaemic Stroke

Long-term aspirin therapy was associated with a trend towards a reduction in RR of probable ischaemic stroke by about 23% (95% CI: –15–48%) compared with control (3.85%/yr aspirin vs 5.02%/yr control; RR 0.77, 0.52–1.15; ARR 1.17%) (Antithrombotic Trialists' Collaboration, 2009).

Haemorrhagic Stroke

Long-term aspirin therapy increased RR of haemorrhagic stroke by about 2-fold compared with control (0.32%/yr aspirin vs 0.14%/yr control; RR 1.90, 1.06–3.44; absolute risk increase 0.18% per year) (Antithrombotic Trialists' Collaboration, 2009).

Timing and Severity of Recurrent Stroke

An analysis of the individual patient data from all RCTs of aspirin after ischaemic stroke or TIA has offered insights into the effect of aspirin on the timing and severity of recurrent stroke.

Rothwell and colleagues found that in 12 trials of secondary prevention of stroke in 15,778 patients with TIA or ischaemic stroke randomized to aspirin or control, aspirin reduced the 12-week risk of any stroke by half (hazard ratio [HR] 0.49, 95% CI: 0.40–0.60), disabling or fatal ischaemic stroke by two-thirds (0.34, 0.25–0.46), and acute MI by two-thirds (0.30, 0.17–0.52) (Rothwell et al., 2016).

The effect of aspirin was consistent among the trials and independent of patient characteristics, stroke aetiology, and aspirin dose.

The effect of aspirin was, however, greater in the first 6 weeks after randomization (indeed, greatest in the first 2 weeks) than the second 6 weeks, and attenuated further to be of limited long-term benefit thereafter.

These results suggest that we might have underestimated the effect of aspirin in preventing early

Table 19.1 Summary of the results of randomized controlled trials of long-term antiplatelet therapy in patients with TIA or ischaemic stroke of presumed arterial origin

Drugs compared	Meta-analysis of RCTs	Patient number	Risk ratio (95% confidence interval)				Study reference
			Recurrent stroke	Major vascular events	Haemorrhagic stroke	Major bleed	
Single antiplatelet drugs vs control							
Aspirin vs control	11 RCTs	9469	0.83 (0.72 to 0.96)	0.83 (0.75 to 0.93)	1.90 (1.06 to 3.44)	2.69 (1.25 to 5.76)	Antithrombotic Trialists' Collaboration et al., 2009
Dipyridamole vs control	9 RCTs	11,158	0.82 (0.68 to 1.00) (odds ratio)	0.86 (0.79 to 0.93)		0.76 (0.37 to 1.56)	De Schyrver et al., 2007
Cilostazol vs control	1 RCT	1095	0.58 (0.41 to 0.91)	0.61 (0.41 to 0.91)			Gotoh et al., 2000
Dual antiplatelet drugs vs control							
Aspirin + Dipyridamole vs control		6946	0.61 (0.51 to 0.71)	0.66 (0.57 to 0.75)		8.1% (A+D) vs	Leonardi-Bee et al., 2005
Single antiplatelet drugs vs aspirin							
Dipyridamole vs Aspirin	3 RCTs	3386 (High vascular risk)	1.02 (0.88 to 1.18)				De Schyrver et al., 2007
Ticlopidine vs Aspirin	5 RCTs	7070 (High vascular risk)	0.94 (0.82 to 1.07) (odds ratio)				Sudlow et al., 2009
Clopidogrel vs Aspirin	One RCT	6431	0.92 (0.80 to 1.07)	0.93 (0.82 to 1.06)			CAPRIE Steering Committee, 1996
Cilostazol vs Aspirin	2 RCTs	3477	0.67 (0.52 to 0.86)	0.72 (0.57 to 0.91)	0.26 (0.13 to 0.55)	0.74 (0.61 to 0.90)*	Kamal et al., 2011
Triflusal vs Aspirin	4 RCTs	2944	1.10 (0.86 to 1.40) (odds ratio, A vs T)	1.02 (0.83 to 1.26) (odds ratio, A vs T)	1.94 (0.91 to 4.15) (odds ratio, A vs T)	2.66 (1.55 to 4.56) (odds ratio, A vs T)	Costa et al., 2005
Terutroban vs Aspirin	1 RCT	19,120		1.02 (0.94 to 1.12)		1.11 (1.02 to 1.21) (minor bleeding)	Bousser et al., 2011
Dual antiplatelet drugs vs aspirin							
Clopidogrel & Aspirin vs Aspirin	One RCT	4320	0.80 (0.63 to 1.03)	0.84 (0.69 to 1.03)	1.18 (0.53 to 2.64)	1.11 (0.71 to 1.73)	Hankey et al., 2011

Table 19.1 (cont.)

Drugs compared	Meta-analysis of RCTs	Patient number	Recurrent stroke	Risk ratio (95% confidence interval)		Major bleed	Study reference
				Major vascular events	Haemorrhagic stroke		
Lacunar stroke patients							
	One RCT	3020	0.92 (0.72 to 1.16)	0.89 (0.72 to 1.11)	1.65 (0.83 to 3.31)	1.97 (1.41 to 2.71)	SPS3 Investigators et al., 2012
Dipyridamole & Aspirin vs Aspirin	5 RCTs	7612	0.78 (0.68 to 0.90)	0.82 (0.72 to 0.92)		1.08 (0.75 to 1.54) (high vascular risk)	Halkes et al., 2008 De Schryver et al., 2007
Oral Gp IIb/IIIa inhibitors vs Aspirin	1 RCT	3319		0.94 (0.85 to 1.03)		8.0% vs 2.8%	Topol et al., 2003
Single antiplatelet drug vs clopidogrel							
Prasugrel (3.75 mg daily) vs Clopidogrel	1 RCT	3747 (Japanese)	0.99 (0.72 to 1.36)	1.05 (0.76 to 1.44)	0.44 (0.14 to 1.42)	0.49 (0.09 to 2.66)	Ogawa et al., 2019
Dual antiplatelet drugs vs clopidogrel							
Clopidogrel & Aspirin vs Clopidogrel	One RCT	7599	0.98 (0.85 to 1.13)	0.94 (0.84 to 1.05)	1.60 (0.97 to 2.64)	3.34 (2.1 to 5.4)	Diener et al., 2004
Dipyridamole & Aspirin vs Clopidogrel	One RCT	20,322	1.02 (0.93 to 1.11)	0.99 (0.92 to 1.07)	1.42 (1.11 to 1.83)	1.15 (1.00 to 1.32)	Sacco et al., 2008
Dual antiplatelet drugs vs aspirin or clopidogrel							
Cilostazol & Aspirin or Clopidogrel vs aspirin or clopidogrel	One RCT	1884 (Japanese)	0.51 (0.34 to 0.77)	0.52 (0.35 to 0.77)	0.66 (0.27 to 1.60)	0.66 (0.27 to 1.60)	Toyoda et al., 2019
Dual antiplatelet drugs vs standard antiplatelet prescription							
Vorapaxar & Standard Antiplatelet vs Standard Antiplatelet therapy	1 RCT	4883		1.03 (0.85 to 1.25)	2.52 (1.46 to 4.36) (intracranial haemorrhage)		Morrow et al., 2013

RCT: randomized controlled trial. TIA: transient ischaemic attack of the brain or eye.

*Extracranial haemorrhage

recurrent stroke and MI after TIA and ischaemic stroke, overestimated the effect of aspirin in preventing long-term recurrent stroke, and been unaware of the benefits of aspirin in reducing the severity of early recurrent ischaemic stroke.

Extracranial Haemorrhage

Aspirin was associated with a 2- to 3-fold increase in extracranial bleeding compared with control (0.25%/yr aspirin vs 0.06%/yr control; RR 2.69, 95% CI: 1.25–5.76: absolute risk increase [ARI] 0.19% per year). There was no significant heterogeneity among the 5 trials that recorded extracranial haemorrhage (chi square 3.6; *p* = 0.5) (Antithrombotic Trialists' Collaboration, 2009).

Effects of Aspirin According to Body Weight and Dose

An analysis of the individual patient data from 117,279 participants enrolled in 10 randomized trials of aspirin in primary prevention of cardiovascular events revealed modifying effects of body weight (10-kg bands) on the effects of low doses (≤100 mg) and higher doses (300–325 mg or ≥500 mg) of aspirin (Rothwell et al., 2018).

Low doses of aspirin (75–100 mg) were only effective in preventing vascular events in patients weighing less than 70 kg, and had no benefit in the 80% of men and nearly 50% of all women weighing 70 kg or more. By contrast, higher doses of aspirin were only effective in patients weighing 70 kg or more. The ability of 75–100 mg aspirin to reduce cardiovascular events decreased with increasing weight (*p*-interaction = 0.0072), with benefit seen in people weighing 50–69 kg (HR 0.75 [95% CI 0.65–0.85]) but not in those weighing 70 kg or more (0.95 [0.86–1.04]; 1.09 [0.93–1.29] for vascular death). Higher doses of aspirin (≥325 mg) had the opposite interaction with body weight (difference *p*-interaction = 0.0013), reducing cardiovascular events only at higher weight (*p*-interaction = 0.017).

These data suggest that body weight should be considered when deciding on the dose of aspirin to be prescribed.

Non-responsiveness

The antiplatelet effect of aspirin may be compromised by patient non-adherence, decreased drug absorption, genetic polymorphisms, increased platelet turnover, increased platelet reactivity to other agonists, and exogenous thromboxane A2 from activated leucocytes or endothelium.

Dipyridamole vs Control

TIA and Ischaemic Stroke Patients

Serious Vascular Events

A systematic review of 9 RCTs of long-term dipyridamole versus control in 11,158 patients with previous ischaemic stroke or TIA revealed that long-term dipyridamole reduced the RR of serious vascular events (the composite event of vascular death, non-fatal MI, and non-fatal stroke) by about 14% (95% CI: 7–21%) compared with control (RR 0.86, 95% CI: 0.79–0.93) (De Schryver et al., 2007) (see Table 19.1).

Among 4 RCTs of long-term *extended-release* dipyridamole versus control in 9741 patients, the extended-release form of dipyridamole reduced the RR of serious vascular events by about 17% (95% CI: 9–24%) compared with control (RR, Mantel–Haenszel [M-H], Fixed: 0.83, 95% CI: 0.76–0.91) (De Schryver et al., 2007).

Stroke

A meta-analysis of individual patient data from RCTs of dipyridamole versus control in a total of 4913 patients with TIA and ischaemic stroke reported that, compared with control, assignment to dipyridamole was associated with an 18% (95% CI: 0–32%) reduction in odds of stroke (Leonardi-Bee et al., 2005).

Major Bleeding

Dipyridamole was not associated with an excess risk of major or fatal extracranial bleeding complications, compared with control, among 4 RCTs in a total of 3443 patients (RR: 0.76, 95% CI: 0.37–1.56) (De Schryver et al., 2007).

Headache

Dipyridamole was associated with an excess of headache, compared with control (37.2% dipyridamole vs 22.8% control) and was sufficiently severe to lead to discontinuation of study drug in the European Stroke Prevention Study (ESPS) 2 trial among 8.0% of patients assigned dipyridamole compared with 2.4% assigned placebo (RR 3.20, 95% CI: 2.25–4.54).

The headache is due to vasodilatation and is usually self-limited, but can occasionally last several weeks.

Dipyridamole may also cause gastrointestinal (GI) upset leading to discontinuation of study drug in some cases (placebo 3.6%, dipyridamole 6.2%; RR 1.65, 95%

CI: 1.21–2.26), and may precipitate angina in patients with occlusive coronary artery disease by a steal effect.

Cilostazol vs Control

Ischaemic Stroke Patients

Serious Vascular Events

In one RCT, the Cilostazol Stroke Prevention Study, involving 1095 patients with recent (1–6 months ago) ischaemic stroke, cilostazol 100 mg twice daily reduced the risk of serious vascular events by 38.8% (95% CI: 8.6–59.0) compared with placebo (4.2% per year cilostazol vs 6.8% per year placebo; ARR 2.6% per year; number needed to treat [NNT]: 38) (Gotoh et al., 2000).

Stroke

Cilostazol also reduced the risk of recurrent ischaemic stroke (the primary outcome) by 41.7% (95% CI: 8.6–59.0) in the Cilostazol Stroke Prevention Study (Gotoh et al., 2000).

Adverse Effects

Adverse effects of cilostazol included headache, tachycardia, and palpitations, which were probably related to its vasodilatory properties.

Aspirin and Dipyridamole vs Control

High Vascular Risk Patients

Serious Vascular Events

Among 13,380 high vascular risk patients enrolled in 15 RCTs, the combination of aspirin and dipyridamole significantly reduced the RR of serious vascular events (relative risk reduction [RRR] 26%, 95% CI: 20–32%) compared with control (RR 0.74, 95% CI: 0.68–0.80) (De Schryver et al., 2007).

TIA and Ischaemic Stroke Patients

A total of 6946 patients with TIA and ischaemic stroke have been randomized to the combination of aspirin and dipyridamole vs control in the long term (Leonardi-Bee et al., 2005).

Stroke

The combination of aspirin and dipyridamole was associated with a 39% (95% CI: 29–49%) reduction in odds of stroke compared with control (Leonardi-Bee et al., 2005).

Serious Vascular Events

The combination of aspirin and dipyridamole was associated with a 34% (25–43%) reduction in odds of serious vascular events compared with control (Leonardi-Bee et al., 2005).

Headache

The combination of aspirin and dipyridamole was associated with a greater incidence of headache compared with control (26.7% aspirin and dipyridamole vs 22.8% control).

Major Bleeding

The combination of aspirin and dipyridamole was associated with a greater incidence of any bleeding (8.1% aspirin and dipyridamole vs 4.2% control) compared with control (Leonardi-Bee et al., 2005).

Dipyridamole vs Aspirin

High Vascular Risk Patients

Major Vascular Events

Among 3386 high vascular risk patients enrolled in 3 RCTs, there was no evidence that dipyridamole is more effective in preventing vascular events compared with aspirin (RR 1.02, 95% CI: 0.88–1.18) (De Schryver et al., 2007).

Ticlopidine vs Aspirin

High Vascular Risk Patients

Among 5 RCTs of ticlopidine versus aspirin in high vascular risk patients, ticlopidine did not significantly reduce the risk of serious vascular events compared with aspirin (odds ratio [OR] 0.94, 95% CI: 0.82–1.07) (Figure 19.1) (Sudlow et al., 2009).

Skin Rash

Compared with aspirin, ticlopidine is associated with a 2-fold increase in the odds of skin rash (11.8% ticlopidine vs 5.5% aspirin, OR 2.2, 95% CI: 1.7–2.9)

Diarrhoea

Compared with aspirin, ticlopidine is associated with a 2-fold increase in the odds of diarrhoea (20.4% ticlopidine vs 9.9% aspirin, OR 2.3, 95% CI: 1.9–2.8).

Review: Thienopyridine derivatives versus aspirin for preventing stroke and other serious vascular events in high vascular risk patients
Comparison: 1 Thienopyridine versus aspirin in high vascular risk patients
Outcome: 1 Stroke, MI or vascular death during follow up

Study or subgroup	Thienopyridine n/N	Aspirin n/N	Peto Odds Ratio Peto,Fixed,95% CI	Weight	Peto Odds Ratio Peto,Fixed,95% CI
AAASPS	128/902	110/907		7.6 %	1.20 [0.91, 1.57]
CAPRIE	976/9599	1063/9586		67.2 %	0.91 [0.83, 0.99]
Japanese-B	8/170	16/170		0.8 %	0.49 [0.21, 1.12]
Sadowski 1995	19/154	29/166		1.5 %	0.67 [0.36, 1.24]
Schoop 1983	0/31	2/31		0.1 %	0.13 [0.01, 2.14]
STAMI	18/734	26/736		1.6 %	0.69 [0.38, 1.26]
TASS	370/1529	395/1540		21.2 %	0.93 [0.79, 1.09]
Total (95% CI)	**13119**	**13136**		**100.0 %**	**0.92 [0.85, 0.99]**

Total events: 1519 (Thienopyridine), 1641 (Aspirin)
Heterogeneity: Chi^2 = 9.70, df = 6 (P = 0.14); I^2 = 38%
Test for overall effect: Z = 2.27 (P = 0.023)
Test for subgroup differences: Not applicable

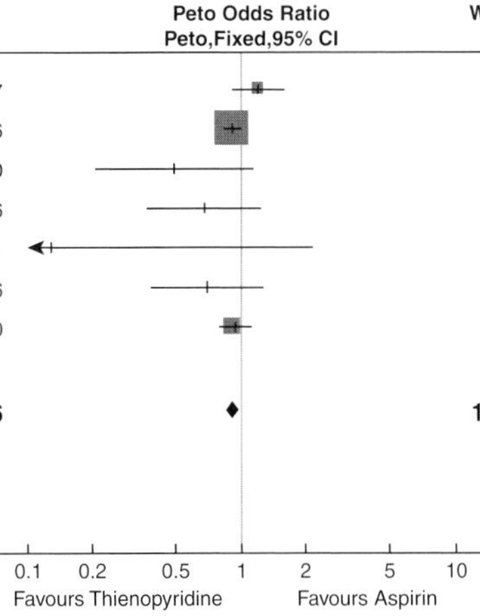

0.1 0.2 0.5 1 2 5 10
Favours Thienopyridine   Favours Aspirin

Figure 19.1 Forest plot showing the effects of *thienopyridine derivatives (ticlopidine, clopidogrel) vs aspirin* in *high vascular risk patients* on *serious vascular events* (stroke, myocardial infarction [MI], or vascular death) at the end of follow-up.

Reproduced from Sudlow et al. (2009) with permission from the authors and John Wiley & Sons Limited. Copyright Cochrane Library, reproduced with permission.

Neutropenia

Compared with aspirin, ticlopidine is associated with a 3-fold excess of neutropenia ($<1.2 \times 10^9$/L) (2.3% ticlopidine vs 0.8% aspirin, OR 2.7, 95% CI: 1.5–4.8).

Thrombocytopenia

There are no published trial data available for the frequency of thrombocytopenia associated with ticlopidine compared with aspirin, but observational data have shown that ticlopidine is associated with a significant excess both of thrombocytopenia and of thrombotic thrombocytopenic purpura.

Clopidogrel vs Aspirin

Clopidogrel is an oral thienopyridine P2Y12 ADP receptor inhibitor.

High Vascular Risk Patients

The CAPRIE trial randomized 19,185 high vascular risk patients to long-term clopidogrel (n = 9599) or aspirin (n = 9586) (CAPRIE Steering Committee, 1996; Sudlow et al., 2009).

Serious Vascular Events

Clopidogrel significantly reduces the odds of serious ischaemic vascular events by about 9% (95% CI: 1–17%) compared with aspirin (see Figure 19.1) (CAPRIE Steering Committee, 1996; Sudlow et al., 2009).

Ischaemic Stroke Patients

The CAPRIE trial randomized 6431 patients with previous ischaemic stroke to long-term clopidogrel (n = 3233) or aspirin (n = 3198) (CAPRIE Steering Committee, 1996; Sudlow et al., 2009).

Stroke

Clopidogrel was associated with a trend towards a reduction in risk of recurrent stroke compared with aspirin (RR 0.92, 95% CI: 0.80–1.07 (Gouya et al., 2014)) and odds of stroke compared with aspirin (OR 0.90, 95% CI: 0.77–1.06) (Sudlow et al., 2009), which is consistent with the effect observed for all thienopyridines (OR 0.90, 95% CI: 0.80–1.00) (see Figure 19.1) (Sudlow et al., 2009).

Serious Vascular Events

For patients with previous TIA or ischaemic stroke, clopidogrel does not significantly reduce the risk of serious vascular events compared with aspirin (RRR: 7.3%, 95% CI: −5.7 to 18.7%; OR 0.90, 0.77–1.06), but the results are consistent with the significant effect of clopidogrel compared with aspirin in all high-risk patients (Figure 19.2) (CAPRIE Steering Committee, 1996; Sudlow et al., 2009). These data are derived from one study, which was not designed to have the statistical power to reliably identify or exclude a modest but important treatment effect of clopidogrel in patient subgroups

Review: Thienopyridine derivatives versus aspirin for preventing stroke and other serious vascular events in high vascular risk patients
Comparison: 2 Thienopyridine versus aspirin in patients with TIA or ischaemic stroke
Outcome: 3 Stroke (of all types) during follow up

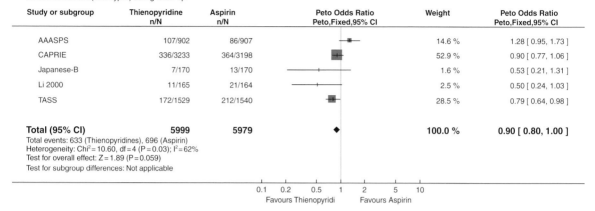

Study or subgroup	Thienopyridine n/N	Aspirin n/N	Peto Odds Ratio Peto,Fixed,95% CI	Weight	Peto Odds Ratio Peto,Fixed,95% CI
AAASPS	107/902	86/907		14.6 %	1.28 [0.95, 1.73]
CAPRIE	336/3233	364/3198		52.9 %	0.90 [0.77, 1.06]
Japanese-B	7/170	13/170		1.6 %	0.53 [0.21, 1.31]
Li 2000	11/165	21/164		2.5 %	0.50 [0.24, 1.03]
TASS	172/1529	212/1540		28.5 %	0.79 [0.64, 0.98]
Total (95% CI)	**5999**	**5979**		**100.0 %**	**0.90 [0.80, 1.00]**

Total events: 633 (Thienopyridines), 696 (Aspirin)
Heterogeneity: Chi^2 = 10.60, df = 4 (P = 0.03); I^2 = 62%
Test for overall effect: Z = 1.89 (P = 0.059)
Test for subgroup differences: Not applicable

0.1　0.2　0.5　1　2　5　10
Favours Thienopyridi　Favours Aspirin

Figure 19.2 Forest plot showing the effects of *thienopyridine derivatives (ticlopidine, clopidogrel) vs aspirin* in patients with previous TIA or ischaemic stroke on *stroke* at the end of follow-up.

Reproduced from Sudlow et al. (2009) with permission from the authors and John Wiley & Sons Limited. Copyright Cochrane Library, reproduced with permission.

according to qualifying diagnoses (e.g. cerebrovascular disease) or outcome events (e.g. stroke) (CAPRIE Steering Committee, 1996). The trial was designed to have the statistical power to reliably identify or exclude a modest but important treatment effect of clopidogrel compared with aspirin in all high-risk patients combined for the composite outcome of major vascular events.

Gastrointestinal Haemorrhage

Clopidogrel was associated with significantly less GI haemorrhage (OR: 0.71, 95% CI: 0.6–0.9) and upper-GI symptoms (OR: 0.84, 95% CI: 0.8–0.9) compared with aspirin. However, these data are derived from one trial (CAPRIE trial) where patients were pre-selected as being tolerant of aspirin, and the dose of aspirin was 325 mg daily.

Skin Rash and Diarrhoea

Clopidogrel was also associated with a significant one-third increased odds of skin rash (OR: 1.32, 95% CI: 1.2–1.5) and diarrhoea (OR: 1.34, 95% CI: 1.2–1.6) compared with aspirin.

Non-reponsiveness

Non-responsiveness to clopidogrel is an issue for some individuals because clopidogrel is a prodrug that requires bioactivation by cytochrome P450 (CYP) iso-enzymes to the active compound. Common reduced-function CYP2C19-2 and CYP2C19-3 polymorphisms and drug–drug interactions (e.g. PPIs) interfere with its

bioactivation and antiplatelet effects. Other limitations of clopidogrel include a delayed onset and irreversibility of its antiplatelet effects.

Cilostazol vs Aspirin

TIA and Ischaemic Stroke Patients

Serious Vascular Events

A meta-analysis of two RCTs involving 3477 Asian participants reported that, compared with aspirin, cilostazol was associated with a significantly lower risk of composite outcome of vascular events (6.77% vs 9.39%, RR 0.72, 95% CI: 0.57–0.91). (Figure 19.3) (Kamal et al., 2011; Dinicolantonio et al., 2013).

Stroke

Cilostazol was associated with a lower risk of all stroke (RR 0.67, 95% CI: 0.52–0.86), and haemorrhagic stroke (0.53% vs 2.01%, RR 0.26, 95% CI: 0.13–0.55), and a non-significant trend towards a reduction in ischaemic stroke (RR 0.80, 95% CI: 0.67–1.07), compared with aspirin (Kamal et al., 2011).

Extracranial Haemorrhage

Cilostazol was associated with less extracranial hae-morrhage during follow-up compared to aspirin (RR 0.74, 95% CI: 0.61–0.90) (Figure 19.4) (Kamal et al., 2011).

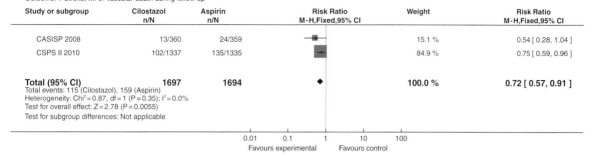

Review: Cilostazol versus aspirin for secondary prevention of vascular events after stroke of arterial origin
Comparison: 1 Cilostazol versus aspirin in patients with ischaemic stroke or TIA
Outcome: 1 Stroke, MI or vascular death during follow-up

Study or subgroup	Cilostazol n/N	Aspirin n/N	Risk Ratio M-H,Fixed,95% CI	Weight	Risk Ratio M-H,Fixed,95% CI
CASISP 2008	13/360	24/359		15.1 %	0.54 [0.28, 1.04]
CSPS II 2010	102/1337	135/1335		84.9 %	0.75 [0.59, 0.96]
Total (95% CI)	**1697**	**1694**		**100.0 %**	**0.72 [0.57, 0.91]**

Total events: 115 (Cilostazol), 159 (Aspirin)
Heterogeneity: Chi² = 0.87, df = 1 (P = 0.35); I² = 0.0%
Test for overall effect: Z = 2.78 (P = 0.0055)
Test for subgroup differences: Not applicable

0.01   0.1   1   10   100
Favours experimental   Favours control

Figure 19.3 Forest plot showing the effects of *cilostazol vs aspirin in patients with previous TIA or ischaemic stroke* on *serious vascular events (stroke, MI, or vascular death)* at the end of follow-up.

Reproduced from Kamal et al. (2011) with permission from the authors and John Wiley & Sons Limited. Copyright Cochrane Library, reproduced with permission.

Review: Cilostazol versus aspirin for secondary prevention of vascular events after stroke of arterial origin
Comparison: 1 Cilostazol versus aspirin in patients with ischaemic stroke or TIA
Outcome: 8 Extracranial haemorrhage during follow-up

Study or subgroup	Cilostazol n/N	Aspirin n/N	Risk Ratio M-H,Fixed,95% CI	Weight	Risk Ratio M-H,Fixed,95% CI
CASISP 2008	10/360	17/359		8.1 %	0.59 [0.27, 1.26]
CSPS II 2010	145/1337	192/1335		91.9 %	0.75 [0.62, 0.92]
Total (95% CI)	**1697**	**1694**		**100.0 %**	**0.74 [0.61, 0.90]**

Total events: 155 (Cilostazol), 209 (Aspirin)
Heterogeneity: Chi² = 0.39, df = 1 (P = 0.53); I² = 0.0%
Test for overall effect: Z = 3.02 (P = 0.0026)
Test for subgroup differences: Not applicable

0.01   0.1   1   10   100
Favours experimental   Favours control

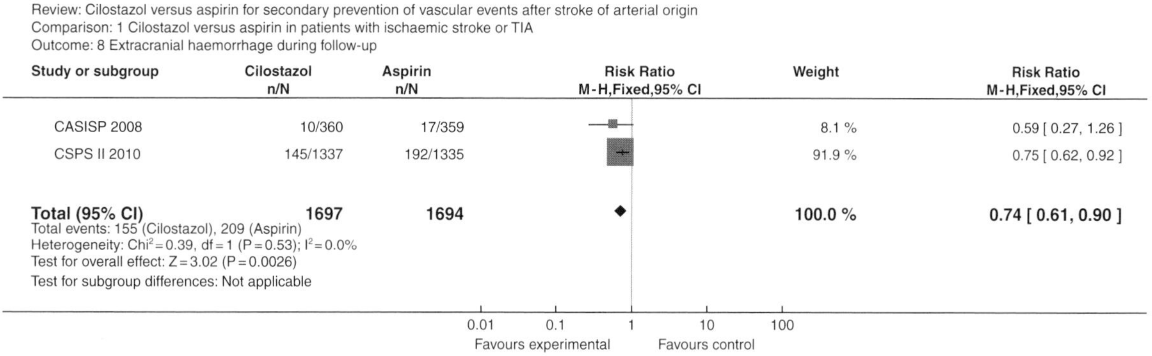

Figure 19.4 Forest plot showing the effects of *cilostazol vs aspirin in patients with previous TIA or ischaemic stroke* on *extracranial haemorrhage* at the end of follow-up.

Reproduced from Kamal et al. (2011) with permission from the authors and John Wiley & Sons Limited. Copyright Cochrane Library, reproduced with permission.

Minor Adverse Effects

Compared with aspirin, cilostazol was significantly associated with minor adverse effects (8.22% vs 4.95%, RR 1.66, 95% CI: 1.51–1.83) (Figure 19.5).

TIA and Ischaemic Stroke Patients with a High Risk of Cerebral Haemorrhage

The prevention of cardiovascular events in ischaemic stroke patients with high risk of cerebral haemorrhage (PICASSO) trial randomized 1534 Asian patients with recent (within the previous 180 days) non-cardioembolic ischaemic stroke ($n = 1433$) or TIA ($n = 79$), who were deemed to be at high risk of bleeding on the basis of magnetic resonance imaging (MRI) findings of previous intracerebral haemorrhage or multiple microbleeds, in a 2 × 2 factorial

design, to receive cilostazol (100 mg twice a day) or aspirin (100 mg once a day), with and without probucol (250 mg twice a day) as a concomitant treatment (Kim et al., 2018).

Probucol is an activator of cholesteryl ester transfer protein, and thus a cholesterol-lowering drug with pleiotropic effects on endothelial function. It was hypothesized that probucol might be beneficial when added to standard lipid-lowering treatment in patients with ischaemic stroke who are prone to haemorrhage.

Participants were followed-up for a median of 1.9 years (interquartile range [IQR] 1.0–3.0) for the co-primary outcomes of a composite of vascular events (stroke, MI, and vascular death; to assess efficacy) and haemorrhagic stroke (to assess safety).

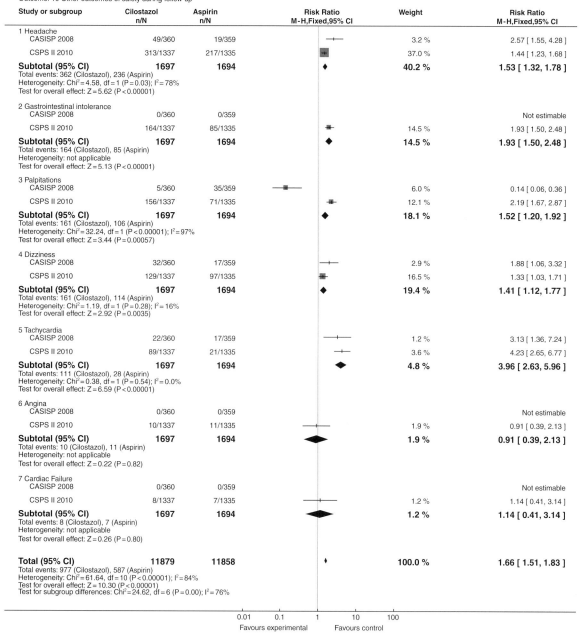

Review: Cilostazol versus aspirin for secondary prevention of vascular events after stroke of arterial origin
Comparison: 1 Cilostazol versus aspirin in patients with ischaemic stroke or TIA
Outcome: 10 Other outcomes of safety during follow-up

Study or subgroup	Cilostazol n/N	Aspirin n/N	Risk Ratio M-H,Fixed,95% CI	Weight	Risk Ratio M-H,Fixed,95% CI
1 Headache					
CASISP 2008	49/360	19/359		3.2 %	2.57 [1.55, 4.28]
CSPS II 2010	313/1337	217/1335		37.0 %	1.44 [1.23, 1.68]
Subtotal (95% CI)	**1697**	**1694**		**40.2 %**	**1.53 [1.32, 1.78]**
Total events: 362 (Cilostazol), 236 (Aspirin)					
Heterogeneity: Chi² = 4.58, df = 1 (P = 0.03); I² = 78%					
Test for overall effect: Z = 5.62 (P < 0.00001)					
2 Gastrointestinal intolerance					
CASISP 2008	0/360	0/359			Not estimable
CSPS II 2010	164/1337	85/1335		14.5 %	1.93 [1.50, 2.48]
Subtotal (95% CI)	**1697**	**1694**		**14.5 %**	**1.93 [1.50, 2.48]**
Total events: 164 (Cilostazol), 85 (Aspirin)					
Heterogeneity: not applicable					
Test for overall effect: Z = 5.13 (P < 0.00001)					
3 Palpitations					
CASISP 2008	5/360	35/359		6.0 %	0.14 [0.06, 0.36]
CSPS II 2010	156/1337	71/1335		12.1 %	2.19 [1.67, 2.87]
Subtotal (95% CI)	**1697**	**1694**		**18.1 %**	**1.52 [1.20, 1.92]**
Total events: 161 (Cilostazol), 106 (Aspirin)					
Heterogeneity: Chi² = 32.24, df = 1 (P < 0.00001); I² = 97%					
Test for overall effect: Z = 3.44 (P = 0.00057)					
4 Dizziness					
CASISP 2008	32/360	17/359		2.9 %	1.88 [1.06, 3.32]
CSPS II 2010	129/1337	97/1335		16.5 %	1.33 [1.03, 1.71]
Subtotal (95% CI)	**1697**	**1694**		**19.4 %**	**1.41 [1.12, 1.77]**
Total events: 161 (Cilostazol), 114 (Aspirin)					
Heterogeneity: Chi² = 1.19, df = 1 (P = 0.28); I² = 16%					
Test for overall effect: Z = 2.92 (P = 0.0035)					
5 Tachycardia					
CASISP 2008	22/360	17/359		1.2 %	3.13 [1.36, 7.24]
CSPS II 2010	89/1337	21/1335		3.6 %	4.23 [2.65, 6.77]
Subtotal (95% CI)	**1697**	**1694**		**4.8 %**	**3.96 [2.63, 5.96]**
Total events: 111 (Cilostazol), 28 (Aspirin)					
Heterogeneity: Chi² = 0.38, df = 1 (P = 0.54); I² = 0.0%					
Test for overall effect: Z = 6.59 (P < 0.00001)					
6 Angina					
CASISP 2008	0/360	0/359			Not estimable
CSPS II 2010	10/1337	11/1335		1.9 %	0.91 [0.39, 2.13]
Subtotal (95% CI)	**1697**	**1694**		**1.9 %**	**0.91 [0.39, 2.13]**
Total events: 10 (Cilostazol), 11 (Aspirin)					
Heterogeneity: not applicable					
Test for overall effect: Z = 0.22 (P = 0.82)					
7 Cardiac Failure					
CASISP 2008	0/360	0/359			Not estimable
CSPS II 2010	8/1337	7/1335		1.2 %	1.14 [0.41, 3.14]
Subtotal (95% CI)	**1697**	**1694**		**1.2 %**	**1.14 [0.41, 3.14]**
Total events: 8 (Cilostazol), 7 (Aspirin)					
Heterogeneity: not applicable					
Test for overall effect: Z = 0.26 (P = 0.80)					
Total (95% CI)	**11879**	**11858**		**100.0 %**	**1.66 [1.51, 1.83]**
Total events: 977 (Cilostazol), 587 (Aspirin)					
Heterogeneity: Chi² = 61.64, df = 10 (P < 0.00001); I² = 84%					
Test for overall effect: Z = 10.30 (P < 0.00001)					
Test for subgroup differences: Chi² = 24.62, df = 6 (P = 0.00); I² = 76%					

0.01 0.1 1 10 100
Favours experimental   Favours control

Figure 19.5 Forest plot showing the effects of *cilostazol vs aspirin* in patients with previous *TIA or ischaemic stroke* on *adverse effects* at the end of follow-up.

Reproduced from Kamal et al. (2011) with permission from the authors and John Wiley & Sons Limited. Copyright Cochrane Library, reproduced with permission.

Serious Vascular Events

The PICASSO trial found that cilostazol reduced the risk of a composite of vascular events by 1.06 per 100 person-years compared with aspirin (HR 0.80, 95% CI: 0.57–1.11; non-inferiority $p = 0.0077$), which met an arbitrary threshold for declaring non-inferiority.

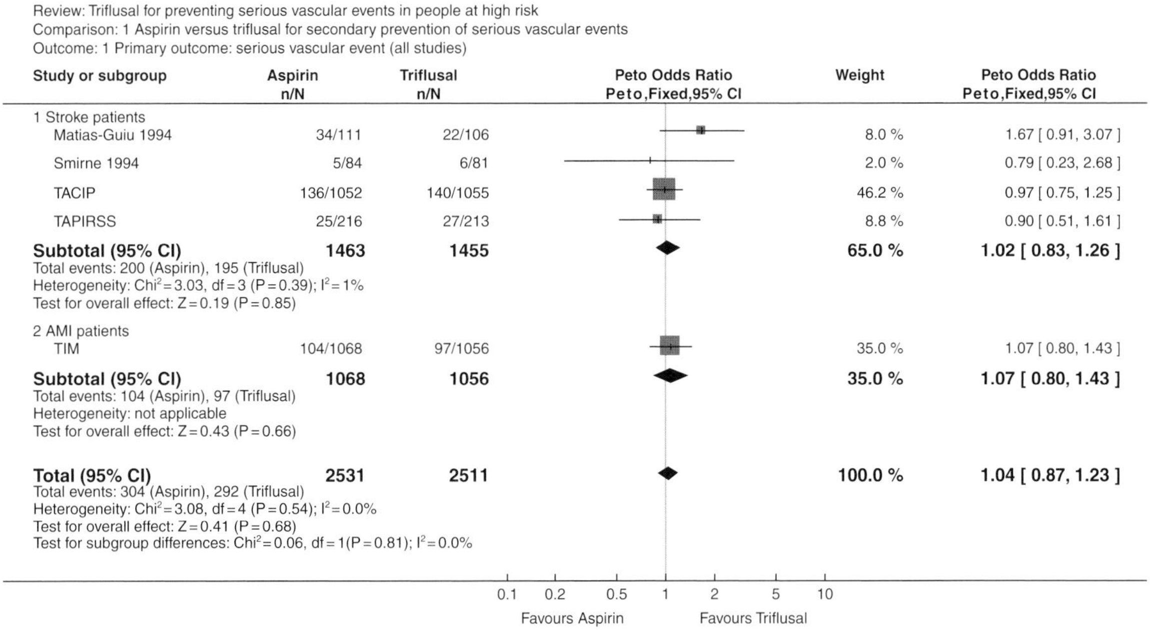

Review: Triflusal for preventing serious vascular events in people at high risk
Comparison: 1 Aspirin versus triflusal for secondary prevention of serious vascular events
Outcome: 1 Primary outcome: serious vascular event (all studies)

Study or subgroup	Aspirin n/N	Triflusal n/N	Peto Odds Ratio Peto,Fixed,95% CI	Weight	Peto Odds Ratio Peto,Fixed,95% CI
1 Stroke patients					
Matias-Guiu 1994	34/111	22/106		8.0 %	1.67 [0.91, 3.07]
Smirne 1994	5/84	6/81		2.0 %	0.79 [0.23, 2.68]
TACIP	136/1052	140/1055		46.2 %	0.97 [0.75, 1.25]
TAPIRSS	25/216	27/213		8.8 %	0.90 [0.51, 1.61]
Subtotal (95% CI)	**1463**	**1455**		**65.0 %**	**1.02 [0.83, 1.26]**
Total events: 200 (Aspirin), 195 (Triflusal)					
Heterogeneity: Chi^2 = 3.03, df = 3 (P = 0.39); I^2 = 1%					
Test for overall effect: Z = 0.19 (P = 0.85)					
2 AMI patients					
TIM	104/1068	97/1056		35.0 %	1.07 [0.80, 1.43]
Subtotal (95% CI)	**1068**	**1056**		**35.0 %**	**1.07 [0.80, 1.43]**
Total events: 104 (Aspirin), 97 (Triflusal)					
Heterogeneity: not applicable					
Test for overall effect: Z = 0.43 (P = 0.66)					
Total (95% CI)	**2531**	**2511**		**100.0 %**	**1.04 [0.87, 1.23]**
Total events: 304 (Aspirin), 292 (Triflusal)					
Heterogeneity: Chi^2 = 3.08, df = 4 (P = 0.54); I^2 = 0.0%					
Test for overall effect: Z = 0.41 (P = 0.68)					
Test for subgroup differences: Chi^2 = 0.06, df = 1(P = 0.81); I^2 = 0.0%					

0.1   0.2   0.5   1   2   5   10
Favours Aspirin   Favours Triflusal

Figure 19.6 Forest plot showing the effects of *triflusal vs aspirin in patients with previous ischaemic stroke* or *acute myocardial infarction* on *serious vascular events* at the end of follow-up.

Reproduced from Costa et al. (2005) with permission from the authors and John Wiley & Sons Limited. Copyright Cochrane Library, reproduced with permission.

However, cilostazol was not significantly superior to aspirin in safety ($p = 0.18$) or in efficacy ($p = 0.18$).

The addition of probucol to cilostazol or aspirin reduced the risk of a composite of vascular events by 1.84 per 100 person-years compared with aspirin or cilostazol alone (HR 0.69, 95% CI: 0.50–0.97; superiority $p = 0.0316$), and thus seemed superior to standard care.

Haemorrhagic Stroke

Probucol did not appear to increase the risk of haemorrhagic stroke (HR 0.65, 97.5% CI: 0.27–1.57; superiority $p = 0.55$).

PICASSO heralds an emerging group of randomized trials of antiplatelet therapy for people with comorbid ischaemic and haemorrhagic diseases (e.g. RESTART [ISRCTN71907627], RESTARTFr [NCT02966119], and STATICH [2014–002636-13]).

Triflusal vs Aspirin

TIA and Ischaemic Stroke Patients

Serious Vascular Events

Among 2944 patients with stroke or TIA who were enrolled in 4 RCTs of triflusal vs aspirin and followed for 6 to 47 months, there was no significant difference in the rate of serious vascular events between triflusal and aspirin; the odds ratio (OR) for serious vascular events among patients assigned aspirin compared to triflusal was 1.02 (95% CI: 0.83–1.26) (Figure 19.6) (Costa et al., 2005).

Stroke

Triflusal was not significantly more effective than aspirin in preventing recurrent stroke in three RCTs; aspirin was associated with a non-significant trend towards a higher rate of ischaemic stroke compared to triflusal in three RCTs involving patients with previous stroke (11.2% aspirin vs 10.3% triflusal; OR 1.10, 95% CI: 0.86–1.40) (Costa et al., 2005).

Haemorrhagic Stroke

Aspirin was associated with a non-significant trend towards a higher rate of haemorrhagic stroke compared with triflusal in three RCTs involving patients with previous stroke (OR 1.94, 95% CI: 0.91–4.15) (Costa et al., 2005).

Major Systemic (extracranial) Haemorrhage

In three RCTs of triflusal vs aspirin in a total of 2753 stroke patients, aspirin was associated with a significant increase in major systemic (extracranial) haemorrhage

Review: Triflusal for preventing serious vascular events in people at high risk
Comparison: 1 Aspirin versus triflusal for secondary prevention of serious vascular events
Outcome: 22 Number of patients with any intracranial haemorrage or other major systemic haemorrhage

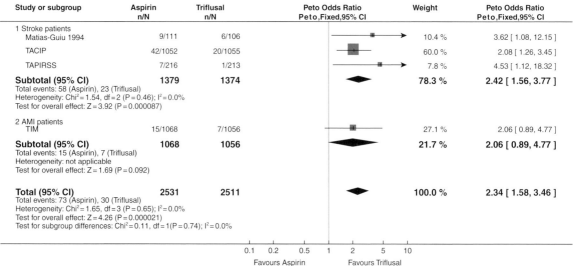

Study or subgroup	Aspirin n/N	Triflusal n/N	Peto Odds Ratio Peto,Fixed,95% CI	Weight	Peto Odds Ratio Peto,Fixed,95% CI
1 Stroke patients					
Matias-Guiu 1994	9/111	6/106		10.4 %	3.62 [1.08, 12.15]
TACIP	42/1052	20/1055		60.0 %	2.08 [1.26, 3.45]
TAPIRSS	7/216	1/213		7.8 %	4.53 [1.12, 18.32]
Subtotal (95% CI)	**1379**	**1374**		**78.3 %**	**2.42 [1.56, 3.77]**

Total events: 58 (Aspirin), 23 (Triflusal)
Heterogeneity: Chi^2=1.54, df=2 (P=0.46); I^2=0.0%
Test for overall effect: Z=3.92 (P=0.000087)

2 AMI patients					
TIM	15/1068	7/1056		27.1 %	2.06 [0.89, 4.77]
Subtotal (95% CI)	**1068**	**1056**		**21.7 %**	**2.06 [0.89, 4.77]**

Total events: 15 (Aspirin), 7 (Triflusal)
Heterogeneity: not applicable
Test for overall effect: Z=1.69 (P=0.092)

| **Total (95% CI)** | **2531** | **2511** | | **100.0 %** | **2.34 [1.58, 3.46]** |

Total events: 73 (Aspirin), 30 (Triflusal)
Heterogeneity: Chi^2=1.65, df=3 (P=0.65); I^2=0.0%
Test for overall effect: Z=4.26 (P=0.000021)
Test for subgroup differences: Chi^2=0.11, df=1(P=0.74); I^2=0.0%

0.1 0.2 0.5 1 2 5 10
Favours Aspirin   Favours Triflusal

Figure 19.7 Forest plot showing the effects of *triflusal vs aspirin* in patients with *previous ischaemic stroke or acute myocardial infarction* on any *intracranial haemorrhage or other major systemic haemorrhage* at the end of follow-up.

Reproduced from Costa et al. (2005) with permission from the authors and John Wiley & Sons Limited. Copyright Cochrane Library, reproduced with permission.

compared with triflusal (OR 2.66, 95% CI: 1.55–4.56) (Costa et al., 2005).

Intracranial Haemorrhage or Other Major Systemic (extracranial) Haemorrhage

In three RCTs of triflusal vs aspirin in a total of 2753 stroke patients, aspirin was associated with a significant increase in the composite outcome of intracranial haemorrhage or major systemic (extracranial) haemorrhage compared to triflusal (OR 2.42, 95% CI: 1.56–3.77) (Figure 19.7) (Costa et al., 2005).

Terutroban vs Aspirin

Terutroban is a selective antagonist of thromboxane–prostaglandin receptors on platelets and the vessel wall.

Ischaemic Stroke Patients

Among 19,120 patients with a recent non-cardioembolic ischaemic stroke (<3 months) or TIA (<8 days), random allocation to terutroban 30 mg per day for a mean of 28.3 months (standard deviation [SD] 7.7) was associated with no reduction in ischaemic stroke, MI, or vascular death (excluding haemorrhagic death) compared with aspirin 100 mg per day (11% vs 11%; HR 1.02, 95% CI: 0.94–1.12) but an increase in minor bleeding (12% vs 11%; HR 1.11, 95% CI: 1.02–1.21) (Bousser et al., 2011).

Clopidogrel Plus Aspirin vs Aspirin

High Vascular Risk Patients

A recent Cochrane systematic review identified 15 RCTs comparing over 30 days' use of aspirin plus clopidogrel with aspirin plus placebo or aspirin alone in 33,970 people with coronary disease, ischaemic cerebrovascular disease, peripheral arterial disease, or at high risk of atherothrombotic disease, but not having a coronary stent (Squizzato et al., 2017; Donadini et al., 2018).

Ischaemic Stroke

Aspirin plus clopidogrel was associated with a reduction in ᴜᴇ risk of fatal and non-fatal ischaemic stroke compared with aspirin (RR 0.73, 95% CI: 0.59–0.91; participants = 4006; studies = 5; moderate quality evidence) (Figure 19.8).

Myocardial Infarction --
There was a lower risk ᴏᴊ fatal and non-fatal MI with clopidogrel plus aspirin compared with aspirin plus placebo or aspirin alone (RR 0.78, 95% CI: 0.69–0.90; participants = 16,175; studies = 6; moderate quality evidence).

Review: Clopidogrel plus aspirin versus aspirin alone for preventing cardiovascular events
Comparison: 1 Clopidogrel (Clo) plus aspirin (ASA) versus aspirin alone
Outcome: 4 Fatal and non-fatal ischaemic stroke

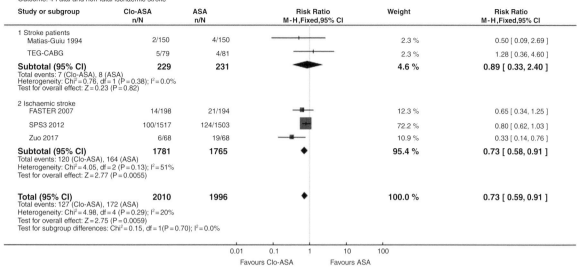

Study or subgroup	Clo-ASA n/N	ASA n/N	Risk Ratio M-H,Fixed,95% CI	Weight	Risk Ratio M-H,Fixed,95% CI
1 Stroke patients					
Matias-Guiu 1994	2/150	4/150		2.3 %	0.50 [0.09, 2.69]
TEG-CABG	5/79	4/81		2.3 %	1.28 [0.36, 4.60]
Subtotal (95% CI)	**229**	**231**		**4.6 %**	**0.89 [0.33, 2.40]**
Total events: 7 (Clo-ASA), 8 (ASA) Heterogeneity: Chi²=0.76, df=1 (P=0.38); I²=0.0% Test for overall effect: Z=0.23 (P=0.82)					
2 Ischaemic stroke					
FASTER 2007	14/198	21/194		12.3 %	0.65 [0.34, 1.25]
SPS3 2012	100/1517	124/1503		72.2 %	0.80 [0.62, 1.03]
Zuo 2017	6/68	19/68		10.9 %	0.33 [0.14, 0.76]
Subtotal (95% CI)	**1781**	**1765**		**95.4 %**	**0.73 [0.58, 0.91]**
Total events: 120 (Clo-ASA), 164 (ASA) Heterogeneity: Chi²=4.05, df=2 (P=0.13); I²=51% Test for overall effect: Z=2.77 (P=0.0055)					
Total (95% CI)	**2010**	**1996**		**100.0 %**	**0.73 [0.59, 0.91]**
Total events: 127 (Clo-ASA), 172 (ASA) Heterogeneity: Chi²=4.98, df=4 (P=0.29); I²=20% Test for overall effect: Z=2.75 (P=0.0059) Test for subgroup differences: Chi²=0.15, df=1(P=0.70); I²=0.0%					

0.01   0.1   1   10   100
Favours Clo-ASA   Favours ASA

Figure 19.8 Forest plot showing the effects of *clopidogrel vs aspirin* in *high vascular risk patients (CHARISMA) or patients with acute myocardial infarction (CURE)* on *serious vascular events* at the end of follow-up.

Reproduced from Squizzato et al. (2017) with permission from the authors and John Wiley & Sons Limited. Copyright Cochrane Library, reproduced with permission.

Mortality

There was no difference in the effectiveness of aspirin plus clopidogrel in preventing cardiovascular mortality (RR 0.98, 95% CI: 0.88–1.10; participants = 31,903; studies = 7; moderate quality evidence), and no evidence of a difference in all-cause mortality (RR 1.05, 95% CI: 0.87–1.25; participants = 32,908; studies = 9; low quality evidence).

Major and Minor Bleeding

There was a higher risk of major bleeding with clopidogrel plus aspirin compared with aspirin plus placebo or aspirin alone (RR 1.44, 95% CI: 1.25–1.64; participants = 33,300; studies = 10; moderate quality evidence) and of minor bleeding (RR 2.03, 95% CI: 1.75–2.36; participants = 14,731; studies = 8; moderate quality evidence).

Net Effect in High Vascular Risk Patients

The addition of clopidogrel to aspirin compared with aspirin alone in people at high risk of cardiovascular disease and people with established cardiovascular disease without a coronary stent was associated with 23 (95% CI: 7–39) fewer cases of ischaemic stroke and 13 (95% CI: 6–19) fewer cases of MI for every 1000 patients treated during a median period of 12 months, but also with an increase of 9 (95% CI: 6–12) cases of major bleeding during a median period of 10.5 months

According to Grading of Recommendations Assessment, Development and Evaluation (GRADE) criteria, the quality of evidence was moderate for all outcomes except all-cause mortality (low-quality evidence) and adverse events (very low-quality evidence).

Prior Ischaemic Stroke or TIA

The Clopidogrel for High Atherothrombotic Risk and Ischemic Stabilization, Management, and Avoidance (CHARISMA) trial randomly assigned 15,603 patients with either clinically evident cardiovascular disease (*n* = 12,153) or multiple atherothrombotic risk factors (*n* = 3284) to receive clopidogrel (75 mg per day) plus low-dose aspirin (75–162 mg per day) or placebo plus low-dose aspirin and followed them for a median of 28 months (Bhatt et al., 2006).

A total of 4320 patients with prior ischaemic stroke (n = 3245) or TIA (1233) within the previous 5 years were enrolled in the CHARISMA trial (Hankey et al., 2011).

Major Vascular Events – The rate of stroke, MI, or death due to vascular causes with clopidogrel plus aspirin was 8.1% (174/2157) compared with aspirin monotherapy of 9.6% (207/2163) (RR 0.84, 95% CI: 0.69–1.03) (Hankey et al., 2011).

Recurrent Stroke – The rate of recurrent stroke with clopidogrel plus aspirin dual antiplatelet therapy was

4.9% (105/2157) compared with aspirin monotherapy of 6.1% (131/2163) (RR 0.80, 95% CI: 0.63–1.03) (Hankey et al., 2011).

Among patients randomized more than 30 days after the qualifying stroke or TIA, of those assigned to placebo plus acetylsalicylic acid (ASA), 85 (5.7%) experienced a stroke compared with 71 (4.8%) patients assigned to clopidogrel plus ASA (HR 0.83, 95% CI: 0.60–1.14) (Hankey et al., 2011).

Any Bleeding – Among patients with prior stroke or TIA assigned clopidogrel plus ASA compared with placebo plus ASA, there was a significant excess of any bleeding (20.5% placebo plus ASA, 37.4% clopidogrel plus ASA, HR 2.08, 95% CI: 1.86–2.34) and moderate bleeding (1.1% placebo plus ASA, 2.4% clopidogrel plus ASA, HR 2.15, 95% CI: 1.32–3.49) (Hankey et al., 2011).

Major Bleeding – Among patients randomized to placebo plus ASA, 37 (1.7%) experienced a severe bleed compared with 41 (1.9%) patients randomized to clopidogrel plus ASA (HR 1.11, 95% CI: 0.71–1.73).

Intracerebral Haemorrhage – Intracerebral haemorrhage was equally uncommon in the treatment groups (0.5% [placebo plus ASA] vs 0.6% [clopidogrel plus ASA], HR 1.18, 95% CI: 0.53–2.64).

Among patients randomized more than 30 days after the qualifying stroke or TIA, of those assigned to placebo plus ASA, 0.4% experienced an intracerebral haemorrhage compared with 0.4% of patients assigned to clopidogrel plus ASA (HR: 1.01, 95% CI: 0.20–5.00) (Hankey et al., 2011).

Carriers of CYP2C19 Polymorphisms in the CHARISMA Trial

Clopidogrel is a thienopyridine prodrug with a 2-stage activation mediated largely by the drug-metabolizing enzyme CYP2C19. The active metabolite of clopidogrel specifically and irreversibly binds to the platelet P2Y12 purinergic receptor, which inhibits ADP-mediated platelet activation and aggregation.

The common *loss*-of-function *2 single nucleotide polymorphism (SNP) in CYP2C19 has been associated with decreased conversion of clopidogrel into its active metabolite, decreased antiplatelet activity based on *ex vivo* platelet reactivity testing in on-treatment patients, and a higher rate of recurrent cardiovascular events in the setting of percutaneous coronary intervention.

The *17 *gain*-of-function SNP in CYP2C19 has been associated in some studies with increased conversion of clopidogrel into its active metabolite, a lower rate of recurrent cardiovascular events, and an increased bleeding risk. This has led to CYP2C19 genetic testing to define clopidogrel treatment in patients following percutaneous coronary intervention in some health systems.

Among a subset of 4819 patients from the CHARISMA trial who consented to genotyping, carriers of CYP2C19 loss-of-function alleles did not have an increased rate of ischaemic events but did have a significantly lower rate of bleeding with clopidogrel (36.1% [240/665] vs 42.5% [681/1601] in non-carriers, HR 0.80, 95% CI: 0.69–0.93, $p = 0.003$ [genotype/treatment interaction, p-value = 0.023]), suggesting less anti-platelet response with clopidogrel in carriers of the loss-of-function allele (Bhatt et al., 2012).

The CYP2C19 gain-of-function alleles did not affect ischaemic or bleeding endpoints.

Lacunar Stroke

The Secondary Prevention of Small Subcortical Strokes (SPS3) trial randomly assigned 3020 patients with recent symptomatic lacunar infarcts identified by MRI to receive 75 mg of clopidogrel or placebo daily (patients in both groups received 325 mg of aspirin daily) and followed them for a mean of 3.4 years for the primary outcome of any recurrent stroke (SPS3 Investigators, 2012).

The SPS3 trial showed that, among patients with recent lacunar strokes, the addition of clopidogrel to aspirin did not significantly reduce the risk of recurrent stroke and did significantly increase the risk of bleeding and death.

Recurrent Stroke – The risk of recurrent stroke was not significantly reduced with aspirin and clopidogrel (dual antiplatelet therapy) (125 strokes; rate, 2.5% per year) as compared with aspirin alone (138 strokes, 2.7% per year) (HR 0.92; 95% CI: 0.72–1.16) (SPS3 Investigators, 2012; Kwok et al., 2015).

Recurrent Ischaemic Stroke – The risk of recurrent ischaemic stroke was not significantly reduced with aspirin and clopidogrel (dual antiplatelet therapy), compared with aspirin (HR 0.82, 95% CI: 0.63–1.09).

Among classifiable recurrent ischaemic strokes, 71% (133 of 187) were lacunar strokes.

Major Vascular Events – The rate of stroke, MI, or death due to vascular causes was similar among participants assigned clopidogrel plus aspirin (3.1% per year) and aspirin (3.4% per year) (HR 0.89, 95% CI: 0.72–1.11) (SPS3 Investigators, 2012).

Intracerebral Haemorrhage – The rate of intracerebral haemorrhage was 0.42% per year among participants assigned clopidogrel plus aspirin and 0.25% per year among participants allocated aspirin (HR 1.65, 95% CI: 0.83–3.31) (SPS3 Investigators, 2012).

Major Bleeding – The risk of major haemorrhage was almost doubled with dual antiplatelet therapy (105 haemorrhages, 2.1% per year) as compared with aspirin alone (56, 1.1% per year) (HR 1.97, 95% CI: 1.41–2.71; $p < 0.001$).

Mortality – All-cause mortality was increased among patients assigned to receive dual antiplatelet therapy (77 deaths in the group receiving aspirin alone vs 113 in the group receiving dual antiplatelet therapy) (HR 1.52, 95% CI: 1.14–2.04; $p = 0.004$); this difference was not accounted for by fatal haemorrhages (9 in the group receiving dual antiplatelet therapy vs 4 in the group receiving aspirin alone) (SPS3 Investigators, 2012).

Carriers of CYP2C19 Polymorphisms in the SPS3 Trial

Among 522 patients with lacunar stroke who were treated with dual antiplatelet therapy in the SPS3 study and in whom CYP2C19*2 and CYP2C19*17 were genotyped and CYP2C19 metabolizer status was inferred from genotype, there were no differences in outcomes by CYP2C19 metabolizer status (recurrent stroke, OR 1.81 [95% CI: 0.76–4.30]; major bleeding, OR 0.67 [95% CI: 0.22–2.03]) (McDonough et al., 2015).

However, there were significant differences in recurrent stroke by CYP2C19 genotype-inferred metabolizer status in white subcortical stroke patients receiving dual antiplatelet therapy with aspirin and clopidogrel. In white participants, those with CYP2C19 intermediate or poor metabolizer status had higher odds of recurrent stroke (OR 5.19 [95% CI: 1.1–24.9]) than those with extensive or ultrarapid metabolizer status, but there was no evidence of difference in major bleeding (McDonough et al., 2015).

Aspirin Plus Dipyridamole vs Aspirin

TIA and Ischaemic Stroke Patients

Serious Vascular Events – A meta-analysis of 5 trials of aspirin plus dipyridamole versus aspirin in a total of 7612 patients with TIA or minor stroke of presumed arterial origin reported that the combination of aspirin plus dipyridamole reduced the risk of serious vascular events by about 18% (95% CI: 8–28%) compared with aspirin (HR 0.82, 95% CI: 0.72–0.92) (Halkes et al., 2008).

The proportional benefits of ASA plus dipyridamole versus ASA were consistent in subgroup analyses based on age, sex, qualifying event, hypertension, diabetes, previous stroke, ischaemic heart disease, aspirin dose, type of vessel disease, and dipyridamole formulation, as well as across baseline risk strata as assessed with two different risk scores.

Stroke – The 5 trials also showed that aspirin plus dipyridamole versus aspirin was more effective than ASA alone in preventing recurrent stroke (HR 0.78, 95% CI: 0.68–0.90) (Halkes et al., 2008).

Timing and Severity of Recurrent Stroke – Rothwell and colleagues reported that among seven trials of dipyridamole plus aspirin versus aspirin in 9437 patients, the addition of dipyridamole to aspirin had no effect on the risk or severity of recurrent ischaemic stroke within 12 weeks (OR 0.90, 95% CI: 0.65–1.25, $p = 0.53$; modified Rankin Scale [mRS] shift OR 0.90, 0.37–1.72, $p = 0.99$), but dipyridamole and aspirin did reduce risk thereafter (0.76, 0.63–0.92, $p = 0.005$), particularly of disabling or fatal ischaemic stroke (0.64, 0.49–0.84, $p = 0.0010$) (Rothwell et al., 2016).

These results suggest that the effect of dipyridamole in preventing long-term recurrent stroke may be underestimated.

Adverse Effects – The combination of dipyridamole and aspirin is associated with about a 6% absolute excess of headache sufficient to precipitate discontinuation of study drug, compared with aspirin alone (8.1% dipyridamole, 1.9% aspirin) (Diener et al., 1996).

Adding dipyridamole to aspirin did not significantly increase the risk of major or fatal extracranial bleeding compared with aspirin alone in 9 RCTs involving a total of 6981 high vascular risk patients (RR 1.08, 95% CI: 0.75–1.54) (De Schryver et al., 2007).

Lacunar Stroke

Major Vascular Events – Among 2645 patients with lacunar stroke enrolled in the ESPRIT and ESPS-2 trials, the rate of major vascular events (any stroke, MI, or death) was reduced among patients assigned aspirin plus extended-release dipyridamole (178/1346 = 13.2%) versus aspirin (207/1299 = 15.9%) (RR 0.83, 95% CI: 0.69–1.00) (Kwok et al., 2015).

Recurrent Stroke – Among 1268 patients with lacunar stroke enrolled in the ESPS-2 trial, the rate of recurrent stroke was reduced among patients assigned aspirin plus extended-release dipyridamole (52/659 = 7.9%) versus aspirin (70/609 = 11.5%) (RR 0.69, 95% CI: 0.49–0.97) (Kwok et al., 2015).

Oral Gp IIb/IIIa Antagonists Plus Aspirin vs Aspirin

Glycoprotein (GP) IIb/IIIa inhibitors are antiplatelet agents that act by antagonizing GP IIb/IIIa receptors on the platelet surface and block the final common pathway to platelet aggregation by preventing the binding of fibrinogen molecules that form bridges between adjacent platelets.

High Vascular Risk Patients

In the BRAVO trial, 9190 patients with vascular disease (recent cerebrovascular disease [ischaemic stroke or TIA, 41%, n = 3319] or cardiovascular disease [MI, unstable angina, or peripheral arterial disease, 59%, n = 4389)]), were randomly assigned to treatment for up to 2 years with lotrafiban, an orally administered IIb/IIIa receptor antagonist, 30 or 50 mg bid on the basis of age and predicted creatinine clearance or placebo, in addition to aspirin at a dose ranging from 75–325 mg/day at the discretion of the physician-investigator.

Major Vascular Events – There was no significant difference in the primary endpoint (the composite of all-cause mortality, MI, stroke, recurrent ischaemia requiring hospitalization, and urgent revascularization) among patients assigned lotrafiban (16.4%) compared with placebo (17.5%) (HR 0.94, 95% CI: 0.85–1.03, $P = 0.19$) (Topol et al., 2003).

Death – Lotrafiban was associated with a one-third increase in death rate; death occurred in 2.3% of placebo-assigned patients and 3.0% of lotrafiban-group patients (HR 1.33, 95% CI: 1.03–1.72; $p = 0.026$). The cause of excess death was vascular related and was not affected by the type of atherosclerotic involvement at entry to the trial.

Serious Bleeding – Serious bleeding was more frequent in the lotrafiban group (8.0% compared with 2.8%; $p < 0.001$). Serious bleeding was more common among patients who received higher doses of aspirin (>162 mg/d), with or without lotrafiban.

Ischaemic Stroke Patients

Stroke, MI, or Death – There was no significant difference or heterogeneity in the rate of stroke, MI, or death among the 3319 patients with cerebrovascular disease who were assigned lotrafiban (5.9%) versus placebo (7.2%) or the 4389 patients with cardiovascular disease who were assigned lotrafiban (6.4%) versus placebo (5.9%).

Prasugrel vs Clopidogrel

Prasugrel is a newer, third-generation, oral thienopyridine P2Y12 ADP receptor inhibitor but, like clopidogrel, also a prodrug. It is hydrolysed rapidly by esterases to an intermediate metabolite, which undergoes CYP-dependent oxidation to the active compound. However, genetic variation in CYP isoenzymes does not retard its biotransformation; hence, prasugrel has a more consistent platelet response than clopidogrel.

Prasugrel at a maintenance dose of 10 mg/day has proven superior to clopidogrel at 75 mg/day in preventing ischaemic events in patients with acute coronary syndromes scheduled for percutaneous coronary intervention, but led to increasing bleeding (Wiviott et al., 2007). Prasugrel at 10 mg/day has not proved superior to clopidogrel in patients with unstable angina or MI without ST-segment elevation treated medically (Roe et al., 2012). Prasugrel has now been compared with clopidogrel for secondary prevention of recurrent stroke in the large, phase 3, non-inferiority PRASTRO-I trial (Ogawa et al., 2019).

Non-cardioembolic Ischaemic Stroke Patients

In the PRASTRO-I trial, 3747 Japanese patients older than 75 years and weighing more than 50 kg with recent (1–26 weeks previously) non-cardioembolic ischaemic stroke were randomly allocated to double-blind treatment with prasugrel at 3.75 mg/day or clopidogrel at 75 mg/day (Ogawa et al., 2019).

The low dose of prasugrel (3.75 mg) was chosen to avoid the bleeding complications reported at higher doses (10 mg).

The target sample size of 3600 patients was based on estimated primary outcome (ischaemic stroke, MI, or death from other vascular cause) event rates of 4.3% with clopidogrel and 3.6% with prasugrel at 2 years (15% relative risk reduction).

Major vascular events

After a median observation period of 96.1 weeks, the primary outcome was similar in the treatment groups (73 [3.9%] of 1885 patients in the prasugrel group vs

69 [3.7%] of 1862 patients in the clopidogrel group, RR 1.05, 95% CI: 0.76–1.44), failing to confirm the non-inferiority of prasugrel to clopidogrel because the upper 95% CI of the RR was 1.44, exceeding the predefined non-inferiority margin of an upper confidence limit of 1.35.

The primary result was consistent among all patient subgroups, including the 20% of participants with reduced function of CYP2C19.

Bleeding

There was also no safety benefit of low-dose prasugrel compared with clopidogrel; the proportions of patients with life-threatening bleeding were similar (HR prasugrel vs clopidogrel 0.77, 95% CI: 0.41–1.42), as for major bleeding (HR 0.49, 95% CI: 0.09–2.66), and life-threatening bleeding plus major bleeding plus clinically relevant bleeding (HR: 1.02, 95% CI: 0.79–1.33).

Interpretation

Clopidogrel therefore remains an antiplatelet regimen of choice for the secondary prevention of recurrent ischaemic stroke in Japan. There appears to be no benefit from routine CYP2C19 genetic testing to guide the selection of prasugrel over clopidogrel. However, the generalizability of the findings to Japanese people older than 75 years or weighing less than 50 kg (the subject of the ongoing PRASTRO-II trial [JapicCTI-121901]), Japanese women (who composed only 21% of the PRASTRO-I trial), or other non-Japanese populations is unclear. Whether the results are applicable to higher doses of prasugrel, as used in other countries, is also unclear.

Aspirin Plus Clopidogrel vs Clopidogrel

TIA and Ischaemic Stroke Patients

The Management of Atherothrombosis with Clopidogrel in High-Risk Patients with Recent TIA or Ischemic Stroke (MATCH) trial enrolled 7599 patients with recent (<3 months) TIA (21%) or ischaemic stroke (79%), a median of 15 days (range 0–119 days) after their qualifying TIA or ischaemic stroke, and randomly allocated patients to the combination of aspirin 75 mg/day and clopidogrel 75 mg/day or clopidogrel 75 mg/day for 18 months (Diener et al., 2004).

Major Vascular Events – The rate of ischaemic stroke, MI, vascular death, and rehospitalization for acute ischaemic events (the primary outcome event) was not significantly different among patients allocated clopidogrel plus aspirin (15.7%) compared with clopidogrel alone (16.7%) at 18 months (RRR: 6.4%, 95% CI: −4.6%–16.3%; *p* = 0.244; ARR 1.0%) (Diener et al., 2004).

The results were consistent among all subgroups examined, including aetiological subtypes of stroke and different vascular risk factors.

Recurrent Stroke – The rate of any stroke was not significantly different among patients allocated clopidogrel plus aspirin (9%) compared with clopidogrel alone (9%) at 18 months (RRR 2.0%, 95% CI: −13.8%–15.6%, *p* = 0.79; ARR 1.0%) (Diener et al., 2004).

Life-threatening Haemorrhage – Compared with clopidogrel alone, the addition of aspirin to clopidogrel was associated with a significant increase in life-threatening haemorrhage (the primary outcome measure of safety) from 1.3% (clopidogrel) to 2.6% (aspirin plus clopidogrel), which is 2-fold increase in RR, and an increase in absolute risk of 1.26% (95% CI: 0.64–1.88%) over 18 months (*p* < 0.001) (Diener et al., 2004).

Life-threatening haemorrhage was intracranial (0.7% clopidogrel, 1.1% clopidogrel plus aspirin) and GI (0.6% clopidogrel, 1.4% clopidogrel plus aspirin) (Diener et al., 2004).

Major Haemorrhage – Combination of antiplatelet therapy was also associated with a significant increase in major haemorrhage (0.6% clopidogrel, 1.9% clopidogrel plus aspirin, RR 3.34, 95% CI: 2.1–5.4; ARI 1.36, 95% CI: 0.86–1.86) compared with clopidogrel alone (Diener et al., 2004).

The risk of bleeding was cumulative over time. The Kaplan–Meier survival curves for survival free of primary intracerebral haemorrhage for each treatment group did not separate until 3–4 months after randomization, suggesting that the benefit–risk ratio of clopidogrel plus aspirin versus clopidogrel may be greatest in the first few months after stroke. Multiple regression analysis failed to identify any key predictors of bleeding that were not also key predictors of ischaemic events.

Aspirin Plus Dipyridamole vs Clopidogrel

Ischaemic Stroke Patients

The Prevention Regimen for Effectively Avoiding Second Strokes (PRoFESS) trial randomly assigned 20,322 patients with recent (<90 days) ischaemic stroke to receive 25 mg of aspirin plus 200 mg of extended-release dipyridamole (ASA-ERDP) twice daily or to receive 75 mg of clopidogrel daily. Patients were followed for a mean of 2.5 years for the primary outcome event, which was first recurrence of stroke (Sacco et al., 2008).

The PRoFESS trial did not meet the predefined criteria for noninferiority but showed similar rates of recurrent stroke with ASA-ERDP and with clopidogrel. There was no evidence that either of the two treatments (extended-release dipyridamole or clopidogrel) was superior to the other in the prevention of recurrent stroke

Recurrent Stroke – Recurrent stroke occurred in 916 patients (9.0%) receiving ASA-ERDP and in 898 patients (8.8%) receiving clopidogrel (HR 1.01, 95% CI: 0.92–1.11).

Major Vascular Events – The composite of stroke, MI, or death from vascular causes occurred in 1333 patients (13.1%) in each group (HR for ASA-ERDP, 0.99; 95% CI: 0.92–1.07).

Major Bleeding – There were more major haemorrhagic events among ASA-ERDP recipients (419 [4.1%]) than among clopidogrel recipients (365 [3.6%]) (HR 1.15, 95% CI: 1.00–1.32), including intracranial haemorrhage (HR 1.42, 95% CI: 1.11–1.83).

The net risk of recurrent stroke or major haemorrhagic event was similar in the two groups (1194 ASA-ERDP recipients [11.7%] vs 1156 clopidogrel recipients [11.4%]; HR 1.03, 95% CI: 0.95–1.11).

Dual Antiplatelet Therapy with Cilostazol plus Aspirin or Clopidogrel vs Aspirin or Clopidogrel Monotherapy

The CSPS.com Trial randomly allocated 1884 (of an anticipated 4000) patients with high-risk noncardioembolic ischaemic stroke to receive aspirin or clopidogrel alone, or a combination of cilostazol with aspirin or clopidogrel at 292 sites in Japan. The patients were required to have ≥50% stenosis of a major intracranial or extracranial artery or two or more vascular risk factors. The primary efficacy outcome was the first recurrence of ischaemic stroke. Safety outcomes included severe or life-threatening bleeding (Toyoda et al., 2019).

The trial was stopped after a median 1.4-year follow-up due to delay in recruiting patients.

Ischaemic Stroke

Ischaemic stroke recurred in 29 of 932 patients (annualized rate, 2.2%) on dual therapy including cilostazol and

64 of 947 patients (annualized rate, 4.5%) on monotherapy (HR 0.49, 95% CI: 0.31–0.76; $p = 0.001$).

Any Recurrent Stroke

Any recurrent stroke was less frequent among participants assigned dual therapy compared with monotherapy (2.6% vs 5.0% per year; HR 0.51, 95% CI: 0.34–0.77).

Intracranial Haemorrhage

Intracranial haemorrhage was similar among participants assigned dual therapy compared with monotherapy (0.9% vs 1.4% per year; HR 0.66, 95% CI: 0.27–1.60).

Severe or Life-threatening Bleeding

Severe or life-threatening bleeding occurred in 8 patients (annualized rate, 0.6%) on dual therapy and 13 patients (annualized rate, 0.9%) on monotherapy (HR 0.66, 95% CI: 0.27–1.60; $p = 0.354$).

It was concluded that in patients at high risk for recurrent ischaemic stroke, the combination of cilostazol with aspirin or clopidogrel had a lower risk of ischaemic stroke recurrence and a similar risk of severe or life-threatening bleeding compared with aspirin or clopidogrel alone.

Vorapaxar Plus Standard Antiplatelet Therapy vs Standard Antiplatelet Therapy

Vorapaxar is an oral antiplatelet agent that antagonizes thrombin-mediated activation of the protease-activated receptor-1 (the main receptor for thrombin) on the surface of platelets.

Ischaemic Stroke Patients

Among 4883 patients with a history of recent (2 weeks to 12 months) ischaemic stroke, adding vorapaxar 2.5 mg daily to standard antiplatelet therapy for 3 years increased the rate of intracranial haemorrhage compared to placebo (2.5% vs 1.0%; HR 2.52, 95% CI: 1.46–4.36) without reducing recurrent ischaemic stroke (HR 0.99, 95% CI: 0.78–1.25) or the composite of stroke, MI, or cardiovascular death (13.0% vs 11.7%; HR 1.03, 95% CI: 0.85–1.25) (Morrow et al., 2013).

Timing and Predictors of Major Bleeding with Antiplatelet Therapy

An analysis of individual patient data from 6 randomized clinical trials (CAPRIE, ESPS-2, MATCH, CHARISMA, ESPRIT, and PRoFESS) investigating antiplatelet therapy after TIA or ischaemic stroke reported that the observed 3-year risk of major bleeding was 4.6% (95% CI: 4.4–4.9%) (Hilkens et al., 2017). Dual antiplatelet therapy was associated with high early risks of major and GI bleeding that decline after the first month in trial cohorts (Hilkens et al., 2018a).

Predictors of major bleeding were male Sex, Smoking, Type of antiplatelet agents (aspirin–clopidogrel), Outcome on mRS $\geq$3, Prior stroke, Blood pressure high (hypertension), Lower body mass index, Elderly, Ethnicity Asian, and Diabetes (S2TOP-BLEED). Major bleeding risk ranged from 2% in patients aged 45–54 years without additional risk factors to more than 10% in patients aged 75–84 years with multiple risk factors (Hilkens et al., 2017).

The S2TOP-BLEED score showed modest performance in an independent population-based cohort of patients with a TIA or ischaemic stroke (Hilkens et al., 2018b).

Anticoagulation

Oral Anticoagulation vs Control

TIA and Ischaemic Stroke Patients

Eleven trials have assessed the effect of prolonged (>1month) anticoagulant therapy compared with placebo or open control following presumed non-cardioembolic ischaemic stroke or TIA in 2487 participants (Sandercock et al., 2009). The quality of the nine trials which pre-dated routine computed tomography (CT) scanning and the use of the international normalized ratio (INR) to monitor anticoagulation was poor.

Major Vascular Events

There was no evidence of an effect of anticoagulant therapy on the composite of non-fatal stroke, MI, or vascular death (four trials, OR 0.96, 95% CI: 0.68–1.37).

Death from any cause (OR 0.95, 95% CI: 0.73–1.24) and death from vascular causes (OR 0.86, 95% CI: 0.66–1.13) were not significantly different between treatment and control.

Recurrent Stroke

There was no evidence of an effect of anticoagulant therapy on the risk of any recurrent stroke (OR 0.92, 95% CI: 0.72–1.16) (Figure 19.9) or recurrent ischaemic stroke (OR 0.85, 95% CI: 0.66–1.09) (Sandercock et al., 2009).

Intracranial Haemorrhage

Anticoagulants increased fatal intracranial haemorrhage compared with no anticoagulant (OR 2.54, 95% CI: 1.19–5.45). This is equivalent to anticoagulant therapy causing about 11 additional fatal intracranial haemorrhages per year for every 1000 patients given anticoagulant therapy.

Major Extracranial Haemorrhage

Anticoagulants increased major extracranial haemorrhage (OR 3.43, 95% CI: 1.94–6.08). This is equivalent to anticoagulant therapy causing about 25 additional major extracranial haemorrhages per year for every 1000 patients given anticoagulant therapy.

Extracranial Carotid and Vertebral Artery Dissection Patients

Anticoagulation is not more effective than antiplatelet therapy in reducing stroke or death at 90 days or 1 year, or rates of recanalization after recent symptomatic carotid and vertebral artery dissection. In the Cervical Artery Dissection in Stroke Study (CADISS) 250 patients with recent (mean 3.65 [1.91] days) dissection of the carotid ($n = 118$) or vertebral artery ($n = 132$) were randomized to open label antiplatelet therapy (AP; aspirin, clopidogrel, or dipyridamole or in dual combination) or anticoagulation (AC; either unfractionated heparin or a therapeutic dose of low-molecular-weight heparin), followed by warfarin aiming for an INR 2 to 3 for 3 months, after which the choice of AP and AC agents was decided by the local clinician. Novel oral anticoagulants were not used. The total rate of recurrent stroke at 1 year was low (2.4%), and there were no significant differences between treatment groups for any outcome. During 1-year follow-up in the intention-to-treat population, there were 4 primary endpoints (ipsilateral stroke) in the AP group and 2 in the AC group. Considering the combined endpoint of stroke, death, or major bleeding, there were 4 events in the AP arm and 3 in the AC arm. Of the 181 patients with confirmed dissection and complete imaging at baseline and 3 months, there was no difference in the presence of residual narrowing or occlusion between those receiving AP (n = 56 of 92) vs those receiving AC (n = 53 of 89) ($p = 0.97$) (Markus et al., 2019).

Review: Anticoagulants for preventing recurrence following presumed non-cardioembolic ischaemic stroke or transient ischaemic attack
Comparison: 1 Anticoagulant versus control
Outcome: 7 Any recurrent stroke or symptomatic intracranial haemorrhage during follow up

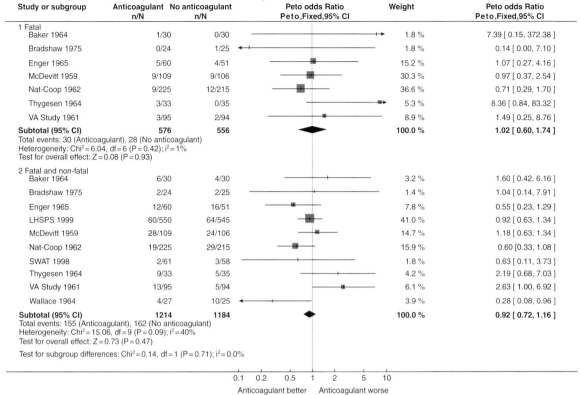

Study or subgroup	Anticoagulant n/N	No anticoagulant n/N	Peto odds Ratio Peto,Fixed,95% CI	Weight	Peto odds Ratio Peto,Fixed,95% CI
1 Fatal					
Baker 1964	1/30	0/30		1.8 %	7.39 [0.15, 372.38]
Bradshaw 1975	0/24	1/25		1.8 %	0.14 [0.00, 7.10]
Enger 1965	5/60	4/51		15.2 %	1.07 [0.27, 4.16]
McDevitt 1959	9/109	9/106		30.3 %	0.97 [0.37, 2.54]
Nat-Coop 1962	9/225	12/215		36.6 %	0.71 [0.29, 1.70]
Thygesen 1964	3/33	0/35		5.3 %	8.36 [0.84, 83.32]
VA Study 1961	3/95	2/94		8.9 %	1.49 [0.25, 8.76]
Subtotal (95% CI)	**576**	**556**		**100.0 %**	**1.02 [0.60, 1.74]**
Total events: 30 (Anticoagulant), 28 (No anticoagulant)					
Heterogeneity: Chi² = 6.04, df = 6 (P = 0.42); i² = 1%					
Test for overall effect: Z = 0.08 (P = 0.93)					
2 Fatal and non-fatal					
Baker 1964	6/30	4/30		3.2 %	1.60 [0.42, 6.16]
Bradshaw 1975	2/24	2/25		1.4 %	1.04 [0.14, 7.91]
Enger 1965	12/60	16/51		7.8 %	0.55 [0.23, 1.29]
LHSPS 1999	60/550	64/545		41.0 %	0.92 [0.63, 1.34]
McDevitt 1959	28/109	24/106		14.7 %	1.18 [0.63, 1.34]
Nat-Coop 1962	19/225	29/215		15.9 %	0.60 [0.33, 1.08]
SWAT 1998	2/61	3/58		1.8 %	0.63 [0.11, 3.73]
Thygesen 1964	9/33	5/35		4.2 %	2.19 [0.68, 7.03]
VA Study 1961	13/95	5/94		6.1 %	2.63 [1.00, 6.92]
Wallace 1964	4/27	10/25		3.9 %	0.28 [0.08, 0.96]
Subtotal (95% CI)	**1214**	**1184**		**100.0 %**	**0.92 [0.72, 1.16]**
Total events: 155 (Anticoagulant), 162 (No anticoagulant)					
Heterogeneity: Chi² = 15.06, df = 9 (P = 0.09); i² = 40%					
Test for overall effect: Z = 0.73 (P = 0.47)					

Test for subgroup differences: Chi² = 0.14, df = 1 (P = 0.71); i² = 0.0%

0.1 0.2   0.5   1   2   5   10
Anticoagulant better   Anticoagulant worse

Figure 19.9 Forest plot showing the effects of *oral anticoagulation vs control* in patients with *previous non-cardioembolic TIA or ischaemic stroke* on *any recurrent stroke or symptomatic intracranial haemorrhage* at the end of follow-up.

Reproduced from Sandercock et al. (2009) with permission from the authors and John Wiley & Sons Limited. Copyright Cochrane Library, reproduced with permission.

Oral Anticoagulation vs Aspirin

TIA and Ischaemic Stroke Patients

There have been eight randomized trials of oral anticoagulant therapy with vitamin K antagonists (warfarin, phenprocoumon, or acenocoumarol) versus antiplatelet therapy for long-term secondary prevention after recent TIA or minor ischaemic stroke of presumed arterial origin in a total of 5762 participants (De Schryver et al., 2012).

Major Vascular Events

Long-term oral anticoagulant therapy with a high INR (3.0–4.5) was associated with a significantly higher rate of recurrent serious vascular events (non-fatal stroke, non-fatal MI, or vascular death) than antiplatelet therapy in the 1316 patients randomized in the SPIRIT trial (OR 1.70, 95% CI:

1.12–2.59), whereas long-term oral anticoagulant therapy with a target INR (2.0–3.6) was associated with a similar rate of recurrent serious vascular events compared with antiplatelet therapy in the 1068 patients randomized in the ESPRIT trial (De Schryver et al., 2012) (Figure 19.10).

Recurrent Stroke

Anticoagulants (in any intensity) are not more efficacious in the prevention of recurrent ischaemic stroke than antiplatelet therapy (medium-intensity anticoagulation: RR 0.80, 95% CI: 0.56–1.14; high-intensity anticoagulation: RR 1.02, 95% CI: 0.49–2.13).

Major Bleeding

Low-intensity anticoagulation (target INR 1.4–2.8) was associated with a similar rate of major bleeding to treatment with antiplatelet agents in one trial

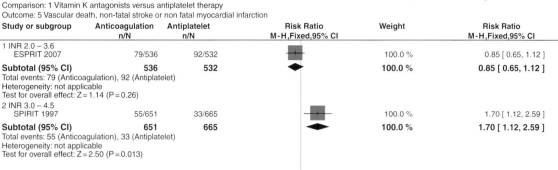

Review: Vitamin K antagonists versus antiplatelet therapy after transient ischaemic attack or minor ischaemic stroke of presumed arterial origin
Comparison: 1 Vitamin K antagonists versus antiplatelet therapy
Outcome: 5 Vascular death, non-fatal stroke or non fatal myocardial infarction

Study or subgroup	Anticoagulation n/N	Antiplatelet n/N	Risk Ratio M-H,Fixed,95% CI	Weight	Risk Ratio M-H,Fixed,95% CI
1 INR 2.0 – 3.6					
ESPRIT 2007	79/536	92/532		100.0 %	0.85 [0.65, 1.12]
Subtotal (95% CI)	**536**	**532**		**100.0 %**	**0.85 [0.65, 1.12]**
Total events: 79 (Anticoagulation), 92 (Antiplatelet)					
Heterogeneity: not applicable					
Test for overall effect: Z = 1.14 (P = 0.26)					
2 INR 3.0 – 4.5					
SPIRIT 1997	55/651	33/665		100.0 %	1.70 [1.12, 2.59]
Subtotal (95% CI)	**651**	**665**		**100.0 %**	**1.70 [1.12, 2.59]**
Total events: 55 (Anticoagulation), 33 (Antiplatelet)					
Heterogeneity: not applicable					
Test for overall effect: Z = 2.50 (P = 0.013)					

0.1   0.2   0.5   1   2   5   10
Favours AC   Favours Antiplatelet

Figure 19.10 Forest plot showing the effects of *oral anticoagulation with VKAs vs antiplatelet therapy* in patients with previous TIA or ischaemic stroke of presumed arterial origin on *serious vascular events* at the end of follow-up.

Reproduced from De Schryver et al. (2012) with permission from the authors and John Wiley & Sons Limited. Copyright Cochrane Library, reproduced with permission.

(WARSS) involving 2206 patients (RR 1.27, 95% CI: 0.79–2.03) (Figure 19.11).

Medium- and high-intensity anticoagulation with vitamin K antagonists, with an INR of 2.0 to 4.5, were not safe because they yielded a higher risk of major bleeding complications (medium-intensity [INR 2.0–3.6] anticoagulation: RR 1.93, 95% CI: 1.27–2.94; high-intensity [INR 3.0–4.5] anticoagulation: RR 9.0, 95% CI: 3.9–21).

Serious Vascular Events or Major Bleeding Complications

Oral anticoagulant therapy with a *high* INR (3.0–4.5) was associated with a significant excess of the composite of recurrent serious vascular events or major haemorrhage compared with antiplatelet therapy (OR 2.30, 95% CI: 1.58–3.35), whereas oral anticoagulant therapy with a medium INR (2.0–3.6) was associated with a similar rate of the composite of recurrent serious vascular events or major haemorrhage compared with antiplatelet therapy (OR 1.00, 95% CI: 0.78–1.29) (Figure 19.12) (De Schryver et al., 2012).

Embolic Stroke of Undetermined Source (ESUS)

Embolic strokes of undetermined source represent 20% of ischaemic strokes and are associated with a high rate of recurrent stroke of about 5% per year despite current antiplatelet therapy.

NAVIGATE-ESUS Trial

The NAVIGATE-ESUS trial compared the efficacy and safety of an oral anticoagulant (factor Xa inhibitor), rivaroxaban (at a daily dose of 15 mg), with aspirin (at a daily dose of 100 mg) for the prevention of recurrent stroke in 7213 patients with recent ischaemic stroke that was presumed to be from cerebral embolism but without arterial stenosis of >50%, lacunar infarction, or an identified major cardioembolic source (Hart et al., 2018). The primary efficacy outcome was the first recurrence of ischaemic or haemorrhagic stroke or systemic embolism in a time-to-event analysis; the primary safety outcome was the rate of major bleeding. The trial was terminated early, when patients had been followed for a median of 11 months because of a lack of benefit with regard to stroke risk and because of bleeding associated with rivaroxaban.

Recurrent Stroke or Systemic Embolism

The primary efficacy outcome occurred in 172 patients in the rivaroxaban group (annualized rate, 5.1%) and in 160 in the aspirin group (annualized rate, 4.8%) (HR 1.07, 95% CI: 0.87–1.33; *p* = 0.52). Recurrent ischaemic stroke occurred in 158 patients in the rivaroxaban group (annualized rate, 4.7%) and in 156 in the aspirin group (annualized rate, 4.7%).

Major Bleeding

Major bleeding occurred in 62 patients in the rivaroxaban group (annualized rate, 1.8%) and in 23 in the aspirin group (annualized rate, 0.7%) (HR 2.72, 95% CI: 1.68–4.39; *p* < 0.001).

Review: Vitamin K antagonists versus antiplatelet therapy after transient ischaemic attack or minor ischaemic stroke of presumed arterial origin
Comparison: 1 Vitamin K antagonists versus antiplatelet therapy
Outcome: 9 Major bleeding complication

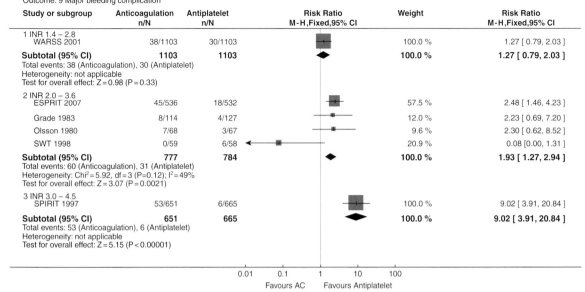

Figure 19.11 Forest plot showing the effects of *oral anticoagulation with VKAs vs antiplatelet therapy* in patients with *previous TIA or ischaemic stroke of presumed arterial origin* on *major bleeding* at the end of follow-up.

Reproduced from De Schryver et al. (2012) with permission from the authors and John Wiley & Sons Limited. Copyright Cochrane Library, reproduced with permission.

Review: Vitamin K antagonists versus antiplatelet therapy after transient ischaemic attack or minor ischaemic stroke of presumed arterial origin
Comparison: 1 Vitamin K antagonists versus antiplatelet therapy
Outcome: 1 The composite vascular death, non-fatal stroke, non-fatal myocardial infarction or major bleeding complication

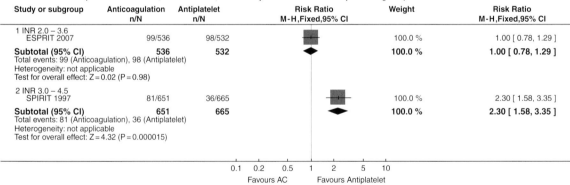

Figure 19.12 Forest plot showing the effects of *oral anticoagulation with VKAs vs antiplatelet therapy* in patients with *previous TIA or ischaemic stroke of presumed arterial origin* on *serious vascular events or major bleeding* at the end of follow-up.

Reproduced from De Schryver et al. (2012) with permission from the authors and John Wiley & Sons Limited. Copyright Cochrane Library, reproduced with permission.

Conclusions

Rivaroxaban was not superior to aspirin with regard to the prevention of recurrent stroke after an initial embolic stroke of undetermined source and was associated with a higher risk of bleeding.

RE-SPECT ESUS Trial

The Randomized, double-blind, Evaluation in secondary Stroke Prevention comparing the EfficaCy and safety of the oral Thrombin inhibitor dabigatran etexilate versus ASA in patients with Embolic Stroke of

Undetermined Source (RE-SPECT ESUS) trial randomly assigned 5390 patients with recent (<6 months) ESUS to either 150 mg or 110 mg of dabigatran twice daily depending on their age and renal function or 100 mg of aspirin daily, a median of 44 days after their index stroke (Diener et al., 2015). The primary efficacy outcome is time to first recurrent stroke (ischaemic, haemorrhagic, or unspecified).

Recurrent Stroke

During a median 19 months' follow-up, the incidence of a recurrent stroke of any type was 4.1%/year among the patients on dabigatran and 4.8%/year among those on aspirin, a difference that was not statistically significant.

A *post hoc* landmark analysis showed a significant reduction in second strokes with dabigatran treatment after the first year, suggesting that anticoagulation may become more effective than aspirin in these patients over time, perhaps because of incident atrial fibrillation.

A *post hoc* subgroup analysis showed that, among patients aged at least 75 years, treatment with dabigatran was linked with a statistically significant 37% reduction in second strokes, compared with treatment with aspirin. These results raise the hypothesis that an anticoagulant might be effective for patients at least 75 years old, possibly because they have a high incidence of atrial fibrillation.

Major Bleeding

The primary safety endpoint of major bleeds, as defined by the International Society on Thrombosis and Haemostasis, occurred in 1.7%/year of patients on dabigatran and 1.4%/year of those on aspirin, a difference that was not statistically significant.

Patients on dabigatran had a significant excess of major bleeds combined with clinically significant nonmajor bleeds: 3.3%/year versus 2.3%/year among those on aspirin.

Interpretation

There may be caveats to the recommendation for antiplatelet therapy in patients with ESUS.

Patients in the NAVIGATE-ESUS trial were only followed for a median of 11 months, as the trial was terminated prematurely. Hence, possible longer-term benefits of rivaroxaban versus aspirin cannot be excluded. The high rate of recurrent stroke of about 5% per year in both treatment groups suggests that the source of embolic stroke was not optimally treated by rivaroxaban 15 mg daily or aspirin. Among many potential sources of embolism in patients with ESUS (arterial, cardiac, paradoxical), it was hypothesized in NAVIGATE-ESUS that covert atrial fibrillation would be common and that recurrent, predominantly cardioembolic, strokes would be effectively treated with rivaroxaban 15 mg daily. This was not substantiated. Further, the mild nature of both the qualifying strokes (median National Institutes of Health Stroke Scale [NIHSS] score = 1) and the recurrent strokes (79% non-disabling) in NAVIGATE-ESUS also suggests that cardiogenic embolism was not a major cause of ESUS; most cardioembolic strokes are large, and disabling or fatal. It is likely that most qualifying strokes and recurrent strokes in NAVIGATE-ESUS were caused by small, platelet thromboemboli from non-stenosing atherosclerosis (<50% diameter stenosis), as is common also in acute coronary syndromes.

Pending the published results of the ongoing randomized trials testing alternative anticoagulants (dabigatran, apixaban) versus aspirin over longer periods of follow-up in patients with ESUS (ClinicalTrials.gov numbers NCT02239120 and NCT02427126), the recent COMPASS trial results in patients with known atherosclerosis (see below, and Sharma et al., 2019), and the results of other trials of non-vitamin K antagonist oral anticoagulant use versus aspirin (Huang et al., 2018), suggest that the safety and effectiveness of the combination of low-dose oral anticoagulation and antiplatelet therapy should also be studied in patients with ESUS.

Oral Anticoagulation vs Clopidogrel Plus Aspirin

TIA and Ischaemic Stroke Patients with Severe Atherosclerosis in the Aortic Arch

The Aortic Arch Related Cerebral Hazard (ARCH) Trial was a prospective randomized controlled, open-labelled trial, with blinded endpoint evaluation (PROBE design) that tested superiority of aspirin 75 to 150 mg/day plus clopidogrel 75 mg/day (A+C) over warfarin therapy (INR 2–3) in patients with ischaemic stroke, TIA, or peripheral embolism with plaque in the thoracic aorta >4 mm and no other identified embolic source (Amarenco et al., 2014).

The trial was stopped after 349 patients were randomized during a period of 8 years and 3 months.

Major Vascular Events

After a median follow-up of 3.4 years, the primary endpoint of cerebral infarction, MI, peripheral embolism, vascular death, or intracranial haemorrhage occurred in 7.6% (13/172) and 11.3% (20/177) of patients on A+C and on warfarin, respectively (log-rank, p = 0.2). The adjusted hazard ratio was 0.76 (95% CI: 0.36–1.61; p = 0.5). Time in therapeutic range (67% of the time for INR 2–3) analysis by tertiles showed no significant differences across groups.

Vascular deaths occurred in 0 patients in the A+C arm compared with 6 (3.4%) patients in the warfarin arm (log-rank, p = 0.013).

Major Bleeding

Major haemorrhages including intracranial haemorrhages occurred in 4 and 6 patients in the A+C and warfarin groups, respectively.

Oral Anticoagulation (low dose) Plus Aspirin vs Aspirin

The Cardiovascular OutcoMes for People using Anticoagulation StrategieS (COMPASS) trial randomized 27,395 participants with stable atherosclerotic vascular disease to receive rivaroxaban (2.5 mg twice daily) plus aspirin (100 mg once daily), rivaroxaban (5 mg twice daily), or aspirin (100 mg once daily) (Eikelboom et al., 2017). The primary outcome was a composite of cardiovascular death, stroke, or MI (major vascular events). The study was stopped for superiority of the rivaroxaban-plus-aspirin group after a mean follow-up of 23 months.

Stable Atherosclerotic Vascular Disease

Major Vascular Events

The composite of cardiovascular death, stroke, or MI occurred in fewer patients in the rivaroxaban-plus-aspirin group than in the aspirin-alone group (379 patients [4.1%] vs 496 patients [5.4%]; HR 0.76; 95% CI: 0.66–0.86; p < 0.001; z = −4.126).

The primary outcome did not occur in significantly fewer patients in the rivaroxaban-alone group than in the aspirin-alone group.

Stroke

Stroke outcome events were slower among 9152 participants assigned rivaroxaban plus aspirin (0.9% per year) versus 9117 participants assigned rivaroxaban (1.3% per year) and 9126 patients assigned aspirin (1.6% per year).

For the comparison of stroke rates of rivaroxaban plus aspirin vs aspirin, the stroke rate was significantly reduced by 42% (HR 0.58, 95% CI: 0.44–0.76; p < 0.001).

For the comparison of stroke rates of rivaraxaban alone versus aspirin alone, the stroke rate was not significantly reduced (HR 0.82, 95% CI: 0.65–1.05).

Independent predictors of stroke were prior stroke, hypertension, systolic blood pressure at baseline, age, diabetes, and Asian ethnicity. Prior stroke was the strongest predictor of incident stroke (HR 3.63, 95% CI: 2.65–4.97; p < 0.0001) and was associated with a 3.4% per year rate of stroke recurrence on aspirin.

Ischaemic/Uncertain Strokes

Ischaemic/uncertain strokes were reduced by nearly half (0.7% per year vs 1.4% per year) (HR 0.51, 95% CI: 0.38–0.68; p < 0.0001) by the combination of rivaroxaban plus aspirin compared with aspirin alone.

Haemorrhagic Transformation of Ischaemic Stroke

Haemorrhagic transformation of ischaemic stroke was less common with the combination of rivaroxaban and aspirin than aspirin alone (<0.1% per year vs 0.2% per year; HR 0.35, 95% CI: 0.13–0.99; p = 0.04).

Fatal and Disabling Stroke

The occurrence of fatal and disabling stroke (mRS 3–6) was decreased by the combination of rivaroxaban and aspirin (32 [0.3% per year] vs 55 [0.6% per year], HR 0.58, 95% CI: 0.37–0.89; p = 0.01).

Major Bleeding

Major bleeding events occurred in more patients in the rivaroxaban-plus-aspirin group compared with the aspirin group alone (288 patients [3.1%] vs 170 patients [1.9%]; HR 1.70, 95% CI: 1.40–2.05; p < 0.001).

Major bleeding events also occurred in more patients in the rivaroxaban-alone group versus the aspirin group.

Intracranial or Fatal Bleeding

There was no significant difference in intracranial or fatal bleeding between the groups.

Deaths

There were 313 deaths (3.4%) in the rivaroxaban-plus-aspirin group as compared with 378 (4.1%) in the aspirin-alone group (HR 0.82, 95% CI:

0.71–0.96; p = 0.01; threshold p-value for significance, 0.0025).

Carotid Artery Disease

The COMPASS trial randomized 1919 patients with carotid artery disease (previous carotid endarterectomy or stent [revascularization procedure] or asymptomatic carotid artery stenosis of at least 50% diagnosed by duplex ultrasound or angiography) to received low-dose rivaroxaban plus aspirin (n = 617), rivaroxaban alone (n = 622), or aspirin alone (n = 680).

The effects of low-dose rivaraxoban plus aspirin on the efficacy outcomes were consistently better than aspirin alone across various subgroups of peripheral artery disease, including carotid artery disease (Anand et al., 2018).

Prior Stroke Patients with Stable Atherosclerotic Disease

Among the 27,395 participants enrolled in the COMPASS trial with stable atherosclerotic disease, 1032 (4%) had prior stroke more than 1 month previously, of whom 502 (49%) had peripheral artery disease and 797 (77%) had coronary artery disease.

Major Vascular Events

Among the 1032 participants with prior stroke, the annualized rate of the composite outcome of cardiovascular death, stroke, or MI was 6.6% in those assigned to aspirin and was reduced to 3.7% in those assigned aspirin and rivaroxaban (HR 0.57, 95% CI: 0.34–0.96; p = 0.04, interaction p = 0.27, NNT = 36 for 1 year) (Sharma et al., 2019).

Ischaemic/Unknown Stroke

Among the 1032 participants with prior stroke, the rate of ischaemic/unknown stroke averaged 3.4% per year among aspirin-assigned patients and was reduced by 67% with rivaroxaban plus aspirin (HR 0.33, 95% CI: 0.14–0.77; p = 0.01, interaction p = 0.28). The absolute stroke reduction in these participants was 2.3% per year with rivaroxaban plus aspirin (NNT for 1 year to prevent one stroke = 43).

Haemorrhagic Stroke

The total number of haemorrhagic stroke outcome events was small in the population with prior stroke (rivaroxaban plus aspirin = 2, rivaroxaban alone = 3, aspirin alone = 0).

Participants with a prior stroke had a higher annualized rate of haemorrhagic stroke of 0.3% than 0.09% for those without prior stroke (HR 3.12, 95% CI: 1.22–7.98; p = 0.02).

Major Bleeding

Major bleeding was not significantly increased in individuals with previous stroke, occurring at an annualized rate of 1.5%, compared with 1.4% in those without a history of previous stroke (HR 1.06, 95% CI: 0.72–1.56; p = 0.76, interaction p = 0.19).

Interpretation

The combination of rivaroxaban and aspirin significantly reduced stroke by 42% compared with aspirin alone in a large population with stable atherosclerotic peripheral and coronary artery disease. The effect was driven by a 49% relative reduction in ischaemic stroke partially offset by a non-significant increase in haemorrhagic stroke. The treatment effect was consistent in the small subgroup of patients with prior stroke, calling for a clinical trial of the use of 2.5 mg rivaroxaban twice daily plus aspirin once daily versus standard care for secondary prevention of stroke in these patients. Rivaroxaban alone did not significantly reduce stroke, and increased haemorrhagic stroke, making this an unattractive treatment option.

Summary

Interpretation of the Evidence

Aspirin reduces the risk of recurrent stroke and other major vascular events by about 13% compared with control. Aspirin increases major bleeding (RR 1.71, 95% CI: 1.41–2.08; absolute annual increase [AAI] 0.13%, 95% CI: 0.08–0.20), mainly caused by major gastrointestinal bleeding (RR 2.07, 95% CI: 1.61–2.66; AAI 0.12%, 95% CI: 0.07–0.19) and intracranial bleeding (RR 1.65, 95% CI: 1.06–5.99; AAI 0.03%, 95% CI: 0.01–0.08).

Terutroban 100 mg twice daily is not more effective than aspirin at preventing recurrent stroke (HR 1.01, 95% CI: 0.92–1.12) and increases minor bleeding (1.11, 1.02–1.21).

Triflusal has similar efficacy to aspirin in preventing stroke and other vascular events (aspirin vs triflusal, RR 1.03, 95% CI: 0.89–1.20), whereas aspirin causes more haemorrhagic strokes than does triflusal (OR 2.15, 95% CI: 1.15–4.04).

In patients of Asian descent, cilostazol (a phosphodiesterase III inhibitor) 100 mg twice daily reduces recurrent ischaemic stroke by 19% (RR 0.81, 95% CI: 0.62–1.06, I^2 = 0%), haemorrhagic stroke by 73% (RR 0.27, 95% CI: 0.13–0.54, I^2 = 0%), and major vascular events by 28% (RR 0.72, 95% CI: 0.57–0.89, I^2 = 0%) compared with aspirin. The addition of probucol to cilostazol or aspirin may reduce the risk of major vascular events in patients with ischaemic stroke at high risk of intracerebral haemorrhage.

Clopidogrel reduces the risk of stroke and other major vascular events by about 9% compared with aspirin. Clopidogrel causes less gastrointestinal bleeding than does 325 mg aspirin daily (RR 0.69, 95% CI: 0.48–1.00). Prasugrel 3.75 mg daily is not non-inferior to clopidogrel 75 mg daily in preventing recurrent major vascular events among Japanese patients with non-cardioembolic ischaemic stroke.

Aspirin 25 mg and extended-release dipyridamole 200 mg twice daily reduces recurrent stroke by about 22% compared with aspirin.

Aspirin 25 mg and extended-release dipyridamole 200 mg twice daily is of similar efficacy to clopidogrel 75 mg daily in preventing recurrent stroke.

Long-term aspirin plus clopidogrel combined is not more effective than clopidogrel alone (RR 1.01, 95% CI: 0.93–1.08) in preventing recurrent stroke. Among patients with recent lacunar strokes, the addition of clopidogrel to aspirin dose not significantly reduce the risk of recurrent stroke but does significantly increase the risk of bleeding and death. However, in people at high risk of cardiovascular disease and people with established cardiovascular disease without a coronary stent, the addition of clopidogrel to aspirin compared with aspirin alone is associated with fewer cases of ischaemic stroke and myocardial infarction but also with more cases of major bleeding during a median period of about a year of follow-up.

The addition of vorapaxar 2.5 mg daily to standard antiplatelet treatment increases intracranial haemorrhage (HR 2.52, 95% CI: 1.46–4.36) without reducing recurrent ischaemic stroke (0.99, 0.78–1.25). The addition of cilostazol to aspirin or clopidogrel is a promising antiplatelet regimen, as it was more effective, and at least as safe, as aspirin or clopidogrel alone among Japanese patients in the CSPS.com trial, and awaits evaluation in other populations.

Long-term oral anticoagulation is not more effective than no anticoagulation in preventing recurrent stroke and other major vascular events in people with presumed non-cardioembolic ischaemic stroke or transient ischaemic attack (TIA), but there is a significant bleeding risk with long-term oral anticoagulation compared with no anticoagulation

Long-term oral anticoagulation with vitamin K antagonists in any dose is not more efficacious than antiplatelet therapy for the secondary prevention of recurrent ischaemic stroke after TIA or minor stroke of presumed arterial origin. Medium- and high-intensity anticoagulation leads to a significant increase in major bleeding complications.

Long-term oral anticoagulation with rivaroxaban or dabigatran was not superior to aspirin in preventing recurrent stroke after an initial embolic stroke of undetermined source and was associated with a higher risk of bleeding.

Implications for Practice

All patients with ischaemic stroke or TIA of presumed arterial origin or embolic stroke of undetermined source should be prescribed antiplatelet therapy.

Aspirin 50–325 mg daily, clopidogrel 75 mg daily, or the combination of aspirin (25 mg) and extended-release dipyridamole (200 mg) twice daily are all appropriate options.

Analysis of individual patient data from the antiplatelet trials suggests that, in the long term, the efficacy of aspirin may attenuate whereas the efficacy of extended-release dipyridamole plus aspirin may be maintained or increase. This hypothesis requires external validation

Cilostazol is more effective and safer than aspirin in secondary stroke prevention among Japanese. The position of cilostazol is not yet established outside Japan.

Triflusal is a second-line alternative.

The long-term use (for >3 months) of aspirin and clopidogrel combined is more effective than aspirin alone in reducing the risk of ischaemic stroke among high vascular risk patients but is also associated with cumulative risks of bleeding that may offset any benefits in preventing recurrent ischaemic events, particularly in patients with lacunar ischaemic stroke.

The COMPASS trial results in patients with predominantly coronary and peripheral artery atherosclerosis raise the exciting possibility that long-term dual pathway inhibition by low-dose anticoagulation (e.g. rivaroxaban 2.5 mg twice daily bid) combined with low-dose antiplatelet therapy (e.g. aspirin 100 mg once daily) may be acceptably safe and substantially more effective than current single pathway inhibition by antiplatelet therapy alone in preventing recurrent vascular events in the long term among patients with atherosclerotic TIA and ischaemic stroke.

References

Amarenco P, Davis S, Jones EF, Cohen AA, Heiss WD, Kaste M, et al.; Aortic Arch Related Cerebral Hazard Trial Investigators. (2014). Clopidogrel plus aspirin versus warfarin in patients with stroke and aortic arch plaques. *Stroke*, **45**, 1248–57

Anand SS, Bosch J, Eikelboom JW, Connolly SJ, Diaz R, Widimsky P, et al.; COMPASS Investigators. (2018). Rivaroxaban with or without aspirin in patients with stable peripheral or carotid artery disease: an international, randomised, double-blind, placebo-controlled trial. *Lancet*, **391**, 219–29.

Antithrombotic Trialists' (ATT) Collaboration, Baigent C, Blackwell L, Collins R, Emberson J, Godwin J, Peto R, et al. (2009). Aspirin in the primary and secondary prevention of vascular disease: collaborative meta-analysis of individual participant data from randomised trials. *Lancet*, **373**, 1849–60.

Bhatt DL, Fox KA, Hacke W, Berger PB, Black HR, Boden WE, et al.; CHARISMA Investigators. (2006). Clopidogrel and aspirin versus aspirin alone for the prevention of atherothrombotic events. *N Engl J Med*, **354**,1706–17

Bhatt DL, Paré G, Eikelboom JW, Simonsen KL, Emison ES, Fox KA, et al.; CHARISMA Investigators. (2012). The relationship between CYP2C19 polymorphisms and ischaemic and bleeding outcomes in stable outpatients: the CHARISMA genetics study. *Eur Heart J*, **33**, 2143–50.

Bousser MG, Amarenco P, Chamorro A, Fisher M, Ford I, Fox KM, et al., for the PERFORM Study Investigators. (2011). Terutroban versus aspirin in patients with cerebral ischaemic events (PERFORM): a randomised, double-blind, parallel-group trial. *Lancet*, **377**, 2013–22. Erratum in: *Lancet*, 378, 402.

CAPRIE Steering Committee. (1996) A randomised, blinded trial of clopidogrel versus aspirin in patients at risk of ischaemic events (CAPRIE). *Lancet*, **348**, 1329–39.

Costa J, Ferro J, Matias-Guiu J, Alvarez-Sabin J, Torres F. (2005). Triflusal for preventing serious vascular events in people at high risk. *Cochrane Database Syst Rev*, 3. CD004296.

De Schryver ELLM, Algra A, vanGijn J. (2007). Dipyridamole for preventing stroke and other vascular events in patients with vascular disease. *Cochrane Database Syst Rev*, 3. CD001820. doi:10.1002/14651858.CD001820.pub3.

De Schryver ELLM, Algra A, Kappelle LJ, van Gijn J, Koudstaal PJ. (2012). Vitamin K antagonists versus antiplatelet therapy after transient ischaemic attack or minor ischaemic stroke of presumed arterial origin. *Cochrane Database Syst Rev*, 9. CD001342. doi:10.1002/14651858.CD001342.pub3.

Diener HC, Bogousslavsky J, Brass LM, Cimminiello C, Csiba L, Kaste M, et al.; MATCH Investigators. (2004).

Aspirin and clopidogrel compared with clopidogrel alone after recent ischaemic stroke or transient ischaemic attack in high-risk patients (MATCH): randomised, double-blind, placebo-controlled trial. *Lancet*, **364**, 331–7.

Diener HC, Cunha L, Forbes C, Sivenius J, Smets P, Lowenthal A. (1996). European Stroke Prevention Study. 2. Dipyridamole and acetylsalicylic acid in the secondary prevention of stroke. *J Neurol Sci*, 143, 1-13.

Diener HC, Easton JD, Granger CB, Cronin L, Duffy C, Cotton D, et al.; RE-SPECT ESUS Investigators. (2015). Design of Randomized, double-blind, Evaluation in secondary Stroke Prevention comparing the EfficaCy and safety of the oral Thrombin inhibitor dabigatran etexilate vs. acetylsalicylic acid in patients with Embolic Stroke of Undetermined Source (RE-SPECT ESUS). *Int J Stroke*, **10**, 1309–12.

Dinicolantonio JJ, Lavie CJ, Fares H, Menezes AR, O'Keefe JH, Bangalore S, et al. (2013). Meta-analysis of cilostazol versus aspirin for the secondary prevention of stroke. *Am J Cardiol*, **112**, 1230–4.

Donadini MP, Bellesini M, Squizzato A. (2018). Aspirin plus clopidogrel vs aspirin alone for preventing cardiovascular events among patients at high risk for cardiovascular events. *JAMA*, **320**, 593–4. doi:10.1001/jama.2018.9641.

Eikelboom JW, Connolly SJ, Bosch J, Dagenais GR, Hart RG, Shestakovska O, et al.; COMPASS Investigators. (2017). Rivaroxaban with or without aspirin in stable cardiovascular disease. *N Engl J Med*, **377**, 1319–30.

Gotoh F, Tohgi H, Hirai S, Terashi A, Fukuuchi Y, Otomo E, et al. (2000). Cilostazol Stroke Prevention Study: a placebo-controlled double-blind trial for secondary prevention of cerebral infarction. *J Stroke Cerebrovasc Dis*, **9**, 147–57.

Gouya G, Arrich J, Wolzt M, Huber K, Verheugt FW, Gurbel PA, et al. (2014). Antiplatelet treatment for prevention of cerebrovascular events in patients with vascular diseases: a systematic review and meta-analysis. *Stroke*, **45**, 492–503.

Halkes PH, Gray LJ, Bath PM, Diener HC, Guiraud-Chaumeil B, Yatsu FM, et al. (2008). Dipyridamole plus aspirin versus aspirin alone in secondary prevention after TIA or stroke: a meta-analysis by risk. *J Neurol Neurosurg Psychiatry*, **79**, 1218–23.

Hankey GJ, Johnston SC, Easton JD, Hacke W, Mas JL, Brennan D, et al.; CHARISMA Trial Investigators. (2011). Effect of clopidogrel plus ASA vs. ASA early after TIA and ischaemic stroke: a substudy of the CHARISMA trial. *Int J Stroke*, **6**, 3–9.

Hart RG, Sharma M, Mundl H, Kasner SE, Bangdiwala SI, Berkowitz SD, et al.; NAVIGATE ESUS Investigators. (2018) Rivaroxaban for stroke prevention after embolic stroke of undetermined source. *N Engl J Med*, **378**, 2191–2201.

Hilkens NA, Algra A, Kappelle LJ, Bath PM, Csiba L, Rothwell PM, Greving JP; CAT Collaboration. (2018a). Early time course of major bleeding on antiplatelet therapy after TIA or ischemic stroke. *Neurology*, **90**, e683–9.

Hilkens NA, Algra A, Diener HC, Reitsma JB, Bath PM, Csiba L, et al.; Cerebrovascular Antiplatelet Trialists' Collaborative Group. (2017). Predicting major bleeding in patients with noncardioembolic stroke on antiplatelets: S2TOP-BLEED. *Neurology*, **89**, 936–43.

Hilkens NA, Li L, Rothwell PM, Algra A, Greving JP. (2018b). External validation of risk scores for major bleeding in a population-based cohort of transient ischemic attack and ischemic stroke patients. *Stroke*, **49**, 601–06.

Huang WY, Singer DE, Wu YL, Chiang CE, Weng HH, Lee M, Ovbiagele B. (2018). Association of intracranial hemorrhage risk with non-vitamin K antagonist oral anticoagulant use vs aspirin use: a systematic review and meta-analysis. *JAMA Neurol*, **75**(12), 1511–18. doi:10.1001/jamaneurol.2018.2215.

Kamal AK, Naqvi I, Husain MR, Khealani BA. (2011). Cilostazol versus aspirin for secondary prevention of vascular events after stroke of arterial origin. *Cochrane Database Syst Rev*, 1. CD008076. doi:10.1002/14651858. CD008076.pub2.

Kim BJ, Lee E-J, Kwon SU, Park JH, Kim YJ, Hong KS, et al. (2018). Prevention of cardiovascular events in Asian patients with ischaemic stroke at high risk of cerebral haemorrhage (PICASSO): a multicentre, randomised controlled trial. *Lancet Neurol*, **17**, 509–18.

Kwok CS, Shoamanesh A, Copley HC, Myint PK, Loke YK, Benavente OR. (2015). Efficacy of antiplatelet therapy in secondary prevention following lacunar stroke: pooled analysis of randomized trials. *Stroke*, **46**, 1014–23.

Leonardi-Bee J, Bath PM, Bousser MG, Davalos A, Diener HC, Guiraud-Chaumeil B, et al.; Dipyridamole in Stroke Collaboration (DISC). (2005). Dipyridamole for preventing recurrent ischemic stroke and other vascular events: a meta-analysis of individual patient data from randomized controlled trials. *Stroke*, **36**, 162–8.

Markus HS, Levi C, King A, Madigan J, Norris J; Cervical Artery Dissection in Stroke Study (CADISS) Investigators. (2019). Antiplatelet therapy vs anticoagulation therapy in cervical artery dissection: the Cervical Artery Dissection in Stroke Study (CADISS) Randomized Clinical Trial Final Results. *JAMA Neurol*, 76, 657-64.

McDonough CW, McClure LA, Mitchell BD, Gong Y, Horenstein RB, Lewis JP, et al. (2015). CYP2C19 metabolizer status and clopidogrel efficacy in the Secondary Prevention of Small Subcortical Strokes (SPS3) study. *JAHA*, **4**, e001652.

Morrow DA, Alberts MJ, Mohr JP, Ameriso SF, Bonaca MP, Goto S, Hankey GJ, et al.; Thrombin Receptor Antagonist in Secondary Prevention of Atherothrombotic Ischemic Events–TIMI 50 Steering Committee and Investigators.

(2013). Efficacy and safety of vorapaxar in patients with prior ischemic stroke. *Stroke*, **44**, 691–8.

Ogawa A, Toyoda K, Kitagawa K, Kitazono T, Nagao T, Yamagami H, et al. (2019). Comparison of prasugrel and clopidogrel in patients with non-cardioembolic ischaemic stroke: the PRASTRO-I randomised trial. *Lancet Neurol*, **18**, 238–47.

Roe MT, Armstrong PW, Fox KA, White HD, Prabhakaran D, Goodman SG, et al. (2012). Prasugrel versus clopidogrel for acute coronary syndromes without revascularization. *N Engl J Med*, **367**, 1297–309.

Rothwell PM, Algra A, Chen Z, Diener HC, Norrving B, Mehta Z. (2016). Effects of aspirin on risk and severity of early recurrent stroke after transient ischaemic attack and ischaemic stroke: time-course analysis of randomised trials. *Lancet*, **388**, 365–75

Rothwell PM, Cook NR, Gaziano JM, Price JF, Belch JFF, Roncaglioni MC, et al. (2018). Effects of aspirin on risks of vascular events and cancer according to bodyweight and dose: analysis of individual patient data from randomised trials. *Lancet*, **392**, 387–99.

Sacco RL, Diener H-C, Yusuf S, Cotton D, Ounpuu S, Lawton WA, et al. (2008). Aspirin and extended-release dipyridamole versus clopidogrel for recurrent stroke. The Prevention Regimen for Effectively Avoiding Second Strokes (PRoFESS) trial. *N Engl J Med*, **359**, 1238–51.

Sandercock PAG, Gibson LM, Liu M. (2009). Anticoagulants for preventing recurrence following presumed non-cardioembolic ischaemic stroke or transient ischaemic attack. *Cochrane Database Syst Rev*, 2. CD000248. doi:10.1002/14651858.CD000248. pub2.

Sharma M, Hart RG, Connolly S, Bosch J, Shestakovska O, Ng KH, et al. (2019). Stroke Outcomes in the Cardiovascular OutcoMes for People using Anticoagulation StrategieS (COMPASS) trial. *Circulation*, **139**(9), 1134–45. doi 10.1161/CIRCULATIONAHA.118.035864.

SPS3 Investigators, Benavente OR, Hart RG, McClure LA, Szychowski JM, Coffey CS, Pearce LA. (2012). Effects of clopidogrel added to aspirin in patients with recent lacunar stroke. *N Engl J Med*, **367**, 817–25.

Squizzato A, Bellesini M, Takeda A, Middeldorp S, Donadini MP. (2017). Clopidogrel plus aspirin versus aspirin alone for preventing cardiovascular events. *Cochrane Database Syst Rev*, 12. CD005158.

Sudlow CLM, Mason G, Maurice JB, Wedderburn CJ, Hankey GJ. (2009). Thienopyridine derivatives versus aspirin for preventing stroke and other serious vascular events in high vascular risk patients. *Cochrane Database Syst Rev*, 4. CD001246. doi:10.1002/14651858.CD001246. pub2.

Topol EJ, Easton D, Harrington RA, Amarenco P, Califf RM, Graffagnino C, et al.; Blockade of the Glycoprotein IIb/IIIa Receptor to Avoid Vascular

Occlusion Trial Investigators. (2003). Randomized, double-blind, placebo-controlled, international trial of the oral IIb/IIIa antagonist lotrafiban in coronary and cerebrovascular disease. *Circulation*, **108**, 399–406.

Toyoda K, Uchiyama S, Yamaguchi T, Easton JD, Kimura K, Hoshino H, et al., for the CSPS.com Trial Investigators. (2019). Dual antiplatelet therapy using cilostazol for secondary prevention in high-risk ischaemic stroke: a multicentre randomised controlled trial. *Lancet Neurol*, **18** (6), 539–48.

Wiviott SD, Braunwald E, McCabe CH, Montalescot G, Ruzyllo W, Gottlieb S, et al. (2007). Prasugrel versus clopidogrel in patients with acute coronary syndromes. *N Engl J Med*, **357**, 2001–15.

Chapter 20

Carotid and Vertebral Artery Revascularization

Mandy D. Müller
Leo H. Bonati
Martin M. Brown

Carotid Stenosis as a Cause of Ischaemic Stroke

This chapter will cover only the revascularization treatment of patients with recently symptomatic carotid stenosis, except in the section on carotid artery stenting (CAS) where some of the relevant studies have mixed symptomatic and asymptomatic patients.

The fact that moderate or severe stenosis is responsible for most cases of ipsilateral stroke was demonstrated by randomized trials that showed that removing the extracranial internal carotid artery (ICA) stenosis at its origin, by means of carotid endarterectomy (CEA), significantly reduces the risk of subsequent ipsilateral carotid territory ischaemic stroke (European Carotid Surgery Trial [ECST] Collaborative Group, 1991; North American Symptomatic Carotid Endarterectomy Trial [NASCET] Collaborators, 1991a,b).

Observational studies in white populations done 30 years ago suggested that about one-quarter of all first-ever ischaemic strokes and transient ischaemic attacks (TIAs) were caused by atherothromboembolism from the origin of the extracranial ICA (Sandercock et al., 1989). More recent studies report an around 8% prevalence of stenosis measuring >50% thought to be causative of ipsilateral ischaemic stroke, with an additional 11% of patients found to have contralateral asymptomatic stenosis (Cheng et al., 2019).

Mechanisms

The mechanisms by which extracranial ICA atherosclerosis causes ischaemic stroke are listed in Table 20.1.

Risk Factors for Ischaemic Stroke Caused by Carotid Stenosis

Degree of Carotid Stenosis

The risk of stroke ipsilateral to a carotid stenosis increases with the degree of symptomatic carotid stenosis until the artery distal to the stenosis begins to collapse (ECST Collaborative Group, 1991; NASCET Collaborators, 1991; Rothwell and Warlow, 2000; Rothwell et al., 2000). A group of symptomatic patients with 'collapse' or 'abnormal post-stenotic narrowing' of the ICA resulting in near-occlusion of the artery was separately identified in NASCET. This was because it was not possible to measure the degree of stenosis using the NASCET method when the post-stenotic ICA was severely narrowed as a result of markedly reduced post-stenotic blood flow (Morgenstern et al., 1997). In NASCET, such patients were therefore arbitrarily allocated a stenosis of 95%. The ECST subsequently also separately analysed such patients, and both trials reported consistent results that these patients had a paradoxically low risk of stroke on best medical treatment alone to the extent that they did not benefit from CEA (Morgenstern et al., 1997; Rothwell and Warlow, 2000; Rothwell et al., 2000). The low risk of stroke in patients with collapse of the ICA distal to a severe stenosis, selected for the trials because of recent TIA or minor stroke, was most probably due to the presence of a good collateral circulation, which is visible on angiography in the vast majority of such patients. Without a good collateral circulation, these patients would most likely have had a major stroke and would not have been eligible for the trials.

Table 20.1 Mechanisms by which extracranial ICA atherosclerosis causes ischaemic stroke

'Vulnerable' atherosclerotic plaque lesions usually situated close to the carotid bifurcation undergo endothelial erosion, fissuring, or rupture, which exposes the subendothelial tissue to circulating blood, resulting in local thrombus formation. This can cause infarction in the territory of the brain supplied by the ICA by the following mechanisms (Torvik et al., 1989; Ogata et al., 1990):

1. Plaque debris or thrombus may embolize and block a more distal vessel, commonly the middle cerebral artery or its branches, occasionally the anterior cerebral, and rarely the ipsilateral posterior cerebral artery in patients with a widely patent posterior communicating artery.
2. Atherosclerotic plaque and/or thrombus may encroach upon the lumen of the ICA sufficiently to cause severe stenosis or occlusion, which may lead to hypoperfusion of distal brain regions, particularly in arterial border zones, and thus to border zone infarction (also known as watershed infarction).
3. Thrombosis at the site of stenosis may propagate up the ICA to occlude its distal branches.

ICA: internal carotid artery.

Recent Neurological Symptoms of Carotid Territory Ischaemia

The risk of stroke ipsilateral to a carotid stenosis is greater in patients with recent neurological symptoms from carotid territory ischaemia than in those with more distant symptoms (Lovett et al., 2003, 2004; Coull et al., 2004). The risk is time dependent, being highest in the few weeks after the presenting event, reasonably high for the first year, and falling quickly over the next 2 years to that of neurologically asymptomatic carotid stenosis (ECST Collaborative Group, 1991; NASCET Collaborators, 1991; Rothwell et al., 2000; Coull et al., 2004). The high early risk of recurrence probably represents the presence of an active unstable atherosclerotic plaque, and the rapid decline in risk over the subsequent year most likely reflects 'healing' of the unstable atheromatous plaque or possibly in some cases an increase in collateral blood flow to the symptomatic hemisphere (ECST Collaborative Group, 1998; NASCET Collaborators, 1998; Rothwell and Warlow, 2000; Rothwell et al., 2000a).

Other Factors

In addition to the severity of carotid stenosis, the presence of neurological symptoms, and the time since symptom onset, a number of other factors have been associated with an increased risk of stroke in the presence of carotid stenosis. These include increasing age, stroke as opposed to a single TIA, multiple TIAs (suggesting an active, unstable plaque), an irregular and ulcerated plaque surface morphology (which is pathologically unstable), absence of angiographic collateral flow, impaired cerebral reactivity, a high frequency of transcranial Doppler (TCD)-detected emboli to the brain, hypertension, and coronary heart disease (Table 20.2) (Rothwell and

Warlow, 1999; Rothwell et al., 2000, 2005). Of all the possible symptoms associated with carotid stenosis, amaurosis fugax (transient monocular blindness) is associated with the lowest risk of recurrence.

More recent research has concentrated on the use of imaging to identify 'vulnerable' plaque and predict those at increased risk of stroke from carotid stenosis. These plaque imaging techniques include ultrasound imaging, single-photon emission computed tomography (SPECT) scanning, and magnetic resonance imaging (MRI) (Liem et al., 2017). Although there is good evidence that plaque characteristics, such as the presence of plaque haemorrhage identified by MRI, identify patients at higher risk of recurrence, these techniques have yet to be shown to be useful in clinical practice and have not entered routine clinical practice.

The purpose of revascularization of a symptomatic extracranial ICA stenosis is to reduce the risk of recurrent ipsilateral carotid territory ischaemic stroke by removing the source of carotid occlusion or thromboembolism. The two most commonly used strategies are CEA and CAS.

Carotid Endarterectomy

Evidence of Overall Risks and Benefits

There have been five randomized controlled trials (RCTs) comparing the effect of endarterectomy for symptomatic carotid stenosis combined with best medical therapy with the effect of best medical therapy alone (Fields et al., 1970; Shaw et al., 1984; Mayberg et al., 1991; ECST Collaborative Group, 1998; NASCET Collaborators, 1998).

The first two trials were small and are now largely ignored as not reflecting later standards of practice (Fields et al., 1970; Shaw et al., 1984). The larger

Table 20.2 Independent prognostic factors for risk of ipsilateral ischaemic stroke in patients with recently symptomatic carotid stenosis who were randomized to best medical treatment alone in the ECST (Rothwell and Warlow, 1999; Rothwell et al., 2005)

Risk factor	Hazard ratio	95% CI	P-value
Stenosis (per 10% increase)	1.18	1.10–1.25	<0.0001
Time since last event (per 7 days)	0.96	0.93–0.99	0.004
Presenting event			0.007
Ocular event	1.0		
Single TIA	1.41	0.75–2.66	
Multiple TIAs	2.05	1.16–3.60	
Minor stroke	1.82	0.99–3.34	
Major stroke	2.54	1.48–4.35	
Previous MI	1.57	1.01–2.45	0.047
Irregular/ulcerated plaque	2.03	1.31–3.14	0.0015
Diabetes	1.35	0.86–2.11	0.19
Near occlusion	0.49	0.19–1.24	0.14

ECST: European Carotid Surgery Trial. CI: confidence interval. TIA: transient ischaemic attack. MI: myocardial infarction.

Veterans Administration (VA#309) trial (Mayberg et al., 1991) showed a non-significant trend in favour of surgery, but was stopped prematurely when the initial results of the two largest trials were published (ECST Collaborative Group, 1991; NASCET Collaborators, 1991). The analyses of these trials were stratified by the severity of stenosis of the symptomatic carotid artery, but the degree of stenosis on pre-randomization angiograms was measured using different methods. It is notable that these trials were started more than 30 years ago at a time when medical therapy was much less intensive than contemporary 'best' medical therapy. Nevertheless, their results continue to provide the main basis for current practice in the treatment of carotid stenosis.

Methods of Measuring Carotid Stenosis

The NASCET method underestimated stenosis compared with the ECST method. Stenoses reported to be 70–99% in the NASCET were equivalent to 82–99% by the ECST method, and stenoses reported to be 70–99% by the ECST method were 55–99% by the NASCET method (Rothwell et al., 1994).

Analysis of ECST Using the NASCET Method of Measurement of Carotid Stenosis

The ECST group re-measured the degree of carotid stenosis on their original angiograms using the method

adopted by the NASCET group, and also redefined their outcome events to match those of NASCET, for comparability (Rothwell et al., 2003a).

Re-analysis of the ECST using NASCET measurements of stenosis showed that endarterectomy reduced the 5-year risk of *any stroke or surgical death* by 5.7% (95% confidence interval [CI]: 0–11.6) in patients with 50–69% stenosis ($n = 646$, $p = 0.05$) and by 21.2% (95% CI: 12.9–29.4) in patients with 70–99% stenosis without 'near occlusion' ($n = 429$, $p < 0.0001$). Surgery was harmful in patients with <30% stenosis ($n = 1321$, $p = 0.007$) and of no benefit in patients with 30–49% stenosis or near-occlusion ($n = 478$, $p = 0.6$ and $n = 78$, $p = 0.7$, respectively). These results of ECST, when analysed in the same way as NASCET, were consistent with the NASCET results (Rothwell et al., 2003a).

Analysis of Pooled Data from RCTs of Endarterectomy for Symptomatic Carotid Stenosis

A pooled analysis of data from the ECST, NASCET and VA#309 trials, which included over 95% of patients with symptomatic carotid stenosis ever randomized to endarterectomy vs medical treatment, showed that there was no statistically significant heterogeneity between the trials in the effect of the randomized treatment allocation on the relative risks (RRs) of any of the main outcomes in any of the stenosis groups

(Rothwell et al., 2003b). Data were therefore merged on 6092 patients with 35,000 patient-years of follow-up.

Risks

It is ironic that the precise purpose of CEA is to prevent stroke (and death), and paradoxically its major potential complication is peri-operative stroke (and death).

Peri-operative Stroke or Death

In the three trials of endarterectomy for symptomatic carotid stenosis, where postoperative complications were systematically reviewed, the overall pooled operative mortality was 1.1% (95% CI: 0.8–1.5), and the operative risk of stroke and death within 30 days of surgery was 7.1% (95% CI: 6.3–8.1) (Rothwell et al., 2003b).

A systematic review of 57 surgical case series, involving a total of 13,285 CEAs, indicated that the *reported* peri-operative risk of stroke and death varied widely from <1% to more than 30%, but was usually about 3–8%, and was on average 5.1% (95% CI: 4.6–5.6%) (Rothwell et al., 1996a,b; Goldstein et al., 1997). The risk was higher in surgical case series in which patients were assessed postoperatively by a neurologist (7.7% [95% CI: 5.0–10.2%], odds ratio [OR]: 1.62 [95% CI: 1.45–1.81]) (Rothwell, 1996a).

Based on the results from the trials, about one in 14 patients undergoing CEA for symptomatic carotid stenosis experiences a peri-operative stroke or dies in the peri-operative period. However, this risk cannot be generalized to one's own institution, surgeons, or patients. In particular, personal experience, and recent case series, suggest that operative rates of CEA for symptomatic patients have declined considerably since NASCET and ECST were published (Matsen et al., 2006). A recent local prospective audit of a large number of patients undergoing CEA by each surgeon and centre is therefore required, and referring doctors (and patients) should have access to the peri-operative stroke and death rate of their prospective surgeon(s) and centres, derived from such an independent and rigorous audit (Goldstein et al., 1997). However, interpretation of unusually high or low operative risks must take into account the effects of chance and case mix. Otherwise, over-simplistic interpretation of crude results may lead to unjustified criticism of individual surgeons, and not to improvements in patient care.

There are several other important prognostic factors for stroke, and peri-operative stroke and death associated with CEA which may influence the decision to operate.

Prognostic Factors for Peri-operative Stroke or Death

Patient factors The risk of peri-operative stroke is greater in patients with *symptomatic* carotid stenosis than asymptomatic carotid stenosis. However, patients with *symptoms* of minor stroke lasting less than 7 days have a lower risk than those with stroke lasting longer, while patients with ocular ischaemia due to carotid stenosis (e.g. amaurosis fugax) have the *lowest* risk of peri-operative stroke or death (Rothwell et al., 1996b).

Other patient factors which have been associated with an increased risk of peri-operative stroke and death in trials of CEA for symptomatic carotid stenosis (Table 20.3) are as follows:

1. Female gender (perhaps because of smaller carotid arteries, perhaps more difficult to operate on).
2. Systolic blood pressure (SBP) >180 mm Hg (perhaps increased risk of reperfusion injury and cerebral haemorrhage).
3. Peripheral arterial disease (a marker of atherosclerotic plaque burden).
4. Occlusion of the contralateral ICA (indicates poor collateral cerebral circulation).
5. Stenosis of the ipsilateral external carotid artery (poor collateral circulation) (Rothwell et al., 1997). The risk of peri-operative stroke or death associated with CEA does not appear to be related to the degree of ipsilateral internal carotid stenosis (Table 20.4).

Table 20.3 Independent predictors of risk of peri-operative major stroke or death within 30 days of CEA in the ECST (Rothwell et al., 1997; Rothwell and Warlow, 1999)

Prognostic variable	Hazard ratio	95% CI	*p*-value
Female gender	2.05	1.29–3.24	0.002
SBP >180 mm Hg	2.21	1.29–3.79	0.004
Peripheral arterial disease	2.48	1.51–4.13	0.0004

Table 20.4 Pooled peri-operative risks of stroke and death within 30 days of CEA according to degree of symptomatic carotid stenosis in patients who underwent CEA in the three RCTs of CEA

Outcome	Carotid stenosis	Risk (%)	95% CI
Stroke or death	<50%	6.7	5.6–8.0
	50–69%	8.4	6.6–10.5
	≥70%	6.2	4.4–8.5
	Near occlusion	5.4	2.4–10.4
	Total	7.1	6.3–8.1
Death	<50%	1.0	0.6–1.6
	50–69%	1.4	0.8–2.5
	≥70%	0.9	0.3–2.0
	Near occlusion	0.7	0–3.7
	Total	1.1	0.8–1.5

Importantly, the operative risk of stroke and death is unrelated to the risk of stroke with best medical treatment alone (Rothwell et al., 2003b, 2005) (see Tables 20.2, 20.3, 20.4).

Surgical factors The surgical factors which may be associated with an increased risk of peri-operative stroke or death are: (a) inexperience due to low surgeon and hospital case volumes (Feasby et al., 2002); and (b) undertaking CEA in the very acute phase of stroke in evolution and crescendo TIAs, and during coronary artery surgery for patients with angina whose carotid stenosis was discovered during preparation for coronary artery surgery (Bond et al., 2003). For neurologically stable patients, such as those enrolled into the trials, there was no evidence of any increase in operative risk in patients operated on within 2 weeks of their last event (Rothwell et al., 2004). Moreover, in a systematic review of surgical case series, early surgery in neurologically stable patients was not associated with an increased operative risk (Bond et al., 2003). These data have led to pressure on surgeons to operate very soon after the onset of symptoms. However, operating on patients with unstable plaque might be hazardous and recent registry data have suggested that the risk is significantly increased in patients operated on within 2 days of symptoms (Strömberg et al., 2012). Thus, the optimal time to operate is probably on the third day after minor symptoms, which allows time for antiplatelet therapy to become active.

Local Adverse Effects of CEA

Other specific adverse effects of CEA, besides those inherent in any operation, include:

1. lower cranial nerve palsy (about 5–9% of patients),
2. peripheral nerve palsy (about 1% of patients),
3. major neck haematoma requiring surgery or extended hospital stay (about 5–7% of patients), and
4. wound infection (3%).

Prognostic Factors for Peri-operative Cranial Nerve Palsy

Patients undergoing CEA for *recurrent* carotid stenosis have an increased risk of cranial nerve injury and wound haematoma (Bond et al., 2003).

The risk of functionally disabling bilateral vagal and hypoglossal nerve palsies is also increased in patients who have already had an endarterectomy on one side or are undergoing *bilateral* CEAs.

Net Benefits and Risks Overall

Because CEA carries a significant risk of peri-operative stroke and death, CEA is only superior to medical therapy alone when the risks of stroke over time on medical therapy are significantly higher than the combined peri-operative risk from CEA plus any stroke that occurred thereafter despite CEA. As discussed above, these risks vary from one individual to another. The peri-operative risks of surgery after randomization in the RCTs for recently symptomatic carotid stenosis initially exceeded the risk of stroke on medical treatment for a period of time and it is only after the risks of the two treatments cross over for a similar period of time that surgery shows a net benefit over medical therapy. The way in which the long-term risk of events on medical treatment alone varies with stenosis severity, while the long-term risk of events after surgery remains fairly constant with stenosis severity, is illustrated in Figure 20.1.

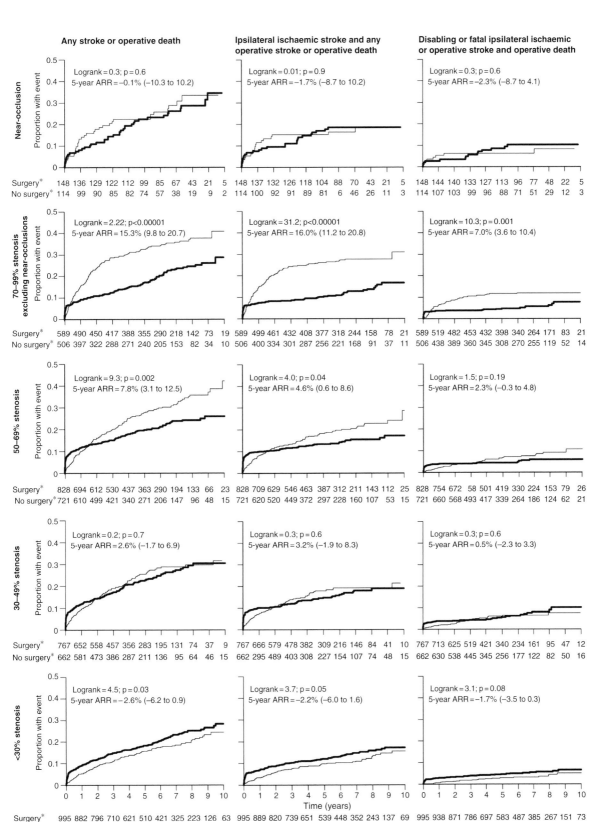

Figure 20.1 Effects of carotid endarterectomy (thick line) vs medical treatment alone (thin line) over 10-year follow-up at different degrees of symptomatic carotid stenosis analysed by intention-to-treat using data pooled from ECST, NASCET, and VA309.

Reproduced from Rothwell et al. (2003b) with permission.

It is a striking feature of patients with severe (70–99%) recently symptomatic carotid stenosis that although the risk of recurrent stroke is higher than attributable to lesser degrees of stenosis, the long-term risk of stroke on medical treatment alone flattens off over time, being much higher in the first 2 years after the index symptom than it is in subsequent years (Figure 20.1). This effect is less pronounced in patients with <70% stenosis. Thus, the net benefit of surgery is greatest in patients with severe stenosis (excluding near-occlusion) but the absolute risk reduction does not increase beyond 3 years of follow-up (Rothwell et al., 2003b). In contrast, the absolute risk reduction achieved by surgery for moderate degrees of stenosis (50 to 79%) increases over time up to at least 8 years after randomization (Figure 20.2).

Evidence from the Cochrane Library

The most recent systematic review for the Cochrane Library was published in 2017 and included data from the 6343 patients enrolled in the NASCET, ECST, and VA trials. No new completed studies were identified. The authors performed a pooled analysis of 6092 participants in whom individual data were available using a re-analysis of all the baseline angiograms for stenosis severity using the NASCET method and a uniform definition of outcome events (Orrapin and Rerkasem, 2017).

Mild carotid stenosis (NASCET <50%) For patients with very mild stenosis measuring <30%, surgery increased the 5-year risk of any stroke or operative death with a risk ratio (RR) of 1.25 (95% CI: 0.99–2.01). For patients with mild stenosis measuring 30–49%, there was no evidence of benefit or harm, with a risk ratio of 0.97 (95% CI: 0.79–1.19). The assumed event rates for this degree of stenosis were 21% with best medical treatment alone and 20% with additional carotid surgery (Figure 20.3).

Moderate carotid stenosis (NASCET: 50–69%) For patients with moderate stenosis, surgery significantly reduced the risk of any stroke or operative death by 23% (RR 0.77, 95% CI: 0.63–0.94). This corresponded to a reduction from an assumed 5-year risk of 23% to 18% with surgery and a number needed to treat (NNT) of around 20 to prevent one event (Figure 20.3).

Severe carotid stenosis (NASCET 70–99%) For patients with severe stenosis, excluding those with near-occlusion, surgery reduced the risk of any stroke or operative death by 47% (RR 0.53, 95% CI: 0.42–0.67%). This corresponds to a reduction from an assumed 5-year risk of 29% to 15% with surgery and a NNT of around 7 to prevent one event (Figure 20.3).

Near-occlusion In patients with near occlusion (defined as very severe stenosis associated with distal luminal collapse of the ICA), there was no evidence of overall benefit or harm from surgery (RR 0.95, 95% CI: 0.59–1.53).

Other outcome measures The Cochrane review also analysed several other outcomes, including ipsilateral carotid territory stroke or operative stroke or death, and disabling or fatal ipsilateral ischaemic stroke or operative stroke or death. The conclusions in relation to the benefit of surgery at different degrees of stenosis were very similar to those discussed above in relation to any stroke or operative death.

Benefits in Clinical Subgroups and Timing of Surgery

Although endarterectomy reduces the RR of stroke or operative death by 47% over the next 5 years in patients with a recently symptomatic severe (70–99%) carotid stenosis, the absolute risk reduction (ARR) is relatively small (14%), because only 29% of these patients have a stroke on medical treatment alone (and 15% have a stroke after CEA).

The operation is therefore of no value for at least two-thirds (71%) of patients who, despite having a severe (70–99%), recently symptomatic carotid stenosis, are destined to remain stroke free for the next 5 years with best medical therapy alone (i.e. without surgery) and can only be harmed by surgery.

It would, therefore, be useful to be able to identify in advance, and operate on, only the 14% of patients (one in seven) with severe symptomatic carotid stenosis who are going to benefit over the next 5 years.

We therefore need to be able to more precisely identify those patients with severe symptomatic carotid stenosis who have a very high risk of stroke on medical treatment alone, coupled with a relatively low operative risk. Simply relying on the presence or absence of recent carotid territory ischaemic symptoms and the degree of carotid stenosis is not good enough (although a good start).

When a systematic review of RCTs reveals a substantially significant overall treatment effect of several standard deviations, as is the case of CEA for severe symptomatic carotid, there is sufficient statistical power to perform subgroup analyses with some confidence in the results (other than purely hypothesis-generating 'data dredging') (see 'Subgroup analyses', Chapter 2, page 17).

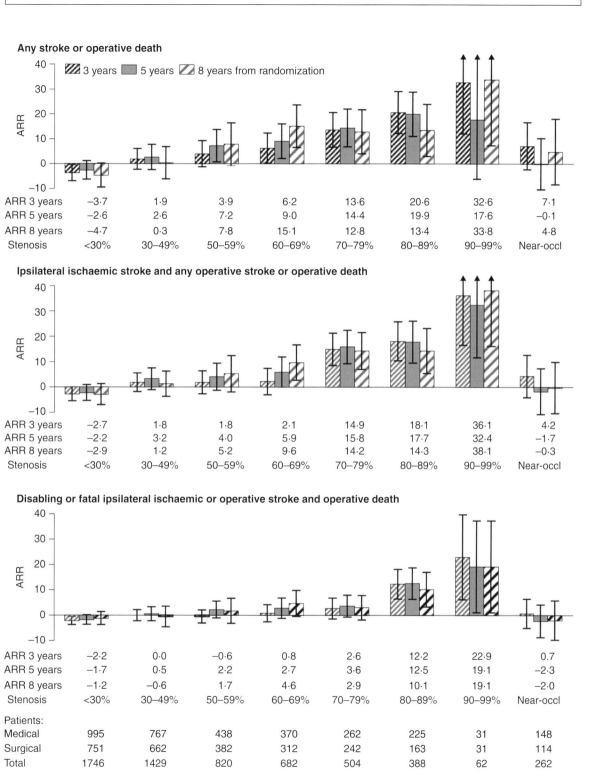

Figure 20.2 Net benefit of carotid endarterectomy treatment above that of medical treatment alone shown as absolute risk reduction for various trial outcomes at different degrees of symptomatic carotid stenosis and follow-up times, analysed by intention-to-treat using data pooled from ECST, NASCET, and VA309. Near-occl = near-occlusion.

Reproduced from Rothwell et al. (2003b) with permission.

Review: Carotid endarterectomy for symptomatic carotid stenosis

Comparison: I Surgery versus no surgery

Outcome: I Any stroke or operative death

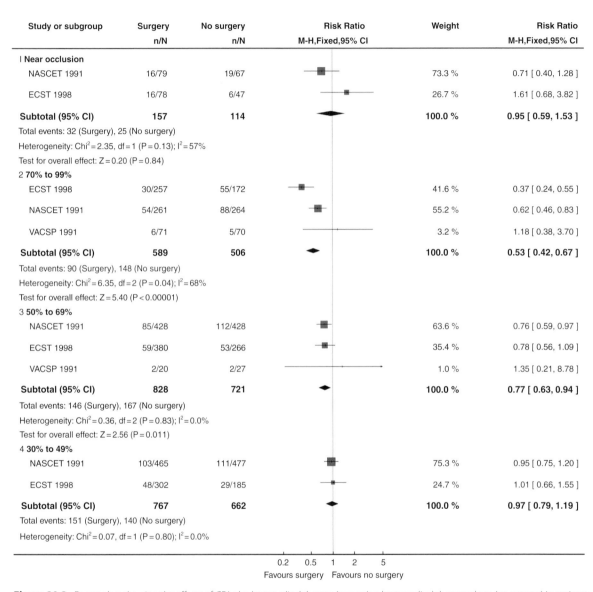

Study or subgroup	Surgery n/N	No surgery n/N	Risk Ratio M-H,Fixed,95% CI	Weight	Risk Ratio M-H,Fixed,95% CI
I Near occlusion					
NASCET 1991	16/79	19/67		73.3 %	0.71 [0.40, 1.28]
ECST 1998	16/78	6/47		26.7 %	1.61 [0.68, 3.82]
Subtotal (95% CI)	**157**	**114**		**100.0 %**	**0.95 [0.59, 1.53]**
Total events: 32 (Surgery), 25 (No surgery)					
Heterogeneity: Chi² = 2.35, df = 1 (P = 0.13); I² = 57%					
Test for overall effect: Z = 0.20 (P = 0.84)					
2 70% to 99%					
ECST 1998	30/257	55/172		41.6 %	0.37 [0.24, 0.55]
NASCET 1991	54/261	88/264		55.2 %	0.62 [0.46, 0.83]
VACSP 1991	6/71	5/70		3.2 %	1.18 [0.38, 3.70]
Subtotal (95% CI)	**589**	**506**		**100.0 %**	**0.53 [0.42, 0.67]**
Total events: 90 (Surgery), 148 (No surgery)					
Heterogeneity: Chi² = 6.35, df = 2 (P = 0.04); I² = 68%					
Test for overall effect: Z = 5.40 (P < 0.00001)					
3 50% to 69%					
NASCET 1991	85/428	112/428		63.6 %	0.76 [0.59, 0.97]
ECST 1998	59/380	53/266		35.4 %	0.78 [0.56, 1.09]
VACSP 1991	2/20	2/27		1.0 %	1.35 [0.21, 8.78]
Subtotal (95% CI)	**828**	**721**		**100.0 %**	**0.77 [0.63, 0.94]**
Total events: 146 (Surgery), 167 (No surgery)					
Heterogeneity: Chi² = 0.36, df = 2 (P = 0.83); I² = 0.0%					
Test for overall effect: Z = 2.56 (P = 0.011)					
4 30% to 49%					
NASCET 1991	103/465	111/477		75.3 %	0.95 [0.75, 1.20]
ECST 1998	48/302	29/185		24.7 %	1.01 [0.66, 1.55]
Subtotal (95% CI)	**767**	**662**		**100.0 %**	**0.97 [0.79, 1.19]**
Total events: 151 (Surgery), 140 (No surgery)					
Heterogeneity: Chi² = 0.07, df = 1 (P = 0.80); I² = 0.0%					

0.2   0.5   1   2   5

Favours surgery   Favours no surgery

Figure 20.3 Forest plots showing the effects of *CEA plus best medical therapy (surgery)* vs best medical therapy alone (no surgery) in patients with recently symptomatic carotid stenosis *in subgroups of severity of carotid stenosis* (1, near occlusion; 2, 70–99%; 3, 50–69%; and 4, 30–49%). Reproduced from Orrapin and Rerkasem (2017) with permission.

Subgroup analyses of pooled data from ECST and NASCET revealed that the effectiveness of CEA in patients with severe symptomatic carotid stenosis was modified significantly by three clinical variables: the patients' sex (P = 0.003), age (p = 0.03), and time from the last symptomatic event to randomization (p = 0.009) (Rothwell et al., 2004). Benefit from surgery was greatest in men, patients aged ≥75 years, and patients randomized within 2 weeks after their last ischaemic event, and fell rapidly with increasing delay. For patients with ≥50% stenosis, the number of patients needed to undergo surgery (NNT) to prevent one ipsilateral stroke in 5 years was 9 for men versus 36 for women, 5 for age ≥75 versus 18 for age <65 years, and 5 for patients randomized within 2 weeks after their last ischaemic event versus 125 for patients randomized at >12 weeks (Rothwell, 2005). These observations were consistent across the 50–69% and ≥70% stenosis groups and similar trends were present in both ECST and NASCET (Figure 20.4).

Sex

Women had a lower risk of ipsilateral ischaemic stroke on medical treatment and a higher operative risk in comparison to men. For recently symptomatic carotid stenosis, surgery is very clearly beneficial in women with ≥70% stenosis, but not in women with 50–69% stenosis (Figure 20.5). In contrast, surgery reduced the 5-year absolute risk of stroke by 8.0% (3.4–12.5) in men with 50–69% stenosis. This sex difference was statistically significant even when the analysis of the interaction was confined to the 50–69% stenosis group.

Age

Benefit from CEA increased with age in patients with recently symptomatic stenosis, particularly in patients aged over 75 years because of their high risk of stroke on medical treatment without a substantially increased risk of peri-operative stroke (Figure 20.4). These findings are consistent with a systematic review of all published surgical case series which reported no increase in the operative risk of stroke and death in older age groups (Rothwell, 2005).

There is therefore no justification for withholding CEA in patients aged over 75 years who are deemed to be medically fit to undergo surgery.

Timing of CEA

Given the high early risk of stroke on medical treatment alone after a TIA or minor stroke in patients with carotid disease (Lovett et al., 2003, 2004; Coull et al., 2004) and the lack of an increased operative risk in neurologically stable patients (see above), early surgery is likely to be most effective. The pooled analysis of data from the trials shows that the benefit from endarterectomy is greatest in patients randomized within 2 weeks of their last event (Figures 20.4 and 20.5). This was particularly important in patients with 50–69% stenosis, where the reduction in the 5-year risk of stroke with surgery was considerable in those who were randomized within 2 weeks of their last event (14.8%, 95% CI: 6.2–23.4), but minimal in patients randomized later (Figure 20.5). It should be borne in mind that surgery was often delayed by up to a week or two after patients were randomized in the RCTs and therefore the benefit of surgery might extend for a week or two longer between symptoms and the date of surgery.

Other Prognostic Factors

Benefit from surgery is probably also greatest in patients presenting with stroke, intermediate in those with cerebral TIA, and lowest in those with retinal events (see Figure 20.4). There was also a trend in the trials towards greater benefit in patients with irregular plaque than a smooth plaque.

The outcome within the ECST of individuals with different characteristics that influence future risk of stroke have been incorporated into a model that predicts the 5-year ipsilateral risk of stroke on medical treatment alone in patients with recently symptomatic carotid stenosis. Although this model was derived from the ECST, it was validated externally using data from NASCET after the ECST angiograms and outcome event definitions were re-analysed to match NASCET (Rothwell and Warlow, 1999; Rothwell et al., 2005). The ECST model showed an excellent fit with the NASCET data (Figure 20.6).

Rothwell and colleagues (2005) provided colour-coded tables to allow clinicians to quickly assess an individual patient's 5-year risk of ipsilateral stroke treated medically from five clinically important variables (Figure 20.7). It should be noted that because the data used to calculate the risk of stroke plotted in Figures 20.6 and 20.7 was derived from ECST, the results are likely to overestimate the current risks of stroke on modern medical therapy in patients being considered for surgery in the current era. Various stands of evidence suggest that current rates of stroke in patients with carotid stenosis treated optimally are now at least half those recorded in ECST and NASCCET (Cheng and Brown, 2017).

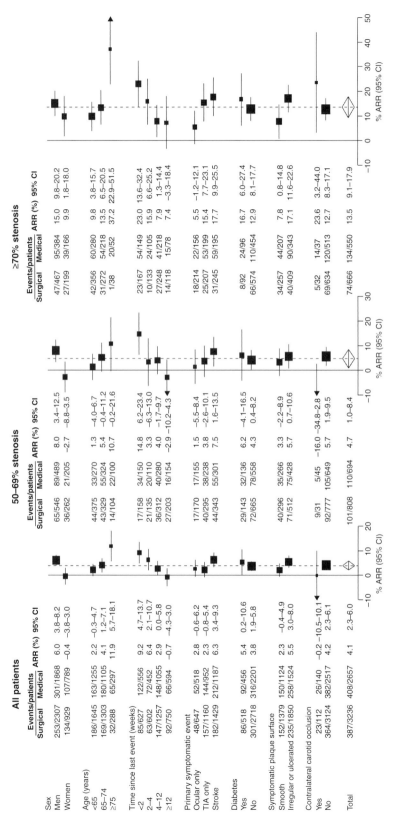

Figure 20.4 Numbers of events and absolute risk reduction (ARR) in 5-year actuarial risk of ipsilateral carotid territory ischaemic stroke or any stroke or death within 30 days after trial surgery according to pre-defined subgroups in all patients, patients with 50–69% stenosis, and those with ≥70% stenosis.

Reproduced from Rothwell et al. (2004), with permission from the authors and Elsevier Limited, publishers of the *Lancet*.

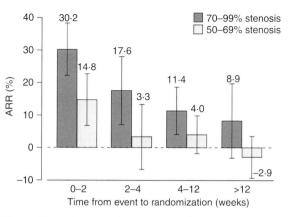

Figure 20.5 Absolute risk reduction (ARR) in 5-year cumulative risk of ipsilateral carotid territory ischaemic stroke or any stroke or death within 30 days after surgery plotted separately for patients with 70–99% stenosis (excluding near-occlusion) and those with 50–69% stenosis stratified by the time from last symptomatic event to randomization. Numbers above bars indicate actual absolute risk reduction. Vertical bars are 95% CIs.

Reproduced from Rothwell et al. (2004), with permission.

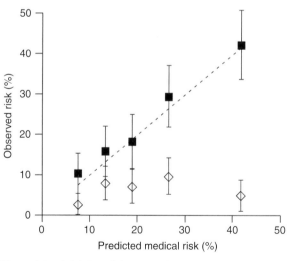

Figure 20.6 Reliability of the ECST risk model in predicting the 5-year rate of ipsilateral ischaemic stroke on medical treatment alone in patients with 50–99% stenosis included in NASCET (filled squares). The 30-day risk of operative stroke in patients randomized to surgery in NASCET stratified by predicted risk on medical treatment is shown to demonstrate that patients at high risk when treated medically did not have a high risk from surgery.

Reproduced from Rothwell et al. (2005) with permission.

Types of CEA

Local vs General Anaesthetic for CEA: Evidence

Although CEA dramatically reduces the risk of stroke in patients with recently symptomatic severe ICA stenosis, the benefit is dependent on maintaining a lower peri-operative stroke risk. For many years, the optimal anaesthetic technique during CEA was controversial. Those favouring local or regional anaesthesia argued that it was safer in terms of medical complications and allowed the patient to be monitored for neurological deficits during surgery. The issue was resolved by the results of a large randomized trial (General Anaesthetic vs Local Anaesthetic, GALA), which showed no significant difference in major outcomes between patients allocated to either anaesthetic technique (GALA Trial Collaborative Group, 2008). A slight reduction in stroke with local anaesthesia was offset by an increase in myocardial infarction. Thus, the choice between the two techniques is a matter for the individual surgeon taking into account their own and the patient's preference.

Eversion vs Conventional CEA

CEA is conventionally undertaken by a longitudinal arteriotomy. Eversion CEA, which employs a transverse arteriotomy and reimplantation of the carotid artery, has been reported to be associated with low peri-operative stroke and restenosis rates but an increased risk of complications associated with a distal intimal flap.

Evidence

A Cochrane review of 5 RCTs evaluating whether eversion CEA was safe and more effective than conventional CEA in a total of 2465 patients reported no significant differences between eversion and conventional CEA techniques in the rate of peri-operative stroke and/or death (1.7% eversion CEA vs 2.6% conventional CEA, OR 0.44, 95% CI: 0.10–1.82), and stroke during follow-up (1.4% vs 1.7%; OR 0.84, 95% CI: 0.43–1.64) (Cao et al., 2001).

Although eversion CEA was associated with a significantly lower rate of restenosis >50% during follow-up than conventional CEA (2.5% eversion vs 5.2% conventional, Peto OR 0.48, 95% CI: 0.32–0.72), there was no evidence that the eversion technique for CEA was associated with a lower rate of neurological events when compared to conventional CEA.

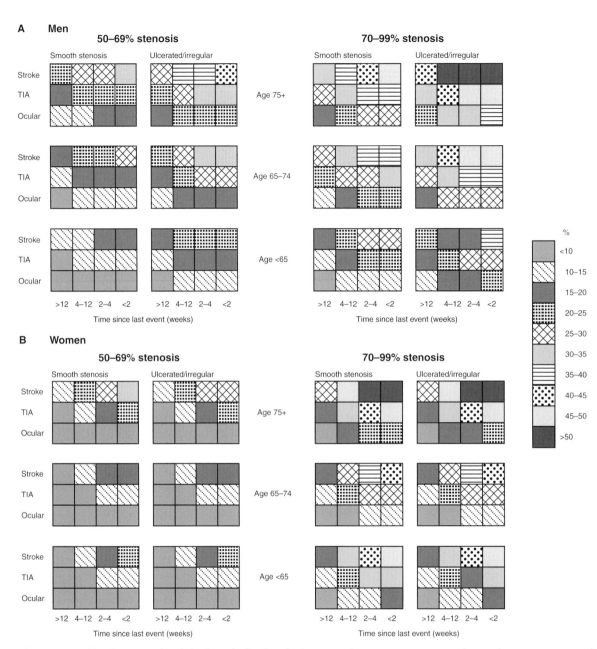

Figure 20.7 Tables showing predicted absolute risk of ipsilateral ischaemic stroke at 5 years in patients with recently symptomatic carotid stenosis treated with medical therapy alone according to five clinically important patient characteristics in (A) men and (B) women. This table was derived from ECST data using a Cox regression model. The terms Stroke, TIA, and Ocular in the tables refer to the most severe symptomatic ipsilateral ischaemic event in the past 6 months.

Reproduced from Rothwell et al. (2005) with permission.

There were no statistically significant differences in local complications between the eversion and conventional group.

A more recent systemic review came to very similar conclusions from the 5 available RCTs, but also included published case series comparing outcomes of eversion with conventional CEA. Among the case series ($N = 20,270$ patients), eversion CEA was associated with significantly lower rates of peri-operative 30-day rates of stroke or death (2.26% vs 4.32%, OR 0.52, 95% CI: 0.44–0.61) and late restenosis >50% (2.34% vs 4.68%, OR 0.49, 95% CI: 0.25–0.94)

(Paraskevas et al., 2018). There were no significant differences in cranial nerve injury or neck haematoma rates.

Conventional CEA included patients undergoing either primary closure or patch closure of the arteriotomy after removal of the plaque. In a separate analysis of both the RCTs and the case series, the authors found no difference between outcome event rates when eversion CEA was compared with the conventional CEA patients who had patch closure (30-day stroke or death rate: 2.35% vs 3.31%, OR 0.64, 95% CI: 0.35–1.18) (Paraskevas et al., 2018).

Comment

Interpretation of the Evidence

There is insufficient evidence from randomized trials to reliably determine the RRs and benefits of eversion and conventional CEA. It is possible that carotid eversion is associated with a lower risk of long-term carotid occlusion and restenosis, but it is still unclear whether this is associated with a lower rate of subsequent neurological events. The recent meta-analysis of case series suggests that eversion CEA is safer and more durable than conventional CEA with primary closure, but eversion CEA has similar outcomes to conventional patched CEA. Patching is discussed in more detail below.

Implications for Practice

Until more reliable evidence is available, the choice of the surgical technique for CEA should depend on the experience and preference of the operating surgeon.

Implications for Research

Further randomized trials are needed to more precisely define the relative and absolute benefits and risks of eversion and conventional CEA, and establish the clinically relevance (or not) of restenosis of the carotid artery (that was previously operated on) as a cause of subsequent stroke. Studies analysing the costs of eversion and conventional CEA are also needed.

Routine or Selective Carotid Artery Shunting for CEA (and different methods of monitoring in selective shunting)

One of the limitations of CEA is the risk of peri-operative stroke, usually ipsilateral carotid territory ischaemic stroke. Peri-operative stroke can result from temporary interruption of cerebral blood flow while the carotid artery is clamped during CEA if collateral flow from the contralateral carotid artery or via the vertebrobasilar circulation is compromised. The duration of interrupted blood flow to the brain can be minimized by bridging the clamped section of the artery with a shunt. Potential disadvantages of shunting include complications such as air and plaque embolism and carotid artery dissection, and an increased risk of local complications such as nerve injury, haematoma, infection, and long-term restenosis. However, reliable data on these risks and the potential benefits are limited. Consequently, some surgeons advocate routine shunting, whereas others prefer to use shunts selectively or avoid them altogether.

Evidence

A Cochrane systematic review of the effect of routine vs selective, or never, shunting during CEA identified six trials involving 1270 patients (Chongruksut et al., 2014). Three trials with 686 patients compared routine shunting with no shunting, one trial with 200 patients compared routine shunting with selective shunting, one trial with 253 patients compared selective shunting with and without near-infrared refractory spectroscopy monitoring, and the other trial with 131 patients compared shunting with a combination of electroencephalographic and carotid pressure measurement with shunting by carotid pressure measurement alone. In general, the authors considered that the trial quality was poor.

For routine versus no shunting, there was no significant difference in the rate of all stroke, ipsilateral stroke or death up to 30 days after surgery, although data were limited.

No significant difference was found between selective shunting with and without near-infrared refractory spectroscopy monitoring, although again the numbers were small.

There was no significant difference in the risk of ipsilateral stroke in patients selected for shunting with the combination of electroencephalogram (EEG) and carotid pressure assessment compared with pressure assessment alone, although again the data were limited.

Comment

Implications for Practice

There is insufficient evidence from RCTs to support or refute the use of routine or selective shunting during CEA and there is little evidence to support the use of one form of monitoring over another in selecting patients requiring a shunt. The use of EEG monitoring combined with carotid pressure assessment may reduce the number of shunts required without increasing the stroke rate, but more data are required to prove this.

Implications for Research

A large, multicentre randomized trial is required to assess whether shunting reduces the risk of peri-operative and long-term death and stroke. Even a modest 25% reduction in the RR of peri-operative stroke or death would result in approximately 15 fewer strokes and deaths per 1000 patients undergoing endarterectomy. However, to detect this reliably (80% power, 5% significance level) would require between 3000 and 5000 patients.

Two policies could be considered: routine shunting for all patients undergoing CEA or selective shunting in those at high risk of intra-operative cerebral ischaemia. The trial needs to be truly randomized, have long-term follow-up (several years), and have blinded outcome assessment, preferably by neurologists. Patients should be stratified by age, sex, degree of ipsilateral and contralateral internal carotid stenosis, the experience of the surgeon, the use of patching, and, in selective shunting, the method of monitoring of cerebral ischaemia.

As regards the method of monitoring in selective shunting, until the efficacy of shunting has been demonstrated, further trials of the method of monitoring are probably not merited. However, a systematic review of the sensitivity and specificity of the various methods of monitoring for cerebral ischaemia would be worthwhile to identify the best method of monitoring to be used in any trial of selective shunting.

Patch Angioplasty vs Primary Closure for CEA

When undertaking a CEA, many surgeons use a patch of autologous vein, or synthetic material, to close the artery, to enlarge the lumen, and, so they hope, to reduce the risk of restenosis and stroke. However, it remains uncertain whether carotid patch angioplasty (with either a venous or a synthetic patch) reduces the risk of carotid artery restenosis and subsequent ischaemic stroke compared with primary closure of the ICA.

Evidence

A Cochrane systematic review of RCTs assessing the safety and efficacy of routine or selective carotid patch angioplasty compared with CEA with primary closure identified 7 trials involving 1967 patients undergoing 2157 operations (Rerkasem and Rothwell, 2009). Follow-up varied from hospital discharge to 5 years. The quality of trials included in the review was judged to be generally poor. Nevertheless, use of a carotid patch was associated with a reduction in the risk of ipsilateral stroke both during the peri-operative period (OR 0.31, 95% CI: 0.15–0.63) and over long-term follow-up (OR 0.32, 95% CI: 0.16–0.63). Patching was also associated with a lower risk of peri-operative carotid occlusion (OR 0.18, 95% CI: 0.08–0.41), and decreased restenosis during long-term follow-up (OR 0.24, 95% CI: 0.17–0.34).

Very few arterial complications, including haemorrhage, infection, cranial nerve palsies and pseudoaneurysm formation, were recorded with either patch or primary closure.

No significant correlation was found between use of patch angioplasty and the risk of either peri-operative or long-term all-cause death rates.

Comment

Interpretation of the Evidence

Limited evidence suggests that carotid patch angioplasty might reduce the risk of peri-operative arterial occlusion and restenosis, and longer-term stroke or death.

Implications for Practice

Although some vascular surgeons do not routinely use patching in patients undergoing CEA, the present data from RCTs (albeit based on small numbers) appear to support a recommendation in favour of routine patching.

The use of selective patching (e.g. for very narrow arteries) has not been studied in RCTs, so no evidence-based recommendations can be made.

Implications for Research

The potential benefit of routine patching could be clinically important (up to 40 strokes prevented per 1000 patients treated) but in order to have reliable evidence on the risks and benefits of patching compared to primary closure, a large multicentre RCT will be required.

This trial should concentrate on clinical outcomes (deaths, all strokes, particularly fatal or disabling strokes, and ipsilateral strokes) as opposed to restenosis and have long-term follow-up (perhaps 5 years).

Assuming a 30-day risk of stroke or death of 5%, the trial would need to recruit about 3000 patients to have an 90% chance of detecting a reduction in the absolute risk of death or stroke to 2.5% (this number would also give a >90% chance of detecting a reduction in the risk of stroke or death at 5 years from 25% to 20%). Such a trial should use a secure method of randomization and be performed on a truly intention-to-treat basis with complete follow-up of all patients. Patients rather than arteries should be randomized so that the number of deaths and strokes is reported on a patient basis rather than an artery basis. Clinical follow-up should be blinded with independent assessment of strokes, preferably by neurologists. The results should be analysed according to the degree of narrowing of the artery and whether the patient had had a previous stroke or TIA or not. It would be possible to use a factorial design for such a trial so that some other procedure could be tested simultaneously, such as routine shunting. Until the benefit of carotid patching in terms of clinical outcomes for the patient is established, any future trials should include a control group of primary closure.

Patches of Different Types for Carotid Patch Angioplasty during Carotid Endarterectomy

Although CEA is effective in patients with symptomatic carotid stenosis, it is not clear whether different surgical techniques affect the outcome, and whether the use of carotid patch angioplasty is superior to primary closure in reducing the risk of restenosis and improving both short- and long-term clinical outcome. Consequently, many vascular surgeons use carotid patching either routinely or selectively. Among those who do use carotid patching, however, there is debate over the choice of patch material. Vein patching (usually harvested from the saphenous vein and sometimes from the jugular vein) is favoured by some because it is easily available, easy to handle and possibly has a greater resistance to infection. Synthetic material, such as Dacron or polytetrafluoroethylene (PTFE), is favoured by others who feel that it offers a lower risk of patch rupture and aneurysmal dilatation, and also that it spares the morbidity associated with saphenous vein harvesting and leaves the vein which may be required for coronary bypass grafting at a later date. It is also possible that one type of synthetic material is better than the other. Furthermore, there are less commonly used materials such as bovine pericardium which have yet to be widely accepted.

Evidence

A systematic review of 13 RCTs of the safety and efficacy of different materials for carotid patch angioplasty in 2083 operations identified seven trials comparing vein closure with PTFE closure, and six comparing Dacron grafts with other synthetic materials (Rerkasem and Rothwell, 2010). In most of the trials a patient could be randomized twice so that each carotid artery was randomized to a different treatment group.

There were no significant differences in the outcomes between vein patches and synthetic materials, except that there were fewer pseudoaneurysms associated with synthetic patches than vein patches (OR 0.09, 95% CI: 0.02–0.49). However, the numbers were small and the clinical significance of this finding uncertain.

Compared to other synthetic patches, Dacron was associated with a higher risk of peri-operative stroke or TIA ($p = 0.03$); restenosis at 30 days ($p = 0.004$); peri-operative stroke ($p = 0.07$); and peri-operative carotid thrombosis ($p = 0.1$). During follow-up for more than 1 year, there were also significantly more strokes ($p = 0.03$) and arterial restenoses ($p < 0.0001$) with Dacron, but again the numbers of outcomes were small and the significance uncertain.

Comment

Interpretation of the Evidence

It is likely that the differences between different types of patch material are very small. Consequently, more data than are currently available will be required to establish whether any differences do exist.

Some evidence exists that PTFE patches may be superior to collagen impregnated Dacron grafts in terms of peri-operative stroke rates and restenosis. However, the evidence is limited and more studies that compare different types of synthetic graft are required to make firm conclusions.

Pseudo-aneurysm formation might be more common after use of a vein patch compared with a synthetic patch.

Implications for Practice

There is no evidence to support the use of vein over synthetic patch material in CEA. The decision of which type of patch to use, if any, remains a matter of individual preference. However, if synthetic material is used, the currently available (limited) evidence from a single trial appears to show benefits from PTFE as opposed to Dacron material.

Implications for Research

Further trials comparing one type of patch with another are required, but they will need large numbers of patients. Further, more trials are required which compare different types of synthetic graft material.

Adjunct Medical Therapies after Carotid Endarterectomy

Antiplatelet Therapy

Antiplatelet drugs are effective and safe for TIA and ischaemic stroke patients in preventing recurrent vascular events, and for patients undergoing vascular surgical procedures in reducing the risk of graft or native vessel occlusion. However, this does not necessarily mean they are effective and safe after CEA.

Evidence

Antiplatelet vs Control

A systematic review of RCTs evaluating whether antiplatelet agents are safe and beneficial after CEA (Engelter and Lyrer, 2003, 2004) identified six trials of antiplatelet therapy administered for at least 30 days after CEA in a total of 907 patients who were followed up for at least 3 months. Most trials used high dose aspirin alone or in combination with other antiplatelet drugs.

Antiplatelet therapy was associated with a significant reduction in the odds of stroke of any type during follow-up (OR 0.58, 95% CI: 0.34–0.98; $p = 0.04$) but not death (OR 0.77, 95% CI: 0.48–1.24), intracranial haemorrhage (OR 1.71, 95% CI: 0.73–4.03), or other serious vascular events.

Aspirin Plus Clopidogrel vs Aspirin

Given the high risk of recurrence in patients with recent symptoms despite aspirin therapy, it is logical to try to improve medical therapy in patients waiting for CEA. One such approach is to use combined antiplatelet therapy. In one study, 100 patients were assigned aspirin 150 mg per day for 4 weeks prior to CEA and then, on the night before CEA, they were randomized to placebo plus long-term aspirin 150 mg per day ($n = 54$) or clopidogrel 75 mg per day plus long-term aspirin 150 mg per day ($n = 46$) (Payne et al., 2004). Compared with placebo plus aspirin, assignment to clopidogrel plus aspirin was associated with a small (8.8%) but significant reduction in platelet response to adenosine diphosphate (ADP) ($p = 0.05$), a 10-fold reduction in the RR of patients having >20 emboli detected by TCD within 3 hours of CEA (OR 10.23, 95% CI: 1.3–83.3; $P = 0.01$), and a significantly increased time from flow restoration to skin closure (an indirect marker of haemostasis) ($P = 0.04$). Surgeons often report increased bleeding in patients taking combined aspirin and clopidogrel, but in this study there was no increase in bleeding complications or blood transfusions.

These results are supported by the Clopidogrel and Aspirin for Reduction of Emboli in Symptomatic carotid Stenosis (CARESS) trial, which has shown that among patients with symptomatic carotid stenosis (before, not after, CEA), that the addition of clopidogrel to aspirin reduces the incidence of cerebral microemboli before (not after) CEA. The CARESS study was a randomized, double-blind, controlled trial comparing clopidogrel plus aspirin versus aspirin in 107 patients with recently (past 3 months) symptomatic carotid artery stenosis >50% and at least one characteristic microembolic signal (MES) detected during a 1-hour TCD recording of the ipsilateral middle cerebral artery (MCA) before randomization. At randomization, patients were assigned either a 300 mg loading dose of clopidogrel (four tablets), followed by 75 mg clopidogrel once daily from day 2 to day 7 ± 1, or a matching placebo loading dose, and once daily placebo from day 2 to day 7 ± 1. Patients in both arms also received 75 mg aspirin (ASA) once daily from day 1 to day 7 ± 1 (on top of clopidogrel or placebo). All study drugs were administered orally. The primary efficacy endpoint was the occurrence of ≥ 1 MES versus none (MES positive or negative patient), detected by off-line analysis (by central reading centre) of the 1-hour recording carried out on day 7 ± 1. Intention-to-treat analysis revealed a significant reduction in the primary endpoint: 43.8% of dual-therapy patients were MES positive on day 7, as compared with 72.7% of monotherapy patients (relative risk reduction 39.8%, 95% CI: 13.8–58.0; $p = 0.0046$) (Markus et al., 2005).

Comment

Interpretation of the Evidence

Antiplatelet drugs reduce the odds of stroke after CEA, but not other major outcomes. However, a statistically significant hazardous effect of antiplatelet therapy may have been missed because of the relatively small sample size.

There is some evidence that the combination of clopidogrel and aspirin might be more effective than aspirin alone in reducing post-operative thromboemboli, as detected by TCD (Payne et al., 2004). Data from several studies suggest that the presence of asymptomatic embolization, as measured by TCD evidence of MESs, might predict future strokes or TIAs in patients with symptomatic stenosis; the risk is reported to be 8- to 31-fold higher in patients who are MES positive (or who have ≥1 MES per TCD recording) than patients who have MES negative ICA stenosis (Valton et al., 1998; Molloy and Markus, 1999).

Implications for Practice

Antiplatelet therapy should be prescribed for all patients after CEA. Aspirin should probably be the first-line agent. Other antiplatelet agents such as clopidogrel and extended-release dipyridamole plus aspirin have also been shown to be effective in patients with TIA and ischaemic stroke not undergoing CEA (Chapter 9), and are likely (based on reasoning [Chapter 2], but not evidence) to also be effective after CEA. Many physicians and surgeons routinely prescribe the combination of aspirin and clopidogrel after TIA or stroke up to the time of CEA and then continue single therapy after surgery.

Implications for Research

Further research should focus on the effectiveness and safety of combinations of aspirin with other antiplatelet drugs.

There is preliminary evidence to suggest that a short period of treatment with aspirin and clopidogrel, for perhaps 1 month, might be more effective than aspirin during the acute phase of the event when patients with symptomatic carotid stenosis are at high risk of recurrent ischaemic events (Payne et al., 2004; Markus et al., 2005). This requires confirming in an adequately powered, dedicated study in a large number of patients with the occurrence of recurrent stroke, other serious vascular events, and bleeding complications as the primary outcome measure.

Anticoagulation

Evidence

There is no evidence to support the use of anticoagulation in patients with recently symptomatic carotid stenosis who are in sinus rhythm (Chapter 10). Warfarin with a target international normalized ratio (INR) of 3–4.5 was harmful in the Stroke Prevention in Reversible Ischaemia Trial (SPIRIT) Study Group (1997), and there was no additional benefit over aspirin from warfarin at a mean INR of 1.8 (target INR 1.4–2.8) in the WARSS trial (Warfarin Aspirin Recurrent Stroke Study Group, 2001) (Chapter 19).

No trials have evaluated warfarin vs aspirin specifically in patients with carotid disease (carotid stenosis [>50%] was an exclusion criterion in the WARSS trial).

Comment
Implications for Practice

As the effect of warfarin in patients with symptomatic carotid stenosis undergoing CEA is likely to be qualitatively similar to that seen in other patients with TIA and ischaemic stroke due to arterial disease (based on reasoning [Chapter 18], not evidence), there is no indication to use oral anticoagulation after CEA. However, an exception can be patients with TIA or ischaemic stroke who have both an apparently symptomatic carotid stenosis *and* atrial fibrillation.

Warfarin is effective and indicated in patients with TIA or ischaemic stroke who are in atrial fibrillation (Chapter 18). The decision to recommend anticoagulation and/or endarterectomy in these patients depends to some extent on whether the recent TIA or stroke is thought to be cardioembolic or due to carotid thromboembolism. This is can be difficult, if not impossible, to determine sometimes. But if the computed tomography (CT) or magnetic resonance imaging (MRI) (diffusion-weighted imaging, DWI) brain scan shows multiple recent infarcts in multiple vascular territories, or echocardiography reveals apical thrombus or atrial enlargement, the source is likely to be the heart and anticoagulation is probably indicated. Alternatively, if echocardiography is normal and perhaps if any ischaemic lesions on brain imaging are confined to the ipsilateral carotid territory, it may be more appropriate to recommend endarterectomy and antiplatelet therapy.

Lowering Blood Pressure

Evidence

Lowering blood pressure effectively reduces the risk of recurrent stroke and other serious vascular events

(Chapter 15) (PROGRESS Collaborative Group, 2001), but the effect in different aetiological subtypes of ischaemic stroke, such as symptomatic carotid stenosis, is unknown.

Among patients with bilateral severe, flow-limiting (≥70%) carotid stenosis who were randomized to best *medical* treatment alone in ECST and NASCET, the risk of subsequent stroke was significantly increased if their SBP at randomization was <130 mm Hg (hazard ratio [HR] 6.0, 95% CI: 2.4–14.7) or 130–149 mm Hg (HR 2.5, 95% CI: 1.5–4.4) compared with patients with bilateral non-flow-limiting carotid stenosis <70% (Rothwell et al., 2003c). There was no increase in stroke risk with higher SBP of 150 mm Hg or more. The 5-year risk of stroke in patients with bilateral ≥70% stenosis was 64.3% in those with SBP <150 mm Hg (median value) versus 24.2% in those with higher blood pressures (p = 0.002).

However, among patients with bilateral severe, flow-limiting (≥70%) carotid stenosis who were randomized to CEA (plus best medical treatment) in ECST and NASCET, the 5-year risk of stroke in patients with bilateral ≥70% stenosis was not significantly different in those with SBP <150 mm Hg (median value) at randomization compared with higher blood pressures (13.4% vs 18.3%, P = 0.6).

Comment

Interpretation of the Evidence

The data from the ECST and NASCET suggest that aggressive lowering of SBP might be harmful in patients with bilateral severe carotid stenosis or severe symptomatic stenosis with contralateral occlusion if they have not undergone CEA. Otherwise, blood pressure lowering is likely to be safe and beneficial in patients with only unilateral ≥70% stenosis (and following endarterectomy on one side in patients with bilateral severe carotid stenosis or severe symptomatic stenosis with contralateral occlusion) (Rothwell et al., 2003c).

Implications for Practice

It is likely that most patients with symptomatic carotid stenosis will benefit from gradual blood pressure lowering. However, the data from the ECST and NASCET suggest that aggressive lowering of SBP without endarterectomy might be harmful in patients with bilateral severe carotid stenosis or severe symptomatic stenosis with contralateral

occlusion (Rothwell et al., 2003c). These patients often also have disease of the vertebral arteries, the carotid siphon and the cerebral arteries (Thiele et al., 1980; Gorelick, 1993); a loss of the normal autoregulatory capacity of the cerebral circulation, such that cerebral blood flow is directly dependent on perfusion pressure (Van der Grond et al., 1995; Grubb et al., 1998); and a high risk of recurrent stroke (Spence, 2000).

Lowering Blood Cholesterol

Evidence

Lowering blood cholesterol, by means of statin drugs, significantly reduces the risk of all serious vascular events, especially myocardial infarction, in patients with a history of symptomatic cardiovascular disease, including stroke or TIA (Heart Protection Study Collaborative Group, 2004). Initially, the extent to which statins reduced recurrent stroke rates was uncertain, but then the Stroke Prevention by Aggressive Reduction in Cholesterol Levels (SPARCL) study convincingly demonstrated that high dose statin therapy (atorvastatin 80 mg daily) significantly reduced the rate of recurrent stroke in patients with recent TIA or stroke (Stroke Prevention by Aggressive Reduction in Cholesterol Levels [SPARCL] Investigators, 2006). Statins also slow the progression of atheroma progression in patients with carotid plaque (Mercuri et al., 1996). In keeping with these observations, a subgroup analysis of the SPARCL study showed that in patients known to have carotid artery stenosis, treatment with atorvastatin was associated with a 33% reduction in the risk of any stroke (HR 0.67, 95% CI: 0.47, 0.94), as well as a 43% reduction in risk of major coronary events (HR 0.57, 95% CI: 0.32–1.00). Carotid revascularization procedures were also reduced by 56% (HR 0.44, 95% CI: 0.24–0.79) in the group randomized to atorvastatin (Sillesen et al., 2008).

Comment

Implications for Practice

Given the evidence that high-dose statin therapy reduces the risk of recurrent stroke in patients with cerebrovascular disease and also specifically in patients with carotid disease, treatment with statin at a dose equivalent to at least 80 mg atorvastatin daily is clearly indicated in patients with symptomatic carotid stenosis before and after CEA.

Implications for Research

Medical therapy in general has improved considerably since the first ECST and NASCET were completed, and specifically, the widespread use of statins, fewer patients smoking, and better blood pressure control have reduced rates of recurrent stroke by about half in most studies. Thus, it can no longer be assumed that surgery is better than optimal modern medical therapy at preventing recurrent stroke, especially in patients with characteristics (e.g. moderate degrees of stenosis), suggesting a lower risk of recurrent stroke. Only one ongoing trial is currently investigating surgery and stenting for patients with symptomatic carotid stenosis, the Second European Carotid Surgery Trial (ECST-2). This RCT compares revascularization by endarterectomy or stenting versus optimized medical therapy alone in patients with asymptomatic or low-to-intermediate risk symptomatic carotid stenosis. ECST-2 is therefore selecting patients using the Carotid Artery Risk (CAR) score that identifies patients eligible to participate with a 5-year risk of ipsilateral stroke on medical therapy alone estimated as being <20%. The trial will therefore provide data validating the CAR score. ECST-2 also incorporates MRI brain and MR plaque imaging at baseline, with MRI follow-up at 2 and 5 years after randomization, which will allow investigation of MRI markers of risk and the use of silent brain infarction as an outcome measure.

Carotid Artery Stenting

Transluminal angioplasty was initially undertaken in the 1960s in the limbs (Dotter et al., 1967) and later in the renal, coronary, and then cerebral arteries. Despite apprehension about the risks of plaque rupture and embolism to the brain causing stroke, angioplasty, and later on primary stenting, at the carotid bifurcation has increased in the past 20 years. Advantages of endovascular treatment of carotid stenosis over endarterectomy were perceived to be the avoidance of general discomfort associated with surgery, a lower rate of access complications (haematoma, wound infection, cranial nerve palsy), and a reduction in general side effects of cardiovascular surgery such as myocardial infarction. In recent years, several large RCTs have therefore compared CAS to the standard surgical treatment (CEA) for carotid stenosis. Until quite recently, little had been known on the long-term safety and efficacy of CAS. CEA on the

other hand, has been shown to be effective in preventing ipsilateral stroke in symptomatic and asymptomatic carotid stenosis over long-term follow-up periods of 10 years or longer. In the last few years, however, several trials published results of extended follow-up providing more detailed insight into how the two treatments compare with regard to their efficacy to prevent stroke in the long term.

In the present chapter, we have summarized the main results of the large trials and updated our previous meta-analysis including all published RCT data (Bonati et al., 2012). We separately provide results for patients with symptomatic or asymptomatic carotid stenosis, and those at normal or elevated perceived surgical risk.

Evidence

Symptomatic Carotid Stenosis

In the past few years, most of the trials comparing CAS with CEA for treatment of symptomatic carotid stenosis completed their long-term follow-up. So far there have been eight RCTs which compared CAS with CEA in patients with symptomatic carotid stenosis (Naylor et al., 1998; Alberts, 2001; Mas et al., 2006; Ringleb et al., 2006; Hoffmann et al., 2008; Steinbauer et al., 2008; International Carotid Stenting Study Investigators et al., 2010), and five trials including both symptomatic and asymptomatic patients (CAVATAS Investigators, 2001; Ling, 2006; Brott et al., 2010; Kuliha et al., 2015).

The first trial on a larger scale was the *Carotid And Vertebral Artery Transluminal Angioplasty Study* (CAVATAS) which randomly assigned 504 patients with mainly symptomatic, severe carotid stenosis to endovascular treatment ($n = 251$) or CEA ($n = 253$) (CAVATAS Investigators, 2001). Among the patients assigned to endovascular treatment, stents were only used in 55 (26%) and balloon angioplasty alone in 158 (74%). Short-term and mid-term results were published in 2001: the rates of major outcome events within 30 days of treatment did not differ significantly between endovascular treatment and surgery (6.4% vs 5.9%, respectively, for disabling stroke or death; 10.0% vs 9.9% for any stroke lasting more than 7 days, or death). Cranial neuropathy was reported in 22 (8.7%) surgery patients, but not after endovascular treatment ($p < 0.0001$). Major groin or neck haematoma occurred less often after endovascular treatment than after surgery (3 [1.2%] vs 17 [6.7%], $p < 0.0015$ [CAVATAS Investigators, 2001]). Patients were followed for a median of 5 years. The 8-year incidence of ipsilateral non-procedural stroke was 11.3% in the endovascular group versus 8.6% in the endarterectomy group (HR 1.22, 95% CI: 0.78–2.14 [Ederle et al., 2009a]).

The first results from large trials investigating primary stenting versus endarterectomy in patients with symptomatic carotid stenosis were published in 2006. The *Endarterectomy versus Angioplasty in Patients with Symptomatic Severe Carotid Stenosis* (EVA-3S) trial included patients with recently symptomatic (within 120 days prior to enrolment) carotid stenosis of >60%, as determined by NASCET criteria (NASCET Collaborators, 1991). The trial was stopped early by the data monitoring committee after inclusion of 527 patients, because the 30-day stroke or death rate was significantly higher in the CAS arm (9.6%) than in the CEA arm (3.9%, $p = 0.01$; [Mas et al., 2006]). Patients were followed for a median of 7.1 and a maximum of 12.4 years. The long-term risk of recurrent ipsilateral stroke beyond the procedural period was similar in both treatment groups. The cumulative risk for the primary endpoint (composite of any ipsilateral stroke after randomization or any procedural stroke or death) was 11.5% in the CAS group versus 7.6% in the CEA group (HR 1.7, 95% CI: 0.95–9.06; $p = 0.07$ [Mas et al., 2014]).

The *Stent-Supported Percutaneous Angioplasty of the Carotid Artery versus Endarterectomy* (SPACE) trial, which also included patients with symptomatic carotid stenosis of ≥50% (according to the NASCET criteria or ≥70% according to ECST criteria), published short-term outcomes in the same year. The trial was stopped after inclusion of 1214 patients for both reasons of futility and lack of funding. Risks of death or stroke between randomization and 30 days after treatment were 7.4% in the CAS group and 6.6% in the CEA group. However, the trial was unable to prove its primary hypothesis that CAS was not inferior to CEA by a predefined margin (Ringleb et al., 2006). Unlike in EVA-3S, patients in SPACE were only followed up for 2 years. The rate of ipsilateral stroke within 2 years including any procedural stroke or death in the intention-to-treat population was 9.5% in the CAS group and 8.8% in the CEA group (Hazard ratio 1.1, 95% CI: 0.75–1.61 [Eckstein et al., 2008]).

In 2010, the *International Carotid Stenting Study* (ICSS) the largest trial comparing CAS versus CEA for symptomatic carotid stenosis with a total of 1713 patients randomized, reported interim findings. ICSS

included patients with symptomatic carotid stenosis of >50% measured according to NASCET criteria. Symptoms attributable to the randomized artery needed to have occurred within 12 months prior to randomization. Patients were randomized in a 1:1 ratio to CAS or CEA. Within the first 120 days of randomization, the primary short-term outcome measure, the combination of stroke, myocardial infarction, or death, occurred in 8.5% of patients randomized to CAS and 5.2% of patients randomized to CEA ($p = 0.006$). Risks of any stroke and all-cause death were both higher in the stenting group than in the endarterectomy group (HR 1.92, 95% CI: 1.27–2.89 and HR 2.76, 95% CI: 1.16–6.56, respectively). This difference was mostly attributable to an excess of non-disabling strokes in the CAS group. Long-term results were published in 2015, showing that stenting was as effective as endarterectomy in preventing fatal or disabling stroke in patients with symptomatic carotid stenosis for up to 10 years after treatment, with cumulative 5-year risks of 6.4% in the CAS group and 6.5% in the CEA group (Bonati et al., 2015). Importantly, the long-term functional outcome as expressed by the level of functional ability measured with the modified Rankin Scale did not differ between the two groups despite the difference in procedural stroke (van Swieten et al., 1988).

In 2011, the North American *Carotid Revascularization Endarterectomy vs Stenting Trial* (CREST), which enrolled 1321 patients with symptomatic and 1181 patients with asymptomatic stenosis, published its results of up to 4 years after randomization (Brott et al., 2010). CREST initially enrolled only patients with symptomatic carotid stenosis, but due to slow enrolment, the eligibility criteria were changed in 2005 to include asymptomatic patients in addition to symptomatic patients. The primary composite endpoint of death, stroke, or myocardial infarction between randomization and 30 days after treatment, or ipsilateral stroke within 4 years after randomization, occurred in 7.2% of CAS and in 6.8% of CEA patients. Among patients with symptomatic carotid stenosis, procedural rates of death or stroke in the CAS arm (6.0%) were lower than in the European trials, but still almost twice as high as in the CEA arm of CREST (3.2%, $p = 0.02$). Long-term follow-up was concluded in 1607 patients with a median duration of follow-up of 7.4 years. There was no significant difference with regard to the primary long-term endpoint which was defined as post-procedural ipsilateral stroke over 10-year follow-up

(6.9% in the CAS group and 5.6% in the CEA group). In addition, no significant difference was found between CAS and CEA with regard to the primary long-term endpoint when asymptomatic and symptomatic patients were analysed separately (Brott et al., 2016).

Asymptomatic Carotid Stenosis

Compared to the wealth of data from RCTs available for patients with symptomatic carotid stenosis, evidence on endovascular treatment for asymptomatic carotid stenosis is limited.

To date there are only two trials, which compared CAS to endarterectomy for treatment of asymptomatic carotid stenosis (CREST [Brott et al., 2016], and ACT-1 [Rosenfield et al., 2016]), while a third, the *Asymptomatic Carotid Surgery Trial 2* (ACST-2 [Bulbulia and Halliday, 2013]), is still ongoing. A fourth trial investigating whether medical therapy alone was equivalent to invasive treatment by CAS or CEA in terms of stroke prevention in patients with asymptomatic carotid stenosis (SPACE-2) was stopped early due to slow recruitment (Eckstein et al., 2016).

In CREST, 1181 patients with asymptomatic carotid stenosis were randomized between CAS and CEA. The risk of procedural stroke or death did not differ significantly between treatments (CAS 2.5%, CEA 1.4%) but the hazard ratio for this outcome, 1.88 (95% CI: 0.79–4.42), was almost identical to the hazard ratio among symptomatic patients in the same trial (1.89, 1.11–3.21). Combining procedural events with ipsilateral strokes during follow-up of up to 10 years after treatment, risks were 8.6% for CAS and 7.9% for CEA in patients with asymptomatic carotid stenosis (HR 1.23, 95% CI: 0.75–2.02 [Brott et al., 2016]).

The *Stent-Protected Angioplasty in asymptomatic patients versus Carotid Endarterectomy* trial (SPACE-2) was intended as a three-armed trial with a 2:2:1 randomization to CAS plus best medical treatment (BMT) versus CEA plus BMT versus BMT alone and a planned sample size of 3640 patients. However, due to slow recruitment the three-armed study design was amended in 2013 to become two parallel RCTs: in one, patients were randomly assigned to CAS versus BMT alone. In a second trial patients were randomly assigned to CEA versus BMT alone. However, the amendment did not result in a significant increase in recruitment and the trial was stopped early after enrolment of 513 patients (CEA vs BMT $n = 203$; CAS vs BMT $n = 197$ and BMT alone $n = 113$). Comparing the risks between CAS and CEA in the first phase of the trial, the combined endpoint of stroke or death within 30 days after treatment occurred in 1.97% of patients treated with CEA and in 2.54% of patients treated with CAS (Eckstein et al., 2016).

The *Randomized Trial of Stent versus Surgery for Asymptomatic Carotid Stenosis* (ACT-1) was a non-inferiority trial, which compared CAS with embolic protection to CEA in patients suffering from asymptomatic carotid stenosis. A total of 1453 patients were randomly allocated in a 3:1 ratio to CAS or CEA. The 30-day rate of death or any stroke was 2.9% in the stenting group and 1.7% in the endarterectomy group, resulting in no significant difference between the two treatment options. Stenting was non-inferior to endarterectomy with regard to the primary composite endpoint (death, stroke, or myocardial infarction within 30 days after the procedure or ipsilateral stroke within 1 year), with an event rate of 3.8% versus 3.4%, respectively. During long-term follow-up of up to 5 years, the cumulative 5-year rate of stroke-free survival was 93.1% in the CAS group and 94.7% in the CEA group ($p = 0.44$ [Rosenfield et al., 2016]).

Carotid Stenosis in Patients at Elevated Surgical Risk

To date, there are only two trials which compared CAS versus CEA in patients with perceived elevated risk for complications with surgery, including SAPPHIRE (Yadav et al., 2004; Wang et al., 2013). Both of those trials included symptomatic as well as asymptomatic patients.

The *Stenting and Angioplasty with Protection in Patients at High Risk for Endarterectomy* (SAPPHIRE) trial aimed to determine whether CAS was not inferior to CEA, for patients with severe carotid artery stenosis and coexisting conditions that would have excluded them from previous trials of CEA (Yadav et al., 2004). The trial randomized 334 patients with neurologically symptomatic carotid stenosis of >50% or asymptomatic carotid stenosis of >80%, who had at least one coexisting condition that potentially increased the risk posed by CEA (e.g. cardiac or pulmonary disease, contralateral carotid occlusion, recurrent stenosis after endarterectomy, previous radiation therapy, or radical surgery to the neck), to carotid stenting with the use of an emboli-protection device (167 patients, of whom 159 received the treatment) or to CEA (167 patients, of whom 151 received the assigned treatment). After 3 years of follow-up, the primary outcome event (the cumulative incidence of death, stroke, or myocardial infarction within 30 days after the procedure or death or ipsilateral stroke between 31 days and 1 year) occurred in 20 of the 167 patients randomly assigned to stenting (cumulative incidence: 12.2%) and in 32 of the 167 patients randomly assigned to endarterectomy (cumulative incidence: 20.1%). This is an absolute difference of 7.9% (95% CI: −0.7%–16.4%, p = 0.004 for non-inferiority, p = 0.053 for superiority). Long-term follow-up over 3 years was completed in 260 patients. The major secondary endpoint at 3 years (the composite of death, stroke, or myocardial infarction within 30 days after the procedure or death or ipsilateral stroke between 31 days and 3 years) occurred in 24.6% in the CAS group and 26.9% in the CEA group, resulting in no significant difference in long-term outcomes between the two treatment options (Gurm et al., 2008).

The second trial was a small, two-centre study conducted in China, which included both symptomatic and asymptomatic patients. In total, 63 patients were randomized to endarterectomy (n = 35) or stenting (n = 28). The primary endpoint (composite of cardiovascular event, death or stroke within 30 days after treatment) occurred only in two patients in the CAS group and in two patients in the CEA group (Wang et al., 2013).

Meta-analysis

We have updated the results of our systematic review and meta-analysis (Bonati et al., 2012) of published RCTs comparing endovascular treatment versus endarterectomy for carotid stenosis, including earlier trials (Naylor et al., 1998; Alberts, 2001; Zhao et al., 2003; Ling, 2006; Hoffmann et al., 2008; Steinbauer et al., 2008; Ederle et al., 2009b; Liu et al., 2009), long-term follow-up results of previously reported trials (Eckstein et al., 2008; Brooks et al., 2014; Mas et al., 2014; Bonati et al., 2015; Brott et al., 2016), as well as new trials (Wang et al., 2013; Kuliha et al., 2015; Eckstein et al., 2016; Rosenfield et al., 2016). We aggregated summary data of all randomized patients in the included studies with Mantel–Haenszel random-effect models, calculating treatment effects as odds ratios (OR) and 95% confidence intervals (CI), with endarterectomy as the reference group. We quantified heterogeneity using the I^2 statistic (Higgins et al., 2011). We considered a value greater than 50% as representing substantial heterogeneity. Review Manager Software, version 5.3 was used.

Death and Stroke Outcomes in Patients with Symptomatic Carotid Stenosis

Death or Stroke between Randomization and 30 Days after Treatment in Symptomatic Patients

This endpoint was available in 12 trials including 5865 patients. Overall, death or stroke occurred in 8.1% (n = 238) of 2935 patients within 30 days of endovascular treatment and in 4.9% (n = 145) of 2930 patients within 30 days of CEA. This difference was highly statistically significant (random effects OR 1.71, 95% CI: 1.30–2.25; Figure 20.8).

Death or Stroke between Randomization and 30 Days after Treatment in Symptomatic Patients according to Age

This endpoint was available in 7 trials including a total of 4009 patients. Death or stroke between randomization and 30 days after treatment occurred in 6.4% (n = 66) of 1029 patients <70 years of age in the CAS group and in 5.7% (n = 58) of 1022 patients <70 years of age in the CEA group. In patients ≥70 years of age, death or stroke between randomization and 30 days after treatment occurred in 11.8% (n = 115) in the CAS group and in 5.7% (n = 56) in the CEA group. Hence, age significantly modified the treatment effect on the rate of death or any stroke between randomization and 30 days after treatment (Figure 20.9).

Death or Major or Disabling Stroke between Randomization and 30 Days after Treatment in Symptomatic Patients

This endpoint was available in 9 trials including 5452 patients in total. Death or major or disabling stroke between randomization and 30 days after treatment occurred in 3.7% (n = 101) of 2723 patients in the CAS group and in 2.8% (n = 77) of 2729 patients in the CEA group (Figure 20.10).

Death or Any Stroke between Randomization and 30 days after Treatment or Ipsilateral Stroke until the End of Follow-up in Symptomatic Patients

This endpoint could be extracted from 9 trials including a total of 5532 patients. Death or any stroke between randomization and 30 days after treatment or ipsilateral stroke until the end of follow-up occurred in 11.0% (n = 306) of 2780 patients in the endovascular group and in 7.7% (n = 212) of 2752 patients in the endarterectomy group (random effects OR 1.48, 95% CI: 1.23–1.79, p < 0.0001; Figure 20.11)

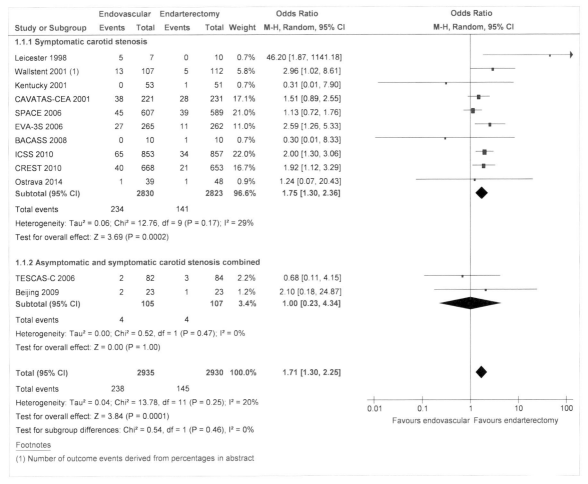

Figure 20.8 Forest plot showing the comparison between *endovascular treatment and CEA for symptomatic carotid artery stenosis* on the *outcome of any stroke or death* between randomization and 30 days after treatment in 12 RCTs.
Updated from Bonati et al. (2012) with permission.

Death and Stroke Outcomes in Patients with Asymptomatic Carotid Stenosis

Death or Any Stroke between Randomization and 30 Days after Treatment in Asymptomatic Patients

Overall, in 6 RCTs including 3201 patients, death or stroke occurred within 30 days of endovascular treatment in 2.7% ($n = 54$) of 1974 patients and within 30 days of CEA in 1.6% ($n = 20$) of 1227 patients (random effects OR 1.63, 95% CI: 0.95–2.79).

Death or Any Stroke between Randomization and 30 Days after Treatment or Ipsilateral Stroke until the End of Follow-up in Asymptomatic Patients

This endpoint could be extracted from 4 trials including a total of 2771 patients. Overall, death or any stroke between randomization and 30 days after treatment or ipsilateral stroke until the end of follow-up occurred in 4.2% ($n = 75$) of 1756 patients in the endovascular group and in 3.8% ($n = 39$) of 1015 patients in the endarterectomy group (random effects OR 1.3, 95% CI: 0.86–1.95; Figure 20.12).

Other Procedural Outcomes

MI between Randomization and 30 Days after Treatment in Symptomatic or Asymptomatic Patients

This endpoint could be extracted from 14 trials including a total of 8507 patients. Overall, myocardial infarction between randomization and 30 days after treatment occurred in 0.6% ($n =$

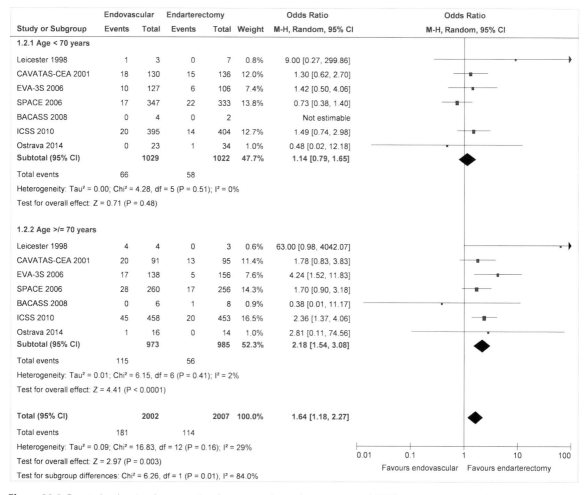

Figure 20.9 Forest plot showing the comparison between *endovascular treatment and CEA for symptomatic carotid artery stenosis* on the outcome of *any stroke or death* between randomization and 30 days after treatment, grouped according to age (<70 years vs ≥70 years). Updated from Bonati et al. (2012) with permission.

27) of 4635 of patients in the endovascular group and in 1.4% (*n* = 53) of 3872 patients in the endarterectomy group (random effects OR 0.45, 95% CI: 0.28–0.72; *p* = 0.0009; Figure 20.13).

Cranial Nerve Palsy within 30 Days of Procedure in Symptomatic or Asymptomatic Patients

This endpoint was available in 13 trials including a total of 8539 symptomatic and asymptomatic patients. In total, cranial neuropathy occurred within 30 days of endovascular treatment in 0.8% (*n* = 13) of 4650 patients, compared with 5.1% (*n* = 199) of 3889 patients assigned to CEA (random effects OR 0.08, 95% CI: 0.05–0.14).

Subgroup Analysis

A better understanding of the determinants of an increased risk from CAS compared to CEA might help to identify patients who could be safely treated by stenting instead of CEA. A number of subgroup analyses have therefore been conducted trying to provide data to guide clinicians in the choice between CAS and CEA.

Effects of Age and Sex

We have already described above the striking effect of age on the risk of stenting compared to endarterectomy in the updated Cochrane analysis (see Figure 20.9). A recent pooled individual data analysis

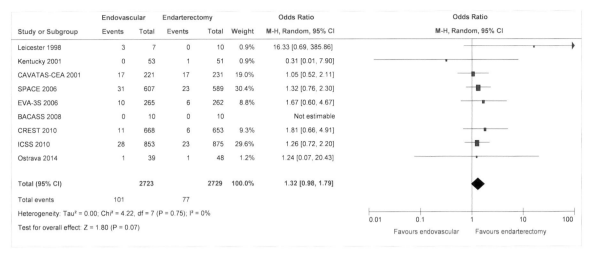

Figure 20.10 Forest plot showing the comparison between *endovascular treatment and CEA for symptomatic carotid artery stenosis* on the outcome of *death or major or disabling stroke* between randomization and 30 days after treatment, in nine RCTs.

Updated from Bonati et al. (2012) with permission.

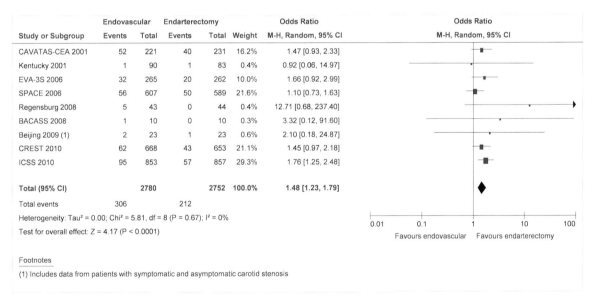

Figure 20.11 Forest plot showing the comparison between *endovascular treatment and CEA for symptomatic carotid artery stenosis* on the outcome of *death or any stroke* between randomization and 30 days after treatment or ipsilateral stroke until the end of follow-up.

Updated from Bonati et al. (2012) with permission.

performed by the Carotid Stenosis Trialists' Collaboration (CSTC) investigated the effect of age in more detail in an analysis confined to the four more recent large trials of CAS versus CEA (ICSS, SPACE, EVA-3S, and CREST). The CSTC analyses showed a pattern of increasing CAS-versus-CEA peri-procedural difference in treatment risk for symptomatic patients across the whole age range (Howard et al., 2016). In patients allocated CAS, the risk of peri-procedural stroke or death for patients treated with CAS increased with age, with only a 2.1% risk for those aged <60 years and

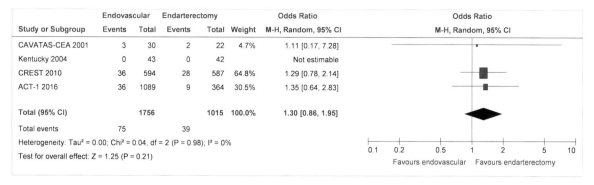

Study or Subgroup	Endovascular Events	Total	Endarterectomy Events	Total	Weight	Odds Ratio M-H, Random, 95% CI	Odds Ratio M-H, Random, 95% CI
CAVATAS-CEA 2001	3	30	2	22	4.7%	1.11 [0.17, 7.28]	
Kentucky 2004	0	43	0	42		Not estimable	
CREST 2010	36	594	28	587	64.8%	1.29 [0.78, 2.14]	
ACT-1 2016	36	1089	9	364	30.5%	1.35 [0.64, 2.83]	
Total (95% CI)		1756		1015	100.0%	1.30 [0.86, 1.95]	
Total events	75		39				

Heterogeneity: Tau² = 0.00; Chi² = 0.04, df = 2 (P = 0.98); I² = 0%
Test for overall effect: Z = 1.25 (P = 0.21)

Favours endovascular   Favours endarterectomy

Figure 20.12 Forest plot showing the comparison between *endovascular treatment and CEA for asymptomatic carotid artery stenosis* on the outcome of *death or any stroke* between randomization and 30 days after treatment or ipsilateral stroke until the end of follow-up. Updated from Bonati et al. (2012) with permission.

a monotonic increase in risk to about 11% for those aged 70–74 years, with little change in stroke or death risk for age groups thereafter above 70 years ($p < 0.0001$). In contrast, the peri-procedural risk of CEA did not increase with age. As a consequence, there was little difference in risk of CAS versus CEA at young ages (<65 years), but above age 70 years, CEA was clearly safer than CAS.

It was striking that in the CSTC analysis, age was not associated with an increase in post-procedural stroke risk after the acute treatment period, either within treatment group or between treatment groups (Howard et al., 2016).

Sex did not influence the difference between CAS and CEA with similar treatment effect ORs (men 1.86, 95% CI: 1.19–2.91; women 1.53, 95% CI: 1.02–2.29) (Bonati et al., 2015).

Effect of White-Matter Lesions

Abnormalities in white matter are a common finding on CT and MRI scans of the brain, especially in patients with stroke. In NASCET, white-matter lesions were associated with a higher peri-operative risk of stroke or death in patients assigned to CEA (Streifler et al., 2002). Patients with widespread white-matter changes allocated to the best medical management group also had an increased risk of stroke or death. Only one RCT comparing CAS and CEA, ICSS, has examined the influence of white-matter lesion severity on baseline imaging and outcomes (Ederle et al., 2013). The 1036 patients included in ICSS had baseline imaging available. The severity of white-matter disease was measured on these scans using the age-related white-matter changes (ARWMC)

score. Median ARWMC score was 7, and patients were dichotomized into those with a score of 7 or more indicating more than average severity of white-matter lesions and those with a score of less than 7. In patients treated with CAS, those with an ARWMC score of 7 or more had an increased risk of peri-procedural stroke within 30 days of treatment compared with those with a score of less than 7 (HR for any stroke 2.76, 95% CI: 1.17–6.51). In patients treated by CEA, there was no significant relationship between the ARWMC score and peri-procedural stroke. CAS was associated with a higher risk of stroke compared with CEA in patients with an ARWMC score of 7 or more (HR for any stroke 2.98, 1.29–6.93). However, there was no difference in peri-procedural risk of stroke comparing CAS with CEA in patients with an ARWMC score of less than 7.

Recent Developments in Carotid Artery Stenting: Cerebral Protection Devices and Alternative Access Routes

Since the introduction of CAS as a new technique, there has been concern regarding the risk of debris being dislodged from the atheromatous plaque during catheterization and stent deployment, resulting in cerebral emboli causing neurological deficit. This apprehension has led to the introduction and increasing use of cerebral protection devices. The concept was first described in a series by Theron and colleagues in 1996 (Theron et al., 1996). Since then, there have been many case series reporting experience of endovascular treatment with temporary cerebral protection (Reimers et al., 2001, 2004; Guimaraens et al.,

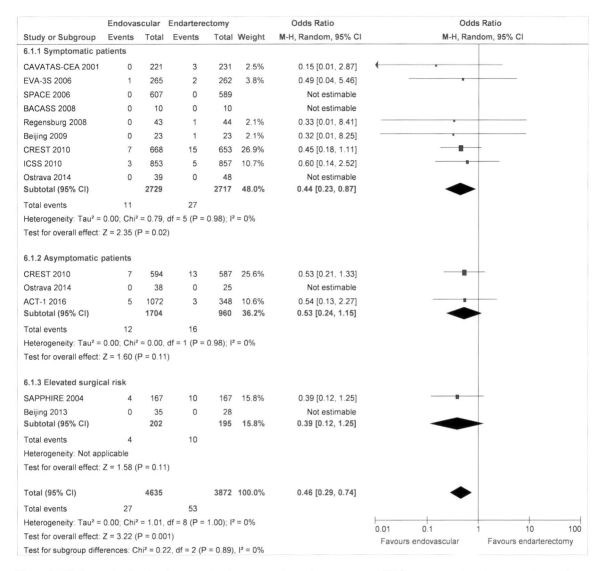

Figure 20.13 Forest plot showing the comparison between *endovascular treatment and CEA for asymptomatic and symptomatic carotid artery stenosis* on the outcome of *myocardial infarction* between randomization and 30 days after treatment.
Updated from Bonati et al. (2012) with permission.

2002; Lin et al., 2004; Gray et al., 2006, 2007; Safian et al., 2010). A systematic review of non-randomized studies reported higher rates of silent ischaemic brain lesions on diffusion-weighted magnetic resonance imaging (MRI) with unprotected stenting than with protected stenting (Schnaudigel et al., 2008). However, some of the included studies used historical control groups or were prone to selection bias. In addition, these comparisons might have been biased by a learning curve effect.

Newer RCTs comparing stenting with embolic protection devices to unprotected stenting contradicted those findings. In the MRI substudy of ICSS, patients were randomly assigned to endovascular treatment or endarterectomy. Brain MRI, including DWI to detect ischaemic brain lesions, was performed in all patients before and after treatment. A subgroup analysis showed that patients who received endovascular treatment with cerebral protection devices of the distal filter type showed a higher incidence of new ischaemic brain lesions seen on DWI after treatment than patients treated with unprotected stenting (Bonati et al., 2010). Two small randomized studies comparing stenting with embolic filter protection to unprotected stenting confirmed these results (Barbato et al., 2008; MacDonald et al., 2010). In light of the discrepant findings mentioned above, considerable uncertainty remains whether distal filter devices truly increase the safety of carotid stenting. The filters might capture some emboli during the procedure. However, in order to deploy the device, the interventionist has to first cross the stenosis with the device, which in turn possibly dislodges debris from the atherosclerotic plaque before the protection is in place. In addition, one must also consider that distal filter devices cannot prevent embolic events originating from the aortic arch occurring during the navigation of the arch in order to reach the lesion at the carotid bifurcation during CAS with a femoral approach. In order to avoid this problem, trans-cervical approaches, where the common carotid artery is directly catheterized, have been proposed.

Proximal balloon occlusion devices constitute an alternative method of cerebral protection during endovascular treatment. A reversal of blood flow across the stenosis is installed before the lesion is crossed with the catheter. Because the flow reversal is installed before the lesion is crossed, it should in theory lower the risk of embolism to the brain. However, not all patients tolerate flow reversal in the carotid artery.

Only a small amount of randomized evidence comparing the different cerebral protection systems exists. The *Prevention of Cerebral Embolization by Proximal Balloon Occlusion Compared To Filter Protection During Carotid Artery Stenting* (PROFI) trial was a prospective, randomized, single-centre trial which enrolled 62 patients with asymptomatic or symptomatic carotid stenosis who were randomly assigned to CAS with proximal balloon occlusion (*n* = 31) and CAS with distal filter protection (*n* = 31). Patients were followed clinically and with MRI including DWI before and after treatment. The incidence of new ischaemic brain lesions seen on DWI after treatment was significantly higher in the distal filter group than in the balloon occlusion group (87.1% vs 45.2%, *p* = 0.001). This finding was independent of the symptom status of the treated patients (Bijuklic et al., 2012).

A systematic review and meta-analysis of eight randomized and non-randomized studies comparing distal filter devices with proximal balloon occlusion published in 2014 found a significantly lower incidence of new ischaemic brain lesion on DWI after treatment in patients treated with proximal balloon occlusion (effect size –0.43, 95% CI: –0.8; –0.02, I^2 = 70.08% [Stabile et al., 2014]). However, the studies included in this meta-analysis show substantial heterogeneity and potential bias caused by different experience levels of the interventionist or stent design cannot be excluded. To date, there is insufficient evidence to support the superiority of one protection device over the other and a larger RCT is warranted to answer this question.

Comment

Interpretation of the Evidence

In summary, RCTs consistently showed an increased procedural risk of stroke or death associated with endovascular therapy (including balloon angioplasty in the early years and, more recently, primary stenting) compared to endarterectomy for treatment of symptomatic carotid stenosis. However, the excess risk associated with stenting is largely limited to elderly patients of about 70 years or older. In patients younger than 70 years, stenting seems to be a safe alternative to endarterectomy (Bonati et al., 2012). Beyond the procedural period, long-term follow-up data from RCTs show that stenting is as effective as endarterectomy in preventing recurrent ipsilateral stroke. Observed restenosis rates were also very similar in both treatment groups, a finding which confirms that stenting is a durable alternative to endarterectomy.

In asymptomatic patients, there is to date insufficient data to support the superiority of one treatment over the other. The existing data so far show no difference in the rate of procedural stroke or death and both treatments seem to be equally effective in preventing stroke in the long term. However, due to the lack of data, the confidence intervals are wide and henceforth compatible with both a significant reduction and increase in stroke risk. Additional data from asymptomatic patients in the ongoing trials might help resolve this uncertainty in the future.

One of the main advantages of endovascular therapy is that a surgical incision in the neck is not necessary. This leads to a reduction in the risk of cranial nerve palsy, cutaneous nerve injury, or access site haematoma, and possibly results in a shorter hospital stay when patients are treated with CAS. CAS also exhibits a lower risk of myocardial ischaemia than endarterectomy, but this effect was mostly shown in randomized trials where patients were screened with heart enzyme measurement or ECG before and after treatment, which led to the inclusion of asymptomatic coronary events (Yadav et al., 2004; Brott et al., 2010; Kuliha et al., 2015).

In order to lower procedural risk associated with endovascular therapy alternative access routes such as direct carotid catheterization and novel cerebral protection devices (flow reversal) have been developed.

Implications for Practice

According to current evidence, stenting may be considered a safe and effective alternative to endarterectomy to treat symptomatic carotid stenosis of ≥50% (according to the NASCET measurement of degree) in patients who are younger than 70 years. In addition, stenting may be considered in patients who are at increased surgical risk due to coexisting conditions, patients in whom carotid stenosis occurred after previous CEA or after neck irradiation, or in patients with surgically inaccessible carotid stenosis, as long as these patients are considered to benefit from revascularization compared to medical therapy alone.

In patients with asymptomatic carotid stenosis, there is to date insufficient data to justify stenting as an alternative to endarterectomy. However, the existing data support the continuing inclusion of patients with asymptomatic carotid stenosis in currently ongoing RCTs comparing the two treatment options (ACST-2) or comparing endovascular treatment to best medical therapy alone (CREST-2).

Implications for Research

Ongoing clinical trials comparing short- and long-term benefits and risks of stenting versus endarterectomy need to be large enough to minimize random error in the estimates of the overall safety and effectiveness of stenting compared with endarterectomy, and to enable meaningful pre-specified subgroup analyses.

The data available are still insufficient in patients with asymptomatic carotid stenosis. Three trials are currently running: the *Asymptomatic Carotid Surgery Trial 2* (ACST-2) had recruited over 3500 patients by February 2020. This trial aims to randomize a total of 3600 patients before the end of 2020. Second, the

Carotid Revascularization and Medical Management for Asymptomatic Carotid Stenosis Trial (CREST-2) had recruited 1600 patients by February 2020 and recruitment of 2480 patients in the United States and Canada in the next 2 years is intended. This trial consists of two independent multicentre RCTs, both of which recruit patients with asymptomatic high-grade carotid stenosis. In the first, patients are randomized in a 1:1 ratio between CAS with embolic protection versus BMT alone. In the second, patients are randomized to CEA versus BMT alone. Finally, the *Second European Carotid Surgery Trial* (ECST-2) completed recruitment of more than 400 patients in 2019, but follow-up is ongoing. This trial includes both asymptomatic and symptomatic patients, assessed as having a low or intermediate risk of future stroke, who are randomized between optimized medical therapy alone and CEA.

Vertebral Stenosis as a Cause of Ischaemic Stroke

Atherosclerosis of the vertebral artery is a less common cause of stroke than carotid atherosclerosis, accounting for only about 5% of all ischaemic stroke (Markus et al., 2013). Patients with recently symptomatic stenosis in the vertebrobasilar circulation have risk of recurrent stroke, which has been reported to be similar to that of carotid stenosis, especially in the first month (Gulli et al., 2013).

Angioplasty and Stenting for Vertebral Artery Stenosis

Surgery for vertebral artery disease is rarely performed, but stenting is technically relatively straightforward and in case series stenting has a low procedural stroke rate of around 1–1.5% when performed for extracranial stenosis (Stayman et al., 2011). However, stenting for intracranial vertebral artery stenosis is more hazardous with stroke rates reported of up to 10% (Eberhardt et al., 2006). Few RCTs have been performed to assess the value of vertebral artery stenting in comparison with medical therapy alone and those that have been done have all been stopped before more than a small number of patients had been recruited.

Evidence

The first RCT to investigate the revascularization treatment of vertebral artery stenosis was the

Carotid and Vertebral Artery Transluminal Angioplasty Study (CAVATAS), which was performed before stenting entered widespread use. This trial was only able to randomize 16 patients with extracranial vertebral artery stenosis to angioplasty or best medical therapy, despite randomizing over 500 patients with carotid artery stenosis during the same time period. Vertebral angioplasty was shown to be a safe treatment with no deaths or strokes in any arterial territory within the first 30 days. However, during a mean follow-up period of 4.7 years, no patient in either treatment group experienced a vertebrobasilar territory stroke (Coward et al., 2007).

The Stenting and Aggressive Medical Management for Preventing Recurrent Stroke in Intracranial Stenosis (SAMMPRIS) trial compared stenting using a self-expandable stent plus intensive medical therapy, versus intensive medical therapy alone, for symptomatic intracranial stenosis. A variety of different sites of intracranial stenosis were included, mostly in the anterior circulation, and only a small number of patients with intracranial vertebral artery stenosis were randomized (Chimowitz et al., 2011). In keeping with the results of the trial as a whole, in the 60 patients with symptomatic intracranial stenosis of a vertebral artery, the 2-year primary event rate (30-day stroke or death plus subsequent stroke in the territory of the qualifying artery) was 9.5% (95% CI: 2.5–33.0) in the medical group and 21.1% (95% CI: 11.1–37.7) in the stenting group, which clearly favoured intensive medical therapy in these patients.

The Vitesse Intracranial Stent Study for Ischemic Therapy (VISSIT) randomized 112 patients with symptomatic intracranial stenosis at a variety of intracerebral sites between stenting using a balloon-expandable stent or best medical therapy (Zaidat et al., 2015). This trial reported overall results similar to that of SAMMPRIS, favouring medical therapy alone, but neither the number nor the results in patients with intracranial vertebral artery stenosis have been reported.

The Vertebral Artery Stenting Trial (VAST) included 115 patients with symptomatic vertebral artery stenosis and compared stenting with BMT (Compter et al., 2015). Almost all the patients had extracranial stenosis and only 19 patients had intracranial vertebral artery stenosis. The patients could be treated with any type of stent. The trial was stopped early after the death of a patient from a complication of stenting led to new regulatory requirements, for which no funding was available. The primary composite outcome event of vascular death, myocardial infarction, or any stroke occurred within 30 days of treatment in only 3 patients (5%) in the stenting group and one patient (2%) in the medical group. During a median follow-up of 3 years, seven (12%, 95% CI: 6–24) patients in the stenting group and four (7%, 95% CI: 2–17) in the medical treatment group had a stroke in the territory of the symptomatic vertebral artery. The authors noted that the risk of recurrent vertebrobasilar stroke was low and questioned the need for another larger RCT.

The Vertebral Artery Ischaemia Stenting Trial (VIST) is the most recent trial to be published and followed up 179 patients with symptomatic vertebral stenosis for a mean of 3.5 years (Markus et al., 2017). The patients were randomized between vertebral angioplasty or stenting plus best medical therapy or best medical therapy alone with randomization stratified by site of stenosis. There were 148 patients who had extracranial stenosis and 31 who had intracranial vertebral artery stenosis. Only 3 patients had angioplasty alone and the remainder of vascularized patients had stenting. Recruitment was stopped because of cessation of funding. No peri-procedural complications occurred with extracranial stenting; 2 strokes occurred during intracranial stenting. There was no significant difference in the primary outcome event of fatal or nonfatal stroke at any time, which occurred in 5 patients in the stent group and 12 in the medical group (HR 0.40, 95% CI: 0.14–1.13).

The authors of the report of VIST conducted a meta-analysis of SAMMPRIS, VAST, and VIST, published only as an online supplement to the paper (Markus et al., 2017). This showed no advantage for stenting or angioplasty versus BMT alone in extracranial or intracranial vertebral artery stenosis combined or analysed separately (Figure 20.14).

Comment

Interpretation of the Evidence

Taken together, the RCTs comparing angioplasty or stenting for vertebral artery stenosis show that the risks of the procedure are low, but medical therapy appears equally effective at preventing recurrent stroke. The risks of stenting are higher in patients with intracranial vertebral artery stenosis. None of the trials have

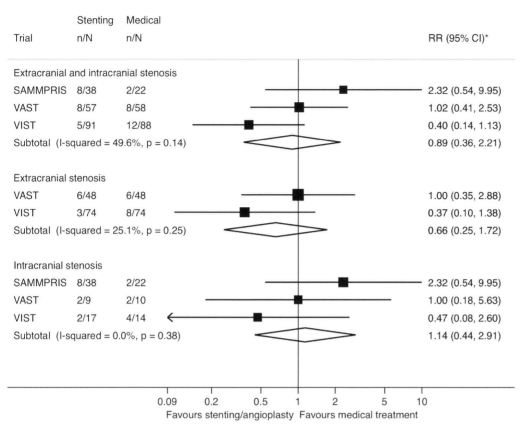

Figure 20.14 Forest plot showing the *comparison between stenting and medical treatment alone for symptomatic vertebral artery stenosis* on the outcome of *any stroke in any arterial territory* during follow-up according to site of vertebral artery stenosis, in three RCTs. CAVATAS was not included.

Reproduced from Markus et al. (2017) with permission.

recruited patients sufficiently early after onset of symptoms to show whether stenting is more effective if performed within 2 weeks of a vertebral artery event.

Implications for Practice

Stenting should not be offered as a routine treatment for patients with intracranial vertebral artery stenosis. In patients with extracranial stenosis, stenting has a low procedural risk and therefore should be considered for patients who have recurrent symptoms in the territory of the stenosis despite optimum medical therapy.

Implications for Research

Further RCTs are needed to establish whether early stenting within 2 weeks of symptoms from extracranial vertebral artery stenosis is beneficial in preventing early recurrence of stroke.

Summary

Carotid Endarterectomy

Interpretation of the Evidence

With the exception of near-occlusion, carotid endarterectomy (CEA) is of overall benefit in the long term for selected patients with recent symptomatic carotid stenosis measured as greater than 50%, using the North American Symptomatic Carotid Endarterectomy Trial (NASCET) method, provided that the surgical risk of stroke and death is low.

The benefit is greater in patients with greater degrees of stenosis (until the artery distal to the stenosis begins to collapse), men, the elderly (aged 75 years or older), and those operated on within 2 weeks after the last ischaemic event, and falls rapidly with increasing delay.

For patients with ≥70% stenosis, the number of patients needed to undergo surgery to prevent one ipsilateral stroke in 5 years is around 7, assuming the results of the old trials still apply. For patients with 50–69% stenosis, the number needed to treat is around 20, but because medical therapy has improved considerably since the trials were completed, the evidence supporting this estimate is poor.

Implications for Practice

Patients with recent symptomatic carotid territory ischaemic events should be screened for the presence of carotid stenosis by Doppler ultrasonography, contrast enhanced magnetic resonance angiography, or computed tomography (CT) angiography, depending on local availability and imaging expertise. It is desirable to confirm results suggesting stenosis sufficient to warrant intervention with a second non-invasive investigation. Catheter angiography may be required to confirm uncertain results or demonstrate near-occlusion.

For individual patients in whom symptomatic carotid stenosis has been detected, the following should be considered when deciding whether to offer the patient CEA:

- Patient's absolute risk of an ipsilateral carotid territory ischaemic stroke (which can be prevented by CEA) – this is, on average, about 5–7% per year over 5 years, but is higher with more severe degrees of symptomatic stenosis, in men, in the elderly, within the first few weeks of symptom onset, and in the presence of irregular plaque surface morphology and impaired collateral flow and cerebral perfusion reserve.

- The surgical peri-operative stroke and death rate – this was about 7% on average in the randomized controlled trials (RCTs), and is likely to be higher in women, and in patients with systolic hypertension, peripheral arterial disease, and occlusion of the contralateral internal carotid artery (ICA) and ipsilateral external carotid artery. However, recent data suggest that operative rates of CEA for symptomatic patients have declined considerably since the NASCET and European Carotid Surgery Trial (ECST) were published. The experience of both the surgeon and hospital is a crucial factor, and the results of a recent prospective audit of local surgical peri-operative stroke and death rates should be widely available and consulted.

- The patient's risk of other disabling and fatal events, and life expectancy.
- The effectiveness compared with best medical therapy alone, and compared with best medical therapy combined with other alternative strategies of recanalizing the carotid stenosis, such as carotid stenting.

Carotid Stenting

Carotid stenting is less invasive than CEA and causes fewer local complications (cranial neuropathy and neck haematoma), but in general carries a higher procedural risk of stroke than CEA. Stenting should be considered as an alternative to CEA in younger patients, or those at increased risk from CEA, so long as an experienced interventionist is available to perform the stenting.

Vertebral Stenting

Optimized medical therapy should be considered first-line treatment for vertebral artery stenosis. Stenting should not be offered as a routine treatment for patients with intracranial vertebral artery stenosis because of the high risk of procedural stroke. In patients with extracranial stenosis, stenting has a low procedural risk and therefore should be considered for patients who have recurrent symptoms in the territory of the stenosis despite optimum medical therapy.

References

Alberts MJ. (2001). Results of a multicentre prospective randomized trial of carotid artery stenting vs. carotid endarterectomy. *Stroke*, **32**, 325.

Barbato JE, Dillavou E, Horowitz MB, Jovin, TG, Kanal E. (2008). A randomized trial of carotid artery stenting with and without cerebral protection. *J Vasc Surg*, **47**, 760–5. doi:10.1016/j.jvs.2007.11.058.

Bijuklic K, Wandler A, Hazizi F, Schofer J. (2012). The PROFI study (prevention of cerebral embolization by proximal balloon occlusion compared to filter protection during carotid artery stenting): a prospective randomized trial. *J Am Coll Cardiol*, **59**, 1383–9.

Bonati LH, Dobson J, Featherstone RL, Ederle J, van der Worp HB, de Borst GJ, et al.; International Carotid Stenting Study Investigators. (2015). Long-term outcomes after stenting versus endarterectomy for treatment of symptomatic carotid stenosis: the International Carotid Stenting Study (ICSS) randomised trial. *Lancet* 385: 529–538

Bonati LH, Jongen LM, Haller S, Flach HZ, Dobson J, Nederkoorn PJ, et al. (2010). New ischaemic brain lesions on MRI after stenting or endarterectomy for symptomatic carotid stenosis: a substudy of the International Carotid Stenting Study (ICSS). *Lancet Neurol*, **9**, 353–62.

Bonati LH, Lyrer P, Ederle J, Featherstone R, Brown MM. (2012). Percutaneous transluminal balloon angioplasty and stenting for carotid artery stenosis. *Cochrane Database Syst Rev*, 9. CD000515. doi:10.1002/14651858.CD000515.pub4.

Bond R, Rerkasem K, Rothwell PM. (2003). A systematic review of the risks of carotid endarterectomy in relation to the clinical indication and the timing of surgery. *Stroke*, **34**, 2290–2301.

Brooks WH, Jones MR, Gisler P, McClure RR, Coleman TC, Breathitt L, et al. (2014). Carotid angioplasty with stenting versus endarterectomy: 10-year randomized trial in a community hospital. *JACC*, **7**. 163–8.

Brott TG, Hobson RW, Howard G, Roubin GS, Clark WM, Brooks W, et al. (2010). Stenting versus endarterectomy for treatment of carotid-artery stenosis. *N Engl J Med*, **363**, 11–23.

Brott TG, Howard G, Roubin GS, Meschia JF, Mackey A, Brooks W, et al. (2016). Long-term results of stenting versus endarterectomy for carotid-artery stenosis. *N Engl J Med*, **374**, 1021–31.

Bulbulia R, Halliday A. (2013). ACST-2 – an update. A large, simple randomised trial to compare carotid endarterectomy versus carotid artery stenting to prevent stroke in asymptomatic patients. *Gefasschirurgie*, **18**, 626–32.

Cao PG, De Rango P, Zannetti S, Giordano G, Ricci S, Celani MG . (2001). Eversion versus conventional carotid endarterectomy for preventing stroke. *Cochrane Database Syst Rev*, 1. CD001921.

CAVATAS Investigators. (2001). Endovascular versus surgical treatment in patients with carotid stenosis in the Carotid and Vertebral Artery Transluminal Angioplasty Study (CAVATAS): a randomised trial. *Lancet*, **357**, 1729–37.

Cheng SF, Brown MM. (2017). Contemporary medical therapies of atherosclerotic carotid artery disease. *Semin Vasc Surg*, **30**, 8–16

Cheng SF, Brown MM, Simister RJ, Richards T. (2019). Contemporary prevalence of carotid stenosis in patients presenting with ischaemic stroke. *Br J Surg*, **106**, 872–8.

Chimowitz MI, Lynn MJ, Derdeyn CP, Turan TN, Fiorella D, Lane BF, et al. (2011). Stenting versus aggressive medical therapy for intracranial arterial stenosis. *N Engl J Med*, **365**, 993–1003.

Chongruksut W, Vaniyapong T, Rerkasem K. (2014). Routine or selective carotid artery shunting for carotid endarterectomy (and different methods of monitoring in selective shunting). *Cochrane Database Syst Rev*, 6. CD000190. doi:10.1002/14651858.CD000190.pub3.

Compter A, van der Worp HB, Schonewille WJ, Schonewille WJ, Vos JA, Boiten J, et al; VAST Investigators. (2015). Stenting versus medical treatment in patients with symptomatic vertebral artery stenosis: a randomised open-label phase 2 trial. *Lancet Neurol*, **14**, 606–14.

Coull AJ, Lovett JK, Rothwell PM, on behalf of the Oxford Vascular Study. (2004). Population based study of early risk of stroke after transient ischemic attack or minor stroke: implications for public education and organisation of services. *BMJ*, **328**, 326–8.

Coward LJ, McCabe DJ, Ederle J, Featherstone RL, Clifton A, Brown MM; CAVATAS Investigators. (2007). Long-term outcome after angioplasty and stenting for symptomatic vertebral artery stenosis compared with medical treatment in the Carotid and Vertebral Artery Transluminal Angioplasty Study (CAVATAS): a randomized trial. *Stroke*, **38**, 1526–30.

Dotter CT, Judkins MP, Rosch J. (1967). Nonoperative treatment of arterial occlusive disease: a radiologically facilitated technique. *Radiol Clin North Am*, 5, 531–42.

Eberhardt O, Naegele T, Raygrotzki S, Weller M, Ernemann U. (2006). Stenting of vertebrobasilar arteries in symptomatic atherosclerotic disease and acute occlusion: case series and review of the literature. *J Vasc Surg*, **43**, 1145–54.

Eckstein H-H, Ringleb P, Allenberg J-R, Berger J, Fraedrich G, Hacke W, et al. (2008). Results of the Stent-Protected Angioplasty versus Carotid Endarterectomy (SPACE) study to treat symptomatic stenoses at 2 years: a multinational, prospective, randomised trial. *Lancet Neurol*, 7, 893–902

Eckstein, H-H, Reiff, T, Ringleb, P, Jansen, O, Mansmann, U, Hacke, W. (2016). SPACE-2: a missed opportunity to compare carotid endarterectomy, carotid stenting, and best medical treatment in patients with asymptomatic carotid stenosis. *Eur J Vasc Endovasc Surg*, **51**, 761–5. doi:10.1016/j.ejvs.2016.02.005.

Ederle J, Davagnanam I, van der Worp HB, Venables GS, Lyrer PA, Featherstone RL, et al. (2013). Effect of white-matter lesions on the risk of periprocedural stroke after carotid artery stenting versus endarterectomy in the International Carotid Stenting Study (ICSS): a prespecified analysis of data from a randomised trial. *Lancet Neurol*, **12**, 866–72.

Ederle, J, Featherstone, RL, Brown, MM. (2009a). Long-term outcome of endovascular treatment versus medical care for carotid artery stenosis in patients not suitable for surgery and randomised in the Carotid and Vertebral Artery Transluminal Angioplasty study (CAVATAS). *Cerebrovasc Dis*, **28**, 1–7. doi:10.1159/000215936.

Ederle J, Bonati LH, Dobson J, Featherstone RL, Gaines PA, Beard JD. (2009b). Endovascular treatment with angioplasty or stenting versus endarterectomy in patients with carotid artery stenosis in the Carotid and Vertebral Artery Transluminal Angioplasty Study (CAVATAS): long-term follow-up of a randomised trial. *Lancet Neurol*, **8**, 898–907. doi:10.1016/S1474-4422(09)70228-5.

Engelter S, Lyrer P (2003). Antiplatelet therapy for preventing stroke and other vascular events after carotid endarterectomy. *Cochrane Database Syst Rev*, 2. CD001458. doi:10.1002/14651858.CD001458.

Engelter S, Lyrer P. (2004). Antiplatelet therapy for preventing stroke and other vascular events after carotid endarterectomy (Cochrane Corner). *Stroke*, **35**, 1227–8

European Carotid Surgery Trialists' Collaborative Group. (1991). MRC European Carotid Surgery Trial. Interim results for symptomatic patients with severe (70–99%) or with mild (0–29%) carotid stenosis. *Lancet*, **337**, 1235–43.

European Carotid Surgery Trialists' Collaborative Group. (1998). Randomised trial of endarterectomy for recently symptomatic carotid stenosis: final results of the MRC European Carotid Surgery Trial (ECST). *Lancet*, **351**, 1379–87.

Feasby TE, Quan H, Ghali WA. (2002). Hospital and surgeon determinants of carotid endarterectomy outcomes. *Archiv Neurol*, **59**, 1877–81.

Fields WS, Maslenikov V, Meyer JS, Hass WK, Remington RD, MacDonald M. (1970). Joint study of extracranial arterial occlusion. V. Progress report on prognosis following surgery or non- surgical treatment for transient cerebral ischaemic attacks and cervical carotid artery lesions. *JAMA*, **211**, 1993–2003.

GALA Trial Collaborative Group, Lewis SC, Warlow CP, Bodenham AR, Colam B, Rothwell PM, Torgerson D, et al. (2008). General anaesthesia versus local anaesthesia for carotid surgery (GALA): a multicentre, randomised controlled trial. *Lancet*, **372**, 2132–42.

Goldstein LB, Moore WS, Robertson JT, Chaturvedi S. (1997). Complication rates for carotid endarterectomy: a call for action. *Stroke*, **28**, 889–90.

Gorelick PB. (1993). Distribution of atherosclerotic cerebrovascular lesions. Effects of age, race, and sex. *Stroke*, **24**, 116–19

Gray WA, Hopkins LN, Yadav S, Davis T, Wholey M, Atkinson R. (2006). Protected carotid stenting in high-surgical-risk patients: the ARCHeR results. *J Vasc Surg*, **44**, 258–68. doi:10.1016/j.jvs.2006.03.044.

Gray WA, Yadav JS, Verta P, Scicli A, Fairman R, Wholey M. (2007). The CAPTURE registry: predictors of outcomes in carotid artery stenting with embolic protection for high surgical risk patients in the early post-approval setting. *Catheter Cardiovasc Interv*, **70**, 1025–33. doi:10.1002/ccd.21359.

Grubb Jr RL, Derdeyn CP, Fritsch SM, Carpenter DA, Yundt KD, Videen TO, et al. (1998). Importance of hemodynamic factors in the prognosis of symptomatic carotid occlusion. *JAMA*, 280, 1055–60.

Guimaraens L, Sola MT, Matali A, Arbelaez A, Delgado M, Soler L. (2002). Carotid angioplasty with cerebral protection and stenting: report of 164 patients (194 carotid percutaneous transluminal angioplasties). *Cerebrovasc Dis*, **13**, 114–19.

Gulli G, Marquardt L, Rothwell PM, Markus HS. (2013). Stroke risk after posterior circulation stroke/transient ischemic attack and its relationship to site of vertebrobasilar stenosis: pooled data analysis from prospective studies. *Stroke*, 44, 598–604.

Gurm HS, Yadav JS, Fayad P, Katzen BT, Mishkel GJ, Bajwa TK. (2008). Long-term results of carotid stenting versus endarterectomy in high-risk patients. *N Engl J Med*, **358**, 1572–9. doi:10.1056/NEJMoa0708028.

Heart Protection Study Collaborative Group. (2004). Effects of cholesterol-lowering with simvastatin on stroke and other major vascular events in 20,536 people with cerebrovascular disease or other high-risk conditions. *Lancet*, **363**, 757–67.

Higgins JP, Altman DG, Gotzsche PC, Juni P, Moher D, Oxman AD. (2011). The Cochrane Collaboration's tool for assessing risk of bias in randomised trials. *BMJ*, **343**, d5928. doi:10.1136/bmj.d5928.

Hoffmann A, Taschner C, Mendelowitsch A, Merlo A, Radue EW. (2008). Carotid artery stenting versus carotid endarterectomy – a prospective randomised controlled single-centre trial with long-term follow-up (BACASS). *Schweizer Archiv fur Neurologie und Psychiatrie*, **159**, 84–9.

Howard G, Roubin GS, Jansen O, Hendrikse J, Halliday A, Fraedrich G, et al. (2016). Association between age and risk of stroke or death from carotid endarterectomy and carotid stenting: a meta-analysis of pooled patient data from four randomised trials. *Lancet*, **387**, 1305–11.

International Carotid Stenting Study Investigators. (2010). Carotid artery stenting compared with endarterectomy in patients with symptomatic carotid stenosis (International Carotid Stenting Study): an interim analysis of a randomised controlled trial. *Lancet*, **375**, 985–97.

Kuliha M, Roubec M, Prochazka V. (2015). Randomized clinical trial comparing neurological outcomes after carotid endaterectomy or stenting. *J Vasc Surg*, 62, 519.

Liem MI, Kennedy F, Bonati LH, van der Lugt A, Coolen BF, Nederveen A, et al. (2017). Investigations of carotid stenosis to identify vulnerable atherosclerotic plaque and determine individual stroke risk. *Circ J*, **81**, 1246–53.

Lin PH, Bush RL, Lubbe DF, Cox MM, Zhou W, McCoy SA (2004). Carotid artery stenting with routine cerebral protection in high-risk patients. *Am J Surg*, **188**, 644–52. doi:10.1016/j.amjsurg.2004.08.035.

Ling F. (2006). Preliminary report of trial of endarterectomy versus stenting for the treatment of carotid atherosclerotic stenosis in China (TESCAS-C). *Chinese J Cerebrovasc Dis*, **3** 4–8.

Liu CW, Liu B, Ye W, Wu WW, Li YJ, Zheng YH. (2009). Carotid endarterectomy versus carotid stenting:

a prospective randomized trial. *Zhonghua Wai Ke Za Zhi*, 47, 267–70.

Lovett JK, Coull A, Rothwell PM, on behalf of the Oxford Vascular Study. (2004). Early risk of recurrent stroke by aetiological subtype: implications for stroke prevention. *Neurology*, **62**, 569–74.

Lovett J, Dennis M, Sandercock PAG, Bamford J, Warlow CP, Rothwell PM. (2003). The very early risk of stroke following a TIA. *Stroke*, **34**, e138–e140.

MacDonald S, Evans DH, Griffiths PD, McKevitt FM, Venables GS, Cleveland TJ, et al. (2010). Filter-protected versus unprotected carotid artery stenting: a randomised trial. *Cerebrovasc Dis*, **29**, 282–9.

Markus HS, Droste DW, Kaps M, Larrue V, Lees K, Siebler M, Ringelstein EB (2005). Dual antiplatelet therapy with clopidogrel and aspirin in symptomatic carotid stenosis evaluated using doppler embolic signal detection. The Clopidogrel and Aspirin for Reduction of Emboli in Symptomatic carotid Stenosis (CARESS) trial. *Circulation*, **111**, 2233–40.

Markus HS, Larsson SC, Kuker W, Schulz UG, Ford I, Rothwell PM, Clifton A; VIST Investigators. (2017). Stenting for symptomatic vertebral artery stenosis: The Vertebral Artery Ischaemia Stenting Trial. *Neurology*, **89**, 1229–36.

Markus HS, van der Worp HB, Rothwell PM. (2013). Posterior circulation ischaemic stroke and transient ischaemic attack: diagnosis, investigation, and secondary prevention. *Lancet Neurol*, **12**, 989–98.

Mas J-L, Chatellier G, Beyssen B, Branchereau A, Moulin T, Becquemin JP, et al. (2006). Endarterectomy versus stenting in patients with symptomatic severe carotid stenosis. *N Engl J Med*, **355**, 1660–71.

Mas JL, Arquizan C, Calvet D, Viguier A, Albucher JF, Piquet P (2014). Long-term follow-up study of endarterectomy versus angioplasty in patients with symptomatic severe carotid stenosis trial. *Stroke*, **45**, 2750–6. doi:10.1161/STROKEAHA.114.005671.

Matsen SL, Chang DC, Perler BA, Roseborough GS, Williams GM. (2006). Trends in the in-hospital stroke rate following carotid endarterectomy in California and Maryland. *J Vasc Surg*, **44**, 488–95.

Mayberg MR, Wilson E, Yatsu F, Weiss DG, Messina L, Hershey LA, et al. (1991). Carotid endarterectomy and prevention of cerebral ischemia in symptomatic carotid stenosis. Veterans Affairs Cooperative Studies Program 309 Trialist Group. *JAMA*, **266**, 3289–94.

Mercuri M, Bond MG, Sirtori CR, Veglia F, Crepaldi G, Feruglio FS, et al. (1996). Pravastatin reduces carotid intima-media thickness progression in an asymptomatic hypercholesterolemic Mediterranean population: the Carotid Atherosclerosis Italian Ultrasound Study. *Am J Med*, **101**, 627–34.

Molloy J, Markus HS. (1999). Asymptomatic embolization predicts stroke and TIA risk in patients with carotid artery stenosis. *Stroke*, 30, 1440–3.

Morgenstern LB, Fox AJ, Sharpe BL, Eliasziw M, Barnett HJ, Grotta JC, for the North American Symptomatic Carotid Endarterectomy Trial (NASCET) Group. (1997). The risks and benefits of carotid endarterectomy in patients with near occlusion of the carotid artery. *Neurology*, **48**, 911–15.

Naylor AR, Bolia A, Abbott RJ, Pye IF, Smith J, Lennard N. (1998). Randomized study of carotid angioplasty and stenting versus carotid endarterectomy: a stopped trial. *J Vasc Surg*, 28, 326–334.

North American Symptomatic Carotid Endarterectomy Trial Collaborators. (1991a). Beneficial effect of carotid endarterectomy in symptomatic patients with high-grade carotid stenosis. *N Engl J Med*, **325**, 445–53.

North American Symptomatic Carotid Endarterectomy Trial Collaborators. (1991b). North American Symptomatic Carotid Endarterectomy Trial. Methods, patient characteristics, and progress. *Stroke*, **22**, 711–20.

North American Symptomatic Carotid Endarterectomy Trial Collaborators (1998). Benefit of carotid endarterectomy in patients with symptomatic moderate or severe stenosis. *N Engl J Med*, **339**, 1415–25.

Ogata J, Masuda J, Yutani C, Yamaguchi T. (1990). Rupture of atheromatous plaque as a cause of thrombotic occlusion of stenotic internal carotid artery. *Stroke*, **21**, 1740–45.

Orrapin S, Rerkasem K. (2017). Carotid endarterectomy for symptomatic carotid stenosis. *Cochrane Database Syst Rev*, 6. CD001081. doi:10.1002/14651858.CD001081. pub3.

Paraskevas KI, Robertson V, Saratzis AN, Naylor AR. (2018). An updated systematic review and meta-analysis of outcomes following eversion vs. conventional carotid endarterectomy in randomised controlled trials and observational studies. *Eur J Vasc Endovasc Surg*, **55**, 465–73. doi.org/10.1016/j.ejvs.2017.12.025

Payne DA, Jones CI, Hayes PD, Thompson MM, London NJ, Bell PR, et al. (2004). Beneficial effects of clopidogrel combined with aspirin in reducing cerebral emboli in patients undergoing carotid endarterectomy. *Circulation*, **109**, 1476–81.

PROGRESS Collaborative Group. (2001). Randomised trial of a perindopril-based blood-pressure- lowering regimen among 6,105 individuals with previous stroke or transient ischaemic attack. *Lancet*, **358**, 1033–41.

Reimers B, Corvaja N, Moshiri S, Sacca S, Albiero R, Di Mario C. (2001). Cerebral protection with filter devices during carotid artery stenting. *Circulation*, **104**, 12–15.

Reimers B, Schluter M, Castriota F, Tubler T, Corvaja N, Cernetti C. (2004). Routine use of cerebral protection during carotid artery stenting: results of a multicenter registry of 753 patients. *Am J Med*, **116**, 217–22. doi:10.1016/j.amjmed.2003.09.043

Rerkasem K, Rothwell PM. (2009). Patch angioplasty versus primary closure for carotid endarterectomy. *Cochrane Database Syst Rev*, 4. CD000160. doi:10.1002/14651858. CD000160.pub3.

Rerkasem K, Rothwell. PM (2010). Patches of different types for carotid patch angioplasty. *Cochrane Database Syst Rev*, 3. CD000071. doi:10.1002/14651858.CD000071. pub3.

Ringleb PA, Allenberg J, Bruckmann H, Eckstein HH, Fraedrich G, Hartmann M. (2006). 30 day results from the SPACE trial of stent-protected angioplasty versus carotid endarterectomy in symptomatic patients: a randomised non-inferiority trial. *Lancet*, **368**, 1239–47. doi:10.1016/ S0140-6736(06)69122-8.

Rosenfield K, Matsumura JS, Chaturvedi S, Riles T, Ansel GM, Metzger DC. (2016). Randomized trial of stent versus surgery for asymptomatic carotid stenosis. *N Engl J Med*, **374**, 1011–20.

Rothwell PM. (2005). With what to treat which patient with recently symptomatic carotid stenosis? *Pract Neurol*, **5**, 68–83.

Rothwell P, Slattery J, Warlow C. (1997). Clinical and angiographic predictors of stroke and death from carotid endarterectomy: systematic review. *BMJ*, **315**, 1571–7.

Rothwell PM, Eliasziw M, Gutnikov SA, Fox AJ, Taylor W, Mayberg MR, et al., for the Carotid Endarterectomy Trialists' Collaboration. (2003b). Pooled analysis of individual patient data from randomised controlled trials of endarterectomy for symptomatic carotid stenosis. *Lancet*, **361**, 107–16.

Rothwell PM, Eliasziw M, Gutnikov SA, Warlow CP, Barnett HJ, for the Carotid Endarterectomy Trialists' Collaboration. (2004). Endarterectomy for symptomatic carotid stenosis in relation to clinical subgroups and the timing of surgery. *Lancet*, **363**, 915–24.

Rothwell PM, Gibson R, Warlow CP. (2000). Interrelation between plaque surface morphology and degree of stenosis on carotid angiograms and the risk of ischemic stroke in patients with symptomatic carotid stenosis. *Stroke*, **31**, 615–21.

Rothwell PM, Gibson RJ, Slattery JM, Sellar RJ, Warlow CP. (1994). Equivalence of measurements of carotid stenosis: a comparison of three methods of 1001 angiograms. *Stroke*, **25**, 2435–9.

Rothwell PM, Gutnikov SA, Warlow CP, for the ECST. (2003a). Re-analysis of the final results of the European Carotid Surgery Trial. *Stroke*, **34**, 514–23.

Rothwell PM, Howard SC, Spence D. (2003c). Relationship between blood pressure and stroke risk in patients with symptomatic carotid occlusive disease. *Stroke*, **34**, 2583–90.

Rothwell PM, Mehta Z, Howard SC, Gutnikov SA, Warlow CP. (2005). From subgroups to individuals: general principles and the example of carotid endarterectomy. *Lancet*, **365**, 256–65.

Rothwell PM, Slattery J, Warlow CP. (1996a). A systematic comparison of the risk of stroke and death due to carotid endarterectomy. *Stroke*, 27, 260–5.

Rothwell PM, Slattery J, Warlow CP. (1996b). A systematic comparison of the risk of stroke and death due to carotid endarterectomy for symptomatic and asymptomatic carotid stenosis. *Stroke*, **27**, 266–9.

Rothwell PM, Warlow CP, for the European Carotid Surgery Trialists' Collaborative Group. (2000). Low risk of ischaemic stroke in patients with collapse of the internal carotid artery distal to severe carotid stenosis: cerebral protection due to low post-stenotic flow? *Stroke*, **31**, 622–30.

Rothwell PM, Warlow CP, on behalf of the ECST Collaborators. (1999). Prediction of benefit from carotid endarterectomy in individual patients: a risk-modelling study. *Lancet*, **353**, 2105–10.

Safian RD, Jaff MR, Bresnahan JF, Foster M, Bacharach JM, Yadav J. (2010). Protected carotid stenting in high-risk patients: results of the SpideRX arm of the carotid revascularization with ev3 arterial technology evolution trial. *J Interv Cardiol*, **23**, 491–8.

Sandercock PA, Warlow CP, Jones LN, Starkey IR. (1989). Predisposing factors for cerebral infarction: the Oxfordshire community stroke project. *BMJ*, **298**, 75–80.

Schnaudigel S, Groschel K, Pilgram SM, Kastrup A. (2008). New brain lesions after carotid stenting versus carotid endarterectomy: a systematic review of the literature. *Stroke*, **39**, 1911–19. doi:10.1161/strokeaha.107.500603.

Shaw DA, Venables GS, Cartilidge NE, Bates D, Dickinson PH. (1984). Carotid endarterectomy in patients with transient cerebral ischaemia. *J Neurol Sci*, **64**, 45–53.

Sillesen H, Amarenco P, Hennerici MG, Callahan A, Goldstein LB, Zivin J, et al. (2008). Atorvastatin reduces the risk of cardiovascular events in patients with carotid atherosclerosis: a secondary analysis of the Stroke Prevention by Aggressive Reduction in Cholesterol Levels (SPARCL) trial. *Stroke*, **39**, 3297–3302.

Spence JD. (2000). Management of resistant hypertension in patients with carotid stenosis: high prevalence of renovascular hypertension. *Cerebrovasc Dis*, **10**, 249–54.

Stabile E, Sannino A, Schiattarella GG, Gargiulo G, Toscano E, Brevetti L. (2014). Cerebral embolic lesions detected with diffusion-weighted magnetic resonance imaging following carotid artery stenting: a meta-analysis of 8 studies comparing filter cerebral protection and proximal balloon occlusion. *JACC*, **7**, 1177–83.

Stayman AN, Nogueira RG, Gupta R. (2011). A systematic review of stenting and angioplasty of symptomatic extracranial vertebral artery stenosis. *Stroke*, **42**, 2212–16.

Steinbauer MG, Pfister K, Greindl M, Schlachetzki F, Borisch I, Schuirer G. (2008). Alert for increased long-term follow-up after carotid artery stenting: results of a prospective, randomized, single-center trial of carotid artery stenting vs carotid endarterectomy. *J Vasc Surg*, **48**, 93–8. doi:10.1016/j.jvs.2008.02.049.

Streifler JY, Eliasziw M, Benavente OR, Alamowitch S, Fox AJ, Hachinski V, et al. (2002). Prognostic importance of leukoaraiosis in patients with symptomatic internal carotid artery stenosis. *Stroke*, **33**, 1651–5.

Stroke Prevention by Aggressive Reduction in Cholesterol Levels (SPARCL) Investigators. (2006). High-dose atorvastatin after stroke or transient ischemic attack. *N Engl J Med*, 355, 549–59.

Stroke Prevention in Reversible Ischaemia Trial (SPIRIT) Study Group. (1997). A randomised trial of anticoagulants versus aspirin after cerebral ischaemia of presumed arterial origin. *Annals of Neurology*, **42**, 857–65.

Strömberg S, Gelin J, Osterberg T, Bergström GM, Karlström L, Osterberg K; Swedish Vascular Registry (Swedvasc) Steering Committee. (2012). Very urgent carotid endarterectomy confers increased procedural risk. *Stroke*, **43**, 1331–5.

Theron JG, Payelle GG, Coskun O, Huet HF, Guimaraens L. (1996). Carotid artery stenosis: treatment with protected balloon angioplasty and stent placement. *Radiology*, **201**, 627–36. doi:10.1148/radiology.201.3.8939208

Thiele BL, Young JV, Chikos PM, Hirsch JH, Strandness DE. (1980). Correlation of arteriographic findings and symptoms in cerebrovascular disease. *Neurology*, **30**, 1041–6.

Torvik A, Svindland A, Lindboe CF. (1989). Pathogenesis of carotid thrombosis. *Stroke*, **20**, 1477–83.

Valton L, Larrue V, Le Traon AP, Massabuau P, Geraud G. (1998). Microembolic signals and risk of early recurrence in patients with stroke or transient ischemic attack. *Stroke*, **29**, 2125–8.

Van der Grond J, Balm R, Kappelle J, Eikelboom BC, Mali WP. (1995). Cerebral metabolism of patients with stenosis or occlusion of the internal carotid artery. *Stroke*, **26**, 822–8.

van Swieten JC, Koudstaal PJ, Visser MC, Schouten HJ, van Gijn J. (1988). Interobserver agreement for the assessment of handicap in stroke patients. *Stroke*, **19**, 604–7.

Wang P, Liang C, Du J, Li J. (2013). Effects of carotid endarterectomy and carotid artery stenting on high-risk carotid stenosis patients. *Pakistan J Med Sci*, **29**.

Warfarin Aspirin Recurrent Stroke Study Group. (2001). A comparison of warfarin and aspirin for the prevention of recurrent ischemic stroke. *N Engl J Med*, **345**, 1444–51.

Yadav JS, Wholey MH, Kuntz RE, Fayad P, Katzen BT, Mishkel GJ. (2004). Protected carotid-artery stenting versus endarterectomy in high-risk patients. *N Engl J Med*, **351**, 1493–1501. doi:10.1056/NEJMoa040127.

Zaidat OO, Fitzsimmons BF, Woodward BK, Wang Z, Killer-0berphalzer M, Wakhloo A, et al; VIS-SIT Trial Investigators. (2015). Effect of a balloon-expandable intracranial stent vs medical therapy on risk of stroke in patients with symptomatic intracranial stenosis: the VISSIT randomized clinical trial. *JAMA*, **313**, 1240–8.

Zhao XL, Ji XM, Peng M, Ling F. (2003). A follow-up: stroke in patients with bilateral severe carotid stenosis after intervention treatment. *Chinese J Clin Rehab*, 7, 2714–15.

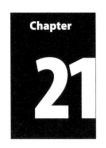

Cervical Artery Dissection and Cerebral Vasculitis

Philippe A. Lyrer
Christopher Traenka
Stefan T. Engelter

Extracranial cervical artery dissection and cerebral vasculitis are uncommon causes of ischaemic stroke. Both may occur at any age. Intracranial artery dissection is even less common and less well defined (Debette et al., 2015).

Cervical Artery Dissection

Cervical artery dissection (CAD) of the internal carotid or the vertebral artery is characterized by an intramural haematoma which is thought to be caused by a subintimal tear into the arterial wall (Engelter et al., 2017). CAD accounts for up to 2.5% of all ischaemic strokes (Debette and Leys, 2009). However, it is a major cause (up to 25%) of ischaemic stroke in young and middle-aged adults (Leys et al., 2002; Nedeltchev et al., 2005). The mean age at occurrence of CAD is about 45 years (Debette et al., 2011a; Bejot et al., 2014). There is a slight male predominance among CAD patients (A. J. Metso et al., 2012), and men are on average 5 years older than women when experiencing CAD (Schievink et al., 1993; Bejot et al., 2014). CAD may occur spontaneously or subsequent to mechanical trigger events (e.g. minor [sports associated] trauma, cervical manipulation or severe [poly-] trauma) (Engelter et al., 2013). Putative risk factors for spontaneous CAD have been identified in large cohort studies. Recent infection (Grau et al., 1999; Kloss et al., 2012), hypertension (Debette et al., 2011b), and migraine (T. M. Metso et al., 2012) have been associated with spontaneous CAD. In rare cases, CAD may occur in patients with hereditary connective tissue disorders, with vascular Ehlers–Danlos syndrome being the most common among these patients (Grond-Ginsbach and Debette, 2009).

CAD may present with ischaemic stroke, transient ischaemic attack, or local symptoms (e.g. Horner's syndrome, cranial nerve palsy, tinnitus, or cervical root impairment) (Schievink, 2001; Debette et al.,

2011a). Most commonly, CAD patients suffer from cervical pain or headache (Schievink, 2001). The mural blood accumulation in CAD may be located subadventitially, thereby causing local compression syndromes (such as Horner's syndrome) or – in very rare cases of arterial rupture – it may result in subarachnoid haemorrhage. Stenosis or occlusion of the dissected artery may occur due to the intramural haematoma and subsequent arterial narrowing. This may lead to cerebral ischaemic events, which are more often embolic rather than due to haemodynamic compromise (Engelter et al., 2007).

If suspected, the diagnosis of CAD can be confirmed by the presence of at least one of the following, widely used and established neurovascular criteria: Visualization of a mural haematoma, aneurysmal dilatation, long tapering stenosis, intimal flap, double lumen or occlusion >2 cm above the carotid bifurcation revealing an aneurysmal dilatation or a long tapering stenosis after recanalization in the internal carotid or vertebral artery (Debette and Leys, 2009). Both internal carotid and vertebral artery dissection may be visualized by magnetic resonance imaging (MRI), computed tomography (CT), or neurosonography. Specific fat-suppressed T1 sequences in MRI can most accurately depict the mural haematoma in CAD (Figure 21.1). Although neurosonography in general has a lower sensitivity in the diagnosis of CAD, it can detect a mural haematoma at very early stages of the vascular changes (Figure 21.2), when MRI can be falsely negative (Nebelsieck et al., 2009).

Intravenous Thrombolysis in Cervical Artery Dissection

Acute therapies such as intravenous thrombolysis (IVT) or endovascular recanalization therapy (EVT) have to be considered in CAD patients presenting

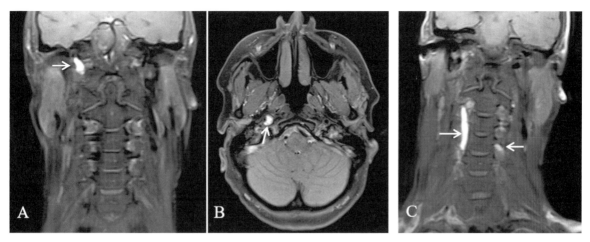

Figure 21.1 Fat-suppressed T1-weighted MRI showing a mural haematoma of the right internal carotid artery (Patient 1, A+B) and the right vertebral artery (Patient 2, C). The arrows indicate the hyperintense signal of the mural haematoma in fat-suppressed T1-weighted imaging.

with ischaemic stroke. Based on the pathophysiology of CAD, there might be the risk of an increasing mural haematoma of the dissected vessel if treated with IVT in the acute setting. This might lead to a haemodynamic worsening and to an infarct growth. However, regarding the existing evidence on IVT in CAD, this seems to be a theoretical concern and there is currently no convincing reason to withhold IVT or EVT in CAD patients. IVT or EVT increase the odds to induce recanalization of an occluded (dissected) artery or of a distal (intracranial) thrombosis in CAD patients, too.

Evidence: Comments

Although established as safe and efficacious in patients with ischaemic stroke from different aetiologies (Emberson et al., 2014; Wardlaw et al., 2014), the evidence for the use of IVT in CAD patients is scarce and based on observational, non-randomized data only. Current guidelines of acute stroke treatment do not recommend against IVT in CAD patients; it is considered reasonably safe within 4.5 hours and is probably recommended (Class IIa; Level of Evidence C) (Jauch et al., 2013; Demaerschalk et al., 2016).

IVT in non-CAD ischaemic stroke patients and in CAD patients was compared in observational, registry-based studies (Engelter et al., 2009; Zinkstok et al., 2011). In one of these studies, CAD patients showed a slightly (but statistically significant after adjustment for age, gender, and stroke severity) lower recovery rate than patients with a stroke attributable to another cause. In this study, only 36% of CAD patients

versus 44% of non-CAD patients (odds ratio [OR]$_{\text{adjusted}}$ 0.50 [95% confidence interval, CI: 0.27–0.95], p = 0.03) reached an excellent outcome at 3 months (i.e. excellent outcome defined as a modified Rankin Scale [mRS] score of 0 or 1) (Engelter et al., 2009). There was a high rate (67.7%) of CAD patients with a large artery occlusion in this study. Known as a negative prognostic factor in IVT treated stroke patients, this higher rate of large artery occlusion might – at least in part – explain the lower recovery rate of CAD patients. Yet another study compared meta-analysed data from observational studies and case reports of IVT-treated CAD patients with data from age- and stroke-severity matched patient data from the Safe Implementation of Thrombolysis in Stroke-International Stroke Thrombolysis Register (SITS-ISTR) (Zinkstok et al., 2011). In this study, 3-month mortality, the rate of symptomatic intracranial haemorrhage (ICH), and the number of patients reaching excellent 3-month outcome did not differ between IVT-treated CAD and non-CAD patients.

Data on comparisons of CAD patients receiving IVT versus those who did not are scarce. Analyses on the data from the Cervical Artery Dissection and Ischemic Stroke Patients (CADISP) consortium showed identical rates of favourable recovery after CAD related ischaemic stroke in both IVT treated and non-IVT treated patients (OR$_{\text{adjusted}}$ 0.95 [95% CI: 0.45–2.00]). A meta-analysis across observational studies (n = 10) identified 174 CAD patients receiving IVT (or some other form of thrombolytic treatment, n = 26) who were compared to 672 CAD patients who

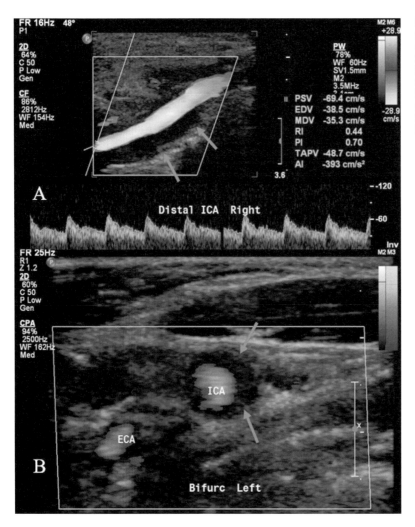

Figure 21.2 A: Colour-coded duplex ultrasound of a right internal carotid artery. Arrows indicate the hypoechogenicity of the arterial wall representing the mural haematoma of an acute cervical artery dissection. B: Transverse ultrasound imaging (power-mode) of an acutely dissected left internal carotid artery. Arrows indicate the hypechogenic mural haematoma.

did not receive thrombolysis. Most importantly, the odds for achieving a favourable 3-month outcome were similar in thrombolyzed and non-thrombolysed CAD patients (OR 0.782 [95% CI: 0.49–1.33], $p = 0.441$). Although there was a higher rate of intracranial haemorrhage in thrombolysed patients (OR 2.65 [95% CI: 0.49–1.33], $p = 0.042$), a symptomatic haemorrhage occurred in one non-thrombolysed patient only (Lin et al., 2016).

Endovascular Therapy in Cervical Artery Dissection

In anterior circulation ischaemic stroke (from any cause) with large vessel occlusion, EVT including mechanical thrombectomy with or without IVT has been shown superior to IVT alone in randomized controlled trials (Berkhemer et al., 2015; Campbell et al., 2015; Goyal et al., 2015; Jovin et al., 2015; Saver et al., 2015). Yet again, data on endovascular therapy specifically in CAD patients are scarce and derived from observational studies only. The endovascular approach seems feasible in CAD although there might be the risk that the false lumen of the dissected artery is chosen for recanalization therapy.

Evidence: Comments

The current evidence on EVT in CAD stroke patients is based on case series and non-randomized, observational studies and should therefore be interpreted very cautiously. In a recent study comparing 38 CAD patients receiving EVT (with or without IVT) to CAD patients receiving IVT, adjusted (age, sex) National Institutes of Health Stroke Scale (NIHSS) excellent outcome (mRS

0–1) was equally frequent in both groups (OR 2.23, 95% CI: 0.52–9.59; p = 0.278) (Traenka et al., 2018). However, partial or complete recanalization of the occluded intracranial artery was (numerically) more frequent in EVT-treated patients (84.2% vs 66.7%) (Traenka et al., 2018). Another study also compared EVT-treated CAD-patients (n = 24) to EVT-treated non-CAD-patients (n = 421) showing no difference in the odds of a favourable 3-month-outcome (OR 0.58 [0.19–1.78], p = 0.34) (Jensen et al., 2017).

In a recent meta-analysis across eight observational studies comparing EVT-treated to IVT-treated CAD patients, the likelihood for a favourable outcome (mRS 0–2) was similar in both groups (OR 0.97 [0.39–2.44], p = 0.96) (Traenka et al., 2018).

Endovascular treatment might be particularly important in patients presenting with tandem occlusion (i.e. occlusion of the dissected artery and a distally located intracranial artery). In a retrospective study of EVT-treated patients, 20 patients with tandem occlusion due to internal carotid artery dissection (ICAD) were compared to non-CAD patients with isolated intracranial artery occlusion. Recanalization rates were similar in both groups (p = 0.23). Likewise, favourable outcome was achieved equally frequent in both groups (CAD-patients 70% vs non-CAD patients 50%, p = 0.093) (Marnat et al., 2016). However, comparisons in this study were not adjusted for confounding variables or differences in baseline characteristics (e.g. stroke severity).

Recurrent Ischaemic Events and Prophylactic Antithrombotic Treatment in CAD

The rate of (recurrent) cerebral ischaemic events or bleeding complications in CAD patients is low while under antithrombotic treatment. In a randomized controlled trial comparing antiplatelet therapy (mostly aspirin) to anticoagulation (mostly warfarin) in CAD patients, the overall rate of ipsilateral (to the dissected artery) ischaemic stroke, death or major bleeding was 2% (4 of 196) in the per-protocol population (CADISS Trial Investigators et al., 2015). There is consensus on the need for any antithrombotic treatment as primary or secondary prophylaxis of (recurrent) cerebral ischaemic events in acute or subacute CAD. Unfortunately, at the current stage, there is still equipoise on the choice of the antithrombotic therapy (anticoagulation or antiplatelets).

Evidence: Comments

There are at least 5 meta-analyses, based on observational data, comparing antiplatelets to anticoagulants in CAD patients (Menon et al., 2008; Lyrer and Engelter, 2010; Kennedy et al., 2012; Sarikaya et al., 2013; Chowdhury et al., 2015). These meta-analyses used different statistical approaches and showed conflicting results. No difference with regard to occurrence of stroke or death was reported by Menon et al. in 2008. A non-significant trend in favour of anticoagulants was reported in a later Cochrane review with regard to the endpoint of death or disability (OR 1.77 [95% CI: 0.98–3.22], p = 0.06) (Lyrer and Engelter, 2010). However, in this analysis major bleeds (symptomatic intracranial haemorrhage [5/627; 0.8%] and major extracranial haemorrhage [7/425; 1.6%]) occurred solely in the anticoagulation group. In turn, Sarikaya et al. showed a beneficial effect of antiplatelets with regard to a composite outcome of ischaemic stroke, intracranial haemorrhage, or death (relative risk [RR] 0.32 [95% CI: 0.12–0.64]). In 2015, the first randomized controlled study comparing antiplatelet treatment to anticoagulants in CAD patients was published. The Cervical Artery Dissection in Stroke Study (CADISS) was designed as a prospective feasibility study randomly assigning CAD patients to either antiplatelet therapy (aspirin, dipyridamole, or clopidogrel alone or in combination) or to anticoagulation therapy (heparin followed by warfarin with a target international normalized ratio [INR] of 2–3) (CADISS TRIAL Investigators et al., 2015). 250 CAD patients, mainly presenting with stroke or transient ischaemic attack (n = 224), were included. With regard to the primary outcome (ipsilateral stroke or death) there was no statistically significant difference between the groups (intention-to-treat population: OR 0.335 [95% CI: 0.006–4.233], p = 0.63). There was one major bleed which occurred in the anticoagulation group. Central reading of the patient baseline imaging confirmed CAD diagnosis in 197 of the 250 study participants. However, the main results of the study did not differ in the per-protocol population. Based on the very low event rates of the purely clinical primary outcome in this study, the authors calculated that 4876 patients per group would be needed to show significant differences between groups. Hence, the use of a surrogate outcome might help to overcome the feasibility issue in a therapy trial in CAD patients. Indeed, there is another prospective, randomized multicentre trial investigating aspirin versus anticoagulation (phenprocoumon) in acute

CAD. The "Biomarkers and Antithrombotic Treatment in Cervical Artery Dissection (TREAT-CAD, NCT0204640, www.clinicaltrials.gov) trial uses a composite primary outcome including both clinical and – more importantly – also imaging surrogate outcome measures. New ischaemic lesions on diffusion weighted imaging (DWI) in CAD patients were observed in up to 25% of patients undergoing repeated brain MRI (Gensicke et al., 2015). The TREAT-CAD study started recruitment in 2013. Study recruitment was completed in December 2018 and results are expected soon.

Cerebral Vasculitis

Cerebral or central nervous system (CNS) vasculitis is defined as the presence of inflammation in the brain-supplying arteries or the veins draining the brain, the spinal cord, or the meninges. It is characterized by the presence of leucocytes in the vessel walls – these leucocytes induce damage to mural structures (Jennette et al., 1994). There is a broad spectrum of clinical manifestations of the disease, going along with a variety of pathological entities. Primary systemic vasculitis is caused by an autoimmune response, while secondary systemic and cerebral vasculitis may be induced by several infectious agents, e.g. measles, human immunodeficiency virus, herpes zoster and varicella zoster viruses, Epstein–Barr virus, or bacterial infections such as listeriosis, syphilis, and many others causing vasculitis with involvement of the brain and the meninges (Ferro, 1998). CNS vasculitis may be referred to small, medium, or large vessels of the CNS. Small and large vessels are in most cases affected by autoimmune disorders, while medium-sized vessels are mainly affected by infectious diseases.

Primary nervous system vasculitis is restricted to the nervous system, and may involve the central as well as the peripheral nervous system (single organ vasculitis, idiopathic). Secondary nervous system vasculitis is caused by a systemic disorder or infection known to cause inflammatory vasculopathy with the presence of systemic vasculitis (multi-organ vasculitis) or may be present in a systemic disorder that is restricted to the nervous system without evidence of further systemic vasculitis (single organ vasculitis with known aetiology) (Siva, 2001).

Primary Angiitis of the Central Nervous System (PACNS)

Primary angiitis of the central nervous system (PACNS, Figure 21.3) is a rare disease. Its incidence rate is estimated to be about 0.24/100,000 per year (Salvarani et al., 2007). The lesions are limited to the small or large vessels of the brain and of the spinal cord. Its neurological presentation can be very heterogeneous.

Some patients will experience acute clinical syndromes such as ischaemic stroke, while others may have a presentation such as a diffuse encephalopathy, or even tumour-like symptoms with clinical progression. Brain biopsy may be crucial to make a histopathological diagnosis confirming segmental inflammation of small arteries and arterioles with intimal proliferation and fibrosis. However, the diagnostic yield of brain biopsy for suspected PACNS is modest and accounts for about 11% of biopsied cases (Torres et al., 2016). A wide range of differential diagnoses consisting of other conditions such as hypertensive subcortical arteriolopathy, cerebral amyloid angiopathy, sarcoidosis, primary brain lymphoma, metastatic brain disease, infectious encephalitis, multiple sclerosis, progressive multifocal leucoencephalopathy, or Creutzfeldt–Jakob disease have to be considered (Alrawi et al., 1999; Torres et al., 2016; Salvarani et al., 2017). To make the diagnosis, history of exposure to vasoactive substances, a postpartum state, history of migraine headaches, thunder-clap headaches, or manifestations typical of reversible cerebral vasoconstriction syndrome (RCVS) have to be excluded (Salvarani et al., 2015). The disease may be progressive over years. Five-year fatality is estimated to be 25%, and for those not dying, progressive disability may occur.

Evidence

To date, there are no data about treatment available based on randomized controlled trials (Salvarani et al., 2017). A recently published large observational series suggested basing therapeutic decisions on the fact of small/distal or large/proximal vessel involvement (Salvarani et al., 2015).

Steroid-induced changes of the patients' mental status may confound the clinical picture of the disease itself, hence some experts suggest avoiding intravenous pulse glucocorticoids. They suggest beginning the patient on oral intake with the equivalent of predisone 1 mg/kg per day (to a maximum of 80 mg/day,

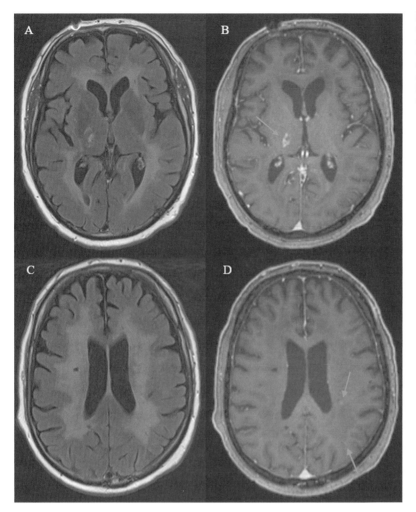

Figure 21.3 MRI of a 62-year-old man with PACNS. A+C: T2-weighted imaging showing confluent T2-hyperintensities of white matter. B+D: T1-weighted contrast-enhanced imaging showing subacute, contrast-enhancing, right thalamic (B) and left subcortical (D) white-matter lesions (arrows) .

or its equivalent) until the diagnostic evaluation is complete. If PACNS can be proven by biopsy, thereby showing a picture of granulomatous inflammation, treatment with a combination of glucocorticoids and cyclophosphamide should be started. Differential diagnoses should be challenged if there is treatment failure with these drugs. Further, rituximab may be used in patients who are intolerant of cyclophosphamide (de Boysson et al., 2014; Salvarani et al., 2015).

The majority of cases in clinical practice will be atypical, non-biopsy-proven PACSN cases. Treatment in these cases should be adapted to the severity and the extent of neurological involvement. These patients should be treated with an initial high dose of glucocorticoids (Salvarani et al., 2015) with a following slow reduction in daily dose. Whether to add cyclophosphamide to the treatment should be decided in each individual case, taking the extent

and the severity of the neurological deficits into account. Alternatively, treatment initiation may be done with intravenous methylprednisone, 15 mg/kg each day for 3 days (Guillevin and Pagnoux, 2003). Peroral prednisone shall then be started on day 4. Well-known, possible treatment-related side effects of glucocorticoids (e.g. bone loss or opportunistic infections) have to be considered and might be encountered by prophylactic treatments. As part of a remission induction strategy, cyclophosphamide can be administered as daily oral or intermittent, monthly intravenous therapy (starting dose for oral therapy: 1.5–2 mg/kg/day; 600 to 750 mg/m^2). As cyclophosphamide might induce leucopenia, the white blood cell count should be monitored closely. Intravenous cyclophosphamide is infused once a month. A dose reduction of cyclophosphamide is mandatory for patients with an estimated glomerular filtration rate less than 20 mL/min. Data on the use of rituximab in PACNS are scarce (De Boysson et al., 2013a; Salvarani et al., 2014). In three cases, improvement of the condition of the patients (radiological and clinical) was reported. Rituximab was used in a dose of either two infusions (each 1 g) separated by 14 days or as 375 mg/m^2 weekly for 4 weeks (de Boysson et al., 2013a; Salvarani et al., 2014).

Comment

The overall incidence of this condition is too low to evaluate a specific therapy against control. Therapeutic recommendations come from case series and are highly empirical. However, there seems to be a clear response rate to immunosuppression with use of steroids. Nevertheless, the proposed doses as well as timed regimens should be evaluated in randomized controlled trials.

Large Artery Vasculitis, Giant Cell Arteritis, and Others

Giant cell arteritis (GCA, Figure 21.4) is the most common vasculitis affecting medium and large cerebral vessels arising from the aortic trunk. GCA occurs at an incidence of 7–18 cases per 100,000 individuals; women are affected twice as often as men. Usually, patients are over 50 years of age at first onset of the disease. GCA was initially described as temporal arteritis (Horton disease), but about 15–27% of patients have extended extracranial involvement, since the entire aorta and all its branches can be affected including the carotid, the subclavian, and the iliac arteries. The most concerning clinical features of the disease are anterior ischaemic optic neuropathy with visual loss and cerebral strokes in the anterior as well as in the posterior circulation (Ruegg et al., 2003) which are the result of vascular inflammation involving cranial arterial branches (Salvarani et al., 2002). Polymyalgia rheumatica (PMR) is an inflammatory disorder that can occur before, and simultaneously with, or develop after, clinical manifestations of GCA. It is two or three times more common than GCA and clinically characterized by girdle pain and stiffness. Population-based studies have shown that PMR occurs in about 50% of patients with GCA, and approximately 15–30% of PMR patients develop GCA (Salvarani et al., 2002; Puppo et al., 2014). In contrast, Takayasu arteritis primarily affects the aorta and its major branches (Figure 21.5). The inflammation and damage are often localized to a portion of the affected vessels, but extensive involvement such as nearly pan-aortitis can be seen. The onset of disease usually occurs before the age of 30 years.

Evidence

Steroids have not been studied against placebo in randomized controlled trials, but the effectiveness is well established by observational studies in which steroids were reported to resolve symptoms. Initial empirical therapy for GCA is recommended as follows: oral prednisolone 40–60 mg daily as a single or divided dose should be started. In cases with recent or impending focal neurological dysfunction, such as visual loss or stroke, pulsed intravenous (i.v.) methylprednisolone 1000 mg every day for the first 3 days may be considered. The oral treatment should be maintained for 2–4 weeks and then gradually reduced every 1–2 weeks by 10% of the total daily dose (about 2.5–5 mg/day) until dose is 10 mg/day. It will be important to frequently monitor clinical symptoms to guide the management. This also comprises the erythrocyte sedimentation rate (ESR) and the C-reactive protein, although they are not always reliable markers of disease activity.

Further maintenance therapy is empirical: prednisolone 5–7.5 mg/day for about 1–2 years should be prescribed. If the patient is asymptomatic and ESR is normal, the dose can be reduced gradually by 1 mg/day every 2–3 months (Myles, 1992; Hayreh et al., 2002; Mazlumzadeh et al., 2006). Adverse effects of steroids are common and related to increasing age at diagnosis, female sex, an initial dose of prednisolone of more than 40 mg/day, a total cumulative dose of at least 2 g of prednisolone, and maintenance doses above 5 mg of prednisolone a day. Calcium and vitamin D supplementation should be given with corticosteroid therapy in all patients. In patients with reduced bone material density, bisphosphonates are indicated (Salvarani et al., 2002). Only sparse data are available on the treatment with further immune-modulating drugs such as methotrexate, azathioprine, cyclophosphamide, or TNF alpha inhibitors. However, limited evidence is also available for the use of biological agents such as tocilizumab, ustekinumab, and abatacept in GCA (Salvarani and Hatemi, 2019). Tocilizumab in combination with prednisolone has recently been tested in a prospective randomized double-blind placebo-controlled trial in 251 GCA patients. Tocilizumab combined with a 26-week prednisolone taper was proven superior to

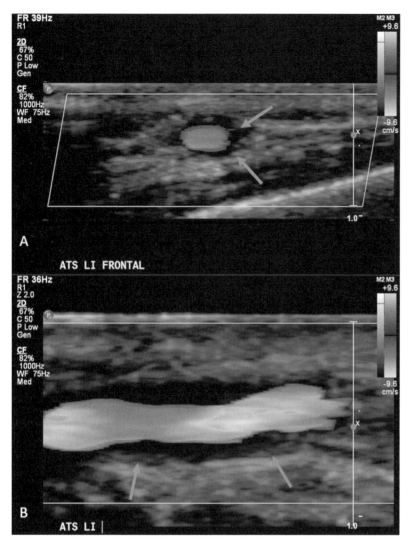

a 26-week or 52-week prednisolone taper and placebo with regard to the primary outcome (sustained remission at week 52) (Stone et al., 2017; Salvarani and Hatemi, 2019). Further evidence from randomized studies with these agents is needed to identify which GCA patients should be treated and for how long they should be treated (Salvarani and Hatemi, 2019). For now, the aforementioned agents may be an opportunity in cases of non-responsiveness to steroids or may be used for their glucocorticoid-sparing effect (Hoffman et al., 2002; Unizony et al., 2012; de Boysson et al., 2013b; Salvarani & Hatemi, 2019). Antiplatelet treatment with acetylic acid 100 mg once daily should be initiated as soon as diagnosis is established. It may prevent visual loss as well as cerebral ischaemic events (de Boysson et al., 2014; Salvarani et al., 2015).

Comment

There are no predictors to guide the duration of corticosteroid therapy. Most patients will have to take glucocorticoids for 2 years or longer. If reduction in corticosteroid dose is not possible (i.e. patients need high doses of steroids to control active disease) or in cases of serious adverse effects, cytotoxic drugs such as methotrexate and azathioprine may allow a dose reduction of steroids (Salvarani et al., 2002). Alternative treatments to steroids have been tested only in small case series or at best in small randomized controlled trials.

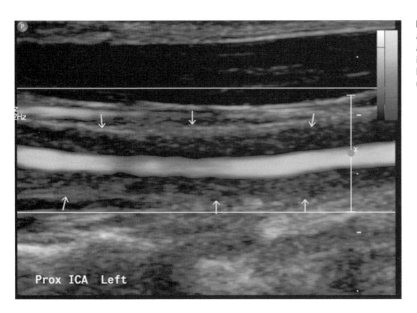

Figure 21.5 Power-mode sonography of a 32-year-old woman with Takayasu arteritis. Longitudinal imaging of the left internal carotid artery shows hypoechogenic vessel wall thickening (arrows).

Overall, data do not allow one to make a definite recommendation beyond individual authors' opinions.

Secondary Vasculitis with Involvement of the CNS: p-ANCA-positive and -negative Systemic Vasculitis

Vasculitides associated with antineutrophil cytoplasmic antibodies (ANCA), also called granulomatosis with polyangiitis (GPA), are considered complex, immune-mediated disorders in which tissue injury results from the interplay of an initiating inflammatory event and a highly specific immune response. Part of this response is directed against previously shielded epitopes of neutrophil granule proteins, leading to high-titre autoantibodies known as ANCA. ANCA are directed against antigens present within the primary granules of neutrophils and endothelial cells (Falk et al., 2011; Mouthon et al., 2014). ANCA are highly specific for a group of disorders associated with vascular inflammation known as the ANCA-associated granulomatis with polyangiitis (formerly Wegener's granulomatosis). CNS involvement may be observed in up to 51% of patients at GPA diagnosis. Headache (66%) is one of the main symptoms, followed by sensory (43%) and motor impairment (31%). CNS involvement may be characterized by pachymeningitis, cerebral ischaemic lesions, haemorrhagic lesions, and also involvement of the hypophysis. According to the clinical–radiological presentation, granulomatous (G-CNS) and vasculitic (V-CNS) phenotypes are distinguished. G-CNS patients more frequently have headaches, while V-CNS patients more frequently have motor impairment and renal involvement (Guellec et al., 2015).

Evidence

Induction therapy with corticosteroids, although empirical, is the treatment of first choice. After initial oral prednisolone (1 mg/kg/day – maximum dose 80 mg/day) or i.v. methylprednisolone (10 mg/kg/day) the dose should be reduced by 50% over the first 2 weeks to 0.5 mg/kg/day and by another 50% over the next 6 weeks. At week 8, the patients should be taking a dose of 0.25 mg/kg/day. Adding cyclophosphamide is advised for patients with CNS involvement. It should be used in a dose of 2 mg/kg/day orally, up to a maximum dose of 200 mg/day (reduced dosage if age >60 years, presence of infection or neutropenia). Alternatively, it can be given in 15 mg/kg/day i.v. pulses (e.g. 10 pulses over 25 weeks). Induction therapy produces clinical responses in 86% of patients. Again, further immune-modulating drugs such as methotrexate, azathioprine, or leflunomide may be initiated as glucocorticoid-sparing drugs (Moosig et al., 2013).

Comment

Alternative drugs or interventions that may also be used are mycophenolate mofetil, intravenous immunoglobulins, rituximab, anti-IgE therapy, anti-IL-5 antibodies, or plasma exchange. Data for these types of treatments are available from many case series or small controlled randomized trials.

Summary

Cervical artery dissection (CAD) is characterized by an intramural haematoma due to a subintimal tear and accounts for up to 25% of ischaemic strokes in young and middle-aged adults. Data regarding intravenous thrombolysis and endovascular thrombectomy in CAD are scarce and observational – both are reasonably safe and probably recommended. Based on observational evidence, antithrombotic therapy is used to prevent first or recurrent cerebral ischaemic events in acute or subacute CAD, and event rates are low with either antiplatelet or anticoagulant therapy. The long-term rate of recurrent cerebral ischaemic events or bleeding complications in CAD patients is low while under antithrombotic treatment. Cerebral vasculitis treatment is based on observational series. When primary angiitis of the central nervous system is confirmed by biopsy, a combination of glucocorticoids and cyclophosphamide should be started. Rituximab may be used in patients who are intolerant of cyclophosphamide. In atypical, non-biopsy-proven cases, treatment should be adapted to the severity of neurological involvement. For giant cell arteritis, initial high-dose prednisolone is recommended, beginning a slow taper after 2–4 weeks and continuing at a low dose for 1–2 years. Treatment of p-ANCA-positive and -negative systemic vasculitis with cerebral involvement includes induction corticosteroid therapy followed by addition of cyclophosphamide or other glucocorticoid-sparing drugs.

References

Alrawi A, Trobe JD, Blaivas M, Musch DC. (1999). Brain biopsy in primary angiitis of the central nervous system. *Neurology*, **53**(4), 858–60.

Bejot Y, Daubail B, Debette S, Durier J, Giroud M. (2014). Incidence and outcome of cerebrovascular events related to cervical artery dissection: the Dijon Stroke Registry. *Int J Stroke*, **9**(7), 879–82. doi:10.1111/ijs.12154.

Berkhemer OA, Fransen PS, Beumer D, van den Berg LA, Lingsma HF, Yoo AJ, et al; MR CLEAN Investigators. (2015). A randomized trial of intraarterial treatment for acute ischemic stroke. *N Engl J Med*, **372**(1), 11–20. doi:10.1056/NEJMoa1411587.

CADISS Trial Investigators, Markus HS, Hayter E, Levi C, Feldman A, Venables G, Norris J. (2015). Antiplatelet treatment compared with anticoagulation treatment for cervical artery dissection (CADISS): a randomised trial. *Lancet Neurol*, **14**(4), 361–7. doi:10.1016/S1474-4422(15)70018-9.

Campbell BC, Mitchell PJ, Kleinig TJ, Dewey HM, Churilov L, Yassi N, et al., for the EXTEND-IA Investigators. (2015). Endovascular therapy for ischemic stroke with perfusion-imaging selection. *N Engl J Med*, **372**(11), 1009–18. doi:10.1056/NEJMoa1414792.

Chowdhury MM, Sabbagh CN, Jackson D, Coughlin PA, Ghosh J. (2015). Antithrombotic treatment for acute extracranial carotid artery dissections: a meta-analysis. *Eur J Vasc Endovasc Surg*, **50**(2), 148–56. doi:10.1016/j.ejvs.2015.04.034.

de Boysson H, Arquizan C, Guillevin L, Pagnoux C. (2013a). Rituximab for primary angiitis of the central nervous system: report of 2 patients from the French COVAC cohort and review of the literature. *J Rheumatol*, **40**(12), 2102–03. doi:10.3899/jrheum.130529

de Boysson H, Boutemy J, Creveuil C, Ollivier Y, Letellier P, Pagnoux C, et al. (2013b). Is there a place for cyclophosphamide in the treatment of giant-cell arteritis? A case series and systematic review. *Semin Arthritis Rheum*, **43**(1), 105–12. doi:10.1016/j.semarthrit.2012.12.023.

de Boysson H, Zuber M, Naggara O, Neau JP, Gray F, Bousser, MG, et al; French Vasculitis Study Group and the French NeuroVascular Society. (2014). Primary angiitis of the central nervous system: description of the first fifty-two adults enrolled in the French cohort of patients with primary vasculitis of the central nervous system. *Arthritis Rheumatol*, **66**(5), 1315–26. doi:10.1002/art.38340.

Debette S, Compter A, Labeyrie MA, Uyttenboogaart M, Metso TM, Majersik JJ, et al. (2015). Epidemiology, pathophysiology, diagnosis, and management of intracranial artery dissection. *Lancet Neurol*, **14**(6), 640–54. doi:10.1016/S1474-4422(15)00009-5

Debette S, Grond-Ginsbach C, Bodenant M, Kloss M, Engelter S, Metso T, et al.; Cervical Artery Dissection Ischemic Stroke Patients Group. (2011a). Differential features of carotid and vertebral artery dissections: the CADISP study. *Neurology*, **77**(12), 1174–81. doi:10.1212/WNL.0b013e31822f03fc.

Debette S, Leys D. (2009). Cervical-artery dissections: predisposing factors, diagnosis, and outcome. *Lancet Neurol*, **8**(7), 668–78. doi:10.1016/S1474-4422(09)70084-5.

Debette S, Metso T, Pezzini A, Abboud S, Metso A, Leys D, et al.; Ischemic Stroke Patients Group. (2011b). Association of vascular risk factors with cervical artery dissection and ischemic stroke in young adults. *Circulation*, **123**(14), 1537–44. doi:10.1161/CIRCULATIONAHA.110.000125.

Demaerschalk BM, Kleindorfer DO, Adeoye OM, Demchuk AM, Fugate JE, Grotta JC, et al.; American Heart Association Stroke Council and Council on Epidemiology and Prevention. (2016). Scientific rationale for the inclusion and exclusion criteria for intravenous alteplase in acute ischemic stroke: a statement for healthcare professionals from the American Heart Association/American Stroke Association. *Stroke*, **47**(2), 581–641. doi:10.1161/STR.0000000000000086.

Emberson J, Lees KR, Lyden P, Blackwell L, Albers G, Bluhmki E, et al.; Stroke Thrombolysis Trialists' Collaborative Group (2014). Effect of treatment delay, age, and stroke severity on the effects of intravenous thrombolysis with alteplase for acute ischaemic stroke: a meta-analysis of individual patient data from randomised trials. *Lancet*, **384** (9958), 1929–35. doi:10.1016/S0140-6736(14)60584-5.

Engelter ST, Brandt T, Debette S, Caso V, Lichy C, Pezzini A, et al.; Cervical Artery Dissection in Ischemic Stroke Patients Study Group. (2007). Antiplatelets versus anticoagulation in cervical artery dissection. *Stroke*, **38**(9), 2605–11. doi:10.1161/STROKEAHA.107.489666.

Engelter ST, Grond-Ginsbach C, Metso TM, Metso AJ, Kloss M, Debette S, et al.; Ischemic Stroke Patients Study, G. (2013). Cervical artery dissection: trauma and other potential mechanical trigger events. *Neurology*, **80**(21), 1950–7. doi:10.1212/WNL.0b013e318293e2eb.

Engelter ST, Rutgers MP, Hatz F, Georgiadis D, Fluri F, Sekoranja L, et al. (2009). Intravenous thrombolysis in stroke attributable to cervical artery dissection. *Stroke*, **40** (12), 3772–6. doi:10.1161/STROKEAHA.109.555953.

Engelter ST, Traenka C, Lyrer P. (2017). Dissection of cervical and cerebral arteries. *Curr Neurol Neurosci Rep*, **17** (8), 59. doi:10.1007/s11910-017-0769-3.

Falk RJ, Gross WL, Guillevin L, Hoffman GS, Jayne DR, Jennette JC, et al.; American College of Rheumatology; American Society of Nephrology; European League Against Rheumatism. (2011). Granulomatosis with polyangiitis (Wegener's): an alternative name for Wegener's granulomatosis. *Arthritis Rheum*, **63**(4), 863–4. doi:10.1002/art.30286.

Ferro JM. (1998). Vasculitis of the central nervous system. *J Neurol*, **245**(12), 766–76.

Gensicke H, Ahlhelm F, Jung S, von Hessling A, Traenka C, Goeggel Simonetti B, et al. (2015). New ischaemic brain lesions in cervical artery dissection stratified to antiplatelets or anticoagulants. *Eur J Neurol*, **22**(5), 859–65, e861. doi:10.1111/ene.12682.

Goyal M, Demchuk AM, Menon BK, Eesa M, Rempel JL, Thornton J, et al.; ESCAPE Trial Investigators. (2015). Randomized assessment of rapid endovascular treatment of ischemic stroke. *N Engl J Med*, **372**(11), 1019–30. doi:10.1056/NEJMoa1414905.

Grau AJ, Brandt T, Buggle F, Orberk E, Mytilineos J, Werle E, et al. (1999). Association of cervical artery dissection with recent infection. *Arch Neurol*, **56**(7), 851–6.

Grond-Ginsbach C, Debette S. (2009). The association of connective tissue disorders with cervical artery dissections. *Curr Mol Med*, **9**(2), 210–14.

Guellec D, Cornec-Le Gall E, Groh M, Hachulla E, Karras A, Charles P, et al., the French Vasculitis Study Group. (2015). ANCA-associated vasculitis in patients with primary Sjogren's syndrome: detailed analysis of 7 new cases and systematic literature review. *Autoimmun Rev*, **14**(8), 742–750. doi:10.1016/j.autrev.2015.04.009

Guillevin L, Pagnoux C. (2003). When should immunosuppressants be prescribed to treat systemic vasculitides? *Intern Med*, **42**(4), 313–17.

Hayreh SS, Zimmerman B, Kardon RH. (2002). Visual improvement with corticosteroid therapy in giant cell arteritis. Report of a large study and review of literature. *Acta Ophthalmol Scand*, **80**(4), 355–67.

Hoffman GS, Cid MC, Hellmann DB, Guillevin L, Stone JH, Schousboe J, et al.; International Network for the Study of Systemic Vasculitides (INSSYS). (2002). A multicenter, randomized, double-blind, placebo-controlled trial of adjuvant methotrexate treatment for giant cell arteritis. *Arthritis Rheum*, **46**(5), 1309–18. doi:10.1002/art.10262.

Jauch EC, Saver JL, Adams HP Jr, Bruno A, Connors JJ, Demaerschalk BM, et al.; (2013). Guidelines for the early management of patients with acute ischemic stroke: a guideline for healthcare professionals from the American Heart Association/American Stroke Association. *Stroke*, **44** (3), 870–947. doi:10.1161/STR.0b013e318284056a.

Jennette JC, Falk RJ, Milling DM. (1994). Pathogenesis of vasculitis. *Semin Neurol*, **14**(4), 291–9. doi:10.1055/s-2008-1041088.

Jensen J, Salottolo K, Frei D, Loy D, McCarthy K, Wagner J, et al. (2017). Comprehensive analysis of intra-arterial treatment for acute ischemic stroke due to cervical artery dissection. *J Neurointerv Surg*, **9**(7), 654–8. doi:10.1136/neurintsurg-2016-012421.

Jovin TG, Chamorro A, Cobo E, de Miquel MA, Molina CA, Rovira A, et al.; REVASCAT Trial Investigators. (2015). Thrombectomy within 8 hours after symptom onset in ischemic stroke. *N Engl J Med*, **372**(24), 2296–2306. doi:10.1056/NEJMoa1503780.

Kennedy F, Lanfranconi S, Hicks C, Reid J, Gompertz P, Price C, et al.; CADISS Investigators. (2012). Antiplatelets vs anticoagulation for dissection: CADISS nonrandomized arm and meta-analysis. *Neurology*, **79**(7), 686–9. doi:10.1212/WNL.0b013e318264e36b.

Kloss M, Metso A, Pezzini A, Leys D, Giroud M, Metso TM, et al. (2012). Towards understanding seasonal variability in cervical artery dissection (CeAD). *J Neurol*, **259**(8), 1662–7. doi:10.1007/s00415-011-6395-0.

Leys D, Bandu L, Henon H, Lucas C, Mounier-Vehier F, Rondepierre P, et al. (2002). Clinical outcome in 287 consecutive young adults (15 to 45 years) with ischemic stroke. *Neurology*, **59**(1), 26–33.

Lin J, Sun Y, Zhao S, Xu J, Zhao C. (2016). Safety and efficacy of thrombolysis in cervical artery dissection-related ischemic stroke: a meta-analysis of observational studies. *Cerebrovasc Dis*, **42**(3–4), 272–9. doi:10.1159/000446004.

Lyrer P, Engelter S. (2010). Antithrombotic drugs for carotid artery dissection. *Cochrane Database Syst Rev*, 10. CD000255. doi:10.1002/14651858.CD000255.pub2.

Marnat G, Mourand I, Eker O, Machi P, Arquizan C, Riquelme C, et al. (2016). Endovascular management of tandem occlusion stroke related to internal carotid artery dissection using a distal to proximal approach: insight from the RECOST Study. *AJNR Am J Neuroradiol*, **37**(7), 1281–8. doi:10.3174/ajnr.A4752.

Mazlumzadeh M, Hunder GG, Easley KA, Calamia KT, Matteson EL, Griffing WL, et al. (2006). Treatment of giant cell arteritis using induction therapy with high-dose glucocorticoids: a double-blind, placebo-controlled, randomized prospective clinical trial. *Arthritis Rheum*, **54** (10), 3310–18. doi:10.1002/art.22163.

Menon R, Kerry S, Norris JW, Markus HS. (2008). Treatment of cervical artery dissection: a systematic review and meta-analysis. *J Neurol Neurosurg Psychiatry*, **79**(10), 1122–7. doi:10.1136/jnnp.2007.138800

Metso AJ, Metso TM, Debette S, Dallongeville J, Lyrer, PA, Pezzini A, et al. (2012). Gender and cervical artery dissection. *Eur J Neurol*, **19**(4), 594–602. doi:10.1111/j.1468-1331.2011.03586.x.

Metso TM, Tatlisumak T, Debette S, Dallongeville J, Engelter ST, Lyrer PA, et al. (2012). Migraine in cervical artery dissection and ischemic stroke patients. *Neurology*, **78** (16), 1221–8. doi:10.1212/WNL.0b013e318251595 f

Moosig F, Bremer JP, Hellmich B, Holle JU, Holl-Ulrich K, Laudien M, et al. (2013). A vasculitis centre based management strategy leads to improved outcome in eosinophilic granulomatosis and polyangiitis (Churg-Strauss, EGPA): monocentric experiences in 150 patients. *Ann Rheum Dis*, **72**(6), 1011–17. doi:10.1136/annrheumdis-2012-201531.

Mouthon L, Dunogue B, Guillevin L. (2014). Diagnosis and classification of eosinophilic granulomatosis with polyangiitis (formerly named Churg-Strauss syndrome). *J Autoimmun*, **48–49**, 99–103. doi:10.1016/j.jaut.2014.01.018

Myles, AB. (1992). Steroid treatment in giant cell arteritis. *Br J Rheumatol*, **31**(11), 787.

Nebelsieck J, Sengelhoff C, Nassenstein I, Maintz D, Kuhlenbaumer G, Nabavi DG, et al. (2009). Sensitivity of neurovascular ultrasound for the detection of spontaneous cervical artery dissection. *J Clin Neurosci*, **16**(1), 79–82. doi:10.1016/j.jocn.2008.04.005.

Nedeltchev K, der Maur TA, Georgiadis D, Arnold M, Caso V, Mattle HP, et al. (2005). Ischaemic stroke in young adults: predictors of outcome and recurrence. *J Neurol Neurosurg Psychiatry*, **76**(2), 191–5. doi:10.1136/jnnp.2004.040543

Puppo C, Massollo M, Paparo F, Camellino D, Piccardo A, Shoushtari Zadeh Naseri M, et al. (2014). Giant cell arteritis: a systematic review of the qualitative and semiquantitative methods to assess vasculitis with 18 F-fluorodeoxyglucose positron emission tomography. *Biomed Res Int*, **2014**, 574248. doi:10.1155/2014/574248.

Ruegg S, Engelter S, Jeanneret C, Hetzel A, Probst A, Steck AJ, Lyrer P. (2003). Bilateral vertebral artery occlusion resulting from giant cell arteritis: report of 3 cases and review of the literature. *Medicine (Baltimore)*, **82**(1), 1–12.

Salvarani C, Brown RD, Jr, Calamia KT, Christianson TJ, Weigand SD, Miller DV, et al. (2007). Primary central nervous system vasculitis: analysis of 101 patients. *Ann Neurol*, **62**(5), 442–51. doi:10.1002/ana.21226.

Salvarani C, Brown RD Jr, Christianson T, Miller DV, Giannini C, Huston J 3rd, et al. (2015). An update of the Mayo Clinic cohort of patients with adult primary central nervous system vasculitis: description of 163 patients. *Medicine (Baltimore)*, **94**(21), e738. doi:10.1097/MD.0000000000000738

Salvarani C, Brown RD, Jr, Hunder GG. (2017). Adult primary central nervous system vasculitis. *Isr Med Assoc J*, **19**(7), 448–53.

Salvarani C, Brown RD, Jr., Huston J, 3rd, Morris J M, Hunder GG. (2014). Treatment of primary CNS vasculitis with rituximab: case report. *Neurology*, **82**(14), 1287–8. doi:10.1212/WNL.0000000000000293.

Salvarani C, Cantini F, Boiardi L, Hunder GG. (2002). Polymyalgia rheumatica and giant-cell arteritis. *N Engl J Med*, **347**(4), 261–71. doi:10.1056/NEJMra011913.

Salvarani C, Hatemi G. (2019). Management of large-vessel vasculitis. *Curr Opin Rheumatol*, **31**(1), 25–31. doi:10.1097/BOR.0000000000000561.

Sarikaya H, da Costa BR, Baumgartner RW, Duclos K, Touze E, de Bray JM, et al. (2013). Antiplatelets versus anticoagulants for the treatment of cervical artery dissection: Bayesian meta-analysis. *PLoS One*, **8**(9), e72697. doi:10.1371/journal.pone.0072697.

Saver JL, Goyal M, Bonafe A, Diener HC, Levy EI, Pereira VM, et al.; SWIFT PRIME Investigators. (2015). Stent-retriever thrombectomy after intravenous t-PA vs. t-PA alone in stroke. *N Engl J Med*, **372**(24), 2285–95. doi:10.1056/NEJMoa1415061.

Schievink WI. (2001). Spontaneous dissection of the carotid and vertebral arteries. *N Engl J Med*, **344**(12), 898–906. doi:10.1056/NEJM200103223441206.

Schievink WI, Mokri B, Whisnant JP. (1993). Internal carotid artery dissection in a community. Rochester, Minnesota, 1987–1992. *Stroke*, **24**(11), 1678–80.

Siva A. (2001). Vasculitis of the nervous system. *J Neurol*, **248**(6), 451–68.

Stone JH, Tuckwell K, Dimonaco S, Klearman M, Aringer M, Blockmans D, et al. (2017). Trial of Tocilizumab in Giant-Cell Arteritis. *N Engl J Med*, **377**(4), 317–28. doi:10.1056/NEJMoa1613849.

Torres J, Loomis C, Cucchiara B, Smith M, Messe S. (2016). Diagnostic yield and safety of brain biopsy for suspected primary central nervous system angiitis. *Stroke*, **47**(8), 2127–9. doi:10.1161/STROKEAHA.116.013874.

Traenka C, Jung S, Gralla J, Kurmann R, Stippich C, Simonetti BG, et al. (2018). Endovascular therapy versus intravenous thrombolysis in cervical artery dissection ischemic stroke – results from the SWISS registry. *Eur Stroke J*, **3**(1), 47–56. doi:10.1177/2396987317748545.

Unizony S, Arias-Urdaneta L, Miloslavsky E, Arvikar S, Khosroshahi A, Keroack B, et al. (2012). Tocilizumab for the treatment of large-vessel vasculitis (giant cell arteritis, Takayasu arteritis) and polymyalgia rheumatica. *Arthritis Care Res (Hoboken)*, **64**(11), 1720–9. doi:10.1002/acr.21750.

Wardlaw JM, Murray V, Berge E, del Zoppo GJ. (2014). Thrombolysis for acute ischaemic stroke. *Cochrane Database Syst Rev*, 7. CD000213. doi:10.1002/14651858.CD000213.pub3.

Zinkstok SM, Vergouwen MD, Engelter ST, Lyrer PA, Bonati LH, Arnold M, et al. (2011). Safety and functional outcome of thrombolysis in dissection-related ischemic stroke: a meta-analysis of individual patient data. *Stroke*, **42**(9), 2515–20. doi:10.1161/STROKEAHA.111.617282.

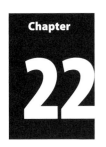

Chapter

22

Prevention of Intracerebral and Subarachnoid Haemorrhage

James P. Klaas
Robert D. Brown, Jr.

Intracerebral haemorrhage (ICH) and subarachnoid haemorrhage (SAH) can be associated with considerable morbidity and mortality despite the most aggressive contemporary management strategies. Too often in medicine the focus is on treatment strategies after an event has occurred. With worldwide case fatality rates still approaching 50%, the ideal 'treatment' for ICH and SAH is prevention.

Intracerebral Haemorrhage

ICH accounts for 10–15% of all strokes, with a worldwide incidence of 10–20 haemorrhages per 100,000 people. As the current population ages, this incidence is expected to increase (Krishnamurthi et al., 2014). The mortality rate is staggering – less than 50% of individuals survive the first 30 days following an ICH (Sacco et al., 2009). Even those who survive often have significant morbidity; roughly 80% of survivors are functionally dependent 6 months after the haemorrhage (Kase and Kurth, 2011). Such dire outcomes highlight the importance of primary prevention. However, secondary prevention is also important for survivors of an ICH, as the recurrence rate is 2.1/100 in the first year and 1.2/100/year thereafter (Hanger et al., 2007).

Primary, non-traumatic ICH accounts for more than 80% of all ICHs, and results from damage to the blood vessels from either chronic hypertension or cerebral amyloid angiopathy. Secondary ICH is due to an underlying structural lesion such as an arteriovenous malformation (AVM) or neoplasm. Most of the literature pertains to primary, non-traumatic ICH. Therefore, this will be the primary focus of the chapter, although secondary ICH due to arteriovenous and cavernous malformations (CMs) will also be covered.

Prevention of primary, non-traumatic ICHs principally rests on risk factor management and judicious use of antithrombotic medications.

Risk Factors

Multiple risk factors for ICH have been identified. Several risk factors are non-modifiable, such as increasing age, male sex, and presence of either the ε2 or ε4 apolipoprotein E (APOE) polymorphism (Biffi et al., 2010; An et al., 2017). Modifiable risk factors include hypertension, smoking, excessive alcohol intake, diet, psychosocial factors, and antithrombotic and sympathomimetic drugs (Feldmann et al., 2005; O'Donnell et al., 2016; An et al., 2017). In the INTERSTROKE international study comparing 3059 ICH patients and case–controls, modifiable risk factors accounted for 87% of the population attributable risk of ICH (O'Donnell et al., 2016).

Evidence

Hypertension

Elevated blood pressure is a well-established risk factor for primary, non-traumatic ICH (Rapsomaniki et al., 2014; O'Donnell et al., 2016), including recurrent ICH (Rodriguez-Torres et al., 2018). In a population attributable risk analysis of the 32-country INTERSTROKE case–control study, hypertension was the single most important risk factor, contributing to fully 56.5% (95% confidence interval [CI]: 52.0–60.6) of all ICH cases (O'Donnell et al., 2016).

The major randomized trials of blood pressure lowering have unfortunately often reported only outcome event rates for all strokes, without distinguishing between ischaemic and haemorrhagic stroke. Blood pressure lowering does have a substantial benefit for prevention of all stroke. In a systematic review of 54 mixed primary and secondary prevention RCTs enrolling 265,323 individuals, every 10 mm Hg reduction in systolic blood pressure (SBP) significantly reduced stroke occurrence, relative risk (RR) 0.73 (95% CI: 0.68–0.77) (Ettehad et al., 2016). However, few trials have separately reported ICH as an endpoint. One large trial that did distinguish among outcome stroke subtypes found magnified relative benefit for ICH prevention. The PROGRESS trial enrolled 6105 patients with an index cerebrovascular event, including ICH in 11%, cerebral ischaemia in 84%, and unknown stroke type in 4% (PROGRESS Collaborative Group, 2001). All patients received standard long-term blood pressure control, and were randomly allocated to additional fixed-dose angiotensin-converting enzyme (ACE) inhibitor and thiazide diuretic or additional placebo. Assignment to additional fixed-dose antihypertensives was associated with a reduction in ICH over the mean 3.9-year follow-up period: 1.2% versus 2.4%, RR 0.50 (95% CI: 0.26–0.67). In contrast, for recurrent ischaemic stroke, the RR was 0.76 (95% CI: 0.65–0.90).

Smoking

For primary, non-traumatic ICH, a systematic review of 14 case–control and 11 cohort studies reported a combined RR of 1.31 (95% CI: 1.09–1.58) for current smokers (Ariesen et al., 2003). In the international INTERSTROKE case–control study, in a population attributable risk analysis, current smoking contributed to 3.6% (95% CI: 0.9–13.0) of all ICH cases (O'Donnell et al., 2016).

While no randomized trial has evaluated the effect of tobacco cessation interventions on ICH occurrence, observational studies suggest benefit. In a meta-analysis of nine case–control studies and three cohort studies, former smokers did not have increased risk of ICH, RR of 1.06 (95% CI: 0.89–1.26) (Ariesen et al., 2003).

Alcohol

Multiple studies have identified excess alcohol intake (variously defined) as an independent risk factor for ICH (Feldmann et al., 2005; Zhang et al., 2011; Larsson et al., 2016; O'Donnell et al., 2016; Bell et al., 2017). In a meta-analysis of 11 prospective cohort studies following 487,000 individuals over a total 9.9 million person-years, light and moderate alcohol drinking (up to 2 drinks/day) was not associated with ICH, high alcohol drinking (2–4 drinks/day) showed a non-significant trend towards association (RR 1.25, 95% CI: 0.93–1.67), and heavy alcohol drinking (>4 drinks/day) was associated (RR 1.67, 95% CI: 1.25–2.23) (Larsson et al., 2016). In the large international case–control study, INTERSTROKE, population attributable risk analysis

indicated high or heavy episodic alcohol intake contributed to 9.8% (95% CI: 6.4–14.8) of all ICH cases (O'Donnell et al., 2016).

While no randomized trial has evaluated the effect of alcohol cessation or moderation interventions on ICH occurrence, the finding in observational studies of associations only with excessive, not moderate or abstinent, alcohol drinking suggests prevention benefit.

Diet

A systematic review identified longitudinal cohort studies evaluating the association of dietary fruits (seven studies) and dietary vegetables (five studies) with haemorrhagic stroke. In dose–response analyses, each 100 g/day increase in daily fruit intake was associated with reduced haemorrhagic stroke, RR 0.66 (95% CI: 0.50–0.86) and each 100 g/day increase in daily vegetable intake showed a non-significant trend towards reduced haemorrhagic stroke, RR 0.76 (95% CI: 0.55–1.06) (Aune et al., 2017). In the large, 32-country INTERSTROKE case–control study, diet quality was assessed using the modified alternative healthy eating index. Higher scores indicated greater adherence to dietary recommendations, including high intake of fruits, vegetables, whole grains, and nuts and a higher intake of fish relative to meat, poultry, and eggs. Population attributable risk analysis indicated that unhealthy diet contributed to 24.5% (95% CI: 16.5–34.8) of all ICH cases (O'Donnell et al., 2016).

Diabetes

Epidemiological studies have suggested, but not confirmed, a possible mild association of diabetes mellitus with ICH. In a systematic review, 19 case–control studies in aggregate indicated a mild increased risk of ICH with diabetes mellitus (odds ratio [OR] 1.23, 95% CI: 1.04–1.45), and 3 longitudinal studies qualitatively showed the same association (RR 1.27, 95% CI: 0.68–2.36) (Boulanger et al., 2016). However, in the later, larger, 32-country INTERSTROKE case–control study, diabetes mellitus was not a risk factor for ICH (O'Donnell et al., 2016).

Additional Modifiable Risk Factors and Relative Contributions

In addition to hypertension, tobacco, alcohol, and diet, the large, 32-country INTERSTROKE case–control study identified as independent risk factors for ICH: elevated waist-to-hip ratio (OR 1.33, 95% CI:

1.09–1.62); reduced regular physical activity (OR 1.59, 95% CI: 1.23–2.08); and psychosocial stress/depression (OR 2.84, 95% CI: 1.98–4.08) (O'Donnell et al., 2016).

Implications for Clinical Practice

Intracerebral haemorrhage is a highly preventable disease. Observational epidemiological studies suggest that up to 5 of every 6 ICHs can be prevented by optimal treatment of the seven modifiable risk factors of elevated blood pressure, unhealthy diet, sedentary physical activity, abdominal obesity, psychosocial stress/depression, tobacco use, and excessive alcohol use.

Among these, hypertension stands out as the single most important risk factor for ICH, contributing to more than half of all cases, and with confirmed benefit of treatment in at least one randomized clinical trial. This evidence supports an intensive approach to long-term blood pressure reduction in both primary and secondary prevention. The framework for management should be the contemporary definition of high blood pressure, which designates as normal less than 120/80; elevated SBP between 120 and 129 and diastolic blood pressure (DBP) less than 80; stage 1 hypertension SBP between 130 and 139 or DBP between 80 and 89; stage 2 hypertension SBP being 140–180 or DBP 90–120; and hypertensive crisis being SBP >180 or DBP >120 (Whelton et al., 2018). Individuals with elevated blood pressure within the normal range (SBP 120–129 and DBP <80) may be treated with nonpharmacological blood pressure management, including healthy diet, weight loss, physical activity, and moderate alcohol intake. Individuals with stage 1 hypertension (SBP 130–139 or DBP 80–89) who have no major risk factors for cardiovascular disease may also be treated with nonpharmacological management; those with stage 1 hypertension with age, diabetes, tobacco, cholesterol, or other risk factors placing them at a 10-year risk of cardiovascular events of 10% or more, or a first ICH, are best additionally treated with start of single-agent pharmacological antihypertensive therapy. Individuals with stage 2 hypertension (SBP ≥140 or DBP ≥90) should be treated with a combination of nonpharmacological management plus antihypertensive drug therapy, using two agents of different pharmacological classes. When pharmacological therapy is indicated, consideration should be given to including a calcium channel antagonist and to avoiding a beta-blocker to maximize stroke reduction (Whelton et al., 2018).

The additional modifiable risks factors for ICH should also be attentively treated. For obesity and physical activity, ideal goals have been defined in the Life's Simple 7 programme for maintenance of neurovascular and cardiovascular health (Lloyd-Jones et al., 2010; Saver and Cushman, 2018): attaining a body mass index < 5 kg/m^2 and participating in moderate-intensity physical activity 2.5 hours or more a week or vigorous-intensity physical activity 1.25 hours or more a week. For diet, the component of the Life's Simple 7 ideal eating recommendations most relevant to ICH prevention is consuming ≥4.5 cups/day of fruits and vegetables. Tobacco abstinence and alcohol moderation or abstinence should be obtained with use of behavioural and, if needed, pharmacotherapies (Meschia et al., 2014).

Medications/Drugs

Antithrombotics

Agents that block thrombus formation, while helpful in averting ischaemic vascular disease, necessarily carry a risk of bleeding, including at intracranial sites. The use of both antiplatelet and anticoagulant medications is associated with an increased risk of ICH (Hemphill et al., 2015). During the past several decades, randomized trials have serially expanded the prevention antithrombotic indications so that a greater proportion of middle-aged and elderly individuals are taking antiplatelet agents to avert ischaemic events of atherosclerotic origin and anticoagulant agents to avert ischaemic events from atrial fibrillation. Correspondingly, the incidence of antithrombotic-associated ICH has increased as well, especially in the elderly (Flaherty et al., 2007; Krishnamurthi et al., 2014). From 1990–2010, the age-standardized incidence rate for haemorrhagic stroke worldwide increased from 69.4 to 85.2 per 100,000 person-years (Krishnamurthi et al., 2014). In addition to occurring more frequently, anticoagulant-associated and antiplatelet-related haemorrhages also are more severe, with larger haematoma volumes and higher mortality rates (Lopes et al., 2017; Inohara et al., 2018). Therefore, prevention of ICH requires judicious use of these medications.

Evidence

Antiplatelet Agents

The Antithrombotic Trialists' Collaboration performed an individual participant data pooled analysis

465

of aspirin use aggregating data from primary prevention trials (6 RCTs, 95,000 individuals followed for 660,000 person-years) and secondary prevention trials (16 RCTs, 17,000 individuals followed for 43,000 person-years) (Antithrombotic Trialists' Collaboration et al., 2009). In primary prevention trials, allocation to aspirin was associated with increased haemorrhagic stroke, 0.04% versus 0.03% per year, RR 1.32 (95% CI: 1.00–1.76). A qualitatively similar effect was seen in the more recent, large ASPREE primary prevention trial of 19,114 individuals followed for a mean 4.7 years, with haemorrhagic stroke rates of 0.1% versus 0.08% per year, hazard ratio (HR) 1.27 (95% CI: 0.81–2.00) (McNeil et al., 2018). In secondary prevention trials, a similar non-significant trend towards increased haemorrhagic stroke occurred with allocation to aspirin, 0.16% versus 0.08% per year, RR 1.67 (95% CI: 0.97–2.90) (Antithrombotic Trialists' Collaboration et al., 2009). Overall, in contemporary primary prevention trials undertaken in the statin era, the benefit–risk ratio for prophylactic aspirin is exceptionally small, with reduced ischaemic vascular events not clearly outweighing increased haemorrhagic events (Ridker, 2018). In contrast, for secondary prevention after a first atherosclerotic ischaemic vascular event, the benefits of aspirin do outweigh the increased risks of bleeding.

Among patients who have had an ICH, the safety and benefits of resuming or starting antiplatelet agents to avert coronary or other ischaemic vascular events are uncertain. Observational series have not shown a higher rate of recurrent ICH among ICH survivors treated with antiplatelet therapy (Ding et al., 2018), but are prone to confounding by indication and cannot be considered to provide reliable guidance. Randomized trials are under way that will provide useful guidance when completed, including the RESTART trial (ISRCTN71907627).

Anticoagulants

In large randomized trials for stroke prevention in atrial fibrillation, the annual rate of intracranial haemorrhage ranges from 0.3% to 0.6% in patients taking warfarin or other vitamin K antagonists (VKAs) and from 0.1% to 0.2% in those taking direct oral anticoagulants (DOACs) (Steiner et al., 2017). The DOACs include direct thrombin inhibitors (e.g. dabigatran) and factor Xa inhibitors (e.g. rivaroxaban and apixaban). Large randomized controlled trials (RCTs)

have generally reported rates of intracranial haemorrhage as a general category, subsuming not only haemorrhagic strokes (spontaneous ICHs and spontaneous SAHs) but also non-stroke bleeding (subdural haemorrhages, epidural haemorrhages, and also traumatic intracerebral and SAHs). However, a few trials have provided more detailed analyses, finding that, among all the intracranial bleeds, about half or a little more are haemorrhagic strokes (41–56% spontaneous ICHs and 3–6% spontaneous SAHs) (Hart et al., 2012; Hankey et al., 2014; Lopes et al., 2017).

Despite these risk elevations, the benefit–risk ratio of anticoagulation is favourable for the preponderance of patients with anticoagulation-responsive conditions placing them at high risk of thromboembolic events, such as atrial fibrillation, mechanical cardiac valves, and hypercoagulable states.

The lesser risk of ICH with DOACs compared with VKAs has been shown in DOAC class-specific systematic reviews. A systematic review in the Cochrane Library analysing factor Xa inhibitors compared with VKAs in atrial fibrillation identified 13 RCTs enrolling 67,688 patients (Bruins Slot and Berge, 2018). Random allocation to factor Xa inhibitors, compared with VKAs, was associated with fewer intracranial haemorrhages during trial follow-up, 0.6% versus 1.3%, OR 0.50 (95% CI: 0.42–0.59) (Figure 22.1). Similarly, a different systematic review analysing direct thrombin inhibitors identified 3 RCTs enrolling 25,442 patients (Providência et al., 2014). Random allocation to direct thrombin inhibitors, compared with VKAs, tended to be associated with fewer intracranial haemorrhages during trial follow-up, 0.5% versus 1.1%, RR 0.64 (95% CI: 0.28–1.48).

A common clinical question is whether or not to resume anticoagulation following an ICH in a patient with atrial fibrillation or other enduring indication for anticoagulation. Observational series have not shown a higher rate of recurrent ICH among ICH survivors treated with anticoagulant therapy (Biffi et al., 2017), but are prone to confounding by indication and cannot be considered to provide reliable guidance. Randomized trials are under way that will provide useful guidance when completed, including the RESTART trial (ISRCTN71907627). An alternative to resuming lifelong anticoagulation is to perform left atrial appendage occlusion with devices that completely fill the appendage (e.g. the Watchman device) or devices that seal the

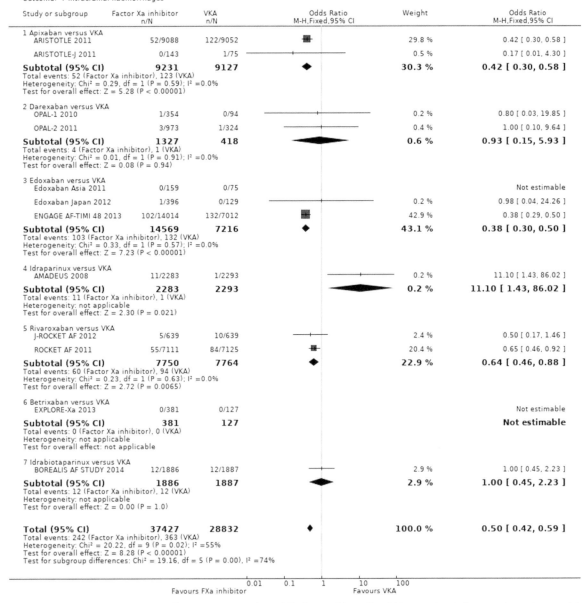

Review: Factor Xa inhibitors versus vitamin K antagonists for preventing cerebral or systemic embolism in patients with atrial fibrillation
Comparison: 1 Factor Xa inhibitors versus VKA
Outcome: 7 Intracranial haemorrhages

Figure 22.1 Forest plot showing the effects in patients with atrial fibrillation of *factor Xa inhibitors vs vitamin K antagonists* on *intracranial haemorrhages*. Typically, about half or a little more of these intracranial haemorrhages are haemorrhagic strokes (41–56% spontaneous intracerebral haemorrhages and 3–6% spontaneous subarachnoid haemorrhages).

appendage off from the circulation (e.g. the Lariat device). The devices frequently do require an abbreviated period of anticoagulation when they are first placed. A systematic review identified five RCTs enrolling 1285 patients with atrial fibrillation comparing left atrial appendage occlusion (LAAO) with medical therapies (antiplatelet, anticoagulant, or placebo) (Hanif et al., 2018). Random allocation to LAAO was associated with a non-significant decrease in stroke (RR 0.78, 95% CI: 0.47–1.29) and reduced mortality (RR 0.71, 95% CI: 0.51–0.99).

Statins – The use of HMG-COA reductase inhibitor medications (statins) that lower cholesterol levels and prevent ischaemic cerebral and cardiac events of atherosclerotic origin is widespread. In addition to cholesterol lowering, statins additionally exert anti-thrombotic effects, including inhibiting platelet activation and reducing procoagulant protein tissue factor expression (Owens and Mackman, 2014). The antithrombotic actions of statins have been recognized as mediating part of their benefits in reducing ischaemic cerebral and coronary events, but also raise the possibility that they could increase the frequency of ICH.

In a meta-analysis of 31 RCTs, no broad, statistically significant effect of statins on ICH was observed (OR 1.08, 95% CI: 0.88–1.32) (McKinney and Kostis, 2012). However, there does seem to be a small increase in ICH risk when statins are given at high dose or to patients with a history of cerebrovascular injury (stroke or transient ischaemic attack [TIA]). A systematic review of high-statin-dose RCTs identified 7 trials enrolling 62,204 patients (Pandit et al., 2016). During trial follow-up, ICH occurred more often in patients allocated to high-dose statin compared with no statin, 0.41% versus 0.27%, RR 1.53 (95% CI: 1.16–2.01). Similarly, a systematic review of statin treatment in patients with a history of cerebrovascular disease identified 2 trials enrolling 8011 patients reporting the occurrence of haemorrhagic stroke events (Vergouwen et al., 2008). During trial follow-up, haemorrhagic stroke occurred more often among patients allocated to statin compared with no statin, 1.9% versus 1.1%, RR 1.73 (95% CI: 1.19–2.50).

Despite the potential minor increase in ICH with high-dose statins or treatment of patients with prior stroke, the net benefit of statin therapy in patients with atherosclerotic disease or risk factors is well established. In a meta-analysis of 19 RCTs, statin therapy was associated with decreased all-cause mortality (RR 0.86, 95% CI: 0.80–0.93); stroke (RR 0.71, 95% CI: 0.62–0.82); and myocardial infarction (RR 0.64, 95% CI: 0.57–0.71) (Chou et al., 2016).

In patients at very high risk for ICH who require lipid-lowering therapy, treatment with PCSK9 inhibitors in lieu of statins is an option. PCSK9 inhibitors do not show similar off-target antithrombotic effects in physiological studies. In the FOURIER randomized clinical trial, enrolling 25,982 patients, allocation to a PCSK9 inhibitor (with lowering of low-density lipoprotein cholesterol from 92 mg/dL to 30 mg/dL) was not associated with an increase in haemorrhagic stroke, 0.21% versus 0.18%, HR 1.16 (95% CI: 0.68–1.98) (Sabatine et al., 2017).

Vitamin E

Vitamin E (alpha-tocopherol) is a lipid-soluble anti-oxidant widely taken as a dietary supplement. While its cytoprotective and anti-atherogenic properties potentially could confer benefits for varied medical conditions, vitamin E also has antiplatelet effects that could increase haemorrhagic stroke. Large trials evaluating vitamin E have generally shown overall disappointing results for primary aims of reducing cardiovascular disease, dementia, cancer, and other conditions. In addition, a potential adverse effect of increasing haemorrhagic stroke has been noted. A meta-analysis of 5 randomized trials involving 100,748 participants found that vitamin E supplementation was associated with more frequent haemorrhagic stroke during trial course, 0.44% versus 0.36%, RR 1.22 (95% CI: 1.00–1.48; p = 0.045). In terms of absolute risk, these findings indicate supplementation would result in one additional ICH for every 1250 individuals using vitamin E (Schurks et al., 2010).

Arteriovenous Malformations

Cerebral AVMs are congenital blood vessel anomalies characterized by a nidus of abnormal vessels that forms a direct connection between arteries and veins without an interposed capillary network. While cerebral AVMs have a prevalence of 0.05% as incidental findings on magnetic resonance imaging (MRI), their annual population-based symptomatic presentation (incidence) rate is about 1.3 per 100,000 persons (Morris et al., 2009; Derdeyn et al., 2017). The most common modes of presentation are with ICH, occurring in a little more than one-half of patients, and with seizures, occurring in one-third, with headache, progressive neurological deficits, or other symptoms occurring in one-tenth (Derdeyn et al., 2017). Annual bleeding rate estimates for AVMs range from 1 to 4% per year (Mohr et al., 2014).

Various interventions, including neurosurgical excision, endovascular occlusion, and radiation therapies, are used to obliterate an AVM and thus prevent haemorrhage. However, each carries risk of procedural complications and also of destabilizing an AVM leading to haemorrhage if incomplete obliteration occurs. An important predictor of future ICH under medical therapy is having had a prior ICH; the risk of recurrent ICH among patients with previously ruptured AVMs is 4-fold higher than of first-ever ICH among patients with unruptured AVMs (Kim et al., 2014).

Evidence

Among patients with unruptured AVMs, one randomized trial of treatment strategies has been performed, comparing interventional therapy (neurosurgery, embolization, or stereotactic radiotherapy, alone or in combination) added to medical management with medical management alone (pharmacological therapy for neurological symptoms as needed). Among 223 enrolled patients with mean follow-up of 2.8 years, allocation to medical management alone was associated with decreased death or symptomatic stroke: 10.1% versus 30.7%, HR 0.27 (95% CI: 0.14–0.54) (Mohr et al., 2014).

Among patients with ruptured AVMs, no randomized trial comparing broad treatment strategies for prevention of recurrent ICH has been performed. The frequency of recurrent ICH under medical management is high, about 5% per year, and is further increased by older age, female sex, a deep venous drainage pattern, and coexisting arterial aneurysms in feeding arteries (Derdeyn et al., 2017).

Implications for Practice

For unruptured AVMs, the ARUBA study is the only randomized trial to date, and, therefore, provides the best evidence for management. However, there were several criticisms of the trial. First, because the trial was halted early, the mean follow-up was only 33 months. This length of time does not capture an individual's lifetime risk of AVM rupture. Furthermore, shorter duration of follow-up favours medical management, as the risks of intervention are immediate. Second, as the intervention(s) utilized were at the discretion of the treating physician, there was significant treatment heterogeneity. Finally, the exclusion criteria eliminated individuals with AVMs that were potentially at higher risk of rupture or for which treatment was not feasible (Knopman and Stieg, 2014). Nonetheless, initial medical management is a reasonable treatment strategy for most patients.

For ruptured AVMs, in the absence of randomized trials, treatment decisions must be guided by estimates of individual risk under medical and under different interventional strategies and their combinations (Derdeyn et al., 2017). Given the high rate of recurrent ICH under medical therapy, for many patients an interventional approach, if anatomically feasible, is reasonable.

Cavernous Malformations

Cavernous malformations are closely packed, enlarged blood vessels lacking muscular and elastic layers without interposed neural tissue. Occurring in sporadic and familial form, they are the second most common type of cerebrovascular anomaly. Based on autopsy and MRI series, they have a prevalence of about 0.5% in the general population, and comprise 10–15% of all vascular malformations (Flemming et al., 2017). The hereditary forms are more likely to develop multiple lesions and the preponderance arise from mutations in three genes, *CCM1*, *CCM2*, and *CCM3*, encoding proteins involved in junction formation between vascular endothelial cells (Spiegler et al., 2018). Most CM are asymptomatic and found incidentally. When symptomatic, seizure is the most common presenting symptom, followed by ICH.

Haemorrhages from CMs tend to be less severe compared with primary ICHs or AVM-associated haemorrhages, reflecting the reduced perfusion pressure within the vascular anomalies, but can cause severe deficits depending on the location of the CM (Brown et al., 2005). In an individual participant data pooled meta-analysis of 1620 patients from seven cohorts, the annual bleeding rate under medical management alone was 3.16% (95% CI: 2.74–3.58%). Factors increasing bleeding risk were prior ICH (HR 5.6, 95% CI: 3.2–9.7) and brainstem location (HR 4.4, 95% CI: 2.3–8.6) (Horne et al., 2016).

Leading interventional options to prevent ICH include surgical resection and stereotactic radiosurgery. There have been no randomized trials of these approaches. In a meta-analysis of 63 observational cohorts, neurosurgical excision was associated with a combined rate of subsequent non-fatal ICH, new neurological deficit without ICH, or death of 6.6% (95% CI: 5.7–7.5%) per year, over a median follow-up of 3.3 years. Stereotactic radiosurgery was associated with a combined rate of subsequent non-fatal ICH, new neurological deficit without ICH, or death of 5.4% (95% CI: 4.5–6.4%) per year, over a median follow-up of 4.1 years (Poorthuis et al., 2014). Accordingly, indirect comparison suggests that interventional treatment, compared with medical therapy alone, is associated with lower subsequent stroke and death rates in patients who have had a prior ICH, but higher stroke and death rates in patients with no history of ICH. As a result, complete surgical resection is a reasonable strategy in patients with a CM that has bled and is accessible (Akers et al., 2017). Stereotactic radiation is a reasonable option in patients with a CM that has bled but is surgically inaccessible due to location in deep-seated or eloquent brain regions. For patients with a CM that has not bled, medical therapy is a reasonable initial management strategy.

Subarachnoid Haemorrhage

Aetiologies for non-traumatic SAH are divided into aneurysmal or non-aneurysmal. There are numerous causes of non-aneurysmal SAH, including cerebral amyloid angiopathy, cerebral venous sinus thrombosis, cerebral vasculitides, reversible cerebral vasoconstriction syndrome, vascular malformations, intracranial arterial dissections, perimesencephalic (pre-truncal) hemorrhage sickle cell disease, pituitary apoplexy, and cerebral hyperperfusion following carotid endarterectomy. Despite having multiple aetiologies, non-aneurysmal SAHs account for only a minority of all non-traumatic SAHs. More than 80% of SAHs are due to rupture of an intracranial aneurysm (Brown, 2010). Hence, the focus of this section is the prevention of aneurysmal SAH (aSAH).

Unruptured intracranial aneurysms (UIAs) are not uncommon – roughly 2–5% of the general population harbours an aneurysm (Thompson et al., 2015). However, aneurysm rupture is uncommon, with an estimated annual incidence of aSAH around 6 per 100,000, though with substantial geographical regional variation in bleeding rates (Etminan et al., 2019). Although most aneurysms do not rupture, when one does the resultant morbidity and mortality is substantial. Mortality rates range from 25–50%, and roughly 15% of patients die before reaching a hospital. Even among survivors, a substantial proportion will have permanent neurological deficits.

Even in advance of identifying patients harbouring a saccular aneurysm, broad, population-directed treatment of vascular risk factors that promote aneurysm formation and rupture, such as high blood pressure and smoking, likely substantially reduces aSAH

rates. Between 1980 and 2010, the incidence of SAH was reduced by one-third, from 10.2 to 6.1 per 100 000 person-years, in tandem with improved blood pressure control and tobacco abstinence (Etminan et al., 2019). Prevention is importantly furthered by targeted strategies to prevent aSAH, consisting of identification and treatment of intracranial aneurysms prior to rupture. Several modifiable and non-modifiable factors have been identified for the development, growth, and rupture of intracranial aneurysms. The presence/absence of these factors can be used to guide which patients to screen for an UIA, and help predict which aneurysms are at risk for rupture. This information can further be used to decide whether or not to treat, and, if so, whether surgical or endovascular management is indicated.

Non-modifiable Factors

Age

Aneurysms are acquired lesions, so the risk of developing an aneurysm increases with age, especially after age 30 (Vlak et al., 2011). Correspondingly, the risk of aSAH increases with age, reaching a peak in the fifth or sixth decade of life, with a median age of 51.3 years in a prospective Finnish cohort study (Korja et al., 2014; Etminan et al., 2019).

Sex

The prevalence of UIAs is more than 1.6-fold higher in woman compared with men (Vlak et al., 2011). Women also have a higher incidence of aSAH, and female sex has been identified in several studies to be an independent risk factor for aSAH (Korja et al., 2014; Etminan et al., 2019), but large cohort studies have not found gender to be a risk factor for UIA rupture (International Study of Unruptured Intracranial Aneurysms Investigators, 1998; Morita et al., 2012).

Geographical Region

The prevalence of UIA does not vary significantly across countries (Vlak et al., 2011). In contrast, the incidence and risk of aSAH is higher in both the Finnish and Japanese populations (Greving et al., 2014; Etminan et al., 2019).

Genetic/Congenital Syndromic Conditions

Several genetic and congenital disorders are associated with an increased risk of developing intracranial aneurysms, including autosomal dominant polycystic kidney disease, type IV Ehlers–Danlos syndrome, Marfan syndrome, fibromuscular dysplasia, hereditary haemorrhagic telangiectasia, neurofibromatosis type 1, pseudoxanthoma elasticum, microcephalic osteodysplastic primordial dwarfism, coarctation of the aorta, and bicuspid aortic valve (Thompson et al., 2015).

Family or Personal History of UIA or SAH

First-degree relatives of an individual with a known UIA or previous aSAH are at somewhat higher risk for both compared to the general population. Reported familial occurrence of UIA ranges from 7 to 20% (Thompson et al., 2015). Based on a study conducted in the Netherlands, an estimated 4% of first-degree relatives of patients with aSAH harbour a UIA, and these individuals have a 3–7 times higher risk of aSAH (Raaymakers, 1999). The risk may be higher for siblings compared to children (Raaymakers, 1999). A UIA may be at slightly greater risk of rupture if there is a family history of a UIA (Broderick et al., 2009) but family history of UIA was not noted to be a risk factor for UIA haemorrhage in large UIA cohort studies (Wiebers et al., 2003). There are some data suggesting that a personal history of a prior aSAH increases the risk of rupture of small UIAs (Wiebers et al., 2003).

Modifiable Factors

Hypertension

A systematic review of longitudinal and case–control epidemiological studies investigating risk factors for aSAH identified hypertension (no defined blood pressure cut-point) as a statistically significant risk factor, with an OR of 2.6 (95% CI: 2.0–3.1) (Feigin et al., 2005b). An analysis of 26 cohort studies from the Asia-Pacific region also found hypertension (defined as SBP ≥140 mm Hg) to be a major risk factor for aSAH (HR 2.0 [95% CI: 1.5–2.7]), and the continuous variable analysis calculated a 31% (95% CI: 23–38%) increase in risk of aSAH for every 10 mm Hg increase in SBP (Feigin et al., 2005b). In an individual participant data pooled analysis of six prospective cohort studies with 29,166 person-years of follow-up, hypertension was an independent risk factor for rupture, with HR 1.4 (95% CI: 1.1–1.8) (Greving et al., 2014). Hypertension also increases the risk of rupture of small (<7 mm) aneurysms, with a HR of 2.6 (95% CI: 2.1–3.3) as reported in a prospective cohort study from Finland (Guresir et al., 2013).

There have been no randomized trials that have assessed whether treatment of hypertension prevents development or rupture of intracranial aneurysms. Based on the strong epidemiological associations and pathophysiological rationale, maintenance of normotension in patients with unruptured aneurysms is indicated. Evidence regarding whether aggressive, rather than conventional, long-term blood pressure control targets would further reduce aSAH will come from randomized trials, including the currently enrolling PROTECT-U study (NCT03063541) randomizing unruptured aneurysm patients to intensive blood pressure treatment (SBP <120 mm Hg) plus low-dose aspirin versus conventional blood pressure treatment (SBP <140 mm Hg) and no aspirin.

Tobacco

A systematic review identified 23 case–control and 14 cohort studies evaluating the relation of smoking and SAH. The longitudinal studies included 892 SAH incident cases during a cumulative 9.2 million person-years of follow-up, and the case–control studies added another 3936 SAH cases. In combined analysis, the overall RR for SAH was 2.2 (95% CI: 1.3–3.6) for current smokers (Feigin et al., 2005a). Among patients with known saccular aneurysms, continued smoking of tobacco is an important risk factor for aneurysm growth and rupture, and more than doubles the risk of aSAH (Brinjikji et al., 2016).

While no randomized trial has evaluated the effect of tobacco cessation interventions on SAH occurrence, observational studies suggest benefit in primary prevention. The worldwide decline in tobacco use between 1980 and 2010 coincided with a worldwide decline in SAH incidence. In a meta-analysis of 34 studies from 18 countries, smoking prevalence declined from 27% to 12%, and with every 1% decline, the age- and sex-adjusted incidence of SAH decreased by 2.4% (95% CI: 1.6–3.3) (Etminan et al., 2019).

Alcohol

A meta-analysis of 23 case–control and 14 cohort studies found no association of SAH with light and moderate drinking, but an association with heavy alcohol drinking (>1.8 drinks/day), with longitudinal studies showing RR 2.1 (95% CI: 1.5–2.8) and case–control studies RR 1.5 (95% CI: 1.3–1.8) (Feigin et al., 2005a).

While no randomized trial has evaluated the effect of alcohol cessation or moderation interventions on SAH occurrence, the finding in observational studies of associations only with excessive, not moderate or abstinent, current alcohol drinking suggests prevention benefit.

Medications/Drugs

Several medications/drugs have been implicated as factors influencing development of UIA and/or risk of aSAH.

Aspirin – Preclinical, pathological, and imaging studies suggest that chronic inflammation in the arterial wall contributes to aneurysm development and rupture (Tulamo et al., 2018; Wang et al., 2018). Accordingly, aspirin, despite its antithrombotic properties, has the potential to reduce aSAH through anti-inflammatory effects.

Several large observational studies have suggested a potential protective effect of aspirin therapy. For example, in a nested case–control study of the prospective International Study of Unruptured Intracranial Aneurysms (ISUIA), 58 cases developing aneurysm rupture were matched to 213 controls without rupture (Hasan et al., 2011). On multivariate analysis, taking aspirin ≥ 3 times/week, compared with never taking aspirin, was associated with reduced odds of aSAH, OR 0.27 (95% CI: 0.11–0.67). In another study, patients harbouring 1302 ruptured aneurysms were compared with those harbouring 5109 unruptured aneurysms (Can et al., 2018). In multivariate analysis, aspirin use was associated with decrease rupture (OR 0.60, 95% CI: 0.45–0.80), and the relationship showed an inverted dose–response. In contrast, among patients who had a rupture, aspirin use was associated with increased risk of re-rupture before surgical or endovascular treatment (OR 8.15, 95% CI: 2.22–30.0).

There are no large-scale randomized trials of aspirin use to avert aSAH. One small, imaging-endpoint, trial randomized 11 patients with unruptured intracranial aneurysms to aspirin 81 mg daily or control (Hasan et al., 2013). After 3 months of allocated therapy, all patients underwent vessel wall imaging MRI and then aneurysm clipping with aneurysm dome tissue harvest. Allocation to aspirin was associated with imaging findings of reduced aneurysm wall enhancement and histological findings of reduced macrophage infiltration and decreased expression of pro-inflammatory molecules. No difference in clinical course was noted. Large, clinical endpoint trials are needed, including the currently enrolling PROTECT-U study (NCT03063541) randomizing unruptured aneurysm patients to intensive blood pressure treatment (SBP <120 mm Hg) plus low-dose aspirin versus conventional blood pressure treatment (SBP <140 mm Hg) and no aspirin.

Oral Contraceptives – Women are more prone than men to intracranial aneurysm formation and rupture, with 1.5-fold increased frequency. Oestrogen accordingly has been hypothesized to potentially contribute to aSAH, although in different animal models it shows protective as well as pathogenic effects. Findings in epidemiological studies have shown variable findings, and a meta-analysis of 1 longitudinal and 7 case–control studies did not show a statistically significant increase in risk (RR 5.4, 95% CI: 0.7–43.5) (Feigin et al., 2005b).

Sympathomimetic Agents – Multiple studies have shown an increased risk of a SAH with the use of various sympathomimetic agents. These include phenylpropanolamine, a drug formerly commonly used in appetite suppressants and cough/cold remedies (Kernan et al., 2000), and illicit substances, such as cocaine (Chang et al., 2013) and methamphetamines (Lappin et al., 2017; Darke et al., 2018). Caffeine-containing medications have been reported to increase the risk of aSAH (Lee et al., 2013), but not beverages containing caffeine, such as coffee or tea (Larsson et al., 2008).

Diet

Diet may play a role in the risk of aSAH, although evidence is limited. Data regarding consumption of 15 common foods were gathered as part of the Australasian Cooperative Research on Subarachnoid hemorrhage Study (ACROSS), a multicentre population-based case–control study of patients with first-ever aSAH in Australia and New Zealand. In addition to smoking and hypertension, multivariate analysis identified eating the fat on meat or chicken skin >4 times/week (OR 1.75 [95% CI: 1.19–2.57]), drinking skim/reduced fat milk (OR 1.71 [95% CI: 1.23–2.36]), and eating fruit (OR 1.68 [95% CI: 1.17–2.40]) <4 times/week as significant independent risk factors for aSAH (Shiue et al., 2012). Additionally, analysis of a dietary questionnaire, completed as part of a randomized placebo-controlled trial assessing whether vitamin E or beta-carotene reduced cancer risk among male Finnish smokers, observed that yogurt intake (range 0–86 g/day) was associated with higher risk of aSAH (RR 1.83 [95% CI: 1.20–2.80]) for highest intake compared with no intake (Larsson et al., 2009a), whereas vegetable intake was associated with a lower risk (RR 0.62 [95% CI: 0.40–0.98]) for highest quintile (median intake 153.7 g/day) compared with the lowest quintile (25.4 g/day) (Larsson et al., 2009b). These data suggest that increased consumption of skim/reduced fat milk, fruit, and vegetables, and reduced intake of animal fat and yogurt may reduce the risk of aSAH.

Screening

Detecting unruptured intracranial aneurysms enables enhanced prevention targeted on patients with known vulnerable lesions. Awareness of aneurysm presence provides impetus to greater adherence to medical therapies, including blood pressure control and tobacco cessation, and allows neuroendovascular and surgical interventions to be undertaken in patients with particularly high-risk lesions.

Although incidental discovery of UIAs has increased with the development and widespread utilization of non-invasive imaging studies, especially computed tomography (CT) and MR angiography, most patients harbouring UIAs remain unaware of their presence. Screening the general population is unfeasible and cost-ineffective (Li et al., 2012). Therefore, algorithms have been explored to guide selective screening imaging, among individuals at high risk of harbouring a UIA.

Evidence

Determining who to screen is guided by cost-effectiveness models that have shown that magnetic resonance angiography (MRA) or computed tomography angiography (CTA) screening is generally not cost-effective in individuals with risk of harbouring UIAs equal to the general population (2–5%), is of uncertain cost-effectiveness in individuals with mildly increased risk (5–10%), and is cost-effective in individuals with moderately to highly increased risk (11–100%) (Takao et al., 2008; Bor et al., 2010). Features that increase likelihood of presence of a UIA include a personal history of a syndromic genetic/congenital disorder often associated with the development of an intracranial aneurysm or a family history of a UIA and/or aSAH. Using genetic disorders/family history to guide screening is additionally supported by the more severe phenotype of UIA in these patients, including: greater likelihood of having multiple UIAs; UIAs with greater rupture risk than in sporadic

cases; UIAs that tend to rupture at an earlier age; and UIAs that tend to rupture at smaller sizes (Hitchcock and Gibson, 2017).

Genetic/congenital syndromic disorders associated with sufficiently high rates of UIA rates to support screening include: (1) type IV Ehler–Danlos syndrome (all individuals [12% risk] – modestly cost-effective); (2) coarctation of the aorta (all individuals [10% risk] – borderline cost-effective); (3) polycystic kidney disease (patients with one or more family members with history of UIA/SAH [16–23% risk] – cost-effective; patients without family history of UIA/SAH [6–11% risk] – uncertain cost-effectiveness).

While having a single affected family member does not sufficiently increase risk to justify screening, having two or more first-degree relatives further increases the risk towards cost-effective levels. For example, in a case–control study in Sweden, among 5282 SAH patients and 26,402 matched controls, the odds of SAH increased modestly for individuals with one affected first-degree relative (OR 2.15, 95% CI: 1.77–2.59) but increased sharply for individuals with two affected first-degree relatives (OR 51.0, 95% CI: 8.56–1117). The yield of screening will be further magnified by the presence of strong family aggregation and a history of hypertension or smoking. In the Familial Intracranial Aneurysm Study in the USA, MRA screening in individuals with at least 2 affected siblings or ≥3 affected family members, who also had either history of hypertension or smoking, identified UIAs in 19.1% of individuals (Brown et al., 2008).

Screening for UIA in families with ≥2 first-degree relatives with a history of aSAH is cost-effective and beneficial. Two separate studies, utilizing Markov models, reported that screening such individuals resulted in longer life expectancy (from 39.44 to 39.55 years), reduced morbidity (from 0.28% to 0.18%) and mortality (from 0.43% to 0.05%), with an incremental cost-effectiveness ratio of $37,400–38,410 per quality-adjusted life-year (QALY) (Takao et al., 2008; Bor et al., 2010). Based on one of these models, the optimal strategy would be to screen such individuals every 7 years from ages 20–80 years (Bor et al., 2010).

The optimal screening strategy to detect new or recurrent aneurysms in patients who have had a first aneurysm identified and treated is uncertain. Patients who had a first aSAH with successful clipping or coiling of the aneurysm that ruptured do have an elevated risk of subsequent de novo development of an additional aneurysm at a remote arterial site or of a recurrent aneurysm at the original site. In a study of 610 aSAH patients who underwent surgical clipping, follow-up CTAs, performed at a median 8.9 years, identified new aneurysms in 16% (95% CI: 13–19%), of which 81% were at a new site and 19% at the clip site. Whether routine screening after 5 years would be beneficial was not clear, as the findings were highly sensitive to the degree to which a patient's quality of life would be lowered by being told that they had a small, low-risk recurrent aneurysm not requiring treatment (Wermer et al., 2008).

Implications for Clinical Practice

Based on the evidence, screening of individuals with ≥2 family members with a UIA and/or aSAH is recommended, but it is less clear whether to screen patients with a prior aSAH or members of a family with only one affected first-degree relative. Further, it is reasonable to screen select patients with syndromic genetic/congenital conditions that predispose to aneurysm formation and aSAH, especially polycystic kidney disease, coarctation of the aorta, and vascular Ehler–Danlos syndrome (Thompson et al., 2015). The yield of aneurysm detection increases if additional risk factors are present, which should be considered in deciding whether or not to screen an individual.

Identifying Aneurysms at High Risk of Rupture

As the majority of intracranial aneurysms never rupture, and preventive surgical clipping and endovascular coiling therapies carry peri-procedural risks and expense, it is neither feasible nor appropriate to treat all UIAs. Surgical and endovascular preventive occlusion will confer benefit only in patients with UIAs at higher risk for rupture under medical therapy alone. Accordingly, extensive observational studies have been undertaken to identify features that identify which aneurysms are at greater risk of rupture (Wiebers et al., 2003; Wermer et al., 2007; Morita et al., 2012; Villablanca et al., 2013; Greving et al., 2014; Mehan et al., 2014).

Evidence

Baseline Features

A collaborative study pooled individual patient data from 6 prospective cohort studies, including the large

International Study of Unruptured Intracranial Aneurysms (ISUIA), performed at 60 centres in the USA, Canada, and Europe and the Unruptured Cerebral Aneurysm Study (UCAS) performed at 283 centres in Japan (Wiebers et al., 2003; Morita et al., 2012; Greving et al., 2014). Collectively, data were available regarding 8382 patients with 10,272 UIAs followed for 29,166 person-years, among whom 230 patients experienced rupture, with an overall 1-year risk of 1.4% (95% CI: 1.1–1.6%) and 5-year risk of 3.4% (95% CI: 2.9–4.0%).

Independent predictors of aneurysm rupture were younger age, hypertension, larger aneurysm size, aneurysm location, and geographical region (Table 22.1). In addition, history of prior SAH from another aneurysm nearly reached statistical significance. For aneurysm size, risk increased monotonically with larger aneurysm diameter, with particularly elevated hazard with aneurysms 10–19.9 mm and ≥20 mm. For aneurysm location, compared with middle cerebral artery aneurysms, rupture risk was increased for anterior cerebral, posterior

Table 22.1 Independent predictors of aneurysm rupture in pooled analysis of 8382 patients

Characteristic	Hazard ratio (95% CI)
Age (per 5 years)	0.7 (0.5–0.9)
Hypertension	1.4 (1.1–1.8)
Size of aneurysm	
<5.0 mm	Reference
5.0–6.9 mm	1.1 (0.7–1.7)
7.0–9.9 mm	2.4 (1.6–3.6)
10.0–19.9 mm	5.7 (3.9–8.3)
≥20.0 mm	21.3 (13.5–33.8)
Aneurysm location	
Middle cerebral artery	Reference
Internal carotid artery	0.5 (0.3–0.9)
Anterior cerebral artery	1.7 (1.1–2.6)
Posterior cerebral artery	1.9 (1.2–2.9)
Posterior communicating artery	2.1 (1.4–3.0)
Prior SAH from other aneurysm	1.4 (0.9–2.2)
Geographical region	
N America + Eur (not Finland)	Reference
Japan	2.8 (1.8–4.2)
Finland	3.6 (2.0–6.3)

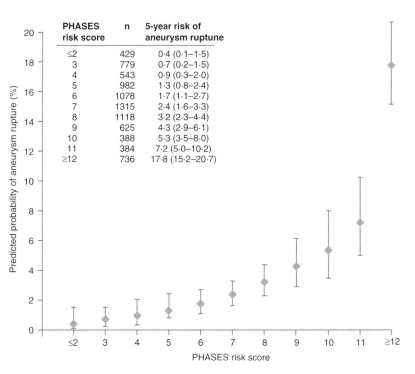

PHASES risk score	n	5-year risk of aneurysm rupture
≤2	429	0·4 (0·1–1·5)
3	779	0·7 (0·2–1·5)
4	543	0·9 (0·3–2·0)
5	982	1·3 (0·8–2·4)
6	1078	1·7 (1·1–2·7)
7	1315	2·4 (1·6–3·3)
8	1118	3·2 (2·3–4·4)
9	625	4·3 (2·9–6·1)
10	388	5·3 (3·5–8·0)
11	384	7·2 (5·0–10·2)
≥12	736	17·8 (15·2–20·7)

Figure 22.2 Predicted 5-year rate of aneurysm rupture based on the PHASES score. Reproduced from Greving et al. (2014), with permission from Elsevier Limited.

Copyright Elsevier Limited.

communicating, and posterior cerebral artery aneurysms, and decreased for internal carotid artery aneurysms. With regard to geographical region, rupture hazard was increased in Japanese and Finnish populations. The model showed a c statistic of 0.82 (95% CI: 0.79–0.85), indicating good predictive performance. However, it has not been extensively validated in independent populations.

Based on the results, the collaborative group developed a simple scoring system for prediction of aneurysmal rupture: PHASES (Population/ Hypertension/Age/Size/Earlier bleed/Site) (Greving et al., 2014) (Table 22.2). The risk score assigns weighted points based on the presence or absence of the identified independent predictors and ranges from 0 to 22, with higher scores indicating increased risk. For example, a score of 3 corresponds to a 5-year risk of rupture of 0.7% compared to 7.2% for a score of 11 (Figure 22.2) (Greving et al., 2014).

Morphological characteristics of aneurysms that increase rupture risk may allow additional stratification of patients into higher or lower risk groups. These aneurysm characteristics were not systematically assessed in all of the pooled prospective studies. However, a systematic study-level meta-analysis of prospective cohort, retrospective cohort, and case–

control studies of aneurysm morphological features identified 102 investigations analysing a total of 28,812 aneurysms (Kleinloog et al., 2018). Five morphological factors showed strong association with aneurysm rupture: (1) irregular shape (including multilobulated and presence of blebs); (2) higher aspect ratio (aneurysm height divided by neck diameter); (3) large relative size (aneurysm height divided by parent artery diameter); (4) greater bottleneck shape (aneurysm width divided by neck diameter); and (5) greater height-to-width ratio (aneurysm height divided by aneurysm width). For two of these features, data were poolable across studies. For irregular shape, across 10 studies (8736 unruptured, 1122 ruptured aneurysms), the OR was 4.80 (95% CI: 2.67–8.66). For higher aspect ratio, across 3 studies (3655 unruptured, 2453 ruptured aneurysms), the OR was 10.22 (95% CI: 4.25–24.58).

MR imaging evidence of aneurysm wall inflammation is an additional potential biomarker of aneurysm instability and heightened rupture risk. A systematic review collating 5 studies of 492 UIA patients found a strong association of aneurysm wall enhancement with aneurysm rupture, OR 34.26, 95% CI: 10.20– 115.07 (Wang et al., 2018). In studies reporting results distinguished by aneurysm size, among smaller (<7 mm) aneurysms, abnormal wall enhancement

Patient	Age (single)	< 40 years	4
		40–60 years	3
		61–70 years	2
		71–80 years	1
		>80 years	0
	Risk factor incidence (multiple)	Previous SAH from a different aneurysm	4
		Familial intracranial aneurysms or SAH	3
		Japanese, Finnish, Inuit ethnicity	2
		Current cigarette smoking	3
		Hypertension (systolic BP > 140 mm Hg)	2
		Autosomal-polycystic kidney disease	2
		Current drug abuse (cocaine, amphetamine)	2
		Current alcohol abuse	1
	Clinical Symptoms related to UIA (multiple)	Cranial nerve deficit	4
		Clinical or radiological mass effect	4
		Thromboembolic events from the aneurysm	3
		Epilepsy	1
	Other (multiple)	Reduced quality of life due to fear of rupture	2
		Aneurysm multiplicity	1
	Life expectancy due to chronic and/or malignant Diseases (single)	< 5 years	4
		5–10 years	3
		> 10 years	1
	Comorbid disease (multiple)	Neurocognitive disorder	3
		Coagulopathies, thrombophilic diseases	2
		Psychiatric disorder	2
Aneurysm	Maximum diameter (single)	≤ 3.9 mm	0
		4.0–6.9mm	1
		7.0–12.9 mm	2
		13.0–24.9 mm	3
		≥ 25 mm	4
	Morphology (multiple)	Irregularity or lobulation	3
		Size ratio > 3 or aspect ratio > 1.6	1
	Location (single)	BasA bifurcation	5
		Vertebral/basilar artery	4
		AcomA or PcomA	2
	Other (multiple)	Aneurysm growth on serial imaging	4
		Aneurysm de novo formation on serial imaging	3
		Contralateral stenoocclusive vessel disease	1
Treatment	Age-related risk (single)	< 40 years	0
		41–60years	1
		61–70years	3
		71–80years	4
		> 80 years	5
	Aneurysm size-related risk (single)	< 6.0 mm	0
		6.0–10.0 mm	1
		10.1–20.0 mm	3
		> 20 mm	5
	Aneurysm complexity-related risk	High	3
		Low	0
	Intervention-related risk	Constant*	5

Favors UIA repair   Favors UIA conservative management

Figure 22.3 The unruptured intracranial aneurysm treatment score. Reproduced from Etminan et al. (2015), with permission from Wolters Kluwer Health, Inc.

Table 22.2 PHASES risk score to grade future rupture risk of unruptured aneurysm

PHASES aneurysm risk score	Points
(P) Population	
North American, European (other than Finnish)	0
Japanese	3
Finnish	5
(H) Hypertension	
No	0
Yes	1
(A) Age	
<70 years	0
≥70 years	1
(S) Size of aneurysm	
<7.0 mm	0
7.0–9.9 mm	3
10.0–19.9 mm	6
≥20 mm	10
(E) Earlier SAH from another aneurysm	
No	0
Yes	1
(S) Site of aneurysm	
ICA	0
MCA	2
ACA/Pcom/posterior	4

To calculate the PHASES risk score for an individual, the number of points associated with each indicator can be added up to obtain the total risk score. For example, a 55-year-old North American man with no hypertension, no previous SAH, and a medium-sized (8 mm) posterior circulation aneurysm will have a risk score of 0+0+0+3+0+4=7 points. According to figure 3, this score corresponds to a 5-year risk of rupture of 2.4%. SAH=subarachnoid haemorrhage. ICA=internal carotid artery. MCA=middle cerebral artery. ACA=anterior cerebral arteries (including the anterior cerebral artery, anterior communicating artery, and pericallosal artery). Pcom=posterior communicating artery. posterior=posterior circulation (including the vertebral artery, basilar artery, cerebellar arteries, and posterior cerebral artery).

was similarly associated with rupture, OR 26.12, 95% CI: 6.11–111.76.

Aneurysm Growth

In addition to baseline features, growth over time of an unruptured aneurysm is associated with increased rupture risk. In a pooled analysis of serially imaged patients from 3 prospective cohorts, 12% of the 734 UIAs (in 557 patients) showed growth during a mean 2.7 year follow-up, and those with growth had a 12-fold increased risk of rupture (Backes et al., 2015). In another pooled study of 10 prospective cohorts (1507 patients, 1909 aneurysms), during a median follow-up of 2.5 years, aneurysm growth occurred in 14% of aneurysms (17% of patients). Among the 1.2% of patients with aneurysm rupture during follow-up, preceding aneurysm growth occurred in 8/18 (44%) (Backes et al., 2017). Independent predictors of aneurysm growth were older age, prior SAH, Japanese or Finnish population, larger size of aneurysm, and irregular aneurysm shape. From these predictors, the ELAPSS score was devised to grade aneurysm growth risk (Table 22.3).

Implications for Clinical Practice

Across studies, larger aneurysm size and posterior circulation location, and Japanese or Finnish ethnicity are consistently identified as potent predictors of aneurysm rupture, with hypertension and age also contributing. The PHASES score is a tool that can be used to calculate an estimated 5-year risk of rupture for a given UIA from clinical features, size, and location alone. Irregular aneurysm shape and presence of abnormal enhancement in the aneurysm wall likely further increase risk. The predicted risk can be weighed against the risk of surgical and endovascular intervention, and help guide providers and patients regarding management of a UIA. In patients initially managed medically, features predicative of aneurysm growth, assessed with the ELAPSS score, may identify individuals in whom monitoring with serial imaging for aneurysm stability could be cost-effective.

Treatment Options

If a procedural management approach is pursued, options include either surgical clipping or endovascular treatment. Surgical clipping involves an open craniotomy and placement of a metallic clip at the base of the aneurysm. Endovascular treatment, now the most commonly utilized method, usually involves the placement of platinum coils within the aneurysm leading to thrombosis and occlusion of the aneurysm. However, other endovascular treatments exist, including flow diverters and liquid embolic agents.

Table 22.3 ELAPSS risk score to grade future growth risk of unruptured aneurysm

Risk factor	Points
Earlier subarachnoid haemorrhage	
Yes	0
No	1
Location of aneurysm	
ICA, ACA, AComA	0
MCA	3
PCA, PComA	5
Age	
≤60 years	0
>60 years	1
Population	
N America, China, Europe (not Finland)	0
Japan	1
Finland	7
Size of aneurysm	
1.0–2.9	0
3.0–4.9	4
5.0–6.9	10
7.0–9.9	13
≥10.0	22
Shape of aneurysm	
Regular	0
Irregular	4

Predicted risk of growth		
ELAPSS score	3-y risk of growth (%)	5-y risk of growth (%)
<5	5	8
5–9	8	13
10–14	12	19
15–19	18	28
20–24	26	40
≥25	43	61

Evidence

Randomized Trials

Only two randomized trials of modest size provide information regarding the relative advantages of medical, surgical, and endovascular therapies for UIAs.

An international randomized trial comparing endovascular coiling to medical therapy alone was planned to have a large sample size, but was terminated early due to slow recruitment. Compared with the planned 2000 patients followed for 10 years, the achieved 80 patients followed for 1.1 years was insufficient to provide substantial insight. Among the enrolled patients (42 endovascular, 38 medical), no patient in either treatment group experienced the primary outcome of death or dependency (modified Rankin Scale [mRS] 3–6) as a result of SAH, ischaemic stroke, or procedural complications (Raymond et al., 2011).

A Canadian–European RCT compared endovascular coiling with surgical clipping among patients with unruptured aneurysms (Darsaut et al., 2017). Patients with UIAs 3–25 mm in diameter were enrolled, and the primary outcome was treatment failure, defined as the composite of: (1) initial failure to achieve aneurysm occlusion with the assigned modality, (2) intracranial haemorrhage during follow-up, or (3) residual aneurysm on 1-year imaging. Among 104 randomized patients with data available through 1 year of follow-up, there was no statistically significant difference in the treatment failure primary endpoint for clipping compared with coiling (10.4% vs 17.9%, OR 0.54, 95% CI: 0.13–1.90; $p = 0.40$). New neurological deficits (23.1% vs 8.7%, OR 3.12, 95% CI: 1.05–10.57) and hospitalizations beyond 5 days (46.2% vs 8.7%, OR: 8.85, 95% CI: 3.22–28.59) were more frequent after clipping.

Given the paucity of RCT data, decision-making perforce continues to take into consideration non-randomized comparison of observational studies of the course under medical therapy (reviewed above – *Identifying aneurysms at high risk of rupture*), and of the rates of technical success, peri-procedural complications, and long-term outcomes under surgical and endovascular approaches.

Observational Studies

Historically, the international, multicentre ISUIA observational study reshaped patterns of care after suggesting that: (1) complication rates of both clipping and coiling procedures were high enough to outweigh benefit for patients at low risk of rupture, and (2) among the preventive obliteration strategies, coiling had less morbidity than clipping. Among 4060 prospectively followed patients, 1917 were treated surgically and 451 were treated endovascularly (Wiebers et al., 2003). Overall, among interventionally treated UIA patients with no history of SAH from any aneurysm, death and dependency (mRS 3–6) at 1 year was 12.6% with surgical clipping and 9.8% with endovascular coiling. Among UIA patients with a history of past SAH from a different aneurysm, death and dependency at 1 year was 10.1%% with surgical clipping and 7.1% with coiling. In the surgery group, peri-procedural complications included aneurysm rupture during surgery in 6%, intracranial haemorrhage in 4%, and cerebral infarction in 11%. In the endovascular group, peri-procedural complications included peri-operative haemorrhage in 2% and cerebral infarction in 5%. The degree of immediate aneurysm obliteration was not assessed in the surgical cohort. With endovascular treatment, complete obliteration was accomplished in 55%, incomplete in 24%, and no obliteration in 3%.

Subsequent to the ISUIA study, important further technical advances in procedural interventions have occurred, most notably the development for endovascular treatment of stent-assisted coiling and of flow diverter stents to treat wide-necked aneurysms (Becske et al., 2013).

For surgical clipping, an updated systematic review collated 60 studies with 9845 patients harbouring 10,845 aneurysms (Kotowski et al., 2013). Technical success evaluation indicated that 91.8% (99% CI: 90–93.2%) of aneurysms were completely occluded, 3.9% (99% CI: 2.9–5.2%) had a neck remnant, and 4.3% (99% CI: 3.3–5.7%) were incompletely occluded. The mortality rate was 1.7% (99% CI: 0.9–3.0%), and the rate of death or dependency (mRS 3–6 or nearest equivalent) up to 1 year post-surgery was 6.7% (99% CI: 4.9–9.0). Interpretive caution of the clinical outcomes is indicated as funnel plot analysis suggested the presence of substantial publication bias. Features associated with death or dependent outcome with surgical intervention were posterior circulation aneurysm location (RR 4.1, 99% CI: 2.3–7.6) and aneurysm diameter >10 mm (RR 3.5, 95% CI: 1.4–8.9), while older patient age (>55 years) did not reach statistical significance (RR 2.6, 95% CI: 0.4–17.7).

For endovascular coiling, an updated systematic review collated 97 studies with 7172 patients (Naggara et al., 2012). Rates of death or dependency (mRS 3–6 or nearest equivalent) at 1 month declined over time, from 5.6% (99% CI: 4.7–6.6%) among patients treated through the year 2000, to 3.1% (99% CI: 2.4–4.0%) among patients treated after 2004. Non-significant increases in risk of death or dependency were noted with larger aneurysm size (RR 2.83, 99% CI: 0.81–9.91) and posterior aneurysm location (RR 2.30, 99% CI: 0.31–16.98). In an earlier meta-analysis from the same group of the first 71 studies, initial technical success in achieving aneurysm occlusion was attained in 86.1% of aneurysms. However, 24.4% of treated aneurysms recurred, necessitating retreatment in 9.1% of patients (Naggara et al., 2012).

Implications for Clinical Practice

In the absence of decisive randomized trials, decision-making regarding whether and how to pursue preventive obliteration of unruptured intracranial haemorrhages can be challenging. Procedural intervention is reasonable in UIA patients with clinical and aneurysm features indicating a high risk of rupture under medical therapy and relatively low risk of complications with endovascular or surgical therapy. In these patients, among individuals who are technical candidates for either coiling or clipping, endovascular coiling is associated with a reduction in procedural morbidity and mortality but has a higher risk of recurrence (Thompson et al., 2015). Conversely, initial conservative medical management is reasonable in UIA patients with clinical and aneurysm features indicating a low risk of rupture under medical therapy and relatively low risk of complications with endovascular or surgical therapy. Features that favour consideration of preventive occlusion include younger patient age, prior SAH from a different aneurysm, familial intracranial aneurysms, large aneurysm size, irregular shape, basilar or vertebral artery location, and aneurysm growth on serial imaging. Using a Delphi consensus-building approach, an international multidisciplinary group of experts developed a treatment score to help clinicians decide whether or not to pursue treatment (Etminan et al., 2015) (see Figure 22.3). The score is helpful in identifying important features to be considered in decision-making, though variations from it are reasonable and not infrequent in practice (Ravindra et al., 2018).

Summary

Intracerebral haemorrhage and subarachnoid haemorrhage are associated with considerable morbidity and mortality. Too often the focus is on acute treatment after a haemorrhage has occurred, instead of primary and secondary prevention. Medical therapies to control hypertension, achieve tobacco abstinence, and avoid excessive alcohol consumption can confer broad reductions in haemorrhage risk across pathophysiological subtypes. Judicious restriction of antiplatelet and anticoagulant therapies to only those individuals and those intensities for which they are indicated also can substantially reduce haemorrhagic stroke frequency. Specific endovascular and surgical therapies, judiciously employed, will further reduce risk of first or recurrent haemorrhage from structural vascular anomalies, including arteriovenous malformation, cavernous malformations, and saccular aneurysms.

References

Akers A, Al-Shahi Salman R A, Awad I, Dahlem K, Flemming K, Hart B, et al. (2017). Synopsis of guidelines for the clinical management of cerebral cavernous malformations: consensus recommendations based on systematic literature review by the Angioma Alliance Scientific Advisory Board Clinical Experts Panel. *Neurosurgery*, **80**(5), 665–80.

An SJ, Kim TJ, Yoon B-W. (2017). Epidemiology, risk factors, and clinical features of intracerebral hemorrhage: an update. *J Stroke*, 19(1), 3–10.

Antithrombotic Trialists' Collaboration, Baigent C, Blackwell L, Collins R, Emberson J, Godwin J, Peto R, et al. (2009). Aspirin in the primary and secondary prevention of vascular disease: collaborative meta-analysis of individual participant data from randomised trials. *Lancet*, **373**(9678), 1849–60.

Ariesen MJ, Claus, SP, Rinkel GJ, Algra A. (2003). Risk factors for intracerebral hemorrhage in the general population: a systematic review. *Stroke*, **34**(8), 2060–5.

Aune D, Giovannucci E, Boffetta P, Fadnes LT, Keum N, Norat T, et al. (2017). Fruit and vegetable intake and the risk of cardiovascular disease, total cancer and all-cause mortality – a systematic review and dose-response meta-analysis of prospective studies. *Int J Epidemiol*, **46**(3), 1029–56.

Backes D, Vergouwen MD, Tiel Groenestege AT, Bor AS, Velthuis BK, Greving JP, et al. (2015). PHASES score for prediction of intracranial aneurysm growth. *Stroke*, **46**, 1221–6.

Backes D, Rinkel GJE, Greving JP, Velthuis BK, Murayama Y, Takao H, et al. (2017). ELAPSS score for prediction of risk of growth of unruptured intracranial aneurysms. *Neurology*, **88**(17), 1600–06.

Becske T, Kallmes, DF, Saatci I, McDougal CG, Szikora I, Lanzino G, et al. (2013). Pipeline for uncoilable or failed aneurysms: results from a multicenter clinical trial. *Radiology*, **267**(3), 858–68.

Bell S, Daskalopoulou M, Rapsomaniki E, George J, Britton A, Bobak M, et al. (2017). Association between clinically recorded alcohol consumption and initial presentation of 12 cardiovascular diseases: population based cohort study using linked health records. *BMJ*, **356**, j909.

Biffi A, Kuramatsu JB, Leasure A, Kamel H, Kourkoulis C, Schwab K, et al. (2017). Oral anticoagulation and functional outcome after intracerebral hemorrhage. *Ann Neurol*, **82**(5), 755–65.

Biffi A, Sonni A, Anderson CD, Kissela B, Jagiella JM, Schmidt H, et al.; International Stroke Genetics Consortium. (2010). Variants at APOE influence risk of deep and lobar intracerebral hemorrhage. *Ann Neurol*, **68**(6), 934–43.

Bor AS, Koffijberg H, Wermer MJ, Rinkel GJ. (2010). Optimal screening strategy for familial intracranial aneurysms: a cost-effectiveness analysis. *Neurology*, **74**(21), 1671–9.

Boulanger M, Poon MT, Wild SH, Al-Shahi Salman R. (2016). Association between diabetes mellitus and the occurrence and outcome of intracerebral hemorrhage. *Neurology*, **87**(9), 870–8.

Brinjikji W, Zhu Y-Q, Lanzino B, Cloft HJ, Murad MH, Wang Z, Kallmes DF. (2016). Risk factors for growth of intracranial aneurysms: a systematic review and meta-analysis. *AJNR*, **37**(4), 615–20.

Broderick JP, Brown, RD Jr, Sauerbeck L, Hornung R, Huston J III, Woo D, et al. (2009). Greater rupture risk for familial as compared to sporadic unruptured intracranial aneurysms. *Stroke*, **40**(6), 1952–7.

Brown RD. (2010). Unruptured intracranial aneurysms. *Semin Neurol*, **30**(5), 537–44.

Brown RD Jr, Flemming KD, Meyer FB, Cloft HJ, Pollock BE, Link MJ, et al. (2005). Natural history, evaluation, and management of intracranial vascular malformations. *Mayo Clin Proc*, **80**(2), 269–81.

Brown RD Jr, Huston J, Hornung R, Foroud T, Kallmes DF, Kleindorfer D, et al. (2008). Screening for brain aneurysm in the Familial Intracranial Aneurysm study: frequency and predictors of lesion detection. *J Neurosurg*, **108**(6), 1132–8.

Bruins Slot KM, Berge E. (2018). Factor Xa inhibitors versus vitamin K antagonists for preventing cerebral or systemic embolism in patients with atrial fibrillation. *Cochrane Database Syst Rev*, 3. doi:10.1002/14651858.CD008980.pub3.

Can A, Rudy RF, Castro VM, Yu S, Dligach D, Finan S, et al. (2018). Association between aspirin dose and subarachnoid hemorrhage from saccular aneurysms: a case-control study. *Neurology*, **91**(12), e1175–e1181. doi:10.1212/WNL.0000000000006200.

Chang TR, Kowalski RG, Caserta F, Carhuapoma JR, Tamargo RJ, Naval NS. (2013). Impact of acute cocaine use on aneurysmal subarachnoid hemorrhage. *Stroke*, **44**(7), 1825–9.

Chou R, Dana T, Blazina I, Daeges M, Jeanne TL. (2016). Statins for prevention of cardiovascular disease in adults: evidence report and systematic review for the US Preventive Services Task Force. *JAMA*, **316**(19), 2008–24.

Darke S, Lappin J, Kaye S, Duflou J (2018). Clinical characteristics of fatal methamphetamine-related stroke: a national study. *J Forensic Sci*, **63**(3), 735–9.

Darsaut TE, Findlay JM, Magro E, Kotowski M, Roy D, Weill A, et al. (2017). Surgical clipping or endovascular coiling for unruptured intracranial aneurysms: a pragmatic randomised trial. *J Neurol Neurosurg Psychiatry*, **88**(8), 663–8.

Derdeyn CP, Zipfel GJ, Albuquerque FC, Cooke DL, Feldmann E, Sheehan JP, Torner JC; American Heart Association Stroke Council. (2017). Management of brain arteriovenous malformations: a scientific statement for healthcare professionals from the American Heart Association/American Stroke Association. *Stroke*, **48**(8), e200–e224.

Ding X, Liu X, Tan C, Yin M, Wang T, Liu Y, et al. (2018). Resumption of antiplatelet therapy in patients with primary intracranial hemorrhage-benefits and risks: a meta-analysis of cohort studies. *J Neurol Sci*, **384**, 133–8.

Etminan N, Chang HS, Hackenberg K, de Rooij NK, Vergouwen MDI, Rinkel GJE, Algra A. (2019). Worldwide incidence of aneurysmal subarachnoid hemorrhage according to region, time period, blood pressure, and smoking prevalence in the population: a systematic review and meta-analysis. *JAMA Neurol*, **76** (5), 588–97. doi:10.1001/jamaneurol.2019.0006. [Epub ahead of print]

Etminan N, Brown RD Jr, Beseoglu K, Juvela S, Raymond J, Morita A, et al. (2015). The unruptured intracranial aneurysm treatment score: a multidisciplinary consensus. *Neurology*, **85**(10), 881–9.

Ettehad D, Emdin CA, Kiran A, Anderson SG, Callender T, Emberson J, et al. (2016). Blood pressure lowering for prevention of cardiovascular disease and death: a systematic review and meta-analysis. *Lancet*, **387**(10022), 957–67.

Feigin V, Parag, V, Lawess CMM, Rogers A, Suh II, Woodward M, et al. (2005a). Smoking and elevated blood pressure are the most important risk factors for subarachnoid hemorrhage in the Asia-Pacific region: an overview of 26 cohorts involving 306,620 participants. *Stroke*, **36**(7), 1360–5.

Feigin VL, Rinkel, GJ, Lawes CM, Algra A, Bennett DA, van Gijn J, et al. (2005b). Risk factors for subarachnoid hemorrhage: an updated systematic review of epidemiological studies. *Stroke*, **36**(12)., 2773–80.

Feldmann E, Broderick JP, Kernan WN, Viscoli CM, Brass LM, Brott T, et al. (2005). Major risk factors for intracerebral hemorrhage in the young are modifiable. *Stroke*, **36**(9), 1881–5.

Flaherty ML, Kissela B, Woo D, Kleindorfer D, Alwell K, Sekar P, et al. (2007). The increasing incidence of anticoagulant-associated intracerebral hemorrhage. *Neurology*, **68**(2), 116–21.

Flemming KD, Graff-Radford J, Aakre J, Kantarci K, Lanzino G, et al. (2017). Population-based prevalence of cerebral cavernous malformations in older adults: Mayo Clinic Study of Aging. *JAMA Neurol*, **74**, 801–05.

Greving JP, Wermer MJ, Brown RD, Morita A, Juvela S, Yonekura M, et al. (2014). Development of the PHASES score for prediction of risk of rupture of intracranial aneurysms: a pooled analysis of six prospective cohort studies. *Lancet Neurol*, **13**(1), 59–66.

Guresir E, Vatter H, Schuss P, Platz J, Konczalla J, de Rochement Rdu M, et al. (2013). Natural history of small unruptured anterior circulation aneurysms: a prospective cohort study. *Stroke*, **44**(11), 3027–31.

Hanger HC, Wilkinson TJ, Fayez-Iskander N, Sainsbury R. (2007). The risk of recurrent stroke after intracerebral haemorrhage. *J Neurol Neurosurg Psychiatry*, **78**(8), 836–40.

Hanif H, Belley-Cote EP, Alotaibi A, Dvirnik N, Neupane B, Beyene J, et al. (2018). Left atrial appendage occlusion for stroke prevention in patients with atrial fibrillation: a systematic review and network meta-analysis of randomized controlled trials. *J Cardiovasc Surg (Torino)*, **59**(1), 128–39.

Hankey GJ, Stevens SR, Piccini JP, Lokhnygina Y, Mahaffey KW, Halperin JL, et al. ROCKET AF Steering Committee and Investigators. (2014). Intracranial hemorrhage among patients with atrial fibrillation anticoagulated with warfarin or rivaroxaban: the rivaroxaban once daily, oral, direct factor Xa inhibition compared with vitamin K antagonism for prevention of stroke and embolism trial in atrial fibrillation. *Stroke*, **45**, 1304–12.

Hart RG, Diener HC, Yang S, Connolly SJ, Wallentin L, Reilly PA, et al. (2012). Intracranial hemorrhage in atrial fibrillation patients during anticoagulation with warfarin or dabigatran: the RE-LY trial. *Stroke*, **43**, 1511–17.

Hasan DM, Mahaney KB, Brown RD, Meissner I, Piepgras DG, Huston J, et al. (2011). Aspirin as a promising agent for decreasing incidence of cerebral aneurysm rupture. *Stroke*, **42**(11), 3156–62.

Hasan DM, Chalouhi N, Jabbour P, Dumont AS, Kung DK, Magnotta VA, et al. (2013). Evidence that acetylsalicylic acid attenuates inflammation in the walls of human cerebral aneurysms: preliminary results. *J Am Heart Assoc*, **2**(1), e000019. doi:10.1161/JAHA.112.000019.

Hemphill JC 3rd, Greenberg SM, Anderson CS, Becker K, Bendok BR, Cushman M, et al. (2015). Guidelines for the management of spontaneous intracerebral hemorrhage: a guideline for healthcare professionals from the American Heart Association/American Stroke Association. *Stroke*, **46** (7), 2032–60.

Hitchcock E, Gibson WT. (2017). A review of the genetics of intracranial berry aneurysms and implications for genetic counseling. *J Genet Couns*, **26**(1), 21–31.

Horne MA, Flemming KD, Su IC, Stapf C, Jeon JP, Li D, et al.; Cerebral Cavernous Malformations Individual Patient

Data Meta-analysis Collaborators. (2016). Clinical course of untreated cerebral cavernous malformations: a meta-analysis of individual patient data. *Lancet Neurol*, **15**(2), 166–73.

Inohara T, Xian Y, Liang L, Matsouaka RA, Saver JL, Smith EE, et al. (2018). Association of intracerebral hemorrhage among patients taking non-vitamin K antagonist vs vitamin K antagonist oral anticoagulants with in-hospital mortality. *JAMA*, **319**(5), 463–73. doi:10.1001/jama.2017.21917.

International Study of Unruptured Intracranial Aneurysms Investigators. (1998). Unruptured intracranial aneurysms – risk of rupture and risks of surgical intervention. *N Engl J Med*, **339**(24), 1725–33.

Kase CS, Kurth T. (2011). Prevention of intracerebral hemorrhage recurrence. *Continuum (Minneap Minn)*, **17**(6), 1304–17. doi:10.1212/01.CON.0000410037.64971.e3.

Kernan WN, C. M. Viscoli, CM, Brass LM, Broderick JP, Brott T, Feldmann E, et al. (2000). Phenylpropanolamine and the risk of hemorrhagic stroke. *N Engl J Med*, **343**(25), 1826–32.

Kim H, Al-Shahi Salman R, McCulloch CE, Stapf C, Young WL; MARS Coinvestigators. (2014). Untreated brain arteriovenous malformation: patient level meta-analysis of hemorrhage predictors. *Neurology*, **83**, 590–7.

Kleinloog R, de Mul N, Verweij BH, Post JA, Rinkel GJE, Ruigrok YM. (2018). Risk factors for intracranial aneurysm rupture: a systematic review. *Neurosurgery*, **82**(4), 431–40.

Knopman J, Stieg PE. (2014). Management of unruptured brain arteriovenous malformations. *Lancet*, **383**(9917), 581–3.

Korja M, Lehto H, Juvela S. (2014). Lifelong rupture risk of intracranial aneurysms depends on risk factors: a prospective Finnish cohort study. *Stroke*, **45**(7), 1958–63.

Kotowski M, Naggara O, Darsaut TE, Nolet S. (2013). Safety and occlusion rates of surgical treatment of unruptured intracranial aneurysms: a systematic review and meta-analysis of the literature from 1990 to 2011. *J Neurol Neurosurg Psychiatry*, **84**(1), 42–8.

Krishnamurthi RV, Moran AE, Forouzanfar MH, Bennett DA, Mensah GA, Lawes CM, et al.; Global Burden of Diseases, Injuries, and Risk Factors 2010 Study Stroke Expert Group. (2014). The global burden of hemorrhagic stroke: a summary of findings from the GBD 2010 study. *Glob Heart*, **9**(1), 101–6.

Lappin JM, Darke S, Farrell M. (2017). Stroke and methamphetamine use in young adults: a review. *J Neurol Neurosurg Psychiatry*, **88**(12), 1079–91.

Larsson S C, Mannisto S, Virtanen MJ, Kontto J, Albanes D, Virtamo J. (2008). Coffee and tea consumption and risk of stroke subtypes in male smokers. *Stroke*, **39**(6), 1681–7.

Larsson SC, Mannisto S, Virtanen, MJ, Kontto J, Albanes D, Virtamo J. (2009a). Dairy foods and risk of stroke. *Epidemiology*, **20**(3), 355–60.

Larsson SC, Mannisto S, Virtanen MJ, Kontto J, Albanes D, Virtamo J. (2009b). Dietary fiber and fiber-rich food intake in relation to risk of stroke in male smokers. *Eur J Clin Nutr*, **63**(8), 1016–24.

Larsson SC, Wallin A, Wolk A, Markus HS. (2016). Differing association of alcohol consumption with different stroke types: a systematic review and meta-analysis. *BMC Med*, **14**(1), 178.

Lee SM, Choi NK, Lee B-C, Cho K-H, Yoon B-W, Park B-J. (2013). Caffeine-containing medicines increase the risk of hemorrhagic stroke. *Stroke*, **44**(8), 2139–43.

Li LM, Bulters, DO, Kirollos R. (2012). A mathematical model of utility for single screening of asymptomatic unruptured intracranial aneurysms at the age of 50 years. *Acta Neurochirurgica*, **154**(7), 1145–52.

Lloyd-Jones DM, Hong Y, Labarthe D, Mozaffarian D, Appel LJ, Van Horn L, et al., on behalf of the American Heart Association Strategic Planning Task Force and Statistics Committee. (2010). Defining and setting national goals for cardiovascular health promotion and disease reduction: the American Heart Association's Strategic Impact Goal through 2020 and beyond. *Circulation*, **121**, 586–613.

Lopes RD, Guimarães PO, Kolls BJ, Wojdyla DM, Bushnell CD, Hanna M, et al. (2017). Intracranial hemorrhage in patients with atrial fibrillation receiving anticoagulation therapy. *Blood*, **129**(22), 2980–7.

McKinney JS, Kostis WJ. (2012). Statin therapy and the risk of intracerebral hemorrhage: a meta-analysis of 31 randomized controlled trials. *Stroke*, **43**(8), 2149–56.

McNeil JJ, Wolfe R, Woods RL, Tonkin AM, Donnan GA, Nelson MR, et al.; ASPREE Investigator Group. (2018). Effect of aspirin on cardiovascular events and bleeding in the healthy elderly. *N Engl J Med*, **379**(16), 1509–1518.

Mehan WA Jr, Romero, JM, Hirsch JA, Sabbag DJ, Gonzalez RG, Heit JJ, et al. (2014). Unruptured intracranial aneurysms conservatively followed with serial CT angiography: could morphology and growth predict rupture? *J Neurointerv Aurg*, **6**(10), 761–6.

Meschia JF, Bushnell C, Boden-Albala B, Braun LT, Bravata DM, Chaturvedi S, et al. (2014). Guidelines for the primary prevention of stroke: a statement for healthcare professionals from the American Heart Association/American Stroke Association. *Stroke*, **45**(12), 3754–832.

Mohr JP, Parides MK, Staph C, Moquete E, Moy CS, Overbey JR, et al. (2014). Medical management with or without interventional therapy for unruptured brain arteriovenous malformations (ARUBA): a multicentre, non-blinded, randomised trial. *Lancet*, **383**(9917), 614–21.

Morita A, Kirino T, Hashi K, Aoki N, Fukuhara S, Hashimoto N, et al. (2012). The natural course of unruptured cerebral aneurysms in a Japanese cohort. *N Engl J Med*, **366**(26), 2474–82.

Morris Z, Whiteley WN, Longstreth WT Jr, Weber F, Lee YC, Tsushima Y, et al. (2009). Incidental findings on brain magnetic resonance imaging: systematic review and meta-analysis. *BMJ*, **339**, b3016.

Naggara ON, Lecler A, Oppenheim C, Meder JF, Raymond J. (2012). Endovascular treatment of intracranial unruptured aneurysms: a systematic review of the literature on safety with emphasis on subgroup analyses. *Radiology*, **263**(3), 828–35.

O'Donnell MJ, Chin SL, Rangarajan S, Xavier D, Liu L, Zhang H, et al.; INTERSTROKE investigators. (2016). Global and regional effects of potentially modifiable risk factors associated with acute stroke in 32 countries (INTERSTROKE): a case-control study. *Lancet*, **388**(10046), 761–75. doi:10.1016/S0140-6736(16)30506-2. Epub 2016 Jul 16.

Owens AP 3rd, Mackman N. (2014). The antithrombotic effects of statins. *Annu Rev Med*, **65**, 433–45.

Pandit AK, Kumar P, Kumar A, Chakravarty K, Misra S, Prasad K (2016). High-dose statin therapy and risk of intracerebral hemorrhage: a meta-analysis. *Acta Neurol Scand*, **134**(1), 22–8.

Poorthuis MH, Klijn CJ, Algra A, Rinkel GJ, Al-Shahi Salman R. (2014). Treatment of cerebral cavernous malformations: a systematic review and meta-regression analysis. *J Neurol Neurosurg Psychiatry*, **85**(12), 1319–23.

PROGRESS Collaborative Group. (2001). Randomised trial of a perindopril-based blood-pressure-lowering regimen among 6,105 individuals with previous stroke or transient ischaemic attack. *Lancet*, **358**(9287), 1033–41.

Providência R, Grove EL, Husted S, Barra S, Boveda S, Morais J. (2014). A meta-analysis of phase III randomized controlled trials with novel oral anticoagulants in atrial fibrillation: comparisons between direct thrombin inhibitors vs. factor Xa inhibitors and different dosing regimens. *Thromb Res*, **134**(6), 1253–64.

Raaymakers TW. (1999). Aneurysms in relatives of patients with subarachnoid hemorrhage: frequency and risk factors. MARS Study Group. Magnetic Resonance Angiography in Relatives of patients with Subarachnoid hemorrhage. *Neurology*, **53**(5), 982–8.

Rapsomaniki E, Timmis A, George J, Pujades-Rodriguez M, Shah AD, Denaxas S, et al. (2014). Blood pressure and incidence of twelve cardiovascular diseases: lifetime risks, healthy life-years lost, and age-specific associations in 1·25 million people. *Lancet*, **383**(9932), 1899–911.

Ravindra VM, de Havenon A, Gooldy TC, Scoville J, Guan J, Couldwell WT, et al. (2018). Validation of the unruptured intracranial aneurysm treatment score: comparison with real-world cerebrovascular practice. *J Neurosurg*, **129**(1), 100–06. doi:10.3171/2017.4.JNS17548.

Raymond J, Darsaut TE, Molyneux AJ; TEAM Collaborative Group. (2011). A trial on unruptured intracranial aneurysms (the TEAM trial): results, lessons from a failure and the necessity for clinical care trials. *Trials*, **12**(64). doi:10.1186/1745-6215-12-64.

Ridker PM. (2018). Should aspirin be used for primary prevention in the post-statin era? *N Engl J Med*, **379**(16), 1572–4.

Rodriguez-Torres A, Murphy M, Kourkoulis C, Schwab K, Ayres AM, Moomaw CJ, et al. (2018). Hypertension and intracerebral hemorrhage recurrence among white, black, and Hispanic individuals. *Neurology*, **91**(1), e37–e44.

Sacco S, Marini C, Toni C, Olivieri L, Carolei A. (2009). Incidence and 10-year survival of intracerebral hemorrhage in a population-based registry. *Stroke*, **40**(2), 394–9

Sabatine MS, Giugliano RP, Keech AC, Honarpour N, Wiviott SD, Murphy SA, et al.; FOURIER Steering Committee and Investigators. (2017). Evolocumab and clinical outcomes in patients with cardiovascular disease. *N Engl J Med*, **376**(18), 1713–22.

Saver JL, Cushman M. (2018). Striving for ideal cardiovascular and brain health: it is never too early or too late. *JAMA*, **320**(7), 645–7.

Schurks M, Glynn RJ, Rist PM, Tzourio C, Kurth T. (2010). Effects of vitamin E on stroke subtypes: meta-analysis of randomised controlled trials. *BMJ*, **341**, c5702.

Shiue I, Arima H, Hankey GJ, Anderson C. (2012). Modifiable lifestyle behaviours account for most cases of subarachnoid haemorrhage: a population-based case-control study in Australasia. *J Neurol Sci*, **313**(1–2), 92–4.

Spiegler S, Rath M, Paperlein C, Felbor U. (2018). Cerebral cavernous malformations: an update on prevalence, molecular genetic analyses, and genetic counselling. *Mol Syndromol*, **9**(2), 60–9.

Steiner T, Weitz JI, Veltkamp R. (2017). Anticoagulant-associated intracranial hemorrhage in the era of reversal agents. *Stroke*, **48**(5), 1432–7.

Takao H, Nojo T, Ohtomo K. (2008). Screening for familial intracranial aneurysms: decision and cost-effectiveness analysis. *Acad Radiol*, **15**(4), 462–71.

Thompson BG, Brown RD Jr., Amin-Hanjani S, Broderick JP, Cockroft KM, Connolly ES Jr, et al. (2015). Guidelines for the management of patients with unruptured intracranial aneurysms: a guideline for healthcare professionals from the American Heart Association/American Stroke Association. *Stroke*, **46**(8), 2368–400.

Tulamo R, Frösen J, Hernesniemi J, Niemelä M. (2018). Inflammatory changes in the aneurysm wall: a review. *J Neurointerv Surg*, **10**(Suppl 1), i58–i67.

Vergouwen MD, de Haan R, Vermeulen M, Roos YB. (2008). Statin treatment and the occurrence of hemorrhagic stroke in patients with a history of cerebrovascular disease. *Stroke*, **39**(2), 497–502.

Villablanca JP, Duckwiler, GR, Jahan R, Tateshima S, Martin NA, Frazee J, et al. (2013). Natural history of asymptomatic unruptured cerebral aneurysms evaluated at CT angiography: growth and rupture incidence and correlation with epidemiologic risk factors. *Radiology*, **269**(1), 258–65.

Vlak MH, Algra, A, Brandenburg R, Rinkel GJ. (2011). Prevalence of unruptured intracranial aneurysms, with emphasis on sex, age, comorbidity, country, and time period: a systematic review and meta-analysis. *Lancet Neurol*, **10**(7), 626–36.

Wang X, Zhu C, Leng Y, Degnan AJ, Lu J. (2018). Intracranial aneurysm wall enhancement associated with aneurysm rupture: a systematic review and meta-analysis. *Acad Radiol*, **26**(5), 664–73. doi:10.1016/j.acra.2018.05.005.

Wermer MJ, Koffijberg H, van der Schaaf I. (2008). Effectiveness and costs of screening for aneurysms every 5 years after subarachnoid hemorrhage. *Neurology*, **70**(22), 2053–62.

Wermer MJ, van der Schaaf, IC, Algra A, Rinkel GJ. (2007). Risk of rupture of unruptured intracranial aneurysms in relation to patient and aneurysm characteristics: an updated meta-analysis. *Stroke*, **38**(4), 1404–10.

Whelton PK, Carey RM, Aronow WS, Casey DE Jr, Collins KJ, Dennison Himmelfarb C, et al. (2018). 2017 ACC/AHA/AAPA/ABC/ACPM/AGS/APhA/ASH/ASPC/NMA/PCNA Guideline for the Prevention, Detection, Evaluation, and Management of High Blood Pressure in Adults: a report of the American College of Cardiology/American Heart Association Task Force on Clinical Practice Guidelines. *Hypertension*, **71**(6), e13–e115.

Wiebers DO, Whisnant, JP, Huston J 3rd, Meissner I, Brown RD Jr, Piepgras DG, et al. (2003). Unruptured intracranial aneurysms: natural history, clinical outcome, and risks of surgical and endovascular treatment. *Lancet*, **362**(9378), 103–10.

Zhang Y, Tuomilehto J, Jousilahti P, Wang Y, Antikainen R, Hu G. (2011). Lifestyle factors on the risks of ischemic and hemorrhagic stroke. *Arch Intern Med*, **171**(20), 1811–18.

Chapter

23

Evidence-based Motor Rehabilitation after Stroke

Gert Kwakkel

Janne M. Veerbeek

Introduction

About 10.3 million people worldwide have a new stroke every year and about 25.7 million stroke survivors and 6.5 million stroke-related deaths are reported (Feigin et al., 2015), making stroke the second most common cause of death and one of the main causes of acquired adult disability (Langhorne et al., 2011; Feigin et al., 2015). The main goal of stroke rehabilitation is to restore patients' independence in their activities of daily living (ADL) and with that health-related quality of life (HR-QoL). Thrombolysis applied within the first 4.5 hours post-stroke (Kohrmann et al., 2006; Prabhakaran et al., 2015) and endovascular stroke treatment such as thrombectomy (Berkhemer et al., 2015; Saver et al., 2016) are both aimed to restrict the consequences of irreversible brain damage very early post-stroke. Evidence-based stroke rehabilitation is seen as the next most effective option to minimize the disabling consequences of stroke (Langhorne et al., 2011). Rehabilitation has a rather non-specific definition: 'A problem solving process aiming at reducing the disability and handicap resulting from a disease' (Langhorne and Legg, 2003). The interventions delivered have different levels of complexity and may be classified at level of services involved (i.e. service level), type of discipline that delivered the therapy (i.e. operator level), or more specific type of intervention applied (i.e. treatment level) (Langhorne and Legg, 2003). These different levels in which therapists need to be educated to implement new protocols are assumed to be better than the usual care, but make the experimental intervention a black box and designing trials to evaluate the effectiveness of rehabilitation interventions rather complex. Effective stroke rehabilitation allows patients to cope with the existing neurological deficits and entails a cyclic process of: (1) assessing to identify and quantify patients' needs and wishes; (2) defining realistic and attainable goals for improvement; (3) applying the most effective intervention for achieving set goals; and (4) monitoring the improvements in light of set goals (Langhorne et al., 2011).

Classification of Stroke Outcome

Disabling disorders such as stroke can be classified within the World Health Organization's (WHO) International Classification of Functioning, Disability, and Health model (ICF) (WHO, 2001) (www.who.int/classifications/icf), which provides a framework for the effect of stroke on the individual (Figure 23.1) in terms of pathology (disease or diagnosis), impairment (symptoms and signs), activity limitations (disability), and participation restriction (handicap) (Langhorne et al., 2011). This commonly accepted framework of the ICF is used across all medical specialties involved in stroke care for assessment of impairments such as high blood pressure, glycaemia, hemiplegia, pain, visuospatial neglect, memory deficits, fatigue, and depression. Assessing its second and third domains (activity and participation) is less common in medicine, but fundamental in stroke rehabilitation (Langhorne et al., 2011). Indeed, the final purpose of rehabilitation is to improve patients' functioning, i.e. the activities that patients perform in their home environment, and their participation in social life. The different domains of ICF should be separately and specifically measured, in order to obtain a comprehensive assessment of the patient (Lejeune and Stoquart, 2015).

Mechanisms Underlying Stroke Recovery

Motor recovery is a heterogeneous and complex process that probably occurs through a combination of spontaneous neurological recovery and learning-dependent processes, including restitution (i.e. restoring the functionality of damaged neural tissue), substitution (i.e. reorganization of partly spared neural pathways to relearn lost functions), and

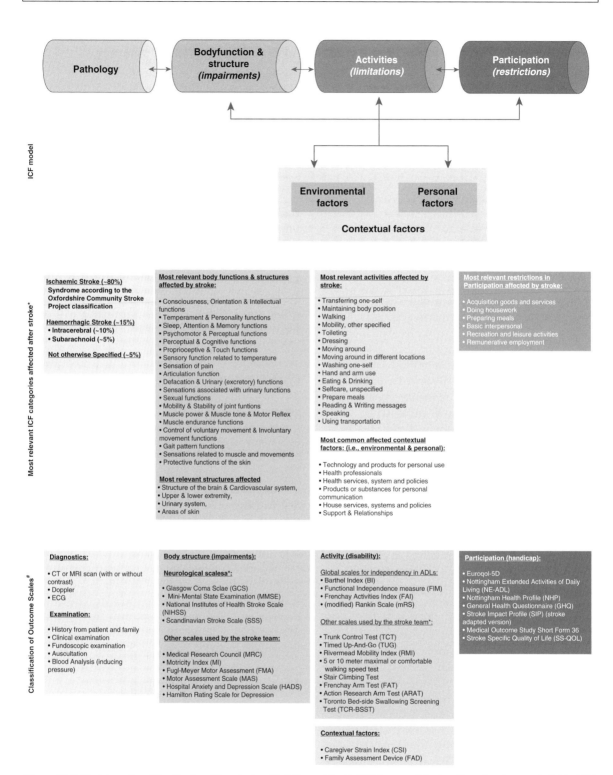

Figure 23.1 The International Classification of Functioning, Disability, and Health (ICF) framework for the effect of stroke on an individual. This figure summarizes key features of WHO's ICF model and includes the most relevant categories affected after stroke and examples of measurement scales used in those categories. ADL = activities of daily living, ECG = electrocardiograph. With permission from the *Lancet* (Langhorne et al., 2011).

compensation (i.e. improvement of the disparity between the impaired skills of a patient and the demands of their environment) (Langhorne et al., 2011; Buma et al., 2013). Several longitudinal studies with repeated measurements in time have shown that about 70–80% of most observed neurological improvements can be explained by spontaneous neurological recovery in the first 3 months (Kwakkel et al., 2006b). Due to the logistic pattern of neurological recovery, meaningful activities return, such as walking ability, upper limb capacity, and performing ADL. However, next to these underlying mechanisms, there is growing evidence that intensive, context- and task-specific motor training has a surplus value beyond expected levels of spontaneous recovery. Estimates from several meta-analyses show that the contribution of rehabilitation on top of this non-linear improvement ranges from 5 to 15% of the variance of outcome (Kwakkel et al., 2004; Veerbeek et al., 2014; Kwakkel et al., 2015). This finding shows that the added value of motor rehabilitation interventions should be seen as ways to enhance the pattern of (spontaneous) neurological recovery in the first 3 months post-stroke, making patients earlier independent in their environment than when therapies are postponed or inadequate (Kwakkel et al., 1999).

Despite growing evidence from a number of animal studies (Murphy and Corbett, 2009), the underlying mechanisms that drive motor recovery early post-stroke are still poorly understood (Cramer 2008a, 2008b). The evidence that motor learning is able to interact with early mechanisms of spontaneous neurological recovery is limited (Buma et al., 2013). Findings from several longitudinal kinematic studies suggest that improvements are mainly based on learning adaptation strategies in which patients learn to optimize the still intact or spontaneously recovered end-effectors after stroke (Buma et al., 2013; van Kordelaar et al., 2013; Kwakkel et al., 2015b; Cortes et al., 2017). Recently, a number of studies suggest that this amount of spontaneous neurological recovery is highly predictable within the first 72 hours post-stroke, which follows a proportional amount of change in motor outcome (Prabhakaran et al., 2008; Winters et al., 2015; Veerbeek et al., 2018; van der Vliet et al., 2020, in press), neglect (Nijboer et al., 2013), and aphasia (Lazar et al., 2010).

Predictability of Stroke Recovery

Due to spontaneous mechanisms of neurological recovery, the time course after stroke follows a logistic pattern, which is characterized by larger improvements in neurological impairments such as synergistic motor control, strength, and visuospatial attention during the first 10 weeks post-stroke (Kwakkel et al., 2006b; Kwakkel and Kollen, 2013). This subacute phase is followed by a gradual levelling off in observed improvements in the months that follow. After 3 to 6 months, recovery of most activities such as dexterity and walking ability plateaus (Kwakkel and Kollen, 2013).

Several cohort studies have shown that final outcomes of the upper (Kwakkel and Kollen, 2007) and lower limb (Kwakkel et al. 2006b; Smith et al., 2017), as well as independency in ADL (Veerbeek et al., 2011b), are highly predictable within the first days post-stroke. In particular, the initial severity of neurological deficits, often assessed with the National Institutes of Health Stroke Scale (NIHSS), and, with that, initial disability (Veerbeek et al., 2011b; Kwakkel and Kollen, 2013) are important indicators of final outcome 6 months after stroke onset (Kwakkel and Kollen, 2013; Scrutinio et al., 2017). In addition, patients of older age have poorer outcomes in ADL when compared with younger subjects. However, it remains unclear to what extent this determinant is modified by the pre-morbidities before stroke (Kwakkel and Kollen, 2013). Important determinants for motor recovery of the upper limb are the voluntary control of finger extension and shoulder abduction (i.e., SAFE model) (Nijland et al., 2010), reflecting the integrity of the corticospinal tract (CST), and the presence of motor evoked potentials (MEPs) (Stinear et al., 2017, Stinear, 2017). However, testing the intactness of CST by transcranial magnetic stimulation (TMS) of the abductor digiti minimi (ADM) (TMS-ADM) within the first 48 hours and 11 days post-stroke showed no added prognostic value when compared with the clinical SAFE model alone for the upper limb (Hoonhorst et al., 2018). For outcome of walking ability, patients' ability to sit independently without any support for at least 30 seconds and severity of lower limb paresis within the first 72 hours post-stroke are seen as important prognostic indicators (Veerbeek et al., 2011c).

Evidence-based Practice in Stroke Motor Rehabilitation

In the present chapter, we will review the evidence of the most used rehabilitation interventions aimed at improving meaningful activities such as upper limb capacity, balance control, gait, and other (basic) ADL post-stroke. For this purpose, we restricted what we investigated to the pooled and summarized evidence from randomized clinical trials (RCTs) as presented in well-conducted phase III trials that obey the ONSORT statement (Schulz et al., 2010) (www.consort-statement.org/), Cochrane reviews of trials, and meta-analyses that obey key criteria of the PRISMA (Schulz et al., 2010) (www.prisma-statement.org/).

In the next paragraphs, we will look mainly at interventions that have shown strong or moderate evidence in terms of body functions and activities. Therapies with **strong** evidence for improving body functions and meaningful activities (**i.e., Level 1**) were based on generally consistent findings in multiple, relevant, high-quality RCTs (PEDRO scores >3) (Veerbeek et al., 2014) and analysed in meta-analyses (preferably Cochrane reviews) that after pooling of individual phase II trials of high quality showed significant overall effects favouring the experimental intervention. Alternatively, a single phase III or IV trial of sufficient methodological quality was also considered as strong evidence. **Moderate evidence (i.e., Level 2)** was based on evidence that was provided in one relevant trial of high quality.

The evidence of (neuro)pharmacological interventions combined with motor rehabilitation as well as studies that used transcranial direct current stimulation (tDCS) or repetitive transcranial magnetic stimulation (rTMS) are beyond the scope of the present chapter and are discussed elsewhere in this book.

Evidence for Very Early Mobilization within 24 Hours Post-stroke

Very early rehabilitation, in which patients are mobilized out-of-bed in the first 48 hours after stroke and during which they are stimulated to be physically active, was strongly believed to contribute to the effectiveness of stroke-unit care. This belief was built on four neutral, phase II trials (N = 218), making the evidence for very early mobilization post-stroke rather weak (Bernhardt et al., 2015a).

The recently conducted phase III trial (Bernhardt et al., 2015b), involving 2104 stroke patients, showed that fewer patients in the very early mobilization group (6.5 times 30 minutes within 24–48 hours post-stroke) had a favourable outcome on the modified Rankin Scale (mRS) when compared with those in the

usual care group (who were mobilized 3 times for 10 minutes within the first 24 hours) (N = 480 [46%] vs N = 525 [50%]). Eighty-eight (8%) of all patients died in the very early mobilization group compared with 72 (7%) patients in the usual care group. No differences were found with respect to non-fatal serious adverse events and immobility-related complications in the AVERT study (Bernhardt et al., 2015b; Langhorne et al., 2018). In other words, the intervention tested was not simply earlier, but was also more frequent and of a higher dose than usual care. Indeed, the difference achieved in frequency and dose was greater than the difference in timing of first mobilization (median 18 hours vs 22 hours after stroke onset).

The AVERT study suggests that a higher dose of early mobilization (201 minutes versus 31 minutes) is accompanied by a reduction in the odds of a favourable outcome at 3 months following the mRS. Although not significant, subgroup analysis showed a trend disfavouring early mobilization of severe strokes (NIHSS ≥16 points) and those with a haemorrhagic stroke, suggesting higher risk for poor outcome according to the mRS (mRS >2) when compared with usual care (Bernhardt et al., 2015b). In fact, the findings of the AVERT study suggest that very early mobilization of stroke patients should be restricted to a few times in the first 24 hours and limited to small doses of 10 minutes at most. The AVERT study raises several essential questions to be addressed in future research. First, why is applying a higher dose of out-of-bed therapy in the first 2 days after onset more harmful than a lower dose of shorter duration in patients with severe stroke? Second, is the impaired regional cerebral blood flow in penumbral areas sensitive to orthostatic variation? One may assume that, especially in severe and haemorrhagic strokes, the cerebrovascular autoregulation needed to sustain sufficient regional cerebral blood flow is impaired. High doses of long-duration mobilization very early after stroke, which often result in tired and drowsy patients slumping in their chair, may further reduce the regional cerebral blood flow in critical penumbral and oligaemic brain areas and increase neurological damage. Further research is now needed into the longitudinal association between body and head position and cardiac output on the one hand, and impaired cerebral haemodynamics and reduced cerebral perfusion on the other, in patients with (hyper)acute stroke (Kwakkel, 2015a;

Krakauer and Carmichael, 2018). Although the AVERT study suffers from some minor methodological problems such as contamination, as the usual care group started mobilization earlier each year, the indirect message of this groundbreaking trial is that sufficiently powered phase III trials are possible in complex interventions such as stroke rehabilitation (Bernhardt et al., 2015b; Kwakkel, 2015a).

Evidence for Intensive, Task-oriented Practice beyond the Acute Phase Post-stroke

There is no clear definition of the term 'intensity' of practice. In the literature, 'dose' or 'intensity' of practice has often been described as 'frequency of repetitions of desired movement', 'amount of external work', or 'amount of time that is dedicated to practice' (Kwakkel, 2006a). Preferable measures of dose would be active time in therapy or number of repetitions of an exercise (Lohse et al., 2014). However, actual valid measures of intensity, besides behavioural mapping techniques (Bernhardt et al., 2004), are still lacking. Future trials should use portable activity monitors and/or robotics to offer better estimates of the actual amount of practice applied.

One Cochrane review of 33 trials ($N = 1853$) showed that repetitive practice of functional mobility-related and upper limb tasks, or parts of these tasks, is favourable for patients after stroke when compared with usual care (French et al., 2016). These findings were most pronounced for improvement of gait and regardless of timing post-stroke. The post-intervention effects of intensive practice did sustain up until a 6-month follow-up (French et al., 2016).

Time dedicated to practice may be a simple surrogate for the actual intensity of practice applied in trials (Kwakkel et al., 1999; Kwakkel et al., 2004; Veerbeek et al., 2011a; Lohse et al., 2014). In the present chapter, we defined intensity as 'the number of hours spent in exercise therapy' (Kwakkel et al., 2004; Lohse et al., 2014; Veerbeek et al., 2014). Various systematic reviews and meta-analyses have shown that more time spent in exercise therapy has beneficial effects for patients after stroke (Kwakkel et al., 2004; Veerbeek et al., 2011a; Lohse et al., 2014; Veerbeek et al., 2014). This finding is regardless of timing post-stroke and type of motor rehabilitation intervention. However, the optimal dose of exercise therapy is still unknown after stroke. Systematic reviews with meta-analysis suggest that additional therapy time

of ≈17 hours over 10 weeks results in favourable outcomes on all three domains of the ICF (Veerbeek et al., 2014). In the same vein, Lohse and colleagues found after pooling 30 trials ($N = 1750$) there was a positive relationship between the time scheduled for therapy and therapy outcomes such as ADL and gait. These data suggest that larger doses of therapy may lead to better outcomes post-stroke. Based on cumulative meta-analyses of trials and as a rule of thumb, it is recommended that patients should exercise at least 45 minutes on working days as long as there are rehabilitation goals (Veerbeek et al., 2014).

It is, however, unclear when exactly intensive rehabilitation should be started post-stroke. At least, the AVERT study indicates that the paradigm 'more is better' is not the case when starting within the first 24 hours. Generally, there is consensus that rehabilitation services should be start within the first days post-stroke and be based on the patient's ability. The intensity should be progressive when the first vulnerable days have passed and target meaningful activities such as making transfers, gait, and dressing.

Evidence for Fitness Training and Sports Post-stroke

There is growing interest in fitness training after stroke, although this type of training is still not common in rehabilitation medicine, when compared with other cardiovascular diseases such as myocardial infarction (Saunders et al., 2016). Physical fitness training can be defined as 'a subset of physical activity which is planned, structured, repetitive, and deliberately performed to train (improve) one or more components of physical fitness' (Saunders et al., 2016). These components include cardiorespiratory fitness, muscle strength, muscle power, flexibility, balance, and body composition (Saunders et al., 2016). As patients after stroke often are less physically active and frequently have a reduced physical fitness, physical fitness training has the potential to improve these aspects. In general, three types of physical fitness training can be distinguished: (1) cardiorespiratory training; (2) resistance training; and (3) mixed training forms in which cardiorespiratory and resistance training are combined.

In a Cochrane review by Saunders and colleagues (2016), a total of 58 trials ($N = 2797$) was identified, in which mainly ambulatory stroke patients in the chronic phase were included. Physical fitness training appeared to be safe (Saunders et al., 2016). Meta-analyses showed clear evidence that fitness training including cardiorespiratory training involving functional tasks such as walking is beneficial for patients after stroke in terms of walking performance. There was some evidence that cardiorespiratory training has the ability to improve cardiorespiratory fitness, and that mixed training may improve measures of walking performance. In line with another Cochrane review, no evidence was found to support resistance training or strengthening exercises alone (Saunders et al., 2016). In addition, most benefits disappeared at follow-up, except for walking distance and maximal gait speed. The effects of cardiorespiratory training and mixed training on quality of life, mood, death, and dependency are still unclear (Saunders et al., 2016).

Evidence-based Interventions to Improve the Upper Limb

Around 80% of the stroke survivors have motor impairments of the upper limb that affect their ability to perform, and participate in, activities of daily living (ADL). The severity of upper limb paresis and in particular the patients' ability to extend wrist and fingers are the strongest determinants that define upper limb capacity at 3 and 6 months post-stroke (Nijland et al., 2010; Stinear, 2010; Coupar et al., 2013; Kwakkel and Kollen, 2013). Therapies that are targeting these patients with an initial favourable prognosis at baseline of their trial have also shown beneficial effects on outcome of upper limb capacity. In contrast, rehabilitation interventions trials that selected patients without voluntary motor control of wrist and finger extension have shown that their beneficial effects are restricted to improvements in motor impairments alone. This finding further supports the notion that evidence-based therapies for the upper limb strongly depend on ability of the patients to voluntarily control the hand (i.e. have a favourable prognosis) (Langhorne et al., 2011). With that, next to the therapy, selecting patients for a specific intervention is an important part of adequate rehabilitation care post-stroke.

Significant effects are found for: (1) constraint-induced movement therapy (CIMT) and its modified versions (mCIMT); (2) electromyography-triggered neuromuscular stimulation (EMG-NMS) of wrist and finger extensors; (3) mental practice; and (4) virtual reality training of the upper limb (Veerbeek et al., 2014). Next to these interventions, positive effects have also been found for the body functions and/or activities level for (5) bilateral arm training (BAT) with rhythmic auditory cueing (BATRAC); (6) mirror therapy; and (7) robot-assisted therapy for the upper limb. The evidence for these interventions will be discussed below.

(Modified) Constraint-Induced Movement Therapy

Constraint-induced movement therapy was developed to overcome upper limb impairments after stroke and is the most investigated intervention for the rehabilitation of patients with upper limb limitations (Figure 23.2).

Practices include: (A) cutting bread, (B) pouring water, (C) picking up and replacing money, and (D) playing a game. Use of the unaffected limb is restricted by a padded mitt.

The signature protocol for the original form of CIMT contains (1) intensive, graded practice of the paretic upper limb to enhance task-specific use of the affected limb for up to 6 hours a day for 2 weeks; (2) constraint or forced use therapy, wearing a mitt on the non-paretic hand to promote the use of the impaired limb during 90% of the total hours awake; and (3) adherence-enhancing behavioural methods designed to transfer the gains obtained in the clinical setting or the laboratory to patients' real-world environment (i.e. a transfer package) (Kwakkel et al., 2015b). Modified versions of CIMT often apply only the first two elements of CIMT with a limited intensity. CIMT or modified versions of this treatment use operant training techniques to enhance upper limb capacity. However, for this behavioural therapy some preservation of finger and wrist extension of the paretic upper limb is needed.

A recent meta-analysis of 51 trials ($N = 1784$) showed beneficial effects on motor function, arm–hand activities, and self-reported arm–hand functioning in daily life of both types (i.e. CIMT or mCIMT) immediately after treatment and at follow-up (20 weeks), whereas no evidence was found for the efficacy of constraint alone (as used in forced use therapy) (Kwakkel et al., 2015b). Figures 23.3 and 23.4 show forest plots of overall effect sizes of CIMT, modified versions of CIMT (mCIMT), and forced use therapy.

Sensitivity analyses showed no significant differences in effect sizes between original CIMT and mCIMT, dose of CIMT (additional time spent in exercise therapy between 5 hours and 60 hours), or timing

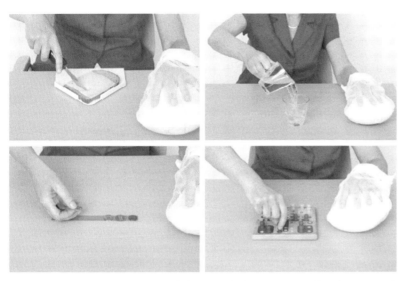

Figure 23.2 Task-oriented practices with the paretic limb in constraint-induced movement therapy (CIMT). With permission from the *Lancet Neurology* (Kwakkel et al., 2015).

of CIMT (trials started within or after the first 3 months after stroke onset) (Kwakkel et al., 2015b).

In summary, (m)CIMT is found to be the most effective therapy to enhance upper arm function and arm–hand activities post-stroke (Kwakkel et al., 2015b). In contrast, meta-analyses showed no evidence for grip strength, sensibility, or pain, while for patients beyond 3 months post-stroke, no effects were found for motor function of the paretic arm. These findings strongly suggest that with (m)CIMT patients learn to optimize motor performance (Buma et al., 2013; van Kordelaar et al., 2013; Kwakkel et al., 2015b).

EMG-NMS of Wrist and Finger Extensors

With electromyography-triggered neuromuscular stimulation (EMG-NMS), peripheral nerves and muscles are stimulated with electrodes (Pomeroy et al., 2006). In this chapter, only stimulation with external electrodes is discussed. Electrostimulation can be applied during training of activities (i.e. functional electrical stimulation [FES]) or in a non-functional manner (e.g. performing wrist and finger extension without a functional purpose) (Veerbeek et al., 2014). Stimulation in EMG-NMS is only activated when the patient actively attains an individualized, pre-set threshold value of muscle activity (Veerbeek et al., 2014). It was found that EMG-NMS of the wrist and finger extensors of the paretic arm has significant positive effects on synergy independent motor control of the paretic arm and arm–hand activities (Veerbeek

et al., 2014). These findings were based on 25 trials (N = 492) (Veerbeek et al., 2014). Application of EMG-NMS of the wrist and finger extensors should be considered in patients with some voluntary wrist and/or finger extension. In addition, it should be noticed that application of EMG-NMS is mainly investigated in patients who are beyond 1 month and quite often beyond 6 months after stroke onset. The optimal frequency and intensity of the stimulation are unclear (Veerbeek et al., 2014).

Mental Practice with Motor Imagery

Mental practice of motor actions and/or activities for the upper limb aims to improve their performance (Barclay-Goddard et al., 2011; Langhorne et al., 2011a; Veerbeek et al., 2014) and is often combined with physical practice. Based on a meta-analysis of 14 RCTs (N = 424), mental practice combined with physical practice has significant beneficial effects for outcome of arm–hand activities at termination of the intervention period, but the sustainability is unclear (Barclay-Goddard et al., 2011). No effects have been found for synergy independent motor control of the paretic arm, nor for muscle strength or basic ADL (Veerbeek et al., 2014). To participate in this type of training, patients needed to be able to have some active movement abilities in the paretic arm. However, it should be noted that testing the patient's ability to perform mental imaging is difficult and therefore implementation in daily practice is hampered.

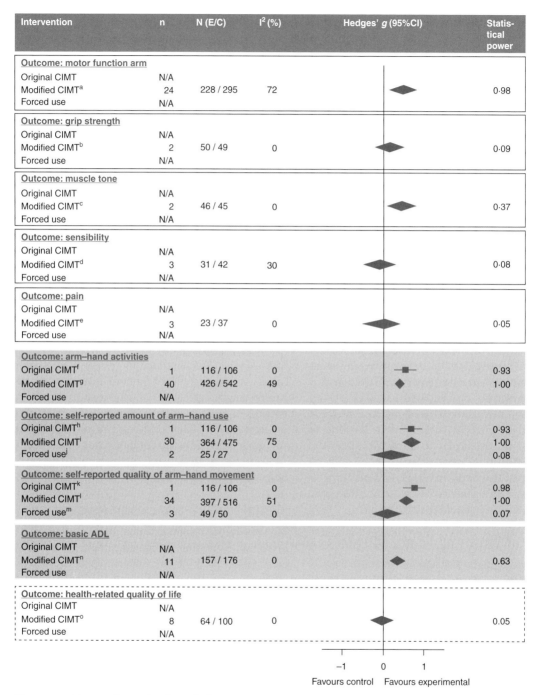

Intervention	n	N (E/C)	I^2 (%)	Hedges' g (95%CI)	Statistical power
Outcome: motor function arm					
Original CIMT	N/A				
Modified CIMT[a]	24	228 / 295	72		0·98
Forced use	N/A				
Outcome: grip strength					
Original CIMT	N/A				
Modified CIMT[b]	2	50 / 49	0		0·09
Forced use	N/A				
Outcome: muscle tone					
Original CIMT	N/A				
Modified CIMT[c]	2	46 / 45	0		0·37
Forced use	N/A				
Outcome: sensibility					
Original CIMT	N/A				
Modified CIMT[d]	3	31 / 42	30		0·08
Forced use	N/A				
Outcome: pain					
Original CIMT	N/A				
Modified CIMT[e]	3	23 / 37	0		0·05
Forced use	N/A				
Outcome: arm–hand activities					
Original CIMT[f]	1	116 / 106	0		0·93
Modified CIMT[g]	40	426 / 542	49		1·00
Forced use	N/A				
Outcome: self-reported amount of arm–hand use					
Original CIMT[h]	1	116 / 106	0		0·93
Modified CIMT[i]	30	364 / 475	75		1·00
Forced use[j]	2	25 / 27	0		0·08
Outcome: self-reported quality of arm–hand movement					
Original CIMT[k]	1	116 / 106	0		0·98
Modified CIMT[l]	34	397 / 516	51		1·00
Forced use[m]	3	49 / 50	0		0·07
Outcome: basic ADL					
Original CIMT	N/A				
Modified CIMT[n]	11	157 / 176	0		0·63
Forced use	N/A				
Outcome: health-related quality of life					
Original CIMT	N/A				
Modified CIMT[o]	8	64 / 100	0		0·05
Forced use	N/A				

−1   0   1

Favours control   Favours experimental

Figures 23.3 & 23.4 Forest plot of overall effect sizes of constraint-induced movement therapy (CIMT), modified CIMT, and forced use therapy post intervention (Figure 23.3) and at follow-up (Figure 23.4). Effects classified in accordance with the International Classification of Functioning, Disability, and Health (ICF; WHO). Diamonds represent the overall effect sizes after pooling the standardized mean differences (SMD). The SMD was based on adjusted Hedges' g (95% CI) model. If pooling was not possible, the individual SMD is shown based on an adjusted Hedges' g analysis. The SMD Hedges' g model is a model calculated on the basis of the difference between the means of the experimental and the control groups divided by the *pooled standard deviation of both groups in a trial and multiplied by a correction factor* called J for the degrees of freedom. The different ICF categories: body functions (black outline), activities (grey), and participation (dotted outline). ADL = activities of daily living. E = experimental group. C = control group. N/A = no data available. *Sufficient statistical power (1−β ≥0.80). With permission from the *Lancet Neurology* (Kwakkel et al., 2015).

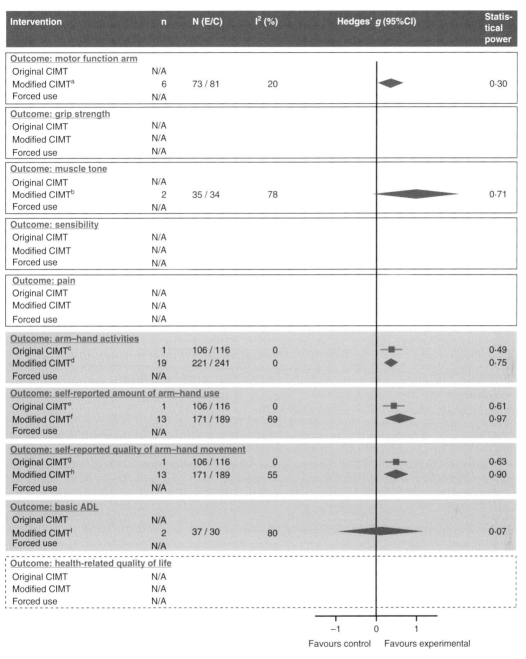

Intervention	n	N (E/C)	I^2 (%)	Hedges' g (95%CI)	Statis-tical power
Outcome: motor function arm					
Original CIMT	N/A				
Modified CIMT[a]	6	73 / 81	20		0·30
Forced use	N/A				
Outcome: grip strength					
Original CIMT	N/A				
Modified CIMT	N/A				
Forced use	N/A				
Outcome: muscle tone					
Original CIMT	N/A				
Modified CIMT[b]	2	35 / 34	78		0·71
Forced use	N/A				
Outcome: sensibility					
Original CIMT	N/A				
Modified CIMT	N/A				
Forced use	N/A				
Outcome: pain					
Original CIMT	N/A				
Modified CIMT	N/A				
Forced use	N/A				
Outcome: arm–hand activities					
Original CIMT[c]	1	106 / 116	0		0·49
Modified CIMT[d]	19	221 / 241	0		0·75
Forced use	N/A				
Outcome: self-reported amount of arm–hand use					
Original CIMT[e]	1	106 / 116	0		0·61
Modified CIMT[f]	13	171 / 189	69		0·97
Forced use	N/A				
Outcome: self-reported quality of arm–hand movement					
Original CIMT[g]	1	106 / 116	0		0·63
Modified CIMT[h]	13	171 / 189	55		0·90
Forced use	N/A				
Outcome: basic ADL					
Original CIMT	N/A				
Modified CIMT[i]	2	37 / 30	80		0·07
Forced use	N/A				
Outcome: health-related quality of life					
Original CIMT	N/A				
Modified CIMT	N/A				
Forced use	N/A				

−1   0   1

Favours control   Favours experimental

Figures 23.3 & 23.4 (cont).

Virtual Reality Training for the Upper Limb

Virtual reality and interactive video gaming are new types of therapy being provided to people after having a stroke (Laver et al., 2017). The therapy involves using computer-based programs that are designed to simulate real-life objects and events.

Therefore, some voluntary movement of the upper limb is required.

A Cochrane review of 72 trials ($N = 2470$) investigating virtual reality training of the upper paretic limb showed evidence that the use of virtual reality and interactive video gaming is equal to conventional therapy for improving arm function but better when added to conventional therapy to increase therapy intensity (Laver et al., 2017). Virtual reality training is also beneficial for ADL when compared with the same dose of conventional therapy. No effects for gait speed and quality of life could be demonstrated. The long-term effects are unclear (Laver et al., 2017). No differences between phases post-stroke or system (specialized virtual reality system or commercial gaming consoles) used could be detected. The included trials used different virtual reality programs and most interventions were delivered in a hospital or clinic setting; only five applied a home-based telerehabilitation approach (Laver et al., 2017).

Mirror Therapy for the Upper Limb

During mirror therapy, a mirror is placed in the patient's midsagittal plane, thus reflecting movements of the non-paretic side as if it were the affected side. Sixty-two trials ($N = 1982$) did investigate effects of mirror therapy after stroke. Pooling these phase II trials showed significant effects in terms of improved upper limb capacity and ADL, and a reduction in pain; no effects on visuospatial neglect were found (Thieme et al., 2018). The above effects were not maintained at follow-up for most trials; however, phase III trials are lacking in this field.

Robot-assisted Therapy for the Upper Limb

Robot-assisted therapies for the upper limb (RT-UL) is a promising, fast-growing field in stroke rehabilitation. Mehrholz and colleagues (2018) showed in their Cochrane review involving 45 trials ($N= 1619$) that patients who received robot-assisted arm training after stroke are more likely to improve in motor function and muscle strength, as well as their generic ADL. However, in this Cochrane review it was also stated that variation between trials in duration and amount of training, type of treatment, and differences in patient characteristics did hamper comparison and proper interpretation of claimed effects (Mehrholz et al., 2018).

Another systematic review (reflecting 43 trials, $N = 1348$) found that the improvements in upper limb motor function as measured with the Fugl–Meyer Assessment (FMA) were not clinically relevant (Veerbeek et al., 2017). Furthermore, the evidence for better outcomes in terms of upper limb capacity is lacking when compared with non-robotic treatment or usual care. In particular, shoulder–elbow robotics were shown to be more effective in enhancing

synergistic-independent motor control of the (proximal part of the) upper limb than usual care, whereas wrist–hand robotics were shown to be effective in improving motor control of the paretic wrist–hand function when compared with usual care. No evidence was found for robot type, suggesting that more expensive upper limb robots allowing control of more degrees of freedom are not superior to simpler models (Kwakkel and Meskers, 2014). More importantly, displayed effects of RT-UL with respect to motor function did not generalize to meaningful improvements in upper limb capacity post-stroke (Kwakkel and Meskers, 2014).

Depending on prognosis for arm recovery, future assist-as-needed robots and their training protocols should allow compensation with the trunk and synergy-dependent adaptation strategies of the paretic arm during meaningful tasks. In addition, future trials in patients with chronic impairment after stroke should have a primary outcome measure that includes improvements of arm function by using compensation strategies (Kwakkel and Meskers, 2014).

Simultaneous Bilateral Training for Improving Arm Function

Bilateral arm training with or without rhythmic auditory or visual cueing (using a metronome) is a promising method to enhance the use of the paretic arm; however, the underlying working mechanisms are still poorly understood. It is assumed that the impaired paretic arm may improve by exploiting interhemispheric interactions (van Delden et al., 2013; van Delden et al., 2015). In particular, based on the principle of interhemispheric recruitment from the non-affected hemisphere (i.e. exercise-induced neuroplasticity by means of 'neural cross-talk'), BAT with rhythmic auditory cueing (BATRAC) may serve as an effective therapy for patients in whom the CST system is seriously affected. Several meta-analyses of 23 trials ($N = 830$) of simultaneous BAT with or without rhythmic cueing showed limited evidence for improving upper limb motor function when compared with usual or no care (Coupar et al., 2010; van Delden et al., 2012). No evidence was found when BAT or BATRAC were compared with an equally dosed, modified version of CIMT (van Delden et al., 2012; van Delden et al., 2013). However, meta-analysis suggests that patients with a mild motor impairment benefit more from mCIMT when compared with BAT(RAC) (van Delden et al., 2012).

Evidence-based Interventions to Improve Mobility, Gait Performance, and Walking Competency

Circuit Class Training

A resource-efficient way of delivering intensive rehabilitation is circuit class therapy (CCT) focused on gait and mobility-related activities. In this group therapy, patients are treated simultaneously in small groups and perform functional activities in various working stations with a staff-to-patient ratio of 1:3–6. CCT is mostly compared with face-to-face individual care (van de Port et al., 2012; English and Hillier, 2017).

A Cochrane review published in 2017 found 17 phase II trials (N = 1297) and yielded significant beneficial effects post-intervention for walking distance, gait speed, mobility, independency in walking, activities-specific balance confidence, and health-related quality of life when compared with other interventions (English and Hillier, 2017). CCT did not significantly influence length of stay, and, importantly, did not induce an increased fall risk, implying it is a safe way to exercise after stroke (English and Hillier, 2017).

CCT has been tested in both stroke survivors who live at home and patients who receive inpatient rehabilitation. In most studies, patients were able to walk 10 metres without support of another person. Interestingly, depending on the size of classes, CCT needed 2 to 3 times fewer staff members (physical and occupation therapists) than individual care, making this intervention cost-effective.

Body-Weight-Supported Treadmill Training

Task-specific training that included stepping on a treadmill with partial-body-weight support (BWSTT) was seen as a promising therapy that may enhance independent gait and improve performance. In recent years, one phase III trial (N = 408) (Duncan et al., 2011) and two Cochrane reviews have been conducted in this field (Moseley et al., 2005; Mehrholz et al., 2017).

In the Locomotor Experience Applied Poststroke (LEAPS) trial, patients received 36 sessions of 90 minutes of BWSTT starting 2 months post-stroke and were compared with an equally dosed home-based therapy or compared with delayed BWSTT starting beyond 6 months post-stroke. The LEAPS

trial showed that patients who received early BWSTT have a faster recovery in their gait speed when compared with those that were allocated to a delayed amount of BWSTT, which started after 6 months. However, no differences were observed between the early BWSTT when compared with the home-based therapy programme during the trial period of 1 year (Duncan et al., 2011). After 1 year, no differences were found between the three treatment arms, suggesting that BWSTT is not superior to progressive exercise at home when managed by a physical therapist.

Generally, the above findings are in line with the Cochrane review of Mehrholz and colleagues dedicated to the effectiveness treadmill training in general and the role of body support to enhance walking performance (Mehrholz et al., 2017). This Cochrane review involved 56 trials (N = 3105) and showed no superior effects of treadmill training with or without body weight support with respect to improvement of independent gait when compared with other interventions. However, moderate evidence was found that walking speed and walking endurance improve (Mehrholz et al., 2017). Furthermore, treadmill training was found to be safe, with no more adverse events in the group of patients receiving BWSTT than in those in the control group.

Robot-assisted Gait Training

With robotic-assisted gait training (RAGT), an apparatus which guides the walking cycle by electromechanical driven footplates or exoskeleton is used (Veerbeek et al., 2014). Electromechanical devices for RAGT can be differentiated into end-effector devices in which a patient's feet are placed on foot-plates and exoskeleton types of device in which the different upper and lower segments of the lower limb are controlled around the knees and hips during the gait circle (Mehrholz et al., 2017).

A Cochrane review involving 36 phase II trials (N = 1472) showed higher post-intervention odds for achieving independent gait for those who were treated with RAGT in combination with physical therapy. However, no significant differences were found for other parameters such as gait speed and walking distance. This review suggests that RAGT is more effective for patients in the first 3 months after stroke who are not able to walk independently. No significant differences between end-effector devices and exoskeleton devices were found (Mehrholz et al., 2017).

Evidence for Early Supported Discharge

One Cochrane review of 17 trials (N = 2422), mainly conducted in the UK, Denmark, Sweden, and Norway, showed strong evidence for early supported discharge (ESD) of stroke patients with mild to moderate disability (Barthel Index ranging from 10 to 17 out of 20 points) from hospitals with support of services in their own community (Langhorne and Baylan, 2017). In most trials, ESD was provided by coordinated multidisciplinary teams that included therapists, nurses, and doctors. ESD resulted in a significant reduction in length of stay of 6 days next to an overall significant reduction for death or institutionalization at the end of scheduled follow-up favouring ESD. Patients discharged early did not have an increased risk of re-hospitalization. There were small, positive effects for extended ADL and patient satisfaction with the services. In addition, caregiver strain did not increase significantly nor was harm found in caregivers' subjective health status (Langhorne and Baylan, 2017). No effects were found for ADL, self-reported health status, and mood by patients and caregivers, and caregivers' satisfaction with the services. The effects were smaller at 1- and 5-year follow-up.

The above findings suggest that ESD services provided for patients with some deficits in basic ADL can reduce long-term dependency and admission to institutional care as well as reducing the length of hospital stay. The combination of ESD with support at home is found without adverse effects on mood or subjective health status of patients or caregivers. The effects were most pronounced for those with a mild disability receiving high-quality services at home.

Evidence for Caregiver- or Family-mediated Exercises

Several meta-analyses show that intensity of training and repetitive task training are crucial aspects of stroke rehabilitation, concluding that more exercise therapy improves outcomes (Langhorne et al., 2011; Veerbeek et al., 2014; French et al., 2016). Guidelines recommend that patients admitted to a rehabilitation facility should have the opportunity to receive a daily dose of 45 minutes of exercise therapy in the first 3 months after stroke (Veerbeek

et al., 2014). However, most patients admitted to hospital stroke units, rehabilitation centres, or nursing homes are physically inactive or involved in activities that contribute little to their recovery. Acknowledging that the resources (mostly staff) in rehabilitation settings are limited, caregiver- or family-mediated exercises may be a novel method to increase the intensity of exercise therapy with minimal use of resources (Vloothuis et al., 2016). One such novel method could be to actively involve caregivers in mediating exercises. In particular, when caregiver-mediated exercises (CME) are combined with e-health/telerehabilitation services, easy contact with and monitoring by the rehabilitation team is promoted (Vloothuis et al., 2015; Kwakkel and van Wegen, 2017). Theoretically, CME may enhance ESD by providing a smoother transition from inpatient setting to the home situation. In addition, CME can easily continue in the community setting. Based on 9 trials involving 333 patient–caregiver couples, some evidence was found in a recently conducted Cochrane review that CME could have a positive effect on patients' standing balance (low-quality evidence) and quality of life (very low-quality evidence) directly after the intervention (Vloothuis et al., 2016). In the long term, low-quality evidence was found for a positive effect on walking distance, without significant side effects or beneficial effects in terms of caregiver strain (Vloothuis et al., 2016). No significant effects were found for basic ADL, such as dressing and bathing, after intervention (moderate-quality evidence) or follow-up (low-quality evidence) and no significant effects for extended ADL, such as cooking and gardening. Based on these findings, it was concluded that CME may be a promising form of therapy to add to usual care (Vloothuis et al., 2016); however, phase III trials were lacking. Recently, the ATTEND Collaborative Group conducted the first phase III trial on the effectiveness of family-mediated exercises postacute stroke in the low- to middle-income country India (ATTEND Collaborative Group, 2017). In this trial, 1250 stroke patients were discharged from 14 hospitals in India and randomly assigned to receive additional structured rehabilitation training in family-mediated exercises compared with usual care (ATTEND, 2017). Family-mediated exercises were delivered in three 1-hour sessions in hospital and continued in up to six home visits for up to 2 months after discharge. With that, the experimental group in the ATTEND trial received about 18 hours of CME therapy (ATTEND, 2017). It is important to note that usual care in India often indicates no care. The primary outcome was assessed using the mRS, with death or dependency (mRS 3–6) at 6 months post-stroke. Unfortunately, the results of this pragmatic phase III trial showed no favourable benefits when the proportion of disabled and deceased patients (285 [47%] of 607 patients) in the intervention group was compared with that in the control group (287 [47%] of 605 patients) at 6 months after stroke (odds ratio 0.98, 95% confidence interval [CI]: 0.78–1.23; $p = 0.87$). In addition, no surplus value was found in terms of secondary outcomes such as length of hospital stay, basic and extended ADL, perceived anxiety, depression, and quality of life of patients and burden on their caregivers. These results render the ATTEND trial neutral, without any positive trends to suggest that family-delivered rehabilitation services at home when compared with no therapy or a very limited number of sessions of outpatient care is not more effective. However, the trial may be criticized with respect to lack of treatment contrast between experimental and control group. As a consequence, the focus of therapy may have been too diluted and too limited to cause significant differences in term of mRS, in particular, acknowledging that exercise therapy does not follow a 'one-size-fits-all principle' to achieve clinically meaningful improvements post-stroke. Overall, one may conclude that family- or care-mediated exercise is still in its infancy and may improve if the therapy is applied in combination with e-health services to facilitate transfer to a patient's own home environment (Vloothuis et al., 2015; Kwakkel & van Wegen, 2017).

Summary

Unfortunately, there is just one dose–response trial in stroke rehabilitation (Lang et al., 2016). Therefore, the optimal amount of therapy in the different phases post-stroke is still unknown. Recently, there is strong evidence that rehabilitation services should be applied with care very early post-stroke. Based on the AVERT study, it is recommended to restrict patients in the amount of out-of-bed therapy very early post-stroke and to offer exercise therapy in small doses of maximally 10 minutes per bout in the first 2 days. In contrast, due to the exponentially growing number of trials in the field of stroke rehabilitation, there is moderate to strong evidence that augmented, task-specific

training may enhance the pattern of recovery in the first 6 months post-stroke. In addition, there is strong evidence that these programmes may prevent deterioration and learned non-use in the chronic phase post-stroke. In particular, forced use paradigms such as constraint-induced movement therapy as well as fitness training programmes for improving mobility show strong evidence. However, this evidence is based on pooling a number of small phase II trials, whereas large pragmatic trials in the field of stroke rehabilitation are still scarce. The reason for the lack of large pragmatic trials is that investigating complex rehabilitation interventions in randomized controlled trials following CONSORT guidelines is difficult. Factors such as inadequate blinding procedures, prognostic imbalance at baseline in phase II trials, lack of treatment contrast between experimental and control arms, lack of clarity about the exact treatment protocol, and insufficient statistical power, as well as contamination of the treatment arm that should serve as a control, are important factors that may bias outcome. For this reason, recently we raised a task force to improve stroke recovery research and to set standards and agreement for using a uniform set of definitions and outcomes and a common vision for accelerating progress in stroke recovery research (Bernhardt, et al., 2017).

Declaration of Interests

GK has received grants from the European Research Council, Dutch National Institutes of Health (ZonMw), the Dutch Brain Foundation (Hersenstichting Nederland), the Dutch Heart Foundation, and the Royal Dutch Society for Physical Therapy (grant number 8091.1), the Netherlands Organisation for Health and Development for conducting the EXPLICIT-stroke trial (ZonMw; grant number 89000001), and an ERC advanced grant (number 291339-4D-EEG) for the 4D-EEG project from the European Commission. The funders had no role in design, conduct, data collection, data management, data analysis, data interpretation, or preparation of the manuscript. JMV did not receive grants.

Acknowledgements

We thank Hans Ket for his cooperation in the literature search, Mark van den Brink for the figures, and Jan Klerkx for his support in linguistically editing this chapter.

References

ATTEND Collaborative Group. (2017). Family-led rehabilitation after stroke in India (ATTEND): a randomised controlled trial. *Lancet*, **390**(10094), 588–99. doi:10.1016/S0140-6736(17)31447-2. Epub 2017 Jun 27. Erratum in: *Lancet*, 2017, 390(10094), 554. PubMed PMID: 28666682.

Barclay-Goddard R, Stevenson T, Poluha W, Thalman L. (2011). Mental practice for treating upper extremity deficits in individuals with hemiparesis after stroke. *Cochrane Database Syst Rev*, 5. CD005950. available from: PM:21563146

Berkhemer O, Fransen P, Beumer D, van den Berg L, Lingsma H, Yoo A, et al. (2015). A randomized trial of intraarterial treatment for acute ischemic stroke. *N Engl J Med*, 372(1), 11–20. available from: PM:25517348

Bernhardt J, Dewey H, Thrift A, Donnan G. (2004). Inactive and alone: physical activity within the first 14 days of acute stroke unit care. *Stroke*, **35**(4), 1005–09.

Bernhardt J, English C, Johnson L, Cumming T. (2015a). Early mobilization after stroke: early adoption but limited evidence. *Stroke*, **46**(4), 1141–6 available from: PM:25690544

Bernhardt J, Langhorne P, Lindley R, Thrift A, Ellery F, Collier J, et al. (2015b). Efficacy and safety of very early mobilisation within 24 h of stroke onset (AVERT): a randomised controlled trial. *Lancet*, **386**, (9988), 46–55. available from: PM:25892679

Bernhardt J, Hayward KS, Kwakkel G, Ward NS, Wolf SL, Borschmann K, et al. (2017). Agreed definitions and a shared vision for new standards in stroke recovery research: The Stroke Recovery and Rehabilitation Roundtable Taskforce. *Neurorehabil Neural Repair*, 31(9), 793–9. doi:10.1177/1545968317732668. PubMed PMID: 28934920.

Buma F, Kwakkel G, Ramsey N. (2013). Understanding upper limb recovery after stroke. *Restor Neurol Neurosci*, **31**(6) 707–22. available from: PM:23963341

Cortes JC, Goldsmith J, Harran MD, Xu J, Kim N, Schambra HM, et al. (2017). A short and distinct time window for recovery of arm motor control early after stroke revealed with a global measure of trajectory kinematics. *Neurorehabil Neural Repair*, 31(6), 552–60. available from: PM 28506149

Coupar F, Pollock A, Rowe P. Weir C, Langhorne P. (2013). Predictors of upper limb recovery after stroke: a systematic review and meta-analysis. *Clin Rehabil*, **26**(4), 291–313.

Coupar F, Pollock A, van Wijck F, Morris J, Langhorne P. (2010). Simultaneous bilateral training for improving arm function after stroke. *Cochrane Database Syst Rev*, 4. CD006432. available from: PM:20393947

Cramer S. 2008a. Repairing the human brain after stroke. II. Restorative therapies. *Annul Neurol*, **63**(5) 549–60.

Cramer S. 2008b. Repairing the human brain after stroke: I. Mechanisms of spontaneous recovery. *Ann Neurol*, **63**(3) 272–87.

Duncan, P., Sullivan, K., Behrman, A., Azen, S., Wu, S., Nadeau, S., et al. (2011). Body-weight-supported treadmill rehabilitation after stroke. *N Engl J Med*, **364**(21), 2026–36. available from: PM:21612471

English C, Hillier S. (2017). Circuit class therapy for improving mobility after stroke. *Cochrane Database Syst Rev*, 7. CD007513. available from: PM: 28573757

Feigin VL, Krishnamurthi RV, Parmar P, Norrving B, Mensah GA, Bennett DA, et al.; GBD 2013 Writing Group; GBD 2013 Stroke Panel Experts Group. (2015). Update on the global burden of ischemic and hemorrhagic stroke in 1990–2013: the GBD 2013 Study. *Neuroepidemiology*, **45**(3), 161–76. available from: PM 26505981

French B, Thomas LH, Coupe J, McMahon NE, Connell L, Harrison J, et al. (2016). Repetitive task training for improving functional ability after stroke. *Cochrane Database Syst Rev*, 11. CD006073. available from: PM 27841442

Hoonhorst MHJ, Nijland RHM, van den Berg PJS, Emmelot CH, Kollen BJ, Kwakkel G. (2018). Does transcranial magnetic stimulation have an added value to clinical assessment in predicting upper-limb function very early after severe stroke? *Neurorehabil Neural Repair*, 32(8), 682–90.

Kohrmann M, Juttler E, Fiebach J, Huttner H, Siebert S, Schwark C, et al. (2006). MRI versus CT-based thrombolysis treatment within and beyond the 3 h time window after stroke onset: a cohort study. *Lancet Neurol*, **5**(8), 661–7. available from: PM:16857571

Krakauer JW, Carmichael ST. (2018). *Broken Movement: The Neurobiology of Motor Recovery after Stroke.* Cambridge, MA: MIT Press.

Kwakkel G, Wagenaar R, Twisk J, Lankhorst G, Koetsier J. (1999). Intensity of leg and arm training after primary middle-cerebral-artery stroke: a randomised trial. *Lancet*, **354**(9174), 191–6.

Kwakkel G. (2006a). Impact of intensity of practice after stroke: issues for consideration. *Disabil Rehabil*, **28**(13–14), 823–30. available from: PM:16777769

Kwakkel, G. (2015a). Very early mobilisation within 24 hours results in a less favorable outcome at 3 months [commentary 2]. *Physiotherapy*, **61**(4), 220.

Kwakkel G, Kollen B. (2007). Predicting improvement in the upper paretic limb after stroke: a longitudinal prospective study. *Restor Neurol Neurosci*, **25**(5–6), 453–60. available from: PM:18334763

Kwakkel G, Kollen B. (2013). Predicting activities after stroke: what is clinically relevant? *Int J Stroke*, **8**(1) 25–32. available from: PM:23280266

Kwakkel G, Kollen B, Twisk J. (2006b). Impact of time on improvement of outcome after stroke. *Stroke*, **37**(9), 2348–53. available from: PM:16931787

Kwakkel G, Meskers C. (2014). Effects of robotic therapy of the arm after stroke. *Lancet Neurol*, **13**(2), 132–3. available from: PM:24382581

Kwakkel G, van Peppen R, Wagenaar R, Wood Dauphinee S, Richards C, Ashburn A, et al. (2004). Effects of augmented exercise therapy time after stroke: a meta-analysis. *Stroke*, **35**(11), 2529–39. available from: PM:15472114

Kwakkel G, van Wegen EEH. (2017). Family-delivered rehabilitation services at home: is the glass empty? *Lancet*, **390**(10094), 538–9. doi:10.1016/S0140-6736(17)31489-7. Epub 2017 Jun 27. PubMed PMID: 28666681.

Kwakkel G, Veerbeek J, van Wegen E, Wolf S. (2015b). Constraint-induced movement therapy after stroke. *Lancet Neurol*, **14**(2), 224–34. available from: PM:25772900

Lang CE, Strube MJ, Bland MD, Waddell KJ, Cherry-Allen KM, Nudo RJ, Dromerick AW, Birkenmeier RL. (2016). Dose response of task-specific upper limb training in people at least 6 months poststroke: a phase II, single-blind, randomized, controlled trial. *Ann Neurol*, **80**(3), 342–54. Available from PM: 27447365

Langhorne P, Baylan S. (2017). Early Supported Discharge Trialists. Early supported discharge services for people with acute stroke. *Cochrane Database Syst Rev*, 7. CD000443. available from: PM: 28703869

Langhorne P, Bernhardt J, Kwakkel G. (2011). Stroke rehabilitation. *Lancet*, **377**(9778), 1693–1702. available from: PM:21571152

Langhorne P, Collier JM, Bate PJ, Thuy MN, Bernhardt J. (2018). Very early versus delayed mobilisation after stroke. *Cochrane Database Syst Rev*, 10. CD006187. doi:10.1002/14651858.CD006187.pub3.

Langhorne P. Legg L. (2003). Evidence behind stroke rehabilitation. *J Neurol Neurosurg Psychiatry*, **74**(Suppl 4), iv18–iv21.

Laver KE, Lange B, George S, Deutsch JE, Saposnik G, Crotty M. (2017). Virtual reality for stroke rehabilitation. Cochrane Database Syst Rev, 11. CD008349. available from: PM 29156493

Lazar R, Minzer B, Antoniello D, Festa J, Krakauer J, Marshall R. (2010). Improvement in aphasia scores after stroke is well predicted by initial severity. *Stroke*, **41**(7), 1485–8. available from: PM:20538700

Lejeune T., Stoquart G. (2015). The challenge of assessment in rehabilitation. *J Rehabil Med*, **47**, 672. available from: PM:26074394

Lohse K, Lang C, Boyd L. (2014). Is more better? Using metadata to explore dose-response relationships in stroke rehabilitation. *Stroke*, **45**(7), 2053–8. available from: PM:24867924

Mehrholz J, Pohl M, Platz T, Kugler J, Elsner B. (2018). Electromechanical and robot-assisted arm training for improving activities of daily living, arm function, and arm muscle strength after stroke. *Cochrane Database Syst Rev*, 9, CD006876. available from: PM:30175845

Mehrholz J, Thomas S, Elsner B. (2017). Treadmill training and body weight support for walking after stroke. *Cochrane Database Syst Rev*, 8. CD002840. available from: PM:28815562

Moseley A, Stark A, Cameron I, Pollock A. (2005). Treadmill training and body weight support for walking after stroke. *Cochrane Database Syst Rev*, 4. CD002840. available from: PM:16235304

Murphy T, Corbett D. (2009). Plasticity during stroke recovery: from synapse to behaviour. *Nat Rev Neorosci*, **10** (12), 861–72.

Nijboer T, van de Port I, Schepers V, Post M, Visser-Meily A. (2013). Predicting functional outcome after stroke: the influence of neglect on basic activities in daily living. *Front Hum Neurosci*, 7, 182.

Nijland R, van Wegen E, Harmeling-van der Wel B, Kwakkel G. (2010). Presence of finger extension and shoulder abduction within 72 hours after stroke predicts functional recovery: early prediction of functional outcome after stroke: the EPOS cohort study. *Stroke*, **41**(4), 745–50. available from: PM:20167916

Pomeroy V, King L, Pollock A, Baily-Hallam A, Langhorne P. (2006). Electrostimulation for promoting recovery of movement or functional ability after stroke. *Cochrane Database Syst Rev*, 2. CD003241. available from: PM:16625574

Prabhakaran S, Zarahn E, Riley C, Speizer A, Chong J, Lazar R, et al. (2008). Inter-individual variability in the capacity for motor recovery after ischemic stroke. *Neurorehabil Neural Repair*, **22**(1), 64–71. available from: PM:17687024

Prabhakaran S, Ruff I, Bernstein RA. (2015). Acute stroke intervention: a systematic review. *JAMA*, **313**(14), 1451–62. Available from: PM: 25871671

Saver JL, Goyal M, van der Lugt A, et al. (2016). Time to treatment with endovascular thrombectomy and outcomes from ischemic stroke: a meta-analysis. *JAMA*, **316** (12),1279–88. Available from: PM: 27673305

Saunders DH, Sanderson M, Hayes S, Kilrane M, Greig CA, Brazzelli M, Mead GE. (2016). Physical fitness training for stroke patients. *Cochrane Database Syst Rev*, 3. CD003316. available from: PM 27010219

Schulz K, Altman D, Moher D. (2010). CONSORT 2010 statement: updated guidelines for reporting parallel group randomised trials. *J Clin Epidemiol*, **63**(8), 834–40. available from: PM:20346629

Scrutinio D, Lanzillo B, Guida P, Mastropasqua F, Monitillo V, Pusineri M, et al. (2017). Development and validation of a predictive model for functional outcome after stroke rehabilitation: the Maugeri model. *Stroke*, 48 (12), 3308–15. available from: PM:29051222

Smith MC, Barber PA, Stinear CM. (2017). The TWIST algorithm predicts time to walking independently after stroke. *Neurorehabil Neural Repair*, **31**(10–11), 955–64. available from: PM 29090654

Stinear, C. (2010). Prediction of recovery of motor function after stroke. *Lancet Neurol*, **9**(12), 1228–32. available from: PM:21035399

Stinear CM, Byblow WD, Ackerley SJ, Smith MC, Borges VM, Barber PA. (2017). PREP2: A biomarker-based algorithm for predicting upper limb function after stroke. *Ann Clin Transl Neurol*, **4**(11), 811–20. available from: PM 29159193

Stinear CM. (2017). Prediction of motor recovery after stroke: advances in biomarkers. *Lancet Neurol*, **16**(10), 826–36. available from: PM:28920888

Thieme H, Morkisch N, Mehrholz J, Pohl M, Behrens J, Borgetto B, Dohle C. (2018). Mirror therapy for improving motor function after stroke. *Cochrane Database Syst Rev*, 7, CD008449. available from: PM:22419334

van de Port I, Wevers L, Lindeman E, Kwakkel G. (2012). Effects of circuit training as alternative to usual physiotherapy after stroke: randomised controlled trial. *BMJ*, **344**, e2672. available from: PM:22577186

van Delden A, Beek PJ, Roerdink M, Kwakkel G, Peper C. (2015). Unilateral and bilateral upper-limb traning interventions after stroke have similar effects on bimanual coupling strength. *Neurorehabil Neural Repair*, **29**(3) 255–67.

van Delden A, Peper C, Beek P, Kwakkel G. (2012). Unilateral versus bilateral upper limb exercise therapy after stroke: a systematic review. *J Rehabil Med*, **44** (2), 106–117. available from: PM:22266762

van Delden A, Peper C, Nienhuys K, Zijp N, Beek J, Kwakkel G. (2013). Unilateral versus bilateral upper limb training after stroke: the Upper Limb Training After Stroke clinical trial. *Stroke*, **44**(9), 2613–16.

van Kordelaar J, van Wegen E, Nijland R, Daffertshofer A, Kwakkel G. (2013). Understanding adaptive motor control of the paretic upper limb early poststroke: the EXPLICIT-stroke program. *Neurorehabil Neural Repair*, **27** (9), 854–63. available from: PM:23884015

van der Vliet R, Selles RW, Andrinopoulou ER, Nijland R, Ribbers GM, Frens MA, Meskers C, Kwakkel G. (2020). Predicting upper limb motor impairment recovery after stroke: a mixture model. *Ann Neurol*, 2020 (in press). Available at PM: 31925838

Veerbeek J, Koolstra M, Ket J, van Wegen E, Kwakkel G. (2011a). Effects of augmented exercise therapy on outcome of gait and gait-related activities in the first 6 months after stroke: a meta-analysis. *Stroke*, **42**(11), 3311–15. available from: PM:21998062

Veerbeek J, Kwakkel G, van Wegen E, Ket J, Heymans M. (2011b). Early prediction of outcome of activities of daily living after stroke: a systematic review. *Stroke*, **42**(5), 1482–8. available from: PM:21474812

Veerbeek J, van Wegen E, Harmeling-van der Wel B, Kwakkel G. (2011c). Is accurate prediction of gait in nonambulatory stroke patients possible within 72 hours poststroke? The EPOS study. *Neurorehabil Neural Repair*, **25**(3), 268–74. available from: PM:21186329

Veerbeek J, van Wegen E, van Peppen R, Van der Wees P, Hendriks E, Rietberg M, et al. (2014). What is the evidence for physical therapy poststroke? A systematic review and meta-analysis. *PLoS One*, **9**(2), e87987. available from: PM:24505342

Veerbeek JM, Langbroek-Amersfoort AC, van Wegen EE, Meskers CG, Kwakkel G. (2017). Effects of robot-assisted therapy for the upper limb after stroke. *Neurorehabil Neural Repair*, **31**(2), 107–21. doi:10.1177/1545968316666957. Review. PubMed PMID: 27597165.

Veerbeek JM, Winters C, van Wegen EEH, Kwakkel G. (2018). Is the proportional recovery rule applicable to the lower limb after a first-ever ischemic stroke? *PLoS One*, **13**(1), e0189279. available from: PM:29329286

Vloothuis JDM, Mulder M, Nijland RHM, Goedhart QS, Konijnenbelt M, Mulder H, Hertogh CMPM, van Tulder M, van Wegen EEH, Kwakkel G. (2019). Caregiver-mediated exercises with e-health support for early supported discharge after stroke (CARE4STROKE): a randomized controlled trial. *PLoS One*, **14**(4), e0214241. Available from PM: 30958833

Vloothuis JDM, Mulder M, Veerbeek JM, Konijnenbelt M, Visser-Meily JMA, Ket JCF, et al. (2016). Caregiver-mediated exercises for improving outcomes after stroke. *Cochrane Database Syst Rev*, 12. CD011058. doi:10.1002/14651858.CD011058.pub2.

Wang X, You S, Sato S, Yang J, Carcel C, Zheng D, Yoshimura S, Anderson CS, Sandset EC, Robinson T, Chalmers J, Sharma VK. (2018). Current status of intravenous tissue plasminogen activator dosage for acute ischaemic stroke: An updated systematic review. *Stroke Vasc Neurol*, **3**(1), 28–33. Available from PM: 29600005

Winters C, van Wegen E, Daffertshofer A, Kwakkel G. (2015). Generalizability of the proportional recovery model for the upper extremity after an ischemic stroke. *Neurorehabil Neural Repair*, **29**(7), 614–22. available from: PM:25505223

World Health Organization. (2001). *International Classification of Functioning, Disability and Health (ICF)*. Geneva: WHO.

Chapter 24

Language and Cognitive Rehabilitation after Stroke

Marian C. Brady

Jonathan J. Evans

Introduction: Language and Cognition after Stroke

Language Impairment after Stroke

Aphasia[1] is an acquired loss or impairment of language as a consequence of brain damage. Importantly, it excludes other communication difficulties attributed to confusion, dementia, or motor deficits (such as dysarthria). About a third of people who experience their first ischaemic stroke also experience aphasia (30% of people admitted with their first ischaemic stroke [Engelter et al., 2006]; 35% of adults admitted after stroke [Dickey et al., 2010]). Language impairment profiles can be very individualistic as measured by the severity and the degree of involvement across the comprehension and expression of spoken and written language. Functional impacts may include a prolonged hospital stay, poorer functional recovery and abilities in activities of daily living, reduced quality of life, reduced social networks, and difficulty returning to work compared to stroke survivors without aphasia (Black-Schaffer and Osberg, 1990; Paolucci et al., 2005; Gialanella and Prometti, 2009; Gialanella, 2011). Aphasia can persist after stroke with 61% of stroke survivors still experiencing communication problems a year after onset (Pedersen et al., 2004). Effective and timely rehabilitation of aphasia is crucial to an individual's recovery after stroke.

Cognitive Impairment after Stroke

Impairment of cognitive domains such as memory, perception, attention, and executive functions is also common after stroke. Estimates of incidence/prevalence vary widely depending on assessment method, but Jokinen and colleagues (2015) reported that in a consecutive

sample of 409 patients from an acute stroke unit, 83% were found to have impairment in at least one cognitive domain and 50% were impaired in at least three domains. Even in the patients with good clinical recovery at 3 months, 71% had some form of cognitive impairment. Furthermore, cognitive impairment was found to be associated with functional dependence at 15 months, independent of stroke severity. Others have found similar levels of impairment and evidence of a relationship with functional status (Tatemichi et al., 1994; Middleton et al., 2014). Thus, cognitive impairments are an important therapeutic target.

Language Rehabilitation and Speech and Language Therapy

Speech and language therapy (SLT) seeks to maximize an individuals' communication activities and participation. The design of an SLT intervention is dictated by careful assessment of language abilities and theoretical approach (such as semantic, phonological, melodic intonation, or constraint-induced language therapy, to name a few). The treatment intervention can also vary in the delivery model (group, 1-to-1, or facilitated by computer or volunteer) and the therapy regimen (intensity, dosage, duration, timing of the intervention). Speech and language therapy for people with aphasia following stroke is beneficial, but the evidence to support this has been widely dispersed (Brady et al., 2016).

Speech and Language Therapy or No Therapy for People with Aphasia

Study Design and Patients

A systematic review of 22 randomized controlled trials (RCTs) compared the communication abilities of 1620 people, some of whom received SLT while

---

[1] Historically referred to as dysphasia

others were randomly allocated to receive no SLT (Brady et al., 2016). Five trials randomized people across two SLT interventions and a no treatment group and so the evidence summary is based on 27 paired 'randomized comparisons'. Participants' age ranged from 28 to 94 years, they were between 2 days to 29 years post-stroke onset, and their aphasia ranged from mild to severe.

Interventions

Among the SLT interventions contributing to this evidence include groups that received 'conventional' SLT, computer-mediated SLT, group SLT, functional SLT, intensive SLT, language enrichment therapy, constraint-inducted aphasia therapy, melodic intonation therapy (MIT), independent training, and volunteer-facilitated SLT.

Functional Communication

Based on pooled data from 10 trials, patients who received SLT performed better on measures of functional language abilities compared with those who did not receive SLT (standardized mean difference [SMD] 0.28, 95% confidence interval [CI]: 0.06–0.49; P = 0.01) (Brady et al., 2016). At 6 months follow-up (based on a small amount of pooled data from 111 participants in two trials) there was no longer any evidence of this effect. In contrast, the RATs-3 trial (n = 152; completed after the Cochrane review was published) found no benefit on measures of functional communication measures for patients within 2 weeks of aphasia onset following 1 hour daily cognitive-linguistic SLT over 4 weeks compared with no therapy access (Nouwens et al., 2017).

Receptive Language

Eleven trials measured participants' receptive language (Brady et al., 2016). Pooled statistical data from 6 trials (9 randomized comparisons), comparing the auditory comprehension of participants who received SLT to those who did not, showed no evidence of a difference between the groups (SMD 0.06, 95% CI: −0.15–0.26; P = 0.42). Five trials compared the groups' reading comprehension. Those participants who received SLT performed better on tests of reading comprehension than those who did not receive SLT (SMD 0.31, 95% CI: 0.03–0.59; P = 0.03). In one trial the participants receiving SLT also received an acupuncture co-intervention.

Expressive Language

Seven randomized comparisons evaluated the naming abilities of participants who received SLT compared with those who had not received SLT, but there was no evidence of a difference between the groups (Brady et al., 2016). In contrast, eight randomized comparisons compared participants' writing abilities and found that the participants who had received SLT performed better on measures of writing abilities than those who had received no SLT (SMD 0.41, 95% CI: 0.14–0.67; P = 0.0003). There was some evidence of statistical heterogeneity in this meta-analysis (heterogeneity: chi^2 = 11.15, degrees of freedom [df] = 7 [P = 0.13]; I^2 = 37%). This was no longer evident when the data from two Chinese randomized comparisons were removed from the meta-analysis (I^2 = 0%), but the overall effect remained (SMD 0.27, 95% CI: 0.03–0.56; P = 0.08). Other measures of expressive language, such as copying, repetition, and fluency, which are less relevant to the functional use of language, were reported by a small number of trials, and did not show any indication of a difference between the groups. At 6 months follow-up there was no evidence of a difference in a group's expressive language naming skills based on the pooled data from 3 small trials (Brady et al., 2016).

Severity of Language Impairment

Seven trials compared a group that received SLT with one that did not by measuring the severity of the participants' aphasia impairment using a range of multilingual aphasia test batteries. Based on the pooled data available, there was no evidence of a significant difference between the groups (SMD 0.55, 95% CI: −0.14–1.25; P = 0.12).

Evidence Overview

People with aphasia who received SLT had higher scores on measures of functional communication, receptive language (reading comprehension), and expressive language (general) than people who had no SLT. Significant differences were not evident across all measures nor at follow-up. Sample sizes were small. For ethical reasons, random allocation of patients within the early stages of stroke to groups that have no access to SLT are unlikely in the future, with more recent trials of SLT making comparisons to participants who had access to deferred therapy (e.g. the FCET2EC trial, Breitenstein et al., 2017) or an alternative approach to therapy (the VERSE 3 trial, Godecke et al., 2018).

SLT or Social Support for People with Aphasia

Study Design and Patients

Nine RCTs involving 447 people with aphasia compared SLT interventions (conventional, group, or telerehabilitation interventions) with interventions providing social support (Brady et al., 2016). Aphasia onset ranged from 12 days (an average of those participating in one intervention trial [Bowen et al., 2012]) up to 28 years. Four trials recruited participants within 4 weeks of stroke onset. The remainder of the trials recruited after this acute phase. Description of the participants varied. Their ages ranged from 18 to 97 years. The people who received SLT in one trial (David et al., 1982) were significantly older (mean age [± SD] 70 [± 8.7]) years) compared to those who received social support (65 [± 10.6] years). All trials reported the severity of participants' aphasia, which ranged from mild to severe.

Interventions

Providing people with social support stimulates conversation and augments functional language use. Interventions in this category included participation in art, dance, or music classes or other non-language-orientated therapeutic interventions (e.g. art, physical or music therapy). Other social interventions typically included providing regular conversational stimulation or alternative informal, unstructured communicative interactions. These interventions did not include targeted 'therapy' designed to resolve expressive or receptive language impairments. In some cases, such interventions were included in a trial of SLT as an attention control. However, providing regular (additional) language stimulation is likely to benefit functional language use. Conversational stimulation could be easily implemented and supported by family members or volunteers and is an important adjunct to formal SLT (Brady et al., 2018). Hence, we have presented these data separately.

Social support considered within one Cochrane review was provided by volunteer visitors, nurses, a psychologist, SLT students, research assistants, or in a group manner through external movement classes, arts groups, or church or support groups (Brady et al., 2016). Providers were given training and (in three trials) a manual of permitted activities. Interventions were provided for between 1 and 3 hours weekly for between 1 and 12 months. Most were face-to-face support, although two used an internet-supported videoconferencing tool.

Functional Communication

Using a range of tools, five trials (involving 247 people) found no evidence of a difference in participants' functional communication based on whether they had access to SLT or social support activities.

Receptive, Expressive, and Severity of Language Impairment

Few data were available to inform our understanding of the benefits of SLT versus social support on participants' receptive language. Pooled summary data from two small trials (involving 23 people) found no evidence of a difference between the groups' receptive language skills. Similarly, data based on three small randomized comparisons ($n = 33$) showed no evidence of a difference in naming skills between the groups. At individual trial level, significant effects were observed favouring both social support and SLT. Other aspects of expressive language such as sentences, picture description, writing, and fluency were informed by even smaller trials (often in isolation), limiting confidence in their findings (Brady et al., 2016).

Adherence to Interventions

A total of 40 people stopped participating in SLT in the trials considered within this comparison compared to 65 participants lost to the social support groups (odds ratio [OR] 0.51, 95% CI: 0.32–0.81; $P = 0.005$), confounding the findings described above. We identified more participants ($n = 45$) who did not adhere to their social support intervention than those who failed to adhere to their allocated SLT ($n = 11$) (OR 0.18, 95% CI: 0.09 to 0.37; $P < 0.00001$). Thus, social support interventions (or the rationale in their use) were less acceptable for some people with aphasia than SLT interventions, resulting in systematic difference in the groups' adherence rates (Brady et al., 2018).

Evidence: Overview

Seven trials compared 447 people who received SLT with groups who received social support and stimulation. Differences in language measures observed (favouring the group that received social support over those that received SLT) were derived mainly from one small trial and confounded by significantly higher losses and non-adherence rates in the social support groups (Brady et al., 2018). In contrast, a large rigorously conducted trial found no evidence of a significant difference (Bowen et al., 2012). Additional research should confirm whether social support and stimulation provide benefits to some aspects of language skills and why more people fail to adhere to this intervention. In the meantime, rehabilitation guidelines recommend social stimulation for people with aphasia in the form of conversational support from people with training in supporting impaired language skills and referral to support groups alongside formal SLT interventions (Intercollegiate Stroke Working Party, 2016).

High- or Low-Intensity Speech and Language Therapy for Aphasia

Study Design and Patients

A Cochrane systematic review of eight RCTs (involving 263 people with aphasia) compared the delivery of high-intensity SLT interventions to a lower intensity of intervention (Brady et al., 2016).

Interventions

Higher-intensity interventions were quantified by number of hours of direct therapy per week (ranging from 4 to 15 hours). These high-intensity therapies were compared with therapy delivered at a lower intensity (ranging from 1.5 to 5 hours weekly). Home-based practice activities or tasks were not included in this calculation of intensity (Brady et al., 2016).

Functional Communication

Two trials compared high- (7.5 to 10 hours therapy weekly) to low- (1.5 to 2 hours therapy weekly) intensity interventions by measuring participants' performance on the Functional Communication Profile (Sarno, 1969). Those who received the higher-intensity SLT ($n = 45$) had better functional communication than those who received SLT at a lower intensity ($n = 39$) (mean difference [MD] 11.75, 95% CI: 4.09 to 19.40; $P = 0.003$) (Brady et al., 2016). These benefits were still evident on follow-up at 40 weeks. The FCET2EC trial randomly allocated people ($n = 158$, aged 70 years or younger) with chronic aphasia (of at least 6 months in duration) to receive 3 weeks of intensive SLT of at least 10 hours weekly versus deferred intensive therapy (but continued usual SLT access). Measuring functional communication, the intensive SLT group significantly improved from baseline compared to the usual care group who did not (Breitenstein et al., 2017).

Receptive Language

Data from two trials compared high- (10 hours weekly) to low-intensity (2 to 5 hours weekly) SLT regimens and, where possible, data were pooled. Performance on measures of auditory comprehension and reading did not differ between the groups.

Expressive Language

There was no evidence of a difference in expressive language skills (measured using naming, repetition, fluency, and writing subtests) between the groups across three trials that had access to high- (10 hours weekly) or low-intensity (2 to 5 hours weekly) SLT. The recent Big CACTUS trial found benefit in measures of word finding among a chronic group of patients (more than 4 months after aphasia onset) but not functional communication when they had access to self-managed, computer-based therapy software (up to 30 minutes' practice daily over 6 months) compared to usual care (which averaged approximately 1 hour every 2 weeks) (Palmer et al., 2015).

Severity of Language Impairment

Based on the meta-analysis of five RCTs, people who received high-intensity SLT ($n = 96$; ranging from 5 to 10 hours weekly) experienced a lower severity of aphasia at the end of treatment period compared to people who received low-intensity SLT ($n = 91$; 1.5 to 5 hours) (SMD 0.38, 95% CI: 0.07–0.69; $P = 0.02$). One recently completed small trial ($n = 30$; Stahl et al., 2017) found that intensity of intervention may not be as important in the context of a chronic patient population. Among that trial's patients who were at least 1 year after aphasia onset, overall language benefits were observed in the context of SLT but there was no additional benefit with the higher-intensity therapy (4 hours daily) compared to the moderate-intensity approach (2 hours daily). In contrast, the VERSE trial compared acute patients' ($n = 246$, 12 weeks following index stroke) overall language severity following usual care and two experimental SLT approaches but found no evidence of a difference between the groups' recovery on overall measures of aphasia severity (Godecke et al., 2018).

Adherence to Interventions

Information on therapy adherence was available for four trials. More people failed to complete the higher-intensity SLT interventions ($n = 35/114$; 4 to 10 hours SLT weekly) compared to those who received SLT at a lower intensity ($n = 17/102$; 1.5 to hours SLT weekly). Intensive SLT interventions may not be acceptable or feasible for all people with aphasia after stroke. The data contributing to measures of functional language and severity of impairment only reflect the participants who remained in the trials. Interestingly, all the individuals who dropped out of the intervention were recruited within a few months of stroke onset. Two trials that recruited participants who were 2 or more years after stroke onset did not report any dropouts. Importantly, the three trials that recruited people within 3 months of stroke onset found benefit of high-intensity SLT (measured by aphasia severity) for those participants who remained within the trials (SMD 0.47, CI: 95% 0.05–088). In contrast, the participants recruited several years after stroke did not demonstrate similar evidence of effect of high- compared to lower-intensity SLT (SMD 0.06 95%, CI: −0.67– +0.78).

Evidence: Overview

Functional language and aphasia severity improved following access to high-intensity SLT (compared to SLT at a lower intensity), but the findings were confounded by the greater number of participants dropping out from the therapy delivered at a higher intensity. There is some indication that timing of intensive SLT for aphasia after stroke may be important for tolerance of high-intensity interventions (and perhaps benefit), though numbers of trials and participants informing these meta-analyses were small.

Speech and Language Therapy Delivery

A range of approaches to providing SLT is available to therapists, including delivery of SLT to a group or on a 1-to-1 basis, face-to-face SLT, computer-based SLT, or SLT delivered by a professional therapist or a trained volunteer.

Study Design: SLT Delivery Models

Few RCTs compare group SLT, 1-to-1 SLT, computer-facilitated, or volunteer-facilitated SLT to SLT delivered directly by a professional therapist.

Evidence Overview: SLT Delivery Models

There is no evidence of a difference in the functional communication skills (3 trials involving 43 people with aphasia) or severity of aphasia (4 trials involving 122 people with aphasia) of people who received SLT on a 1-to-1 versus group basis. A small number of trials based on small numbers of participants found no evidence of a difference in the provision of SLT interventions facilitated by volunteers or computers (under the direction of professional therapists, where volunteers received appropriate training and had access to relevant therapy materials and therapeutic intervention plans) compared to SLT delivered by a professional therapist. Clinical guidelines support the provision or augmentation of therapy provision by trained volunteers, family members, and computer programs (Intercollegiate Stroke Working Party, 2016).

Theoretical Approaches to Speech and Language Therapy

A wide range of theoretical approaches to SLT exist, including constraint-induced aphasia therapy (e.g. Pulvermuller et al., 2001), MIT (Albert et al., 1973), and semantic-based therapy (e.g. Howard et al., 1985).

Constraint-induced Aphasia Therapy

Constraint-induced aphasia therapy (CIAT) involves creating 'constraints' on the use of communication components that would naturally support verbal expression (e.g. visual feedback, gesture, or facial expressions). Constraints are created by placing a physical barrier or screen between speaker and listener and 'forcing' the use of specific verbal output to communicate meaning. CIAT is usually provided in a group format and at a high level of intensity. Five RCTs (174 people) compared CIAT with conventional 1-to-1 SLT, other group therapy, or a semantic approach to SLT. In most cases, the durations of therapies were matched. Only two trials controlled for the intensity, duration, and dose (total number of therapy hours provided) across the two arms of the trials (Sickert et al., 2014) (Wilssens et al., 2015). A third controlled for the duration and dose of therapy (Ciccone et al., 2016.). Meta-analyses of four trials (where data permitted) showed no evidence of a difference between CIAT and other theoretical approaches to SLT provision on measures of functional communication, receptive language, expressive language, severity of aphasia, or quality of life.

Melodic Intonation Therapy

Melodic intonation therapy (Albert et al., 1973) involves the repetitive singing of short phrases while tapping the rhythm of the phrase. MIT is generally thought optimal for the language rehabilitation of severe non-fluent aphasia. The rationale for this approach is based on melody activating regions of the right hemisphere of the brain that could support language use and the use of rhythm in language. The current evidence base for this approach is poor and based primarily on case studies and case series (Hurkmans et al., 2012; van der Meulen et al., 2012). One small RCT ($n = 27$) compared the use of MIT with conventional SLT approaches but found no evidence of a difference between the groups (van der Meulen et al., 2014).

Semantic-based SLT

Semantic approaches to the rehabilitation of people with aphasia are based on the cognitive neuropsychological model of language processing in the brain (Whitworth et al., 2005). Semantic therapy aims to improve processing at the level of word *meaning*, which will in turn lead to improved use and comprehension of language. Four small RCTs ($n = 177$) compared participants who received semantic SLT interventions to participants who received an alternative SLT (phonologically based, communicative SLT, a repetition in the presence of a picture approach, or CIAT approach). There was no evidence of a difference between the participants on any language measures.

Evidence Overview: Theoretical Approaches to SLT

Some trials addressing such comparisons have recently been reported or are ongoing. To date, comparisons are based on a small number of trials involving few participants (typically fewer than 20). No one theoretical approach has been demonstrated to be more effective than another. Similarly, national clinical guidelines do not as yet recommend one theoretical approach over another (unlike many other aspects of stroke rehabilitation). Additional large, rigorous, well-funded trials are required to further inform our understanding.

Cognitive Rehabilitation after Stroke

Cognitive rehabilitation (CR) has been defined as 'a process whereby people with brain injury work together with health service professionals and others to remediate or alleviate cognitive deficits arising from a neurological insult' (Wilson, 2002, p. 99). This definition highlights that CR interventions may aim to reduce a cognitive deficit caused by damage to the brain, with the intention of restoring normal, or at least improved, cognitive functioning. However, it also includes interventions where the aim is to improve the ability to perform everyday activities by compensating for a cognitive deficit that cannot be improved.

The past two to three decades have seen the evidence base in relation to CR increase to the point that clinical guidelines have begun to emerge that are based on systematic reviews of the literature (e.g. Cicerone et al., 2011). However, much of this evidence relates to studies with patients with a range of different forms of acquired brain injuries and therefore may include not only patients who have suffered a stroke but also patients who have suffered traumatic brain injury (TBI), anoxia, encephalitis, and so on. The stroke-specific CR literature is relatively small. Some Cochrane reviews exist, but the methodological quality of the stroke-specific CR evidence base is generally quite low, and as a result few studies survive the rigorous inclusion criteria of a Cochrane review. Clinical guideline writers therefore have had to decide whether to write guidelines based only upon the most rigorous RCT evidence relating specifically to stroke, or to make recommendations on the wider, but lower quality, evidence, which may not be specific to stroke. This almost certainly accounts for the substantial differences in conclusions drawn in different guideline documents.

Memory after Stroke

Background to Interventions

Memory impairments appear to be the most common form of cognitive deficit after stroke. Jokinen and colleagues (2015) found that 60% of patients had impairment of memory 3 months after stroke. The presence of memory impairment has been found to be specifically associated with dependence and functioning in everyday life (Tatemichi et al., 1994; Middleton et al., 2014). Memory is not a unitary system and specific forms of memory difficulty may occur (e.g. visual vs verbal impairment), but the major distinction is between working memory (holding and manipulating information in mind) and long-term memory (remembering information and events anywhere from a few minutes ago to many years ago). In addition, a distinction is drawn between forgetting what has happened ('retrospective memory' – e.g. what I did yesterday; what I was told this morning; how to find a place I visited last week) and forgetting to do things ('prospective memory' – e.g. forgetting to pay a bill, go to an appointment, pass on a message or take medication; das Nair and Lincoln, 2007). In terms of everyday functioning, while impairments in retrospective and prospective memory may both cause difficulties, deficits in prospective memory are likely to have the most serious consequences for everyday life (Evans, 2013).

Interventions

Reflecting the different types of memory impairment, interventions for memory deficits have taken several forms. Most work is in relation to long-term memory, but recently there has also been a focus on working memory, though the latter tends to be included with attention training because of the overlap between the constructs of attention and working memory. In relation to long-term memory, some interventions are aimed at enhancing initial learning of information so that it will be better retained. Other interventions are focused on improving the likelihood that a person will carry out an intended task. For enhancing learning, one intervention that has been investigated relatively extensively in people with acquired brain injury, albeit not extensively in people with stroke, is errorless learning. This refers to a general principle of attempting to avoid making errors while learning something new. The rationale is that if a person with a memory impairment makes an error while learning something new, they will find it difficult to remember that the response was an error, but also be more likely to make the same error again as a result of implicit memory processes (Baddeley and Wilson, 1994). Hence, errorless learning techniques aim to minimize the likelihood that a mistake is made during learning. There is a range of other mental strategies that are designed to improve the encoding of information into memory, with the intention that the information will be stored, retained, and retrieved more effectively (Evans, 2009). The other major approach to memory rehabilitation involves the use of external memory aids of some form. These include diaries, notebooks, wall charts, and electronic reminding devices such as pagers, personal digital assistants, and smart phones (Evans et al., 2003).

Study Designs

Although the number of studies of memory rehabilitation has increased somewhat over the last decade, there are still very few high-quality RCTs of memory rehabilitation interventions for stroke. In their original Cochrane review of CR for memory impairment in stroke, das Nair and Lincoln (2007) identified just two trials that met inclusion criteria. In the updated Cochrane review (das Nair et al., 2016), 13 studies were included, but most were graded as moderate in quality and reporting quality was judged to be poor in many studies. Sample sizes were typically small, and outcome measures varied considerably between studies. The current NICE guideline (National Institute for Health and Care Excellence [NICE], 2013) included two RCTs. Cicerone and colleagues' (2011) series of three systematic reviews of CR (for TBI and stroke) considered 70 papers relating to memory interventions, but of these only 7 were considered to be well-designed prospective RCTs and most of the studies included mainly patients with TBI. Of the rest of the studies, 3 were quasi-randomized trials, 7 were cohort studies without randomization, and 53 were case series or studies using single subject methods. One might, in fact, argue that the class allocation for well-conducted single-case experimental design studies ought to be higher (Tate et al., 2014), but even then very few studies would be considered high-quality single-case experimental designs examining memory interventions in stroke.

Evidence and Overview

Conclusions with regard to which, if any, memory interventions are recommended vary between reviews and guideline documents. The Cochrane review (das Nair et al., 2016) and other reviews (e.g. Gillespie et al., 2015) that draw upon well-conducted RCTs conclude that there is limited evidence to support or refute the effectiveness of memory rehabilitation for stroke. Gillespie and colleagues (2015) note one report on data relating to stroke patients from an RCT of a pager-based reminding system, but argue this needs replicating before making recommendations. Das Nair and colleagues (2016) conclude that subjective measures of memory show some benefit of memory rehabilitation interventions but only at the first assessment point following intervention and no benefit is shown at longer-term follow-up (at least 3 months). No specific recommendation is made therefore with regard to specific interventions. On the other hand, Cicerone and colleagues (2011) recommend use of external compensations with direct application to functional activities for people with severe memory deficits after TBI or stroke, albeit the level of this recommendation is not at the strongest level. The NICE guideline (2013) notes the limited evidence to draw upon and suggests that one should use interventions for memory and cognitive functions that focus on relevant functional tasks, taking into account the underlying impairment. The NICE guideline also notes a range of possible interventions including interventions to increase awareness of the memory deficit; enhancing learning using errorless learning and elaborative techniques; using external aids (e.g. diaries, lists, calendars, and alarms); and making changes to the environment that will support memory.

Non-spatial Attention Interventions

Background to Interventions

Deficits in attention are common after stroke (Loetscher and Lincoln 2013). Prevalence estimates vary and depend upon time since stroke, but in terms of longer-term outcomes up to 50% of people may experience attention deficits (Barker-Collo et al., 2010; Loetscher and Lincoln, 2013). There are several forms of attention dependent upon different anatomical systems, and therefore a person may have a deficit in one system but not another. Although conceptualizations of attention differ, the systems are commonly described as arousal, alertness, selective attention, sustained attention, divided attention, and spatial orienting (dealt with later in terms of unilateral neglect).

Interventions

Interventions for attention deficits have mainly involved attempts to improve, or restore, normal attention functions through practising attention-demanding tasks, sometimes using computerized training programmes (Gillespie et al., 2015). Other interventions have involved learning mental strategies to manage attention in functional situations, but these interventions have not been the focus of RCTs in stroke patients.

Study Designs

As with memory, there are very few RCTs of attention training interventions in stroke. Loetscher and Lincoln's (2013) Cochrane review includes six studies, four of which were parallel group studies and two were cross-over designs. The NICE guideline (2013) includes two RCTs (Westerberg et al., 2007; Barker-Collo et al., 2009). Most studies had small sample sizes and methodological limitations. Cicerone and colleagues (2011) included eight studies, with six of them being Class III level of evidence.

Evidence and Overview

Six studies including 223 participants compared CR with usual care (no treatment) (Loetscher and Lincoln, 2013). Meta-analyses demonstrated no significant long-term effect of CR on subjective measures of attention (two studies, 99 participants; SMD 0.16, 95% CI: −0.23–0.56; $P = 0.41$). In terms of effects at end of treatment, there was a borderline significant effect for subjective measures of attention (two studies, 53 participants, SMD 0.53, 95% CI: −0.03–1.08; $P = 0.06$). A statistically significant effect was found in favour of CR for immediate effects on standardized measures of divided attention (four studies, 165 participants; SMD 0.67, 95% CI: 0.35–0.98; $P < 0.0001$). No significant effects were found for other domains of attention including alertness (four studies, 136 participants, SMD 0.14, 95% CI: −0.20–0.48; $P = 0.41$), selective attention (six studies, 223 participants, SMD −0.08, 95% CI: −0.35–0.18; $P = 0.53$), or sustained attention (four studies, 169 participants, SMD 0.39, 95% CI: −0.16–0.94; $P = 0.16$). There were no significant effects on functional abilities in daily living (two studies, 75 participants, SMD 0.29, 95% CI: −0.16–0.75; $P = 0.21$). Loetscher and Lincoln concluded that the effectiveness of CR remains unconfirmed.

Cicerone and colleagues (2011) concluded that computer-based interventions could be considered as an adjunct to clinician-guided treatment of attention deficits after stroke. But relying on repeated practice on computer-based tasks without some involvement and intervention by a therapist was not recommended. SIGN 118 (2010) notes that there is not yet sufficient evidence to support or refute the benefits of CR for patients with problems of attention. NICE 162 (2013) suggests that 'attention training' may be considered, and alternatively interventions should focus on training people on functional tasks, and use strategies to manage the environment including using prompts that are relevant to the task.

Spatial Attention

Background to Interventions

Unilateral neglect refers to the failure to attend to one side of space, more commonly the left side. Patients with unilateral neglect may ignore one side of their body, they may groom one side of their face, they may eat food from only one side of a plate, have difficulty reading, and bump into people or objects when moving around their environment. Prevalence figures vary widely across studies, something that may arise from the fact that neglect is more prevalent in the acute phase post-stroke than later stages. Neglect is an important predictor of long-term outcome after stroke (Bowen et al., 2013).

Interventions

Many interventions for unilateral neglect have been developed. Luauté (2006) identified 18 different approaches, dating back to the 1940s, but with most interventions being developed in the 1980s and 1990s. Many interventions have a strong theoretical basis and have emerged out of studies that have examined the underlying causes of the condition. Bowen and colleagues (2013) note that approaches to the rehabilitation of unilateral neglect can be classified as 'bottom up' or 'top down'. They state that bottom-up approaches are aimed specifically at the impairment with the intention of modifying the underlying deficit. Top-down approaches aim to teach a person to compensate for the impairment so as to improve everyday functioning, without necessarily affecting the underlying deficit. Most interventions that have been developed are top down, and include scanning training in which the person is trained to scan to the left in order to increase the likelihood of noticing stimuli in left hemi-space. Interventions described as visual scanning training may vary considerably, from computer-training programmes to use of specific anchoring techniques such as placing a red marker to the left of text when reading using an instruction to find the red line before reading each line. Examples of bottom-up interventions include use of prism glasses (e.g. Mizuno et al., 2011), eye-patching (e.g. Fong et al., 2007), and limb activation (Robertson et al., 2002). Prism glasses shift the visual field to the right so that stimuli on the left are more likely to be perceived, but the key therapeutic effect is that the shift of the visual field rightwards appears to persist for a period of time after the glasses are removed (Frassinetti et al., 2002). Limb activation involves the patient being prompted to make some form of movement of the left limb in left hemi-space, with the aim that activation of sensory and motor systems in the right hemisphere will stimulate increased attention to the left side of visual space.

Study Designs

Studies of interventions for unilateral neglect are challenging to conduct because neglect is often transitory, is variable between people, and fluctuates considerably within individuals. Thus, while it is a common problem, the number of people in one location with specific forms of stable, persistent neglect who are willing to participate in an intervention trial is always likely to be modest. There have been many studies investigating interventions, but very few high-quality RCTs. There is a small number of well-conducted single-case experimental design studies (e.g. Tunnard and Wilson, 2014), but these are typically excluded from systematic reviews and meta-analyses. Therefore, the recommendations that arise from systematic reviews vary considerably, depending on the level of evidence included for consideration.

Evidence and Overview

Luauté and colleagues (2006) concluded that there was insufficient evidence to provide their strongest level of recommendation, but did recommend use of visual scanning training, mental imagery, feedback training, and prism adaptation. They acknowledge, however, that most follow-up periods post-intervention were relatively short. Cicerone and colleagues (2011) gave visual scanning training their highest level of recommendation (practice standard). Bowen and colleagues (2013) included 23 papers with a total of 628 participants, but only 18 studies compared an intervention with a control (either an attention control or treatment as usual). They note that, overall, the methodological quality of studies included was poor. They found a significant effect in favour of CR compared with any control (10 with attention control, 6 with usual care), for immediate effects on standardized neglect assessments (16 studies, 437 participants, SMD 0.35, 95% CI: 0.09–0.62; $P = 0.0092$). However, sensitivity analyses including only studies of high methodological quality removed evidence of a significant effect. They also found no evidence of immediate effects on activities of daily living (ADL), or persisting effects on either standardized measures or ADL. Thus Bowen and colleagues (2013) conclude that 'there is still insufficient evidence to draw generalized conclusions about the effect of CR interventions on functional ability in ADL or on standardized neglect assessments' (p. 18). SIGN 118 (2010) provides only a good practice suggestion that patients with neglect should be assessed and taught compensatory strategies. NICE 162 (2013) recommends that people are screened and provided with education and support, and that interventions for neglect focus on functional tasks and may include interventions to help people scan to the neglected side, such as brightly coloured lines or highlighter on the edge of the page; alerting techniques such as auditory cues; repetitive task performance such as dressing; and altering the perceptual input using prism glasses.

The most consistent recommendation across reviews is for visual scanning training, with an emphasis on this training being implemented in functional situations or with a pathway to generalization clearly built in to the training programme.

Perception Interventions

Background to Interventions

In addition to spatial neglect, there is a range of other forms of visual and perceptual disorders that may arise following stroke. Visual field defects are estimated to affect 20–57% of people who have had a stroke (Pollock et al., 2011). Bowen and colleagues (2011) note that perceptual disorders include visual object agnosia, prosopagnosia, spatial, visuospatial, tactile, body, sensation, location, motion, colour processing, and auditory perceptual disorders (p. 5). Prevalence figures for perceptual disorders appear to be around 50–70% (Rowe et al., 2013). Visual perceptual disorders have a major impact on ADL. If a person has a hemianopia, the consequences for some may be similar to those for someone with neglect, though people with hemianopia are more likely to be aware of, and adjust to, their impairment than those with neglect. A person with Balint's syndrome will have difficulty reaching accurately to locate an object in space. A person who has difficulty perceiving individual objects from the background will have difficulties finding objects in a kitchen, such as the utensils in a drawer. Visual object agnosia means that familiar objects are not recognized, and prosopagnosia means that a familiar person such as a spouse or friend is not recognized. A person with depth perception, or impairment in the ability to perceive motion, will have difficulty crossing roads. Other forms of perceptual disorders may lead to difficulties navigating in the environment.

Interventions

Pollock and colleagues (2011, 2019) included interventions aimed at either improving a visual field defect or improving the ability of a person to cope with the visual field loss. Bowen and colleagues (2011) classified interventions for perceptual disorders into four forms: functional training; sensory stimulation; strategy training; and repetition (of a task), though these are rather broad and to some extent overlapping ideas. Functional training refers to simply practising everyday tasks (e.g. dressing, cooking) with the aim that performance will improve despite the presence of a perceptual impairment. Repetition is similar in referring to practising perceptual tasks, but the tasks are not typically functional tasks. Sensory stimulation also refers to undertaking training tasks, but here the emphasis is on making judgements about basic perceptual features such as colour, shape, and length. Strategy training involves learning a mental strategy that facilitates perception, though it does not change the underlying impairment.

Study Designs

As with other domains, there are very few high-quality RCTs in the literature. In their original Cochrane review, Pollock and colleagues (2011), identified 13 studies (344 participants, of whom 285 were participants with stroke) but only six studies compared an intervention with a control group of some form. In the updated review, Pollock and colleagues (2019) included 19 studies (702 randomized participants, with data for 520 participants with stroke); however, only nine of these studies compared the effect of an intervention with a placebo, control, or no treatment group and eight had data which could be included in meta-analyses. Bowen and colleagues (2011) identified six studies with a total of 338 participants, with just three studies able to provide data for analysis.

Evidence and Overview

In people with visual field loss, Pollock and others (2019) concluded that there was insufficient evidence to draw any conclusions regarding the effectiveness of interventions aiming for restitution when compared with a control group. They reported that there was low-quality evidence that compensatory scanning training was more beneficial than control or placebo on quality of life (two studies, 96 participants, MD 9.36, 95% CI: 3.10–15.62). They also concluded that there was low- or very low-quality evidence of no effect of scanning training on measures of visual field, extended activities of daily living, reading, and scanning ability. Pollock and colleagues (2019) also examined substitutive studies (use of a prism), finding that three studies (166 participants) compared a type of prism with a control. They noted that there was low or very low-quality evidence that prisms did not have an effect on measures of activities of daily living, reading, falls, or quality of life, with very low-quality evidence that they may have an effect on scanning ability (one study, 39 participants, MD 9.80, 95% CI: 1.91–17.69).

For other visual perceptual disorders, Bowen and colleagues (2011) found no evidence of a difference in ADL self-care scores (one study, 33 participants, MD 0.9, 95% CI: −1.6–3.5; $P = 0.47$) or in an odds ratio of passing a driving test (one study, 97 participants, OR 1.3, 95% CI: 0.56–3.1). They concluded that there is currently insufficient evidence to support or refute the view that interventions for perceptual problems are effective.

Cicerone and colleagues (2011) argue that systematic training of visuospatial and visual organization skills may be considered for persons with visual perceptual deficits after right hemisphere stroke as part of acute rehabilitation. Exactly what constitutes this training is unclear. They also suggest that computer-based interventions intended to produce an extension of damaged visual fields may be considered. Both of these recommendations are at the level of practice options, so the lowest of their three levels of recommendation.

Executive Function Interventions

Background to Interventions

Executive functions are the abilities that allow us to solve problems, make decisions, formulate plans and intentions, and initiate, monitor, and regulate behaviour (Evans, 2003). They are associated with the frontal lobes, but executive deficits may arise from lesions elsewhere, particularly when these regions are part of a circuit that closely involves the frontal lobes. Vataja and others (2003) found that 34% of their sample of 214 patients with ischaemic stroke showed evidence of executive dysfunction, with lesions in frontal–subcortical circuits (e.g. pallidum, corona radiata, or centrum semiovale) being more frequent in patients with executive dysfunction than in those without. Executive dysfunction, sometimes referred to as a dysexecutive syndrome, is acknowledged to have a major impact on functioning in relation to activities of daily living, work, leisure, and relationships. People with a dysexecutive syndrome may be disorganized, impulsive, fail to think

through actions, and vulnerable to being distracted and not following through with goals/intentions. They may be able to carry out routine activities well but find it difficult to deal with novelty or unstructured situations that rely on self-initiation and task monitoring.

Interventions

Interventions for executive dysfunction include training (or re-training) in problem-solving skills (e.g. Problem Solving Therapy), mental strategies aimed at improving goal or task management (Goal Management Training), or use of an external aid to prompt task initiation and guide task completion. Chung and colleagues (2013) classified the first two approaches as restorative and the latter as compensatory. For example, Problem Solving Therapy (von Cramon et al., 1991) involves teaching people the steps involved in solving a problem and practising each step in a range of tasks. Goal Management Training (Levine et al., 2000; Krasny-Pacini et al., 2014) involves teaching people a STOP:THINK strategy in which participants learn to interrupt ongoing activity to determine whether they are doing what they intended or whether they have drifted off task. They learn to clearly identify the main goal of their current activity; they specify the steps involved, implement the steps, and use the STOP:THINK approach. For many people with executive dysfunction, interventions that rely on the person self-initiating use of a mental strategy or re-learning to problem-solve provide an unrealistic goal. However, checklists or other forms of an external prompting system can be used to enable people to initiate actions and be guided through tasks (Evans, 2003).

Study Designs

Most studies evaluating interventions for executive dysfunction have been conducted with people with TBI or acquired brain injury of mixed aetiologies. Participant groups composed only of people after stroke are not typical. Studies investigating interventions for executive functions have been poor methodologically. The Cochrane review of Chung and colleagues (2013) included 19 RCTs (one a crossover RCT) covering 13 different interventions. Of the 13 interventions, seven were classified as restorative (aimed at improving underlying executive skills) and five were compensatory. There was some uncertainty over intervention classifications, a common issue for interventions broadly described as 'cognitive rehabilitation'. Three studies compared CR with standard care. Six studies compared CR with no treatment or placebo treatment. Ten studies compared experimental CR with standard CR.

Evidence and Overview

There are few high-quality RCTs of interventions for executive function and groups tend to be of mixed aetiology. In the 2013 Cochrane review of Chung and colleagues, around 40% of the total number of participants included in the meta-analyses were stroke patients, and data were not reported separately. Chung and colleagues (2013) concluded that there was insufficient evidence to either support or refute the hypothesis that CR interventions improve executive function. Their primary outcome measure was global executive function, meaning scores on either the Behavioural Assessment of the Dysexecutive Syndrome (BADS) (Wilson et al., 1996) or the Hayling and Brixton test batteries (Burgess and Shallice, 1997). Given the relatively poor test–retest reliability of executive function tests, and the fact that many interventions for executive dysfunction are aimed at improving everyday functioning rather than test performance, a measure of global executive functioning might not be the best primary outcome measure. Only two studies actually included either the BADS or Hayling and Brixton as outcome measures. However, the authors also looked at a range of specific executive function component process outcomes (e.g. planning, flexibility, inhibition, concept formation, working memory) and at measures of activities of daily living, vocational performance, and quality of life. The conclusion for all of these outcome variables was the same – there is no compelling evidence to support interventions.

Cicerone and colleagues (2011) made no recommendations in relation to people after stroke but concluded that there was sufficient evidence to recommend that meta-cognitive strategy training focused on training self-monitoring and emotional regulation be a practice standard for people with executive dysfunction after TBI. Neither the SIGN nor NICE guidelines provide any guidance with regard to interventions for executive dysfunction after stroke.

Interventions for People with Cognitive Deficits after Stroke That Are Not Domain Specific

We have focused so far on literature relating to interventions where there has been an explicit aim to target specific cognitive impairments, albeit the interventions may be compensatory and include functional outcome measures. This potentially means that literature that is not domain-specific in some way is not included, such as studies where everyday functioning is the primary outcome measure, and interventions are focused primarily on ways of improving performance of these specific functional tasks, in people with cognitive impairment following stroke. However, here again the evidence base is very limited. A Cochrane review of occupational therapy for cognitive impairment in stroke (Hoffmann et al., 2010) included only one small RCT and drew no conclusions. A recent large-scale cluster RCT, in which 1042 participants (around 70% of whom had cognitive impairment) were randomly allocated to a 3-month occupational therapy intervention or standard care, found no effect of the intervention on measures of functional ability, mobility, mood, or health-related quality of life in people after stroke who were resident in care homes (Sackley et al., 2015).

Implications for Clinical Practice

Language Rehabilitation

Based on high-quality reviews of effectiveness, SLT benefits the functional communication and language recovery of people with aphasia following stroke. However, the SLT provided within the research context was typically at a higher level of intensity than that which might be expected in usual care. We also have some indication that intensity is an important factor in language rehabilitation both in terms of recovery and acceptability of intervention for people. The lack of evidence of a difference between SLT and social support interventions suggests that such social stimulation may be an 'active' component in language rehabilitation (rather than a passive attention control). The success of many peer support initiatives available for people with aphasia would suggest that people with aphasia find this support beneficial, but more evidence about its effectiveness and the significantly higher non-adherence to this intervention is required. Similarly, the available evidence appears to support the use of trained volunteers and computers in facilitating therapy delivery. Such delivery models are likely to be essential if intensive SLT intervention models are to be feasible within the current healthcare services resources.

Cognitive Rehabilitation

For all domains of cognition, there is insufficient evidence to make very clear recommendations regarding specific intervention techniques. This conclusion is reflected in all of the relevant literature reviews that include only high-quality trials. The inability to make recommendations arises from the absence of (high-quality) evidence rather than evidence of absence of an effect. For this reason, some guideline writers have been content to draw on a wider range of forms of evidence to offer some clinical guidance. For all domains, the most common general principles are that interventions should arise from an assessment process that examines the nature of the cognitive impairment and the functional consequences of that impairment. There is no substantial evidence in any domain that impairment-focused interventions that are not clearly linked to functional tasks will be effective.

In the domain of memory, best practice is to support people to understand their memory difficulties and how they impact on everyday activities. Where someone has something specific to learn, errorless learning and other elaborative learning techniques may be useful. But the most effective approach is use of external memory aids, which can be selected and adapted to specific everyday remembering tasks. In the domain of attention, the evidence suggests that computerised attention training in isolation does not improve functioning. Interventions should identify meaningful activities, determine the impact of attentional difficulties on these activities and implement mental strategies and/or external aids that will support a person to focus and maintain attention to task. For visual neglect, visual scanning training in functional situations with a pathway to generalization clearly built-in to the training programme is recommended. For deficits in visual fields, scanning training is recommended. For other perceptual and executive deficits, there is simply insufficient evidence to make specific recommendations.

Implications for Research

Language Rehabilitation Research

Language rehabilitation is an active field of research with many ongoing trials and international initiatives to support it. Well-supported and well-conducted trials will continue to inform our understanding and optimization of the different models of therapy delivery, theoretical approaches, and therapy regimens. Improvements in the conduct and reporting of that research are also required, such as the recent consensus on a minimum core data set for aphasia research (Wallace et al., 2019). Additional activities seek a greater understanding of the effectiveness of SLT for specific subgroups (for example people differing in aphasia profile or the length of time since their stroke). Some SLT approaches may be more effective for some people (and aphasia profiles) than others. RELEASE (a National Institute for Health Research-funded international collaboration of more than 70 aphasia researchers) has collated 5928 pre-existing individual participant data from 174 primary aphasia research data sets across 28 countries to examine such questions (Brady et al., 2015). Other large-scale collaborative work includes the Predicting Language Recovery and Outcome After Stroke (PLORAS) study that aims to support individualized predictions about recovery from aphasia based on lesion size and location determined by magnetic resonance imaging (MRI) brain images and scores on measures of language (Seghier et al., 2016).

Cognitive Rehabilitation Research

The evidence base in relation to CR after stroke has grown over the last few decades, but not to the point that we can make confident recommendations about interventions in most domains of cognition. More high-quality RCTs are needed. Funders, researchers, literature reviewers, and guideline writers need to think carefully about the nature of studies that can contribute to the evidence base. Researchers should also consider using high-quality single-case experimental design (SCED) methodology too – quality appraisal tools for SCED studies are available to guide study design and evaluate published studies, and the Oxford Centre for Evidence-Based Medicine has graded systematic reviews of randomized n-of-1 trials as Level 1 evidence.

Summary

Speech and language therapy offers benefit to people with aphasia after stroke. Intensive intervention, if tolerated by the person with aphasia, is also likely to augment benefits. We need more information to gain further insights into the optimal intervention regimen, delivery model, and theoretical approach and how these factors interact with the characteristics of the person with aphasia, the nature of their language impairments, and their stroke.

In relation to cognitive rehabilitation, studies of the prevalence of cognitive impairments post-stroke are consistent in identifying that deficits in most domains of cognition are common and affect everyday functioning. The evidence base relating specifically to interventions in stroke is limited. While the evidence base has reached the point at which conducting systematic reviews, including Cochrane reviews, is a reasonable exercise, few firm conclusions can be drawn. Such reviews do, however, serve to highlight that interventions for cognitive deficits in all domains exist and need refining and evaluating more thoroughly with a wider range of methodologies.

References

Albert ML, Sparks RW, Helm NA. (1973). Melodic intonation therapy for aphasia. *Arch Neurol*, 29(2)130–1.

Baddeley AD, Wilson BA. (1994). When implicit learning fails: amnesia and the problem of error elimination. *Neuropsychologia*, **32**, 53–68.

Barker-Collo S, Feigin VL, Lawes CM, Parag V, Senior H, Rodgers A. (2009). Reducing attention deficits after stroke using attention process training: a randomized controlled trial. *Stroke*, 40(10), 3293–8

Barker-Collo S, Feigin VL, Parag V, Lawes CMM, Senior H. (2010). Auckland Stroke Outcomes Study Part 2: Cognition and functional outcomes 5 years poststroke. *Neurology*, **75**, 1608–18.

Black-Schaffer RM, Osberg JS. (1990). Return to work after stroke: development of a predictive model. *Arch Phys Med Rehabil*, **71**(5), 285–90.

Bowen A, Hazelton C, Pollock A, Lincoln NB. (2013). Cognitive rehabilitation for spatial neglect following stroke. *Cochrane Database Syst Rev*, 7. CD003586. doi:10.1002/14651858.CD003586.pub3.

Bowen A, Hesketh A, Patchick E, Young A, Davies L, Vail A, et al. (2012). Clinical effectiveness, cost effectiveness and service users' perceptions of early, well-resourced communication therapy following a stroke: a randomised controlled trial (the ACT NoW Study). *Health Technol Assess*, **16**(26), 1–160.

Bowen A, Knapp P, Gillespie D, Nicolson DJ, Vail A. (2011). Non-pharmacological interventions for perceptual disorders following stroke and other adult-acquired, non-progressive brain injury. *Cochrane Database Syst Rev*, 4. CD007039.

Brady MC, Ali M, VandenBerg K, Williams J, Williams LR, Abo M, et al. (2020). RELEASE: a protocol for a systematic review based, individual participant data, meta- and network meta-analysis, of complex speech-language therapy interventions for stroke-related aphasia. *Aphasiology*, **34**, (2), 137–57.

Brady MC, Godwin J, Kelly, Enderby P, Elders A, Campbell P. (2018). Attention control comparisons with SLT for people with aphasia following stroke: methodological concerns raised following a systematic review. *Clin Rehabil*, **32**(10), 1383–95. doi 0269215518780487.

Brady MC, Kelly H, Godwin J, Enderby P, Campbell P. (2016). Speech and language therapy for aphasia following stroke. *Cochrane Database Syst Rev*, 6. CD000425. doi:10.1002/14651858.CD000425.pub4.

Breitenstein C, Grewe T, Flöel A, Ziegler W, Springer L, Martus P, et al., for the FCET2EC study group. (2017). Intensive speech and language therapy in patients with chronic aphasia after stroke: a randomized, open-label, blinded-endpoint, controlled trial in a health-care setting. *Lancet*, **389**(10078), 1528–38.

Burgess PW, Shallice T. (1997). *The Hayling and Brixton Tests*. Bury St. Edmunds: Thames Valley Test Company.

Chung CSY, Pollock A, Campbell T, Durward BR, Hagen S. (2013). Cognitive rehabilitation for executive dysfunction in adults with stroke or other adult non-progressive acquired brain damage. *Cochrane Database Syst Rev*, 4. CD008391. doi:10.1002/14651858.CD008391.pub2.

Ciccone N, West D, Cream A, Cartwright J, Rai T, Granger A, et al. (2016) Constraint-induced aphasia therapy (CIAT): a randomised controlled trial in very early stroke rehabilitation. *Aphasiology*, **30**(5), 566–84.

Cicerone KD, Langenbahn DM, Braden C, Malec JF, Kalmar K, Fraas M, et al. (2011). Evidence-based cognitive rehabilitation: updated review of the literature from 2003 through 2008. *Arch Phys Med Rehabil*, **92**, 519–30.

das Nair R, Cogger H, Worthington E, Lincoln NB. (2016). Cognitive rehabilitation for memory deficits after stroke. *Cochrane Database Syst Rev*, 9. CD002293. doi:10.1002/14651858.CD002293.pub3.

das Nair R, Lincoln N. (2007). Cognitive rehabilitation for memory deficits following stroke. *Cochrane Database Syst Rev*, 3. CD002293. doi:10.1002/14651858.CD002293.pub2.

David R, Enderby P, Bainton D. (1982). Treatment of acquired aphasia: speech therapists and volunteers compared. *J Neurol Neurosurg Psychiatry*, **45**(11), 957–61.

Dickey L, Kagan A, Lindsay MP, Fang J, Rowland A, Black S. (2010). Incidence and profile of inpatient stroke-induced aphasia in Ontario, Canada. *Arch Phys Med Rehabil*, **91**(2), 196–202.

Engelter ST, Gostynski M, Papa S, Frei M, Born C, Ajdacic-Gross, V, et al. (2006). Epidemiology of aphasia attributable to first ischemic stroke: incidence, severity, fluency, etiology, and thrombolysis. *Stroke*, **37**(6), 1379–84.

Evans JJ. (2003). Rehabilitation of executive deficits. In BA Wilson, ed., *Neuropsychological Rehabilitation*. Abingdon: Swets and Zeitlinger.

Evans JJ. (2009). The cognitive group, Part 2: Memory. In BA Wilson, F Gracey, JJ Evans, A. Bateman, eds., *Neuropsychological Rehabilitation: Theory, Therapy and Outcomes*. Cambridge: Cambridge University Press.

Evans JJ. (2013). Disorders of memory. In LH Goldstein, JE McNeil, eds., *Clinical Neuropsychology: A Practical Guide to Assessment and Management for Clinicians*. 2nd ed. Chichester: Wiley.

Evans JJ, Needham P, Wilson, BA, Brentnall S. (2003). Which memory impaired people make good use of memory aids? Results of a survey of people with acquired brain injury. *J Int Neuropsychol Soc*, **9**, 925–935.

Fong KNK, Chan MKL, Ng PPK, Tsang MHN, Chow KKY, Lau, CWL, et al. (2007). The effect of voluntary trunk rotation and half-field eye-patching for patients with unilateral neglect in stroke: a randomized controlled trial. *Clin Rehabil*, **21**, 729–41.

Frassinetti F, Angeli V, Meneghello F, Avanzi S, Ladavas E. (2002) Long-lasting amelioration of visuospatial neglect by prism adaptation. *Brain*, **125**, 608–23.

Gialanella B. (2011) Aphasia assessment and functional outcome prediction in patients with aphasia after stroke. *J Neurol*, **258**(2), 343–9.

Gialanella B, Prometti P. (2009). Rehabilitation length of stay in patients suffering from aphasia after stroke. *Top Stroke Rehabil*, **16**(6):437–44.

Gillespie DC, Bowen A, Chung, CS. Cockburn J, Knapp P, Pollock A. (2015) Rehabilitation for post-stroke cognitive impairment: an overview of recommendations arising from systematic reviews of current evidence. *Clin Rehabil*, **29**(2), 120–8.

Godecke E, Rai T, Cadilhac DA, Armstrong E, Middleton S, Ciccone N, et al., (2018). Statistical analysis plan (SAP) for the Very Early Rehabilitation in Speech (VERSE) after stroke trial: an international 3-arm clinical trial to determine the effectiveness of early, intensive, prescribed, direct aphasia therapy. *Int J Stroke*, **13**(8), 863–80.

Hoffmann T, Bennett S, Koh CL, McKenna KT. (2010). Occupational therapy for cognitive impairment in stroke

patients. *Cochrane Database Syst Rev*, 9. CD006430. doi:10.1002/14651858.CD006430.pub2.

Howard D, Patterson K, Franklin S, Orchard-lisle V, Morton J. (1985). The facilitation of picture naming in aphasia. *Cogn Neuropsychol*, **2**(1), 49–80.

Hurkmans J, de Bruijn M, Boonstra AM, Jonkers R, Bastiaanse R, Arendzen H, et al. (2012). Music in the treatment of neurological language and speech disorders: A systematic review. *Aphasiology*, **26**(1), 1–19.

Intercollegiate Stroke Working Party. (2016). National Clinical Guideline for Stroke. 5th ed. Royal College of Physicians. Available at: https://www.rcplondon.ac.uk/guide lines-policy/stroke-guidelines. Accessed 24th January 2020.

Jokinen H, Melkas S, Ylikoski R, Pohjasvaara T, Kaste M, Erkinjuntti T, et al. (2015). Post-stroke cognitive impairment is common even after successful clinical recovery. *Eur J Neurol*, **22**, 1288–94.

Krasny-Pacini A, Chevignard M, Evans JJ. (2014). Goal management training for rehabilitation of executive functions: a systematic review of effectiveness in patients with acquired brain injury. *Disabil Rehabil*, **36**, 105–16.

Levine B, Robertson IH, Clare L, Carter G, Hong J, Wilson BA, et al. (2000). Rehabilitation of executive functioning: an experimental-clinical validation of goal management training. *J Int Neuropsychol Soc*, **6**, 299–312.

Loetscher T, Lincoln NB. (2013). Cognitive rehabilitation for attention deficits following stroke. *Cochrane Database Syst Rev*, 5. CD002842.

Luauté J, Halligan P, Rode G, Rossetti Y, Boisson D. (2006). Visuo-spatial neglect: a systematic review of current interventions and their effectiveness. *Neurosci Biobehav Rev*, **30**(7), 961–82.

Middleton LE, Lam B, Fahmi H, Black SE, McIlroy WE, Stuss DT, et al. (2014). Frequency of domain-specific cognitive impairment in sub-acute and chronic stroke. *Neurorehabilitation*, **34**(2), 305–12.

Mizuno K, Tsuji T, Takebayashi T, Fujiwara T, Hase K, Liu M. (2011). Prism adaptation therapy enhances rehabilitation of stroke patients with unilateral spatial neglect: a randomized, controlled trial. *Neurorehabil Neural Repair*, **25**, 711–20.

National Institute for Health and Care Excellence (NICE). (2013). Stroke rehabilitation: long-term rehabilitation after stroke. Retrieved from www.nice.org.uk/guidance/cg162.

Nouwens F, de Lau LM, Visch-Brink EG, van de Sandt-Koenderman WM, Lingsma HF, Goosen S, et al. (2017). Efficacy of early cognitive-linguistic treatment for aphasia due to stroke: a randomised controlled trial (Rotterdam Aphasia Therapy Study-3). *Eur Stroke J*, **2**(2), 126–36.

Palmer R, Dimairo M, Cooper C, Enderby P, Brady M, Bowen A, Latimer N, Julious S, Cross E, Alshreef A , Harrison M, et al. (2019). Self-managed, computerised speech and language therapy for patients with chronic aphasia post-stroke compared with usual care or attention control (Big CACTUS) : a multicentre, single-blinded, randomised controlled trial. *Lancet Neurol*, **18**(9), 821–33.

Paolucci S, Matano A, Bragoni M, Coiro P, De Angelis D, Fusco FR, et al. (2005). Rehabilitation of left brain-damaged ischemic stroke patients: the role of comprehension language deficits. *Cerebrovasc Dis*, **20**(5), 400–06.

Pedersen PM, Vinter K, Olsen TS. (2004). Aphasia after stroke: type, severity and prognosis. The Copenhagen Aphasia Study. *Cerebrovasc Dis*, **17**(1), 35–43.

Pollock A, Hazelton C, Henderson CA, Angilley J, Dhillon B, Langhorne P, et al. (2011). Interventions for visual field defects in patients with stroke. *Cochrane Database Syst Rev*, 10. CD008388. doi:10.1002/14651858. CD008388.pub2.

Pollock A, Hazelton C, Rowe FJ, Jonuscheit S, Kernohan A, Angilley J, et al. (2019). Interventions for visual field defects in patients with stroke. *Cochrane Database Syst Rev*, 5. CD008388. doi:10.1002/14651858.CD008388.pub3.

Pulvermuller F, Neininger B, Elbert T, Mohr B, Rockstroh B, Koebbel P, Taub E. (2001). Constraint-induced therapy of chronic aphasia after stroke. *Stroke*, **32**(7): 1621–6.

Robertson IH, McMillan TM, MacLeod E, Edgeworth J, Brock D. (2002). Rehabilitation by limb activation training reduces left-sided motor impairment in unilateral neglect patients: a single-blind randomised control trial. *Neuropsychol Rehabil*, **12**, 439–54.

Rowe FJ, Wright D, Brand D, Jackson C, Harrison S, Maan T, et al. (2013). A prospective profile of visual field loss following stroke: prevalence, type, rehabilitation, and outcome. *Biomed Res Int*, **2013**, 719096.

Sackley CM, Walker MF, Burton CR, Watkins CL, Mant J, Roalfe AK, et al. (2015). An occupational therapy intervention for residents with stroke related disabilities in UK care homes (OTCH): cluster randomised controlled trial. *BMJ*, **350**, h468.

Sarno, MT. (1969). *The Functional Communication Profile: Manual of Directions*. Vol. 42. New York: Institute of Rehabilitation Medicine, New York University Medical Center.

Seghier ML, Patel E, Prejawa S, Ramsden S, Selmer A, Li L, et al. (2016). The PLORAS database: a data repository for predicting language outcome and recovery after stroke. *Neuroimage*, **124**(Pt B), 1208–12.

Sickert A, Anders LC, Munte TF, Sailer M. (2014). Constraint-induced aphasia therapy following sub-acute stroke: a single-blind, randomised clinical trial of a modified therapy schedule. *J Neurol Neurosurg Psychiatry*, **85**(1), 51–5.

SIGN. (2010). 118 Management of patients with stroke: rehabilitation, prevention and management of complications, and discharge planning. A national clinical guideline. Edinburgh: Scottish Intercollegiate Guidelines Network. ISBN 978 1 905813 63 6. www.sign.ac.uk/assets/sign118.pdf

Stahl B, Mohr B, Büscher V, Dreyer FR, Lucchese G, Pulvermüller F. (2017) Efficacy of intensive aphasia therapy in patients with chronic stroke: a randomised controlled trial. *J Neurol Neurosurg Psychiatry*, **89**, 586–92.

Tate RL, Perdices M, McDonald S, Togher L, Rosenkoetter U. (2014). The design, conduct and report of single-case research: resources to improve the quality of the neurorehabilitation literature. *Neuropsychol Rehabil*, **24**, 315–31.

Tatemichi TK, Desmond DW, Stern Y, Paik M, Sano M, Bagiella E. (1994). Cognitive impairment after stroke – frequency, patterns, and relationship to functional abilities. *J Neurol Neurosurg Psychiatry*, **57**, 202–07.

Tunnard C, Wilson BA. (2014). Comparison of neuropsychological rehabilitation techniques for unilateral neglect: an ABACADAEAF single-case experimental design. *Neuropsychol Rehabil*, **24**, 382–99.

van der Meulen I, van de Sandt-Koenderman ME, Ribbers GM. (2012). Melodic Intonation Therapy: present controversies and future opportunities. *Arch Phys Med Rehabil*, **93**(1 Suppl), S46–52.

van der Meulen I, van de Sandt-Koenderman WM, Heijenbrok-Kal MH, Visch-Brink EG, Ribbers GM. (2014). The efficacy and timing of melodic intonation therapy in subacute aphasia. *Neurorehabil Neural Repair*, **28**(6),36–44.

Vataja R, Pohjasvaara T, Mäntylä R, Ylikoski R, Leppävuori A, Leskelä M, et al. (2003). MRI correlates of executive dysfunction in patients with ischaemic stroke. *Eur J Neurol*, 10, 625–31.

von Cramon DY, von Cramon GM, Mai N. (1991). Problem-solving deficits in brain-injured patients: a therapeutic approach. *Neuropsychol Rehabil*, **1**, 45–64.

Wallace SJ, Worrall L, Rose T, Le Dorze G, Breitenstein C, Hilari K, et al. (2019). A core outcome set for aphasia treatment research: the ROMA consensus statement. *Int J Stroke*, 14(2), 180–5. doi:1747493018806200.

Whitworth A, Webster J, Howard D. (2005). *A Cognitive Neuropsychological Approach to Assessment and Intervention in Aphasia: A Clinician's Guide*. Hove: Psychology Press.

Wilson BA. (2002). Towards a comprehensive model of cognitive rehabilitation. *Neuropsychol Rehabil*, **12**, 97–110.

Wilson BA, Alderman N, Burgess PW, Emslie H, Evans JJ. (1996). *The Behavioural Assessment of Dysexecutive Syndrome*. Flempton: Thames Valley Test Company.

Wilssens I, Vandenborre D, van Dun K, Verhoeven J, Visch-Brink E, Marien P. (2015). Constraint-induced aphasia therapy versus intensive semantic treatment in fluent aphasia. *Am J Speech Lang Pathol*, **24**(2), 281–94.

Westerberg H, Jacobaeus H, Hirvikoski T, Clevberger P, Ostensson ML, Bartfai A, et al. (2007). Computerized working memory training after stroke – a pilot study. *Brain Inj*, **21**(1), 21–9.

Chapter 25

Using Pharmacotherapy to Enhance Stroke Recovery

Larry B. Goldstein

Introduction

Preclinical studies show that a variety of systemically administered drugs can affect post-stroke functional recovery; however, data from prospective clinical trials are inconsistent. There are likely many reasons for these failures of translational medicine, yet there is reason to believe that the identification of effective pharmacological approaches for improving functional outcomes after stroke may be possible (Cramer, 2011). Novel strategies include stem cell transplantation, hormonal therapy, and the administration of exogenous growth factors; statins hold promise. This discussion focuses on the potential effects of medications acting on central neurotransmitters on the recovery process.

Preclinical Studies

Amphetamine is among the most extensively studied, systemically administered drugs with the potential to modulate the recovery process after stroke and traumatic brain injury. Experiments indicating that the administration of amphetamine beneficially affects functional outcome date to at least the 1940s (Maling and Acheson, 1946). Nearly 40 years later, the drug's therapeutic potential was highlighted by a series of experiments by Feeney and coworkers (Feeney et al., 1981, 1982). Their work showed that when combined with task-relevant training, a single dose of d-amphetamine given 24 hours following unilateral sensorimotor cortex ablation in the rat increased the rate of locomotor recovery, an observation confirmed in other laboratories (Dunbar et al., 1989; Goldstein and Davis, 1990b; Goldstein, 1995; Goldstein and Bullman, 1999). Additional studies found that post-injury administration of amphetamine not only accelerated the rate of recovery, but also could promote the recovery of otherwise permanent neurological deficits, extending the data from rodents to other species. For example, in cats, amphetamine given after unilateral or bilateral frontal motor cortex ablations leads to a restoration of both locomotor ability (Meyer et al., 1963; Hovda and Feeney, 1984; Sutton et al., 1989) and tactile placing (Feeney and Hovda, 1983). After occipital lobe injury, amphetamine combined with visual experience leads to the recovery of stereoscopic vision (Feeney and Hovda, 1985; Hovda et al., 1989) in addition to tactile placing (Hovda et al., 1987) and to the recovery of sensory function after ischaemic injury to the barrel cortex in rats (Hurwitz, et al., 1989, 1990; Dietrich et al., 1990). Improved recovery of motor function with amphetamine administration was also found after middle cerebral artery distribution infarction (Stroemer et al., 1994), traumatic brain injury (Prasad et al., 1995), and skilled reaching after both cortical ischaemia (Adkins & Jones, 2005) and ablation injury (Ramic et al., 2006). In a primate model, d-amphetamine combined with training led to a long-term improvement in motor task performance after cortical infarction in squirrel monkeys (Barbay et al., 2006). Although largely positive, there are reports of other studies that failed to find a benefit of amphetamine, possibly due to differences in experimental conditions (Schmanke et al., 1996; Dose et al., 1997; Brown et al., 2004; Alaverdashvili et al., 2007).

Amphetamine may affect the release and activity of several neurotransmitters including dopamine, serotonin, and norepinephrine (Fuxe and Ungerstedt, 1970), but several lines of evidence suggest its action on recovery is mediated through epinephrine. Intraventricular infusion of norepinephrine in rats facilitates motor recovery, mimicking the amphetamine effect (Boyeson and Feeney, 1990). Similar infusion of dopamine is ineffective if its conversion to norepinephrine is blocked by the administration of a dopamine-beta-hydroxylase inhibitor (Boyeson and Feeney, 1990). Selective depletion of central norepinephrine with (N-[(2-chloroethyl)]-N-ethyl-2-bromobenzylamine; DSP-4) impairs motor recovery after a later injury to the cerebral cortex (Goldstein et al., 1991; Boyeson et al., 1992a). Selective injury to the locus coeruleus, the primary source of central noradrenergic projection fibres, also has a detrimental effect on motor recovery after a subsequent injury to the rat sensorimotor cortex, although the effect varies among experiments (Weaver et al., 1988; Boyeson et al., 1992b; Boyeson et al., 1993; Goldstein, 1997). When performed at least 2 weeks before a unilateral sensorimotor cortex ablation, bilateral, contralateral, and ipsilateral locus coeruleus lesions block locomotor recovery (Goldstein, 1997).

Because each locus coeruleus has widespread projections, selective lesions of the ipsilateral and contralateral dorsal noradrenergic bundle were used to determine whether norepinephrine levels in the damaged or undamaged hemisphere correlated with recovery. Locomotor recovery was impaired by contralateral but not ipsilateral dorsal noradrenergic bundle lesions and the overall rate of recovery correlated with norepinephrine content in the contralateral, but not ipsilateral, cerebral hemisphere (Goldstein and Bullman, 1997). The observation is consistent with functional magnetic resonance imaging (MRI) studies in humans that find changes in the cerebral hemisphere contralateral to a stroke that correlate with motor recovery (Cramer et al., 1997; Bütefisch et al., 2005).

The neurobiological processes underlying amphetamine (i.e. norepinephrine) modulated recovery remain uncertain. One theme that arises from laboratory experiments is that the effect of d-amphetamine on recovery depends on concomitant training. In the original experiments by Feeney and colleagues (1982), the amphetamine effect was blocked if the rats were not allowed to walk rather than being trained in conjunction with drug administration. There was no drug effect if rats were handled rather than trained, suggesting that specific locomotor experience was required (Goldstein and Davis, 1990c). Motor recovery in cats was not enhanced with d-amphetamine administration in the absence of training, and there was no reinstatement of depth perception in cats after visual cortex ablation if they were kept in the dark after being given d-amphetamine (Hovda and Feeney, 1984; Feeney and Hovda, 1985).

d-Amphetamine given in addition to training leads to neuronal changes in both the ipsilateral and contralateral cerebral cortex (Stroemer et al., 1995). The combination of post-injury training and amphetamine administration is associated with an increase in projection fibres from the contralateral, non-

injured cerebral cortex to the pontine motor nuclei (Ramic et al., 2006). Therefore, amphetamine may induce long-term changes in neuronal structure that could, in part, underlie its impact on recovery.

d-Amphetamine's effect on locomotor recovery after sensorimotor cortex injury in the rat is dose dependent (Goldstein, 1990). There is increasing benefit as the dose is increased to 2.6 mg/kg base weight, but decreasing benefit as the dose is increased further. In cats, motor recovery after cortex injury is facilitated when a series of amphetamine/training sessions are carried out every 4 days for 2 weeks as compared with a single session (Hovda and Feeney, 1984). Amphetamine improves binocular depth perception in visually decorticated cats when given beginning 10 days after injury, but there is no benefit if treatment is delayed for 3 months (Feeney and Hovda, 1985).

Several principles arise from these experimental studies. Some systemically administered drugs such as d-amphetamine may modulate post-brain injury recovery. The effect depends on concomitant behavioural experience/training. Timing and dosing are critical. For d-amphetamine, at least part of the drug effect appears to be exerted in the cerebral hemisphere contralateral to the injury.

Preclinical Pharmacology

Table 25.1 summarizes the effects of selected drugs on recovery after focal brain injury (Goldstein, 1998).

Noradrenergic Agents

Given the hypothesis that d-amphetamine acts through norepinephrine, other centrally acting noradrenergic drugs would be anticipated to affect post-brain injury recovery. Motor recovery is accelerated by the norepinephrine precursor, L-threo-3,4-dihydroxyphenylserine (L-DOPS) (Kikuchi et al., 1999, 2000). Effects on recovery similar to amphetamine also occur after administration of phenylpropanolamine (Chen et al., 1986), phentermine (Hovda et al., 1983), and, depending on dosing regimen, methylphenidate (Kline et al., 1994). Further illustrating the complex interaction of dose and experience, the effect of methylphenidate depends on the number and timing of treatment sessions (Kline et al., 1994). Single doses of the α_2-adrenergic receptor antagonists idazoxan and yohimbine, which increase synaptic norepinephrine release, facilitate motor recovery when given to rats after unilateral sensorimotor cortex injury (Goldstein et al., 1989; Feeney and Westerberg, 1990; Sutton and Feeney, 1992).

Table 25.1 Selected laboratory and clinical studies of drug effects on recovery after focal brain injury

Transmitter or drug class/drug	Action	Recovery effect	
		Laboratory	Clinical
Norepinephrine bitartrate	...	+	...
Amphetamine sulfate	Sympathomimetic	+	+/Neutral
Phentermine	Sympathomimetic	+	...
Phenylpropanolamine	Sympathomimetic	+	...
Methylphenidate	Sympathomimetic	+	?
Yohimbine	α_2-AR antagonist	+	...
Idazoxan	α_2-AR antagonist	+	...
Clonidine	α_2-AR agonist	–	(–)
Haloperidol	α_1–AR antagonist	–	(–)
Prazosin	α_1-AR antagonist	–	(–)
Propranolol	β-AR antagonist	Neutral	...
GABA	...	–	...
Diazepam	GABA agonist	–	(–)
Muscimol	GABA agonist	–	...
Antiseizure medications			
Phenytoin	...	–	(–)
Phenobarbital	...	–	...
Dizoclipine maleate	...	–/Neutral	...
Carbamazepine	...	Neutral	...
Vigabatrin	...	Neutral	...
Antidepressants			
Trazodone	5-HT reuptake blocker	–	+
Fluoxetine	5-HT reuptake blocker	Neutral	+/Neutral
Desipramine	NE reuptake blocker	+	...
Amitriptyline	Mixed 5-HT and NE reuptake blocker	–/Neutral	...
Dopamine			
Haloperidol	Butyrophenone	–	(–)
Fluanisone	Butyrophenone	–	...
Droperidol	Butyrophenone	–	...
Spiroperidol	Antagonist	–	...
Apomorphine	Agonist	+	...

* The effects of selected drugs on recovery in laboratory animal models and in preliminary clinical studies in humans recovering from stroke. GABA indicates γ-aminobutyric acid; AR, adrenergic receptor; 5-HT, serotonin; NE, norepinephrine; +, a beneficial effect; ?, the drug has been insufficiently tested in humans to reach preliminary conclusions about its effect on recovery; –, a detrimental effect; symbols in parentheses, drugs that were included in the list of potentially harmful agents in 2 retrospective studies but have not been examined separately; and ellipses, lack of data.

Revised from Goldstein (1998).

Antihypertensives

Antihypertensives crossing the blood–brain barrier that act on noradrenergic receptors have the potential to affect post-brain injury recovery. The α_2-adrenergic receptor agonist clonidine (Goldstein and Davis, 1990a) and the α_1-adrenergic receptor antagonists phenoxybenzamine (Feeney and Westerberg, 1990) and prazosin (Feeney and Westerberg, 1990; Sutton and Feeney, 1992) interfere with locomotor recovery after cortex injury. Deficits also transiently re-emerge in animals that recovered motor function when given either clonidine or prazosin (Sutton and Feeney, 1992). In contrast to drugs active at α-adrenergic receptors, the β-adrenergic receptor antagonist propranolol has no effect on locomotor recovery (Feeney and Westerberg, 1990).

Major Tranquillizers and Related Drugs

Feeney and colleagues (1982) reported not only that *d*-amphetamine coupled with training facilitated locomotor recovery in rats, but also that even a single dose of haloperidol was harmful. Haloperidol administration also blocked *d*-amphetamine-facilitated recovery of stereoscopic vision in visually decorticated cats (Hovda et al., 1989). Butyrophenones such as fluanisone and droperidol reinstate neurological deficits in rats that recovered motor function after cortex injury (Van Hasselt, 1973). Although these observations raise the possibility that dopamine, in addition to norepinephrine, might modulate post-brain injury recovery, as noted above, intraventricular administration of norepinephrine improves recovery similar to *d*-amphetamine, but intraventicular dopamine is neutral (Boyeson and Feeney, 1990). Because haloperidol and other major tranquillizers also have effects at noradrenergic receptors (Peroutka et al., 1977; Cohen and Lipinski, 1986), it is hypothesized that their impact on recovery is noradrenergically mediated. The relative dose-dependent detrimental effects of haloperidol and clozapine on post-sensorimotor cortex injury in rats is correlated with their relative potencies at noradrenergic receptors (Goldstein and Bullman, 2002).

Antidepressants

Antidepressants affect the reuptake and metabolism of a variety of central neurotransmitters, including norepinephrine. Serotonin, a target of several antidepressants, modulates the release of norepinephrine through activation of 5-HT3 and possibly 5-HT1C receptors in rat hippocampal neurones (Blandina et al., 1991). In addition, various antidepressants, including fluoxetine, induce neurogenesis in the hippocampus, an effect thought to underlie their delayed impact on depression (Santarelli et al., 2003). The administration of a single dose of trazodone, however, transiently slows motor recovery in rats with cortical

injury and reinstates the hemiparesis in recovered animals (Boyeson and Harmon, 1993). In contrast, desimpramine facilitates, whereas fluoxetine and amitriptyline had no effect on, motor recovery in experimental animal studies (Boyeson and Harmon, 1993; Boyeson et al., 1994). Another study found the administration of fluoxetine after traumatic brain injury in rats had no impact on memory, balance, or gait (Wilson and Hamm, 2002), and chronic fluoxetine negatively affected memory and had no effect on electrophysiological measures after dentate gyrus injury in rats (Keith et al., 2007). Thus, preclinical data supporting a direct effect of antidepressants on post-stroke recovery are inconsistent.

Anxiolytics

Diazepam, an indirect γ-amino butyric acid (GABA) agonist, has a permanent and severe detrimental impact on recovery of sensory function when given after anteromedial neocortex damage in the rat, an action associated with neuroanatomical changes in the thalamus and substantia nigra (Schallert et al., 1986; Jones and Schallert, 1992). Co-administration of a benzodiazepine antagonist blocks this detrimental effect (Hernandez et al., 1989). Because anxiolytics that do not act through the GABA/benzodiazepine receptor are neutral with respect to recovery, the harmful actions of benzodiazepines seem to be due to a specific, receptor-mediation action (Schallert et al., 1992).

Anticonvulsants

The negative effects of diazepam and other benzodiazepines on post brain injury recovery raise concern for similar actions of other anticonvulsants. Phenobarbital delays recovery from somatosensory deficits after unilateral injury to the cerebral cortex in rats (Hernandez and Holling, 1994) and phenytoin administration worsens sensorimotor deficits after cortical injury (Brailowsky et al., 1986). In contrast, chronic administration of carbamazepine does not affect recovery (Schallert et al., 1992).

Possible Mechanisms of Neurotransmitter-modulated Recovery

Diaschisis, remote metabolic depression in brain structures anatomically and functionally linked, but not adjacent to the area of primary injury, can be demonstrated in both animal models (Jaspers et al.,

1990; Feeney, 1991; Theodore et al., 1992) and humans (Lenzi et al., 1982; Martin and Raichle, 1983; Fiorelli et al., 1991; Tanaka et al., 1992). Because *d*-amphetamine's effect on recovery is evident within hours in some animal models, it was hypothesized that drugs that prolong or worsen diaschisis would be detrimental, whereas those that reverse diaschisis would be beneficial (Feeney, 1991). Resolution of crossed cerebellar diaschisis in humans, however, is not associated with recovery after hemispheric stroke-related hemiparesis (Infeld et al., 1995).

Long-term potentiation (LTP) refers to changes in synaptic efficiency following specific types of neurotransmitter exposure and is considered a physiological mechanism for learning and memory (Bliss and Collingridge, 1993). Because the initial effects of *d*-amphetamine on post-brain injury recovery occur within hours, and because of the need for concomitant training, induction of LTP is an attractive potential mechanism underlying the effects of at least certain classes of drugs on recovery. LTP is mediated through the *N*-methyl-D-aspartate (NMDA) receptor complex and leads to activation of both pre- and postsynaptic mechanisms, resulting in a long-lasting effect on synaptic strength. In addition to the hippocampus, LTP (and its correlate, long-term depression) occurs in a variety of brain regions, including the motor (Iriki et al., 1989; Keller et al., 1990) and visual cortex (Artola and Singer, 1989; Aroniadou and Teyler, 1991). In addition to amphetamine (Dunwiddie et al., 1982; Delanoy et al., 1983; Gold et al., 1984), neurotransmitters including norepinephrine (Dunwiddie et al., 1982; Gold et al., 1984; Stanton and Sarvey, 1985; Burgard et al., 1989; Dahl and Sarvey, 1989; Bröcher et al., 1992), serotonin (Kulla and Manahan-Vaughan, 2002), dopamine (Manahan-Vaughan and Kulla, 2003), GABA (Wigstrom and Gustafsson, 1985; Satoh et al., 1986; Olpe and Karlsson, 1990), and acetylcholine (Ito et al., 1988; Williams and Johnston, 1988; Burgard and Sarvey, 1990; Bröcher et al., 1992) can affect the induction of LTP. Consistent with this possible mechanism, the impact on recovery of a variety of drugs acting on central neurotransmitters can be predicted based on their effect on LTP (Goldstein, 1998, 2000, 2006). The effects of norepinephrine on synaptic function and plasticity, however, are complex and can vary in different brain regions (Marzo et al., 2009).

Pharmacological Effects on Post-stroke Recovery in Humans

Disability and Dependence

There have been several clinical studies assessing the effects of amphetamine on post-stroke recovery in humans (Table 25.2). The studies were small and have important differences in methodologies. An initial 'proof-of-concept' study randomized eight subjects with stable post-stroke motor deficits to receive either 10 mg of *d*-amphetamine or placebo coupled with physical therapy within 10 days of ischaemic stroke (Crisostomo et al., 1988). As assessed 24 hours later, the *d*-amphetamine-treated group had a significant improvement in motor performance compared with the placebo-treated group. The study, however, involved only a small number of highly selected patients, and the clinical significance of the effect was uncertain.

A second double-blind, placebo-controlled trial included 5 *d*-amphetamine-treated and 5 placebo-treated patients with treatment given in conjunction with physical therapy once every 4 days for 10 sessions beginning 15 to 30 days after stroke (Walker-Batson et al., 2001). Amphetamine-treated patients had significantly greater improvements in motor scores compared with placebo-treated patients with a consolidation of the benefit after treatment was completed.

Other studies using different or similar trial designs have failed to confirm these observations. One randomized 24 subjects to receive 10 mg of amphetamine daily for 14 days, followed by 5 mg for 3 days or placebo (Reding et al., 1995). The subjects were enrolled more than 1 month after stroke and there was not a tight coupling between drug administration and physical therapy. Compared with the previous studies, there was a longer delay between stroke and treatment, and physical therapy was not temporally linked to drug exposure. Other negative studies evaluated *dl*- rather than *d*-amphetamine (Sonde et al., 2001), or used different dosing regimes or intervals between treatment sessions and treatment durations, or only included subjects with severe deficits (Martinsson et al., 2003). Two additional trials using a treatment and dosing regimen similar to the single positive study with longer-term follow-up also failed to find benefit (Treig et al., 2003; Gladstone et al., 2006).

Overall, the results of clinical trials evaluating the effect of *d*-amphetamine combined with physical

Table 25.2 Comparative clinical trials of the effects of amphetamine on post-stroke motor recovery

Study	N	Stroke-treatment interval	d-amphetamine dose / treatment frequency	Drug-therapy session interval (duration)	Outcome assessment
Crisostomo et al., 1988	8	<10 days	10 mg, one session	<3 hour (45 min)	1 day
Reding et al., 1995	21	>1 month	10 mg daily for 14 days, then 5 mg daily for 3 days	Same day (? Duration)	1 month
Walker-Batson et al., 1995	10	16–30 days	10 mg every 4 days for 10 sessions	"Peak of drug action" (? Duration)	1 week and 1 year
Sonde et al., 2001	39	5–10 days	10 mg twice weekly*	1 hour (30 min)	3 months
Martinsson et al., 2003	30	<96 hours	5 or 10 mg once or twice daily for 5 days	Same day (15 min vs 30–45 min)	3 months and 1 year
Treig et al., 2003	24	<6 weeks	10 mg every 4 days for 10 sessions	1 hour (45 min)	90 days and 1 year
Gladstone et al., 2006	71	5–10 days	10 mg twice weekly for 10 sessions	90 min (1 hour)	6 weeks and 3 months

* dl-amphetamine

** Duration of physiotherapy varied (both groups received d-amphetamine)

From Goldstein (2009).

therapy on post-stroke motor recovery have been disappointing and have not been consistent with the available extensive preclinical data. A meta-analysis including data from 3 small trials noted a trend towards more deaths at the end of follow-up among subjects randomized to amphetamine (Figure 25.1; OR 2.8, 95% confidence interval [CI]: 0.9–8.6), which may have been due to baseline imbalances between the groups (Martinsson et al., 2007). Including data from 9 trials ($n = 114$ amphetamine, $n = 112$ controls), the same meta-analysis found no overall effect on motor recovery (Figure 25.2) or activities of daily living (Figure 25.3; 4 trials, $n = 58$ amphetamine, $n = 55$ controls). As reflected above, it was concluded that 'too few patients have been studied to draw any definite conclusions about the effects of amphetamine treatment on recovery from stroke'.

Methylphenidate is used as a psychostimulant in apathetic patients to improve their participation in physiotherapy (Kaplitz, 1975; Johnson et al., 1992). The preclinical data reviewed above suggested benefit in improving post-brain injury motor recovery, but the dosing and treatment schedule is critical (Kline et al., 1994). Two clinical studies did not find any treatment-associated improvement in motor recovery with methylphenidate, although there were cardiovascular side effects (Larsson et al., 1988; Grade et al., 1998).

An uncontrolled study of L-DOPS combined with physiotherapy was conducted in a group of subjects with chronic, stroke-related motor deficits (Nishino et al., 2001). The subjects' average Fugl-Meyer motor score improved by 4.4 points ($p < 0.001$), and 10-minute walk time was shortened by 16% ($p < 0.001$) after 28 days of drug administration. Because the study was not controlled and physiotherapy alone can improve motor function even in the setting of established deficits (Wade et al., 1992; Green et al., 2002), the clinical significance of the observation is not certain.

Post-stroke depression is common, and antidepressants of various classes are used not only to treat the attendant psychiatric symptoms but also to improve the patient's participation in rehabilitative interventions (El Husseini et al., 2012). The effects of two norepinephrine reuptake blockers (i.e. nortriptyline [Lipsey et al., 1984], maprotiline [Dam et al., 1996]) on post-stroke disability were neutral when given chronically. Dosing, however, may be critical. Brain norepinephrine content is reduced after chronic, but not acute, administration of desipramine (Roffler-Tarlov et al., 1973). Trazadone is an antidepressant that blocks α_1-adrenergic receptors and interferes with motor recovery after cortex injury in rats (Boyeson and Harmon, 1993). A small clinical trial, however, found that chronic administration of

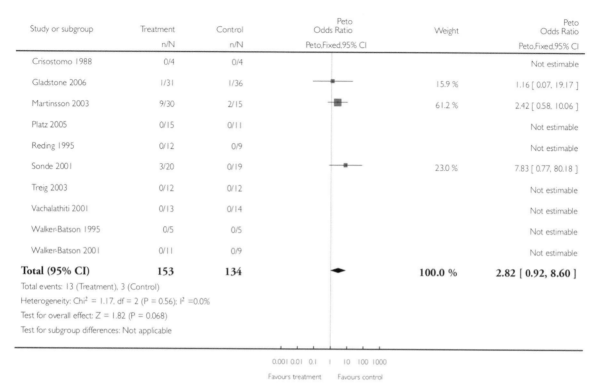

Figure 25.1 Meta-analysis of effects of *post-stroke treatment with amphetamines on mortality.*

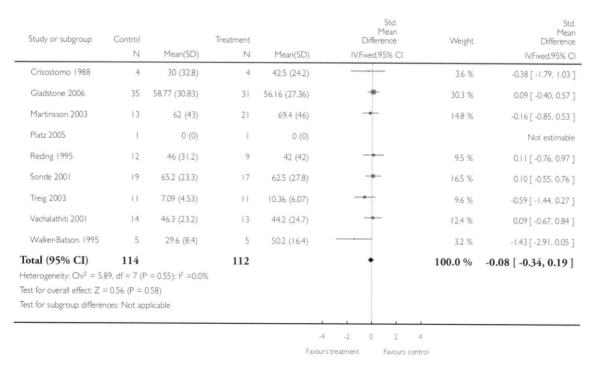

Figure 25.2 Meta-analysis of effects of *post-stroke treatment with amphetamines on motor recovery.*

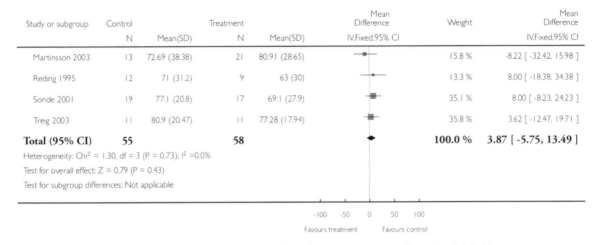

Figure 25.3 Meta-analysis of effects of *post-stroke treatment with amphetamines on recovery of activities of daily living.*

trazadone to depressed stroke patients receiving physical therapy led to improvements in their activities of daily living (Reding et al., 1986). The discrepancy could be due to different pharmacological effects of one-time versus chronic administration on norepinephrine levels, related to its action on serotonin levels, or to its antidepressant effects.

As noted above, there are scant preclinical data showing an effect of serotonergic drugs on post-brain injury recovery. Despite this, a small clinical study suggested that the selective serotonin reuptake inhibitor (SSRI) fluoxetine might facilitate post-stroke recovery (Dam et al., 1996). This was followed by the Fluoxetine for Motor Recovery after Acute Ischemic Stroke (FLAME) trial that randomly assigned 118 subjects with stroke-related moderate to severe hemiparesis to fluoxetine 20 mg daily or placebo for 3 months beginning 5 to 10 days after symptom onset (Chollet et al., 2011). Improvement at 90 days was greater in the fluoxetine (adjusted mean 34.0 points [95% CI: 29.7–38.4]) than in the placebo group (24.3 points [19.9–28.7]; p = 0.003). There was also benefit as assessed by the modified Rankin score (mRS) at 90 days with 26% of those treated with fluoxetine compared with 9% of those who received placebo being independent (mRS 0–2, p = 0.015). The effect was independent of depression. The trial, however, included only a small number of subjects; whether the benefit is sustained over time is not known.

A meta-analysis of the effects of SSRIs on post-stroke disability included data from 13 trials of

fluoxetine, 1 trial of sertraline, 3 trials of citalopram, and 5 trials of paroxetine (n = 1310) (Mead et al., 2013). Treatment with an SSRI was superior to controls (standard mean difference 0.92, 95% CI: 0.62–1.23; number needed to treat = 3) with no evidence of differences among the antidepressants (Figure 25.4). Many of the trials were small and there was significant heterogeneity among the studies. It was concluded that SSRIs might be associated with improved post-stroke recovery, but that much of the evidence is of poor quality, and larger, high-quality studies are needed.

The TALOS study (The Efficacy of Citalopram Treatment in Acute Stroke) was a Danish placebo-controlled, randomized, double-blind study in which 642 nondepressed patients with recent (<7 days) first-ever ischaemic stroke were randomized to either citalopram (n = 319) or placebo (n = 323) for 6 months as add-on to standard medical care. Improvement in functional recovery on the mRS from 1 to 6 months occurred in 160 (50%) patients on citalopram and 136 (42%) on placebo (odds ratio, 1.27; 95% CI: 0.92–1.74; p = 0.057). When dropouts before 31 days were excluded (n = 90), the analysis population showed an odds ratio of 1.37 (95% CI: 0.97–1.91; p = 0.07). It was concluded that early citalopram treatment did not improve functional recovery in nondepressed ischaemic stroke patients within the first 6 months, although a borderline, statistically significant effect was observed in the analysis population. The risk of cardiovascular events was similar between treatment groups, and citalopram treatment was well tolerated (Kraglund et al., 2018).

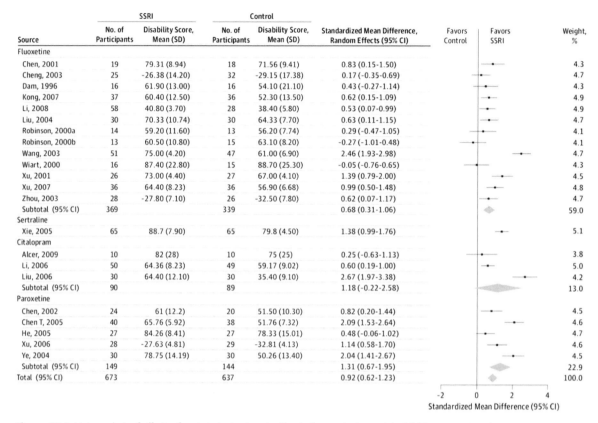

	SSRI		Control					
Source	No. of Participants	Disability Score, Mean (SD)	No. of Participants	Disability Score, Mean (SD)	Standardized Mean Difference, Random Effects (95% CI)	Favors Control	Favors SSRI	Weight, %
Fluoxetine								
Chen, 2001	19	79.31 (8.94)	18	71.56 (9.41)	0.83 (0.15-1.50)			4.3
Cheng, 2003	25	-26.38 (14.20)	32	-29.15 (17.38)	0.17 (-0.35-0.69)			4.7
Dam, 1996	16	61.90 (13.00)	16	54.10 (21.10)	0.43 (-0.27-1.14)			4.3
Kong, 2007	37	60.40 (12.50)	36	52.30 (13.50)	0.62 (0.15-1.09)			4.9
Li, 2008	58	40.80 (3.70)	28	38.40 (5.80)	0.53 (0.07-0.99)			4.9
Liu, 2004	30	70.33 (10.74)	30	64.33 (7.70)	0.63 (0.11-1.15)			4.7
Robinson, 2000a	14	59.20 (11.60)	13	56.20 (7.74)	0.29 (-0.47-1.05)			4.1
Robinson, 2000b	13	60.50 (10.80)	15	63.10 (8.20)	-0.27 (-1.01-0.48)			4.1
Wang, 2003	51	75.00 (4.20)	47	61.00 (6.90)	2.46 (1.93-2.98)			4.7
Wiart, 2000	16	87.40 (22.80)	15	88.70 (25.30)	-0.05 (-0.76-0.65)			4.3
Xu, 2001	26	73.00 (4.40)	27	67.00 (4.10)	1.39 (0.79-2.00)			4.5
Xu, 2007	36	64.40 (8.23)	36	56.90 (6.68)	0.99 (0.50-1.48)			4.8
Zhou, 2003	28	-27.80 (7.10)	26	-32.50 (7.80)	0.62 (0.07-1.17)			4.7
Subtotal (95% CI)	369		339		0.68 (0.31-1.06)			59.0
Sertraline								
Xie, 2005	65	88.7 (7.90)	65	79.8 (4.50)	1.38 (0.99-1.76)			5.1
Citalopram								
Alcer, 2009	10	82 (28)	10	75 (25)	0.25 (-0.63-1.13)			3.8
Li, 2006	50	64.36 (8.23)	49	59.17 (9.02)	0.60 (0.19-1.00)			5.0
Liu, 2006	30	64.40 (12.10)	30	35.40 (9.10)	2.67 (1.97-3.38)			4.2
Subtotal (95% CI)	90		89		1.18 (-0.22-2.58)			13.0
Paroxetine								
Chen, 2002	24	61 (12.2)	20	51.50 (10.30)	0.82 (0.20-1.44)			4.5
Chen T, 2005	40	65.76 (5.92)	38	51.76 (7.32)	2.09 (1.53-2.64)			4.6
He, 2005	27	84.26 (8.41)	27	78.33 (15.01)	0.48 (-0.06-1.02)			4.7
Xu, 2006	28	-27.63 (4.81)	29	-32.81 (4.13)	1.14 (0.58-1.70)			4.6
Ye, 2004	30	78.75 (14.19)	30	50.26 (13.40)	2.04 (1.41-2.67)			4.5
Subtotal (95% CI)	149		144		1.31 (0.67-1.95)			22.9
Total (95% CI)	673		637		0.92 (0.62-1.23)			100.0

Standardized Mean Difference (95% CI)

Figure 25.4 Meta-analysis of effects of *post-stroke treatment with selective serotonin reuptake inhibitors on post-stroke recovery.*

The UK-based Fluoxetine Or Control Under Supervision (FOCUS) trial randomized 3127 patients with a clinical diagnosis of recent (2–15 days previously) stroke to fluoxetine 20 mg once daily (*n* = 1564) or matching placebo (*n* = 1563) for 6 months. For the primary outcome measure, the mRs at 6 months, which was available in 1553 (99.3%) patients in each treatment group, random allocation to fluoxetine did not alter the distribution across mRs categories at 6 months compared with placebo (common OR, adjusted for minimization variables, 0.951; 95% CI: 0.839–1.079; *p* = 0.439).

Among secondary outcomes, allocation to fluoxetine did reduce the frequency of new depression by 6 months compared with placebo (13.0% fluoxetine vs 16.9% placebo, absolute difference 3.78%, 95% CI of difference: 1.26–6.30%; *p* = 0.0033),

However, allocation to fluoxetine also increased the frequency of bone fractures (2.9% fluoxetine vs 1.5% placebo, absolute difference 1.41%, 95% CI of diff: 0.38–2.43; *p* = 0.0070).

There were no significant differences in other events or outcomes at 6 or 12 months.

These results suggest that fluoxetine 20 mg given daily for 6 months after acute stroke does not improve functional outcome, but it likely reduces the occurrence of depression (although a secondary outcome, this is a well-recognized effect of fluoxetine), and also likely increases bone fractures (noted in some observational studies, but again, a secondary outcome) (FOCUS Trial Collaboration, 2019).

Recovery from Aphasia

Clinical studies have also evaluated pharmacological approaches for reducing stroke-related language impairments (Albert et al., 1988; Bachman and Morgan, 1988). A double-blind study randomized 21 subjects who had post-stroke aphasia to 10 mg *d*-amphetamine or placebo between 16 and 45 days after stroke using a treatment schedule similar to the trial that was found beneficial for motor recovery (Walker-Batson et al., 2001). Improvement, assessed with the Porch Index of Communicative Ability, was greater 1 week after treatment was completed in those who received *d*-amphetamine (*p* = 0.015). The difference between the groups, however, was no longer significant after 6 months. Two randomized trials found no benefit of bromocriptine on any measure of aphasia (Gupta et al., 1995; Sabe et al., 1995). Although there is a variety of potential explanations for this negative finding, the results are not surprising because preclinical studies suggested that recovery is mediated through noradrenergic rather than dopaminergic mechanisms.

Piracetam is a derivative of GABA that has no effect on the synthesis, release, or uptake of GABA and has no effect on GABA post-synaptic binding, but does have effects on the cholinergic system and increases synaptic norepinephrine release (Masotto et al., 1985). It also has diverse effects on blood flow and platelet reactivity, but its specific mechanism of action is unknown, and there are virtually no preclinical studies assessing its potential impact on post-stroke recovery. Despite this, several trials have been conducted assessing its impact on recovery after stroke in humans. A small trial found a transient improvement in aphasia in subjects randomized to receive piracetam (Enderby et al., 1994), with a second small study finding benefits in some language subtests at the end of 6 weeks of treatment (Kessler et al., 2000). A third found only trends toward benefit (Huber et al., 1997). It remains unclear whether piracetam treatment results in a clinically meaningful, long-term benefit.

Impaired Recovery

Several of the centrally acting drugs with the capacity to negatively affect post-stroke recovery are commonly given to patients who had an ischaemic stroke to treat comorbid and concomitant medical problems (Goldstein and Davis, 1988). These include various antihypertensives, anti-epileptics, anxiolytics, and major tranquillizers. Whether these drugs have a detrimental effect on recovery in humans can only be assessed in retrospective studies, which have several inherent limitations, including unmeasured confounding. With this caveat, a retrospective cohort study (*n* = 58) found that the motor recoveries of stroke patients who received one or a combination of the antihypertensives clonidine or prazosin, major tranquillizers, benzodiazepines, or the anticonvulsant phenytoin had poorer recoveries

than those who did not receive one of these drugs, even after adjustment for other factors, including initial stroke severity (Goldstein et al., 1990). Similar results were found in a retrospective analysis of data from a prospective clinical trial focused on post-stroke recovery in which nearly 40% of 96 control subjects received one or a combination of potentially harmful drugs (72% in the 'detrimental' group received a benzodiazepine, 22% a major tranquillizer or related drug, 14% an α_2-adrenergic receptor agonist, 8% an α_1-adrenergic receptor antagonist, and 6% phenobarbital or phenytoin) (Goldstein et al., 1995). There were significant differences in recovery based on the drugs the subjects had received, with recovery being impaired in those who had been given a 'detrimental' drug. The finding was replicated in an analysis of a third independent cohort (Troisi et al., 2002). This study included 154 patients admitted to a rehabilitation hospital within 2 months of stroke. In this group, 19% received a benzodiazepine, 13% a major tranquillizer or related drug, 3% an α_2-adrenergic receptor agonist, 8% phenobarbital, and 3% phenytoin. After multivariable adjustment, those who received a potentially detrimental drug were found to have significantly poorer recoveries.

Summary

Extensive laboratory studies provide evidence for the rationale of pharmacological approaches for improving post-stroke functional recovery. Although a proven pharmacological approach resulting in a clinically meaningful improvement in post-stroke recovery remains elusive, it is reasonable to avoid medications that may have harmful effects in patients who have had a stroke.

References

Adkins DL, Jones TA. (2005). D-amphetamine enhances skilled reaching after ischemic cortical lesions in rats. *Neurosci Lett*, **380**, 214–18.

Alaverdashvili M, Lim DH, Whishaw IQ. (2007). No improvement by amphetamine on learned non-use, attempts, success or movement in skilled reaching by the rat after motor cortex stroke. *Eur J Neurosci*, **25**, 3442–52.

Albert ML, Bachman DL, Morgan A, Helm-Estabrooks N. (1988). Pharmacotherapy for aphasia. *Neurology*, **38**, 877–9.

Aroniadou VA, Teyler TJ. (1991). The role of NMDA receptors in long-term potentiation (LTP) and depression (LTD) in rat visual cortex. *Brain Res*, **562**, 136–43.

Artola A, Singer W. (1989). NMDA receptors and developmental plasticity in visual neocortex. In GL Collingridge JC Watkins, eds., *The NMDA Receptor.* Oxford: Oxford University Press, pp. 153–66.

Bachman DL, Morgan A. (1988). The role of pharmacotherapy in the treatment of aphasia. *Aphasiology*, **3–4**, 225–8.

Barbay S, Zoubina EV, Dancause N, Frost SB, Eisner-Janowicz I, Stowe AM, et al. (2006). A single injection of D-amphetamine facilitates improvements in motor training following a focal cortical infarct in squirrel monkeys. *Neurorehabil Neural Repair*, **20**, 455–8.

Blandina P, Goldfarb J, Walcott J, Green JP. (1991). Serotonergic modulation of the release of endogenous norepinephrine from rat hypothalamic slices. *J Pharmacol Exp Ther*, **256**, 341–7.

Bliss TV, Collingridge GL. (1993). A synaptic model of memory: long-term potentiation in the hippocampus. *Nature*, **361**, 31–9.

Boyeson MG, Callister TR, Cavazos JE. (1992a). Biochemical and behavioral effects of a sensorimotor cortex injury in rats pretreated with the noradrenergic neurotoxin DSP-4. *BehavNeurosci*, **106**, 964–73.

Boyeson MG, Feeney DM. (1990). Intraventricular norepinephrine facilitates motor recovery following sensorimotor cortex injury. *Pharmacol BiochemBehav*, **35**, 497–501.

Boyeson MG, Harmon RL. (1993). Effects of trazodone and desipramine on motor recovery in brain-injured rats. *Am J Phys Med Rehabil*, **72**, 286–93.

Boyeson MG, Harmon RL, Jones JL. (1994). Comparative effects of fluoxetine, amitriptyline and serotonin on functional motor recovery after sensorimotor cortex injury. *Am J Phys Med Rehabil*, **73**, 76–83.

Boyeson MG, Krobert KA, Grade CM, Scherer PJ. (1992b). Unilateral, but not bilateral, locus coeruleus lesions facilitate recovery from sensorimotor cortex injury. *Pharmacol Biochem Behav*, **43**, 771–7.

Boyeson MG, Scherer PJ, Grade CM, Krobert KA. (1993). Unilateral locus coeruleus lesions facilitate motor recovery from cortical injury through supersensitivity mechanisms. *Pharmacol Biochem Behav*, **44**, 297–305.

Brailowsky S, Knight RT, Efron R. (1986). Phenytoin increases the severity of cortical hemiplegia in rats. *Brain Res*, **376**, 71–7.

Bröcher S, Artola A, Singer W. (1992). Agonists of cholinergic and noradrenergic receptors facilitate synergistically the induction of long-term potentiation in slices of rat visual cortex. *Brain Res*, **573**, 27–36.

Brown AW, Bjelke B, Fuxe K. (2004). Motor response to amphetamine treatment, task-specific training, and limited motor experience in a postacute animal stroke model. *Exp Neurol*, **190**, 102–08.

Burgard EC, Decker G, Sarvey JM. (1989). NMDA receptor antagonists block norepinephrine-induced long-lasting potentiation and long-term potentiation in rat dentate gyrus. *Brain Res*, **482**, 351–5.

Burgard EC, Sarvey JM. (1990). Muscarinic receptor activation facilitates the induction of long-term potentiation (LTP) in the rat dentate gyrus. *Neurosci Lett*, **116**, 34–39.

Bütefisch CM, Kleiser R, Körber B, Müller K, Wittsack HJ, Hömberg V, et al. (2005). Recruitment of contralesional motor cortex in stroke patients with recovery of hand function. *Neurology*, **64**, 1067–9.

Chen MJ, Sutton RL, Feeney DM. (1986). Recovery of function after brain injury in rat and cat: beneficial effects of phenylpropanolamine. *Abstracts Soc Neurosci*, **12**, 881.

Chollet F, Tardy J, Albucher, JF, Thalamas C, Berard E, Lamy C, et al. (2011). Fluoxetine for motor recovery after acute ischaemic stroke (FLAME): a randomised placebo-controlled trial. *Lancet Neurol*, **10**, 123–30.

Cohen BM, Lipinski JF. (1986). In vivo potencies of antipsychotic drugs in blocking alpha 1 noradrenergic and dopamine D2 receptors: implications for drug mechanisms of action. *Life Sci*, **39**, 2571–80.

Cramer SC. (2011). An overview of therapies to promote repair of the brain after stroke. *Head Neck*, **33**, (Suppl 1), S5–7.

Cramer SC, Nelles G, Benson RR, Kaplan JD, Parker RA, Kwong KK, et al. (1997). A functional MRI study of subjects recovered from hemiparetic stroke. *Stroke*, **28**, 2518–27.

Crisostomo EA, Duncan PW, Propst MA, Dawson DB, Davis JN. (1988). Evidence that amphetamine with physical therapy promotes recovery of motor function in stroke patients. *Ann Neurol*, **23**, 94–7.

Dahl D, Sarvey JM. (1989). Norepinephrine induces pathway-specific long-lasting potentiation and depression in the hippocampal dentate gyrus. *Proc Natl Acad Sci USA*, **86**, 4776–80.

Dam M, Tonin P, De Boni A, Pizzolato G, Casson S, Ermani M, et al. (1996). Effects of fluoxetine and maprotiline on functional recovery in poststroke hemiplegic patients undergoing rehabilitation therapy. *Stroke*, **27**, 1211–14.

Delanoy RL, Tucci DL, Gold PE. (1983). Amphetamine effects on long term potentiation in dentate granule cells. *Pharmacol Biochem Behav*, **18**, 137–9.

Dietrich WD, Alonso O, Busto R, Ginsberg MD. (1990). Influence of amphetamine treatment on somatosensory function of the normal and infarcted rat brain. *Stroke*, **21** (Suppl. III), III-147-III-150.

Dose JM, Dhillon HS, Maki A, Kraemer PJ, Prasad RM. (1997). Lack of delayed effects of amphetamine, methoxamine, and prazosin (adrenergic drugs) on

527

behavioral outcome after lateral fluid percussion brain injury in the rat. *J Neurotrauma*, 14, 327–37.

Dunbar GL, Smith GA, Look SK, Whalen RJ. (1989). d-Amphetamine attenuates learning and motor deficits following cortical injury in rats. *Abstracts Soc Neurosci*, 15, 132.

Dunwiddie TV, Roberson NL, Worth T. (1982). Modulation of long-term potentiation: effects of adrenergic and neuroleptic drugs. *Pharmacol Biochem Behav*, 17, 1257–64.

El Husseini N, Goldstein LB, Peterson ED, Zhao X, Pan W, Olson D.M, et al. (2012). Depression and antidepressant use after stroke and transient ischemic attack. *Stroke*, 43, 1609–16.

Enderby P, Broeckx J, Hospers W, Schildermans F, Deberdt W. (1994). Effect of piracetam on recovery and rehabilitation after stroke: a double-blind, placebo-controlled study. *Clin Neuropharmacol*, 17, 320–31.

Feeney DM. (1991). Pharmacologic modulation of recovery after brain injury: a reconsideration of diaschisis. *J Neurol Rehabil*, 5, 113–28.

Feeney DM, Gonzalez A, Law WA. (1981). Amphetamine restores locomotor function after motor cortex injury in the rat. *Proc West Pharmacol Soc*, 24, 15–17.

Feeney DM, Gonzalez A, Law WA. (1982). Amphetamine, haloperidol, and experience interact to affect the rate of recovery after motor cortex injury. *Science*, 217, 855–7.

Feeney DM, Hovda DA. (1983). Amphetamine and apomorphine restore tactile placing after motor cortex injury in the cat. *Psychopharmacology*, 79, 67–71.

Feeney DM, Hovda DA. (1985). Reinstatement of binocular depth perception by amphetamine and visual experience after visual cortex ablation. *Brain Res*, 342, 352–6.

Feeney DM, Westerberg VS. (1990). Norepinephrine and brain damage: alpha noradrenergic pharmacology alters functional recovery after cortical trauma. *Can J Psychol*, 44, 233–52.

Fiorelli M, Blin J, Bakchine S, Laplane D, Baron JC. (1991). PET studies of cortical diaschisis in patients with motor hemi-neglect. *J Neurol Sci*, 104, 135–42.

FOCUS Trial Collaboration. (2019). Effects of fluoxetine on functional outcomes after acute stroke (FOCU): a pragmatic, double-blind, randomized, controlled trial. *Lancet*, 393, 265–74.

Fuxe K, Ungerstedt U. (1970). Histochemical, biochemical and functional studies on central monoamine neurons after acute and chronic amphetamine administration. In E Costa, S Garattini, eds., *Amphetamines and Related Compounds*. New York: Raven Press, pp. 257–288.

Gladstone DJ, Danells CJ, Armesto A, McIlroy WE, Staines WR, Graham SJ, et al. (2006). Physiotherapy coupled with dextroamphetamine for motor rehabilitation after hemiparetic stroke: a randomized, double-blind, placbo-controlled trial. *Stroke*, 37, 179–85.

Gold PE, Delanoy RL, Merrin J. (1984). Modulation of long-term potentiation by peripherally administered amphetamine and epinephrine. *Brain Res*, 305, 103–07.

Goldstein LB. (1990). Pharmacology of recovery after stroke. *Stroke*, 21 (Suppl. III), III-139–III-142.

Goldstein LB. (1995). Right vs. left sensorimotor cortex suction-ablation in the rat: no difference in beam-walking recovery. *Brain Res*, 674, 167–70.

Goldstein LB. (1997). Effects of bilateral and unilateral locus coeruleus lesions on beam-walking recovery after subsequent unilateral sensorimotor cortex suction-ablation in the rat. *Restor Neurol Neurosci*, 11, 55–63.

Goldstein LB. (1998). Potential effects of common drugs on stroke recovery. *Arch Neurol*, 55, 454–6.

Goldstein LB. (2000). Effects of amphetamines and small related molecules on recovery after stroke in animals and man. *Neuropharmacology*, 39, 852–9.

Goldstein LB. (2006). Neurotransmitters and motor activity: effects on functional recovery after brain injury. *NeuroRx*, 3, 451–7.

Goldstein LB. (2009). Amphetamine trials and tribulations. *Stroke*, 40 (Suppl. 1), S133–S135.

Goldstein LB, Bullman S. (1997). Effects of dorsal noradrenergic bundle lesions on recovery after sensorimotor cortex injury. *Pharmacol Biochem Behav*, 58, 1151–7.

Goldstein LB, Bullman S. (1999). Age but not sex affects motor recovery after unilateral sensorimotor cortex suction-ablation in the rat. *Restor Neurol Neurosci*, 15, 39–43.

Goldstein LB, Bullman S. (2002). Differential effects of haloperidol and clozapine on motor recovery after sensorimotor cortex injury in the rat. *Neurorehabil Neural Repair*, 16, 321–5.

Goldstein LB, Coviello A, Miller GD, Davis, JN. (1991). Norepinephrine depletion impairs motor recovery following sensorimotor cortex injury in the rat. *Restor Neurol Neurosci*, 3, 41–7.

Goldstein LB, Davis JN. (1988). Physician prescribing patterns following hospital admission for ischemic cerebrovascular disease. *Neurology*, 38, 1806–09.

Goldstein LB, Davis JN. (1990a). Clonidine impairs recovery of beam-walking in rats. *Brain Res*, 508, 305–09.

Goldstein LB, Davis JN. (1990b). Influence of lesion size and location on amphetamine-facilitated recovery of beam-walking in rats. *Behav Neurosci*, 104, 318–25.

Goldstein LB, Davis J.N. (1990c). Post-lesion practice and amphetamine-facilitated recovery of beam-walking in the rat. *Restor Neurol Neurosci*, 1, 311–14.

Goldstein LB, Hasselblad V, McCrory DC, Matchar DB. (1995). Meta-analysis and comparison of randomized trials of endarterectomy for symptomatic carotid stenosis. *Neurology*, **45** (Suppl 4), A375.

Goldstein LB, Matchar DB, Morgenlander JC, Davis JN. (1990). Influence of drugs on the recovery of sensorimotor function after stroke. *J NeuroloRehabi*, **4**, 137–44.

Goldstein LB, Poe HV, Davis JN. (1989). An animal model of recovery of function after stroke: Facilitation of recovery by an a2-adrenergic receptor antagonist. *Ann Neurol*, **26**, 157.

Grade C, Redford B, Chrostowski J, Toussaint L, Blackwell B. (1998). Methylphenidate in early poststroke recovery: a double-blind, placebo-controlled study. *Arch Phys Med Rehabil*, **79**, 1047–50.

Green J, Forster A, Bogle S, Young J. (2002). Physiotherapy for patients with mobility problems more than 1 year after stroke: a randomised controlled trial. *Lancet*, **359**, 199–203.

Gupta SR, Mlcoch AG, Scolaro C, Moritz T. (1995). Bromocriptine treatment of nonfluent aphasia. *Neurology*, **45**, 2170–3.

Hernandez TD, Holling LC. (1994). Disruption of behavioral recovery by the anti-convulsant phenobarbital. *Brain Res*, **635**, 300–06.

Hernandez TD, Jones GH, Schallert T. (1989). Co-administration of Ro 15–1788 prevents diazepam-induced retardation of recovery of function. *Brain Res*, **487**, 89–95.

Hovda DA, Bailey B, Montoya S, Salo AA, Feeney DM. (1983). Phentermine accelerates recovery of function after motor cortex injury in rats and cats. *FASEB J*, **42**, 1157.

Hovda DA, Feeney DM. (1984). Amphetamine with experience promotes recovery of locomotor function after unilateral frontal cortex injury in the cat. *Brain Res*, **298**, 358–61.

Hovda DA, Sutton RL, Feeney DM. (1987). Recovery of tactile placing after visual cortex ablation in cat: a behavioral and metabolic study of diaschisis. *Exp Neurol*, **97**, 391–402.

Hovda DA, Sutton RL, Feeney DM. (1989). Amphetamine-induced recovery of visual cliff performance after bilateral visual cortex ablation in cats: measurements of depth perception thresholds. *Behav Neurosci*, **103**, 574–84.

Huber W, Willmes K, Poeck K, Van Vleymen B, Deberdt W. (1997). Piracetam as an adjuvant to language therapy for aphasia: a randomized double-blind placebo-controlled pilot study. *Arch Phys Med Rehabil*, **78**, 245–50.

Hurwitz BE, Dietrich WD, McCabe PM, Watson BD, Ginsberg MD, Schneiderman N. (1989). Amphetamine-accelerated recovery from cortical barrel-field infarction: pharmacological treatment of stroke. In MD. Ginsberg, WD Dietrich, eds., *Cerebrovascular Diseases. The Sixteenth Research (Princeton) Conference*. New York: Raven Press, pp. 309–318.

Infeld B, Davis SM, Lichtenstein M, Mitchell PJ, Hopper JL. (1995). Crossed cerebellar diaschisis and brain recovery after stroke. *Stroke*, **26**, 90–5.

Iriki A, Pavlides C, Keller A, Asanuma H. (1989). Long-term potentiation in the motor cortex. *Science*, **245**, 1385–7.

Ito T, Miura Y, Kadokawa T. (1988). Effects of physostigmine and scopolamine on long-term potentiation of hippocampal population spikes in rats. *Can J Physiol Pharmacol*, **66**, 1010–16.

Jaspers RMA, Van Der Sprenkel JWB, Tulleken CAF, Cools AR. (1990). Local as well as remote functional and metabolic changes after focal ischemia in cats. *Brain Res Bull*, **24**, 23–32.

Johnson ML, Roberts MD, Ross AR, Witten CM. (1992). Methylphenidate in stroke patients with depression. *Am J Phys Med Rehabil*, **71**, 239–41.

Jones TA, Schallert T. (1992). Subcortical deterioration after cortical damage: effects of diazepam and relation to recovery of function. *Behav Brain Res*, **51**, 1–13.

Kaplitz SE. (1975). Withdrawn, apathetic geriatric patients responsive to methylphenidate. *J Am Geriatr Soc*, **23**, 271–6.

Keith JR, Wu Y, Epp JR, Sutherland RJ. (2007). Fluoxetine and the dentate gyrus: memory, recovery of function, and electrophysiology. *Behav Pharmacol*, **18**, 521–31.

Keller A, Iriki A, Asanuma H. (1990). Identification of neurons producing long-term potentiation in the cat motor cortex: intracellular recordings and labeling. *J Comp Neurol*, **300**, 47–60.

Kessler J, Thiel A, Karbe H, Heiss WD. (2000). Piracetam improves activated blood flow and facilitates rehabilitation of poststroke aphasic patients. *Stroke*, **31**, 2112–16.

Kikuchi K, Nishino K, Ohyu H. (1999). L-DOPS-Accelerated recovery of locomotor function in rats subjected to sensorimotor cortex ablation injury: pharmacobehavioral studies. *Tohoku J Exp Med*, **188**, 203–15.

Kikuchi K, Nishino K, Ohyu H. (2000). Increasing CNS norepinephrine levels by the precursor L-DOPS facilitates beam-walking recovery after sensorimotor cortex ablation in rats. *Brain Res*, **860**, 130–5.

Kline AE, Chen MJ, Tso-Olivas DY, Feeney DM. (1994). Methylphenidate treatment following ablation-induced hemiplegia in rat: experience during drug action alters effects on recovery of function. *Pharmacol Biochem Behav*, **48**, 773–9.

Kraglund KL, Mortensen JK, Damsbo AG, Modrau B, Simonsen SA, Iversen HK, et al. (2018). Neuroregeneration and Vascular Protection by Citalopram in Acute Ischemic Stroke (TALOS). *Stroke*, **49**(11), 2568–76. doi:10.1161/STROKEAHA.

Kulla A, Manahan-Vaughan D. (2002). Modulation by serotonin 5-HT(4) receptors of long-term potentiation and depotentiation in the dentate gyrus of freely moving rats. *Cereb Cortex*, **12**, 150–62.

Larsson M, Ervik M, Lundborg P, Sundh V, Svanborg A. (1988). Comparison between methylphenidate and placebo as adjuvant in care and rehabilitation of geriatric patients. *Comp Gerontol*, **2**, 53–9.

Lenzi GL, Frackowiak RSJ, Jones T. (1982). Cerebral oxygen metabolism and blood flow in human cerebral infarction. *J Cereb Blood Flow Metab*, **2**, 321–35.

Lipsey JR, Pearlson GD, Robinson RG, Rao K, Price TR. (1984). Nortriptyline treatment of post-stroke depression: a double-blind study. *Lancet*, **1**, 297–300.

Maling HM, Acheson GH. (1946). Righting and other postural activity in low-decerebrate and in spinal cats after d-amphetamine. *J Neurophysiol*, **9**, 379–86.

Manahan-Vaughan D, Kulla A. (2003). Regulation of depotentiation and long-term potentiation in the dentate gyrus of freely moving rats by dopamine D2-like receptors. *Cereb Cortex*, **13**, 123–35.

Martin WRW, Raichle ME. (1983). Cerebellar blood flow and metabolism in cerebral hemisphere infarction. *Ann Neurol*, **14**, 168–76.

Martinsson L, Eksborg S, Wahlgren NG. (2003). Intensive early physiotherapy combined with dexamphetamine treatment in severe stroke: a randomized, controlled pilot study. *Cerebrovasc Dis*, **16**, 338–45.

Martinsson L, Hardemark H, Eksborg S. (2007). Amphetamines for improving recovery after stroke. *Cochrane Database Syst Rev*, 1. CD002090.

Marzo A, Bai J, Otani S. (2009). Neuroplasticity regulation by noradrenaline in mammalian brain. *Curr Neuropharmacol*, **7**, 286–95.

Masotto, C., Apud, J. A., & Racagni, G. (1985). Neurochemical studies on GABAergic and aminergic systems in the rat brain following acute and chronic piracetam administration. *Pharmacol Res Commun*, **17**, 749–72.

Mead GE, Hsieh CF, Hackett M. (2013). Selective serotonin reuptake inhibitors for stroke recovery. *JAMA*, **310**, 1066–7.

Meyer PM, Horel JA, Meyer DR. (1963). Effects of dl-amphetamine upon placing responses in neodecorticate cats. *J Comp PhysiolPsychol*, **56**, 402–04.

Nishino K, Sasaki T, Takahashi K, Chiba M, Ito T. (2001). The norepinephrine precursor L-threo-3, 4-dihydroxyphenylserine facilitates motor recovery in chronic stroke patients. *J Clin Neurosci*, **8**, 547–50.

Olpe HR, Karlsson G. (1990). The effects of baclofen and two GABA B-receptor antagonists on long-term potentiation. *Naunyn Schmiedeberg Arch Pharmacol*, **342**, 194–7.

Peroutka SJ, U'Pritchard DC, Greenberg DA, Snyder SH. (1977). Neuroleptic drug interactions with norepinephrine alpha receptor binding sites in rat brain. *Neuropharmacology*, **16**, 549–56.

Prasad RM, Dose JM, Dhillon HS, Carbary T, Kraemer PJ. (1995). Amphetamine affects the behavioral outcome of lateral fluid percussion brain injury in the rat. *Restor Neurol Neurosci*, **9**, 65–75.

Ramic M, Emerick AJ, Bollnow MR, O'Brien TE, Tsai SY, Kartje GL. (2006). Axonal plasticity is associated with motor recovery following amphetamine treatment combined with rehabilitation after brain injury in the adult rat. *Brain Res*, **1111**, 176–86.

Reding MJ, Orto LA, Winter SW, Fortuna IM, Di Ponte P, McDowell FH. (1986). Antidepressant therapy after stroke. A double-blind trial. *Arch Neurol*, **43**, 763–5.

Reding MJ, Solomon B, Borucki SJ. (1995). Effect of dextroamphetamine on motor recovery after stroke. *Neurology*, **45** (Suppl. 4), A222.

Roffler-Tarlov S, Schildkraut JJ, Draskoczy PR. (1973). Effects of acute and chronic administration of desmethylimipramine on the content of norepinephrine and other monamines in the rat brain. *Biochem Pharmacol*, **22**, 2923–6.

Sabe L, Salvarezza F, Cuerva AG, Leiguarda R, Starkstein S. (1995). A randomized, double-blind, placebo-controlled study of bromocriptine in nonfluent aphasia. *Neurology*, **45**, 2272–4.

Santarelli L, Saxe M, Gross C, Surget A, Battaglia F, Dulawa S, et al. (2003). Requirement of hippocampal neurogenesis for the behavioral effects of antidepressants. *Science*, **301**, 805–09.

Satoh M, Ishihara K, Iwama T, Takagi H. (1986). Aniracetam augments, and midazolam inhibits, the long-term potentiation in guinea-pig hippocampal slices. *Neurosci Lett*, **68**, 216–20.

Schallert T, Hernandez TD, Barth TM. (1986). Recovery of function after brain damage: Severe and chronic disruption by diazepam. *Brain Res*, **379**, 104–11.

Schallert T, Jones TA, Weaver MS, Shapiro LE, Crippens D, Fulton R. (1992). Pharmacologic and anatomic considerations in recovery of function. *Phys Med Rehabil*, **6**, 375–93.

Schmanke TD, Avery RA, Barth TM. (1996). The effects of amphetamine on recovery of function after cortical damage in the rat depend on the behavioral requirements of the task. *J Neurotrauma*, **13**, 293–307.

Sonde L, Nordström M, Nilsson C-G, Lökk J, Viitanen M. (2001). A double-blind placebo-controlled study of the effects of amphetamine and physiotherapy after stroke. *Cerebrovasc Dis*, **12**, 253–7.

Stanton PK, Sarvey JM. (1985). Blockade of norepinephrine-induced long-lasting potentiation in the hippocampal dentate gyrus by an inhibitor of protein synthesis. *Brain Res*, **361**, 276–83.

Stroemer RP, Kent TA, Hulsebosch CE. (1994). Amphetamines permanently promote recovery following cortical infarction. *Abstracts Soci Neurosci*, **20**, 186.

Stroemer RP, Kent TA, Hulsebosch CE. (1995). Neocortical neural sprouting, synaptogenesis, and behavioral recovery after neocortical infarction in rats. *Stroke*, **26**, 2135–44.

Sutton RL, Feeney DM. (1992). α-Noradrenergic agonists and antagonists affect recovery and maintenance of beam-walking ability after sensorimotor cortex ablation in the rat. *Restor Neurol Neurosci*, **4**, 1–11.

Sutton RL, Hovda DA, Feeney DM. (1989). Amphetamine accelerates recovery of locomotor function following bilateral frontal cortex ablation in cats. *Behav Neurosci*, **103**, 837–41.

Tanaka M, Kondo S, Hirai S. Ishiguro K, Ishihara T, Morimatsu M. (1992). Crossed cerebellar diaschisis accompanied by hemiataxia: a PET study. *J Neurol Neurosurg Psychiatry*, **55**, 121–5.

Theodore DR, Meier-Ruge W, Abraham J. (1992). Microvascular morphometry in primate diaschisis. *Microvasc Res*, **43**, 147–55.

Treig T, Werner C, Sachse M, Hesse S. (2003). No benefit from D-amphetamine when added to physiotherapy after stroke: a randomized, placebo-controlled study. *Clin Rehabil*, **17**, 590–9.

Troisi E, Paolucci S, Silvestrini M, Matteis M, Vernieri F, Grasso MG., et al (2002). Prognostic factors in stroke rehabilitation: the possible role of pharmacological treatment. *Acta Neurol Scand*, **105**, 100–06.

Van Hasselt P. (1973). Effect of butyrophenones on motor function in rats after recovery from brain damage. *Neuropharmacology*, **12**, 245–7.

Wade DT, Collen FM, Robb GF, Warlow CP. (1992). Physiotherapy intervention late after stroke and mobility. *Br Med J*, **304**, 609–13.

Walker-Batson D, Curtis S, Natarajan R, Ford J, Dronkers N, Salmeron E, et al. (2001). A double-blind, placebo-controlled study of the use of amphetamine in the treatment of aphasia. *Stroke*, **32**, 2093–8.

Walker-Batson D, Smith P, Curtis S, Unwin H, Greenlee R. (1995). Amphetamine paired with physical therapy accelerates motor recovery after stroke – further evidence. *Stroke*, **26**, 2254–9.

Weaver MS, Chen MJ, Westerberg VS, Feeney DM. (1988). Locus coeruleus lesions facilitate recovery of locomotor function after sensorimotor cortex contusion in the rat. *Abstracts Soc Neurosci*, **14**, 405.

Wigstrom H, Gustafsson B. (1985). Facilitation of hippocampal long-lasting potentiation by GABA antagonists. *Acta Physiol Scand*, **125**, 159–72.

Williams S, Johnston D. (1988). Muscarinic depression of long-term potentiation in CA3 hippocampal neurons. *Science*, **242**, 84–7.

Wilson MS, Hamm RJ. (2002). Effects of fluoxetine on the 5-HT1A receptor and recovery of cognitive function after traumatic brain injury in rats. *Am J Phys Med Rehabil*, **81**, 364–72.

Chapter 26

Electrical and Magnetic Brain Stimulation to Enhance Post-stroke Recovery

Mark Parsons
Jodie Marquez

Investigation into the merits of non-invasive brain stimulation as a therapeutic tool in stroke has gained momentum over the past two decades. These techniques include transcranial direct current stimulation (tDCS), high-definition tDCS (HD-tDCS), transcranial alternating current stimulation (tACS), transcranial random noise stimulation (tRNS), repetitive transcranial magnetic stimulation (rTMS), and theta burst stimulation (TBS). To date, the most studied modalities used to modulate brain excitability are tDCS and rTMS.

The use of cortical stimulation to facilitate stroke recovery is based on the premise that a focal lesion produces a region of decreased neuronal output and disrupts the balance of interhemispheric inhibition. Therefore, current delivered from an external source may facilitate a shift of this imbalance to a more equal state by increasing excitability of the perilesional areas and/or decreasing inhibition arising from the contralesional hemisphere (Schlaug et al., 2008).

Transcranial Direct Current Stimulation

The Stimulator

tDCS involves applying a weak, direct current of electricity, usually 1–2 mA, to the scalp via two rubber electrodes sheathed in saline-soaked sponges. The current flows in a direction away from the cathode to the anode; therefore, the effects depend on the position and polarity of the electrodes. The tDCS-stimulating device is a 13 cm × 21 cm portable box, which is typically programmed to ramp up the current over several seconds to minimize discomfort. Subjects experience a tingling/itching sensation under the electrodes, which abates in most cases by 1 minute owing to tolerance. The portability, ease of application, and relatively low cost of the device render it a practical therapy option for stroke clinicians.

Mechanisms of Action

Transcranial direct current stimulation is said to be neuromodulatory as it delivers subthreshold stimulation that affects the neuronal firing rate by altering the balance of ions inside and outside the neuronal membrane, producing hyperpolarization in the region of the cathode and depolarization of the resting membrane potential beneath the anode (Nitsche et al., 2003; Giordano et al., 2017). Sustained application (typically 10–30 min) generates changes at the synaptic level that persist transiently following the cessation of stimulation (Nitsche and Paulus, 2000). These effects are similar to those seen in long-term potentiation where there is a lasting increase in postsynaptic potentials. This in turn is capable of inducing cortical reorganization, most likely by increasing local synaptic effectiveness and network processing (Krause et al., 2013) and may be propagated in anatomically or functionally connected distant cortical and subcortical regions (Lang et al., 2005). Computational models have been developed that have improved our understanding of the effects of tDCS on single neurones, yet the mechanisms of how tDCS affects and interacts with a network or neuronal populations, particularly inhibitory interneurones, remain obscure (Radman et al., 2009).

In addition to effecting changes in neuronal membrane polarization, there are also non-neural cells and tissues (such as blood vessels and connective tissue) within the central nervous system that may also influence the effects of tDCS. These may influence physiological mechanisms such as vascular motility, inflammation, and cell migration, which would seem relevant in stroke recovery (Brunoni et al., 2012).

Application of tDCS

Electrode position and orientation will affect the outcome produced by tDCS, as different neuronal populations with different tissue characteristics will be stimulated; therefore, the induced currents may be distorted and unpredictable, particularly in the case of stroke in which the brain tissue may not be anatomically intact.

The most commonly used protocol for tDCS stimulation in stroke is the anodal montage with the anode positioned over the area of the scalp corresponding to the lesioned motor cortex (to increase excitability of the perilesional regions) and the cathode on the contralateral forehead. Conversely, cathodal stimulation involves application of the cathode over the region of the contralesional motor cortex and the anode on the contralateral forehead to downregulate excitability, thus releasing the lesioned hemisphere from excessive transcallosal inhibition (Boggio et al., 2007). A third variation places the anode on the lesioned cortex and the cathode on the non-lesioned cortex with the intent of achieving both anodal and cathodal effects simultaneously and is termed bihemispheric tDCS. Finally, extracephalic tDCS is a montage where the cathode is placed more distally, usually over the contralesional upper arm. This has the proposed advantage of avoiding unwanted excitability changes under the cathode but there is uncertainty regarding safety as current could potentially affect the brainstem (Redfearn et al., 1964) and the increased distance between the electrodes could negatively impact current density and therefore the duration of effects (Moliadze et al., 2010b).

There is an immense range of possible dose parameters (current intensity, duration, number of sessions, etc.) which provides flexibility but also presents a challenge in determining optimal dosage for individual clients (Peterchev et al., 2012).

Safety

Routinely used tDCS protocols appear to be safe with thousands of subjects tested worldwide and very few reported cases of adverse events. Furthermore, the induced effects, both electrophysical and behavioural, appear to be totally reversible (Liebetanz et al., 2009; Bikson et al., 2016; Antal et al., 2017). The exclusion criteria are very general and include unstable medical conditions, epilepsy, acute eczema at the electrode sites, metallic implants near the electrodes (e.g. cochlear implants, aneurysm clips), pacemaker, pregnancy, and neuromodifying medications.

Current density and total charge are the most important parameters for judging safety and must exceed 24 mA/cm^2 before brain tissue is at risk of harm (McCreery et al., 1990). The current density in typical protocols is approximately 0.1 mA/cm^2, well within these limits. Safety considerations have been built into the tDCS unit whereby the operator can programme a predefined upper voltage limit to shut down the unit if high resistance occurs. In this scenario, the operator will add more saline solution/remoisten the electrode pads and recommence the session.

The risk of epileptic seizure is often raised in the literature due to a reported episode in one of the earliest studies (Redfearn et al., 1964), but as tDCS does not cause seizure, nor reduce the seizure threshold in animals, this does not appear to be a valid risk for human subjects with no history of seizure (Nitsche et al., 2008).

Several isolated cases of adverse reactions have been reported; these include skin irritation and breakdown following consecutive applications of tDCS, headache, and fatigue. Yet it should be stated that the safety of prolonged periods of application in stroke patients is relatively unknown; for example, it may produce occult effects, particularly on cognitive function, which have not been anticipated or measured (Fitz and Reiner, 2015). A systematic review of 23 randomized trials, allocating 371 patients to active tDCS and 293 to control, reported dropouts or adverse events in 6 of these studies, with comparable proportions of events in the active and sham conditions, risk difference (RD) 0.01, 95% confidence interval (CI): –0.02 to 0.03 (Figure 26.1) (Elsner et al., 2016a).

Variation in Effects

The physiological effects of tDCS on the cortex in healthy subjects are generally uniform; however, there is wide variation in the size of the effect that cannot be explained purely by stimulation parameters (Kim et al., 2014). This inconsistent effect is likely to be the result of many variables that are known to influence corticomotor plasticity, as listed in Table 26.1, and an interaction between them. The relative contribution of each variable is impossible to determine at this stage as there is a lack of studies which systematically manipulate each factor while controlling for the other parameters (Saiote et al., 2013). Inter-individual variation is even greater in the stroke population due to changes in cortical anatomy, including gliosis with corresponding increases in cerebrospinal fluid, which has a conductance 4–10 times greater than brain tissue (Wagner et al., 2007b).

Review: Transcranial direct current stimulation (tDCS) for improving activities of daily living, and physical and cognitive functioning, in people after stroke
Comparison: 1 tDCS versus any type of placebo or passive control intervention
Outcome: 9 Secondary outcome measure: dropouts, adverse events and deaths during the intervention period

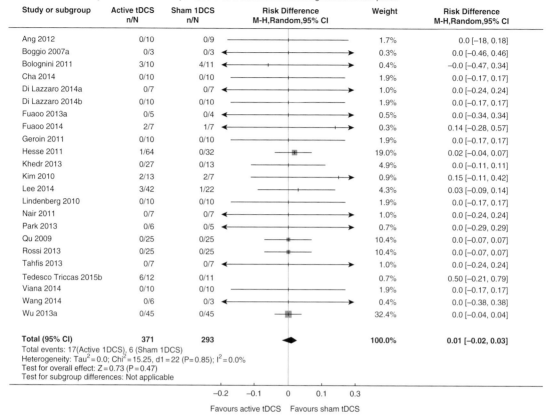

Study or subgroup	Active tDCS n/N	Sham 1DCS n/N	Risk Difference M-H,Random,95% CI	Weight	Risk Difference M-H,Random,95% CI
Ang 2012	0/10	0/9		1.7%	0.0 [−18, 0.18]
Boggio 2007a	0/3	0/3		0.3%	0.0 [−0.46, 0.46]
Bolognini 2011	3/10	4/11		0.4%	−0.0 [−0.47, 0.34]
Cha 2014	0/10	0/10		1.9%	0.0 [−0.17, 0.17]
Di Lazzaro 2014a	0/7	0/7		1.0%	0.0 [−0.24, 0.24]
Di Lazzaro 2014b	0/10	0/10		1.9%	0.0 [−0.17, 0.17]
Fuaoo 2013a	0/5	0/4		0.5%	0.0 [−0.34, 0.34]
Fuaoo 2014	2/7	1/7		0.3%	0.14 [−0.28, 0.57]
Geroin 2011	0/10	0/10		1.9%	0.0 [−0.17, 0.17]
Hesse 2011	1/64	0/32		19.0%	0.02 [−0.04, 0.07]
Khedr 2013	0/27	0/13		4.9%	0.0 [−0.11, 0.11]
Kim 2010	2/13	2/7		0.9%	0.15 [−0.11, 0.42]
Lee 2014	3/42	1/22		4.3%	0.03 [−0.09, 0.14]
Lindenberg 2010	0/10	0/10		1.9%	0.0 [−0.17, 0.17]
Nair 2011	0/7	0/7		1.0%	0.0 [−0.24, 0.24]
Park 2013	0/6	0/5		0.7%	0.0 [−0.29, 0.29]
Qu 2009	0/25	0/25		10.4%	0.0 [−0.07, 0.07]
Rossi 2013	0/25	0/25		10.4%	0.0 [−0.07, 0.07]
Tahfis 2013	0/7	0/7		1.0%	0.0 [−0.24, 0.24]
Tedesco Triccas 2015b	6/12	0/11		0.7%	0.50 [−0.21, 0.79]
Viana 2014	0/10	0/10		1.9%	0.0 [−0.17, 0.17]
Wang 2014	0/6	0/3		0.4%	0.0 [−0.38, 0.38]
Wu 2013a	0/45	0/45		32.4%	0.0 [−0.04, 0.04]
Total (95% CI)	**371**	**293**		**100.0%**	**0.01 [−0.02, 0.03]**

Total events: 17(Active 1DCS), 6 (Sham 1DCS)
Heterogeneity: Tau^2=0.0; Chi^2=15.25, d1=22 (P=0.85); I^2=0.0%
Test for overall effect: Z=0.73 (P=0.47)
Test for subgroup differences: Not applicable

−0.2   −0.1   0   0.1   0.3
Favours active tDCS   Favours sham tDCS

Figure 26.1 Forest plot showing the effects of *transcranial electrical direct stimulation vs control* on the *composite of dropouts, adverse events, and deaths* at the end of the intervention period, in post-stroke patients.

Reproduced from Elsner et al. (2016a), with permission from John Wiley & Sons Limited. Copyright Cochrane Library.

Evidence

Studies in stroke patients have tested tDCS as a potential therapy for several different outcomes of interest, using varied electrode montages, in individuals with diverse stroke characteristics. The M1 hand area has been the therapeutic target used most extensively, due to its superficial location on the cortex and importance for recovery of upper extremity function, but several studies report successfully stimulating the leg area of M1, the language centres, and cerebellum.

Effects of tDCS according to Outcome

Activities of Daily Living (ADL)

A systematic review in the Cochrane Library identified 10 randomized controlled trials (RCTs) with a total of

407 stroke patients assessing the effect of tDCS on ADL functional level, as measured on the Frenchay Activities Index, the Barthel Index, or similar scales (Elsner et al., 2016a). For the outcome of absolute level of ADL function at the end of the intervention period, in nine trials, allocation to tDCS (232 patients), compared with control (164 patients), was associated with higher ADL function at the end of the intervention period: standardized mean difference (SMD) 0.24 (05% CI: 0.0 –0.44; p = 0.02). Effects were consistent across trials, I^2 = 0%. One small additional trial evaluating change in ADL, rather than absolute ADL, function found a qualitatively similar effect (Figure 26.2).

Six of these studies, with 269 participants, assessed the sustained effects of tDCS beyond the intervention period on ADL at end of study follow-up and found evidence of a sustained beneficial effect: SMD 0.31,

Table 26.1 Factors affecting response to tDCS

Stimulation characteristics	Patient characteristics	Stroke characteristics
Mode of stimulation	Age	Location of the lesion
Frequency and intensity of stimulation	Gender	Dominant vs nondominant lesions
Region of the brain stimulated	Concomitant pharmacotherapy	Time since stroke
Interval between sessions	Psychological status	Severity of paresis
Total number of sessions	The extent of skilled hand use	Cortical involvement/motor network integrity
Timing of repeat sessions	Individual morphology, e.g. cranial and brain anatomy; functional organization of circuits	
Time of day	Genetic factors, e.g. polymorphism of neurotrophins	
Motor and cognitive interference	Circadian rhythms	
Adjuvant therapy	Cardiovascular fitness	
Outcome measures used		

Review: Transcranial direct current stimulation (tDCS) for improving activities of daily living, and physical and cognitive functioning, in people after stroke
Comparison: 1 tDCS versus any type of placebo or passive control intervention
Outcome: 2 Primary outcome measure: ADLs until the end of follow-up

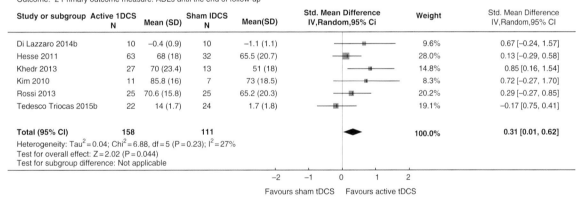

Figure 26.2 Forest plot showing the effects of *transcranial electrical direct stimulation vs control* on *activities of daily living* at the end of the intervention period, in post-stroke patients.
Reproduced from Elsner et al. (2016a), with permission from John Wiley & Sons Limited. Copyright Cochrane Library.

95% CI: 0.01–0.62; $p = 0.04$. However, the confidence interval was wide and there was evidence of moderate heterogeneity across trials ($I^2 = 27\%$) (Figure 26.3).

Upper Limb Function

A systematic review in the Cochrane Library identified 16 RCTs enrolling 484 stroke patients assessing the effect of tDCS on upper limb function, as measured on the Action Research Arm Test, the Fugl-Meyer Score, or similar assessments (Elsner et al., 2016a). For the outcome of absolute amount of improvement in upper limb function scores, in 10

trials, allocation to tDCS (243 patients), compared with control (188 patients), was not associated with a statistically significant difference in arm and hand function at the end of the intervention period: SMD 0.11 (05% CI: –0.17–0.39). Four small, additional trials evaluating change in upper limb, rather than absolute upper limb, function found qualitatively similar effects (Figure 26.4).

Lower Limb Function

Studies investigating the effects of tDCS on lower limb function are fewer, in part because the somatotopy of

Review: Transcranial direct current stimulation (tDCS) for improving activities of daily living, and physical and cognitive functioning, in people after stroke
Comparison: 1 tDCS versus any type of placebo or passive control intervention
Outcome: 1 Primary outcome measure: ADLs at the end of the intervention period

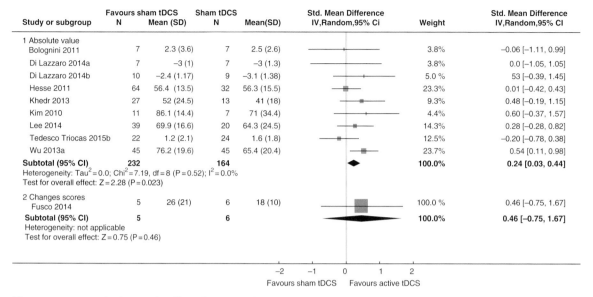

Study or subgroup	Favours sham tDCS N	Mean (SD)	Sham tDCS N	Mean(SD)	Std. Mean Difference IV,Random,95% Ci	Weight	Std. Mean Difference IV,Random,95% Ci
1 Absolute value							
Bolognini 2011	7	2.3 (3.6)	7	2.5 (2.6)		3.8%	−0.06 [−1.11, 0.99]
Di Lazzaro 2014a	7	−3 (1)	7	−3 (1.3)		3.8%	0.0 [−1.05, 1.05]
Di Lazzaro 2014b	10	−2.4 (1.17)	9	−3.1 (1.38)		5.0 %	53 [−0.39, 1.45]
Hesse 2011	64	56.4 (13.5)	32	56.3 (15.5)		23.3%	0.01 [−0.42, 0.43]
Khedr 2013	27	52 (24.5)	13	41 (18)		9.3%	0.48 [−0.19, 1.15]
Kim 2010	11	86.1 (14.4)	7	71 (34.4)		4.4%	0.60 [−0.37, 1.57]
Lee 2014	39	69.9 (16.6)	20	64.3 (24.5)		14.3%	0.28 [−0.28, 0.82]
Tedesco Triocas 2015b	22	1.2 (2.1)	24	1.6 (1.8)		12.5%	−0.20 [−0.78, 0.38]
Wu 2013a	45	76.2 (19.6)	45	65.4 (20.4)		23.7%	0.54 [0.11, 0.98]
Subtotal (95% CI)	232		164			100.0%	0.24 [0.03, 0.44]

Heterogeneity: Tau^2 = 0.0; Chi^2 = 7.19, df = 8 (P = 0.52); I^2 = 0.0%
Test for overall effect: Z = 2.28 (P = 0.023)

2 Changes scores							
Fusco 2014	5	26 (21)	6	18 (10)		100.0 %	0.46 [−0.75, 1.67]
Subtotal (95% CI)	5		6			100.0%	0.46 [−0.75, 1.67]

Heterogeneity: not applicable
Test for overall effect: Z = 0.75 (P = 0.46)

−2 −1 0 1 2
Favours sham tDCS   Favours active tDCS

Figure 26.3 Forest plot showing the effects of *transcranial electrical direct stimulation vs control* on *activities of daily living* at the end of follow-up, in post-stroke patients.
Reproduced from Elsner et al. (2016a), with permission from John Wiley & Sons Limited. Copyright Cochrane Library.

the legs is located deep in the central sulcus and technically difficult to isolate. However, there is consistent evidence that this area can be reached and is a feasible target for tDCS stimulation (Chang et al., 2015). Individual RCTs have provided signals of potential benefit from the use of anodal tDCS to improve postural stability (Sohn et al., 2013; Koyama et al., 2015), lower limb muscle strength (Tanaka et al., 2009; Tanaka et al., 2011), and gait function (Tahtis et al., 2014). Conversely, individual RCTs did not show strong signals of beneficial effects on gait parameters, balance control (Chang et al., 2015), and lower limb biomechanics (Tahtis et al., 2014). These isolated reports from small studies require further validation.

Spasticity

A systematic review identified three RCTs enrolling 206 patients evaluating tDCS compared with control for post-stroke spasticity, as assessed with the Modified Ashworth Scale (Elsner et al., 2016b). Overall, tDS did not significantly alter the absolute amount of improvement in spasticity scores: standardized mean difference −0.61, 95% CI: −1.51–0.30; *p* = 0.19.

Aphasia

A systematic review identified 12 RCTs assessing tDCS for post-stroke aphasia, among which 6 trials, enrolling 66 patients, could be pooled for the outcome of accuracy of picture naming. Allocation to tDCS, compared with control, was not associated with a statistically significant difference in correct picture naming at the end of the intervention period (SMD 0.37, 95% CI: −0.18–0.92; *p* = 0.19) (Elsner et al., 2015) (Figure 26.5). No studies were identified that used a standardized measure of functional communication, that is, an objective measure of real-life communication, rather than a more narrow endpoint like picture naming. Subsequent, modestly larger RCTs have continued to provide mixed positive (Meinzer et al., 2016) and neutral (Spielmann et al., 2018) signals.

Hemispatial Neglect

A systematic review identified two studies, providing three randomized comparisons of 32 patients, assessing tDCS for hemispatial neglect after stroke, as measured by the Line Bisection Test. Allocation to tDCS, compared with control, was associated with a statistically significant greater reduction in

Review: Transcranial direct current stimulation (tDCS) for improving activities of daily living, and physical and cognitive functioning, in people after stroke
Comparison: 1 tDCS versus any type of placebo or passive control intervention
Outcome: 3 Secondary outcome measure: upper extremely function at the end of the intervention period

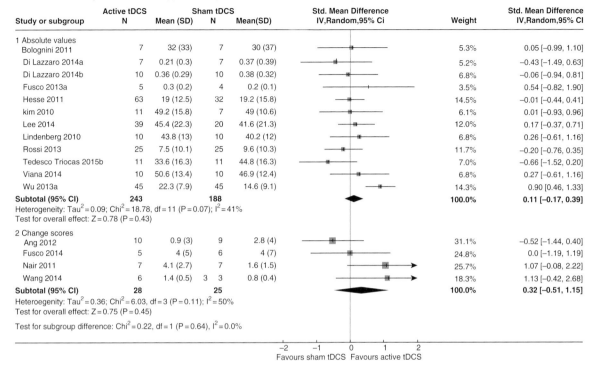

Figure 26.4 Forest plot showing the effects of *transcranial electrical direct stimulation vs control* on *upper limb function* at the end of the intervention period, in post-stroke patients.

Reproduced from Elsner et al. (2016a), with permission from John Wiley & Sons Limited. Copyright Cochrane Library.

Review: Transcranial direct current stimulation (tDCS) for improving aphasia in patients with aphasia after stroke
Comparison: 1 tDCS plus speech and language therapy (SLT) versus sham tDCS plus SLT for improving aphasia
Outcome: 1 Language impairment: accuracy of naming until end of intervention phase

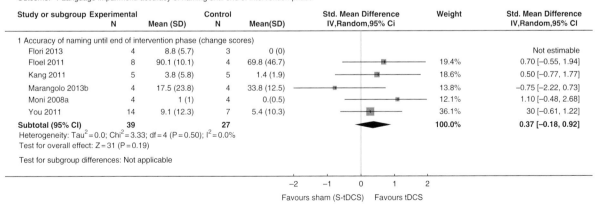

Figure 26.5 Forest plot showing the effects of *transcranial electrical direct stimulation vs control* on *accuracy of picture naming* at the end of the intervention period, in post-stroke patients.

Reproduced from Elsner et al. (2015), with permission from John Wiley & Sons Limited. Copyright Cochrane Library.

hemispatial inattention: SMD −1.07, 95% CI: −1.76 to −0.37; p = 0.003 (Salazar et al., 2018). However, two of the comparisons used a shared control group, warranting interpretive caution.

Additional Cognitive Functions

Studies in healthy adults have suggested tDCS to be capable of improving additional cognitive domains, including attention, memory, and executive functions (Smith and Clithero, 2009). Small RCTs have explored effects of tDCS in elements of these domains in stroke patients, with mixed results (Kang et al., 2009; Yun et al., 2015; Kazuta et al., 2017; Shaker et al., 2018). Due to the prevalence of cognitive impairment post-stroke and its association with poor rehabilitation outcomes, further research in this field is warranted.

Mood

Transcranial direct current stimulation has induced mood improvements in several neuropsychiatric conditions but has been assessed in one modest-sized, controlled trial for post-stroke depression, enrolling 48 patients (Valiengo et al., 2017). Stimulation intensity was 2 mA for 30 minutes daily for 10–12 sessions, centred on left dorsolateral prefrontal cortex. On the primary endpoint, score on the Hamilton Depression Rating Scale, tDCS was associated with less depressed scores at the final 6-week visit (mean difference [MD] 4.7, 95% CI: 2.1–7.3; p < 0.001), but not at the 2-week or 4-week visit. This encouraging initial trial result supports the merit of further investigations.

Dysphagia

A systemic review identified four sham-controlled RCTs, enrolling 109 patients, assessing tDCS for post-stroke swallowing dysfunction (Chiang et al., 2018). Sites of stimulation were ipsilateral or contralateral swallowing or pharyngeal motor and sensory cortices. Allocation to tDCS, compared with sham, was associated with a greater improvement in swallowing scale scores: SMD 0.61 (95% CI: 0.14–1.08). There was substantial variation across trials in stimulation intensity (1 mA and 2 mA), duration of treatment (between 4 days and 10 days), and time from stroke onset to treatment start (between <7 days and >1 month), but the net positive signal supports further studies to confirm benefit and identify optimal treatment parameters.

Effects of tDCS according to Type and Hemisphere of Stimulation

Three broad variations in stimulation paradigm have been evaluated in tDCS studies: (1) anodal tDCS over the lesioned hemisphere; (2) cathodal tDCS over the lesioned hemisphere; and (3) bihemispheric stimulation with anodal tDCS over the lesioned and cathodal tDCS over the non-lesioned hemisphere. For outcomes of improvement in ADL and improvement in motor function, the pattern of trial results is suggestive, but not definitive, that cathodal-ipsilesional and bihemispheric stimulation paradigms are more effective than anodal-ipsilesional.

In the systematic review in the Cochrane Library of tDCS to improve ADL in post-stroke patients, study stimulations were: (1) anodal tDCS over the lesioned hemisphere (5 trials, 164 patients); (2) cathodal tDCS over the lesioned hemisphere (6 trials, 301 patients); and (3) bihemispheric stimulation with anodal tDCS over the lesioned and cathodal tDCS over the non-lesioned hemisphere (2 trials, 33 patients). There was no statistically significant evidence of heterogeneity in the overall positive treatment effect across the three stimulation paradigms (subgroup heterogeneity p = 0.16). However, within-subgroup point estimates were positive for cathodal-lesional (SMD 0.33) and bihemispheric (SMD 0.30) paradigms, compared with neutral for anodal (SMD -0.04) (Elsner et al., 2016a) (Figure 26.6). Similar findings were noted in a systematic review of tDCS for motor performance in stroke patients. Among the 19 RCTs identified, stimulation types studied were: anodal tDCS in 9 trials, cathodal tDCS in 7 trials, and bihemispheric tDCS in 3 trials. None of the stimulation paradigms reached a statistically significant within-subgroup treatment effect, but point estimates were positive for cathodal (SMD 0.39) and bihemispheric (SMD 0.24) paradigms, compared with neutral for anodal (SMD 0.05) (Marquez et al., 2015).

Effects of tDCS according to Stroke Characteristics

Time since Stroke

Preliminary data have provided conflicting signals regarding the effect of time since stroke upon responsiveness to tDCS, and modification may vary by the functional networks being stimulated. In the systematic review in the Cochrane Library of tDCS to improve

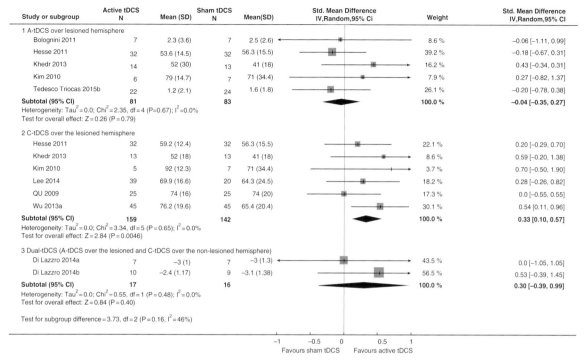

Review: Transcranial direct current stimulation (tDCS) for improving activities of daily living, and physical and cognitive functioning, in people after stroke
Comparison: 3 Subgroup analysis for primary outcome measure: ADLs at the end of the intervention period
Outcome: 2 Planned analysis: effects of type stimulation (A-tDCS/C-tDCS/dual-tDCS) and location of stimulation (lesioned/non-lesioned hemisphere) on
ADLs at the end of the intervention period (study)

Study or subgroup	Active tDCS N	Mean (SD)	Sham tDCS N	Mean(SD)	Std. Mean Difference IV,Random,95% Ci	Weight	Std. Mean Difference IV,Random,95% CI
1 A-tDCS over lesioned hemisphere							
Bolognini 2011	7	2.3 (3.6)	7	2.5 (2.6)		8.6 %	−0.06 [−1.11, 0.99]
Hesse 2011	32	53.6 (14.5)	32	56.3 (15.5)		39.2 %	−0.18 [−0.67, 0.31]
Khedr 2013	14	52 (30)	13	41 (18)		16.2 %	0.43 [−0.34, 0.31]
Kim 2010	6	79 (14.7)	7	71 (34.4)		7.9 %	0.27 [−0.82, 1.37]
Tedesco Triocas 2015b	22	1.2 (2.1)	24	1.6 (1.8)		26.1 %	−0.20 [−0.78, 0.38]
Subtotal (95% CI)	**81**		**83**			**100.0 %**	**−0.04 [−0.35, 0.27]**
Heterogeneity: Tau²=0.0; Chi²=2.35, df=4 (P=0.67); I²=0.0%							
Test for overall effect: Z=0.26 (P=0.79)							
2 C-tDCS over the lesioned hemisphere							
Hesse 2011	32	59.2 (12.4)	32	56.3 (15.5)		22.1 %	0.20 [−0.29, 0.70]
Khedr 2013	13	52 (18)	13	41 (18)		8.6 %	0.59 [−0.20, 1.38]
Kim 2010	5	92 (12.3)	7	71 (34.4)		3.7 %	0.70 [−0.50, 1.90]
Lee 2014	39	69.9 (16.6)	20	64.3 (24.5)		18.2 %	0.28 [−0.26, 0.82]
QU 2009	25	74 (16)	25	74 (20)		17.3 %	0.0 [−0.55, 0.55]
Wu 2013a	45	76.2 (19.6)	45	65.4 (20.4)		30.1 %	0.54 [0.11, 0.96]
Subtotal (95% CI)	**159**		**142**			**100.0 %**	**0.33 [0.10, 0.57]**
Heterogeneity: Tau²=0.0; Chi²=3.34, df=5 (P=0.65); I²=0.0%							
Test for overall effect: Z=2.84 (P=0.0046)							
3 Dual-tDCS (A-tDCS over the lesioned and C-tDCS over the non-lesioned hemisphere)							
Di Lazzro 2014a	7	−3 (1)	7	−3 (1.3)		43.5 %	0.0 [−1.05, 1.05]
Di Lazzro 2014b	10	−2.4 (1.17)	9	−3.1 (1.38)		56.5 %	0.53 [−0.39, 1.45]
Subtotal (95% CI)	**17**		**16**			**100.0 %**	**0.30 [−0.39, 0.99]**
Heterogeneity: Tau²=0.0; Chi²=0.55, df=1 (P=0.48); I²=0.0%							
Test for overall effect: Z=0.84 (P=0.40)							
Test for subgroup difference=3.73, df=2 (P=0.16, I²=46%)							

−1   −0.5   0   0.5   1
Favours sham tDCS   Favours active tDCS

Figure 26.6 Forest plot showing the effects of *transcranial electrical direct stimulation vs control* on *activities of daily living* at the end of the intervention period, in post-stroke patients, according to the type and hemisphere of stimulation.
Reproduced from Elsner et al. (2016a), with permission from John Wiley & Sons Limited. Copyright Cochrane Library.

ADL in post-stroke patients, stimulation time periods analysed were: (1) acute/subacute (first 1–4 weeks post-stroke: 4 trials, 213 patients); (2) late subacute (1–6 months post-stroke: 2 trials, 140 patients); and (3) chronic (>6 months post-stroke: 4 trials, 93 patients) (Elsner et al., 2016a). Although point estimates directionally favoured earlier treatment periods, there was no statistically significant evidence of variation in treatment effects across the timing subgroups (subgroup heterogeneity *p* = 0.59) (Figure 26.7). In a systematic review of tDCS for motor performance in stroke patients, among 11 RCTs with clear chronic stroke populations, stimulation time periods analysed were acute/subacute (3 trials) and chronic (8 trials) (Marquez et al., 2015). Confidence intervals for treatment effects overlapped across the two time intervals, suggesting subgroup differences did not reach statistical significance. However, point estimates directionally favoured the later treatment period, in which benefit reached statistical significance: SMD 0.45 (95% CI: 0.09–0.80) (Figure 26.8).

Stroke Severity

In the systematic review of tDCS for motor performance in stroke patients, among 13 RCTs with clear severity populations, effects were analysed in individuals with mild/moderate impairments (9 trials) and moderate/severe impairments (4 trials) (Marquez et al., 2015). Confidence intervals for treatment effects overlapped across the two time-deficit severity subgroups, suggesting subgroup differences did not reach statistical significance. However, point estimates directionally favoured the mild/moderate severity group, in which benefit reached statistical significance: SMD 0.37 (95% CI: 0.05–0.70) (see Figure 26.8).

Implications for Practice and Research

Currently, there is suggestive, but inconsistent and imprecise, evidence available indicating that tDCS may improve ADL performance, motor function, swallowing, mood, and language and other cognitive functions after stroke. There is insufficient evidence to

Review: Transcranial direct current stimulation (tDCS) for improving activities of daily living, and physical and cognitive functioning, in people after stroke
Comparison: 3 Subgroup analysis for primary outcome measure: ADLs at the end of the intervention period
Outcome: 1 Planned analysis: duration of illness-acute/subacute phase versus postacute phase for ADLs at the intervention period

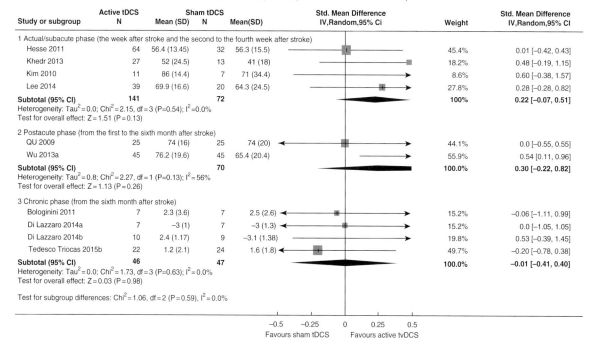

Study or subgroup	Active tDCS N	Mean (SD)	Sham tDCS N	Mean(SD)	Std. Mean Difference IV,Random,95% Ci	Weight	Std. Mean Difference IV,Random,95% CI
1 Actual/subacute phase (the week after stroke and the second to the fourth week after stroke)							
Hesse 2011	64	56.4 (13.45)	32	56.3 (15.5)		45.4%	0.01 [−0.42, 0.43]
Khedr 2013	27	52 (24.5)	13	41 (18)		18.2%	0.48 [−0.19, 1.15]
Kim 2010	11	86 (14.4)	7	71 (34.4)		8.6%	0.60 [−0.38, 1.57]
Lee 2014	39	69.9 (16.6)	20	64.3 (24.5)		27.8%	0.28 [−0.28, 0.82]
Subtotal (95% CI)	141		72			100%	0.22 [−0.07, 0.51]
Heterogeneity: Tau²=0.0; Chi²=2.15, df=3 (P=0.54); I²=0.0%							
Test for overall effect: Z=1.51 (P=0.13)							
2 Postacute phase (from the first to the sixth month after stroke)							
QU 2009	25	74 (16)	25	74 (20)		44.1%	0.0 [−0.55, 0.55]
Wu 2013a	45	76.2 (19.6)	45	65.4 (20.4)		55.9%	0.54 [0.11, 0.96]
Subtotal (95% CI)			70			100.0%	0.30 [−0.22, 0.82]
Heterogeneity: Tau²=0.8; Chi²=2.27, df=1 (P=0.13); I²=56%							
Test for overall effect: Z=1.13 (P=0.26)							
3 Chronic phase (from the sixth month after stroke)							
Bologinini 2011	7	2.3 (3.6)	7	2.5 (2.6)		15.2%	−0.06 [−1.11, 0.99]
Di Lazzaro 2014a	7	−3 (1)	7	−3 (1.3)		15.2%	0.0 [−1.05, 1.05]
Di Lazzaro 2014b	10	2.4 (1.17)	9	−3.1 (1.38)		19.8%	0.53 [−0.39, 1.45]
Tedesco Triocas 2015b	22	1.2 (2.1)	24	1.6 (1.8)		49.7%	−0.20 [−0.78, 0.38]
Subtotal (95% CI)	46		47			100.0%	−0.01 [−0.41, 0.40]
Heterogeneity: Tau²=0.0; Chi²=1.73, df=3 (P=0.63); I²=0.0%							
Test for overall effect: Z=0.03 (P=0.98)							

Test for subgroup differences: Chi²=1.06, df=2 (P=0.59), I²=0.0%

−0.5   −0.25   0   0.25   0.5
Favours sham tDCS   Favours active tvDCS

Figure 26.7 Forest plot showing the effects of *transcranial electrical direct stimulation vs control* on *activities of daily living* at the end of the intervention period, according to time since stroke until treatment period.

Reproduced from Elsner et al. (2016a), with permission from John Wiley & Sons Limited. Copyright Cochrane Library.

clarify the optimal type, targeting, intensity, and duration of tDCS for different functional domains. Clearly, not all stroke patients respond in the same way or benefit from tDCS to the same magnitude, and future research needs to establish well-defined patient selection criteria. If tDCS does work by enhancing neuroplasticity and capacity for reorganization, it is likely that its effects will be maximized if given in tandem with concomitant intensified behavioural rehabilitation therapy in the functional domain targeted for improvement. This expectation, however, requires validation in clinical trials.

There are currently numerous ongoing registered, large-scale RCTs, and this further evidence is necessary to substantiate whether tDCS has merit as a therapeutic adjunct in stroke rehabilitation.

Transcranial Magnetic Stimulation

The Stimulator

Transcranial magnetic stimulation is delivered to the brain by passing a strong, brief electrical current through an insulated wire coil placed on the skull. Several coils are available, with the two most common being circular and figure-8, whereby the latter produces a more focused electric field peak under the centre of the coil (Peterchev et al., 2012). The subject's head is partially immobilized in a padded head- or chinrest to prevent movement, and the coil is generally held in place by the researcher for the duration of the stimulation. In contrast to tDCS, TMS has high focality, and accurate positioning is required and is usually achieved with neuronavigational equipment (Cabrera et al., 2014).

Transcranial magnetic stimulation can be used in several different modes: single-pulse TMS is used to investigate the excitability of the corticospinal system, paired-pulse TMS can be used to assess connectivity within and between cortical regions, and long trains of stimuli can be used to induce excitability changes desired for stroke rehabilitation (rTMS) (Paulus et al., 2013).

Mechanism of Action

Repetitive transcranial magnetic stimulation acts as a neurostimulator. The electric current produced by

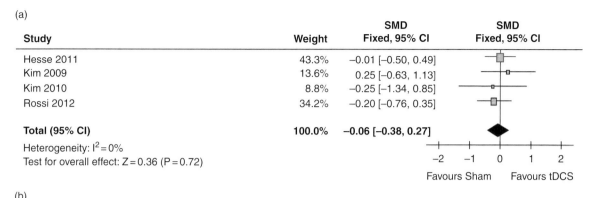

Figure 26.8 Forest plots showing the effects of *transcranial electrical direct stimulation vs control* on *motor performance* at the end of the intervention period, according to time since stroke until treatment period. (a) Chronic period after stroke. (b) Subacute period after stroke. Reproduced from Marquez et al. (2015), with permission from the authors.

the coil generates a transient magnetic field which passes into the brain, where it induces a secondary current in a parallel plane to the plane of the coil, which depolarizes neurones (Bolognini et al., 2009). The induced electric field causes the shift of ions in the brain without the need for current to flow across the skull; therefore, it avoids the skull impedance issues encountered with tDCS. When delivered over the primary motor cortex, it induces efferent volleys along the corticospinal tracts (Barker et al., 1985). Depending on the stimulation duration and frequency, output pulse shape, coil geometry, positioning, and strength of the magnetic field, rTMS can be used to either excite or inhibit areas of the cortex with great temporal precision (Priori et al., 2009).

Application of TMS

Conventional rTMS protocols use trains of evenly spaced pulses usually consisting of stimuli applied at

either low frequency (1–2 Hz) to decrease cortical excitability, or high frequency rTMS (>1 Hz) to increase it. More recently, new rTMS paradigms have been developed in which the train duration and temporal spacing of the bursts are altered. Theta burst stimulation (TBS) uses repeated high-frequency (50 Hz) bursts of pulses applied at a theta frequency (5 Hz) that may produce more enduring changes in excitability at a lower dosage than conventional rTMS (Paulus et al., 2013). Another technique, known as paired associative stimulation (PAS), combines rTMS with peripheral nerve stimulation at fixed time intervals. Excitation or inhibition can be selectively produced depending on the interval between the stimulation (Wolters et al., 2003).

Safety

Protocol guidelines and safety parameters have been well defined for the use of TMS, and the safety of TMS continues to be supported by the literature (Machii et al., 2006). The only absolute contraindication to TMS is the presence of metal in close contact to the coil. Conditions of increased risk are related to the use of novel paradigms and patient characteristics such as a history of epilepsy, severe cardiac disease, and drugs including alcohol and neuromodifying agents.

The occurrence of seizure is the most serious TMS-related, acute adverse effect but reports of this are extremely rare, with occurrences typically reported when the procedure exceeds the guidelines, or when patients are receiving treatment with medications which may lower the seizure threshold (Rossi et al., 2009). Other safety concerns which have been raised include transient hearing changes (a broadband acoustic artefact is produced by the mechanical deformation of the stimulating coil), localized pain/discomfort, headache, and cognitive changes. A systematic review in the Cochrane Library reported that, of the included 327 stroke patients, adverse events were: transient or mild headache in 2.4%, syncope in 0.6%, anxiety in 0.3%, and insomnia exacerbation in 0.3% (Hao et al., 2013). These effects are considered to be mild and transient and do not typically affect patient compliance.

The potential risk of long-term magnetic field exposure for rTMS operators due to daily exposure over prolonged periods of time is an issue that may need to be addressed in the future (Rossi et al., 2009).

Variation in Effects

The response to rTMS is highly variable and dependent on the same intersubject and intrasubject factors as tDCS (Paulus et al., 2013) (see Table 26.1). The effectiveness of TMS is highly dependent on the state of neuronal activation in the targeted brain region at the time of stimulation (Silvanto and Pascual-Leone, 2008). These state-dependent effects are particularly relevant in TMS considering the specificity and focality of effects and the disruption to neuronal activity following stroke.

Activities of Daily Living (ADL)

In a Cochrane Library meta-analysis of 2 randomized trials enrolling 183 stroke patients, a nonsignificant trend was noted to greater improvements on scales assessing ADL among patients allocated to TMS: SMD 15.92 (95% CI: –2.11 to 33.95, $p = 0.08$) (Hao et al., 2013) (Figure 26.9).

Upper Limb Motor Function

A systematic review identified 34 RCTs enrolling 904 post-stroke patients assessing the effect of TMS on manual dexterity, as measured by performance tests such as grip force, keyboard tapping, and movement accuracy (Zhang et al., 2017). There was evidence of both short-term and long-term benefit.

Considering early outcomes, in 27 RCTs enrolling 669 patients, allocation to TMS was associated with a greater improvement in upper limb function at the end of the intervention period: SMD 0.43 (95% CI: 0.30–0.56; $p < 0.001$). There was no evidence of heterogeneity across trials ($I^2 = 0.0\%$), nor of publication bias (Egger's test $p = 0.92$). Considering sustained effects, in 11 RCTs enrolling 310 post-stroke patients, allocation to TMS was associated with a greater improvement in upper limb function at long-term

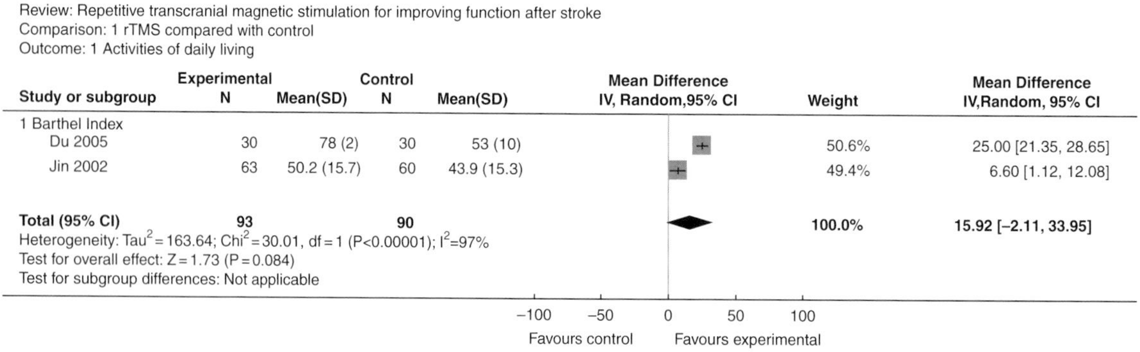

Review: Repetitive transcranial magnetic stimulation for improving function after stroke
Comparison: 1 rTMS compared with control
Outcome: 1 Activities of daily living

Study or subgroup	Experimental N	Mean(SD)	Control N	Mean(SD)	Mean Difference IV, Random,95% CI	Weight	Mean Difference IV,Random, 95% CI
1 Barthel Index							
Du 2005	30	78 (2)	30	53 (10)		50.6%	25.00 [21.35, 28.65]
Jin 2002	63	50.2 (15.7)	60	43.9 (15.3)		49.4%	6.60 [1.12, 12.08]
Total (95% CI)	93		90			100.0%	15.92 [–2.11, 33.95]

Heterogeneity: Tau^2 = 163.64; Chi^2 = 30.01, df = 1 (P<0.00001); I^2=97%
Test for overall effect: Z = 1.73 (P = 0.084)
Test for subgroup differences: Not applicable

-100   -50   0   50   100
Favours control   Favours experimental

Figure 26.9 Forest plot showing the effects of *transcranial magnetic stimulation vs control* on *activities of daily living*, in post-stroke patients. Reproduced from Hao et al. (2013), with permission from John Wiley & Sons Limited. Copyright Cochrane Library.

follow-up 1 month or more after the end of the intervention period: SMD 0.49 (95% CI: 0.29–0.68, $p < 0.001$). However, there was evidence of moderate heterogeneity across trials ($I^2 = 38.7\%$), and weak evidence of publication bias (Egger's test $p = 0.11$).

Walking

A systematic review identified six randomized group and crossover trials, enrolling 166 patients, evaluating TMS to improve gait after stroke, as measured by walking speed (Li et al., 2018). Stimulation parameters varied across trials, with target sites including ipsilesional, contralesional, and bilateral leg motor cortex, stimulation frequencies ranging from 1 to 20 Hz, and duration of stimulation treatment ranging from 1 to 8 weeks. Overall, allocation to TMS was associated with a greater improvement in walking speed at the end of the intervention period: SMD 0.64 (95% CI: 0.32–0.95; $p < 0.0001$). There was no evidence of important heterogeneity across trials ($I^2 = 0\%$). These preliminary positive findings from diverse single-centre studies support further, larger multi-centre studies to confirm benefit and identify optimal treatment parameters.

Aphasia

Low-frequency TMS over the nondominant Broca's region has been proposed to relieve inhibition of the dominant hemisphere and promote language recovery in stroke patients; however, studies to date have provided mixed results. A systematic review of four RCTs with a total of 132 stroke patients found that allocation to TMS was associated with a statistically significant benefit in object naming (SMD 0.51, 95% CI: 0.16–0.86; $p = 0.004$) (Figure 26.10) (Li et al., 2015). Non-significant trends towards benefit were seen for word repetition (SMD 0.31, 95% CI: –0.04 to 0.65; $p = 0.08$) and comprehension (SMD 0.31, 95% CI: –0.14 to 0.75; $p = 0.18$) (Li et al., 2015) (Figures 26.11 and 26.12).

Hemispatial Neglect

A systematic review identified 7 studies, providing 11 randomized comparisons of 184 patients, assessing TMS for hemispatial neglect after stroke, as measured by the Line Bisection Test or Behavioral Inattention Test. Stimulation paradigms varied widely, in laterality (right versus left posterior parietal cortex targets), frequency (including 1, 10, 30,

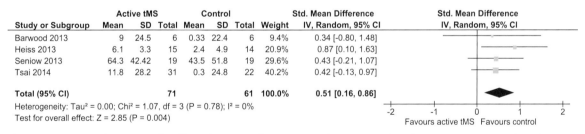

Figure 26.10 Forest plot showing the effects of *transcranial magnetic stimulation vs control* on *object naming*, in post-stroke patients. Figure courtesy of B. Bat-Ordene and JL Saver. Figure freely available under a Creative Commons 4.0 CC-BY use freely with attribution license.

Study or Subgroup	Active tMS Mean	SD	Total	Control Mean	SD	Total	Weight	Std. Mean Difference IV, Random, 95% CI
Barwood 2013	1	3.3	6	0.21	3.5	6	9.3%	0.21 [-0.92, 1.35]
Heiss 2013	3.5	3.4	15	1.3	3.4	14	21.4%	0.63 [-0.12, 1.38]
Seniow 2013	6.8	6.8	19	4.8	8.2	19	29.4%	0.26 [-0.38, 0.90]
Tsai 2014	1	2.4	31	0.4	3.7	22	40.0%	0.20 [-0.35, 0.74]
Total (95% CI)			71			61	100.0%	0.31 [-0.04, 0.66]

Heterogeneity: Tau² = 0.00; Chi² = 0.91, df = 3 (P = 0.82); I² = 0%
Test for overall effect: Z = 1.75 (P = 0.08)

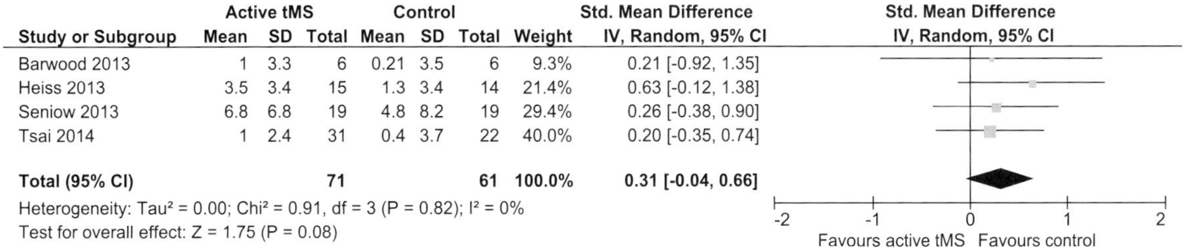

Figure 26.11 Forest plot showing the effects of *transcranial magnetic stimulation vs control* on *word repetition*, in post-stroke patients. Figure courtesy of B. Bat-Ordene and JL Saver. Figure freely available under a Creative Commons 4.0 CC-BY use freely with attribution license.

Study or Subgroup	Active tMS Mean	SD	Total	Control Mean	SD	Total	Weight	Std. Mean Difference IV, Random, 95% CI	Std. Mean Difference IV, Random, 95% CI
Barwood 2013	2	12.3	6	0.17	17.8	6	15.5%	0.11 [-1.02, 1.24]	
Heiss 2013	4.4	3.7	15	1.8	3.72	14	35.2%	0.68 [-0.07, 1.43]	
Seniow 2013	34.6	31.1	19	31.3	28.9	19	49.2%	0.11 [-0.53, 0.74]	
Total (95% CI)			**40**			**39**	**100.0%**	**0.31 [-0.14, 0.76]**	

Heterogeneity: Tau² = 0.00; Chi² = 1.44, df = 2 (P = 0.49); I² = 0%
Test for overall effect: Z = 1.36 (P = 0.17)

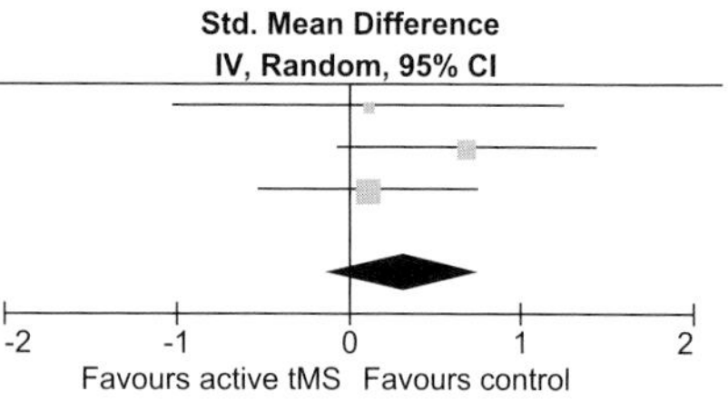

$-2 \quad -1 \quad 0 \quad 1 \quad 2$
Favours active tMS Favours control

Figure 26.12 Forest plot showing the effects of *transcranial magnetic stimulation vs control* on *comprehension*, in post-stroke patients. Figure courtesy of B. Bat-Ordene and JL Saver. Figure freely available under a Creative Commons 4.0 CC-BY use freely with attribution license.

and 50 Hz), and mode (repetitive and theta-burst). Allocation to TMS, compared with control, was associated with a statistically significant greater reduction in hemispatial inattention: SMD −2.16, 95% CI: −3.00 to −1.33, p < 0.0001 (Salazar et al., 2018). However, interpretive caution is warranted as five of the comparisons used shared control groups and there was evidence of substantial heterogeneity across trials (I^2 = 76%).

Additional Cognitive Functions

Studies investigating the merits of TMS for rehabilitation post-stroke of additional domains of cognitive function are limited. Although several studies have reported using TMS in healthy young subjects to facilitate working memory, there are currently few studies reporting TMS-induced ameliorations of memory deficits or executive dysfunction in stroke patients, although at least one small randomized trial suggested potential improvements in memory function (Lu et al., 2015 In a systematic review in the Cochrane Library, across 2 trials enrolling 75 stroke patients, TMS was not associated with a statistically significant greater improvement in global cognition when measured on the Mini-Mental Status Examination (MD 1.87, 95% CI: −5.93–9.68) (Hao et al., 2013).

Mood

Transcranial magnetic stimulation has been approved for the clinical management of general psychiatric patients with major depression who fail to respond to medication (McClintock et al., 2018). Among patients with post-stroke depression, a systematic review identified 22 RCTs enrolling 1764 patients that across outcomes on the Hamilton Depression Rating Scale could be

aggregated (Shen et al., 2017). Stimulation parameters varied widely across studies, with target sites most often left, right, or bilateral dorsolateral prefrontal cortex, frequencies ranging from 0.5 to 15 Hz, and number of treatment sessions varying from 7 to 60. Across all studies, allocation to TMS yielded greater improvements in depression scale scores: mean difference −6.09 (95% CI: −4.45 to −7.74, p < 0.00001). However, interpretive caution is warranted as there was substantial heterogeneity across trials (I^2 = 96%), and visual funnel plot inspection suggested potential presence of some publication bias.

In addition to analysing depression scale score change as a continuous variable, the systematic review evaluated the dichotomous endpoints of depression response (defined as ≥50% reduction in Hamilton Depression Rating Scale score) and complete depression remission. For depression response, across 12 RCTs enrolling 839 patients, allocation to TMS was associated with higher depression response rates, 64.4% versus 39.7%, odds ratio (OR) 3.46 (95% CI: 2.52–4.76). For this outcome, heterogeneity across trials was moderate (I^2 = 39%), and visual inspection of funnel plots did not suggest publication bias. For depression remission, across 11 RCTs enrolling 7710 patients, allocation to TMS did not alter event rates, 28.8% versus 30.2%, OR 0.99 (95% CI: 0.56–1.75).

These findings support a beneficial effect of TMS for post-stroke depression, as for major depression generally, though they are limited by reflecting many single-centre trials, rather than large, multicentre trials, with heterogeneity of stimulation parameters, patient selection, and outcomes. Further, larger trials are needed to clarify optimal target sites, stimulation parameters, and patient characteristics.

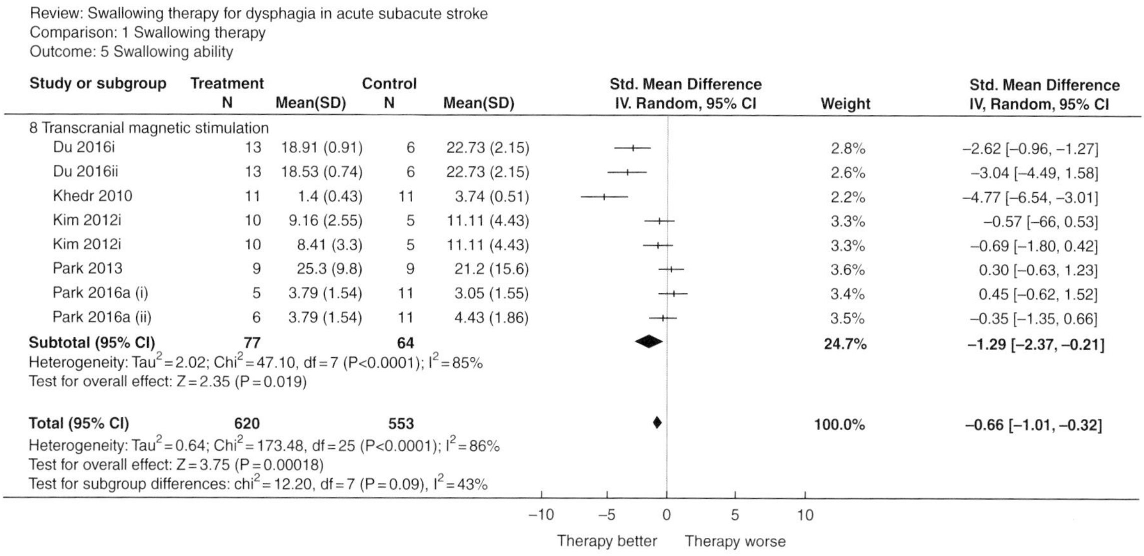

Review: Swallowing therapy for dysphagia in acute subacute stroke
Comparison: 1 Swallowing therapy
Outcome: 5 Swallowing ability

Study or subgroup	Treatment N	Mean(SD)	Control N	Mean(SD)	Std. Mean Difference IV. Random, 95% CI	Weight	Std. Mean Difference IV, Random, 95% CI
8 Transcranial magnetic stimulation							
Du 2016i	13	18.91 (0.91)	6	22.73 (2.15)		2.8%	−2.62 [−0.96, −1.27]
Du 2016ii	13	18.53 (0.74)	6	22.73 (2.15)		2.6%	−3.04 [−4.49, 1.58]
Khedr 2010	11	1.4 (0.43)	11	3.74 (0.51)		2.2%	−4.77 [−6.54, −3.01]
Kim 2012i	10	9.16 (2.55)	5	11.11 (4.43)		3.3%	−0.57 [−66, 0.53]
Kim 2012i	10	8.41 (3.3)	5	11.11 (4.43)		3.3%	−0.69 [−1.80, 0.42]
Park 2013	9	25.3 (9.8)	9	21.2 (15.6)		3.6%	0.30 [−0.63, 1.23]
Park 2016a (i)	5	3.79 (1.54)	11	3.05 (1.55)		3.4%	0.45 [−0.62, 1.52]
Park 2016a (ii)	6	3.79 (1.54)	11	4.43 (1.86)		3.5%	−0.35 [−1.35, 0.66]
Subtotal (95% CI)	**77**		**64**			**24.7%**	**−1.29 [−2.37, −0.21]**

Heterogeneity: Tau^2=2.02; Chi^2=47.10, df=7 (P<0.0001); I^2=85%
Test for overall effect: Z=2.35 (P=0.019)

Total (95% CI)	**620**		**553**			**100.0%**	**−0.66 [−1.01, −0.32]**

Heterogeneity: Tau^2=0.64; Chi^2=173.48, df=25 (P<0.0001); I^2=86%
Test for overall effect: Z=3.75 (P=0.00018)
Test for subgroup differences: chi^2=12.20, df=7 (P=0.09), I^2=43%

−10   −5   0   5   10
Therapy better   Therapy worse

Figure 26.13 Forest plot showing the effects of *transcranial magnetic stimulation vs control* on *swallowing ability*, in post-stroke patients. Reproduced from Bath et al. (2018), with permission from John Wiley & Sons Limited. Copyright Cochrane Library.

Dysphagia

A systematic review in the Cochrane Library identified 5 studies with 8 randomized comparisons of 141 stroke patients, evaluating TMS for post-stroke swallowing dysfunction as measured on the Dysphagia Rating Scale, the Functional Oral Intake Scale, or similar assessment (Bath et al., 2018). Sites of stimulation were ipsilesional, contralesional, or bilateral pharyngeal or esophageal motor cortices. Allocation to TMS, compared with sham, was associated with a greater improvement in swallowing scale scores: SMD −1.29 (95% CI: −0.21 to −2.37; *p* = 0.02). However, substantial heterogeneity across trials was noted (*I*^{2} = 85%), and several trials were rated as having potential risk of bias (Figure 26.13). Overall, the preliminary positive findings support further studies to confirm benefit and identify optimal treatment parameters.

Effects of TMS according to Frequency of Stimulation

High-frequency vs Low-frequency Stimulation

Available evidence suggests similar efficacies of high- and low-frequency TMS for the two therapeutic aims for which large numbers of randomized

trials have been performed in post-stroke patients: improvement in upper limb function and improvement in mood. For upper limb manual dexterity, a meta-analysis evaluated 8 randomized comparisons (258 patients) of high-frequency TMS and 23 randomized comparisons (608 patients) of low-frequency TMS. Both showed similar degree of benefit: high-frequency SMD 0.45 (95% CI: 0.22–0.69), low-frequency SMD 0.42 (95% CI: 0.26–0.58), subgroup heterogeneity *p* = 0.60 (Zhang et al., 2017). For depression, considering 10 trials (735 patients) of high-frequency TMS and 12 trials (833 patients) of low-frequency TMS, both also showed similar magnitudes of benefit: high frequency MD −6.20 (95% CI: −3.19 to −9.21), low-frequency MD −5.40 (95% CI: −3.23 to −7.56) (Shen et al., 2017).

Effects of TMS according to Stroke Characteristics

Time since Stroke

For upper limb function, available evidence does not indicate major differences in the efficacy of TMS when applied at different time intervals since stroke occurrence. A systematic review evaluated 7 randomized comparisons (96 patients) of TMS in the acute period (≤2 weeks); 5 randomized comparisons

(162 patients) of TMS in the subacute period (2 weeks to 6 months); and 8 randomized comparisons (141 patients) in the chronic period (>6 months). Differences in degree of benefit between time periods (SMD point estimates acute 0.69, subacute 043, chronic 0.34) did not reach statistical significance (heterogeneity $p = 0.25$) (Zhang et al., 2017).

Implications for Clinical Practice and Research

Current evidence provides moderate support for the use of TMS as a treatment for patients with post-stroke depression. TMS may particularly be considered for stroke patients with depressed mood not responsive to pharmacological therapy, similar to its use in major depressive disorder generally. However, full remission has not been demonstrated with TMS, and further randomized trials are needed to determine optimal stimulation parameters and patient candidates.

In addition, there is suggestive evidence of potential benefits of TMS to enhance recovery in finger coordination and hand function, walking, hemispatial neglect, and dysphagia. However, the initial positive findings are largely confined to demonstrating improvements in scale scores or laboratory assessments. Demonstration of clinically meaningful improvements in everyday function, and of long-sustained benefits beyond the intervention period, have not yet occurred. Large, multicentre trials with unequivocally functionally important primary outcomes are needed to confirm benefit and provide insight into best stimulation parameters, timing, and patients.

Only limited evidence supports the use of TMS in the management of aphasia after stroke. The effects of TMS on functional language have not been assessed, and further research is required.

If TMS benefits are mediated by enhancing neuroplasticity and capacity for reorganization, it is likely that its effects will be maximized if given concurrently with intensified behavioural rehabilitation therapy in the functional domain targeted for improvement. This supposition, however, requires validation in clinical trials.

Newer Transcranial Electrical and Magnetic Stimulation Modalities

More contemporary modalities have been introduced to the non-invasive stimulation field of stroke research. These are relatively novel and, as such, there is much less available data regarding efficacy,

protocols, and safety. To date, there appears to be consensus that there is minimal cutaneous sensation or discomfort and no reported adverse effects (Chaieb et al., 2014), and the effects are comparable to earlier forms of tDCS and TMS when applied at equivalent intensities and dosage (Moliadze et al., 2010a).

Transcranial Alternating Current Stimulation (tACS)

Transcranial alternating current stimulation refers to electrical stimulation in which the current alternates between the anode and cathode (switching polarity) with a sinusoidal waveform. It can be applied in a wide frequency range and may include a direct current offset (Marshall and Binder, 2013). The hypothesis is that the alternating fields can affect the oscillatory rhythms in the brain in a frequency-dependent manner by synchronizing or desynchronizing neuronal networks (Reato et al., 2013). It is unclear whether tACS induces spikes in fibre tracts or modulates neuronal membrane thresholds in the same way as tDCS.

Transcranial Random Noise Stimulation (tRNS)

Transcranial random noise stimulation is a special form of tACS with frequencies in the range of 0.1 to 100 Hz (low-frequency tACS) and high-frequency ranges from 101 to 640 Hz. It uses an alternating current with random amplitude and frequency variation. In contrast to tDCS, the current flow has no directionality (Terney et al., 2008).

High-definition tDCS

This form of tDCS has been developed in an attempt to improve the anatomical targeting of brain structures and improve focality. It involves the use of small, gel-based electrodes arranged in arrays. For example a 4×1 ring montage uses a centre electrode that determines the polarity of the stimulation and 4 return electrodes in an effort to guide the current flow (Guleyupoglu et al., 2013). Early investigations suggest that this montage can produce a more profound and durable change in motor-evoked potentials than with traditional tDCS (Kuo et al., 2013). Even more sophisticated high-definition montages, using 64 electrodes to focus the current flow, are under investigation (Dmochowski et al., 2011).

Theta Burst Stimulation (TBS)

Theta burst stimulation is a variation of TMS which uses repeated high-frequency (50 Hz) bursts of pulses applied at theta frequency (5 Hz). By varying the train duration and temporal spacing of the bursts, it is possible to use shorter application times and lower intensities than conventional TMS. Several single session studies report promising findings; however, a larger trial with repeated sessions found no beneficial effect for either inhibitory or excitatory TBS (Talelli et al., 2012).

Which Modality? General Comparison of tDCS and TMS

Randomized trials directly comparing tDCS and TMS in post-stroke patients have not yet generally been conducted, as is appropriate, since such active comparator trials are best undertaken only after at least one of the interventions has unequivocally demonstrated benefit for a particular indication and become part of standard care. The two techniques may well have differential advantages and disadvantages for different indications, as the spatial extent, directionality, and intensity of the currents they induce in the brain differ in several important respects (Wagner et al., 2007a) (Table 26.2).

Table 26.2 Comparison of tDCS and TMS modalities

tDCS	TMS
Direct current applied with cathode and anode electrodes	Magnetic field generated by coil
Modifies excitability thresholds	Generates depolarization
Low temporal resolution	High temporal resolution
Diffuse spread of current	Focal current distribution
Skull shunts current	Magnetic field passes through scalp unimpeded
Easy to sham	Difficult to produce sham
Portable	Large and immobile
Inexpensive	10× more expensive than tDCS
No external indicator of effectiveness	Immediate external indicator of effectiveness
Easy to apply with concurrent therapy	Unable to be used with concurrent therapy
Potential to either increase or inhibit excitability	
Able to target various brain tissues	
Intrasubject and intersubject variability in response	

Transcranial direct current stimulation is often criticized for its low spatial resolution. However, in stroke, stimulation of a more distributed network of cortical sites may be desired; therefore, this may be an advantage over TMS (Cabrera et al., 2014). Currently, in indirect comparison of trials of tDCS versus control and trials of TMS versus control, the different modalities show broadly similar magnitudes of effect, but differences in study designs make comparisons difficult. The after-effects of tDCS appear greater than those induced by rTMS, but TBS or other asynchronous rTMS trains may be advantageous and further investigation is required (Romero et al., 2002). Future head-to-head trials will be needed to provide guidance regarding which type of stimulation should be used in which patients.

Summary

Non-invasive brain stimulation to stimulate neuroplasticity, enhance recovery, and improve mood after stroke has made substantial technical advances in the past two decades. The most common neuromodulatory techniques are transcranial direct current stimulation (tDCS), applying a weak electrical current across the brain, and transcranial magnetic stimulation (TMS), inducing an electrical field within the brain.

Currently, the only non-invasive brain stimulation technique and indication for which there is a sufficiently strong evidence base to support routine use in clinical practice is transcranial magnetic stimulation to improve mood in post-stroke depression. TMS applied to dorsolateral prefrontal cortices can substantially reduce depressive symptoms, though not increase complete remission. TMS is a reasonable second-line intervention in patients with post-stroke depressed mood who have been resistant to pharmacotherapy.

For several additional indications in post-stroke patients, both TMS and tDCS have shown signals of potential benefit in randomized trials. The strongest evidence is for enhancement of recovery of upper extremity motor function and hand dexterity with TMS. In addition, there is suggestive evidence for possible benefit in improving recovery of function after stroke in walking (TMS), activities of daily living (tDCS), aphasia (both), hemispatial neglect (both), and swallowing (both).

However, for these and potentially other recovery-enhancing applications, substantial additional larger trials are needed to definitively confirm generalizable benefits and to provide data allowing optimization of stimulatory parameters and patient selection.

References

Antal A, Alekseichuk I, Bikson M, Brockmöller J, Brunoni AR, Chen R, et al. (2017). Low intensity transcranial electric stimulation: safety, ethical, legal regulatory and application guidelines. *Clin Neurophysiol*, **128**(9), 1774–1809.

Barker AT, Jalinous R, Freeston IL. (1985). Non-invasive magnetic stimulation of the human motor cortex. *Lancet*, **1**, 1106–07.

Bath PM, Lee HS, Everton LF. (2018). Swallowing therapy for dysphagia in acute and subacute stroke. *Cochrane Database Syst Rev*, 10. CD000323. doi:10.1002/14651858. CD000323.pub3.

Bikson M, Grossman P, Thomas C, Zannou AL, Jiang J, Adnan T, et al. (2016). Safety of transcranial direct current stimulation: evidence based update 2016. *Brain Stimul*, **9**(5), 641–61.

Boggio PS, Nunes A, Rigonatti SP. (2007). Repeated sessions of non-invasive brain DC stimulation is associated with motor function improvement in stroke patients. *Restor Neurol Neurosci*, **25**, 123–9.

Bolognini N, Pascual-Leone A, Fregni F. (2009). Using non-invasive brain stimulation to augment motor training-induced plasticity. *J Neuroeng Rehabil*, **6**(8).

Brunoni AR, Nitsche MA, Bolognini N, Bikson M, Wagner T, Merabet L, et al. (2012). Clinical research with transcranial direct current stimulation (tDCS): challenges and future directions. *Brain Stimul*, **5**(3), 175–95.

Cabrera LY, Evans EL, Hamilton RH. (2014). Ethics of the electrified mind: defining issues and perspectives on the principled use of brain stimulation in medical research and clinical care. *Brain Topogr*, **27**(1), 33–45.

Chaieb L, Antal A, Pisoni A, Saiote C, Opitz A, Ambrus GG, et al. (2014). Safety of 5 kHz tACS. *Brain Stimul*, **7**(1), 92–6.

Chang MC, Kim DY, Park DH. (2015). Enhancement of cortical excitability and lower limb motor function in patients with stroke by transcranial direct current stimulation. *Brain Stimul*, **8**(3), 561–6.

Chiang CF, Lin MT, Hsiao MY, Yeh YC, Liang YC, Wang TG (2018). Comparative efficacy of noninvasive neurostimulation therapies for acute and subacute poststroke dysphagia: a systematic review and network meta-analysis. *Arch Phys Med Rehabil*, **100**(4), 739–50. doi:10.1016/j.apmr.2018.09.117.

Dmochowski JP, Datta A, Bikson M, Su Y, Parra LC. (2011). Optimized multi-electrode stimulation increases focality and intensity at target. *J Neural Eng*, **8**(4), 046011.

Elsner B, Kugler J, Pohl M, Mehrholz J. (2015). Transcranial direct current stimulation (tDCS) for improving aphasia in patients with aphasia after stroke. *Cochrane Database Syst Rev*, 5. CD009760.

Elsner B, Kugler J, Pohl M, Mehrholz J. (2016a). Transcranial direct current stimulation (tDCS) for improving activities of daily living, and physical and cognitive functioning, in people after stroke. *Cochrane Database Syst Rev*, 3. CD009645. doi:10.1002/14651858. CD009645.pub3.

Elsner B, Kugler J, Pohl M, Mehrholz J. (2016b). Transcranial direct current stimulation for improving spasticity after stroke: a systematic review with meta-analysis. *J Rehabil Med*, **48**(7), 565–70.

Fitz NS, Reiner PB. (2015). The challenge of crafting policy for do-it-yourself brain stimulation. *J Med Ethics*, **41**(5), 410–12.

Giordano, J, Bikson M, Kappenman ES, Clark VP, Coslett HB, Hamblin MR, et al. (2017). Mechanisms and effects of transcranial direct current stimulation. *Dose Response*, **15**(1), 1559325816685467. doi:10.1177/ 1559325816685467. eCollection 2017 Jan-Mar.

Guleyupoglu B, Schestatsky P, Edwards D, Fregni F, Bikson M. (2013). Classification of methods in transcranial electrical stimulation (tES) and evolving strategy from historical approaches to contemporary innovations. *J Neurosci Methods*, **219**(2), 297–311.

Hao Z, Wang D, Zeng Y, Lui M. (2013). Repetitive transcranial magnetic stimulation for improving function after stroke. *Cochrane Database Syst Rev*, 5. CD008862.

Kang EK, Baek MJ, Kim S, Paik NJ. (2009). Non-invasive cortical stimulation improves post-stroke attention decline. *Restor Neurol Neurosci*, **27**(6), 645–50.

Kazuta T, Takeda K, Osu R, Tanaka S, Oishi A, Kondo K, Liu M. (2017). Transcranial direct current stimulation improves audioverbal memory in stroke patients. *Am J Phys Med Rehabil*, **96**(8), 565–71.

Kim JH, Kim DW, Chang WH, Kim YH, Kim K, Im CH. (2014). Inconsistent outcomes of transcranial direct current stimulation may originate from anatomical differences among individuals: electric field simulation using individual MRI data. *Neurosci Lett*, **564**, 6–10.

Koyama S, Tanaka S., Tanabe S, Sadato N. (2015). Dual-hemisphere transcranial direct current stimulation over primary motor cortex enhances consolidation of a ballistic thumb movement. *Neurosci Lett*, **588**, 49–53. doi:20.1016/j. neulet.2014.11.043. epub 2014 Nov 28.

Krause B, Marquez-Ruiz J, Cohen Kadosh R. (2013). The effect of transcranial direct current stimulation: a role for cortical excitation/inhibition balance? *Front Hum Neurosci*, 7, 602.

Kuo HI, Bikson M, Datta A, Minhas P, Paulus W, Kuo M. F, et al. (2013). Comparing cortical plasticity induced by conventional and high-definition 4 x 1 ring tDCS: a neurophysiological study. *Brain Stimul*, **6**(4), 644–8.

Lang N, Siebner HR, Ward NS. Lee L, Nitsche MA. Paulus W., Rothwell JC, et al. (2005). How does transcranial DC stimulation of the primary motor cortex alter regional neuronal activity in the human brain? *Eur J Neurosci*, **22**(2), 495–504.

Li Y, Fan J, Yang J, He C, Li S. (2018). Effects of repetitive transcranial magnetic stimulation on walking and balance function after stroke: a systematic review and meta-analysis. *Am J Phys Med Rehabil*, 97(11), 773–81.

Li Y, Qu Y, Yuan M, Du T. (2015). Low-frequency repetitive transcranial magnetic stimulation for patients with aphasia after stroke: a meta-analysis. *J Rehabil Med*, **47**, 675–81.

Liebetanz D, Koch R, Mayenfels S, Konig F, Paulus W, Nitsche MA. (2009). Safety limits of cathodal transcranial direct current stimulation in rats. *Clin Neurophysiol*, **120**, 1161–7.

Lu H, Zhang T, Wen M, Sun L. (2015). Impact of repetitive transcranial magnetic stimulation on post-stroke dysmnesia and the role of BDNF Val66Met SNP. *Med Sci Monit*, **21**, 761–8. doi:10.12659/MSM.892337.

Machii K, Cohen D, Ramos-Estebanez C, Pascual-Leone A. (2006). Safety of rTMS to non-motor cortical areas in healthy participants and patients. *Clin Neurophysiol*, **117**(2), 455–71.

Marquez J, van Vliet P, McElduff P, Lagopoulos J, Parsons M. (2015). Transcranial direct current stimulation (tDCS): does it have merit in stroke rehabilitation? A systematic review. *Int J Stroke*, **10**(3), 306–16.

Marshall L, Binder S. (2013). Contribution of transcranial oscillatory stimulation to research on neural networks: an emphasis on hippocampo-neocortical rhythms. *Front Hum Neurosci*, 7, 614.

McClintock SM, Reti IM, Carpenter LL, McDonald WM, Dubin M, Taylor SF, et al.; National Network of Depression Centers rTMS Task Group; American Psychiatric Association Council on Research Task Force on Novel Biomarkers and Treatments. (2018). Consensus recommendations for the Clinical Application of Repetitive Transcranial Magnetic Stimulation (rTMS) in the treatment of depression. *J Clin Psychiatry*, **79**(1). pii: 16cs10905. doi:10.4088/JCP.16cs10905.

McCreery DB, Agnew WF, Yuen TG, and Bullara L. (1990). Charge density and charge per phase as cofactors in neural injury induced by electrical stimulation. *IEEE Trans Biomed Eng*, 37, 996–1001.

Meinzer M, Darkow R, Lindenberg R, Flöel A. (2016). Electrical stimulation of the motor cortex enhances treatment outcome in post-stroke aphasia. *Brain*, **139**(Pt 4), 1152–63.

Moliadze V, Antal A, Paulus W. (2010a). Boosting brain excitability by transcranial high frequency stimulation in the ripple range. *J Physiol*, **588**(24), 4891–4904.

Moliadze V, Antal A, Paulus W. (2010b). Electrode-distance dependent after-effects of transcranial direct and random noise stimulation with extracephalic reference electrodes. *Clin Neurophysiol*, **121**, 2165–71.

Nitsche MA, Cohen L, Wassermann EM, Priori A, Lang N, Antal A, et al. (2008). Transcranial direct current stimulation: state of the art 2008. *Brain Stimul*, **1**, 206–23.

Nitsche, MA, Nitsche MS, Klein CC. (2003). Level of action of cathodal DC polarisation induced inhibition of the human motor cortex. *Clin Neurophysiol*, **114**, 600–04.

Nitsche MA, Paulus W. (2000). Excitability changes induced in the human motor cortex by weak transcranial direct current stimulation. *J Physiol*, **527**(3), 633–9.

Paulus W, Peterchev AV, Ridding M. (2013). Transcranial electric and magnetic stimulation: technique and paradigms. *Handb Clin Neurol*, **116**, 329–42.

Peterchev AV, Wagner TA, Miranda PC, Nitsche MA, Paulus W, Lisanby SH, et al. (2012). Fundamentals of transcranial electric and magnetic stimulation dose: definition, selection, and reporting practices. *Brain Stimul*, **5**(4), 435–53.

Priori A, Hallett M, Rothwell JC. (2009). Repetitive transcranial magnetic stimulation or transcranial direct current stimulation? *Brain Stimul*, **2**(4), 241–5.

Radman T, Ramos RL, Brumberg JC, Bikson M. (2009). Role of cortical cell type and morphology in subthreshold and suprathreshold uniform electric field stimulation in vitro. *Brain Stimul*, **2**(4), 215–28.

Reato D, Rahman A, Bikson M, Parra LC. (2013). Effects of weak transcranial alternating current stimulation on brain activity – a review of known mechanisms from animal studies. *Front Hum Neurosci*, 7, 687.

Redfearn JWT, Lippold OC, Constain R. (1964). A preliminary account of the clinical effects of polarizing the brain in certain psychiatric disorders. *Br J Psychiatry*, **110**, 773–85.

Romero JR, Anschel D, Sparing R, Gangitano M, Pascual-Leone A. (2002). Subthreshold low frequency repetitive transcranial magnetic stimulation selectively decreases facilitation in the motor cortex. *Clin Neurophysiol*, **113**, 101–07.

Rossi S, Hallett M, Rossini PM, Pascual-Leone A; Safety of TMS Consensus Group. (2009). Safety, ethical considerations and application guidelines for the use of transcranial magnetic stimulation in clinical practice and research. *Clin Neurophysiol*, **120**, 2008–39.

Saiote C, Turi Z, Paulus W, Antal A. (2013). Combining functional magnetic resonance imaging with transcranial electrical stimulation. *Front Hum Neurosci*, 7, 435.

Salazar APS, Vaz PG, Marchese RR, Stein C, Pinto C, Pagnussat AS. (2018). Noninvasive brain stimulation improves hemispatial neglect after stroke: a systematic review and meta-analysis. *Arch Phys Med Rehabil*, **99**(2), 355–66.e1.

Schlaug G, Renga V, Nair DG. (2008). Transcranial direct current stimulation in stroke recovery. *Arch Neurol*, **65**(12), 1571–6.

Shaker HA, Sawan SAE, Fahmy EM, Ismail RS, Elrahman SAEA. (2018). Effect of transcranial direct current stimulation on cognitive function in stroke patients. *Egypt J Neurol Psychiatr Neurosurg*, **54**(1), 32. doi:10.1186/s41983-018-0037-8.

Shen X, Liu M, Cheng Y, Jia C, Pan X, Gou Q, et al. (2017). Repetitive transcranial magnetic stimulation for the treatment of post-stroke depression: a systematic review and meta-analysis of randomized controlled clinical trials. *J Affect Disord*, **211**, 65–74.

Silvanto, J, Pascual-Leone A. (2008). State-dependency of transcranial magnetic stimulation. *Brain Topogr*, **21**(1), 1–10.

Smith DV, Clithero JA. (2009). Manipulating executive function with transcranial direct current stimulation. *Front Integr Neurosci*, **3**, 26.

Sohn MK, Jee SJ, Kim YW. (2013). Effect of transcranial direct current stimulation on postural stability and lower extremity strength in hemiplegic stroke patients. *Ann Rehabil Med*, **37**(6), 759–65.

Spielmann K, van de Sandt-Koenderman WME, Heijenbrok-Kal MH, Ribbers GM. (2018). Transcranial direct current stimulation does not improve language outcome in subacute poststroke aphasia. *Stroke*, **49**(4), 1018–20.

Tahtis V, Kaski D, Seemungal BM. (2014). The effect of single session bi-cephalic transcranial direct current stimulation on gait performance in sub-acute stroke: a pilot study. *Restor Neurol Neurosci*, **32**(4), 527–32.

Talelli P, Wallace A, Dileone M, Hoad D, Cheeran B, Oliver R, et al. (2012). Theta burst stimulation in the rehabilitation of the upper limb: a semirandomized, placebo-controlled trial in chronic stroke patients. *Neurorehabil Neural Repair*, **26**(8), 976–87.

Tanaka S, Hanakawa T, Honda M, Watanabe K. (2009). Enhancement of pinch force in the lower leg by anodal transcranial direct current stimulation. *Exp Brain Res*, **196**(3), 459–65.

Tanaka S, Takeda K, Otaka Y, Kita K, Osu R, Honda M, et al. (2011). Single session of transcranial direct current stimulation transiently increases knee extensor force in patients with hemiparetic stroke. *Neurorehabil Neural Repair*, **25**(6), 565–9.

Terney D, Chaieb L, Moliadze V, Antal A, Paulus W. (2008). Increasing Human brain excitability by transcranial high-frequency random noise stimulation. *J Neurosci*, **28**, 14147–55.

Valiengo LC, Goulart AC, de Oliveira JF, Benseñor IM, Lotufo PA, Brunoni AR. (2017). Transcranial direct current stimulation for the treatment of post-stroke depression: results from a randomised, sham-controlled, double-blinded trial. *J Neurol Neurosurg Psychiatry*, 8(2), 170–5.

Wagner T, Fregni F, Fecteau S, Grodzinsky A, Zahn M, Pascual-Leone A. (2007a). Transcranial direct current stimulation: a computer-based human model study. *Neuroimage*, **35**, 1113–24.

Wagner T, Valero-Cabre A, Pascual-Leone A. (2007b). Noninvasive human brain stimulation. *Ann Rev Biomed Eng*, **9**, 527–65.

Wolters A, Sandbrink F, Schlottmann A, Kunesch E, Stefan K, Cohen LG, et al. (2003). A temporally asymmetric Hebbian rule governing plasticity in the human motor cortex. *J Neurophysiol*, **89**(5), 2339–45.

Yun GJ, Chun MH, Kim BR. (2015). The effects of transcranial direct-current stimulation on cognition in stroke patients. *J Stroke*, **17**(3), 354–8.

Zhang L, Xing G, Fan Y, Guo Z, Chen H, Mu Q. (2017). Short- and long-term effects of repetitive transcranial magnetic stimulation on upper limb motor function after stroke: a systematic review and meta-analysis. *Clin Rehabil*, 31(9), 1137–53.sss

Index